Total Intravenous Anesthesia and
Controlled Infusions

Anthony R. Absalom • Keira P. Mason
Editors

Total Intravenous Anesthesia and Target Controlled Infusions

A Comprehensive Global Anthology

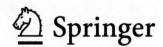 Springer

Editors
Anthony R. Absalom, MBChB, FRCA, MD
Department of Anesthesiology
University Medical Center Groningen
University of Groningen
Groningen, The Netherlands

Keira P. Mason, MD
Department of Anesthesia
Harvard Medical School
Department of Anesthesiology
Perioperative and Pain Medicine
Boston Children's Hospital
Boston, MA, USA

Additional material to this book can be downloaded from
https://link.springer.com/book/10.1007/978-3-319-47609-4

ISBN 978-3-319-83779-6   ISBN 978-3-319-47609-4   (eBook)
DOI 10.1007/978-3-319-47609-4

This Springer imprint is published by Springer Nature
The registered company is Springer International Publishing AG
The registered company address is: Gewerbestrasse 11, 6330 Cham, Switzerland

Dedication by Keira P. Mason

My dedication is foremost to my mother and father, whose sacrifice, love, and encouragement enabled me to pursue my goals and dreams. Leading by example, they showed me to persevere, remain positive, optimistic, and always strive to achieve my personal best. My deepest gratitude and appreciation to my family, Ed, and my two sons, Colin and Tyler. Tyler, you are a tender soul, inventive, hardworking, and brave when faced with challenges beyond your years, and special beyond words. Colin, your tenacity, creativity, and drive make you a unique gem. I am so proud of you both. I hope that I may guide, nurture, and provide for you both as my parents did for me. Never forget your middle name, Jigme….. the name given to monarchs—a reminder for you both to be proud and brave, and to persevere and pursue your dreams, even in the face of adversity and challenges.

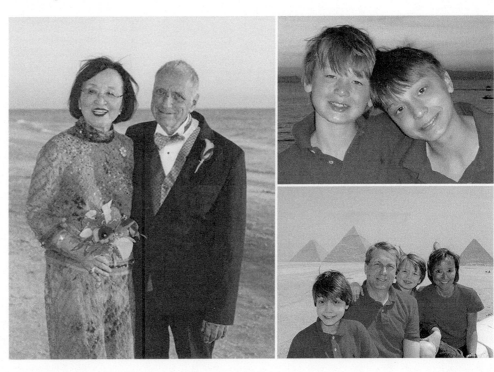

Dedication by Anthony R. Absalom

I dedicate this book to the authors, whose expertise and time made this book possible, and to my family, who have supported me "through thick and thin."

Anthony (Tony) Absalom

Preface

We are honored to present *Total Intravenous Anesthesia and Target Controlled Infusion*. This book is a testament to the passion and expertise of the contributing authors who are all committed to the field of intravenous anesthesia and target controlled infusion. The author list reads like a "Who's who" of anesthetic pharmacology, and includes experts from diverse disciplines and specialties, from 20 countries around the world. We are very appreciative of and honored by their efforts and extend a sincere "thank you" to each author.

This book is a unique contribution to the field. It is the first to address these topics in a comprehensive manner. Each chapter was written by a specialist in that particular area and is intended to be of value to all providers of intravenous sedation and anesthesia. It may be read cover to cover, or read ad hoc, one chapter at a time, out of succession. There is intentional, albeit minimal, repetition of topics. The repetition is intended not only to consolidate important information for the reader but also to convey relevant information for those who may not be reading the book cover to cover. Even when there is "repetition," it is presented in a different style by each of the individual authors, which in most cases masks the repeated elements.

We wish our readers much reading pleasure. Our primary goal is to help improve the care of patients worldwide, and we trust that this book, which represents a true international collaboration among multiple specialists, will be a timeless resource for clinicians and researchers working in the field of intravenous delivery of sedation and anesthesia.

Keira P. Mason
Boston, MA, USA

Anthony R. Absalom
Groningen, The Netherlands

Acknowledgements

We would like to acknowledge our deepest gratitude to Ms. Michelle E. Noonan and Amanda Buckley, the clinical coordinators and administrators who committed themselves to this project, without whom it would never have made it to fruition.

Contents

Contributors

Anthony R. Absalom, MBChB, FRCA, FHEA, MD Department of Anesthesiology, University Medical Center Groningen, University of Groningen, Groningen, The Netherlands

Ram Adapa, MBBS, MD, FRCA, FHEA, PhD Department of Anaesthesia, Cambridge University Hospitals NHS Foundation Trust, Cambridge, UK

Brian J. Anderson, MB ChB, PhD, FANZCA, FCICM Anaesthesia and Intensive Care, Starship Children' Hospital, Auckland, New Zealand

Keith J. Anderson, BSc (Hons), MB, ChB, FRCA Department of Anesthesiology, Foothills Medical Centre, University of Calgary, Calgary, AB, Canada

John N. van den Anker, MD, PhD Division of Paediatric Pharmacology and Pharmacometrics, University of Basel Children's Hospital, Basel, Switzerland

Division of Pediatric Clinical Pharmacology, Children's National Medical Center, Washington, DC, USA

Intensive Care and Department of Pediatric Surgery, Erasmus MC Sophia Children's Hospital, Rotterdam, The Netherlands

Fazil Ashiq, MD Anesthesiology Institute, Cleveland Clinic Abu Dhabi CCAD, Abu Dhabi, United Arab Emirates

Oliver Bagshaw, MB ChB, FRCA Department of Anaesthesia, Birmingham Children's Hospital, Birmingham, West Midlands, UK

Thierry Beths, MRCVS, PhD, Cert VA, CVA, CVPP U-Vet – University of Melbourne, Anesthesiology, Werribee, VIC, Australia

Arno Brouwers, MD Pediatric Intensive Care Unit, Department of Pediatrics, Maastricht University Medical Centre, Maastricht, The Netherlands

Matthew T. V. Chan, MBBS, PhD, FANZCA, FHKCA, FHKAM Department of Anaesthesia and Intensive Care, The Chinese University of Hong Kong, Prince of Wales Hospital, Shatin, Hong Kong

Isabelle Constant, MD, PhD Armand Trousseau Hospital, Anesthesiology and Intensive Care, Paris, France

Luis Ignacio Cortínez, MD Hospital Clinico Pontificia Universidad Catolica De Chile, Anesthesia, Santiago, Chile

Douglas J. Eleveld, PhD Department of Anesthesiology, University Medical Center Groningen, University of Groningen, Groningen, The Netherlands

Frank Engbers, MD, FRCA Department of Anesthesiology, Leiden University Medical Centre, Leiden, The Netherlands

John B. Glen, BVMS, PhD Glen Pharma, Knutsford, Cheshire, UK

Christina J. Hayhurst, MD Division of Anesthesiology Critical Care Medicine, Department of Anesthesiology, Vanderbilt University School of Medicine, Nashville, TN, USA

Wolfgang Heinrichs, MD, PhD AQAI Simulation Center Mainz, Mainz, Germany

Hugh C. Hemmings Jr., MD, PhD, FRCA Department of Anesthesiology and Pharmacology, Weill Cornell Medical College, New York, NY, USA

Karl F. Herold, MD, PhD Department of Anesthesiology, Weill Cornell Medical College, New York, NY, USA

Stefan De Hert, MD, PhD Department of Anesthesiology, Ghent University Hospital, Ghent University, Ghent, Belgium

Christopher G. Hughes, MD Division of Anesthesiology Critical Care Medicine, Department of Anesthesiology, Vanderbilt University School of Medicine, Nashville, TN, USA

Ken B. Johnson, MS, MD Anesthesiology, University of Utah, Salt Lake City, UT, USA

Ross Kennedy, MB, ChB, PhD Department of Anaesthesia, Christchurch Hospital and University of Otago, Christchurch, New Zealand

Gavin N. C. Kenny Department of Anaesthesia, University of Glasgow, Scotland, UK

Susanne Koch, MD Department of Anesthesiology and Intensive Care Medicine, Charité—Universitätsmedizin Berlin, Berlin, Germany

Massimo Lamperti, MD Anesthesiology Institute, Cleveland Clinic Abu Dhabi (CCAD), Abu Dhabi, United Arab Emirates

Piet L. Leroy, MD, PhD Pediatric Intensive Care Unit, Department of Pediatrics, Maastricht University Medical Centre, Maastricht, The Netherlands

Kate Leslie, MD, FRANZCA Department of Anaesthesia and Pain Management, Royal Melbourne Hospital, Parkville, VIC, Australia

Ngai Liu, MD, PhD Department of Anesthesiology, Hôpital Foch, Suresnes, France

Outcomes Research Consortium, Cleveland, OH, USA

Mohamed Mahmoud, MD Department of Anesthesia and Pediatrics, Cincinnati Children's Hospital Medical Center, University of Cincinnati, Cincinnati, OH, USA

Keira P. Mason, MD Department of Anesthesia, Harvard Medical School, Boston, MA, USA

Department of Anesthesiology, Perioperative and Pain Medicine, Boston Children's Hospital, Boston, MA, USA

Kenichi Masui, MD, PhD Anesthesiology Department, National Defense Medical College Hospital, Tokorozawa, Saitama, Japan

Claude Meistelman Department of Anesthesiology and Intensive Care Medicine, Hôpital de Brabois, Faculté de Médecine de Nancy, Vandœuvre, France

Jane Montgomery, MBBS, FRCA, FFICM Department of Anaesthetics, South Devon Healthcare NHS Foundation Trust, Torquay, Devon, UK

Rudolf Mörgeli, MD Department of Anesthesiology and Intensive Care Medicine, Charité—Universitätsmedizin Berlin, Berlin, Germany

Pratik P. Pandharipande, MD, MSCI Division of Anesthesiology Critical Care Medicine, Department of Anesthesiology, Vanderbilt University School of Medicine, Nashville, TN, USA

Johannes Hans Proost, PharmD, PhD Anesthesiology, University Medical Center Groningen, University of Groningen, Groningen, The Netherlands

Johan Ræder, MD, PhD Department of Anaesthesiology—Ullevaal, Oslo University Hospital, Oslo, Norway

Douglas E. Raines, MD Department of Anesthesia, Critical Care, and Pain Medicine, Massachusetts General Hospital, Boston, MA, USA

Philippe Richebe, MD, PhD Maisonneuve Rosemont Hospital, CIUSSS de l'Est-de-l'ile-de-Montreal, Montreal, QC, Canada

Department of Anesthesiology, University of Montreal, Montreal, QC, Canada

Mark G. Roback, MD Department of Pediatrics & Emergency Medicine, University of Minnesota Masonic Children's Hospital, Minneapolis, MN, USA

Janko Samardzic, MD, PhD Medical Faculty, Institute of Pharmacology, Clinical Pharmacology and Toxicology, University of Belgrade, Belgrade, Serbia

Division of Paediatric Pharmacology and Pharmacometrics, University of Basel Children's Hospital, Basel, Switzerland

Jan N.M. Schieveld, MD, PhD Division Child- and Adolescent Psychiatry, Department Psychiatry and Neuro-Psychology, Maastricht University Medical Centre, Maastricht, The Netherlands

The Mutsaersstichting, Venlo, The Netherlands

The Koraalgroep, Sittard, The Netherlands

Stefan Schraag, MD, PhD, FRCA, FFICM Department of Anaesthesia and Perioperative Medicine, Golden Jubilee National Hospital, Scotland, UK

John William Sear, MA, BSc, MBBS, PhD, FFARCS Nuffield Department of Anaesthetics, University of Oxford, Oxford, Oxfordshire, UK

Pablo O. Sepúlveda V., MD German Clinic of Santiago, Anesthesia, Resuscitation and Pain, Santiago, Chile

Frederique S. Servin, MD, PhD APHP HUPNVS Hôpital Bichat, Anesthesia and Intensive Care, Paris, France

Steven L. Shafer, MD Department of Anesthesiology, Perioperative and Pain Medicine, Stanford University School of Medicine, Stanford, CA, USA

Sulpicio G. Soriano Department of Anesthesiology, Perioperative and Pain Medicine, Harvard Medical School, Boston Children's Hospital, Boston, MA, USA

Claudia Spies, MD Department of Anesthesiology and Intensive Care Medicine, Charité—Universitätsmedizin Berlin, Berlin, Germany

Mary Stocker, MA, MBChB, FRCA Department of Anaesthetics, South Devon Healthcare NHS Foundation Trust, Torquay, Devon, UK

Dubravka Svob Strac, PhD Laboratory for Molecular Neuropharmacology, Division of Molecular Medicine, Rudjer Boskovic Institute, Zagreb, Croatia

Michael R. J. Sury, FRCA, PhD Department of Anaesthesia, Great Ormond Street Hospital for Children NHS Foundation Trust, London, UK

Portex Department of Anaesthesia, Institute of Child Health, University College London, London, UK

Nicholas Sutcliffe, BSc Phys, MBChB, MRCP, FRCA Hamad Medical Corporation, Hamad Medical City, Doha, Qatar

Sanne Vaassen, MD Pediatric Intensive Care Unit, Department of Pediatrics, Maastricht University Medical Centre, Maastricht, The Netherlands

Robert A. Veselis, MD Anesthesiology, Memorial Sloan Kettering Cancer Center, New York, NY, USA

Gijs D. Vos, MD, PhD Pediatric Intensive Care Unit, Department of Pediatrics, Maastricht University Medical Centre, Maastricht, The Netherlands

Laszlo Vutskits, MD, PhD Department of Anesthesiology, Pharmacology and Intensive Care, University Hospitals of Geneva, Geneva, Switzerland

Department of Basic Neuroscience, University of Geneva Medical School, Geneva, Switzerland

Jaap Vuyk, MD, PhD Department of Anesthesiology, Leiden University Medical Center (LUMC), Leiden, The Netherlands

Michael Wang, BSc, MSc, PhD Clinical Psychology/Honorary Consultant, Leicester Royal Infirmary, Clinical Psychology Unit, University of Leicester, Leicester, UK

Craig S. Webster, BSc, MSc, PhD Centre for Medical and Health Sciences Education, and Department of Anaesthesiology, University of Auckland, Auckland, New Zealand

Centre for Medical and Health Sciences Education, University of Auckland, Auckland, New Zealand

Björn Weiss, MD Department of Anesthesiology and Intensive Care Medicine, Charité—Universitätsmedizin Berlin, Berlin, Germany

Alissa Wolf, MD Department of Anesthesiology and Intensive Care Medicine, Charité—Universitätsmedizin Berlin, Berlin, Germany

Vivian Man-ying Yuen, MD, MBBS, FANZCA, FHKCA, FHKAM Department of Anaesthesiology, University of Hong Kong Shenzhen Hospital, Shenzhen, Guangdong, China

Part I

Introduction/Background

When and How Did It All Begin? A Brief History of Intravenous Anesthesia

John William Sear

Among the first reports of the intravenous injection of drugs are those describing the studies of Wren and Major [1, 2]. They injected opium dissolved in water into the venous system of a dog, which caused it to be stupefied but did not kill it! Despite this observation made more than 350 years ago, the history of clinical intravenous anesthesia does not really become significant before the late nineteenth century.

The delivery of drugs by the intravenous route requires specific equipment; and for this, we must be grateful for the development of the hollow needle by Francis Rynd in 1845, and the syringe in 1853 by Charles Gabriel Pravaz. The latter was not initially designed for intravenous drug administration but rather for the delivery of perineural and intra-arterial injections. More recently the development of target-controlled infusion delivery regimens aimed at achieving given plasma or effect-site target drug concentrations has usually required dedicated infusion apparatus linked to computer systems that control the rate of drug dosing.

Among the earliest pioneers studying the delivery of intravenous anesthesia to patients was Pierre-Cyprian Ore (Professor of Physiology, University of Bordeaux), who, in 1872, reported 36 cases of anesthesia using chloral hydrate as an intravenous anesthetic in the treatment of patients with tetanus, to the Societe Chirugicale de Paris [3]. Despite his enthusiasm, these early attempts at intravenous anesthesia (IVA) were associated with a high incidence of mortality. As a result, this delayed the further development of IVA until the beginning of the twentieth century.

1909 saw the development of hedonal (a urethane derivative) which was used for the treatment of insomnia. Krawkow and Fedoroff described its role to provide general anesthesia [4, 5]. They described this as the "first

intravenous agent that produced fairly adequate surgical anesthesia with a moderate degree of safety." However, the agent was not sufficiently water soluble, and resulting "weak" solutions acted very slowly to produce anesthesia, and had a long duration of effect. Hence the search for other agents continued with Noel and Souttar examining the possible role of paraldehyde [6]; while Peck and Meltzer described the use of intravenous magnesium sulfate [7]; and ethanol infusions were studied by Naragawa, and Cardot and Laugier [8, 9].

The anesthetic properties of the barbiturates were first observed with diethylbarbituric acid, which was synthesized by Fischer and von Mering [10]. But, again, its low water solubility and prolonged duration of action lead to a delayed further development of the drug. Use of the first barbiturate for intravenous anesthesia was reported in 1921, when Bardet and Bardet studied a mixture of the diethylamines of di-ethyl and di-allyl barbituric acid (Somnifen) [11]. The sodium salt of sec-butyl-(2-bromoallyl)-barbiturate (Pernocton) had greater water solubility, and was introduced into clinical practice in 1927. Further developments lead to the synthesis by Kropp and Taub, and initial clinical studies by Weese and Scharpff of the short-acting, rapid onset hexobarbital (Evipan) [12], although the drug had a high incidence of excitatory side effects. Nevertheless, use of Evipan was recommended as the agent of choice in those individuals with a tendency to bronchospasm.

Barbiturates

The first major development and advance from a clinical viewpoint was the introduction of thiopental, which was administered in separate studies by Lundy, and Waters [13, 14]. At the same time, Tabern and Volwiler had initiated a research program to prepare a series of thiobarbiturates where there was substitution of the oxygen at the C(2) position with a sulfur atom [15]. This led to agents having a

J.W. Sear, MA, BSc, MBBS, PhD, FFARCS (✉)
Nuffield Department of Anaesthetics, University of Oxford, Headington, Oxford, Oxfordshire OX3 9DU, UK
e-mail: john.sear@gtc.ox.ac.uk

© Springer International Publishing AG 2017
A.R. Absalom, K.P. Mason (eds.), *Total Intravenous Anesthesia and Target Controlled Infusions*,
DOI 10.1007/978-3-319-47609-4_1

shorter period of hypnosis. One of these molecules was thiopental. It was devoid of the excitatory side effects seen with hexobarbital. The barbiturate was completely metabolized with only <0.3 % excreted unchanged in the urine. In man, there was a comparatively high rate of metabolism (16–24 % per hour). Thiopental had no analgesic properties, but had the tendency to increase the sensitivity of an individual to pain and touch.

Although it was originally studied in the USA, it was subsequently introduced into the United Kingdom by Jarman and Abel [16]. At this time, maintenance of anesthesia was normally provided by di-ethyl-ether or one of the other volatile agents (all of which had undesirable side effects). As a result, researchers started using infusions of thiopental to maintain anesthesia. However, they found that if the barbiturate was given without opioids or muscle relaxants, large doses of barbiturates were needed to suppress movement, and these doses caused side effects of cardio-respiratory depression and delayed awakening (the pharmacokinetics and metabolism of the barbiturate were not fully defined until much later by Price [17]).

Use of thiopental by infusion has also been cited as the cause of many deaths among the casualties at Pearl Harbor in 1941—with the often quoted, but misconceived and incorrect statement from a surgical colleague "that intravenous anesthesia was an ideal method of euthanasia!!" [18, 19].

Pentobarbital (a metabolite of thiopental) had previously been used as an anesthetic by Lundy in 1932. It caused less laryngospasm than was seen after thiopental, but there was a suggestion that it was associated with an improved recovery profile.

Since the Second World War, further developments have taken place with other drugs being used to provide intravenous anesthesia. Beside thiopental, several other intravenous thio-barbiturates were assessed including thiamylal and thialbarbitone; drugs having the same duration of action and spectrum of activity as thiopental, but lower potency.

Introduction of a methyl thio-ethyl group into the side chain of methitural was aimed at accelerating the breakdown of the drug. Its development led to a drug that was popular in Germany as Thiogenal, and as Neraval in the USA, although the quality of anesthesia was inferior to that of thiopental. Similar comments were made about buthalitone (marketed as Transithal in the UK; as Ulbreval in the USA; and Baytinal in Germany) which was synthesized in the USA in 1936, but not studied until 1954 by Weese and Koss. The potency of buthalitone was about half that of thiopental.

However, a greater advance was seen with the introduction of hexobarbital which causes rapid onset of anesthesia. This property was attributed to the addition of a methyl group at the C1 position. Further development of this molecule led to the introduction in 1957 of methohexital, which was of shorter duration of action and had a shorter half-life

than thiopental [20]. It was irritating to the subcutaneous tissues if accidentally given extravascularly, but more irritant and dangerous if given intra-arterially. Methohexital has two asymmetrical carbon atoms, so existing as four separate isomers. The proprietary drug is a mixture of two of these: α-dl pair (a mixture of all four isomers was shown by Taylor and Stoelting to produce excessive skeletal muscle activity and possible convulsions [21]).

There have been a number of studies described that used the drug by continuous infusion to maintain anesthesia without prolonged recovery times [22, 23]. However, its use was associated with the side effect of pain on injection and a high incidence of involuntary muscle movements. Several other methyl-thiobarbiturates have been studied, but again all had very high incidences of excitatory side effects.

Benzodiazepines

Although a number of benzodiazepines have been studied as sedative drugs since the synthesis of chlordiazepoxide in 1955 (e.g., diazepam, lorazepam), only diazepam has enjoyed any use as an anesthetic induction agent. Titration of the drug to the exact induction dose is difficult, as the drug's profile includes a slow onset of action and prolonged duration. The benzodiazepine is water insoluble, which requires the use of a lipid solvent, but early solvents caused venous irritation. The introduction of an emulsion formulation reduced the incidences of pain on injection and thrombophlebitis, but had no effect on the recovery profile after large doses of diazepam.

More recent advances with the benzodiazepines as agents for the maintenance of anesthesia have revolved around the introduction of firstly midazolam, and more recently remimazolam. The former has been used for the induction and maintenance of intravenous anesthesia [24, 25]. One advantage of these agents is the parallel development of a specific antagonist, flumazenil, which can be given at the termination of anesthesia to facilitate recovery. However, this has not been totally straightforward, as the mismatch between the pharmacokinetics and pharmacodynamics of the agonist and antagonist has resulted in reports of cases showing "rebound hypnotization" after initial recovery [26].

Propanidid

Propanidid (a phenoxyacetic acid derivative of eugenol, the chief constituent of oil of cloves) was a short-acting sedative-hypnotic containing an ester moiety which was broken down by body (pseudochline-esterase) and tissue esterases. It was the first clinically acceptable non-barbiturate intravenous anesthetic when introduced in 1965 but was withdrawn in 1984 because of a high incidence of anaphylactic reactions—again, believed to be due to the poly-oxyethylated castor oil solvent, Cremophor EL (BASF, Ludwigshafen, Germany).

When attempts were made to find an alternative solvent, it was shown that a liposomal formulation had a similar potency in rats to the Cremophor one; it also appeared superior as far as tolerance with a reduced incidence of clonic seizures [27]. A further study was therefore conducted in swine, but this failed to confirm any potential advantage of the liposomal formation over other existing hypnotics [28].

More recently another metabolically active ester with a structure similar to propanidid (AZD 3043) has been evaluated in man—this time, formulated in the lipid emulsion used for propofol [29]. Although the drug had a short context-sensitive half-time, there were some undesirable side effects—water insolubility; low potency; a dose-related increase in heart rate during drug infusion; sporadic episodes of involuntary movements and increased muscle tone (especially during the recovery phase); and in three patients there were episodes of erythema, chest discomfort, and dyspnea after drug dosing. Overall, one or more adverse side effects occurred in 29 % of the patients studied.

Etomidate

This imidazole derivative was discovered in 1964 at Janssen Pharmaceutica in Belgium and introduced into clinical practice in 1974. Unlike many other intravenous agents, etomidate caused little hemodynamic depression, and its use was not associated with histamine release. The agent had the profile of rapid onset and offset, but its use was accompanied by significant adverse side effects: pain on injection—due primarily to the propylene glycol solvent; myoclonic activity; and a high incidence of postoperative nausea and vomiting.

In 1983 it was reported that when the drug was given by continuous infusion to provide ICU sedation to multiply traumatized patients, there was an increase in patient mortality when compared with other sedation regimens [30]. In vitro and in vivo studies have shown that infusions (and single doses) of etomidate result in an inhibition of adrenal steroidogenesis.

As a result, the present role of etomidate in anesthesia practice is confined mainly to use as an induction drug for patients at risk of hemodynamic instability; for those who have shown previous allergic reactions to other induction agents; and electro-convulsive therapy (since etomidate decreases seizure thresholds).

A reformulation of etomidate in a lipid emulsion reduces the incidence of pain on injection, but does not address the issue of reduced cortisol synthesis. More recent attempts at addressing the effects of the imidazole compound on cortisol biosynthesis are further discussed in Chaps. 12 and 16.

Steroids

In 1927, Cashin and Moravek reported the ability of a colloidal suspension of cholesterol to induce anesthesia in cats [31]. Subsequent studies showed no apparent relationship between the hypnotic (anesthetic) and hormonal properties of the steroids, with the most potent anesthetic steroid being pregnan-3,20-dione (pregnanedione) which is virtually devoid of endocrine activity.

Over the next 80 or more years, the anesthetic properties of a large number of steroids were assessed both in vitro, and in vivo in laboratory animals and man. One of the main problems with steroid agents has been their lack of water solubility. Most steroids show high therapeutic indices in animals, but a variable effect in man in terms of the onset of hypnosis, and the rapidity and completeness of recovery.

In 1941, Selye reported that injections of progesterone produced sleep in rodents [32]; however, it was not until the studies by P'An et al., and Murphy and colleagues that the first clinical report of the anesthetic effects of the water soluble steroid hydroxydione was published [33, 34]. However, this drug did not have an ideal profile—as the onset of hypnosis was delayed (not occurring until 3–5 min after drug administration). Was this because the hypnotic effect of hydroxydione was due to a metabolite? It also had a long duration of action; and a high incidence of thrombophlebitis—so requiring the drug to be administered as a high volume, dilute solution. Other side effects included a fall in blood pressure and respiratory depression which also did not occur until sometime after initial drug administration. However, compared with thiopental, hydroxydione had a far greater therapeutic index; other features were an association with a low incidence of postoperative nausea and vomiting.

In the early 1970s, studies were undertaken of a new compound that was a mixture of two steroids (alfaxalone and alfadolone acetate) solvented in polyoxyethylated castor oil (Cremophor EL solution). This resulted in the hypnotic agent Althesin [35]. The main component of the combination was alfaxalone; the alfadolone acetate being added to increase the solubility of the alfaxalone. Althesin was a rapid onset, short-acting drug, which was used to both induce anesthesia, and provide anesthesia when given by repeat intravenous bolus doses or as a continuous infusion. The features of rapid onset and high potency have been associated with the presence of a free-OH group at the C (3) position of the A ring of the pregnane nucleus.

In lower doses, the drug was used to provide sedation during regional anesthetic blocks or to allow controlled ventilation of patients in the intensive care unit. The drug also had advantageous effects on cerebral metabolism with a reduction in cerebral oxygen consumption, and a decrease in cerebral blood flow and CSF pressure leading to a reduction in intracerebral pressure (so making the drug very useful for neuroanesthesia); a low incidence of venous sequelae including thrombophlebitis.

One important facet of its pharmacology was that repeat bolus dosing of Althesin was not associated with a progressive increased duration of effect, as had been seen with barbiturate drugs. This finding led several authors to explore the concept of maintaining anesthesia by a continuous infusion of the steroids [36–40]. These pivotal studies underpin the development of continuous intravenous anesthesia.

However, it was soon found that the use of Althesin was associated with a high incidence of hypersensitivity reactions [41–43]. Research studies aimed at establishing the cause of these reactions were never completely conclusive, and attempts at reformulation were similarly unsuccessful. Hence the drug was withdrawn from clinical practice in 1984, although its use continued in some veterinary species. Recent interest in the use of steroids to provide anesthesia has led to further attempts at reformulation (see Chap. 16).

Other steroid anesthetic agents have been evaluated in animals and man—including minaxolone citrate, eltanolone (5β-pregnanolone), ORG 21465 and ORG 25435—but all have failed to display improved pharmacokinetic or pharmacodynamics profile when compared with other anesthetic agents available at that time.

Phencyclidines

These cyclohexylamine compounds act to produce a different type of anesthesia than that seen with other anesthetic agents—namely, a state of unconsciousness in which the patient appears to be in a cataleptic (or dissociative) state, but able to undergo surgery without any recall of events. Several drugs of this type have been studied, but the first significant compound was phencyclidine (Sernil; or PCP). This is still used today in some veterinary practices; but has been superseded in man because of its high associated incidence of post-anesthetic psychotomimetic side effects and delirium.

The main drug today is ketamine, which was synthesized in 1962 by Stevens at Parke-Davies laboratories, with the first clinical studies undertaken in 1965. Widespread clinical use originates in 1970, and it is still the drug of choice for many clinical scenarios in both human and veterinary practices (this being the case despite evidence of psychotomimetic activity and cardiovascular stimulation in many patients [44, 45]).

There are some data to suggest that the drug (which is a racemic mixture of two optical isomers) may show an improved profile when given as the S (+) isomer alone. Both animal and human studies confirm this to be the more effective isomer, with shorter emergence and faster return of cognitive function. However, its use does not totally abolish the occurrence of the postoperative sequelae.

Propofol

The history underlying the development of the present lead compound (propofol—di-isopropyl phenol) has not been straightforward. Propofol, a substituted derivative of phenol was synthesized by Glen and colleagues at ICI, UK in the early 1970s [46]. Because of the drug's water insolubility, initial studies were conducted with it formulated in three different solvents. The main study programme was conducted with a formulation solvented in Cremophor EL. This resulted in a number of cases of anaphylactoid reactions, and the temporary withdrawal of the drug.

In 1983, a lipid emulsion formulation of the drug was available, with the first dose delivered by my erstwhile colleague, Nigel Kay, in Oxford, UK [47]. The subsequent clinical trials programme showed it to be a drug of great potential, with the drug being licensed for general release in the UK and Europe in 1986 followed by FDA approval in the USA in 1989.

Since that time, the drug has been used worldwide; and the full pharmacokinetic and pharmacodynamics profile of the agent have been defined when used for induction and maintenance of anesthesia; for sedation for minor procedures (with or without regional blockade); and for sedation in the intensive care unit.

The Concept of 'Balanced Anesthesia'

The concept of balanced anesthesia was first introduced by George Crile during the period 1900–1910, with the aim of providing a light general anesthetic with obtunding of the responses to noxious stimuli associated with surgery being achieved by the administration of local anesthetic blocks. In 1926, Lundy used the same term to indicate the balance between a mixture of premedication (often heavy and often excessive), regional anesthesia and general anesthesia [48]. The first use of an intravenous balanced anesthetic technique was thiopental in combination with nitrous oxide and oxygen as reported by Organe and Broad [49]. This concept of using several different components of a total anesthetic was further expanded by Neff et al. with nitrous oxide-oxygen anesthesia being supplemented by intravenous pethidine (meperidine), a neuromuscular relaxant (d-tubocurarine) and sodium thiopental [50].

It is from these roots that present day intravenous anesthesia or total intravenous anesthesia is derived.

Intravenous anesthesia for practice outside the operating theater.

Although anesthesia is usually conducted within the confines of the hospital, office practice, or surgery, there is increasing need for the delivery of anesthesia at various sites of trauma—such as at traffic accidents, other disasters or in the theater of war. The need to develop intravenous anesthesia for these scenarios originates partly from the anesthetic techniques used during the Chaco War (1932–1935) between Bolivia and Paraguay, and the Spanish Civil War (1936–1939).

Apart from hexobarbital, which was introduced in 1932, the medical staff had few other options available, and had to revert to the use of intravenous ethanol and tri-bromomethanol (Avertin). The main advantage of hexobarbital compared to previous barbiturates was its induction of anaesthesia in one arm-brain circulation time.

Again the introduction of thiopental in 1934 by Lundy and Tovell changed practices in these cases. Despite the adverse comments levelled at the use of thiopental at Pearl Harbor by civilian surgical personnel, intravenous agents must remain a key component of anesthesia in these circumstances. The editorial comments of Halford have often overshadowed the truth as presented in the accompanying paper by Adams and Gray. Thankfully suggestion that the use of thiopental was associated with increased adverse outcomes including mortality has not resulted in the abandonment of intravenous anesthesia in the shocked patient.

However, present anesthetic practices outside of the hospital environment have been influenced through the introduction of two key intravenous agents—ketamine in 1970 and Althesin in 1971, together with the availability of a number of short-acting analgesics (initially pentazocine, and later fentanyl, alfentanil, sufentanil, and more recently remifentanil). Examples of successful techniques used by the British army are typified by the studies of Restall and Jago [51, 52]; while American practice was largely based around the use of ketamine, and remains that way to this day. The more recent introduction of propofol into "field anesthesia" represents another new development, which remains to be fully evaluated.

The research and development of new intravenous anesthetic agents continues; but progress is likely to be slower than the rate and pattern of growth seen over the last hundred or so years. Will we see new innovative agents? Only time will tell!

References

1. Wren C. An account of the rise and attempts of a way to convey liquors immediately into the mass of blood. Philos Trans R Soc Lond. 1665;1:128–30.
2. Major DJ. Cirurgia infusoria placidis CL: vivorium dubiis impugnata, cun modesta, ad eadem. Responsione. Kiloni; 1667
3. Ore PC. Etudes, cliniques sur l'anesthesie chirurgicale par la method des injection de chloral dans les veines. Paris: JB Balliere et fils; 1875.
4. Krawkow NF. Ueber die Hedonal-Chloroform-Narkose. Naunyn-Schmiedeberg's Arch. Exp. Pathol. Pharmakol. 1908; Suppl:317–326.
5. Kissin I, Wright AG. The introduction of hedonal: a Russian contribution to intravenous anesthesia. Anesthesiology. 1988;69:242–5.
6. Noel H, Souttar HS. The anaesthetic effects of the intravenous injection of paraldehyde. Ann Surg. 1913;57:64–7.
7. Peck CH, Meltzer SJ. Anesthesia in human beings by intravenous injection of magnesium sulphate. JAMA. 1916;67:1131–3.
8. Naragawa K. Experimentelle studien uber die intravenose infusionsnarkose mittles alkohols. J Exp Med. 1921;2:81–126.
9. Cardot H, Laugier H. Anesthesie par injection intraveineuse d'un melange alcohol-chloroform solution physiologique chez le chien. C R Seances Soc Biol. 1922;87:889–92.
10. Fischer E, von Mering J. Ueber eine neue klasse vonSchlafmitteln. Ther Ggw. 1903;5:97–101.
11. Bardet D, Bardet G. Contribution a l'etude des hypnotiques ureiques; action et utilisation de diethyl-diallyl barbiturate de diethylamine. Bull Gen de Therap. 1921;172:27–33.
12. Weese H, Scharpff W. Evipan, ein neuartiges einschlaffmittel. Dtsch Med Wochenschr. 1932;58:1205–7.
13. Lundy JS, Tovell RM. Some of the newer local and general anesthetic agents: methods of their administration. Northwest Med. 1934;33:308–11.
14. Pratt TW, Tatum AL, Hathaway HR, Waters RM. Sodium ethyl (1-methyl butyl) thiobarbiturate: preliminary experimental and clinical study. Am J Surg. 1934;31:464.
15. Tabern DL, Volwiler EH. Sulfur-containing barbiturate hypnosis. J Am Chem Soc. 1935;57:1961–3.
16. Jarman R, Abel AL. Intravenous anaesthesia with pentothal sodium. Lancet. 1936;1(230):422–4.
17. Price HL. A dynamic concept of the distribution of thiopental ion human body. Anesthesiology. 1960;21:40–5.
18. Halford FJ. A critique of intravenous anesthesia in war surgery. Anesthesiology. 1943;4:67–9.
19. Adams RC, Gray HK. Intravenous anesthesia with pentothal sodium in the case of gunshot wound associated with accompanying severe traumatic shock and loss of blood: report of a case. Anesthesiology. 1943;4:70–3.
20. Stoelting VK. The use of a new intravenous oxygen barbiturate 25398 for intravenous anesthesia (a preliminary report). Anesth Analg. 1957;36:49–51.
21. Breimer DD. Pharmacokinetics of methohexitone following intravenous infusion in humans. Br J Anaesth. 1976;48:643–9.
22. Prys-Roberts C, Sear JW, Low JM, Phillips KC, Dagnino J. Hemodynamic and hepatic effects of methohexital infusion during nitrous oxide anesthesia in humans. Anesth Analg. 1983;62:317–23.
23. Taylor C, Stoelting VK. Methoexital sodium. A new ultrashort acting barbiturate. Anesthesiology. 1960;21:29–34.
24. Nilsson A, Tamsen A, Persson P. Midazolam-fentanyl anesthesia for major surgery. Plasma levels of midazolam during prolonged total intravenous anesthesia. Acta Anaesthesiol Scand. 1986;30:66–9.

25. Nilsson A, Persson MP, Hartvig P, Wide L. Effect of total intravenous anaesthesia with midazolam/alfentanil on the adrenocortical and hyperglycaemic response to abdominal surgery. Acta Anaesthesiol Scand. 1988;32:379–82.

26. Nilsson A, Persson MP, Hartvig P. Effects of the benzodiazepine antagonist flumazenil on postoperative performance following total intravenous anaesthesia with midazolam and alfentanil. Acta Anaesthesiol Scand. 1988;32:441–6.

27. Habazettl H, Vollmar B, Röhrich F, Conzen P, Doenicke A, Baethmann A. Anesthesiologic efficacy of propanidid as a liposome dispersion. An experimental study with rats. Anaesthesist. 1992;41:448–56.

28. Klockgether-Radke A, Kersten J, Schröder T, Stafforst D, Kettler D, Hellige G. Anesthesia with propanidid in a liposomal preparation. An experimental study in swine. Anaesthesist. 1995;44:573–80.

29. Kalman S, Koch P, Ahlén K, Kanes SJ, Barassin S, Björnsson MA, Norberg Å. First human study of the investigational sedative and anesthetic drug AZD3043: a dose-escalation trial to assess the safety, pharmacokinetics, and efficacy of a 30-minute infusion in healthy male volunteers. Anesth Analg. 2015;121:885–93.

30. Ledingham IM, Watt I. Influence of sedation on mortality in critically ill multiple trauma patients. Lancet. 1983;1:1270.

31. Cashin MF, Moravek V. The physiological action of cholesterol. Am J Physiol. 1927;82:294–8.

32. Selye H. Anaesthetic properties of steroid hormones. Proc Soc Exp Biol Med. 1941;46:116.

33. P'An SY, Gardocki JE, Hutcheon DE, Rudel H, Kodet MJ, Laubach GD. General anesthetic and other pharmacological properties of a soluble steroid, 21-hydroxypregnanedione sodium succinate. J Pharmacol Exp Ther. 1955;115:432–7.

34. Murphy FJ, Guadagni N, DeBon FL. Use of steroid anesthesia in surgery. JAMA. 1955;156:1412–4.

35. Child KJ, Currie JP, Davis B, Dodds MG, Pearce DR, Twissell DF. The pharmacological properties in animals of CT1341—a new steroid anaesthetic agent. Br J Anaesth. 1971;43:2–13.

36. Ramsay MAE, Savege TM, Simpson BRJ, Goodwin R. Controlled sedation with alphaxalone-alphadolone. Br Med J. 1974;2:656–9.

37. Savege TH, Ramsay MAE, Curran JPJ, Cotter J, Walling PT, Simpson BR. Intravenous anaesthesia by infusion. A technique using alphaxalone/alphadolone (Althesin). Anaesthesia. 1975;30:757–64.

38. Du Cailar J. The effects in man on infusions of Althesin with particular regard to the cardiovascular system. Postgrad Med J. 1972;48 Suppl 2:72–6.

39. Dechene JP. Alfathesin by continuous infusion supplemented by intermittent pentazocine. Can Anaesth Soc J. 1977;24:702–6.

40. Sear JW, Prys-Roberts C. Dose-related haemodynamic effects of continuous infusions of Althesin in man. Br J Anaesth. 1979;51:867–73.

41. Horton JN. Adverse reaction to Althesin. Anaesthesia. 1973;28:182–3.

42. Avery AF, Evans A. Reactions to Althesin. Br J Anaesth. 1973;43:301–3.

43. Austin TR, Anderson J, Richardson J. Bronchospasm following Althesin anaesthesia. Br Med J. 1973;2:661.

44. Corssen G, Domino EF. Dissociative anesthesia: further pharmacological studies and first clinical experience with phencyclidine derivate CI 581. Anesth Analg. 1966;45:29–40.

45. Dundee JW. Twenty five years of ketamine: a report of an international meeting. Anaesthesia. 1990;45:159–60.

46. James R, Glen JB. Synthesis, biological evaluation and preliminary structure-activity considerations of a series of alkylphenols as intravenous anesthetic agents. J Med Chem. 1980;23:1350–7.

47. Cummings GC, Dixon J, Kay NH, Windsor JP, Major E, Morgan M, Sear JW, Spence AA, Stephenson DK. Dose requirements of ICI 35,868 (propofol, 'Diprivan') in a new formulation for induction of anaesthesia. Anaesthesia. 1984;39:1168–71.

48. Lundy JS. Balanced anesthesia. Minn Med. 1926;9:399.

49. Organe GSW, Broad RJB. Pentothal with nitrous oxide and oxygen. Lancet. 1938;2:1170–2.

50. Neff W, Mayer EC, Perales M. Nitrous oxide and oxygen anesthesia with curare relaxation. Calif Med. 1947;66:67–9.

51. Jago RH, Restall J. Total intravenous anaesthesia. A technique based on alphaxalone/alphadolone and pentazocine. Anaesthesia. 1977;32:904–7.

52. Jago RH, Restall J, Thompson MC. Ketamine and military anaesthesia. The effect of heavy papaveretum premedication and Althesin induction on the incidence of emergence phenomena. Anaesthesia. 1984;39:925–7.

The Development and Regulation of Commercial Devices for Target-Controlled Drug Infusion

2

John B. Glen

Introduction

The mathematical background to the concept of target-controlled infusion (TCI) and its application to the administration of intravenous anaesthetic and analgesic drugs will be discussed elsewhere in this book (see Chap. 25—"Pharmacokinetics and Pharmacodynamics in the Pediatric Patient" by Anderson and Chap. 6—"Basic Pharmacology: Kinetics and Dynamics for Dummies" by Rader). As I was closely involved in the development of propofol, and the clinical trial programme and related studies required to support the introduction of the 'Diprifusor'™ TCI system, this chapter sets out to provide a personal account of the development and regulatory approval of commercial TCI systems.

The Development of Infusion Devices Suitable for Use in Anaesthesia

Propofol, first marketed as an anaesthetic agent for induction and short term maintenance of anaesthesia in 1986, was developed by the Pharmaceuticals Division of Imperial Chemical Industries (ICI, becoming Zeneca in 1993, and in 1999 merging with Astra to form AstraZeneca—these are referred to as ICI or by the generic term "the Company" hereafter). From an early stage in the pharmacological evaluation of the drug, it was apparent that propofol had a pharmacokinetic profile which would allow its use by continuous infusion to maintain anaesthesia, an observation critical to its selection as a candidate drug. Further regulatory approvals were obtained to extend the use of propofol to long term maintenance of anaesthesia and as a sedative, used in association with regional anaesthesia, or to facilitate ventilation in patients requiring intensive care.

J.B. Glen, BVMS, PhD, FRCA (✉)
Glen Pharma, 35 A Bexton Road, Knutsford, Cheshire WA16 0DZ, UK
e-mail: iglen2@compuserve.com

A limiting factor in the clinical development of infusion techniques was the lack of suitable equipment in operating theatres. While anaesthesiologists were familiar with the use of volumetric infusion pumps in the intensive care environment, these devices with their high capital cost and a requirement for expensive disposable cartridges were not suitable for routine theatre use. While some syringe drivers were available, most of these had a maximum delivery rate of 99 ml h^{-1}. In 1986 I wrote to a large number of the infusion device manufacturers to elicit their interest in a collaborative approach to the development of equipment more suitable for routine operating theatre use. Among a small number of positive responses, that from the Ohmeda Company, a subsidiary of BOC Healthcare was the most encouraging. They built a prototype which incorporated a bolus facility for the rapid delivery of loading infusions and could be interfaced with a controller for computer-controlled infusions. Clinical evaluation of this prototype confirmed that it fulfilled all the requirements of an infusion device for anaesthesia, such that the Ohmeda 9000 became the first of a new generation of syringe drivers [1]. This device could provide 'bolus' infusion rates up to 1200 ml h^{-1} suitable for induction of anaesthesia and a continuous infusion rate up to 200 ml h^{-1}. Syringe pumps with similar features were subsequently developed by a range of manufactures around the world.

First Steps Towards Commercial TCI Systems

In the late 1980s I recall a discussion with Walter Nimmo, who was at that time Professor of Anaesthesia at Sheffield University. He had recently returned from a visit to Duke University, North Carolina, where he had been impressed by the work Jerry Reeves and Peter Glass were doing with pharmacokinetic model-driven infusion and suggested that we should consider this approach for the administration of propofol. Studies on the maintenance of anaesthesia in Europe had been done principally with conventional syringe pumps, with depth of anaesthesia adjusted simply by altering the infusion rate in ml per hour to deliver drug within the range of 4–12 mg kg^{-1} h^{-1}. This appeared to be quite satisfactory and was consistent with my experience in laboratory animals, where the response to a change to infusion rate was a prompt change in depth of anaesthesia. As such, I was not convinced at that time that a more sophisticated, 'computer-controlled' system would offer significant benefits to justify the likely cost and added complexity. However, as the various international research groups continued to work with a range of independently developed computer-controlled infusion systems, and began to apply them to the administration of propofol, in early 1990 I persuaded ICI to allow me to organise a workshop on computer simulation and control of i.v. infusions in anaesthesia, with the following objectives:

1. To allow common interest groups to exchange ideas and discuss future developments
2. To promote a degree of standardisation in systems developed for the infusion of propofol
3. To facilitate the development of more convenient systems for the administration of i.v. anaesthetics.

The attendees were mainly academic anaesthesiologists with interests in pharmacokinetics and pharmacodynamics, a number of whom had developed their own prototype computer-controlled systems for the administration of hypnotic or analgesic agents. These included Chris Hull, Cedric Prys-Roberts, Peter Hutton, Gavin Kenny, Martin White and Bill Mapleson from the UK, Luc Barvais, Alain d'Hollander, Frederic Camu and F Cantraine from Belgium, Pierre Maitre and Don Stanski from Switzerland, Jürgen Schüttler and Siggi Kloos from Germany, Xavier Viviand and Bruno Lacarelle from France, Anders Nilsson from Sweden and Peter Glass, Jim Jacobs and Steven Shafer from the USA. Martyn Gray (Ohmeda, UK) and Jim Skakoon (Bard, USA) provided input from infusion device manufacturers, and from the Company, I was accompanied by Ian Cockshott (pharmacokinetics), Philip Arundel (mathematics and electronics) and Katie Hopkins (medical research).

This meeting achieved its objectives in that the participants welcomed the opportunity to share their experience and to seek a route towards wider availability of computer-controlled infusion systems. It was clear that there would need to be a degree of standardisation and discussion of product liability issues highlighted the need for pharmaceutical companies to provide regulatory authorities with more information, before guidance on computer-controlled infusion could be included in drug prescribing information. By the end of this meeting I was convinced that computer-controlled systems could facilitate the administration of propofol for maintenance of anaesthesia but commercial support for a complex and potentially expensive development was yet to be obtained. Together with Jos Heykants of Janssen Pharmaceutica, I organised a second international workshop on 'Target Control Titration in intravenous anesthesia' in the Netherlands just prior to a World Congress of Anaesthesiology congress being held there in June 1992. This meeting was chaired by Carl Hug from the USA and attended by almost 40 academic anaesthesiologists (Fig. 2.1), a number of industry participants and representatives from a regulatory agency (FDA, USA) and a Notified Body (TUV, Germany). I had first suggested the term 'Target Control Titration' as an alternative to the various acronyms that had been used to describe prototype systems developed by different groups when speaking at a Swedish Postgraduate Meeting at Leondahl Castle in October 1991. Gavin Kenny was another speaker at this meeting who agreed that it was desirable to avoid the implication that a computer rather than an anaesthesiologist controls the depth of anaesthesia and thereafter began to refer to Target Controlled Infusion in subsequent papers. In time this terminology, and the acronym TCI, was endorsed by other leaders in the field [2]. The interest of anaesthesiologists and medical device manufacturers in this approach was clearly increasing and possible approaches to commercial development were emerging. The group at Glasgow University had modified their original system [3] to produce a portable system which used a Psion Organiser (POS 200) interfaced with the Ohmeda 9000 syringe pump [4]. Reports of local use of this system, which were later published [5] indicated that 27 of 30 anaesthesiologists who had used the system found that it had changed their use of propofol for maintenance of anaesthesia, the main reasons being greater ease of use and more confidence in the predictability of effects, in comparison with manually controlled infusion. This began to elicit commercial interest within ICI and a project team was constituted in August 1992 to determine the feasibility of developing a TCI system linked to a prefilled syringe presentation of propofol which was already under development.

The 'Diprifusor' TCI Development

The development of the Diprifusor TCI system and associated technology has been described elsewhere [6, 7], but a brief summary is included here to illustrate the strategy adopted. Despite extensive academic experience with TCI, there was no precedent within regulatory agencies for dealing with this kind of drug—device combination, and extensive discussions with drug and device regulatory authorities were held to seek a way forward. A proposal by the Company to link the development to electronically tagged prefilled syringes (Fig. 2.2), to confirm the drug and drug concentration present, was welcomed by these authorities.

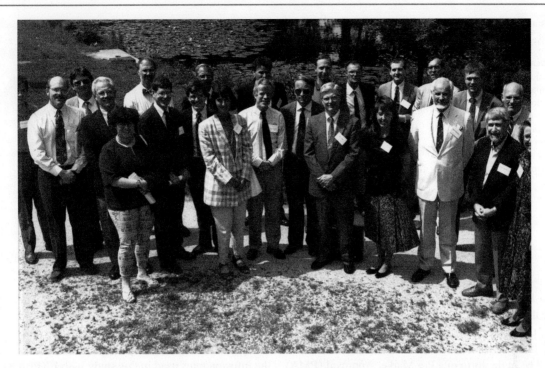

Fig. 2.1 Delegates invited to attend a workshop on 'Target Controlled Titration in Intravenous Anaesthesia', co-sponsored by ICI Pharmaceuticals and Janssen Pharmaceutica in Holland in 1992. Academic delegates from the USA included Julie Barr, Peter Glass, Carl Hug, Jerry Reeves, David Watkins, Steve Shafer and Don Stanski, from the UK Michael Halsey, Cedric Prys-Roberts, Gavin Kenny and Martin White, from Germany Jürgen Schüttler, from Belgium Elisabeth Gepts, Alain D'Hollander and Luc Barvais, from France Frederique Servin, from Australia David Crankshaw and Laurie Mather, from South Africa Johan Coetzee, and a representative of the FDA in the USA, Dan Spyker. (Reproduced with kind permission from Springer Science + Business Media: The Wondrous Story of Anesthesia, EI Eger, II et al. (eds) 2014, Chapter 66, Some examples of industry contributions to the history of anesthesia. Leazer R, Needham D, Glen J, Thomas P, Fig. 66.6, p. 919)

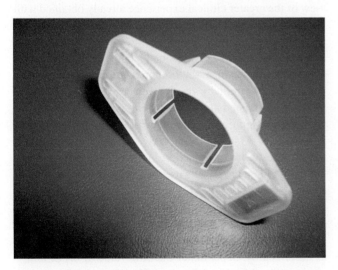

Fig. 2.2 Plastic finger grip with electronic tag utilising Programmed Magnetic Resonance to confirm presence of propofol and identify concentration in glass prefilled syringe (Reproduced with kind permission from AstraZeneca)

This added a significant level of technical complexity to the development but had the commercial benefit to the Company that the new technique would be restricted to use with 'Diprivan'™ the Company's brand of propofol. It is unlikely that commercial support for the development would have been achieved without this approach. It was considered important to separate clearly the responsibilities of the drug company in selecting the pharmacokinetic model and providing guidance on usage, with the addition of target concentration settings to the drug prescribing information, from those of the pump manufacturer. The plan to achieve this involved the development by the Company of the Diprifusor TCI module (Fig. 2.3) containing the TCI control software, with a preferred pharmacokinetic model and software to communicate with the electronic identification tag, the pump display and the pump motor, which could be incorporated by the device manufacturer into a conventional syringe infusion pump. Results of clinical trials with devices containing the preferred model, and proposed guidance on target concentration settings for inclusion in Diprivan labelling, would be submitted to drug regulatory authorities. Within Europe both the Diprifusor TCI module (as an 'Accessory') and integrated devices incorporating the module would be submitted for conformity assessment by a Notified Body (G-MED, France) as designated by EEC Directive 93/42 which came into effect in Jan 1995. The Company spent a considerable time developing a delivery performance specification with a series of test input profiles. Demonstration of conformity with this specification by a device manufacturer, using a final integrated device,

Fig. 2.3 Diprifusor™ TCI
module (8 × 5 × 1 cm)
developed by ICI
Pharmaceuticals (now
AstraZeneca) and containing the
Marsh pharmacokinetic model
and two microprocessors running
independent versions of TCI
control software as developed by
the University of Glasgow
(Reproduced with kind
permission from AstraZeneca)

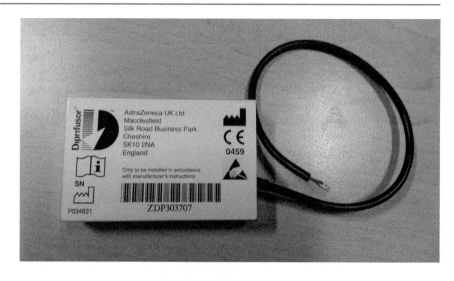

provided a link between the medicines authority assessing the clinical trials submission and the Notified Body evaluating the device. Discussions with the FDA in 1995 concluded that the submission of both clinical and device data should be in the form of a Pre Market Approval (PMA) application, to the group primarily responsible for the assessment of new devices in the USA.

In late 1991, the Ohmeda Company, possibly as a consequence of marketing priority being given to desflurane, decided to stop manufacture of the Ohmeda 9000 pump. As a result, Martyn Gray, an electronics expert who had been collaborating with the Glasgow University group, became available to work as a consultant for the Company. A decision was made to licence the Glasgow University TCI technology as the Company was satisfied that the two processor design incorporated in this system was likely to offer the most robust approach to TCI and Martyn was already familiar with this software. Martyn Gray (Anaesthesia Technology Ltd, Wetherby, UK) played a key role in the design and validation of the Diprifusor TCI module, thus transforming the Glasgow University software into a format that could communicate with and be installed in infusion pumps from a range of manufacturers. The development of the drug concentration identification system also required close collaboration between Martyn Gray and another external consultancy (Scientific Generics Ltd, now Sagentia, Cambridge, UK). An indication of the complexity of this aspect of the development can be seen in the equipment required to manufacture the electronic tag in the syringe finger grip (Fig. 2.4).

To ensure standardisation of drug delivery at a particular target setting, it was important to select a single pharmacokinetic model. Philip Arundel at ICI had developed the pharmacokinetic simulation program EXPLICIT [8] and I selected models described by Dyke and Shafer [9], Tackley

et al. [10], and Marsh [11] for comparison. Detailed information on drug infusion rates and measured blood propofol concentrations were available from healthy control patients in a pharmacokinetic study of propofol [12]. Simulation of the infusion rates used in this study with EXPLICIT showed a degree of positive bias (measured concentrations greater than predicted) with all three models. The degree of positive bias was small and similar with the Tackley and Marsh models and was somewhat greater with the Dyck and Shafer set. Similar results were later obtained in a prospective comparative study with the same three models [13], and in view of the greater clinical experience already obtained with the Marsh model, this was selected for further clinical studies. Meetings continued with academics working in this field and it was agreed that results obtained up to that time would be pooled to obtain a set of population pharmacokinetic parameters. Preliminary results were reviewed in 1993 but the figures obtained at that time using NON-MEM software showed no significant improvement in predictive performance. The Marsh model used in Diprifusor systems incorporates a minor reduction in central volume of distribution but in other respects uses the rate constants described by Gepts and colleagues [14]. A minor typographical error occurred in the description of the adult model given in a study related to the development of a model for children [11] in that Diprifusor systems use a value for k_{12} of $0.114 \, \text{min}^{-1}$ as described by Gepts rather than the value of $0.112 \, \text{min}^{-1}$ given in the Marsh publication. This disparity has a very minor effect on propofol delivery.

For the programme of Company sponsored clinical studies, the Glasgow University software was incorporated in a customised 'Backbar' computer developed by Martyn Gray at Anaesthesia Technology Ltd and linked via a serial port to an Ohmeda 9000 or Graseby 3400 computer compatible syringe pump. Delivery performance tests confirmed that,

Fig. 2.4 Equipment required to manufacture and insert the electronic tag into the plastic fingergrip for glass prefilled syringes of 'Diprivan'™ (Reproduced with kind permission from AstraZeneca)

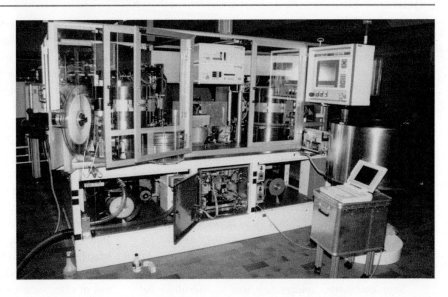

Table 2.1 Example of Diprifusor drug delivery specification in 50 kg subject with an initial target blood propofol concentration of 6 μg ml^{-1}, reduced to 4 μg ml^{-1} at 10 min and increased to 6 μg ml^{-1} at 20 min

Time (min)	1	5	10	20	21	30
Ideal vol (ml)	8.44	15.51	23.59	30.48	34.21	46.41
Min balance vol (ml)	7.60	14.73	22.41	28.96	32.50	44.09
Max balance vol (ml)	8.86	16.29	24.77	32.00	35.92	48.73

at a series of target settings, the delivery of propofol with these two systems was equivalent. Further tests examined inter-syringe and inter-pump variability, linearity of output over a target concentration range of 1–8 μg ml^{-1}, delivery performance over a 6 h period and performance at extremes of body weight accepted by Diprifusor systems (30 and 150 kg). Cumulative volume of drug delivered was measured with an electronic balance and compared with an ideal volume obtained by computer simulation of the same target input using Diprifusor software. At selected time points, infusion error was calculated as follows:

$$\text{Infusion error}\ \% = \frac{(\text{Balance volume} - \text{Ideal volume})}{\text{Ideal volume}} \times 100$$

Initial response time was also calculated as the time required for the predicted target to reach 90 % of the target set when the balance output was fed into Diprifusor software. This work led to a delivery performance specification, with a series of five test protocols, which was supplied to the manufacturers of commercial 'Diprifusor' systems. Initial response times for these test protocols ranged from 0.4 to 1.0 min and infusion error allowed was generally ±5 %. By demonstrating conformity with this specification, manufacturers were able to demonstrate that the Diprifusor module had been correctly installed in their pump and would operate in a manner consistent with the systems used in clinical trials. An example of the specification for one test profile is shown in Table 2.1

Eight prospective clinical studies with the selected TCI control program and using the Marsh pharmacokinetic model for induction and maintenance of anaesthesia in adults were completed and submitted to drug regulatory authorities in Europe and the USA in 1995. The principal objectives of the trial programme were as follows:

1. To determine the target concentration settings required to induce and maintain anaesthesia
2. To examine the influence of premedication [15], analgesic supplementation [16] and mode of ventilation [17] on the target concentrations required.
3. Two studies assessed the predictive performance of the Marsh model using the methods proposed by Varvel and colleagues [18]. Both studies showed an acceptable degree of positive bias (i.e. measured blood propofol concentrations greater than predicted) with median values of 16 % in one study in general surgery patients [19] and 25 % in patients undergoing cardiac surgery [20].
4. To determine the target concentrations required in elderly patients and in patients undergoing cardiac surgery [20]. One unpublished study in cardiac surgery patients was conducted with a double blind study design as requested by FDA and demonstrated no clinically relevant differences between the groups in haemodynamic or safety assessments.
5. To compare the characteristics of anaesthesia and ease of use of the Diprifusor TCI system with manually controlled infusion [21].

Efficacy and safety assessments made in these studies were consistent with previous experience with propofol and the following guidance on target blood propofol concentrations when using Diprifusor TCI systems for induction and maintenance of anaesthesia was proposed as an amendment to 'Diprivan' prescribing information:

In adult patients under 55 years of age anaesthesia can usually be induced with target propofol concentrations in the region of 4 to 8 µg/ml. An initial target of 4 µg/ml is recommended in premedicated patients and in unpremedicated patients an initial target of 6 µg/ml is advised. Induction time with these targets is generally within the range of 60–120 seconds. Higher targets will allow more rapid induction of anaesthesia but may be associated with more pronounced haemodynamic and respiratory depression.

A lower initial target should be used in patients over the age of about 55 years and in patients of ASA grades 3 and 4. The target concentration can then be increased in steps of 0.5 to 1.0 µg/ml at intervals of 1 minute to achieve a gradual induction of anaesthesia

Supplementary analgesia will generally be required and the extent to which target concentrations for maintenance of anaesthesia can be reduced will be influenced by the amount of concomitant analgesia administered. Target propofol concentrations in the region of 3 to 6 µg/ml usually maintain satisfactory anaesthesia.

Drug labelling also highlights the requirement for the target concentration to be titrated to the response of the patient, in view of interpatient variability in propofol pharmacokinetics and pharmacodynamics, and for users to be familiar with the instructions for use in the "'Diprifusor' Guide for Anaesthetists" which provided further information on the concept of TCI and advice on the practical use of the system.

Approvals for amendments to the drug prescribing information and EC certificates of conformance with the requirements of directive 93/42/EEC, allowing CE marks of conformance to be attached to the Diprifusor TCI module and integrated devices containing the module, began to be achieved in the UK and most European countries from 1996 onwards. The first integrated Diprifusor TCI system to gain approval in Europe was the Becton Dickinson Master TCI pump (Vial, later Fresenius, Bresins, France) followed by the Graseby 3500 (Smiths Medical, UK), Alaris IVAC TIVA TCI pump (Alaris Medical, later Carefusion, UK) and later in Japan, the Terumo TE-372 syringe pump.

Further submissions were made to drug authorities to extend the use of Diprifusor TCI systems to conscious sedation for surgical and diagnostic procedures and for intensive care sedation [22], but these submissions have not been made in every country in which approval for induction and maintenance of anaesthesia has been granted. No submission to allow the use of Diprifusor TCI systems in children has been made in any country. Currently used Diprifusor

systems display predicted effect-site propofol concentration using a blood–brain equilibration rate constant (k_{e0}) of 0.26 min^{-1}. This value was obtained from a preliminary analysis of a study in which pharmacodynamic data was obtained by monitoring EEG auditory evoked potentials [23]. A final non-parametric analysis of the study data provided a mean k_{e0} value of 0.2/min [24]. Subsequently, a modified k_{e0} of 1.21 /min was proposed for use with the Marsh model [25] but was not endorsed by AstraZeneca. The opportunity to control effect-site concentration was not incorporated in the original Diprifusor TCI module because of the complexity of the regulatory process, the impossibility of measuring effect-site concentrations and uncertainty about the most appropriate k_{e0} value for use with the Marsh model. More recently the latest version of the Diprifusor TCI module has been modified to allow the control of effect-site concentrations with an intermediate k_{e0} of 0.6 min^{-1}, a value found to be most likely to achieve a stable effect when the target is fixed at a time when a desired effect has been achieved [26]. In a further comparative study the Marsh model and a k_{e0} of 0.6 min^{-1} achieved induction of anaesthesia more rapidly than the Marsh model in blood concentration control or the Schnider model [27, 28] with a k_{e0} of 0.46 min^{-1} in effect-site control with no differences between groups in the magnitude of blood pressure changes or the frequency of apnoea [29].

The clinical trial documentation submitted in Europe was sufficient to gain approval for amendments to Diprivan labelling to allow administration by TCI in most countries in which TCI devices have been approved. Notable exceptions were Japan and the USA. In Japan the 1 % Diprivan Prefilled Syringe with electronic tag drug identification was evaluated and approved as a 1 % Diprivan Injection-Kit following four studies which examined usefulness, benefits, microbiology and use by conventional methods of administration. This was followed by a TCI user study in Japanese patients in which the Graseby 3500 infusion pump with the Diprifusor TCI module was used to assess efficacy, safety and controllability. Predictive performance was also assessed and median bias of 18.8 % was similar to that seen in European studies [30]. Guidance on administration of Diprivan by TCI in Japan recommends the use of slightly lower target settings:

Diprivan should be administered using Diprifusor TCI function of a Diprifusor TCI pump.

(1) Induction

Usually in adults, infusion should be started intravenously with a target blood propofol concentration of 3 µg/ml, which should be increased in steps of 1.0 to 2.0 µg/ml at intervals of one minute if clinical signs do not show onset of anaesthesia in 3 minutes after start of infusion.

In adult patients, anaesthesia can usually be induced with target concentration in the range of 3.0 to 6.0 µg/ml within the range of 1 to 3 minutes.

In elderly patients and in patients of ASA grade 3 and 4, a lower initial target should be used.

(2) Maintenance

The required depth of anaesthesia can usually be maintained by continuous infusion of the drug in combination with oxygen or a mixture of oxygen and nitrous oxide, while the target concentration is titrated against the response of the patient. Target concentrations in the region of 2.5 to 5.0 µg/ml usually maintain satisfactory anaesthesia in adults.

Analgesics (narcotic analgesics, local anaesthetics, etc.) should be used concomitantly.

Despite a lengthy evaluation process during which FDA reviewers and regulatory strategy changed, approval for the Diprifusor TCI system in the USA was not obtained and the agency issued a non-approvable letter in 2001, stating that lack of precision in dosing posed an unacceptable risk. The Company responded that no pharmacokinetic model could be expected to eliminate variability in the concentrations achieved at a particular target setting and that such variability had not been associated with any safety concerns, but approval was not achieved and the Company withdrew the US submission in 2004. A theoretical treatise has since then proved that TCI devices can neither create nor eliminate biological variability, the overall spread of observations being an intrinsic property of the drug [31]. More detailed information on the failure to obtain approval for TCI in the USA is discussed in a recent publication on the history of TCI [32].

'Open' TCI Systems

Around 2002, as 'Diprivan' patents began to expire, a number of medical device manufactures began their independent development of TCI devices without a drug recognition facility which therefore allowed their use with generic preparations of propofol. Among the first of these were the 'Orchestra'® Base Primea introduced by Fresenius Vial in 2003 and the 'Asena'® PK syringe pump (Alaris Medical, now Cardinal Health Care). By this time continuing academic research had led to the publication of an alternative pharmacokinetic model for propofol, developed in volunteers, with covariates for age, weight, height and lean body mass [27]. This study also included characterisation of the relationship between plasma concentration and the time

course of drug effect, and proposed a value for the blood–brain equilibration rate constant (k_{e0}) of propofol of 0.456 min^{-1} and a predicted time of peak effect of 1.7 or 1.6 min when assessed by visual inspection of the EEG [28]. Algorithms to achieve and maintain stable drug concentrations at the site of drug effect had been published earlier [33, 34] and medical device companies came under pressure from academic groups to provide TCI systems which would not only allow the administration of generic propofol with the Marsh model, but would also allow the choice of the alternative pharmacokinetic model, the choice to control plasma or effect-site drug concentrations and the ability to deliver remifentanil or sufentanil by TCI. While these devices refer to plasma rather than blood concentrations, this chapter continues to describe blood concentrations as in the regulatory studies with propofol and remifentanil whole blood concentrations were measured and guidance on target settings in drug labelling is provided in terms of blood concentrations.

In Europe these systems were submitted to a Notified Body to assess conformity with the standards set out in the European Medical Device Directive 93/42 in the same way that the Diprifusor module and integrated Diprifusor TCI pumps were evaluated. As devices intended to deliver anaesthetic (i.e. 'potentially hazardous' substances), these come within Class IIb of the Directive classification and require inspection by a Notified Body with regard to their design, manufacture and quality assurance. A key feature of the Directive is that devices bearing a CE mark, indicating that they have demonstrated a satisfactory assessment of conformity with the requirements of the Directive, can then be marketed throughout Europe and CE marking has also been recognised as a sign of approval by other countries outside Europe. Directive 93/42 provides a series of 'Essential Requirements' which have to be met in relation to safety and performance. In terms of performance, it is sufficient to demonstrate that a device incorporating a particular model at particular target settings will deliver an infusion profile and predict plasma or effect-site drug concentrations in line with mathematical predictions for the same model obtained by computer simulation. Literature publications describing clinical experience with particular models can be used to justify the choice of target settings used in these studies. There is no requirement for the Notified Body to have any contact with the relevant Medicines Authority responsible for the marketing authorisation of the drugs to be infused or the manufacturer of these drugs. A similar approach to device approval has been used by newer entrants in the field. The Perfusor® Space and Infusomat® Space pumps (B Braun, Germany), the Volumed® µVP 7000 and Syramed® µSP600 devices (Arcomed AG, Switzerland) and the Pion® TCI pump (Bionet, Korea) have incorporated the Marsh and Schnider models for propofol, the Minto model for remifentanil and in some cases models for administration of sufentanil, alfentanil, fentanyl, midazolam, ketamine and dexmedetomidine by TCI.

In the case of propofol, the introduction of open TCI systems giving users a choice of pharmacokinetic models and modes of administration has led to a degree of confusion [35] which will be discussed in the section on propofol TCI with open systems. In the following sections the author has used the pharmacokinetic simulation programs TIVAtrainer© (Version 9.1 GuttaBV, Aerdenhout, The Netherlands) and PK-SIM (Specialized Data Systems, Jenkintown, PA, USA) to illustrate, in example subjects, the performance of different pharmacokinetic models or their implementation.

Remifentanil TCI

By the time open TCI systems became available there were already a large number of literature publications on the administration of remifentanil by TCI based on the use of non-approved TCI software and prototypes in research studies. A number of different pharmacokinetic models for remifentanil had been described and I was commissioned by GlaxoSmithKline to assist Professor Jürgen Schüttler with the preparation of a Clinical Overview to support the administration of remifentanil by TCI and to provide guidance on appropriate target remifentanil concentrations for inclusion in drug labelling. This involved a detailed review of 41 published clinical studies involving a total of 2650 subjects, comparison of the performance of the different pharmacokinetic models and the selection of a preferred model, overviews of efficacy and safety and conclusions on risks and benefits. The pharmacokinetic model described by Minto and colleagues [36] was advocated for the following reasons:

1. This model was derived from a composite analysis of data from 65 healthy adults with an age range of 20–85 years
2. A population pharmacokinetic model was developed to account for an observed effect of age and lean body mass on the pharmacokinetics of remifentanil
3. This study also provided a k_{e0} value for remifentanil related to patient age, predicting slower equilibration in patients older than 40 years and faster equilibration in younger patients.
4. Widely used in prototype TCI systems with good clinical results
5. A prospective evaluation of the predictive performance of this model provided acceptable values for bias (−15 %) and inaccuracy (20 %) [37].

Once approved, guidance on the administration of remifentanil by TCI was added to the Statement of Product Characteristics (SPC) for remifentanil ('Ultiva', GlaxoSmithKline) in territories where approved TCI devices were available. Extracts from the SPC include the following:

'Ultiva' may also be given by target controlled infusion (TCI) with an approved infusion device incorporating the Minto pharmacokinetic model with covariates for age and lean body mass. For TCI the recommended dilution of Ultiva is 20–50 micrograms/ml.

Ultiva TCI should be used in association with an intravenous or inhalational hypnotic agent during induction and maintenance of anaesthesia in ventilated adult patients. In association with these agents, adequate analgesia for induction of anaesthesia and surgery can generally be achieved with target blood remifentanil concentrations ranging from 3 to 8 nanograms/ml. Ultiva should be titrated to individual patient response. For particularly stimulating surgical procedures target blood concentrations up to 15 nanograms/ml may be required. At the end of surgery when the TCI infusion is stopped or the target concentration reduced, spontaneous respiration is likely to return at calculated remifentanil concentrations in the region of 1 to 2 nanograms/ml. As with manually-controlled infusion, post-operative analgesia should be established before the end of surgery with longer acting analgesics. There are insufficient data to make recommendations on the use of TCI for spontaneous ventilation anaesthesia and use of TCI for the management of post-operative analgesia is not recommended.

In association with an intravenous or inhalational agent, adequate analgesia for cardiac surgery is generally achieved at the higher end of the range of target blood remifentanil concentrations used for general surgical procedures. Following titration of remifentanil to individual patient response, blood concentrations as high as 20 nanograms/ml have been used in clinical studies

Because of the increased sensitivity of elderly patients to Ultiva, when administered by TCI in this population the initial target concentration should be 1.5 to 4 nanograms/ml with subsequent titration to response.

In obese patients, with the calculation of lean body mass (LBM) used in the Minto model, LBM is likely to be underestimated in female patients with a body mass index (BMI) greater than 35 kg/m2 and in male patients with BMI greater than 40 kg/m2. To avoid underdosing in these patients, remifentanil TCI should be titrated carefully to individual response.

In ASA III/IV patients a lower initial target of 1.5 to 4 nanograms/ml should be used and subsequently titrated to response.

In many respects, the approach adopted for remifentanil TCI was ideal in that a single pharmacokinetic model is recommended and advice on suitable target concentration settings is provided in the drug labelling. Although some studies had used the pharmacodynamic parameters provided by Minto and colleagues to deliver remifentanil by effect-site TCI, GlaxoSmithKline did not wish to recommend this approach. While some of the open TCI systems now available do provide the option to control effect-site concentrations of remifentanil, this mode of administration leads to very minor differences in drug delivery in comparison with plasma concentration control (Fig. 2.5). With a drug with such rapid onset and offset characteristics as remifentanil, it is unlikely that a study comparing the two modes of administration would detect any clinical differences.

One defect in the Minto model is the use of the James equation [38] which underestimates lean body mass in obese patients. However, this was recognised at the time of the regulatory submission and notification of this effect was added to the drug labelling. Estimation of lean body mass will be discussed in more detail in a later section.

Sufentanil TCI

Sufentanil is not marketed in the UK but is used in the USA and a number of European countries and the ability to administer sufentanil by TCI with the pharmacokinetic model described by Gepts and colleagues [39] has been incorporated in some of the open TCI systems now available. In France a brief addendum concerning drug concentrations has been included in the French prescribing information for 'Sufenta'™. Guidance on suggested plasma concentrations includes the following:

Efficient concentration
  – *Anaesthesia. After iv administration, the following plasma concentration of 0.15 to 0.6 ng/ml is usually used to maintain general anaesthesia when combined with hypnotics. Concentrations of 0.4 to 2 ng/ml are requested in cardiac surgery. Plasma and effect site (brain) concentrations equilibrate after 6 min. Spontaneous ventilation is observed at a mean concentration of 0.2 ng/ml.*
  – *Sedation. Combined with a benzodiazepine for long term sedation, the concentration is usually between 0.3 to 2 ng/ml.*

Although a specific pharmacokinetic model is not mentioned, the pharmacokinetics of the drug as described indicates values for Vc (the central volume of distribution) and clearance which are identical to those described by Gepts [39]. Some open TCI systems also provide the

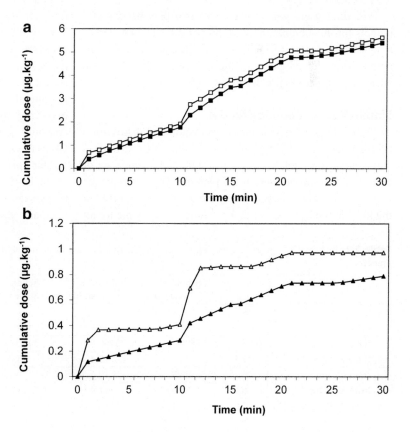

Fig. 2.5 Cumulative dose ($\mu g\ kg^{-1}$) of remifentanil (**a**) and sufentanil (**b**) delivered by blood concentration (Cb_T) or effect site TCI (Ce_T). Remifentanil Cb_T *filled square*, Ce_T *open square* targets 3 ng ml^{-1}, increased to 6 ng ml^{-1} at 10 min, and decreased to 3 ng ml^{-1} at 20 min. Sufentanil Cb_T *filled triangle*, Ce_T *open triangle*, targets 0.5 ng ml^{-1} increased to 1 ng ml^{-1} at 10 min, and decreased to 0.5 ng ml^{-1} at 20 min

opportunity to control effect-site concentrations of sufentanil using the Gepts model combined with a blood–brain equilibration constant (k_{e0}) of 0.112 min^{-1} derived from the mean equilibration half life of 6.2 min described by Scott and colleagues [40]. With a drug such as sufentanil with a relatively slow onset, control of effect-site concentration will lead to the administration of a significantly larger initial dose (Fig. 2.5) and a more rapid onset of effect. One concern with some implementations of the Gepts model is that the model is not weight proportional and without age and weight limits could deliver excessive doses if used in small children.

Propofol TCI with Open TCI Devices

The ability to deliver generic preparations of propofol is possible with open systems which do not require the added security of the electronic identification of the drug and its concentration. Isolated cases have been reported where the wrong concentration of propofol emulsion has been selected [41] or where propofol and remifentanil syringes were mistakenly reversed [42] and in one case led to accidental awareness [43]. Anecdotal reports suggest that such mistakes may occur more frequently than reported. Failure to use the correct syringe brand selection can also lead to errors in drug delivery, in some cases up to almost 20 % of the nominal delivery [44].

Providing users with a choice of two pharmacokinetic models for the administration of propofol by TCI has led to a significant degree of confusion which has probably hindered the wider adoption of the technique [35]. Possible sources of confusion are discussed as follows:

Simple Versus Complex Model
With the Marsh model, as the central volume of distribution (V_1) is related to body weight, both volumes of distribution and clearance are related to body weight and a single set of rate constants can be used for all patients. The consequence is that, at any given target setting, drug delivery in terms of mg kg^{-1} or mg kg^{-1} h^{-1} or μg kg^{-1} min^{-1} is the same for all

patients, independent of body weight, gender or patient age. Although age is requested as an input, this is only to ensure that this adult model is not used in patients younger than 16 years. It is expected that target settings will be titrated to achieve the depth of anaesthesia or sedation desired, and lower targets are recommended in older or debilitated patients. Guidance on recommended target settings is provided in 'Diprivan' labelling and changes in target settings provide proportional changes in the rate of drug delivery. The introduction of this system was accompanied by the provision by the pharmaceutical company of more detailed information on the technique in training materials such as the 'Diprifusor' Guide for Anaesthetists and an extensive programme of training courses provided by local marketing companies with the assistance of local and international experts, often accompanied by demonstrations of the technique achieved with live video links to an operating theatre. The Marsh model has been used extensively and safely for many years since its first introduction in Diprifusor TCI systems in 1996 and it can be estimated that about 25,000 such systems have been introduced to clinical use.

In contrast to the simplicity of the Marsh model the Schnider model is more complex. It is difficult without further calculation to gain much information on the likely performance of a particular pharmacokinetic model from the series of rate constants used as inputs in a TCI program. However, if the volumes and clearances of the three-compartment model are presented in the terms of ml kg^{-1} for volumes and ml kg^{-1} min^{-1} for clearances as in Tables 2.2 and 2.3, some prediction of the differences between models in delivery performance is facilitated. In the Schnider model, V_1 is constant at 4.27 l, age is a covariate for the volume of the second compartment (V_2) and rapid peripheral clearance (Cl_2); and weight, height and lean body mass are all covariates for metabolic clearance (Cl_1). Although gender is not a covariate, it has an influence on Cl_1 as the James equation used to calculate lean body mass is gender specific in such a way that metabolic clearance is about 15–30 % greater in female subjects, the higher figure being seen in heavier patients (Table 2.3). The best way to compare the performance of different pharmacokinetic

Table 2.2 Influence of age and gender on volumes of distribution and clearance with the Marsh and Schnider pharmacokinetic models for propofol

	Marsh	Schnider 30 year, M	Schnider 50 year, M	Schnider 80 year, M	Schnider 30 year, F	Schnider 50 year, F	Schnider 80 year, F
V_1 (ml kg^{-1})	228	61	61	61	61	61	61
V_2 (ml kg^{-1})	473	398	287	119	398	287	119
V_3 (ml kg^{-1})	2895	3400	3400	3400	3400	3400	3400
Cl_1 (ml kg^{-1} min^{-1})	27.1	23.4	23.4	23.4	28.7	28.7	28.7
Cl_2 (ml kg^{-1} min^{-1})	26	26.3	19.5	9.2	26.3	19.5	9.2
Cl_3 (ml kg^{-1} min^{-1})	9.6	11.9	11.9	11.9	11.9	11.9	11.9

All subjects 70 kg, 170 cm

Table 2.3 Influence of body weight and gender on volumes of distribution and clearance with the Marsh and Schnider pharmacokinetic models for propofol

	Marsh	Schnider 50 kg, M	Schnider 70 kg, M	Schnider 110 kg, M	Schnider 50 kg, F	Schnider 70 kg, F	Schnider 110 kg, F
V_1 (ml kg^{-1})	228	85	61	39	85	61	39
V_2 (ml kg^{-1})	473	401	287	182	401	287	182
V_3 (ml kg^{-1})	2895	4760	3400	2164	4760	3400	2164
Cl_1 (ml kg^{-1} min^{-1})	27.1	30	23.4	24	34.4	28.7	31.2
Cl_2 (ml kg^{-1} min^{-1})	26	27.2	19.5	12.4	27.2	19.5	12.4
Cl_3 (ml kg^{-1} min^{-1})	9.6	16.7	11.9	7.6	16.7	11.9	7.6

All subjects 50 year, 170 cm

Fig. 2.6 The influence of patient age on the cumulative dose (mg kg^{-1}) of propofol delivered with the Marsh and Schnider models at a target blood concentration (Cb$_T$) of 4 µg ml^{-1} in 70 kg, 170 cm male subjects. *Filled diamond* Marsh Cb$_T$ all ages, *open square* Schnider Cb$_T$ 30 year, *filled triangle* Schnider Cb$_T$ 50 year, *open triangle* Schnider Cb$_T$ 80 year

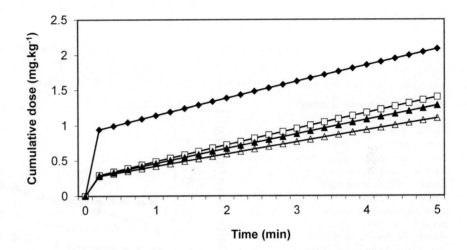

models is to examine delivery performance in terms of the cumulative amount of drug given over the first few minutes (i.e. the induction dose) and thereafter the infusion rate profile delivered in the maintenance phase. The cumulative dose delivered over an extended period can also be useful to give an overall picture of the induction and maintenance phases.

Figure 2.6 shows a comparison of the influence of patient age on the cumulative amount of propofol delivered over 5 min with the Marsh and Schnider models in a 70 kg, 170 cm male subject at a target blood propofol concentration of 4 µg ml^{-1}. It can be seen that the Schnider model, with a much smaller central compartment volume than the Marsh model, delivers a much smaller initial dose by rapid infusion than the Marsh model. By 2 min the Schnider model has delivered only 0.7 mg/kg in the 50-year-old patient whereas the Marsh model has provided 1.4 mg kg^{-1}, independent of patient age. The initial dose delivered by the Schnider model is also independent of patient age but thereafter the slopes of the delivery profiles reflect age related changes in rapid peripheral clearance (Cl$_2$) (Table 2.2). Figure 2.7 shows a comparison of the two models with respect to patient weight in 50 year, 170 cm male subjects. Again, the cumulative dose delivered is much smaller with the Schnider model and as V_1 is constant in this model, the weight related reduction

in V_1 in terms of ml kg^{-1} (Table 2.3) leads to weight related changes in initial dose delivered in terms of mg kg^{-1} with a larger initial dose in lighter patients. Weight related changes in clearance in terms of ml kg^{-1} min^{-1} (Table 2.3) also explain the age related divergence in the cumulative dose lines in the figure.

Because the Schnider model delivers such a small initial dose it has become routine practice in centres which use this model to select an option to control effect-site propofol concentrations. Figure 2.8 shows the cumulative dose of propofol delivered with the Marsh model in blood concentration control mode and the Schnider model in effect control mode (k_{e0} 0.46 min^{-1}) in 50 year, 170 cm male patients of 50, 70 and 110 kg at targets of 4 µg ml^{-1}. In the 70 kg subject, the initial dose delivered with the Schnider model is now similar to that provided by the Marsh model in blood control mode, while that in lighter patients is greater and that in heavier patients is smaller. Once a requested target is reached there is very little difference between blood and effect site modes of control in the infusion rate required to maintain this target. Figure 2.9 shows the infusion rates delivered by the Marsh model in blood concentration control (Cb$_T$) and the Schnider model in blood and effect-site control (Ce$_T$) in 50 year, 170 cm male patients of 50 and 100 kg when propofol target concentrations of 3 µg ml^{-1} have been

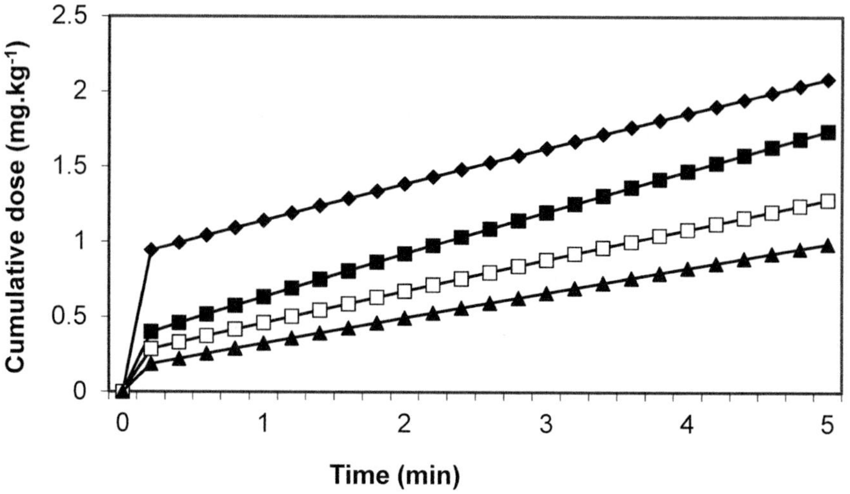

Fig. 2.7 The influence of patient weight on the cumulative dose (mg kg^{-1}) of propofol delivered with the Marsh and Schnider models at a target blood concentration (Cb$_T$) of 4 µg ml^{-1} in 50 year, 170 cm male subjects. *Filled diamond* Marsh Cb$_T$ all weights, *filled square* Schnider Cb$_T$ 50 kg, *open square* Schnider Cb$_T$ 70 kg, *filled triangle* Schnider Cb$_T$ 110 kg

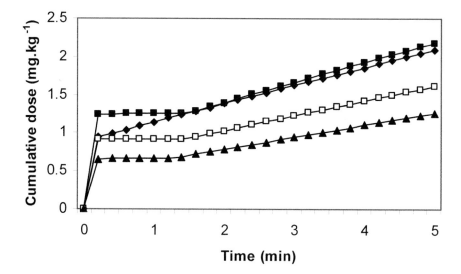

Fig. 2.8 The influence of patient weight on the cumulative dose (mg kg^{-1}) of propofol delivered with Marsh model in blood concentration control (Cb$_T$ 4 µg ml^{-1}) and the Schnider model in effect control (Ce$_T$ 4 µg ml^{-1}) in 50 year, 170 cm male subjects. *Filled square* Schnider Ce$_T$ 50 kg, *filled diamond* Marsh Cb$_T$ all weights, *open square* Schnider Ce$_T$ 70 kg, *filled triangle* Schnider Ce$_T$ 110 kg

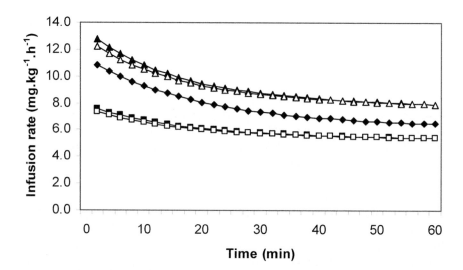

Fig. 2.9 Propofol infusion rates (mg kg^{-1} h^{-1}) delivered with Marsh model in blood concentration control (Cb$_T$ 3 µg ml^{-1}) and the Schnider model in blood concentration (Cb$_T$ 3 µg ml^{-1}) and effect control (Ce$_T$ 3 µg ml^{-1}) in 50 year, 170 cm male subjects weighing 50 or 110 kg. *Filled triangle* 50 kg, Schnider CbT, *open triangle* 50 kg, Schnider CeT, *filled diamond* Marsh Cb$_T$ all weights, *filled square* 110 kg, Schnider Cb$_T$, *open square* 110 kg, Schnider Ce$_T$

set. Infusion rates with the Schnider model in the 50 kg subject are greater than those provided with the Marsh model and those in the 110 kg subject are lower, in both cases reflecting weight related changes in clearance (Table 2.3). In both Schnider simulations, the maintenance infusion rate in effect control mode is only marginally slower than with blood control and this difference disappears over time, in the absence of any change in target setting. Increases in rapid peripheral distribution and clearance (V_2 and Cl_2) in subjects younger than 53 years and decreases in older subjects influence the maintenance infusion rate for the first 30 min but thereafter, in a 70 kg subject, rate is similar to that provided by the Marsh model. The increase in clearance in female subjects seen with the Schnider model leads to greater infusion rates in females and, in terms of mg kg^{-1} h^{-1}, the influence is greater in heavier patients (Fig. 2.10).

The potential attraction of the Schnider model is that the incorporation of covariates for age, body weight and height attempts to explain and reduce inter-individual variability in propofol pharmacokinetics and improve the precision of the model in predicting the blood and effect-site propofol concentrations achieved. Effect-site propofol concentrations

cannot be measured but methodology for the evaluation of predictive performance of TCI systems has been described [18] whereby bias is described by the median performance error (MDPE) for an individual or group of patients and inaccuracy as the median absolute performance error (MDAPE) derived from comparisons of measured and predicted blood propofol concentrations. It has been suggested that MDPE should be no greater than 10–20 % and MDAPE in the region of 20–30 % for a TCI system to be deemed clinically acceptable [45]. While most studies evaluating predictive performance with both the Marsh and Schnider models have found group values for MDPE and MDAPE close to these ranges, group values being medians of medians in an individual patient probably provide an unrealistic picture of the large degree of pharmacokinetic variability between individuals in a group and within an individual over time. This variability becomes evident when one looks at the range of values contributing to the group and individual median values (Table 2.4) [46]. This shows that the benefits of the more complex Schnider model over the simpler Marsh model are limited as considerable inter-individual variability persists with both models. It has been confirmed that the Schnider model produces less

Fig. 2.10 Influence of gender and body weight on propofol infusion rates (mg kg^{-1} h^{-1}) in 50 year, 170 cm subjects with the Schnider model in blood concentration control (Cb_T 3 μg ml^{-1}). *Filled diamond* 50 kg female, *open square* 50 kg male, *filled triangle* 110 kg female, *open triangle* 110 kg male

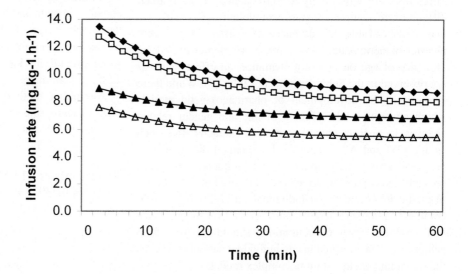

Table 2.4 Predictive performance of the Marsh and Schnider models for propofol as assessed by median performance error (MDPE %) and median absolute performance error (MDAPE %) with values given as the median and range of values encountered for individual patients in each study group

Model	Subjects	n	MDPE %	MDAPE %	Reference
Marsh	Major elective surgery patients	46	16.2 (−21–84)	20.7 (6.3–84)	[19]
Marsh	Orthopaedic or gynaecological surgery	10	−7 (−43–43)[a]	18.2 (8–53)[a]	[13]
Schnider	Healthy adult volunteers	18	1.8 (−34–74)	20.7 (11–74)	[46]
Marsh	Healthy control patients	9	2.3 (−32–33)	24.6 (11–37)	[47]
Schnider	Healthy control patients	9	−0.1 (−22–34)	23.6 (13–43)	[47]
Marsh	Major elective surgery patients	41	16 (−27–84)	26 (11–84)	[48]
Schnider	Major elective surgery patients	41	15 (−23–73)	23 (7–73)	[48]

[a]10–90 percentiles

Fig. 2.11 Influence of body mass index (BMI kg m^{-2}) on lean body mass (LBM kg) in *filled square* male and *open diamond* female subjects, 160 cm height and bodyweight 30–180 kg as calculated with the James equation [38]

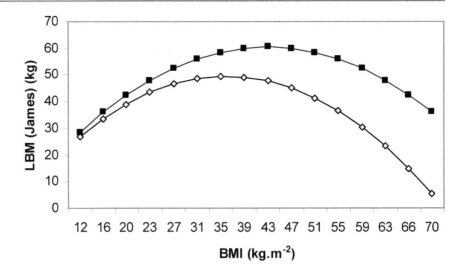

positive bias (measured concentrations greater than predicted) when the target concentration is steady or increasing, but the overall figure in a given patient is influenced by a trend towards negative bias at induction and positive bias at recovery or when a lower target is set [47, 48]. Opposite effects are seen with the Marsh model with positive bias at induction and negative bias during recovery. These differences are most likely a consequence of the marked difference in central compartment volume (V_1) with the two models (Table 2.2) as discussed earlier. More recent pharmacokinetic studies [49, 50] have demonstrated an influence of age on propofol clearance, an effect that was not observed in the Schnider model (Table 2.2). While there is merit in the development of pharmacokinetic models which attempt to take account of age and gender related changes in pharmacokinetics, patient characteristics such as age [28] and ASA status lead to marked differences in propofol pharmacodynamics, which influence the drug concentrations required to achieve a desired effect. On top of predictable trends, inter-individual variability in pharmacokinetics and pharmacodynamics account for the guidance that propofol target concentrations should be titrated to achieve the effect desired in any individual patient and limits the potential benefits of more complex models.

Lean Body Mass Calculation

The Schnider model for propofol, and the Minto model for remifentanil, both incorporate lean body mass (LBM) as a covariate for the calculation of metabolic clearance and both use the equations described by James [38] to determine LBM. However, there are inconsistencies in these equations which in some circumstances lead to erroneous values [51].

The James equations based on weight (kg) and height (cm) for male and female subjects differ as follows:

$$\text{Males}: \text{LBM}\,(\text{kg}) = 1.1 \times \text{weight} - 128 \times (\text{weight/height})^2$$

$$\text{Females}: \text{LBM}\,(\text{kg})$$
$$= 1.07 \times \text{weight} - 148 \times (\text{weight/height})^2$$

Body mass index (BMI) = weight (kg)/height (m^2) increases as body weight increases but increases more slowly if height also increases. Figure 2.11 illustrates the influence of body mass index on lean body mass as calculated by the James equation in male and female subjects of 160 cm height over the weight range of 30–180 kg. It can be seen that LBM reaches a maximum value and begins to decline at a BMI value around 35 kg m^{-2} in female subjects and about 42 kg m^{-2} in males.

Alternative methods to assess LBM based on measurement of antipyrine space or fat free mass (FFM) have been described by Hume [52] and Janmahasatian and colleagues [53], respectively, as follows:

$$\text{Hume}: \text{Males}: \text{LBM}\,(\text{kg})$$
$$= 0.33929 \times \text{height}\,(\text{cm}) + 0.32810 \times \text{weight}\,(\text{kg})$$
$$- 29.533$$

$$\text{Females}: \text{LBM}\,(\text{kg})$$
$$= 0.41813 \times \text{height}\,(\text{cm}) + 0.29569$$
$$\times \text{weight}\,(\text{kg}) - 43.2933$$

$$\text{Janmahasatian and colleagues}: \text{Males}: \text{FFM}$$
$$= \frac{9.27 \times 10^3 \times \text{Body wt}\,(\text{kg})}{6.68 \times 10^3 + 216 \times \text{BMI}}$$

$$\text{Females}: \text{FFM} = \frac{9.27 \times 10^3 \times \text{Body wt}\,(\text{kg})}{8.78 \times 10^3 + 244 \times \text{BMI}}$$

Both of these methods avoid the paradoxical decline in LBM in patients with high values for BMI and can be used to illustrate the differing consequences of the use of the James LBM

Fig. 2.12 Influence of method of calculation of lean body mass on propofol clearance (ml kg^{-1} min^{-1}) in a 160 cm, 40 year female subject. *Filled diamond* James [38], *open triangle* Janmahasatian [53] and *filled square* Hume [52] equations

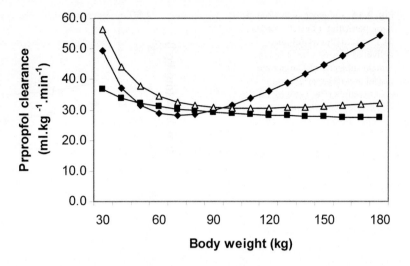

Fig. 2.13 Influence of method of calculation of lean body mass on remifentanil clearance (ml kg^{-1} min^{-1}) in a 160 cm, 40 year female subject. *Filled square* Hume [52], *open triangle* Janmahasatian [53] and *filled diamond* James [38] equations

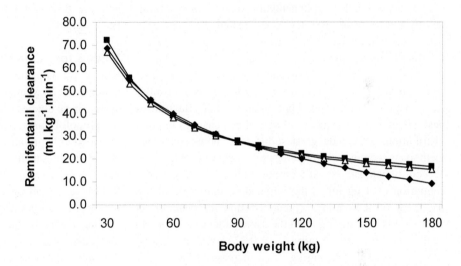

equations in the Schnider model for propofol and the Minto model for remifentanil. In the Schnider model for propofol, clearance is influenced by both LBM and total body weight (TBW): $Cl_1 (1 min^{-1}) = 1.89 + ((TBW - 77) \times 0.0456) + ((LBM - 59) \times -0.0681) + ((Height - 177) \times 0.0264)$. The consequence is that at BMI values greater than 35 kg m^{-2} in female patients, as calculated LBM begins to decrease, metabolic clearance begins to increase again, such that the infusion rates at a given target setting will increase with a potential risk of overdosage.

In the Minto model for remifentanil, age and LBM are covariates for metabolic clearance: $Cl_1 (1 min^{-1}) = 2.6 - 0.0162 \times (Age - 40) + 0.0191 \times (LBM - 55)$. Thus, in patients with high BMI, clearance in terms of l kg^{-1} decreases such that there is a potential risk of underdosage. However, in terms of ml kg^{-1} min^{-1}, the principal influence on infusion rate during maintenance of anaesthesia, the increase in propofol clearance with the Schnider model in a 40 year, 160 cm height, female patient of 180 kg would be 70 % in comparison with values predicted by the Hume and

Janmahasatian equations while the decrease in remifentanil clearance in the same patient would be 40 % (Figs. 2.12 and 2.13). This problem highlights a failure to validate the performance of the proposed models over the whole range of potential patient input characteristics. Once recognised, the manufacturers of the Asena PK and Orchestra Base Primea open TCI systems introduced a compromise solution whereby inputs of body weight and height producing BMI figures above the point where the James equation calculates a declining LBM lead to clearance being calculated based on the maximum LBM for the patient's height. A similar procedure has been implemented in more recently introduced open TCI systems.

Different Implementations of Effect Control Software

At the time of their introduction in 2003 both the Asena PK and the Orchestra Base Primea open TCI pumps provided users with the option of controlling propofol blood or effect-site concentrations with the Schnider pharmacokinetic

Fig. 2.14 Influence of method of implementation of effect control TCI on initial propofol dose delivered in a 20 year, 170 cm female subject with the Schnider model at a target effect site concentration (Ce$_T$) of 4 µg ml^{-1}. *Open square* fixed T peak 1.6 min, *filled diamond* fixed k_{e0} 0.456 min^{-1}

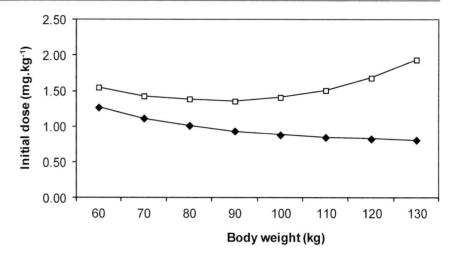

model. However the implementation of the effect control facility in the Asena PK device calculated a k_{e0} for each patient based on a fixed time to peak effect of 1.6 min while the Base Primea pump used a fixed k_{e0} of 0.456 min^{-1}, both figures coming from the original publication by Schnider and colleagues [28]. With both methods, age has an influence on the size of the initial bolus delivered and the time of peak effect as a consequence of age related changes in rapid distribution. As such the greatest difference between the two methods is seen in younger patients. In a 20-year-old, 70 kg, 170 cm female subject, at a propofol effect site target concentration of 4 µg ml^{-1}, the initial dose delivered with a fixed k_{e0} of 0.46 min^{-1} (predicted time to peak effect 1.36 min) is 1.11 mg kg^{-1}. In the same patient with time to peak effect fixed at 1.6 min ($k_{e0} = 0.32$ min^{-1}), the initial dose delivered is 1.43 mg kg^{-1}, an increase of 28 %. The difference between the two methods becomes more marked as body weight increases as shown in Fig. 2.14. In the 60 and 70 kg patients, the difference between the two methods occurs principally because the illustration involves a young patient but, as body weight increases and clearance increases due to the complex influence of body weight and LBM, time to peak effect with a fixed k_{e0} decreases. Thus with the fixed time to peak effect method, a greater reduction in k_{e0} is required to achieve a time to peak of 1.6 min and this slower k_{e0} delivers a greater initial dose at the same target setting. As the disparity between the two methods, in the initial dose delivered over the weight range 80–100 kg increases from 37 to 60 %, while BMI remains below the point at which the James equation provides erroneous values for LBM, it is unlikely that this difference would be abolished by the use of an alternative method of LBM calculation.

The same problem does not occur with the Marsh model as an increase in body weight is not associated with any decrease in the predicted time to peak effect and effect control TCI at a target of 4 µg ml^{-1} with a fixed k_{e0} of 1.2 min^{-1} or a fixed time to peak effect of 1.6 min delivers

an initial dose of 1.4 mg kg^{-1}, independent of patient age or body weight.

Models for TCI in Children

Use of the Diprifusor TCI system is restricted to use in patients of 16 years of age or older as studies with this system have not been conducted in children and no guidance on propofol target concentration for use in children is provided in Diprivan (propofol) labelling. However, a number of studies of the pharmacokinetics of propofol in children have been published and the model described by Kataria and colleagues [54] and the 'Paedfusor' model have been incorporated in some open TCI systems.

The history of the 'Paedfusor' model is as follows: In 1997, discussions with Jürgen Schüttler and Martin White at the time of the ASA meeting in San Diego that year led to the production of a modified Diprifusor system with a pharmacokinetic model which required the calculation of clearance as a power function of body weight on the basis of the preliminary results of a population pharmacokinetic study with propofol which was later published [55]. Central compartment volume (V_1) at 458 ml kg^{-1} was much greater than the value of 228 ml kg used by the Marsh model in adults and to avoid a sudden step change in 16-year-old patients, V_1 is gradually decreased in 13- to 15-year-old patients. This system, which became known as a 'Paedfusor' was provided by Zeneca to Neil Morton in Glasgow who confirmed the ease of use of the system, clinical efficacy and absence of adverse effects when used for induction and maintenance of anaesthesia in healthy children aged 6 months to 16 years [56]. Further studies confirmed good predictive performance when this model was used in children of 1–15 years undergoing cardiac surgery or catheterization [57]. Anaesthesia was induced with an initial propofol target blood concentration of 5 µg ml^{-1} and was supplemented with a TCI infusion of alfentanil. Median performance error (MDPE) and median absolute performance error (MDAPE)

Fig. 2.15 Influence of pharmacokinetic model on propofol infusion rates delivered in a 20 kg child at a target blood concentration (Cb$_T$) of 4 μg ml^{-1} with *filled triangle* Kataria, *open square* Paedfusor and *filled diamond* Marsh adult models

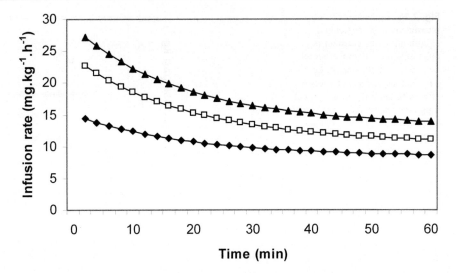

values of 4.1 % and 9.7 %, respectively, were determined. The full details of the Paedfusor model used in this study were provided in a subsequent publication [58]. Both the Kataria and Paedfusor models were found to achieve acceptable predictive performance in a study which compared eight paediatric pharmacokinetic models in healthy young children [59]. At a given target blood propofol concentration both models deliver greater initial doses and subsequent infusion rates than the Marsh adult model with the Kataria model delivering more than the Paedfusor model (Fig. 2.15). Another potential problem with commercial implementations of the Kataria model is that the study publication describes three different models and the same version of the model may not always be selected.

Use of Different Rate Constants to Predict or Control Effect Site Concentration

As mentioned earlier, the original submissions for 'Diprivan' (propofol) and 'Ultiva' (remifentanil) to Medicines Authorities in Europe did not contain information on administration of these drugs by effect control TCI and no guidance on effect-site target concentrations was provided in drug labelling. An early modification of Diprifusor TCI software involved the incorporation of a blood brain equilibration constant (k_{e0}) of 0.26 min^{-1}, but only to allow the prediction of effect site propofol concentration. Despite the lack of regulatory approval from any Medicines Authority at the time in 2003 when open TCI systems began to be marketed, administration of propofol and remifentanil by effect control TCI has become widely practised. Potential confusion arises from the incorporation of different k_{e0} values for effect control with the same drug as has occurred with propofol. The TCI devices provided by Arcomed AG allow a choice of time to peak effect of 1.6 min or 4 min with the Marsh model, Fresenius Kabi use a k_{e0s} of 0.456 min^{-1} for the Schnider model and 1.2 min^{-1} for the Marsh model in

their system, while Carefusion TCI pumps use a time to peak effect of 1.6 min for both models. AstraZeneca considered that a time to peak effect of 4 min was probably too slow, that a time to peak effect of 1.6 min was probably too fast, and only recently a modified version of the Diprifusor module incorporating an intermediate k_{e0} of 0.6 min^{-1} was approved. This value was determined on the basis of a detailed review of published studies in which propofol was given safely by effect control TCI with the Marsh pharmacokinetic model and a range of k_{e0} values. To update the Summary of Product Characteristics for 'Diprivan' with the provision of information on the administration of propofol by effect control TCI a Type II variation was submitted to Medicines Agencies in a selection of European countries. Despite the fact that, with the effect site target recommended for induction with this k_{e0}, the initial dose of propofol delivered would be less than that advised for induction with a manual bolus, and the widespread use of open TCI systems with a range of k_{e0} values, further prospective studies with this k_{e0} were requested. The only exception was Germany where the variation was approved.

The consequences of a range of k_{e0} values for the same drug are as follows:

1. With blood concentration control, the rate of increase in *predicted* effect site concentrations at induction and the rate of decrease in *predicted* effect site concentrations after a reduction in target or during recovery will be influenced. A faster k_{e0} or shorter time to peak effect predicting faster equilibrium between blood and effect site concentrations and vice versa for a slower k_{e0} or longer time to peak effect. However, at any given target setting, the actual rate of onset of effect and rate of recovery will be dependent on the rate of blood brain equilibration in the patient and unaffected by the prediction provided by any model k_{e0}.

Fig. 2.16 Influence of pharmacokinetic model and equilibration rate constant (k_{e0}) on cumulative dose of propofol delivered in a 50 year, 70 kg, 170 cm male subject at a target effect site concentration (Ce_T) of 4 µg ml^{-1}. *Open diamond* Marsh k_{e0} 0.26 min^{-1}, *filled diamond* Marsh k_{e0} 0.6 min^{-1}, *open triangle* Marsh k_{e0} 1.2 min^{-1}, *filled square* Schnider k_{e0} 0.456 min^{-1}

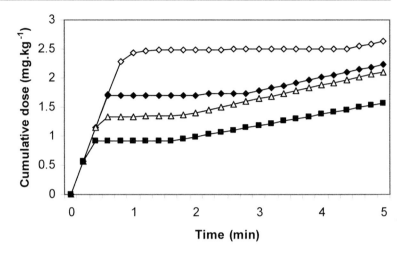

2. With effect control administration, different k_{e0}s can have a marked effect not only on the rate at which predicted effect site concentrations increase and a desired effect-site target is achieved but also on the initial dose delivered at any particular target (Fig. 2.16); and that in return will influence the peak predicted blood concentration (Cb$_{CALC}$) achieved. With the Marsh model and a propofol effect site target of 4 µg ml^{-1} as used in Fig. 2.16, peak Cb$_{CALC}$ ranges from 5.5 µg ml^{-1} with a k_{e0} of 1.2 min^{-1} to 9.4 µg ml^{-1} with a k_{e0} of 0.26 min^{-1}. With the Schnider model and a k_{e0} of 0.456 min^{-1}, despite the administration of a smaller initial dose, peak Cb$_{CALC}$ reaches 13.3 µg ml^{-1}, as a consequence of the smaller central compartment volume in this model. Thus it is imperative in any study which describes effect site concentrations at induction, that information on the model and k_{e0} used is provided to allow meaningful interpretation of any observations [60]. Once equilibrium between predicted blood and brain concentrations is achieved, the infusion rate of drug required to maintain a desired target is essentially similar to that which would be provided with blood concentration control, and the precision of the two systems at that point will be identical.

In summary, the regulatory approach adopted in the approval of second generation, open TCI systems, by providing different models for the same drug, inappropriate methods for the calculation of lean body mass, two different implementations of effect site concentration control, and a choice of different k_{e0} values for effect control, has led to a considerable degree of confusion. The skill of anaesthetists in titrating drug dosage to effect, and dealing with situations where potential overdosage or underdosage could occur, appears to have avoided serious safety issues. Some hospitals adopt a local policy to limit possible confusion by only allowing one model to be used, but problems may arise when trainees move from one institution to another.

Possible Ways Forward

The syringe recognition system used in the development of the Diprifusor TCI system prevents the possibility of the type of 'drug swap' error as described earlier. However, the Diprifusor approach has not been applied to other drugs and electronically tagged syringes are not available for generic preparations of propofol. The use of barcode technology to reduce drug administration errors is showing promising results [61, 62]. Universal compliance with these systems was not achieved, but perhaps one can envisage a future TCI pump where mandatory scanning of the drug to be infused, with a scanner as an integral part of the infusion device, would be required to allow the pump to operate.

It appears that the regulatory approach to clinical use of the technique of TCI and the approval of TCI devices will be dependent on the stage of development of the particular drug involved:

Drug Is Still Being Actively Marketed by the Originating Company

The benefit of the Diprifusor approach, also relevant to remifentanil TCI, is that a single pharmacokinetic model was identified, clinical studies were performed with TCI, and with the involvement of medicines regulatory authorities, guidance on target drug concentrations, appropriate for use with the selected model was included in the drug labelling, now provided as the Summary of Product Characteristics (SPC) in Europe. Key elements in the Diprifusor development were the provision of a delivery performance specification and guidance for device manufacturers on patient age and weight limits deemed suitable for the pharmacokinetic model used. It is suggested that this information should form part of the regulatory submission to a Medicines Authority for any new drug to be given by TCI. The major failing of the current route of approval of 'Open' TCI systems is that the essential requirements of Directive 93/42/EEC can be met, and conformance with full quality assurance procedures demonstrated, and yet TCI devices intended for the same purpose can deliver drug in quite different ways at the same target setting. As such it would seem appropriate that TCI drug delivery devices should be considered as a special case within the Directive and should require the Notified Body evaluating the documentation to consult with the manufacturer of the drug to be infused and a relevant Medical Regulatory Authority to ensure the delivery performance of the device conforms to that held by the Medicines Authority and to avoid the confusion caused by different models for the same drug. Three technical evaluation reports on commercial TCI devices were prepared for the UK Medicines and Healthcare products Regulatory Agency (MHRA) by Craig Davey at the Bath Institute of Medical Engineering. These are available at the following web site: http://nhscep. useconnect.co.uk/CEPProducts/Catalogue.aspx The report on 'Target controlled infusion (TCI) systems part two: Alaris Asena PK' includes the following statements: "It is interesting to note that while a high degree of accuracy is achieved, the different models will actually cause the pump to deliver [propofol] markedly differently from one another … It is beyond the scope of this report to judge the clinical effectiveness for any of the models …" The same comment is made in the report on the Fresenius Vial Base Primea and neither report identified the problems associated with the James calculation of lean body weight or the different implementations of effect control TCI.

Drug Is No Longer Actively Marketed by Originating Company

Propofol

The above approach, while desirable, may not be possible when pharmaceutical companies limit further development effort and expenditure once generic versions of their drug become available and at the same time relevant expertise within the company may have been lost. As such, the driving force for the introduction of TCI for a particular drug comes from the academic community and device manufacturers. In an attempt to resolve the problems highlighted in this chapter, the 'Open TCI initiative' was inaugurated at the time of the 14th World Congress of Anaesthesiologists in Cape Town in 2008, at a meeting hosted by Steve Shafer. This Initiative, now hosted on the web site of the World Society of Intravenous Anaesthesia at www.worldsiva.org has provided a forum for discussion and a focal point for the

collection of study data which has been used in the development of a general purpose pharmacokinetic model for propofol [49]. This model has shown good predictive performance in the subgroups of children, adults, elderly and obese patients contributing data to the study and with further prospective validation may prove to be the preferred model for propofol. If this proves to be the case, there is likely to be a third model added to the options of anaesthetists in Europe, as those familiar with their current preferred model may be reluctant to change their practice, at least in the short term.

On the other hand, in the USA, in the absence of any approved TCI device to date, there may be an opportunity to introduce the technique with a single pharmacokinetic model, thus avoiding the confusion of multiple models for the same drug. Extensive clinical experience has demonstrated that propofol can be safely administered by TCI. In the absence of any approved predicate device, it is likely that a Pre Market Approval (PMA) application will be required and linkage to clinical information in published studies could be provided by device manufacturers in the form of a delivery performance specification linking particular target settings to initial doses delivered ($mg\ kg^{-1}$) and subsequent infusion rate profiles ($mg\ kg^{-1}\ h^{-1}$) recognised as appropriate for propofol. To assist in training and familiarisation with these systems it would be appropriate for such delivery equivalence data to be provided in the device operating manual. Once one device is approved, the requirement for other manufacturers to demonstrate equivalence in a 510 K application would prevent the introduction of different models unless they complied with the approved delivery specification. With propofol now a generic drug, it likely that the onus on funding regulatory submissions and training programs for the introduction of TCI in the USA will fall on the medical device companies. One possible way forward may be for a number of medical device companies to co-fund the more complex PMA submission by one of their number on condition that other subscribers have preferential access to data to facilitate early 510 K submissions.

Other Drugs

For other drugs, both in the USA and elsewhere, it would be desirable for the academic community to reach a consensus on a preferred pharmacokinetic model and, particularly where publications describe different modelling approaches [39, 54], to define the parameters of the model. Again a delivery performance specification should be produced by the first device company developing a system for a particular drug to demonstrate drug delivery rates consistent with existing drug labelling and clinical experience and again this information should be included in the device operating instructions. It is suggested that the evaluation of the first such device submitted to a European Notified body should require that body to consult with the manufacturer of the drug and a relevant Medical Regulatory Authority to ensure the delivery performance of the device conforms to approved drug labelling and subsequent device submissions for the same drug should be required to demonstrate equivalent delivery performance.

Conclusion

While a tightly controlled regulatory approach was adopted in the development of the Diprifusor TCI system, the regulation of open TCI systems in Europe, by allowing duplicate models for the same drug, has probably hindered the wider adoption of TCI by making the technique appear more complex and confusing. With the recent development of a general purpose pharmacokinetic model for propofol, there may be an opportunity for the USA to adopt a sound approach, despite the delay.

References

1. Stokes DN, Peacock JE, Lewis R, Hutton P. The Ohmeda 9000 syringe pump, the first of a new generation of syringe drivers. Anaesthesia. 1990;45:1062–6.
2. Glass PSA, Glen JB, Kenny GNC, Schuttler J, Shafer SL. Nomenclature for computer-assisted infusion devices. Anesthesiology. 1997;86:1430–1.
3. White M, Kenny GNC. Intravenous propofol anaesthesia using a computerised infusion system. Anaesthesia. 1990;45:204–9.
4. Kenny GNC, White M. A portable target controlled propofol infusion system. Int J Clin Monit Comput. 1992;9:179–82.
5. Taylor I, White M, Kenny GNC. Assessment of the value and pattern of use of a target controlled propofol infusion device. Int J Clin Monit Comput. 1993;10:175–80.
6. Glen JB. The development of 'Diprifusor': a TCI system for propofol. Anaesthesia. 1998;53 Suppl 1:13–21.
7. Gray JM, Kenny GNC. Development of the technology for 'Diprifusor' TCI systems. Anaesthesia. 1998;53 Suppl 1:22–7.
8. Arundel PA. Interactive simulation of non-uniform bolus and infusion dosing in linear compartment models. J Pharm Sci. 1989;78:688–90.
9. Dyck JB, Shafer SL. Effects of age on propofol pharmacokinetics. Semin Anesth. 1992;11:2–4.
10. Tackley RM, Lewis GTR, Prys-Roberts C, Coats D, Monk CR. Computer controlled infusion of propofol. Br J Anaesth. 1989;62:46–53.
11. Marsh B, White M, Morton N, Kenny GN. Pharmacokinetic model driven infusion of propofol in children. Br J Anaesth. 1991;67:41–8.
12. Servin F, Cockshott ID, Farinotti R, Haberer JP, Winkler C, Desmonts JM. Pharmacokinetics of propofol infusions in patients with cirrhosis. Br J Anaesth. 1990;65:177–83.
13. Coetzee JF, Glen JB, Wium CA, Boshoff L. Pharmacokinetic model selection for target controlled infusions of propofol. Assessment of three parameter sets. Anesthesiology. 1995;82:1328–45.
14. Gepts E, Camu F, Cockshott ID, Douglas EJ. Disposition of propofol administered as constant rate intravenous infusions in humans. Anesth Analg. 1987;66:1256–63.
15. Struys M, Versichelen L, Rolly G. Influence of pre-anaesthetic medication on target propofol concentration using a 'Diprifusor' TCI system during ambulatory surgery. Anaesthesia. 1998;53 Suppl 1:68–71.
16. Servin FS, Marchand-Maillet F, Desmonts JM. Influence of analgesic supplementation on the target propofol concentrations for anaesthesia with 'Diprifusor' TCI. Anaesthesia. 1998;53 Suppl 1:72–6.
17. Richards AL, Orton JK, Gregory MJ. Influence of ventilator mode on target concentrations required for anaesthesia using a 'Diprifusor' TCI system. Anaesthesia. 1998;53 Suppl 1:77–81.
18. Varvel JR, Donoho DL, Shafer SL. Measuring the predictive performance of computer-controlled infusion pumps. J Pharmacokinet Biopharm. 1992;20:63–94.
19. Swinhoe CF, Peacock JE, Glen JB, Reilly CS. Evaluation of the predictive performance of a 'Diprifusor' TCI system. Anaesthesia. 1998;53 Suppl 1:61–7.
20. Barvais L, Rausin I, Glen JB, Hunter SC, D'Hulster D, Cantraine F, d'Hollander A. Administration of propofol by target-controlled infusion in patients undergoing coronary artery surgery. J Cardiothorac Vasc Anesth. 1996;10:877–83.
21. Russell D, Wilkes MP, Hunter SC, Glen JB, Hutton P, Kenny GNC. Manual compared with target controlled infusion of propofol. Br J Anaesth. 1995;75:562–6.
22. McMurray TJ, Johnston JR, Milligan KR, et al. Propofol sedation using Diprifusor target-controlled infusion in adult intensive care unit patients. Anaesthesia. 2004;59:636–41.
23. White M, Engbers FHM, Schenkels MJ, Burm AGL, Bovill JG. The pharmacodynamics of propofol determined by auditory evoked potentials. Sydney: Abstracts World Congress of Anaesthesiology; 1996. P610.
24. White M, Schenkels MJ, Engbers FHM, et al. Effect-site modelling of propofol using auditory evoked potentials. Br J Anaesth. 1999;82:333–9.
25. Struys MM, De Smet T, Depoorter B, Versichelen LF, Mortier EP, Dumortier FJ, Shafer SL, Rolly G. Comparison of plasma compartment versus two methods for effect compartment–controlled target-controlled infusion for propofol. Anesthesiology. 2000;92:399–406.
26. Thomson AJ, Nimmo AF, Engbers FHM, Glen JB. A novel technique to determine an 'apparent k_{e0}' value for use with the Marsh pharmacokinetic model for propofol. Anaesthesia. 2014;69:420–8.
27. Schnider TW, Minto CF, Gambus PL, et al. The influence of method of administration and covariates on the pharmacokinetics of propofol in adult volunteers. Anesthesiology. 1998;88:1170–82.
28. Schnider TW, Minto CF, Shafer SL, et al. The influence of age on propofol pharmacodynamics. Anesthesiology. 1999;90:1502–16.
29. Thomson AJ, Morrison G, Thomson E, Beattie C, Nimmo AF, Glen JB. Induction of general anaesthesia by effect-site target-controlled infusion of propofol: influence of pharmacokinetic model and k_{e0} value. Anaesthesia. 2014;69:429–35.
30. Kazama T, Ikeda K, Numata K, et al. Assessment of use of "Diprifusor" target controlled infusion (TCI) of 1% Diprivan (ICI 35,868). Anesth Resuscitation. 1998;34:121–39.
31. Hu C, Horstman DJ, Shafer SL. Variability of target-controlled infusion is less than the variability after bolus injection. Anesthesiology. 2005;102:639–45.
32. Struys MM, De Smet T, Glen JB, Vereecke HE, Absalom AR, Schnider TW. The history of target-controlled infusion. Anesth Analg. 2016 (in press)
33. Shafer SL, Gregg KM. Algorithms to rapidly achieve and maintain stable drug concentrations at the site of drug effect with a computer-controlled infusion pump. J Pharmacokinet Biopharm. 1992;20:147–69.

34. Jacobs JR, Williams EA. Algorithm to control "Effect Compartment" drug concentrations in pharmacokinetic model-driven drug delivery. IEEE Trans Biomed Res. 1993;40:993–9.

35. Enlund M. TCI: target controlled infusion or totally confused infusion? Call for an optimised population based pharmacokinetic model for propofol. Ups J Med Sci. 2008;113:161–70.

36. Minto CF, Schnider TW, Egan TD, Youngs E, Lemmens HJ, Gambus PL, et al. Influence of age and gender on the pharmacokinetics and pharmacodynamics of remifentanil. I Model development. Anesthesiology. 1997;86:10–23.

37. Mertens MJ, Engbers FH, Burm AG, Vuyk J. Predictive performance of computer-controlled infusion of remifentanil during propofol/remifentanil anaesthesia. Br J Anaesth. 2003;90:132–41.

38. James WPT. Research on obesity. A report of the DHSS/MRC Group. London: Her Majesty's Stationery Office; 1976.

39. Gepts E, Shafer SL, Camu F, et al. Linearity of pharmacokinetics and model estimation of sufentanil. Anesthesiology. 1995;83:1194–204.

40. Scott JC, Cook JE, Stanski DR. Electroencephalographic quantitation of opioid effect: comparative pharmacodynamics of fentanyl and sufentanil. Anesthesiology. 1991;74:34–42.

41. Chae Y-J, Joe HB, Kim J-A, Lee W-I, Min S-K. Correction of target-controlled infusion following wrong selection of emulsion concentration of propofol. Korean J Anesthesiol. 2014;66:377–82.

42. Sistema Español de Notificación en Seguridad en Anestesia y Reanimación (SENSAR). [Incorrect programming of a target controlled infusion pump. Case SENSAR of the trimester]. Rev Esp Anestesiol Reanim. 2014;61:e27–30.

43. Nimmo AF, Cook TM. Total intravenous anaesthesia; 18:151–8. http://www.nationalauditprojects.org.uk/NAP5_home#pt.

44. Chae Y-J, Kim J-Y, Kim D-W, Moon B-K, Min S-K. False selection of syringe-brand compatibility and the method of correction during target controlled infusion of propofol. Korean J Anesthesiol. 2013;64:251–6.

45. Schüttler J, Kloos S, Schwilden H, Stoeckel H. Total intravenous anaesthesia with propofol and alfentanil by computer-assisted infusion. Anaesthesia. 1988;43(Suppl):2–7.

46. Doufas AG, Bakhshandeh M, Bjorksten AR, Shafer SL. Induction speed is not a determinant of propofol pharmacodynamics. Anesthesiology. 2004;101:1112–21.

47. Glen JB, Servin F. Evaluation of the predictive performance of four pharmacokinetic models for propofol. Br J Anaesth. 2009;102:626–32.

48. Glen JB, White M. A comparison of the predictive performance of three pharmacokinetic models for propofol using measured values obtained during target-controlled infusion. Anaesthesia. 2014;69:550–7.

49. White M, Kenny GNC, Schraag S. Use of target controlled infusion to derive age and gender covariates for propofol clearance. Clin Pharmacokinet. 2008;47:119–27.

50. Eleveld DJ, Proost JH, Cortinez LI, Absalom AR, Struys MMRF. A general purpose pharmacokinetic model for propofol. Anesth Analg. 2014;118:1221–37.

51. Green B, Duffull S. Caution when lean body weight is used as a size descriptor for obese subjects. Clin Pharmacol Ther. 2002;72:743–4.

52. Hume R. Prediction of leanbody mass from height and weight. J Clin Pathol. 1966;19:389–91.

53. Janmahasatian S, Duffull SB, Ash S, Ward LC, Byrne NM, Green B. Quantification of lean bodyweight. Clin Pharmacokinet. 2005;44:1051–65.

54. Kataria BK, Sudha SA, Nicodemus HF, et al. The pharmacokinetics of propofol in children using three different data analysis approaches. Anesthesiology. 1994;80:104–22.

55. Schüttler J, Ihmsen H. Population pharmacokinetics of propofol. Anesthesiology. 2000;92:727–38.

56. Varveris D, Morton NS. Target controlled infusion of propofol for induction and maintenance of anaesthesia using the paedfusor: an open pilot study. Paediatr Anaesth. 2002;12:589–93.

57. Absalom A, Amutike D, Lal A, White M, Kenny GNC. Accuracy of the 'Paedfusor' in children undergoing cardiac surgery or catheterization. Br J Anaesth. 2003;91:507–13.

58. Absalom A, Kenny G. 'Paedfusor' pharmacokinetic data set. Br J Anaesth. 2005;95:110.

59. Sepulveda P, Cortinez LI, Saez C, et al. Performance evaluation of paediatric propofol pharmacokinetic models in healthy young children. Br J Anaesth. 2011;107:593–600.

60. Glen JB. Propofol effect site concentrations: hunt the k_{e0}. Anesth Analg. 2013;117:535–6.

61. Merry AF, Webster CS, Hannam J, et al. Multimodal system designed to reduce errors in recording and administration of drugs in anaesthesia: prospective randomised clinical evaluation. Br Med J. 2011;343.

62. Jelacic S, Bowdle A, Nair BG, Kusulos D, Bower L, Togashi K. A system for anesthesia drug administration using barcode technology: the codonics safe label system and smart anesthesia manager™. Anesth Analg. 2015;121:410–20.

The Memory Labyrinth: Systems, Processes, and Boundaries

3

Robert A. Veselis

Introduction

> The business of life is the acquisition of memories. Carson (Downton Abbey S4E3)

This topical quote was continued as "in the end that's all there is." In a sense this highlights how memory makes us uniquely human. As the human mind is the most complex creation in the universe, it stands to reason that memory embodies to a large extent this complexity. When memory fails in the end for some of us, a large portion of our being human also fails. In dementia some basic forms of memory do still exist and function, and functioning begins to rely more and more on stereotypical unconscious rather than recent autobiographical memories. During our whole lives unconscious memories allow us to function in an ever changing world by, for instance, jumping at a loud (potentially dangerous) noise, moving a piece of food to our mouth, or choosing a candy for unknown reasons from among dozens available. These unconscious memories seem to be implemented in the very core of our brains, and the question of whether consciousness can exist in the absence of memories is one of terminology. Certainly, conscious memories can be absent in the presence of consciousness, but a sine qua non of consciousness is the presence of working memory (memory of the here and now, even if the here and now is never remembered).

From this brief introduction, one can see memory is a complex phenomenon, or more accurately closely interrelated phenomena [1–3]. There are multiple memory systems, the classical division being between conscious and unconscious memory processes, which are supported by different, but not necessarily exclusive neurobiologic processes [4–6]. As will become clear throughout this chapter, the boundaries between these divisions are not as simple as many classification systems (taxonomies) imply. Largely this is a result of trying, as it were, to put memory into a box and it won't fit!

What is a memory? At the most basic level it is a rearrangement of our brains at the synaptic level [7, 8]. Memory is a process that produces a brain different from what it was before, that difference being the memory. Synaptic rearrangement does not occur instantaneously, and the sum of the processes needed to complete these changes is termed "consolidation" [9]. As we can attest to from our daily lives, memory is not a static entity and is constantly evolving over time, although the rate of change may be different over different temporal epochs. Old memories can be re-remembered, and the term re-consolidation describes the process of recalling a memory and then storing a slightly different version. In fact, events similar to this occur every night during sleep, where the neural records of events from the previous day are massaged by waves of the oscillatory activities of the sleeping brain [10–12]. In fact, we are now in an age where it might be possible to manipulate memories at will, the implications of such actions being quite profound and still quite unclear [13].

How does one determine if synaptic changes have occurred? Not being able to visualize synaptic changes in real time (until recently, but with totally impractical methods), a proxy is needed [14]. In the end, the only way one can determine if a memory is present is by observing a change in behavior which is in some way related to the creation of that memory. In this sense memory is a behavior, and therein lies the source of much controversy when memory is discussed. The observations of memory related behaviors are largely undisputed. Everyone agrees, for example, that the reaction time to a stimulus in a particular paradigm has decreased, or that recognition with a given degree of confidence has occurred. However, it is frequently the case that very differing opinions are offered as to how to

R.A. Veselis, MD (✉)
Anesthesiology, Memorial Sloan Kettering Cancer Center, 1275 York Ave, New York, NY 10065, USA
e-mail: veselisr@mskcc.org

© Springer International Publishing AG 2017
A.R. Absalom, K.P. Mason (eds.), *Total Intravenous Anesthesia and Target Controlled Infusions*, DOI 10.1007/978-3-319-47609-4_3

31

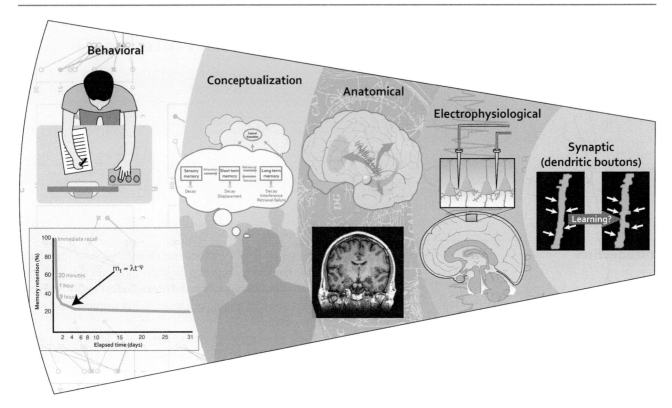

Fig. 3.1 The many levels of memory. Memory can be understood at many different levels, from behavioral changes to synaptic modifications in neurons. Conceptualizations of memory begin with careful behavioral observations in humans or animals, where specific parameters are changed (e.g., time between encoding and recognition), and changes in behavior are measured. A conceptual construct can be created to explain these observations, such as short (working) and long term memory systems. These conceptualizations are then related to underlying neurobiologic mechanisms in terms of anatomy, electrophysiology, and molecular mechanisms [and in some instances physical principles (e.g., quantum mechanics)]. The great challenge is to link changes in, for example, phase changes in oscillatory activity that influences synapse formation with something as complex as recognition memory

these behaviors are explained. Behind every behavioral result, there stands a conceptualization of a memory system, or set of memory systems which allows one to explain why a given behavior resulted [15] (Fig. 3.1, left-most sections).

The best conceptualizations are those that allow one to predict ahead of time what change in behavior will occur under a given set of circumstances [16]. Careful study of behavior under these circumstances will allow more solid acceptance, or lead to more degradation of a given conceptualization. Frequently predictions of a model are tested in a patient with a known brain lesion, e.g. one that affects procedural (e.g., mirror drawing), but not long term memory. Ideally a matching study is done in a patient with an opposite type of lesion, e.g. a patient with a deficit in long term, but not procedural memory [17, 18]. A similar dissociation can be demonstrated between short and long term memory stores [19, 20]. Dissociability along these lines provides strong support of separate memory processes, but one problem is that it may be very difficult to locate a patient with a specific enough lesion that clearly interferes with a single memory function. In this iterative process conceptualizations are

verified or refuted, with new and improved ones being a result. The introduction to a conference on episodic memory written by Baddeley is an excellent example of how this process unfolds [21]. It should be noted that in the 2010s we are still engaged in these iterative processes. Thus, concepts of memory are continually evolving, and certain key ideas are as hotly debated as cherished political beliefs. To best understand memory, one needs to be somewhat familiar with the unfolding of conceptualizations (a.k.a. taxonomies) of memory over time. In this chapter as well, I will describe what is known of anesthetic induced manipulation of memory, though knowledge is still at a somewhat primitive stage.

A History of the Taxonomy of Memory

The noteworthy idea that memory was more than one entity was proposed only in the last half of the last century, really not that long ago. Though in 1949 Hebb presciently suggested a distinction between memory processes with short term memory being defined as evanescent electrical activity, with long term memory being consisting of more permanent neurochemical changes, it was Atkinson and Shiffrin who are most credited with fleshing out the concept of these two major forms of memory [22]. Before then, it was still quite controversial whether memory could be regarded as anything by a unitary process [23]. This argument is eerily similar to the current controversy regarding the nature of recognition in conscious memory, which will be detailed later in this chapter. As usual in these situations, the behaviors which lead to conceptualization of short vs long term memory were well accepted. The now famous 7 ± 2 items capacity of short term memory was established in the 1950s. This was the amount of material that could be recalled immediately after presentation [24, 25]. Fortunately for many generations, telephone numbers fit this bill, especially as alphabetic prefix codes were used. One could easily remember a telephone number after hearing it once. In fact, songs have been written about this (PEnnsylvannia 6-5000, Glen Miller orchestra[1]). Atkinson and Shiffrin (among others) wanted to understand and detail mechanisms to explain this observation. A major insight was to postulate a short term memory store of limited capacity. When the ninth item comes along, item one is pushed out. The interaction of a short term store with recent items in long term memory could explain more complex behaviors, such as the serial position effect, where items from a long (greater than ten item) list are recognized with a U shaped probability [26]. Initial and last items are likely to be remembered better, as items from the start of the list are likely to be rehearsed and incidentally encoded into long term memory, whereas recent items are still present in working memory and easily recalled (more detailed explanations are more complicated, the serial position effect is a whole field of study) [27]. A few decades later, after numerous behavioral/conceptual iterations, short term memory was conceptualized as working memory, itself consisting of different sub-components. Each component was a conceptualization that could explain an associated behavioral or set of behavioral observations. Predictions of previous models broke down when more closely examined, or in patients with specific neurologic lesions. Baddeley improved the concept of short term memory by defining separable components collectively termed working memory [28] (Fig. 3.2). These conceptualizations in turn led to more detailed neurocomputational and neurobiologic conceptualizations that propose how cognitive conceptualizations are instantiated in the brain. It is easy to see how memory can be considered at different scales representative of multiple layers that interact with each other (Fig. 3.1, all sections). For example, a well-accepted neurobiologic

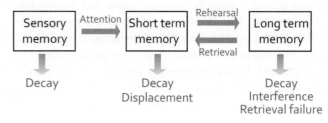

Atkinson and Shiffrin (1968)

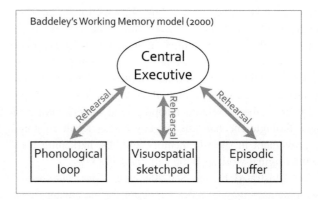

Baddeley's Working Memory model (2000)

Fig. 3.2 Refinement of conceptualizations over time: The figure provides a simple illustration of how a basic conceptualization, of short (STM) and long term memory (LTM), can become more elaborate as more detailed behavioral observations are subject to analysis. A number of observations, such as the inability to remember beyond 7 ± 2 items when rehearsal was prevented, lead to the famous dual store conceptualization, as described by Atkinson and Shiffrin in the 1960s. However, observations predicted by this model (that patients with impaired STM should have broad deficits in LTM) were not actually observed, and a more refined conceptualization of Baddeley resulted, that of working memory with multiple components handling different types of input (phonologic, visuospatial, semantic). It should be remembered that such conceptual elaborations of memory systems are still occurring

conceptualization of working memory is a process embodied in the oscillatory activity of the brain, which provides a capacity as large as the ratio of gamma to theta frequencies (roughly), which happen to be on the order of 7–9 to 1 [29]. Thus, starting with very basic properties of neurons, modeling small world neuronal interactions can serve to explain an observed behavior much removed from this level of detail [30]. Such a reductionist approach lends solid credence to the observation that working memory is fleeting. As mentioned before, a critical requirement of consciousness is working memory, as to be conscious is to be aware of the "here and now," instantiated as working memory [31, 32].

After being processed in working memory, some information does become long term memory. LTM embodies Carson's comments on our being human, as working memory is so evanescent. Not surprisingly the more closely we examine long term memory the more we appreciate that it itself is incredibly complex. As with the dichotomy between

---

[1] http://en.wikipedia.org/wiki/PEnnsylvania_6-5000.

short and long term memory, conceptualizations of LTM began as a dichotomy between conscious and unconscious memory [33]. This dichotomy was best illustrated in the 1950s by the world's most famous neurologic case, H. M. [34]. He was one of a series of seven patients reported by Scoville and Milner describing a peculiar memory deficit after therapeutic surgery to cure intractable epilepsy. Surgery such as this may seem to be a radical approach today, but the concept was founded on the observation from a decade before that if a diseased portion of the brain was removed, this would "liberate" normal functioning brain no longer inhibited by the scarred brain tissue [35]. Interestingly, to this day a similar approach with appropriate refinements still seems to be the best option in some situations, such as drug resistant epilepsy arising from discrete scar tissue in the temporal lobe [36]. With improved surgical methods, seizure mapping, and understanding of neurobiologic mechanisms resection does result in some improvement in specific memory abilities, harkening back to the original work of Hebb and Penfield [37].

As illustrated by the Scoville case series, unexpected consequences may be more important for the advancement of science than dreamed of. After surgical treatment for epilepsy, it did seem that an almost magic cure was found. Before surgery, the patient was essentially incapacitated, sometimes to the point of not being able to leave the house because of relentless seizures or intoxication of too high doses of barbiturates to treat those seizures. After surgery a virtually normal life resulted. Detailed descriptions of the peculiar memory impairment associated with this type of surgery, one that is able to be reproduced in the surgical theater when a patient is given a benzodiazepine, led to eventual knowledge of the key role of the hippocampus in conscious memory. Similarly, one will note that a patient undergoing sedation with light doses of diazepam, midazolam, ketamine, or propofol frequently keeps asking the same question. This is a predictable behavior in patients receiving light doses of these drugs, and results from the fact that patients can't remember the answer to their repetitive questions. It should be noted that after the case reports of Scolville and Milner, it was decades before there was enough evidence to clearly point to the hippocampus as the seat of conscious memory [38]. The reason it took so long to confirm this relationship was that in the original case series not only was the hippocampus removed (bilaterally) during surgery, but the resection also included a complex set of structures closely related to the hippocampus which also resided in the medial temporal lobe [5]. It took many years to determine how these structures were interconnected and how they interacted. The Scolville and Milner case series really re-invigorated the conceptualization of memory systems as being embodied in certain structures of the brain. Not surprisingly a huge amount of basic research on

memory focused on the neuronal architecture of the hippocampus, and related structures [39].

Animals are valuable to study memory, as one can control conditions very closely, manipulate genes, record from individual (giant) neurons, and obtain really fine grained data. For example, a prototypical system is the Aplysia (sea snail/slug), which is a vehicle to study reflex and simple behaviors, such as classical (reflex) and operant (e.g., eating) conditioning. These forms of memory are stereotypical, and though much is known about them, how these systems influence memory processes in humans is still murky. Much of the classical taxonomy of memory relates to these stereotypical, unconscious memory systems. Included in these behaviors are priming, skills and habits, classic conditioning and non-associative behaviors [33]. From the perspective of this chapter, priming is the most important, as it is the type of memory most sought after when studies look for learning during anesthesia. Priming is the preferential response to a previously experienced stimulus, one that is not consciously remembered. Indirect tests to detect these memories must be used, as they are not consciously accessible. The most common task used is word stem completion, where a portion of the stimulus word is presented, and the rate of completion using previously presented words (during anesthesia) is compared with a control list [40]. Habits and skills are stereotypical behaviors that are initially conscious memories that through repetition are incorporated into motor circuits as unconscious memories. Being stereotypical, even small changes in pattern requires new conscious learning (the bane of pianists who initially learn an incorrect note in a passage, for example). Pavlovian conditioning is best known to humans (and maybe dogs) as what occurs when smelling bacon. Non-associative learning embodies habituation or sensitization to a repetitive non-relevant or harmful stimulus, respectively. More complex memories, particularly in animal models, may be difficult to categorize as being conscious or unconscious if the organism cannot provide insight into the experience. For example, in rats a more complex memory is visual object recognition, where a rat will explore a novel object in preference to an object previously seen before. Though some literature equates visual object recognition memory to conscious memory in humans, it seems that the memory systems mediating object recognition may best be related in humans as unconscious memory [41]. The divide between animal neurobiology and human memory becomes wider as more complex memory is considered. In the case of visual object recognition memory, the hippocampus was thought to play a vital role. Hippocampal involvement is considered as a proxy for conscious memory in animal models. A number of studies showed that animals with hippocampal lesions were impaired in object recognition memory. However, when memory paradigms were carefully constructed to not contain spatial cues, it turned out that hippocampal lesions made no difference in object recognition memory. Thus the initial lesion studies were contaminated by subtle environmental cues, highlighting the sensitivity of memory studies to confounding factors. The closest parallel between animal object recognition memory and human memory may be face recognition, which recently has been shown to activate parahippocampal structures [42].

The largest divide between lower animal models and humans occurs in the case of conscious memory, which is the memory referred to by Carson [43]. This is what most people think of as "memory," and is incredibly complex and somewhat hard to pin down, especially in animal models. The history of taxonomy starts with declarative memory, which is a memory we can (consciously) declare we have. Further characterization of conscious memory led to the realization that these memories really occur in a place and in particular a time, best described as episodic memories, episodes that are like frames in a film strip (which in fact is a paradigm used to study this form of memory) [44]. The closer one considers and investigates episodic memory, the more complex it becomes. For example, there is a distinct sense of knowing oneself in episodes of conscious memory, thus best characterized as "autonoetic" memories. In addition, one can envision one's self travelling through time, most critically, into the future (what will happen if I lie about what I did last night …) [45]. It will be very hard to convincingly demonstrate these qualities of conscious memories in animal models. In fact, some authorities do not think animals possess conscious memory as we do, and

that even scientists anthropomorphize their pets. Complex paradigms used in animals are claimed to be representative of higher forms of conscious memory, but other experts consider these memories to be, at best, "episodic like" [46–48]. Thus, even though animal models may provide copious and invaluable information about memory, the ultimate discovery of how human memory works will require study of humans themselves. It will always be a conundrum of how to relate memory from one species to another. Again the observed behaviors in a particular animal model are undisputed, it is the interpretation of how these results relate to human memory that is the source of controversy.

As regards conscious memory, the safest correlate of "conscious memory" in animals is probably spatial memory, which is indisputably mediated by the hippocampus [49–51]. Common paradigms to study this form of memory are paradigms such as the radial maze or the Morris water maze, where the animal depends on extraneous spatial cues to remember previously explored avenues. In fact, the discovery of hippocampal place cells/fields revolutionized concepts of the neurobiology of conscious memory [52, 53]. The divide between animal and human hippocampal neurobiology has been considerably diminished using sophisticated signal analysis methods in epilepsy patients with implanted electrodes, for example [54].

Most readers are probably familiar with the classic taxonomy of memory, which is a distillation of many decades of research founded on centuries of behavioral observations. This classic classification deserves a Figure as a historical starting point (Fig. 3.3). Currently, a

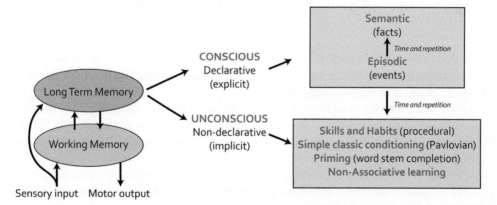

Fig. 3.3 A "classic" conceptualization of human memory systems. Long term memory is classified into various components in Squire's model [55], and is based on much animal work as well as observations in patient lesion cases. These concepts arose after the report of impaired memory in a series of neurologic cases (case HM, reported by Scoville and Milner in 1957), following surgery in the medial temporal lobes. Classically, long term memory was considered in large part as a static entity, which can be classified according to features of the memory (e.g., conscious access vs. unconscious influence). A large body of multiple line evidence obtained over a 30-year period revealed that

the hippocampus was essential for the formation of conscious, episodic memory explaining the observations of Scoville and Milner. A clue to the fact that this classification is just a starting point in understanding memory is illustrated by some "permeability" between categories. For example, at one time the knowledge that George Washington was the first president of the USA was a new and startling memory (an episodic memory), but then it became a "fact," knowledge of the world that we do not recall where and when it was learned (semantic memory). Similarly, patterned behaviors such as skating and playing a musical instrument become unconscious motor memories over time

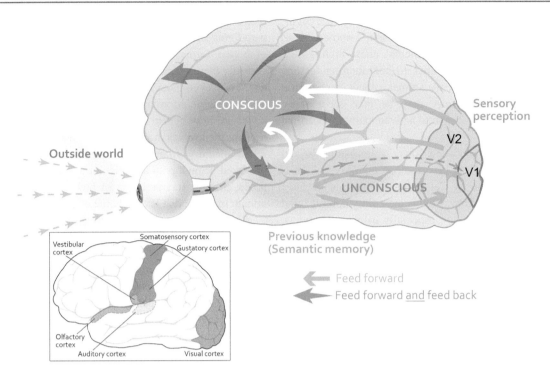

Fig. 3.4 More recent conceptualizations of memory. These conceptualizations build on the concepts presented in Fig. 3.3 using a foundation of neuroanatomical relationships. Memory systems are widely distributed, and interact with each other in somewhat flexible fashions. Those closest to the environment (sensory regions) are "low level" systems which are the most easily understood on a basic physiologic level, and most likely embody portions of unconscious memories. Higher level systems that embody conscious memory likely depend on network activity and distributed processes, though all systems interact with each other in complex fashions to not only subserve memory function, but also consciousness. Higher level interactions are more sensitive to anesthetic effects, and low level systems may still be functional in certain situations during anesthesia, wherein unconscious memories may be formed. However, these memories may simply be perceptual (sensory) priming memories where an enhanced physiologic response occurs to a re-experience of the stimulus. At our current state of knowledge of neurobiology, these sensory memories formed during anesthesia would require the interaction of sensory input regions (e.g., V1 for visual, A1 for auditory) with other multiple brain regions (likely in the medial temporal lobe), with any resulting sensory memories residing in peri-sensory brain regions (V2 or A2). Pathways for sensory processing are shown for the visual modality for clarity, the same principles would apply to auditory or olfactory sensory systems in their respective brain regions

major shift in conceptualization of memory is occurring where taxonomy is changing in nature from a static classification of memory systems to conceptualizations that incorporate information flow from the outside (or inside) world through stages of processing to a conscious or unconscious memory [56] (Fig. 3.4). Information transfer and processing become important components of these conceptualizations, which now include the malleability of memory itself (false memories, eye witness memories, post-traumatic memories, etc.) [57]. Careful readers of the mechanisms of anesthesia literature will no doubt appreciate a close resemblance to similar concepts of consciousness, and the progression of information from sensory and internal sources into a percept that one is consciously aware of [58, 59]. In fact, this is likely no co-incidence, as neurobiology is more than likely parsimonious in implementing solutions for similar problems, be it consciousness, working memory, or long term memory.

A Useful Conceptualization of Memory

One needs to have a working conceptualization of memory that incorporates bits and pieces of different models to avoid getting hopelessly lost. The classic taxonomy is useful in terms of nomenclature, and will be utilized as such. As mentioned, the current direction of memory research is in terms of information processing, and it is best to relate these concepts to the classic nomenclature as a starting point. To simplify, I will only consider information from the outside world, though the same principles, but not necessarily specifics, can be applied to the inner, dreaming world [58, 60]. To begin with, let us consider how a picture frame from the film of our lives becomes a memory, and more. But before this, one should become familiar with the basic construct of a memory study.

Memory as a Behavior: The Ebbinghausen Paradigm, or More Simply, Study-Test Paradigm

About 150 years ago a psychologist, Hermann Ebbinghaus, was interested in quantifying memory. We all know that the most common fate of memory is that it is forgotten [61]. This is a very fortunate state of affairs, for if you pay attention to all the stimuli that are processed in a single day, and then think of what life would be like if you remembered each stimulus for the rest of your life, you would quickly realize you would be living a nightmare. As is common for many "life is stranger than fiction" diseases, there is the rare neurologic case that embodies a form of super-memory [62]. Such people can remember, for example, all the details of the weather on a particular date many years in the past. Not surprisingly, it does turn out that significant psychological distress accompanies such super-memory ability.

Thus, it is no surprise that historically, one might be first interested in quantifying the most basic property of memory, namely how it is lost. Ebbinghaus proceeded to do this in a systematic fashion, where given items were studied, and then recognition for these items was used to quantify memory decay over time. Almost all behavioral observations of memory, both in humans and in animals, use a study-test (encoding, recognition) paradigm, also referred to by those in the field by Ebbinghaus' name. To this day this paradigm is the only way to practically detect and measure a memory, ultimately a result of synaptic re-arrangements in the brain. Another important variable in this paradigm is the time between encoding and recognition [63]. Multiple recognition tasks can be performed, which is what Ebbinghaus did, to define memory decay (or, alternatively, improvement from repeated practice on the task) [64]. There is an almost infinite variety of paradigms available by modifying the three main elements of the study-test paradigm, those being encoding, time to recognition, and recognition. During encoding and recognition tasks, the particular instructions given, including any modification of the environment or context is crucial to interpret the results, as will be exemplified throughout this chapter. Time is the factor that is the most quantifiable, but one must be aware that it is crucially important to know what the person/animal is doing (or more accurately is instructed to do) during the time between encoding and recognition.

What Ebbinghaus quantified was that memory decays very rapidly at first, and then more slowly as time increases (Fig. 3.5a). Eventually, an autobiographical memory remains, those of episodic experiences long ago [65–67]. In closely related circumstances, probably with repeated encoding activity, an episodic experience is transformed into a fact—knowledge about the world. For instance, we know that stoves are hot, but we don't remember how that information got into our memory. This form of memory is termed semantic, a term that embodies perfectly the relatedness to the meaning of words, which is really knowledge of the world. On the other hand, memories associated with motor skills (driving a car, playing a musical instrument) becomes embodied, through repeated encoding, into a primitive (or phylogenetically old) set of neural circuits in our brain which allows automated behavior, and is a form of unconscious memory [68, 69]. But, let's turn back to episodic memory decay. Mathematical modeling of memory decay is possible, and it seems that a power decay function, as opposed to an exponential decay function, fits data the best [70, 71]. Parameters from the power function fit can, for example, quantify memory decay characteristics of common anesthetic sedatives, discussed later in this chapter [72].

Recognition memory is tested by asking the subject to perform matched encoding and recognition tasks. Often the instructions for encoding are thought of as a variation of "remember these items, for you will be asked to name them later." This is certainly a valid encoding paradigm, but more frequently incidental encoding paradigms are used, where the subject follows a relatively easy instruction that on the surface is not related to memory, such as "you will hear a series of words, push one button if the voice is female, and the other if it is male" [73]. No indication is given that the words will be incorporated into a recognition task later. The person pays attention to the task, and normally, the words presented are incorporated into memory automatically, thus the term incidental encoding. Slight modifications of task instructions, such as "push one button if the word is an object that is larger than a bread box, otherwise push the other" will activate different memory systems, and thus result in different memory performance at recognition [74]. In studies of unconscious memory, frequently the length of time of presentation or clarity of the item is varied. For example, a picture may be shown for 33, 50, and 80 ms to determine a perception threshold, and then changes in behavior are measured, those usually being reaction times to stimuli which were presented at longer and shorter time intervals than the perception threshold [75]. Shorter intervals index unconscious memory processes, whereas longer intervals index conscious memory processes. Similarly, words may be degraded by white noise to determine a perception threshold for information content.

During the time interval between encoding and recognition, the environment and instructions to the subject are crucially important. Variations include performing an "interference" task, resting comfortably, sleeping, staring at a cross hair on a computer screen, etc. All will result in differing memory performance, and one should be aware that vagueness about what actually was done during this period would confound results from that study.

There are many recognition paradigms, again with crucial differences in instructions. One main theme is that

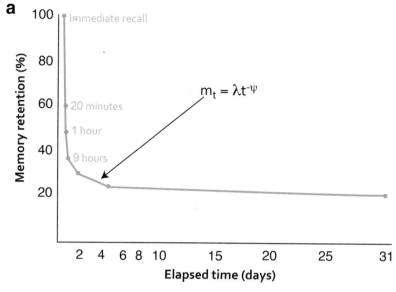

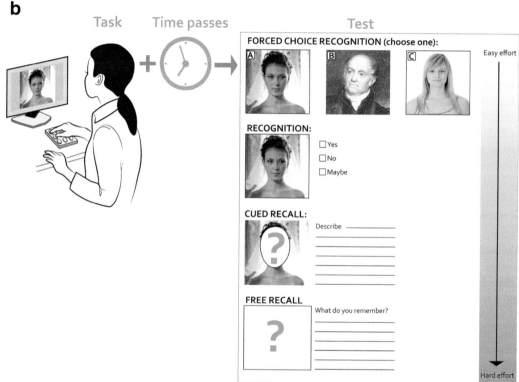

Fig. 3.5 (**a**) The fate of memories is to be forgotten. Ebbinghaus established basic observational principles to quantify memory behavior. An event (stimulus) is experienced (encoded). After a certain time, the presence of memory is tested for by a recognition task. This study-test paradigm (Ebbinghausen paradigm) revealed that most memories are forgotten over time, rapidly at first, and then more and more slowly. A power decay function (as opposed to an exponential decay function) best describes loss of memory over time. (**b**) Depending on specific parameters and instructions for encoding, recognition, etc. many variations of the study-test paradigm are possible. For example, the difficulty in accessing a memory can be varied by giving clues, providing a choice of possibilities, etc. How behavior changes with these modifications provides important insight into how memory operates, and which brain regions are involved with different aspects of memory such as attention and effort needed to retrieve a memory

recognition performance is greatly affected by the effort required to retrieve a memory. It makes sense that if you have to remember a previous item out of the blue, that would be more difficult than choosing between two items after the instruction "you have seen one of these before, which one was it?". This effect is well known, and difficulty of retrieval from hardest to easiest is illustrated by examples as follows: free recall ("what do you remember"), cued recall ("do you remember something that looked like a car"), yes/no recognition ("have you seen this item before, yes/no"), forced choice recognition ("choose the one you have seen before from these three items"), forced choice recognition using two items (Fig. 3.5b). The degree of similarity of the lure items (items given as choices, but not previously presented) will modulate the degree of difficulty, and such variations can be used to determine a "signal strength" of the memory [76].

From these brief examples, one can appreciate the almost infinite variety of paradigms possible in the study-test format. Each small manipulation provides, hopefully, another insight into how memory works.

From Sensation to Memory: Information Flow

This section will focus on conceptualizations of information flow from the outside world into the brain where it can become a memory. These conceptualizations are embodied as distinct memory processes (encoding, storage, recognition, etc.) and are divorced from neurobiologic instantiation [15]. The reader should be aware of this distinction, even though some are closely linked (e.g., hippocampus and conscious memory). One should not get into the habit of freely substituting a neurobiologic mechanism for a conceptualization, or vice versa. Some neurobiologic underpinnings of memory behaviors will be discussed in more detail in the sections on unconscious and recognition memory.

An important differentiation in terminology common to memory and consciousness is needed, particularly for those interested in anesthetic effects on the brain. What is the correct terminology for seeing a light? Some people might say that the light is perceived, whereas others would say that it is sensed. Some would argue that perception is a more complex bit of information than sensation, that perception has some greater structure to it. In fact, in the study of consciousness, a key concept is that of a percept, a unified experience of awareness that incorporates many different threads of information. To avoid confusion, I will use the word "sense" for primary activation of sensory cortices from the outside world (e.g., primary auditory or visual cortices). Terms containing "percept" will relate to a conscious experience of an event from the outside world [31].

The first event of a potential memory is sensation, an activation of primary sensory cortices (Fig. 3.4). Most real world events activate multiple senses, but for research purposes, most stimuli stimulate a single sense. Immediate, unconscious processing occurs of the stimulus to measure basic qualities of the stimulus (e.g., intensity, orientation, frequency, color, etc.). At a very early stage, comparison with a template (a previously experienced stimulus, either at some time in the past, or in the current train of stimuli) is

undertaken [77, 78]. If there is a mismatch, neuronal responses tend to be larger [79–81]. A deviant stimulus may be of interest or importance, and mechanisms come into play to devote attentional resources to the incoming stimulus (aptly named as a "bottom-up" attentional modulating process). Neurophysiologic correlates of the so-called orienting reflex can be measured, e.g. as the mismatch negativity, and can be used to study how sifting through a the constant stream of incoming information directs important details to the most relevant brain systems. As with a Christmas tree, important stimuli are collated with more and more information to elaborate what was just experienced into a conscious percept [56]. As an example, we may jump when we hear a loud noise. Auditory sensation is activated, the characteristics of the sound are automatically extracted (loud, short duration, previous match with an explosion), the flight or fight response may be activated (fear mediated memory), a motor reflex occurs (jump) before further processing occurs. Additional details may then be added, for example from the visual stream (we turn to see a broken plate on the floor). We access previous semantic knowledge (bits of porcelain from a plate, when plates break they make a loud noise) in order to make sense of what just happened. Further fear processing is stopped (it was not a bomb), we collect more details about the plate (pattern completion), and realize it is an anniversary gift from last month, by extracting this information from episodic memory (wherein the fear/anxiety response may be re-activated). Any number of these processes can be influenced pharmacologically, and in this manner the effects of anesthetics on memory can be sorted out [82, 83]. A useful conceptualization (taxonomy) of information flow processing is that proposed by Tulving, the serial-parallel-independent model of memory [43, 57]. This is just one of a number of conceptualizations of memory. but is helpful to know as it incorporates a holistic conceptualization from sensation to long term memory. Anesthetic effects on memory, particularly as regards to unconscious learning during anesthesia, can be thought of in these terms. Some other hierarchical conceptualizations are referenced [84–86].

Serial Parallel Independent (SPI) Model of Memory

The acronym "SPI" is meant to indicate that the interaction among the three major components of this model is dependent on the memory process in play at the time (Fig. 3.6). The three components are arranged in a hierarchical fashion, with input from the outside world coming into the perceptual representation system (PRS). During encoding, information is processed in a Serial fashion, passing from PRS to semantic memory, which collates and decodes sensory input with

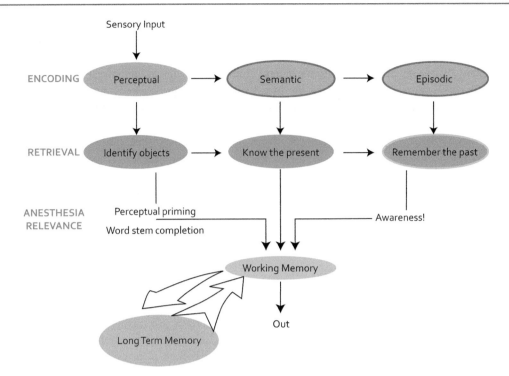

Fig. 3.6 The SPI memory system of Tulving. SPI stands for serial parallel independent model. Three large memory systems representing the perceptual representation system (PRS), semantic, and episodic memory are related in a hierarchical fashion during encoding, where information processing is Serial. Storage of memories is Parallel in each system, and these can be retrieved independently from other systems. Of interest during anesthesia is the PRS, the lowest "rung" of the memory processing, relating to sensory input and perception. If any memory function operates during anesthesia, it would be the PRS. It is likely that perceptual memories, if formed, would be stored in secondary sensory association cortices. On the other hand, if high level episodic memories are present during anesthesia, then "awareness" has occurred, an undesirable event if not expected by either the practitioner or patient

previous knowledge of the world (semantic memory, memory of "facts") to know what just happened. If input is similar to previous experience, it can be processed further incorporating this information (e.g., a red round object may be a ball). Novel qualities of the input are further processed in the higher level of episodic memory, where the experience can be incorporated as a novel event personally relevant in a distinct place and time (episodic memory, such as what we had for dinner last night). Episodic memory contains previous knowledge (I had steak at my favorite restaurant) with novel experiences (this event happened last night at 7 p.m. with a well-known friend). Linking of previous knowledge with novel information is mediated by the hippocampus, notably the spatial and temporal aspects of memory (where I had dinner and when I had dinner) [87]. These qualities are the hallmarks of a conscious (episodic) memory. At each level of processing, distinct forms of memory can be stored in Parallel, with perceptual representations (color, intensity, orientation, etc.) stored in the PRS, factual knowledge (red rubber ball) stored in the semantic system, and personally relevant and novel memories (I threw the red rubber ball against a wall this weekend) in the episodic memory system. A different interaction of this system is defined during recognition, where memories can be retrieved independently

from each system. So red rubber ball is an independent memory of a ball, which could as easily be a blue soft ball. Importantly for understanding the interaction of anesthesia with memory is the fact that memories can be stored in the perceptual system, and then subsequently retrieved independently of the (conscious) semantic and episodic memory systems using techniques such as perceptual priming. The latter is an enhanced reaction (shorter reaction time, greater probability of choosing a previously experienced stimulus over a novel one, etc.) to a stimulus based on its perceptual representation [88].

The beauty of the SPI classification is its simplicity and power to explain diverse phenomena. For example, on the basis of being serial, input into episodic memory is dependent only on input from semantic memory, the memory of facts. However, there is no a priori requirement that these "facts" are indeed "true." Thus, if for whatever reason one has learned the fact that there are Martians who live in Area 51 of New Mexico, then one could have a conscious memory experience of meeting one at dinner last night, and that episodic memory would be as vivid and valid as another person's memory of dining with his wife. Thus, this model is useful to conceptualize how false memories arise and behave [57].

Recognition Memory: Not So Simple— Familiarity and Recollection with a Detour into Déjà vu

Recognition memory is a much more complex process than a binary decision of whether one has experienced a stimulus before. The processes of how someone recognizes that an event or stimulus has been experienced before are still very much being worked out. All authorities agree that there are different qualities present in recognition, and the reader can relate to this as we have all experienced the so-called butcher-on-a-bus phenomenon (a.k.a. "the face is familiar, but I can't remember the name"). We know we have seen someone before (they, the butcher, are familiar), but we

don't remember other details from the episode such as what the person wore, their name, when we saw them, where they were, etc. These qualities are differentiated in the descriptive labels of familiarity and recollection (Fig. 3.7). The ability to remember specific details associated with the familiar face would be to recollect the memory [90, 91].

A tongue twister and key fact to remember is that recollection is not the same as recognition, but recollection is a type of recognition. How best to mechanistically explain recollection is an area of great controversy between two main hypotheses [15]. As this level of detail is now becoming relevant to actions of anesthesia on memory, it is now topical for anesthesiologists to understand these issues.

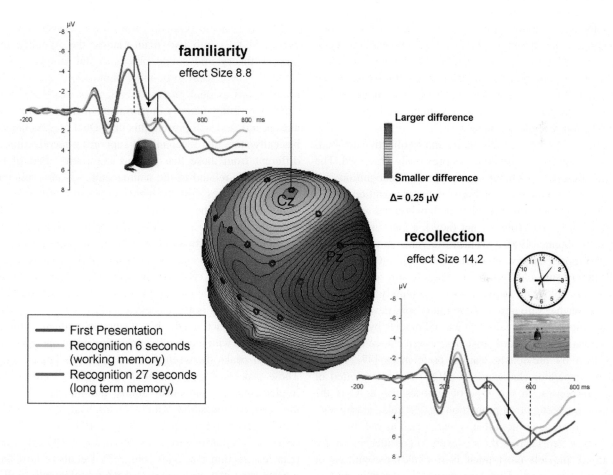

Fig. 3.7 Recognition of a conscious memory produces two different qualities we have all experienced, a fast "familiarity" reaction (I've seen this before, the "fez" is familiar) and a more elaborate recollection reaction of an event located in a time and space in our memories (a day at the beach, for example). Objective measures of brain activity recorded during these intertwined processes can be obtained using the electroencephalogram (EEG). Electrical activity of the brain can be averaged to cancel out "random noise" (EEG activity not related to the recognition task) to reveal the Event-Related Potentials (ERP) of memory processes. The ERP of a memory of a stimulus (*red and green wavy*

lines, versus a new stimulus, *blue wavy line*) is larger in amplitude than a novel stimulus. The familiarity component of recognition occurs earlier than recollection, and is located in a somewhat different brain region (central Cz electrode versus parietal Pz electrode) [Reproduced from Veselis RA, et al. Propofol and midazolam inhibit conscious memory processes very soon after encoding: an event-related potential study of familiarity and recollection in volunteers. Anesthesiology. 2009;110(2):295–312 [89]. With permission from Wolters Kluwer Health, Inc.]

A recent study has shown that previous experience of general anesthesia in young children seems to affect one type of recognition memory, namely recollection, but not the familiarity qualities of recognition [92, 93]. The axiom of "as long as the study is reasonably well done, the attendant observations are rarely disputed" applies to this study. This is one of the few carefully done studies of memory and anesthesia in children. In this study, children who had anesthesia were carefully matched with controls, and both were tested (in the absence of any anesthetic drug) for the recollection and familiarity aspects of recognition memory. Although overall recognition was similar in both groups, a measurable difference in recollection was observed. The question of neurotoxicity of anesthetics, especially in children, is a looming problem, so this concrete observation is most noteworthy [94]. Controversy arises about how best to explain these observations. The authors of the study interpreted their findings using the "dual process" theory of memory. However, one should be aware of other explanations, and be open to different interpretations down the road. To better understand the underpinnings of this study, I will detail how one would study familiarity versus recollection recognition memory.

Differences between familiarity and recollection are studied using study-test paradigms as previously described. The added ingredient to tease out the type of recognition is a measure of confidence (or bias) of the recognition. Thus, during the recognition task, after an item is either recognized as previously seen (old) or not (new), a measure of confidence is obtained [95]. This measure varies among studies, but the most common one is to use a 6 point scale, from "absolutely sure old" (with "moderately sure old,, "somewhat sure old" in between) to "absolutely sure new" (or "somewhat sure new," "moderately sure new"). Similar information can be obtained in animal models by ingenious manipulations of reward strategies, where choice of reward is biased by previously learned preferences [47, 48]. A receiver operator characteristic (ROC) curve is plotted of these responses. In this type of analysis the ROC is the cumulative recognition proportion against false alarms rate (a false alarm is an item that is recognized as old, but is in fact a new item) across the six levels of confidence. So, for example, the left most point is the (old) recognition of highest confidence. Thus, the person is virtually certain they got the right answer, and typically about 20 % of old items are correctly recognized as being old (the y axis), and very few truly new items are incorrectly recognized with high confidence as being old (false alarms, thus, close to 0 % plotted on the x-axis) (Fig. 3.8). Then the next least confidence category is added cumulatively to the previous score, thus the next point is always greater in both axes. As a consequence these graphs generally have 5 unique points (as the last cumulative value is always 100 %). A curve

interpolation graphically describes recognition performance. A set of recognitions that are largely or solely based on familiarity will produce an ROC curve that is characteristically symmetrical along the 45° axis. On the other hand, recognitions based on recollection produce an offset at "sure old" category (at the lowest false alarm rate), and tend to produce a linear response as confidence decreases. Further information can be gained by statistically normalizing scores across a Gaussian distribution (z-scores, which produce a z-ROC). In the case of z-ROC's familiarity recognitions produce a flat line, as the distribution of signal strengths is Gaussian in nature, whereas an inverted curve is present for recollection, which has a non-Gaussian or skewed distribution. Measures of familiarity and recollection as embodied in ROC curves are robustly observed. Controversy rages over what mechanisms produce these observed behaviors.

Mechanisms to explain how these curves may be generated falls into two main camps, the so-called dual process theory and single process/signal strength theory [96, 97]. There seem to be more publications that interpret observations as dual process theories (as was done in the paper describing memory impairments in children receiving anesthesia), so I will present this first. Dual process theories basically state that mechanisms supporting recollection are different from those that support familiarity. Part of this difference is related to the neuroanatomical underpinnings of these processes, with the hippocampus primarily involved in recollection (whereas single process "theorists" posit that the hippocampus is involved in both recollection and familiarity recognitions) [98, 99]. Dual process theorists provide substantial evidence that familiarity based recognition seems to be centered on other medial temporal lobe structures, in particular the parahippocampal regions [100–105]. Familiarity is the easiest to understand conceptually, and is characterized by Gaussian signal strength distributions with recognition occurring when the separation in signal peaks (between different items) is large enough. These processes are thought to be very efficient in their implementation, and occur almost automatically. In fact, this can be measured using electrophysiologic methods such as event-related potentials [89, 104, 106–108]. The onset of familiarity processes occur some 100 ms sooner than recollection processes (Fig. 3.7). Details of how these mechanisms may be instantiated neurobiologically will be presented below. If there is low signal strength or signal peaks are close together (old and new items are very similar to each other), then the confidence in familiarity is low, and the behavioral correlate would be "unsure new/old" i.e., the 3rd or 4th confidence categories. However, if the signal strength is high or signals are well separated, then one might state "sure new" or "sure old." It is important to keep in mind that signal strengths are modeled by Gaussian distribution curves. On the other hand, a recollection

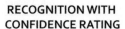
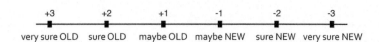

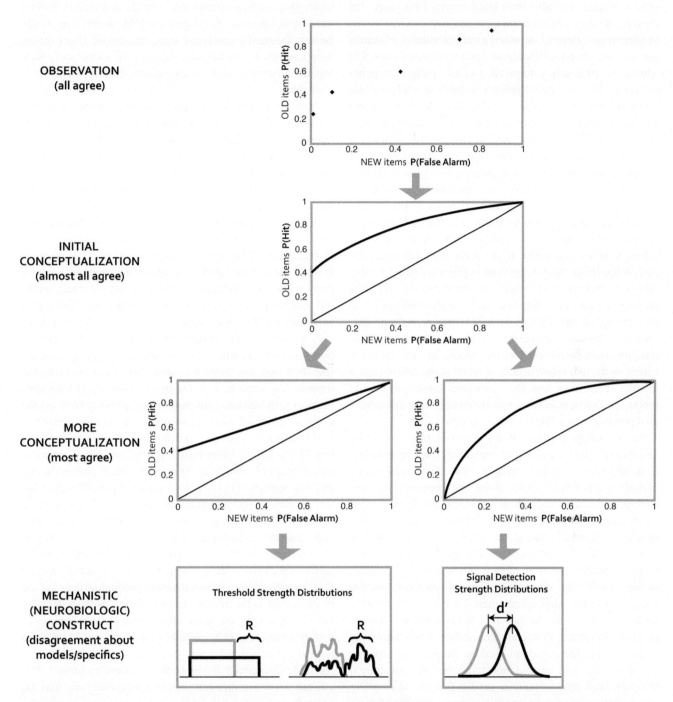

Fig. 3.8 A method to measure the contribution of familiarity versus recollection in recognition memory. This is also an illustrative example of the difficulty in translating observations, which are generally agreed upon, into a conceptualization, which may have a number of alternatives to explain the observations. A receiver operator characteristic curve is created by assessing the confidence of the recognition memory from a surety that the stimulus is old (previously experienced) to surety that it was never experienced (new). See text for details. The methodology to create the ROC curve is fairly standard and widely used. The curve represents the combined contributions of familiarity and recollection to recognition memory. How these contributions are conceptualized is important in understanding memory systems, with two alternative explanations, the dual process versus single process theory, holding sway in different camps. Both conceptualizations use different explanations of why the ROC curve looks the way it does, and why it changes appearance when certain parameters are changed in study paradigms. The dual process theory postulates that familiarity and recollection are separable processes, where familiarity is a process that depends on separation of signals between two Gaussian distributions to separate new and old events, whereas a more complex recognition process is present for recollection. In the latter case, the hippocampus acts as a pattern detector where a certain threshold criterion needs to be met before recognition can occur. The single process theory postulates a single memory process that behaves differently under differing circumstances based on the strength of memories

recognition involves not only the primary stimulus (e.g., the person's face), but also associated details (the party, the clothes, the date). In mechanistic terms one can model this as pattern completion, and when a certain number of details are matched, then recollection of the full pattern occurs. The additional processing required to test pattern matches explains why recollection processes start later and take longer than familiarity processes. On the flip side, if insufficient pattern completion is present then no recollection may occur, i.e. a memory failure. A Gaussian distribution of signal strength will always yield some degree of recognition, be it ever so small. Thus, in the dual process theory recollection is posited as a threshold process (note that the threshold effect applies to the recollection, not the recognition which can also include familiarity processes). Below this threshold no recollection occurs, and any recognition that occurs would be solely based on familiarity. If one is above this pattern completion threshold, then recognition is primarily based on recollection. Recollection would be expected to typically produce a "sure old" response, and the threshold effect is used to explain the offset of the ROC curve at the "sure old" response. Thus two processes (familiarity and recollection, dual processes) are used for recognition. In fact, everyone agrees on the latter statement, however it is emphasized again that the specifics of how these processes come into play in producing a recognition response are thought to be different in dual process versus single process models.

In the single process model theorists posit that both familiarity and recollection processes are continuous expressions of signal strength, but that recollection embodies additional details about the memory. In most experimental paradigms, these additional details are tested by measuring source memory. Thus, instead of just presenting "word" during the study phase, "word" is presented in different locations on the computer screen, with a different color from other words in different locations in the stimulus list. When recognition of word is tested for, the participant is also asked where on the screen or what color the word was. Retrieval of these additional details provides evidence of recollection rather than familiarity (and this was the paradigm used in the study comparing children who had or did not have general anesthesia) [92, 93]. Dual process theories predict that an old recollection response will not occur until a certain number of these details are present, whereas single source theories state that source memory is integral to the memory itself, no matter what strength that memory is.

Needless to say, arguments on either side have not been compelling enough to abate the controversy. The important point the reader has to appreciate is that one needs to be extremely careful not to conflate reliable observations with postulated mechanisms that produce these observations. Thus the findings of Stratmann et al. robustly show some

degree of memory impairment in children who have undergone general anesthesia, which affects recollection out of proportion to familiarity [92]. However, one should be very hesitant to postulate some neurotoxic effect on the hippocampus as a result of anesthesia, be it ever so appealing, until a great deal of additional corroborating evidence is available.

Now, let us take a little detour into the experience of déjà vu to illustrate again the importance of maintaining a divide between observation and explanation. This is a memory feeling we have all likely experienced at one time or another (at least about 80 % of people do). It is the feeling of having experienced a current ongoing event sometime before, with the memory being of excruciating clarity (internally one might think "I know I have experienced these exact events before, I can almost know what will happen next") [109]. There is no accepted explanation for this memory feeling, but a most interesting one is that there is a timing problem between different memory systems, namely working and long term memory. This produces a feeling of experiencing the exact same events (which in fact have only happened once) at different times. Normally information flows in an orderly fashion through working memory (the "here and now") into long term memory (something that happened at some time in the past). However, if long term memory mechanisms somehow simultaneously have access to the contents of working memory, one could experience the same event as happening now and simultaneously in the past [110]. On the other hand, others explain déjà vu as an instantiation of familiarity, or error in pattern completion by the hippocampus [111, 112]. These examples illustrate that there is general agreement on the observations of déjà vu, in no small part due to the fact many of us have personally experienced this. However, when it comes down to explanation of these events, no one knows what particular conceptualization explains these phenomena. It is generally agreed that the neurobiologic mechanisms producing déjà vu are incorporated in the medial temporal lobes, as these feelings can be induced by electrical stimulation of these regions in epileptic patients [112]. Whether the same would occur in normal subjects is unknown, these people would never have electrodes implanted. It may be that the same end result, déjà vu, can arise via different mechanisms, everyone may be correct!

Under the Hood: The Neurobiologic/ Neurocomputational Instantiation of Conscious Memory Processes

The report of HM, who was the key index case in the series of cases reported by Scoville and Milner, began the era of understanding memory processes in terms of neuroanatomical, and subsequently neurobiologic and neurocomputational systems (the terms "in vitro," "in vivo" now include "in computo") [113]. In brief, the famous report of Scoville described a severe impairment in the ability to form new episodic memories (e.g., memorizing a word list) after bilateral removal of a substantial amount of material from the medial temporal lobes. The material contained not only the hippocampi, but many other medial temporal lobe structures, thus it was not until some decades later that the hippocampus was clearly identified as the seat of conscious memory. A combination of animal and patient lesion studies, where neurologic damage was more localized to the hippocampus proper led the way to this insight [38, 114]. During this period, HM had become the most studied neurologic case in history, and really solidified the concept that conscious and unconscious memory are embodied in different processes and neuroanatomy [115]. HM was able to learn unconscious memories as easily as others, e.g. the motor skill of mirror drawing, but had no recollection of any of these experiments immediately after testing. However, over the last few decades it has become equally clear that even though the hippocampus is necessary for conscious memory, it is not sufficient. A complex web of interactions with other brain regions is needed for conscious memory function. As information flow progresses from sensation to long term memory, more and more interactions are needed, and wider and wider regions of brain areas function coherently in networks to support memory function [116, 117].

Interactions between different brain regions occur in the language of oscillations which provide a rich grammar for communication, ranging from frequencies to coherence, to phase shifts [118, 119]. Of particular note is that oscillations in the gamma and theta ranges seem to be very important in memory processes (as well as consciousness, and anesthetic effects thereon) [29, 120–127]. The divisions of the EEG frequency band (i.e., alpha, beta, theta, gamma, etc.) are arbitrary and based on historic interpretations of raw signals in roughly the order of discovery or description [128]. Limits between bands are also arbitrary, and change through time and with the model (human, animal) being studied [113, 129]. Theta ranges approximately from 4 to 7 Hz, whereas gamma frequencies occur at approximately 40–80 Hz. As with many processes, it is not the actual value, but changes in the value itself that are important. Thus, small changes in theta frequency, phase shift, power, etc. can be very significant. As is becoming increasing evident, it is quite a feat to describe with this level of detail how a memory process is embodied in an associated neuroanatomy and the encompassing electrophysiologic milieu. A great deal of progress has been made as details of neuronal physiology have been pinned down, and computational power of computers has increased faithfully following Moore's law. Two memory processes in particular will be considered, those being working and episodic memory as mediated through the medial temporal lobe. The latter will be considered in terms of the qualities of recollection and familiarity. As oscillatory activity in the brain is critically dependent in inter-neuronal connections, which are heavily dependent on GABAergic mechanisms, a key target of anesthetic action on memory may be modulation of electrophysiologic interactions of neuronal networks [130–139].

Working Memory

The first differentiation of memory processes was between short and long term memories. After this insight, short term memory was conceptualized as a series of closely related working memory processes [140, 141]. Working memory is embodied largely in the pre-frontal cortex, richly connected to the medial temporal lobe [142–145]. Details of how information is held in working memory have been worked out in terms of electrophysiology. One can now explain why the capacity of working memory is 7 ± 2 items in terms of oscillatory activity [30]. Purely by using characteristics of neuronal electrophysiology, an underlying slower wave action of frequency theta (hippocampal theta rhythms) can contain information in the form of superimposed faster gamma activity. It turns out that the ratio of gamma to theta (40:4 Hz) is about 7 [146, 147] (Fig. 3.9). As you may note the ratio is closer to 10, but information is contained in only a certain portion of the theta rhythm oscillation cycle. This was one of the first neurocomputational instantiation of memory processes, and others have followed.

Episodic/Conscious Memory

The behavior of more complex systems can be embodied in computational models based on neural networks. A computational neural network structure is created out of interconnected elements, where the rules for response in each element are well defined and usually simple (e.g., when the summation of inputs into the element exceeds a certain threshold value, that element then produces an output, the degree of which can be adjusted according to a weight) [148] (Fig. 3.10). As can be appreciated, each element can be considered a very simple neuron, thus the label of neural network. Most interestingly even simple designs (e.g., two-layer feed-forward network) can learn and reproduce very complex behavior. A set of data, containing input data and output results, is used to train the network to reproduce the behavior sought. Training in this context is a recurrent algorithm wherein the error term between the

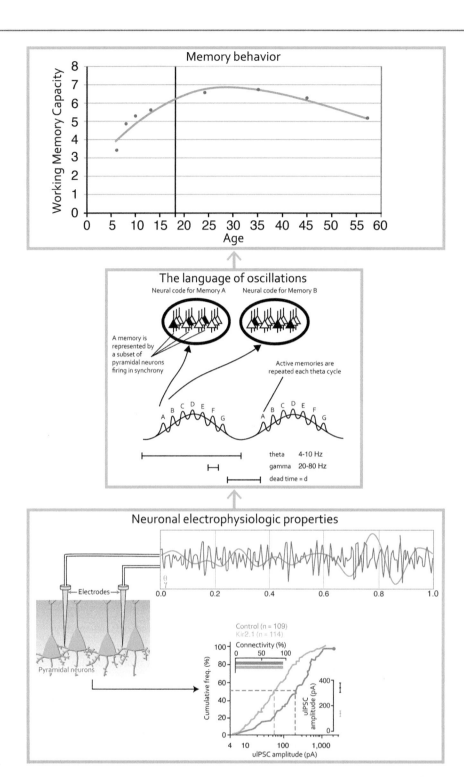

Fig. 3.9 Instantiation of working memory—from electrophysiology to behavior. The brain communicates with itself in the language of oscillations. The electrophysiologic properties of neurons as well as the architecture of their connections determine the frequency of oscillatory activity. Information is contained not only in the frequency of oscillations, but other properties such as phase relationships as well. This is an example of how one can explain why working memory can contain a maximum number of items based on representation of oscillations with differing frequencies (gamma, approximately 40 cycles/s contained within theta oscillations, approximately 7 cycles/s) which are produced by the electrophysiologic properties of neurons. The ratio of gamma to theta oscillations is roughly the capacity of working memory. Many other characteristics of memory can be related to theta and gamma oscillatory activity [middle panel reproduced from Jensen O, Lisman JE. Hippocampal sequence-encoding driven by a cortical multi-item working memory buffer. Trends Neurosci. 2005;28(2):67–72 [147]. With permission from Elsevier Ltd.]

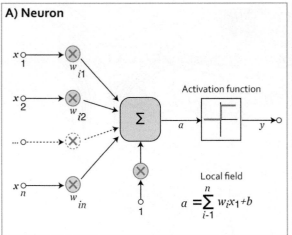

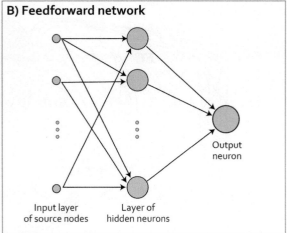

Fig. 3.10 Computational algorithms based on artificial neural networks. Artificial (computational) neural networks are loosely based on neuronal interactions with each other, but greatly simplified, to produce a learned, or trained, output from a series of inputs using Hebbian type learning. Very complex behavior can be modeled with neural networks, even when the input/output rules for each element are simple in nature. Complexity is modeled by the interactions of neural network elements ("w", i=1...n), and a simple two-layer feed-forward fully interconnected network is displayed. Each element processes (e.g., sums, "sigma") inputs from other elements and produces an output based on a rule (e.g., threshold activation, "activation function" in the figure). The strength of the output (inputs into the next layer) can be modified by a weighting factor. Neural networks are trained by matching a set of outputs (e.g., tidal heights) with a series of inputs (date, weather parameters, location, etc.) that are processed by a network with an initial set of weighting parameters (e.g., 0.5). An error term from the output is generated, and weights are modified iteratively to minimize this error term. When a certain acceptable error threshold is achieved, the network is then tested with a set of new (never used before) inputs and the error measured between predicted and actual outputs to assess how well the neural network models real world data. This can be done by training a network on a portion of a data set, and testing on the other part of the data set. Networks can be constructed with more elaborate configurations (e.g., recurrent inputs, more layers, pruned connections) to model even more complex behaviors

output produced by the network and the target output is minimized but adjusting the parameters governing the behavior of the network elements (primarily the weighting of the outputs for each element). For example, inputs can be the power of various EEG frequencies, and the output can be whether the EEG is of a sedated patient or an awake patient [149–152]. The trained network can be used on novel data sets to predict an output with reasonable success. As computational power and algorithms have advanced exponentially "children" of these methods are getting to the point where "the brain," as opposed to the EEG, for example, can be mathematically modeled [153, 154]. In general, there is no deterministic algorithm defined by the training process or modeling. The neural network behaves in a complex manner that is essentially a black box. Practically, neural networks work quite well in many real world situations, for example predicting tidal patterns, automated image/pattern analysis, minimal path finding, and yes, financial applications too. The use of this methodology to model neuroanatomical constructs of conscious memory will now be reviewed.

The Hippocampus

The hippocampus is a set of recurrent looping neural pathways that can very efficiently embody complex information using a sparse encoding [155–157]. The basic structure is presented in Fig. 3.11. The hippocampus is richly connected to the cortex, but the vast majority of connections are indirect. Input from the cortex is received via the entorhinal cortex, and output is through the same structure, but in a different layer (in general the cortex has six layers of neurons). Three major structures comprise the hippocampus, the dentate gyrus, and the cornu ammonis (CA) specifically the CA3 and CA1 subfields (as with many things labels are historic and somewhat poetic). A neural network model representative of hippocampal neurobiology is presented in Fig. 3.12 [158, 159]. As far as neural networks go, this is a fairly complex design. However, this is a very good model for pattern recognition. One of the first insights into the computational abilities of the hippocampus was obtained by measuring individual neuronal responses in behaving rats walking through a maze [53, 160–162]. The same sets of neurons fired when the rat was in a given location, thus the concept of place cells was discovered. The memory of a particular location is embodied in this pattern. One can think of many conscious memories (e.g., words) as a pattern. The neural network model of the hippocampus will produce a threshold type of output when a certain number of elements of a previously learned pattern are present. This is the instantiation of the recollection process, and experimental results from this computational model agree well with

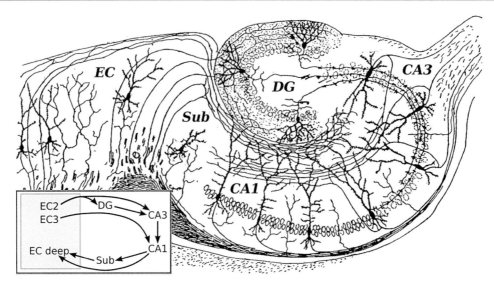

Fig. 3.11 Hippocampal architecture. This Figure is the classic histologic drawing of a rodent hippocampus Santiago Ramon y Cajal published in 1911 (Drawing of the neural circuitry of the rodent hippocampus. Histologie du Système Nerveux de l'Homme et des Vertébrés, Vols. 1 and 2. A. Maloine. Paris. 1911). Such accurate and detailed observations are still very relevant today. Included in this Figure is a conceptualization of information processing through various regions of the hippocampus. Input of information is from close-by regions in the medial temporal lobe (entorhinal cortex, EC). Sensory input via the EC projects to the dentate gyrus (DG), the CA3 and CA1 fields of the hippocampus and the subiculum (Sub) via the perforant pathway. The dentate gyrus projects to the CA3 field of the hippocampus via Mossy fibers. CA3 neurons project to the CA1 field of the hippocampus, which in turn projects back to the subiculum. The subiculum feeds back to the EC. In the EC, superficial and deep layers are arranged to produce a recurrent loop for incoming sensory information. After processing in the hippocampus, output influences information in the entorhinal reverberating circuit, which in turn repetitively activates the hippocampal formation, or is transmitted to other regions of the cerebral cortex. Thus, the hippocampus provides a very complex information processing architecture in a small amount of space, and is ideally suited in terms of pattern completion/recognition

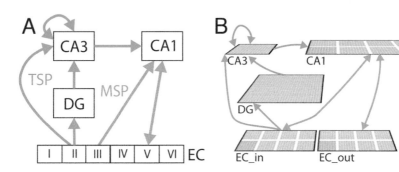

Fig. 3.12 This is a neurocomputational model of the hippocampus (a combination of Figs. 3.10 and 3.11). Most readers are familiar with the terms "in vitro" and "in vivo," and now we can add "in computo" as another way to understand details of physiologic processes. This neural network architecture can be used to understand recognition memory in humans, and can reproduce the observations of recognition memory as described in Fig. 3.8

observations [16, 76, 159]. The reader should be aware that even though this "hangs together nicely," it does not mean this is actually what happens in terms of actual physiologic processes. In a sense this is a mechanistic conceptualization. Adding to this strong circumstantial evidence is the fact that the computational model predicts certain behaviors, that, when actually tested, hold true. Further refinements in mathematical modeling are now being incorporated where, analogous to place cells, there are "time" cells [87]. One of the basic concepts of conscious memory is that an event occurs not only in a particular place, but also in a particular time.

It now seems that a neurocomputational explanation can be proposed for the hippocampus to embody time as well as space.

The Rest of the Brain

A computational model of the non-hippocampally connected cortex is much simpler, where a "simple" two-layer feed-forward network can reproduce signal strength memory behavior (a.k.a. familiarity) (Fig. 3.13). As the reader is likely to appreciate, though this model of familiarity based memory works well to mimic observational results, it is

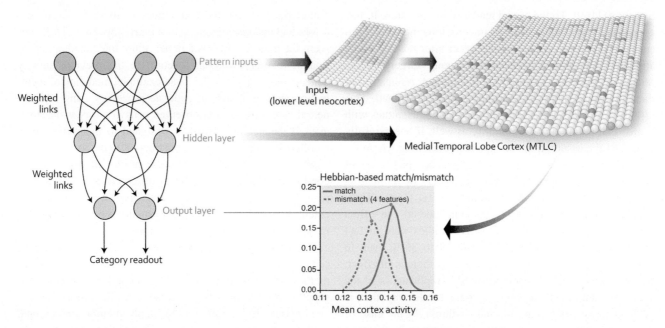

Fig. 3.13 Similar in concept to Fig. 3.12, this is a neural network instantiation of the familiarity component of recognition memory. Such "in computo" modeling can be used to investigate factors important in memory as a bridge between neurobiology and observation. Ideally the model is used to predict a certain outcome when parameters are modified in a predictable fashion. These are then tested "in vivo" to support the validity of such modeling

likely not the way the brain works. Neurons are much more complex than the elements present in a neural network model. However, this modeling is a good starting point for further research, and importantly, may serve well as a basis for investigations of anesthetic effects on memory in terms of electrophysiological mechanisms.

The "Black Box" of Unconscious Memory

To study memory requires some evidence that a memory has been created in the brain, which, as alluded to above, boils down to measuring a change in behavior. This is complex enough in the case of conscious memory, where a simple study-test paradigm can become incredibly complex by manipulation of numerous factors. The same study-test paradigm design is used to study unconscious memory, but with the added caveat that the person or animal in question has to be completely unaware that memory is being created or tested [163, 164]. This requirement is more easily attained in the case of animals, and is the reason I said that many memory behaviors in animals (e.g., object recognition) may best be compared to unconscious memory processes in humans [41]. The change in behavior indicative of the memory cannot be consciously accessible, thus all recognition paradigms mentioned above (recall, forced choice, etc.) cannot be used. To detect unconscious memory requires ingenious methods to measure such a memory. Methods include measuring some improvement in performance (e.g., faster

reaction time to a previously experienced stimulus, when compared to non-experienced stimuli), or a preference for the previously (unconsciously) experienced stimulus. The latter is the basis for the previously popular subliminal advertising campaign [165]. Subliminal advertising is now highly frowned upon by society, but it could be said that if conscious perception of a product occurs in unrelated media (e.g., a movie), then "product placement" has occurred.

A large question about unconscious memory is whether it can influence future behavior. This requires two main criteria to be met, that the person is truly unaware of previous learning, and that the change in behavior is able to be replicated in a number of studies. Closely related questions include publication bias, and statistical "anomalies" where the underlying assumptions of statistical testing are not fully appreciated when conclusions are drawn, namely rejection of the null hypothesis [166, 167]. These topics are of increasing interest as clinical care is driven more and more by major studies published in reputable journals [168]. A typical study of unconscious memory might be as follows. People are asked to read stories about knowledgeable and learned scientists versus stories of sports personalities (presumably not in the running for Nobel Prizes). Then the people who have read these stories are asked to complete a general knowledge questionnaire. A study might demonstrate that people exposed to scientist stories completed the knowledge questionnaires with more correct answers. If the results of the study are positive, it is more likely to be published as being exciting new research (particularly in the psychologic literature) [169]. To the casual reader of the literature it may appear that there is evidence of unconscious memory influence all around us, from walking faster after reading about athletes, to improved outcomes following surgery in the setting of "positive thinking." As it turns out, replication of these studies is more difficult than initially imagined. This difficulty is being appreciated more and more in studies with "hard" end points such as mortality as well. If one carefully considers the assumptions of statistical reasoning where we traditionally accept a $p < 0.05$ as being an acceptable rate of false positives, it turns out that the chance of replicating those results is somewhere around 50 % [168]. Thus, reasons for un-reproducibility may include a) the effect may not exist, and the initial positive studies were in fact false positives (estimated to be from 14 to 36 % even in well-respected peer-reviewed literature) b) there is an effect, but the current study is underpowered to replicate, or c) the study population is different in some subtle way that is difficult to ascertain (e.g., diurnal rhythms). In the case of unconscious learning, an additional problem is that not uncommonly the "unconscious" learning turns out to actually be conscious learning when the appropriate probes (e.g., de-briefing interviews of participants regarding insight) are used. Are the people really unaware that reading a story about a scientist followed by a general knowledge questionnaire has nothing to do with envy for smart people? When general interest in a particular field increases to the level that it becomes important to answer a question definitively, it is more likely that negative studies will be published, and more balanced weight of evidence will ensue. The latter is most important in the case of meta-analyses and Cochrane type reviews. The question of learning during anesthesia seems to have reached this point [170, 171]. All these factors make study of unconscious memory fascinating, while at the same time vexing. More often than not purported evidence of unconscious memory turns out to be a more complex insight into conscious memory. It is still very unclear if learning during anesthesia (if present) truly represents unconscious memory, or some degree of a weak conscious memory.

Memories are not immutable and similarly their categorizations. For example, skills and habits are considered by classical taxonomy to be unconscious memory. For example, one should try singing the national anthem starting with the third line without silently reciting the first two lines (this is a classic situation for musicians who feel compelled to "finish the phrase" when practicing). As we all know, one has had to learn the national anthem somewhere at some time. How did this conscious memory become an unconscious memory of a habit? The same process occurs in conscious memory, where an episodic event (capitals of countries) becomes general knowledge, a semantic memory without time or context (see "time and repetition" interactions Fig. 3.3). I hope I have convinced the reader that the

boundaries between the taxonomies of memory, even conscious and unconscious are at best blurry [56, 88, 117]. It does seem the trend is towards a richer, more integrated appreciation of memory, without a return to the previous unitary concept of memory [172]. As an example, modeling of recollection and familiarity as separate processes using separate neural networks predicts observed behavior very well. However, if the neural network is designed to incorporate both recollection and familiarity constructs into the same network model, lo and behold, very similar results are obtained, the combined network also models observed behavior just as well [76]. As neural networks are "black boxes" to a large extent, how or why this happens remains a mystery. But this may, in fact, be the way our brains work.

Thus, currently, while we know a great deal about conscious memory, the same cannot be said of unconscious memory, particularly in regards to underlying mechanisms supporting these memory processes. Needless to say, this is one reason it is difficult to apply neurocomputational modeling to unconscious memory as has been done for conscious memory. The best conceptualization we have of unconscious memory is that of information flow [43, 56]. Unconscious memories have to be formed from information obtained from the outside world, which by necessity has to get into the brain through sensory cortices. At some point in information collation and processing, unconscious information (e.g., shape, size, intensity, color, orientation, frequency, etc. of a stimulus) becomes a conscious percept. At that point we know we just saw a red rubber ball, maybe one that we used to play with as children. Thus the best we can do with a neurobiologic instantiation of unconscious memory formation is to model information flow from the outside world before it becomes a fully conscious percept, which then has an opportunity to become a conscious memory.

The Neurobiology of Unconscious Memory

The neurobiology of unconscious memory may best be related to the lowest "rung" of the SPI model of memory, the perceptual system (note that "perceptual" is used in the psychological sense, and refers to sensation, not the percept of consciousness). Automatic processing of stimuli, one aspect of which is to filter out extraneous information whilst directing attentional resources to events of interest (orienting reflex), allows one to learn very complex information without being aware of the specifics of that information. In other words, we can learn rules that are complex without ever knowing the rules (subliminal learning) [173]. Compared with conscious memory, very little investigation has been undertaken to understand the basis of unconscious memory. But what little is known reveals a complex underpinning for this behavior. As with conscious memory, information transfer and communication between different brain regions must occur for learning to take place [88, 173]. The type of memory learned as "unconscious" memory during anesthesia is likely different from that studied in humans in the absence of drug during unconscious rule learning. Lower processing power may be needed to form implicit, perceptual memories during anesthesia than unconscious rule learning. The neurobiologic underpinning for rule versus perceptual (sensory) learning may be quite different, though with some overlap of mechanisms likely. Thus, while there is some degree of likelihood of sensory (perceptual) memory formation during anesthesia (as detailed below), there seems to be much less likelihood of the type of learning as embodied in unconscious rule learning, as the latter requires mechanisms such as information transfer across distant

brain regions which are likely to be non-functional during anesthesia.

Anesthetic Effects on Memory

Three large bodies of research exist in this field, those being (1) the effects of anesthetics on conscious memory, which include fear modulation of memory and differential effects on recollection and familiarity processes, (2) the issue of awareness, and (3) the ability to learn unconscious memory during anesthesia (Fig. 3.14). Failure of the "anesthetic system," which includes human system processes as well

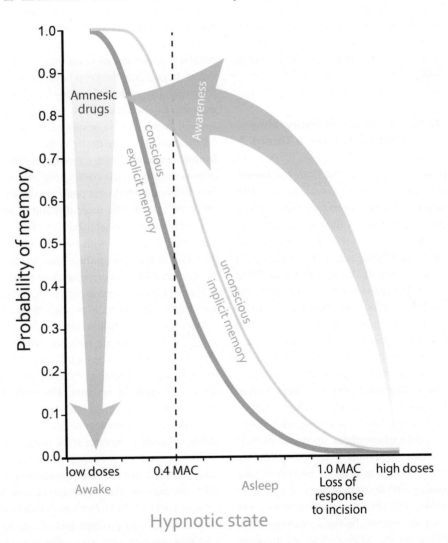

Fig. 3.14 The conceptual relationships between anesthesia and memory. The dose response curve between conscious (explicit) memory and increasing doses of anesthesia is well established, with decreasing probability of memory formation as anesthetic doses increases. When a dose of anesthetic associated with 50 % probability of movement to skin incision (one minimal alveolar concentration—MAC) is present, no chance of conscious memory formation is present. For almost all CNS depressants (most anesthetics), a dose of 0.4 MAC will produce an ~50 % probability of memory impairment on the basis of sedation (inattention to the environment). It is hypothesized that a similar dose

response curve is present for unconscious memory, but is shifted to the right (more resistance to anesthesia). However, this is much less certain, as it is very difficult to quantitate unconscious memory formation. Well established is also the effect of amnesic drugs such as midazolam and propofol, which result in a low probability of conscious memory formation at low doses of drug. When one believes the patient is experiencing 1 MAC of anesthesia, but in fact less anesthetic is present (e.g., technical failure of delivery device), conscious memory is functional when the patient is not expecting this, and awareness results as drugs, to ablate conscious memory when the patient expects no memory is covered by the somewhat vague term "awareness," again not to be confused with the concept of being aware in the sense of consciousness (though, these are closely related). A brief discussion of awareness will be undertaken only to put this huge field of investigation into context regarding memory. The majority of literature of anesthetic effects on unconscious memory relates to the question of whether learning can occur during anesthesia when conscious memory function is not present [174, 175]. Learning during anesthesia is commonly described as implicit memory formation during anesthesia. A much smaller question is the impact of anesthetic drugs on implicit (unconscious) memory during consciousness (i.e., during sedation). The difficulties of differentiating conscious from unconscious memory processes in the setting of mild sedation are formidable, and I will not review this literature, as it is at best confusing.

Anesthetic Effects on Conscious Memory: How Do We Make Patients "Not Remember a Thing!"?

When we're asleep we are disconnected from the outside world [31, 58]. Our brains are busy re-processing memories of the day's events, a portion of which we may experience in our dreams [10, 176–178]. Similarly, during anesthesia we become disconnected from processing sensory input even though sensory input is still being registered, and will be discussed in the section on learning during anesthesia. Thus, information from the outside world cannot become a conscious memory, as not enough processing power is present to form that conscious memory. An unexpected conscious memory that occurs during anesthesia falls under the category of awareness during anesthesia, discussed briefly in the next section. Normally, the practicing anesthetist prevents memory formation by putting their client to sleep. This in itself is not very interesting from a mechanistic point of view, but the transition to this state is, on the other hand, most interesting. If the dose of anesthetic agent can be held to one that produces sedation ("almost sleep"), some degree of conscious memory mechanisms are still functional, and the possibility of memory formation is present.

For sensory information to become a conscious memory (which hereafter in this section will be simply referred to as "memory"), attention must be paid to that information. There is a large body of literature examining the influence of attention on memory formation, and in practice we do use this trick to influence memory formation [179–184]. An example is engaging a patient in conversation while we start an intravenous injection. Most anesthetic agents produce memory impairment in the sedative dose range by interfering with attention (the opposite way of stating this is "producing sedation"). Sedation interferes with information processing in the early stages of memory formation, namely transfer of information from working memory to long term memory [89, 185]. As stated previously, if information disappears from working memory, it is gone forever unless it has been processed into long term memory. Thus, a person who is drunk can walk home in an impaired (sedated), but still barely functional state (for example, stopping before crossing a street with traffic in it), but will have no memory of the excursion back home. Working memory is sufficiently functional to process and react to current events, but these are not subsequently transferred to long term memory. The neurobiologic underpinnings of sedative anesthetic actions, not surprisingly, mimic those of natural sleep, and involve structures in the hypothalamus and other deep brain areas [186–189]. These same neural circuits also seem to be involved in the loss of consciousness that occurs with anesthesia. In practice, the great advantage of preventing memory formation by producing sedation is that we have a real time measure of sedative effect, such as reaction time, slurred speech, eyelid closure, responsiveness, etc. This allows critical titration of drug to desired effect (the clinical end-point of having a patient snoring). Proceeding into a state of sedation/unresponsiveness and coming out of it seems to occur along two different neural/time paths, producing a hysteresis effect [190, 191]. It may be more difficult to arouse a person from sedation once it is established. In other words, the drug concentration associated with awakening may be quite a bit less than that needed to produce unresponsiveness. Sometimes, one can observe an interesting exception to this natural history in that a person can be experiencing concentrations of anesthetic agent that normally produce deep sedation or unresponsiveness, but nevertheless can still respond to external stimuli (e.g., following simple commands) [60]. However, in this state the person may be unable to process other inputs, and be "floating" in a state of "disconnectedness," with various degrees of recall afterwards. The term "dysanesthesia" has been applied to this most interesting state of (un?)consciousness. It is still very unclear if this state is unique to anesthesia, and how best to reproduce it for further study.

As opposed to sedation, some anesthetic agents have unique effects on memory, producing amnesia for events that transpire in the presence of low concentrations of these drugs [192, 193]. Benzodiazepines are the prototypical class of drugs that produce this effect. At concentrations of drug that produce amnesia, sedation is largely absent. Thus the drunkard above becomes the slightly intoxicated person that had their gin and tonic spiked with flunitrazepam (Rohypnol), GHB (gamma hydroxybutyrate), or similar "club" drug. Persons intoxicated in such a fashion may function at a much better level, and seem to be quite awake and unimpaired. Yet, recall of events is much less likely, the amnesia is much more dense [194].

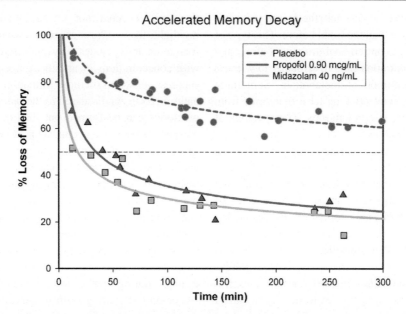

Fig. 3.15 Amnesic drug actions on conscious memory. The low probability of memory formation with amnesic drugs is apparent only after an initial period of memory decay, 15–50 min. Accelerated memory decay occurs when information is learned in the presence of midazolam or propofol. The *top blue line* represents the normal rate of forgetting of information in the placebo group. As Ebbinghaus demonstrated, memory is forgotten over time. These curves represent the loss of memories encoded into long term memory during an encoding task just before time = 0 at which point drug infusion was stopped. When midazolam or propofol were present at low concentrations during the encoding task, those items encoded into long term memory were forgotten at an accelerated rate compared with placebo. Most of the differences in forgetting from placebo happened in the first 45 min. After this time the decay curves are essentially parallel, indicating that consolidation processes that are in play after 45–90 min are not differentially affected by these drugs. The decay of memory can be modeled as a power decay function, and the parameters of this model represent memory impairment due to sedation (lambda in Fig. 3.5a, initial condition) or to lack of consolidation (psi in Fig. 3.5a, accelerated memory decay)

Careful study of memory processes in the presence of low doses of midazolam or propofol reveals the mechanism of this action to be the rapid loss of memories [72]. Details of how amnesic drugs affect memory are best understood in context of information flow from the outside world into a long lasting memory (Fig. 3.15). Terminology is a bit confusing, and one can be led astray by this. As described previously, awareness of the "here and how" occurs in working memory, a limited store of what has just come in from the outside world. Items in working memory can be remembered as long as they are continuously refreshed (rehearsal), think of memorizing a 10 digit phone number. It is easier to remember the first and last digits of the number, the serial position effect. The initial digits are likely already in long term memory, and the last digits heard are in working memory. To critically study the difference between working memory and long term memory processes a paradigm has to be used that prevents rehearsal of any items in working memory, so that one can determine if recognition of an item is truly from working or long term memory. Such a paradigm is the continuous recognition task, where items are presented every few seconds, with items repeated at short (1 or 2 intervening items) or long (10, 20 or 30 intervening items) [72, 82, 89, 195, 196]. The task of the person is to indicate if the item is new (presented the first time) or old (a repeat from the previous set of items). Importantly attention has to be paid to each item as it is presented (is it old or new?), thus preventing rehearsal of any items in working memory. As the capacity of working memory is about 7 items, and if items are presented every 3 s, then an item can reside in working memory no longer than about 20 s. If an item is correctly recognized from more than 10 items previously, then it must be remembered from "long" term memory. This is the confusing part of terminology in that "long" term memory is any time interval longer than working memory, i.e. about 20 s (not very long term in most people's minds). Using this methodology, one can determine if a drug affects working memory (lack of recognition of short interval items), or only long term memory (lack of recognition of longer interval items). Indeed, the sedation effect of drugs affects working memory, whereas amnesic drugs allow long term memories to be formed [89]. However, when these initially recognized items are tested at longer and longer intervals, 10 min, 30 min, 4 h, we find that items initially remembered from long term memory disappear very quickly (in comparison with placebo) [72]. Working and long term memory processes can be indexed by electrophysiologic measurements (event-related potentials), and reveal additional details. This explains the dense amnesia of amnesic drugs. Even if the memory is formed initially, it rapidly disappears. The fact that working memory is largely intact means that behavior in the "here and now" is relatively normal, the person just can't remember what happened at all the night before. This type of amnesia occurs only in the presence of drug, not before, and not after the drug concentration falls to critically low levels on the basis of redistribution of metabolism. Something about the amnesic drug prevents long term memories from being consolidated into lasting memories. The specifics of what happens are still unknown.

The decay characteristics of long term memories formed in the presence of drug can be carefully measured and modeled using a power decay function, and thus the degree of amnesic versus sedative effect of a drug can be quantitated. As mentioned in the previous paragraph, the amnesic effect of a drug must act on some aspect of the sum of processes needed to consolidate a newly formed memory into one that lasts substantially longer. This inhibitory action must occur soon after memory formation, for if it acted much later, then recent memories formed at an earlier time than drug administration would also disappear. Such an effect would be characterized as retrograde amnesia, as depicted in the movies when a traumatic event has occurred. To date no study in humans has documented such a retrograde amnesic effect of any anesthetic drug [197]. In practice, we "ensure" amnesia by administering small doses of these agents, usually midazolam, before noxious events. One should be aware that by giving an amnesic drug, we cannot "erase" previously experienced memories. However, we never know how successful amnesia is until we can debrief the patient some time after the events. It could be that the dose of midazolam used was too low to produce the dense amnesia that was sought.

An interesting field of investigation is how anesthetic effects on memory translate to the pediatric patient population. It is known that working memory doesn't fully develop until quite late, about age 20 or so [198]. Another interesting fact is that most anesthetics influence memory through GABAergic mechanisms, and GABAergic receptor expression changes with age, with different effects in different cortical layers [199]. There are also some animal data that indicate long term memory effects of anesthetics (potentially a marker of neurotoxicity) can be mediated by GABA receptors [133]. Thus, much needs to be clarified regarding anesthetic effects on memory in the pediatric patient population. This will be challenging as this is a difficult age group in which to perform behavioral studies, those being the necessary condition to understand memory.

Awareness During Anesthesia: Interaction with Memory Systems

Awareness during anesthesia represents the ability of conscious memory processes to function in a situation in which they are expected not to be functional. This statement highlights the two "prongs" of this issue. One is fairly straightforward in that episodes of awareness are invariably associated with concentrations of anesthetic agents that are too low to suppress conscious memory formation and retention (consolidation) [200]. As discussed in the previous section conscious memories can be formed but then quickly forgotten in the presence of amnesic agents such as propofol or midazolam. There are ethical dilemmas that revolve around the issue of whether anesthetic practice that depends on lack of consolidation of conscious memories is considered anesthesia [201]. In practical terms this means the patient is "awake" in the presence of an amnesic drug, but has no recollection of events that happened in this state later. One issue that raises ethical concerns in some people's minds may be the duration of this amnesic state. This practice seems to be readily accepted, for example during awake intubations, or the increasingly rare "wake-up test" during neurosurgery, but is frowned upon by some for longer periods of time in a state of "dysanesthesia" where comfortable awareness may be present in a state of dissociation from external stimuli [202]. As mentioned elsewhere in this chapter, multiple states of being may be possible in the presence of anesthetics, and some of these may indeed occur only in the presence of anesthetics rather than having analogs in other situations [31, 58].

The other "prong" of awareness is expectation. It seems that if a complete explanation is provided to the patient of what is likely to happen, awareness is much less distressing, as this was what is expected. This is routinely attested to by the practice of having the patient awake and responsive during critical times during brain surgery ("awake craniotomies"), where preservation of eloquent cortex is the goal of this procedure. In fact, this procedure was standard practice in the era of H. M.s surgery, and now has been rediscovered. as being the best monitor of which part of the brain is important for a certain function, such as language or counting. Analogous to detecting a memory, behavior is the key observation of interest. The importance of patient expectation is attested to by the fact that in situations where sedation is the goal of anesthesia, the occurrence of unexpected awareness can be every bit as distressing as that which occurs during anesthesia where complete unresponsiveness is the goal [203]. Too commonly, patients undergoing sedation for procedures are told by someone that they "won't remember a thing" (which is usually true). This may help reduce anxiety before the procedure, but may also be a dis-service to our patients when sedation is not as deep as the patient was expecting.

Awareness is closely linked with the emotional memory system, mediated through the amygdala. One might consider post-traumatic stress disorder as a "wind-up" phenomenon of the fear mediated memory system. A significant incidence of PTSD can occur with awareness, and it is somewhat unclear how to best capture these events [204–206]. It appears that PTSD can occur at a time quite distant from the inciting event. Routine post-op questioning reveals a very low incidence, by an order of magnitude, of awareness when comparison is made to formal studies of awareness [207, 208]. Why this is the case is unclear, but has been noted in a number of studies. The determine correctly the incidencd of PTSD in the setting of awareness requires longitudinal studies which are excruciatingly difficult and expensive to do, thus data on this are quite sparse at this time. Equally sparse are data on the effects of anesthetics on the fear mediated memory systems [82, 209]. It not only makes sense, but is also a fact that emotive stimuli require higher concentrations of anesthetic agents to prevent them from becoming memories [83]. A few studies have examined the effects of low doses of sevoflurane or propofol on amygdalar function and memory formation, and it does seem that the amygdala is more resistant to the effects of anesthetics. Whether the behavioral observations are linked to the neuroanatomical findings is still an open question.

The goal of reducing "awareness" to zero incidence will require changes in anesthetic practice to eliminate errors in administration (e.g., disconnected IV during TIVA) as well as ensuring appropriate patient expectations. The former can be largely addressed by "being aware of awareness" (e.g., use of checklists, protocolized hand-offs with change in personnel, etc.), and the latter by improving the informed consent process [210, 211].

Learning During Anesthesia, Is It Possible? What Is the Evidence?

The decade of the 1950s was an era of intense stresses with the possibility of global destruction just a button push away. We were surrounded by evidence of this reality from Bikini atoll to Sputnik. The Cold War exploded into full swing and there seemed to be no place to hide. Thus it is no surprise that we looked for answers to unanswerable questions anywhere we could, and one of these places was the unconscious mind. This was the era of "subliminal messages" in advertising [165]. If we could not stop the Manchurian candidate, then why not try to gain some monetary advantage? One wonders if it was just a co-incidence that the first interest in what our minds were doing during anesthesia was born in this cultural context. The first investigations into this issue were quite dramatic, exemplified by statements such as "When questioned at a verbal level he may have no memory at all for the material covered in this [surgical] interval … The next step is to ask permission of the subconscious to release this deeply remembered material." [212]. Thus, under the right circumstances, using specialized hypnotic

techniques, one could peer into the dark unconscious where seemingly every occurrence during the anesthetic experience was faithfully recorded [213]. These concepts fit in quite well with efforts to manipulate the subconscious mind to good and not so good ends. It is no wonder that we continue to this day to desperately seek the truth about what happens in our minds during anesthesia. Despite the multitude of studies that find no evidence of any ability to influence our minds during anesthesia, we hang on to the studies that seem to provide hope that we can influence our unconscious minds which in turn can affect our behavior (positive suggestions, etc.). Are positive results hints of the truth, or, in fact an attempt to assuage a more fundamental need in our human experience?

As the reader can appreciate by now, the evidence to support or refute the formation of memories during anesthesia is roughly equal on both sides of the equation [174, 175]. Over the decades and despite manipulations of, or control for, depth of anesthesia, analgesia, anesthetic regimen, etc. there still is no insight into why there is such variability in results [170, 214–220]. One possibility is a significant "file-drawer" effect, where negative studies are less likely to gain publication, thus it is difficult to weigh the evidence in a Cochrane type analysis [221]. Such publication bias seems to be particularly relevant for social sciences, and one can regard this field as an intersection between these and the "hard" science of mechanisms of anesthesia. One might regard hypnotic methods as a "sociologic" type of approach whereas more recent studies focus on more controlled methods [171, 213]. Just as the presence of memories can only be detected (in practical terms) by looking for changes in behavior after formation of a memory, the only way behavior can be affected by a previous event is by the formation of a memory. Thus the evidence that external events during anesthesia can affect our post-anesthetic behavior is sought in the presence of memories formed during anesthesia. The best methodology to detect unconscious memories is as yet unclear [171]. The behaviors sought must be those not under conscious control (otherwise what is detected is a conscious memory) [163, 164]. Thus, the design of a typical study is to present stimuli (almost always auditory in nature) during clinically adequate anesthesia while the depth of anesthesia is being measured (e.g., using BIS), and then measure a preference for presented versus non-presented stimuli after the anesthesia has worn off. The preference is measured by "the first word that comes to mind" when presented with the first few letters of a word (word stem completion), or by measuring reaction time, for example while reading the words (or a story) [214, 222]. Evidence of unconscious memory is established by a difference in reaction to presented versus non-presented stimuli (at a certain level of statistical likelihood), and some evidence that the memory is not conscious. The latter is usually established by negative recall or recognition tests, or by manipulation of task instructions. For example, the process dissociation procedure incorporates an additional task to "name a word that comes to mind that is *not* the first word you think of." This cognitive procedure requires a conscious manipulation of memory [223]. The results of this task are compared with those of unconsciously mediated word stem completion. There is disagreement on how best to implement the process study procedure when studying learning during anesthesia. Hazadiakos argues that a third category of memory process exists beyond conscious and unconscious, that being guessing. If one re-analyses previous studies that utilized the process dissociation procedure where unconscious memory was detected, then when the possibility of guessing is included these positive results largely disappear [171]. In a sense a more conservative statistical threshold is set by including guessing, and the underlying question is still unanswered as to what the most appropriate threshold should be [166, 167].

Even the same groups of investigators have a hard time replicating their results [219, 220]. This could be a true problem with detection of unconscious memory, or alternatively represent a statistical quandary. If one looks closely at the assumptions underlying probabilistic statistics [as opposed to predictive (e.g., Bayesian) statistics], it is clear that the probability of replication of a result in the original study is on the order of 40 %, when traditional statistical thresholds are used [166, 168]. This seems to agree very well with the historical track record of studies of learning during anesthesia. One way out of this quandary, as suggested by Avidan, is to ask the question of plausibility, is learning during anesthesia a neurobiologic possibility? [224]

There has been much progress made in understanding how anesthesia affects the brain to produce unconsciousness [225, 226]. Needless to say, the story is much more complicated than it seemed even a decade ago. These same principles likely apply to how memory processes work, being as dependent on networks and information transfer as is consciousness. Another approach to the question of learning during anesthesia is a careful consideration of a potential and plausible neurobiologic explanation of this phenomenon. If such a mechanism can be postulated, then efforts can be pursued to identify these processes, and examine anesthetic effects thereon. In short, there is sufficient evidence to support a plausible (if improbable) scenario wherein information from the outside world can be learned by the brain during anesthesia.

At this time, there is overwhelming evidence that information is sensed by the brain during anesthesia. In other words, auditory sensation (perception), though diminished, is still present during unresponsiveness [227–230]. There is really no investigation of visual sensation during anesthesia in humans. Studies focus on auditory perception, as this is the logical entry point of extraneous information of a person whose eyes are taped closed during an anesthetic (one wonders at the incidence of awareness if foam earplugs were used as routinely in the operating room) [231]. The great unknown is what happens to this sensory input after initial sensation during anesthesia? To begin to answer that question one can seek an end result (evidence of implicit memories, which, as described above, has been somewhat unfruitful), or look at processes that support further elaboration of sensory input that could eventually lead to a memory. Local connectivity seems to be intact, thus one could imagine transfer of information from primary sensory cortices to secondary association areas [232–234]. Indeed, in animals, a form of basic memory, visual object recognition memory, does ultimately reside in secondary sensory cortices [235]. This type of memory allows an animal to remember if an object has been seen before, and thus requires no further exploration when new objects are waiting to be discovered. The weight of recent literature supports the nature of this memory to be independent of hippocampal involvement, and thus would not be considered a form of conscious memory [41]. This form of memory may be similar to that sought in implicit memory studies in anesthesia. If these exist, then likely they would reside in secondary sensory cortices, the behavioral instantiation of which would be that of a sensory (perceptual) memory in the lowest rung of the SPI model of Tulving. A question to answer is how is information processed from sensory cortices to become a memory in association cortices? It seems that rather than direct transfer of information from primary to secondary (association) cortices, processing must occur through other brain structures, most likely those of the limbic system [236, 237]. If these nodes are eliminated, primitive or basic memory formation does not occur.

As much as local connectivity is present during anesthesia, connectivity between non-local (distant) regions of brain during anesthesia is severely diminished, if not absent. Feed forward information flow may be preserved, but feedback information flow is not [225, 233, 238–246]. The question that is unclear at this time is where feed forward stops during anesthesia. The critical question is whether sufficient feedforward processing exists through other brain structures to allow transfer of information from sensory to association cortices, which can then become a perceptual (sensory) memory. Initial measures of local connectivity showed that it was preserved. Subsequently, more elegant analytic methods indicated that information content of this connectivity is low or absent [247].

Thus, one can envisage a mechanism by which memories could be formed during anesthesia, but the probability of this occurring seems quite unlikely. At the very least enough functionality of network activity must be present to allow feed-forward processing with at least some feedback to the peri-sensory cortices. At this time very little is known about these processes, even in the absence of anesthesia, let alone during anesthesia. If indeed one could find a situation where implicit memory formation was predictable, the next issue to address is the significance of these memories. Though there is great hope that unconscious memories can influence behavior after anesthesia, at this time the best that can be hoped for is that these memories can be detected. In other research arenas, it is quite controversial whether unconscious memories have an effect on behavior. Replication studies seem to indicate that unconscious memories in fact have little influence on our behavior [164].

Conclusion

As I hope the reader appreciates by now, memory is a very complex set of phenomena, which are still being fleshed out in many directions. The field has gone from a unitary concept to that of multiple memory systems which were considered to be separate. However, as each set of processes is examined closely, they are found to interact with each other more and more closely. The neurobiologic processes supporting memory systems, also considered as separate in the past, are now being revealed as largely separate, but with many mutual interactions and similarities in basic functioning. A given neurobiologic process can be influenced to subserve different higher level systems. Thus, the hippocampus (or portions thereof) function to support some unconscious memories, and unconscious memory systems (e.g., amygdala) modulate conscious memories. Add to this mix the interaction of anesthetics, and one can imagine an almost limitless combinations of effects on memory systems ranging from subtle changes in timing of oscillatory activities in circuits to wholesale blockade of transmission of any information from one part of the brain to another. These are just beginning to be dissected out, and much cross fertilization will occur from the studies of mechanisms of the loss of consciousness from anesthetic drugs. Currently, most of our knowledge resides in the epi-phenomenal realm, i.e. how anesthetics change behavior relevant to memory. We know which drugs are amnesic, which are sedative, and those that have both properties. How these affect cognitive outcomes is just beginning to be investigated (e.g., "triple low" patients, post-operative cognitive dysfunction, delirium, neurotoxicity in children) [248–255]. If there is one thing to remember from this chapter, it is that one needs to approach the field with an open mind, and not be tethered to a particular conceptualization. An open mind in alliance with keen clinical observations will lead to new and better understandings of what we do every day.

References

1. Tulving E. Multiple memory systems and consciousness. Hum Neurobiol. 1987;6(2):67–80.
2. Tulving E, Schacter DL. Priming and human memory systems. Science. 1990;247(4940):301–6.
3. Tulving E. Memory systems and the brain. Clin Neuropharmacol. 1992;15 Suppl 1 Pt A:327A–8A.
4. Zola-Morgan SM, Squire LR. The primate hippocampal formation: evidence for a time-limited role in memory storage. Science. 1990;250(4978):288–90.
5. Squire LR, Zola-Morgan S. The medial temporal lobe memory system. Science. 1991;253(5026):1380–6.
6. Zola-Morgan S, Squire LR. Neuroanatomy of memory. Annu Rev Neurosci. 1993;16:547–63.
7. Cooper SJ, Donald O. Hebb's synapse and learning rule: a history and commentary. Neurosci Biobehav Rev. 2005;28(8):851–74.
8. Hebb DO. The organization of behavior; a neuropsychological theory. New York: Wiley; 1949. p. xix, 335.
9. McGaugh JL. Memory—a century of consolidation. Science. 2000;287(5451):248–51.
10. Rudoy JD, et al. Strengthening individual memories by reactivating them during sleep. Science. 2009;326(5956):1079.
11. Gais S, et al. Sleep transforms the cerebral trace of declarative memories. Proc Natl Acad Sci. 2007;104(47):18778–83.
12. Axmacher N, Haupt S, Fernandez G, Elger CE, Fell J. The role of sleep in declarative memory consolidation: direct evidence by intracranial EEG. Cereb Cortex. 2008;18(3):500–7.
13. Hui K, Fisher CE. The ethics of molecular memory modification. J Med Ethics. 2015;41(7):515–20.
14. Hongpaisan J, Alkon DL. A structural basis for enhancement of long-term associative memory in single dendritic spines regulated by PKC. Proc Natl Acad Sci U S A. 2007;104(49):19571–6.
15. Voss JL, Paller KA. Bridging divergent neural models of recognition memory: introduction to the special issue and commentary on key issues. Hippocampus. 2010;20(11):1171–7.
16. Elfman KW, Parks CM, Yonelinas AP. Testing a neurocomputational model of recollection, familiarity, and source recognition. J Exp Psychol Learn Mem Cogn. 2008;34(4):752–68.
17. Cohen NJ, Squire LR. Preserved learning and retention of pattern-analyzing skill in amnesia: dissociation of knowing how and knowing that. Science. 1980;210(4466):207–10.
18. Heindel WC, et al. Neuropsychological evidence for multiple implicit memory systems: a comparison of Alzheimer's, Huntington's, and Parkinson's disease patients. J Neurosci. 1989;9(2):582–7.
19. Shallice T, Warrington EK. Independent functioning of verbal memory stores: a neuropsychological study. Q J Exp Psychol. 1970;22(2):261–73.
20. Baddeley AD, Warrington EK. Amnesia and the distinction between long- and short-term memory. J Verbal Learn Verbal Behav. 1970;9:176–89.
21. Baddeley A. The concept of episodic memory. Philos Trans R Soc Lond B Biol Sci. 2001;356(1413):1345–50.
22. Atkinson RC, Shiffrin RM. The control of short-term memory. Sci Am. 1971;225(2):82–90.
23. Melton AW. Memory. Science. 1963;140(3562):82–6.
24. Peterson LR, Peterson MJ. Short-term retention of individual verbal items. J Exp Psychol. 1959;58:193–8.
25. Brown J. Some tests of the decay theory of immediate memory. Q J Exp Psychol. 1958;10:12–21.
26. Talmi D, et al. Neuroimaging the serial position curve. A test of single-store versus dual-store models. Psychol Sci. 2005;16(9):716–23.

27. Howard MW, Kahana MJ. A distributed representation of temporal context. J Math Psychol. 2002;46:269.

28. Baddeley A. Working memory. In: Gazzaniga MS, editor. The cognitive neurosciences. Cambridge: MIT Press; 1995. p. 755–64.

29. Lisman JE, Jensen O. The theta-gamma neural code. Neuron. 2013;77(6):1002–16.

30. Lisman JE, Idiart MA. Storage of 7 +/− 2 short-term memories in oscillatory subcycles. Science. 1995;267(5203):1512–5.

31. Pandit JJ. Acceptably aware during general anaesthesia: 'dysanaesthesia'—the uncoupling of perception from sensory inputs. Conscious Cogn. 2014;27:194–212.

32. Baars BJ, Franklin S. How conscious experience and working memory interact. Trends Cogn Sci. 2003;7(4):166–72.

33. Squire LR, Knowlton B, Musen G. The structure and organization of memory. Annu Rev Psychol. 1993;44:453–95.

34. Scoville WB, Milner B. Loss of recent memory after bilateral hippocampal lesions. J Neurol Neurosurg Psychiatry. 1957;20:11–21.

35. Hebb DO, Penfield W. Human behavior after extensive bilateral removal from the frontal lobes. Arch Neurol Psychiatry. 1940;44(2):421–38.

36. Jobst BC, Cascino GD. Resective epilepsy surgery for drug-resistant focal epilepsy: a review. JAMA. 2015;313(3):285–93.

37. Skirrow C, et al. Temporal lobe surgery in childhood and neuroanatomical predictors of long-term declarative memory outcome. Brain. 2014;138:80–93.

38. Zola-Morgan S, Squire LR, Amaral DG. Human amnesia and the medial temporal region: enduring memory impairment following a bilateral lesion limited to field CA1 of the hippocampus. J Neurosci. 1986;6(10):2950–67.

39. Eichenbaum H. The hippocampus and mechanisms of declarative memory. Behav Brain Res. 1999;103(2):123–33.

40. Jacoby LL. Invariance in automatic influences of memory: toward a user's guide for the process-dissociation procedure. J Exp Psychol Learn Mem Cogn. 1998;24(1):3–26.

41. Winters BD, Saksida LM, Bussey TJ. Object recognition memory: neurobiological mechanisms of encoding, consolidation and retrieval. Neurosci Biobehav Rev. 2008;32(5):1055–70.

42. Smith CN, et al. When recognition memory is independent of hippocampal function. Proc Natl Acad Sci. 2014;111(27):9935–40.

43. Tulving E. Episodic memory and common sense: how far apart? Philos Trans R Soc Lond B Biol Sci. 2001;356(1413):1505–15.

44. Gelbard-Sagiv H, et al. Internally generated reactivation of single neurons in human hippocampus during free recall. Science. 2008;322(5898):96–101.

45. Tulving E. Episodic memory: from mind to brain. Annu Rev Psychol. 2002;53:1–25.

46. Clayton NS, Dickinson A. Episodic-like memory during cache recovery by scrub jays. Nature. 1998;395(6699):272–4.

47. Fortin NJ, Wright SP, Eichenbaum H. Recollection-like memory retrieval in rats is dependent on the hippocampus. Nature. 2004;431(7005):188–91.

48. Ergorul C, Eichenbaum H. The hippocampus and memory for "what," "where," and "when". Learn Mem. 2004;11(4):397–405.

49. Shrager Y, et al. Spatial memory and the human hippocampus. Proc Natl Acad Sci U S A. 2007;104(8):2961–6.

50. Pastalkova E, et al. Storage of spatial information by the maintenance mechanism of LTP. Science. 2006;313(5790):1141–4.

51. Broadbent NJ, Squire LR, Clark RE. Spatial memory, recognition memory, and the hippocampus. Proc Natl Acad Sci U S A. 2004;101:14515–20.

52. Poucet B, Save E, Lenck-Santini PP. Sensory and memory properties of hippocampal place cells. Rev Neurosci. 2000;11(2–3):95–111.

53. Alme CB, et al. Place cells in the hippocampus: eleven maps for eleven rooms. Proc Natl Acad Sci U S A. 2014;111:18428–35.

54. Kahana MJ, et al. Human theta oscillations exhibit task dependence during virtual maze navigation. Nature. 1999;399(6738):781–4.

55. Squire LR. Memory and the hippocampus: a synthesis from findings with rats, monkeys, and humans. Psychol Rev. 1992;99(2):195–231.

56. Saksida LM. Neuroscience. Remembering outside the box. Science. 2009;325(5936):40–1.

57. Windhorst C. The slave model of autobiographical memory. Cogn Process. 2005;6(4):253–65.

58. Sanders RD, et al. Unresponsiveness not equal unconsciousness. Anesthesiology. 2012;116(4):946–59.

59. Mashour GA. Integrating the science of consciousness and anesthesia. Anesth Analg. 2006;103(4):975–82.

60. Pandit JJ. Isolated forearm—or isolated brain? Interpreting responses during anaesthesia—or 'dysanaesthesia'. Anaesthesia. 2013;68(10):995–1000.

61. Wixted JT. The psychology and neuroscience of forgetting. Annu Rev Psychol. 2004;55:235–69.

62. Parker ES, Cahill L, McGaugh JL. A case of unusual autobiographical remembering. Neurocase. 2006;12(1):35–49.

63. Lynch MA. Long-term potentiation and memory. Physiol Rev. 2004;84(1):87–136.

64. Hinrichs JV, Ghoneim MM, Mewaldt SP. Diazepam and memory: retrograde facilitation produced by interference reduction. Psychopharmacology (Berl). 1984;84(2):158–62.

65. Medved MI, Hirst W. Islands of memory: autobiographical remembering in amnestics. Memory. 2006;14(3):276–88.

66. Gilboa A. Autobiographical and episodic memory—one and the same? Evidence from prefrontal activation in neuroimaging studies. Neuropsychologia. 2004;42(10):1336–49.

67. Burianova H, Grady CL. Common and unique neural activations in autobiographical, episodic, and semantic retrieval. J Cogn Neurosci. 2007;19(9):1520–34.

68. Fischer S, et al. Motor memory consolidation in sleep shapes more effective neuronal representations. J Neurosci. 2005;25(49):11248–55.

69. Brashers-Krug T, Shadmehr R, Bizzi E. Consolidation in human motor memory. Nature. 1996;382(6588):252–5.

70. Wixted JT. On common ground: Jost's (1897) law of forgetting and Ribot's (1881) law of retrograde amnesia. Psychol Rev. 2004;111(4):864–79.

71. Wixted JT, Carpenter SK. The Wickelgren power law and the Ebbinghaus savings function. Psychol Sci. 2007;18(2):133–4.

72. Pryor KO, et al. Visual P2-N2 complex and arousal at the time of encoding predict the time domain characteristics of amnesia for multiple intravenous anesthetic drugs in humans. Anesthesiology. 2010;113(2):313–26.

73. Kapur S, et al. Neuroanatomical correlates of encoding in episodic memory: levels of processing effect. Proc Natl Acad Sci U S A. 1994;91(6):2008–11.

74. Craik FIM, Lockhart RS. Levels of processing—framework for memory research. J Verbal Learn Verbal Behav. 1972;11(6):671–84.

75. Dehaene S, et al. Imaging unconscious semantic priming. Nature. 1998;395(6702):597–600.

76. Elfman KW, Yonelinas AP. Recollection and familiarity exhibit dissociable similarity gradients: a test of the complementary learning systems model. J Cogn Neurosci. 2014;1–17.

77. Murray MM, Foxe JJ, Wylie GR. The brain uses single-trial multisensory memories to discriminate without awareness. Neuroimage. 2005;27(2):473–8.

78. Busse L, et al. The spread of attention across modalities and space in a multisensory object. Proc Natl Acad Sci U S A. 2005;102(51):18751–6.

79. Shtyrov Y, Hauk O, Pulvermuller F. Distributed neuronal networks for encoding category-specific semantic information:

the mismatch negativity to action words. Eur J Neurosci. 2004;19 (4):1083–92.

80. Picton TW, et al. Mismatch negativity: different water in the same river. Audiol Neurootol. 2000;5(3–4):111–39.

81. Näätänen R. Attention and brain function. Hillsdale, NJ: L. Erlbaum; 1992. p. 494.

82. Pryor KO, et al. Effect of propofol on the medial temporal lobe emotional memory system: a functional magnetic resonance imaging study in human subjects. Br J Anaesth. 2015;115 Suppl 1: i104–13.

83. Pryor KO, et al. Enhanced visual memory effect for negative versus positive emotional content is potentiated at sub-anaesthetic concentrations of thiopental. Br J Anaesth. 2004;93(3):348–55.

84. Henson RN, Gagnepain P. Predictive, interactive multiple memory systems. Hippocampus. 2010;20(11):1315–26.

85. Shimamura AP. Hierarchical relational binding in the medial temporal lobe: the strong get stronger. Hippocampus. 2010;20 (11):1206–16.

86. Cowell RA, Bussey TJ, Saksida LM. Components of recognition memory: dissociable cognitive processes or just differences in representational complexity? Hippocampus. 2010;20 (11):1245–62.

87. Eichenbaum H. Time cells in the hippocampus: a new dimension for mapping memories. Nat Rev Neurosci. 2014;15(11):732–44.

88. Rose M, Haider H, Buchel C. The emergence of explicit memory during learning. Cereb Cortex. 2010;20(12):2787–97.

89. Veselis RA, et al. Propofol and midazolam inhibit conscious memory processes very soon after encoding: an event-related potential study of familiarity and recollection in volunteers. Anesthesiology. 2009;110(2):295–312.

90. Rugg MD, Yonelinas AP. Human recognition memory: a cognitive neuroscience perspective. Trends Cogn Sci. 2003;7(7):313–9.

91. Wais PE, Mickes L, Wixted JT. Remember/know judgments probe degrees of recollection. J Cogn Neurosci. 2008;20 (3):400–5.

92. Stratmann G, et al. Effect of general anesthesia in infancy on long-term recognition memory in humans and rats. Neuropsychopharmacology. 2014;39(10):2275–87.

93. Eichenbaum H. Remember that? Or does it just seem familiar? A sophisticated test for assessing memory in humans and animals reveals a specific cognitive impairment following general anesthesia in infancy. Neuropsychopharmacology. 2014;39(10):2273–4.

94. Hemmings HC, Jevtovic-Todorovic V. Special issue on anaesthetic neurotoxicity and neuroplasticity. Br J Anaesth. 2013;110 Suppl 1:i1–2.

95. Yonelinas AP. Receiver-operating characteristics in recognition memory: evidence for a dual-process model. J Exp Psychol Learn Mem Cogn. 1994;20(6):1341–54.

96. Yonelinas AP, et al. Signal-detection, threshold, and dual-process models of recognition memory: ROCs and conscious recollection. Conscious Cogn. 1996;5(4):418–41.

97. Wixted JT. Dual-process theory and signal-detection theory of recognition memory. Psychol Rev. 2007;114(1):152–76.

98. Sauvage MM, et al. Recognition memory: opposite effects of hippocampal damage on recollection and familiarity. Nat Neurosci. 2008;11(1):16–8.

99. Wais PE, et al. The hippocampus supports both the recollection and the familiarity components of recognition memory. Neuron. 2006;49(3):459–66.

100. Yonelinas AP, et al. Recollection and familiarity deficits in amnesia: convergence of remember-know, process dissociation, and receiver operating characteristic data. Neuropsychology. 1998;12 (3):323–39.

101. Duzel E, et al. Brain activity evidence for recognition without recollection after early hippocampal damage. Proc Natl Acad Sci U S A. 2001;98(14):8101–6.

102. Kahn I, Davachi L, Wagner AD. Functional-neuroanatomic correlates of recollection: implications for models of recognition memory. J Neurosci. 2004;24(17):4172–80.

103. Yonelinas AP, et al. Separating the brain regions involved in recollection and familiarity in recognition memory. J Neurosci. 2005;25(11):3002–8.

104. Curran T, et al. Combined pharmacological and electrophysiological dissociation of familiarity and recollection. J Neurosci. 2006;26(7):1979–85.

105. Daselaar SM, Fleck MS, Cabeza R. Triple dissociation in the medial temporal lobes: recollection, familiarity, and novelty. J Neurophysiol. 2006;96(4):1902–11.

106. Curran T, Cleary AM. Using ERPs to dissociate recollection from familiarity in picture recognition. Brain Res Cogn Brain Res. 2003;15(2):191–205.

107. Opitz B, Cornell S. Contribution of familiarity and recollection to associative recognition memory: insights from event-related potentials. J Cogn Neurosci. 2006;18(9):1595–605.

108. MacKenzie G, Donaldson DI. Dissociating recollection from familiarity: electrophysiological evidence that familiarity for faces is associated with a posterior old/new effect. Neuroimage. 2007;36(2):454–63.

109. Warren-Gash C, Zeman A. Is there anything distinctive about epileptic deja vu? J Neurol Neurosurg Psychiatry. 2014;85 (2):143–7.

110. O'Connor AR, Moulin CJ. Deja vu experiences in healthy subjects are unrelated to laboratory tests of recollection and familiarity for word stimuli. Front Psychol. 2013;4:881.

111. Malecki M. Familiarity transfer as an explanation of the deja vu effect. Psychol Rep. 2015;116(3):955–82.

112. Bartolomei F, et al. Cortical stimulation study of the role of rhinal cortex in deja vu and reminiscence of memories. Neurology. 2004;63(5):858–64.

113. Fuentealba P, Steriade M. The reticular nucleus revisited: intrinsic and network properties of a thalamic pacemaker. Prog Neurobiol. 2005;75(2):125–41.

114. Rempel-Clower NL, et al. Three cases of enduring memory impairment after bilateral damage limited to the hippocampal formation. J Neurosci. 1996;16(16):5233–55.

115. Corkin S. What's new with the amnesic patient H.M.? Nat Rev Neurosci. 2002;3(2):153–60.

116. Varela F, et al. The brainweb: phase synchronization and large-scale integration. Nat Rev Neurosci. 2001;2(4):229–39.

117. Dehaene S, et al. Conscious, preconscious, and subliminal processing: a testable taxonomy. Trends Cogn Sci. 2006;10 (5):204–11.

118. Buzsaki G. Theta oscillations in the hippocampus. Neuron. 2002;33(3):325–40.

119. Buzsaki G, Draguhn A. Neuronal oscillations in cortical networks. Science. 2004;304(5679):1926–9.

120. Fell J, et al. Rhinal-hippocampal theta coherence during declarative memory formation: interaction with gamma synchronization? Eur J Neurosci. 2003;17(5):1082–8.

121. Mormann F, et al. Phase/amplitude reset and theta-gamma interaction in the human medial temporal lobe during a continuous word recognition memory task. Hippocampus. 2005;15 (7):890–900.

122. Canolty RT, et al. High gamma power is phase-locked to theta oscillations in human neocortex. Science. 2006;313 (5793):1626–8.

123. Osipova D, et al. Theta and gamma oscillations predict encoding and retrieval of declarative memory. J Neurosci. 2006;26 (28):7523–31.

124. Nyhus E, Curran T. Functional role of gamma and theta oscillations in episodic memory. Neurosci Biobehav Rev. 2010;34(7):1023–35.

125. Lega B, et al. Slow-theta-to-gamma phase-amplitude coupling in human hippocampus supports the formation of new episodic memories. Cereb Cortex. 2014;26:268–78.
126. Roux F, Uhlhaas PJ. Working memory and neural oscillations: alpha-gamma versus theta-gamma codes for distinct WM information? Trends Cogn Sci. 2014;18(1):16–25.
127. Perouansky M, et al. Slowing of the hippocampal theta rhythm correlates with anesthetic-induced amnesia. Anesthesiology. 2010;113(6):1299–309.
128. La Vaque TJ. The history of EEG Hans Berger. J Neurother. 1999;3(2):1–9.
129. Knoblauch V, et al. Homeostatic control of slow-wave and spindle frequency activity during human sleep: effect of differential sleep pressure and brain topography. Cereb Cortex. 2002;12 (10):1092–100.
130. Baker PM, et al. Disruption of coherent oscillations in inhibitory networks with anesthetics: role of GABA(A) receptor desensitization. J Neurophysiol. 2002;88(5):2821–33.
131. Caraiscos VB, et al. Tonic inhibition in mouse hippocampal CA1 pyramidal neurons is mediated by alpha5 subunit-containing gamma-aminobutyric acid type A receptors. Proc Natl Acad Sci U S A. 2004;101(10):3662–7.
132. Cheng VY, et al. {alpha}5GABAA receptors mediate the amnestic but not sedative-hypnotic effects of the general anesthetic etomidate. J Neurosci. 2006;26(14):3713–20.
133. Saab BJ, et al. Short-term memory impairment after isoflurane in mice is prevented by the alpha5 gamma-aminobutyric acid type A receptor inverse agonist L-655,708. Anesthesiology. 2010;113 (5):1061–71.
134. Lecker I, et al. Potentiation of GABAA receptor activity by volatile anaesthetics is reduced by α5GABAA receptor-preferring inverse agonists. Br J Anaesth. 2013;110 Suppl 1:i73–81.
135. Banks MI, White JA, Pearce RA. Interactions between distinct GABA(A) circuits in hippocampus. Neuron. 2000;25(2):449–57.
136. White JA, et al. Networks of interneurons with fast and slow gamma-aminobutyric acid type A (GABAA) kinetics provide substrate for mixed gamma-theta rhythm. Proc Natl Acad Sci U S A. 2000;97(14):8128–33.
137. Benkwitz C, Banks MI, Pearce RA. Influence of GABAA receptor gamma2 splice variants on receptor kinetics and isoflurane modulation. Anesthesiology. 2004;101(4):924–36.
138. Verbny YI, Merriam EB, Banks MI. Modulation of gamma-aminobutyric acid type A receptor-mediated spontaneous inhibitory postsynaptic currents in auditory cortex by midazolam and isoflurane. Anesthesiology. 2005;102(5):962–9.
139. Burlingame RH, et al. Subhypnotic doses of isoflurane impair auditory discrimination in rats. Anesthesiology. 2007;106(4):754–62.
140. Baddeley AD. Working memory. Science. 1992;255:556–9.
141. Baddeley A. The fractionation of working memory. Proc Natl Acad Sci U S A. 1996;93(24):13468–72.
142. Blumenfeld RS, Ranganath C. Dorsolateral prefrontal cortex promotes long-term memory formation through its role in working memory organization. J Neurosci. 2006;26(3):916–25.
143. Ranganath C, Cohen MX, Brozinsky CJ. Working memory maintenance contributes to long-term memory formation: neural and behavioral evidence. J Cogn Neurosci. 2005;17(7):994–1010.
144. Wager TD, Smith EE. Neuroimaging studies of working memory: a meta-analysis. Cogn Affect Behav Neurosci. 2003;3(4):255–74.
145. Muller NG, Machado L, Knight RT. Contributions of subregions of the prefrontal cortex to working memory: evidence from brain lesions in humans. J Cogn Neurosci. 2002;14(5):673–86.
146. Ward LM. Synchronous neural oscillations and cognitive processes. Trends Cogn Sci. 2003;7(12):553–9.
147. Jensen O, Lisman JE. Hippocampal sequence-encoding driven by a cortical multi-item working memory buffer. Trends Neurosci. 2005;28(2):67–72.
148. Chakrabarti BK, Basu A. Neural network modeling. Prog Brain Res. 2008;168:155–68.
149. Veselis RA, Reinsel R, Wronski M. Analytical methods to differentiate similar electroencephalographic spectra: neural network and discriminant analysis. J Clin Monit. 1993;9(4):257–67.
150. Veselis RA, et al. Use of neural network analysis to classify electroencephalographic patterns against depth of midazolam sedation in intensive care unit patients. J Clin Monit. 1991;7(3):259–67.
151. Kloppel B. Application of neural networks for EEG analysis. Considerations and first results. Neuropsychobiology. 1994;29 (1):39–46.
152. Kloppel B. Neural networks as a new method for EEG analysis. A basic introduction. Neuropsychobiology. 1994;29(1):33–8.
153. Kasabov NK. NeuCube: a spiking neural network architecture for mapping, learning and understanding of spatio-temporal brain data. Neural Netw. 2014;52:62–76.
154. Gulyas A, et al. Navigable networks as Nash equilibria of navigation games. Nat Commun. 2015;6:7651.
155. Duvernoy HM, Bourgouin P. The human hippocampus: functional anatomy, vascularization and serial sections with MRI. 2nd completely rev. and expanded ed. Berlin and New York: Springer; 1998. p. viii, 213.
156. Lisman JE. Hippocampus, II: memory connections. Am J Psychiatry. 2005;162(2):239.
157. Wixted JT, et al. Sparse and distributed coding of episodic memory in neurons of the human hippocampus. Proc Natl Acad Sci U S A. 2014;111(26):9621–6.
158. Rolls ET. A computational theory of episodic memory formation in the hippocampus. Behav Brain Res. 2010;215(2):180–96.
159. Elfman KW, Aly M, Yonelinas AP. Neurocomputational account of memory and perception: thresholded and graded signals in the hippocampus. Hippocampus. 2014;24(12):1672–86.
160. O'Keefe J, Dostrovsky J. The hippocampus as a spatial map. Preliminary evidence from unit activity in the freely-moving rat. Brain Res. 1971;34(1):171–5.
161. O'Keefe J. Hippocampus, theta, and spatial memory. Curr Opin Neurobiol. 1993;3(6):917–24.
162. Samsonovich AV, Ascoli GA. A simple neural network model of the hippocampus suggesting its pathfinding role in episodic memory retrieval. Learn Mem. 2005;12:193–208.
163. Shanks DR, et al. Priming intelligent behavior: an elusive phenomenon. PLoS One. 2013;8(4), e56515.
164. Newell BR, Shanks DR. Unconscious influences on decision making: a critical review. Behav Brain Sci. 2014;37(1):1–19.
165. Bullock A. The secret sales pitch: an overview of subliminal advertising. San Jose, CA: Norwich Publishers; 2004. 272 p.
166. Ioannidis JP. Why most published research findings are false. PLoS Med. 2005;2(8), e124.
167. Johnson VE. Revised standards for statistical evidence. Proc Natl Acad Sci U S A. 2013;110(48):19313–7.
168. Avidan MS, Wildes TS. Power of negative thinking. Br J Anaesth. 2015;114(1):3–5.
169. Yong E. Replication studies: bad copy. Nature. 2012;485 (7398):298–300.
170. Lequeux P-Y, Hecquet F, Bredas P. Does anesthetic regimen influence implicit memory during general anesthesia? Anesth Analg. 2014;119(5):1174–9. doi:10.1213/ANE.0000000000000162.
171. Hadzidiakos D, et al. Analysis of memory formation during general anesthesia (propofol/remifentanil) for elective surgery using the process-dissociation procedure. Anesthesiology. 2009;111 (2):293–301.
172. Nadel L, Hardt O. Update on memory systems and processes. Neuropsychopharmacology. 2011;36(1):251–73.
173. Berns GS, Cohen JD, Mintun MA. Brain regions responsive to novelty in the absence of awareness. Science. 1997;276 (5316):1272–5.

174. Andrade J. Learning during anaesthesia: a review. Br J Psychol. 1995;86(Pt 4):479–506.

175. Ghoneim MM, Block RI. Learning and memory during general anesthesia. Anesthesiology. 1997;87(2):387–410.

176. Genzel L, et al. Light sleep versus slow wave sleep in memory consolidation: a question of global versus local processes? Trends Neurosci. 2014;37(1):10–9.

177. Marshall L, Born J. The contribution of sleep to hippocampus-dependent memory consolidation. Trends Cogn Sci. 2007;11 (10):442–50.

178. Gais S, Born J. Declarative memory consolidation: mechanisms acting during human sleep. Learn Mem. 2004;11(6):679–85.

179. Uncapher MR, Rugg MD. Effects of divided attention on fMRI correlates of memory encoding. J Cogn Neurosci. 2005;17 (12):1923–35.

180. Naveh-Benjamin M, Guez J, Marom M. The effects of divided attention at encoding on item and associative memory. Mem Cognit. 2003;31(7):1021–35.

181. Iidaka T, et al. The effect of divided attention on encoding and retrieval in episodic memory revealed by positron emission tomography. J Cogn Neurosci. 2000;12(2):267–80.

182. Anderson ND, et al. The effects of divided attention on encoding- and retrieval-related brain activity: a PET study of younger and older adults. J Cogn Neurosci. 2000;12(5):775–92.

183. Coull JT. Neural correlates of attention and arousal: insights from electrophysiology, functional neuroimaging and psychopharmacology. Prog Neurobiol. 1998;55(4):343–61.

184. Gardiner JM, Parkin AJ. Attention and recollective experience in recognition memory. Mem Cognit. 1990;18(6):579–83.

185. Veselis RA, et al. Information loss over time defines the memory defect of propofol: a comparative response with thiopental and dexmedetomidine. Anesthesiology. 2004;101(4):831–41.

186. Nelson LE, et al. The alpha2-adrenoceptor agonist dexmedetomidine converges on an endogenous sleep-promoting pathway to exert its sedative effects. Anesthesiology. 2003;98 (2):428–36.

187. Nelson LE, et al. The sedative component of anesthesia is mediated by GABA(A) receptors in an endogenous sleep pathway. Nat Neurosci. 2002;5(10):979–84.

188. Gelegen C, et al. Staying awake—a genetic region that hinders α2 adrenergic receptor agonist-induced sleep. Eur J Neurosci. 2014;40:2311–9.

189. Franks NP. General anaesthesia: from molecular targets to neuronal pathways of sleep and arousal. Nat Rev Neurosci. 2008;9 (5):370–86.

190. Friedman EB, et al. A conserved behavioral state barrier impedes transitions between anesthetic-induced unconsciousness and wakefulness: evidence for neural inertia. PLoS One. 2010;5(7), e11903.

191. Kelz MB, et al. An essential role for orexins in emergence from general anesthesia. Proc Natl Acad Sci U S A. 2008;105 (4):1309–14.

192. Veselis RA, et al. The comparative amnestic effects of midazolam, propofol, thiopental, and fentanyl at equisedative concentrations. Anesthesiology. 1997;87(4):749–64.

193. Ghoneim MM, Hinrichs JV. Drugs, memory and sedation: specificity of effects. Anesthesiology. 1997;87(Oct):734–6.

194. Schwartz RH, Milteer R, LeBeau MA. Drug-facilitated sexual assault ('date rape'). South Med J. 2000;93(6):558–61.

195. Kim M, Kim J, Kwon JS. The effect of immediate and delayed word repetition on event-related potential in a continuous recognition task. Brain Res Cogn Brain Res. 2001;11(3):387–96.

196. Friedman D. ERPs during continuous recognition memory for words. Biol Psychol. 1990;30:61–87.

197. Ghoneim MM, Block RI. Immediate peri-operative memory. Acta Anaesthesiol Scand. 2007;51(8):1054–61.

198. Fandakova Y, et al. Age differences in short-term memory binding are related to working memory performance across the lifespan. Psychol Aging. 2014;29(1):140–9.

199. Datta D, Arion D, Lewis DA. Developmental expression patterns of GABAA receptor subunits in layer 3 and 5 pyramidal cells of monkey prefrontal cortex. Cereb Cortex. 2015;25(8):2295–305.

200. Mashour GA, Avidan MS. Intraoperative awareness: controversies and non-controversies. Br J Anaesth. 2015;115 Suppl 1:i20–6.

201. Glannon W. Anaesthesia, amnesia and harm. J Med Ethics. 2014;40:651–7.

202. Pandit JJ, Russell IF, Wang M. Interpretations of responses using the isolated forearm technique in general anaesthesia: a debate. Br J Anaesth. 2015;115 Suppl 1:i32–45.

203. Kent CD, et al. Psychological impact of unexpected explicit recall of events occurring during surgery performed under sedation, regional anaesthesia, and general anaesthesia: data from the Anesthesia Awareness Registry. Br J Anaesth. 2013;110(3):381–7.

204. Whitlock EL, et al. Psychological sequelae of surgery in a prospective cohort of patients from three intraoperative awareness prevention trials. Anesth Analg. 2015;120(1):87–95.

205. Samuelsson P, Brudin L, Sandin RH. Late psychological symptoms after awareness among consecutively included surgical patients. Anesthesiology. 2007;106(1):26–32.

206. Sandin R. Outcome after awareness with explicit recall. Acta Anaesthesiol Belg. 2006;57(4):429–32.

207. Pollard RJ, et al. Intraoperative awareness in a regional medical system: a review of 3 years' data. Anesthesiology. 2007;106 (2):269–74.

208. Cook TM, et al. 5th National Audit Project (NAP5) on accidental awareness during general anaesthesia: patient experiences, human factors, sedation, consent, and medicolegal issues. Br J Anaesth. 2014;113(4):560–74.

209. Alkire MT, Nathan SV, McReynolds JR. Memory enhancing effect of low-dose sevoflurane does not occur in basolateral amygdala-lesioned rats. Anesthesiology. 2005;103(6):1167–73.

210. Starmer AJ, et al. Changes in medical errors after implementation of a handoff program. N Engl J Med. 2014;371(19):1803–12.

211. Colligan L, Brick D, Patterson ES. Changes in medical errors with a handoff program. N Engl J Med. 2015;372(5):490–1.

212. Cheek DB. Unconscious perception of meaningful sounds during surgical anesthesia as revealed under hypnosis. Am J Clin Hypn. 1959;1(3):101–13.

213. Levinson BW. States of awareness during anaesthesia: preliminary communication. Br J Anaesth. 1965;37(7):544–6.

214. Lubke GH, et al. Dependence of explicit and implicit memory on hypnotic state in trauma patients. Anesthesiology. 1999;90 (3):670–80.

215. Lubke GH, et al. Memory formation during general anesthesia for emergency cesarean sections. Anesthesiology. 2000;92 (4):1029–34.

216. Kerssens C, et al. Memory function during propofol and alfentanil anesthesia: predictive value of individual differences. Anesthesiology. 2002;97(2):382–9.

217. Kerssens C, Gaither JR, Sebel PS. Preserved memory function during bispectral index-guided anesthesia with sevoflurane for major orthopedic surgery. Anesthesiology. 2009;111(3):518–24. doi:10.1097/ALN.0b013e3181b05f0b.

218. Kerssens C, Ouchi T, Sebel PS. No evidence of memory function during anesthesia with propofol or isoflurane with close control of hypnotic state. Anesthesiology. 2005;102(1):57–62.

219. Deeprose C, et al. Unconscious learning during surgery with propofol anaesthesia. Br J Anaesth. 2004;92(2):171–7.

220. Deeprose C, et al. Unconscious auditory priming during surgery with propofol and nitrous oxide anaesthesia: a replication. Br J Anaesth. 2005;94(1):57–62.

221. Franco A, Malhotra N, Simonovits G. Social science. Publication bias in the social sciences: unlocking the file drawer. Science. 2014;345(6203):1502–5.

222. Munte S, et al. Increased reading speed for stories presented during general anesthesia. Anesthesiology. 1999;90(3):662–9.

223. Jacoby LL. A process dissociation framework: separating automatic from intentional uses of memory. J Mem Lang. 1991;33 (1):1–18.

224. Veselis RA. Memory formation during anaesthesia: plausibility of a neurophysiological basis. Br J Anaesth. 2015;115 Suppl 1:i13–9.

225. Mashour GA, Alkire MT. Consciousness, anesthesia, and the thalamocortical system. Anesthesiology. 2013;118(1):13–5. doi:10.1097/ALN.0b013e318277a9c6.

226. Mashour GA. Dreaming during anesthesia and sedation. Anesth Analg. 2011;112(5):1008–10.

227. DiFrancesco MW, et al. BOLD fMRI in infants under sedation: Comparing the impact of pentobarbital and propofol on auditory and language activation. J Magn Reson Imaging. 2013;38 (5):1184–95.

228. Plourde G, et al. Attenuation of the 40-hertz auditory steady state response by propofol involves the cortical and subcortical generators. Anesthesiology. 2008;108(2):233–42.

229. Veselis R, et al. Auditory rCBF covariation with word rate during drug-induced sedation and unresponsiveness: a H2015 PET study. Brain Cogn. 2004;54(2):142–4.

230. Heinke W, et al. Sequential effects of propofol on functional brain activation induced by auditory language processing: an event-related functional magnetic resonance imaging study. Br J Anaesth. 2004;92(5):641–50.

231. Gonano C, et al. Effect of earplugs on propofol requirement and awareness with recall during spinal anesthesia. Minerva Anestesiol. 2010;76(7):504–8.

232. Liu X, et al. Differential effects of deep sedation with propofol on the specific and nonspecific thalamocortical systems: a functional magnetic resonance imaging study. Anesthesiology. 2013;118 (1):59–69. doi:10.1097/ALN.0b013e318277a801.

233. Hudetz AG. General anesthesia and human brain connectivity. Brain Connect. 2012;2(6):291–302.

234. Boveroux P, et al. Breakdown of within- and between-network resting state functional magnetic resonance imaging connectivity during propofol-induced loss of consciousness. Anesthesiology. 2010;113(5):1038–53.

235. Lopez-Aranda MF, et al. Role of layer 6 of V2 visual cortex in object-recognition memory. Science. 2009;325(5936):87–9.

236. Chen X, et al. Encoding and retrieval of artificial visuoauditory memory traces in the auditory cortex requires the entorhinal cortex. J Neurosci. 2013;33(24):9963–74.

237. Baker R, et al. Altered activity in the central medial thalamus precedes changes in the neocortex during transitions into both sleep and propofol anesthesia. J Neurosci. 2014;34(40):13326–35.

238. John ER, Prichep LS. The anesthetic cascade: a theory of how anesthesia suppresses consciousness. Anesthesiology. 2005;102 (2):447–71.

239. John ER, et al. Invariant reversible qEEG effects of anesthetics. Conscious Cogn. 2001;10(2):165–83.

240. Liu X, et al. Propofol disrupts functional interactions between sensory and high-order processing of auditory verbal memory. Hum Brain Mapp. 2012;33(10):2487–98.

241. Hudetz AG, Pearce R. Suppressing the mind: anesthetic modulation of memory and consciousness. Contemporary clinical neuroscience. Totowa, NJ: Humana; 2010. p. x, 252.

242. Hudetz AG, Vizuete JA, Imas OA. Desflurane selectively suppresses long-latency cortical neuronal response to flash in the rat. Anesthesiology. 2009;111(2):231–9. doi:10.1097/ALN.0b013e3181ab671e.

243. Alkire MT, Hudetz AG, Tononi G. Consciousness and anesthesia. Science. 2008;322(5903):876–80.

244. Imas OA, et al. Isoflurane disrupts anterio-posterior phase synchronization of flash-induced field potentials in the rat. Neurosci Lett. 2006;402(3):216–21.

245. Blain-Moraes S, et al. Neurophysiological correlates of sevoflurane-induced unconsciousness. Anesthesiology. 2014;122:307–16.

246. Lee U, et al. Dissociable network properties of anesthetic state transitions. Anesthesiology. 2011;114(4):872–81.

247. Monti MM, et al. Dynamic change of global and local information processing in propofol-induced loss and recovery of consciousness. PLoS Comput Biol. 2013;9(10), e1003271.

248. Sessler DI, et al. Hospital stay and mortality are increased in patients having a "triple low" of low blood pressure, low bispectral index, and low minimum alveolar concentration of volatile anesthesia. Anesthesiology. 2012;116(6):1195–203.

249. Myles PS. Untangling the triple low: causal inference in anesthesia research. Anesthesiology. 2014;121(1):1–3.

250. Kertai MD, White WD, Gan TJ. Cumulative duration of "triple low" state of low blood pressure, low bispectral index, and low minimum alveolar concentration of volatile anesthesia is not associated with increased mortality. Anesthesiology. 2014;121(1):18–28.

251. Monk TG, et al. Predictors of cognitive dysfunction after major noncardiac surgery. Anesthesiology. 2008;108(1):18–30.

252. Rappaport BA, et al. Anesthetic neurotoxicity—clinical implications of animal models. N Engl J Med. 2015;372(9):796–7.

253. Riker RR, et al. Dexmedetomidine vs midazolam for sedation of critically ill patients: a randomized trial. JAMA. 2009;301(5):489–99.

254. MacLaren R, et al. A randomized, double-blind pilot study of dexmedetomidine versus midazolam for intensive care unit sedation: patient recall of their experiences and short-term psychological outcomes. J Intensive Care Med. 2015;30(3):167–75.

255. Hudetz JA, et al. Ketamine attenuates delirium after cardiac surgery with cardiopulmonary bypass. J Cardiothorac Vasc Anesth. 2009;23(5):651–7.

Consciousness and Anesthesia

4

Ram Adapa

There is as yet no generalised theory of anaesthesia. This lack of understanding of the mechanisms underpinning general anaesthesia is partly due to a lack of convergence of the various methodologies employed to explore these. However, this gap is also fundamentally due to the absence of a universally accepted definition of consciousness. Cognitive neuroscience has seen a relatively recent resurgence of interest in the study of consciousness that has successfully brought together sleep and anaesthesia research in an attempt to address this deficiency. Investigations into the neurophysiological mechanisms of consciousness and of general anaesthesia mutually inform each other. Sleep shares behavioural phenotypes with the state of anaesthesia but critically differs in arousal by external stimuli and the rhythmic cycling between different stages. Exploring the relationship of general anaesthesia to sleep has provided substantial insights into the mechanisms of anaesthesia. Basic science, animal and lesion studies over the past several decades provide ample evidence for the fact that anaesthesia and sleep affect key neurochemical circuits in the brainstem, the basal forebrain, the thalamus and the cortex. However, as yet unanswered is the hierarchical organisation in these systems and how disparate pharmacological and pathological entities generate a comparable behavioural state of unconsciousness and unresponsiveness. This chapter will aim to bring together an overview of the current knowledge and recent evidence surrounding the neural, chemical and network substrates underlying consciousness and two common conditions of altered states of consciousness (sleep and anaesthesia).

Brainstem: Basal Forebrain Circuits, Sleep and Anaesthesia

Several brainstem structures have now been well characterised for controlling global sleep states (Fig. 4.1). It is thought that wakefulness is maintained by the action of a collection of cholinergic and monoaminergic nuclei on higher structures [2]. These are now recognised as distinct nuclei found within Moruzzi and Magoun's historical reticular formation [3]. They include the serotonergic dorsal raphe nucleus (DR), the histaminergic tuberomammillary nucleus (TMN), the cholinergic laterodorsal tegmental (LDT) nucleus and the noradrenergic locus coeruleus (LC). These wakefulness promoting nuclei have reciprocal inhibitory connections to the sleep-promoting nuclei, exemplified by the ventrolateral preoptic nucleus (VLPO) of the hypothalamus [2]. The activity in 'wake-promoting' and 'sleep-promoting' nuclei alters depending on level of consciousness [4]. These nuclei have mutually inhibitory projections that produce the necessary conditions for a subcortical 'flip-flop' wake-sleep switch, which can cause rapid transitions between conscious states [2]. Several anaesthetic drugs alter activity in these nuclei at concentrations used clinically to induce anaesthesia [5].

Natural sleep cycles through several stages of non-rapid eye movement (NREM) sleep, switching into rapid eye movement (REM) sleep associated with vivid dreaming. These switches occur several times, with increasing REM sleep periods before the transition to consciousness. A similar mutual inhibition model has been proposed to understand the neural mechanisms underlying REM sleep, the 'REM flip-flop switch'. This consists of mutually inhibitory REM-off and REM-on areas in the mesopontine tegmentum [6]. The REM-on neurons in the pedunculopontine tegmental (PPT) nucleus and the laterodorsal tegmental (LDT) neurons trigger cortical desynchronisation via the thalamus. REM-off neurons (in the LC and raphe) become inactive during REM sleep and inhibit REM-on neurons to terminate

R. Adapa, MBBS, MD, FRCA, PhD (✉)
Department of Anaesthesia, Cambridge University Hospitals NHS
Foundation Trust, Hills Road, Cambridge CB2 0QQ, UK
e-mail: ra342@cam.ac.uk

© Springer International Publishing AG 2017
A.R. Absalom, K.P. Mason (eds.), *Total Intravenous Anesthesia and Target Controlled Infusions*,
DOI 10.1007/978-3-319-47609-4_4

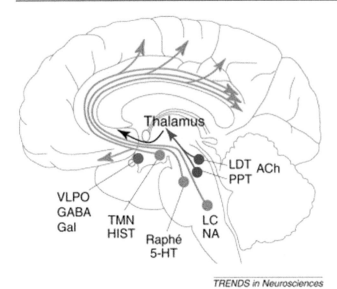

Fig. 4.1 The ascending arousal system sends projections from the brainstem and posterior hypothalamus throughout the forebrain. Neurons of the laterodorsal tegmental nuclei and pedunculopontine tegmental nuclei (LDT and PPT) (*blue circles*) send cholinergic fibres (Ach) to many forebrain targets, including the thalamus, which then regulate cortical activity. Aminergic nuclei (*green circles*) diffusely project throughout much of the forebrain, regulating the activity of cortical and hypothalamic targets directly. Neurons of the tuberomammillary nucleus (TMN) contain histamine (HIST), neurons of the raphe nuclei contain 5-HT and neurons of the locus coeruleus (LC) contain noradrenaline (NA). Sleep-promoting neurons of the ventrolateral preoptic nucleus (VLPO, *red circle*) contain GABA (Reproduced from Saper et al. [1] with permission from Elsevier)

REM sleep. REM sleep may therefore be initiated either by direct excitation of REM-on neurons or by inhibition of REM-off neurons.

The importance of these regions in induction of anaesthesia is evident from microinjection studies where injection of propofol or barbiturates into the medial preoptic area results in potentiation of a natural sleep-like state. Injection of GABA-A agonists into the TMN in rats also causes sedation and hypnosis, and this effect is reversed with GABA-A antagonist injection [7]. Histaminergic neurons in the TMN are also modulated by isoflurane [8] and by propofol through inhibition of histamine release from the TMN [7].

The role of other neurotransmitters such as noradrenaline and acetylcholine in the regulation of the sleep-wake cycle is also important in understanding the effects of commonly used sedative and anaesthetic agents (Table 4.1). For example, dexmedetomidine-induced sedation closely resembles NREM sleep, and this may be the result of inhibition of noradrenaline release from the LC [9]. Reduced inhibitory LC activity on the VLPO in turn increases the inhibitory activity of the VLPO on the ascending arousal circuits. Noradrenergic inhibition in the LC may contribute to anaesthetic-induced unconsciousness; mutant mice lacking

dopamine-B-hydroxylase (which is required to synthesise norepinephrine in the locus coeruleus) have been shown to be more sensitive to anaesthetics [10]. Propofol has been recently demonstrated to be dependent on GABA-A release from the VLPO projections to the LC to cause sedation in rats [11]. Similarly, inhibition of cholinergic activity inhibits sleep-promoting activity in brainstem regions including the LDT, and the sedative effect of opioids may be due to the subsequent reduced acetylcholine release [12]. Conversely, physostigmine administration has been demonstrated to increase local acetylcholine concentrations and partially reverse propofol and inhalational anaesthesia [13, 14]. As such, anaesthesia has traditionally been thought to be mediated by direct activation of the GABA-A receptor in an endogenous sleep pathway [7].

The transition to unconsciousness with anaesthetic agents is unlikely to be mediated exclusively through arousal nuclei. For example, hypothalamic orexinergic neurons do not appear to play a role in anaesthetic-induced unconsciousness; rather, they modulate emergence from general anaesthesia [15]. Ketamine appears to activate the locus coeruleus in association with its hypnotic effects [16] and is dependent, in part, on noradrenergic neurotransmission [17].

Adenosine as a Mediator of Homeostatic Control

Prolonged periods of wakefulness and sleep deprivation are associated with a predisposition to sleep with alterations in sleep architecture, such as a compensatory rebound increase in REM sleep and an increase in extracellular ATP and adenosine [18]. It is postulated that this increase in extracellular adenosine accumulation during wakefulness inhibits LC activity that results in unopposed VLPO activity. Natural sleep can therefore reverse the behavioural and cognitive effects of sleep deprivation (in fact, it is thought this is the primary purpose of natural sleep [19]). In this regard, this aspect of LC-VLPO modulation is essential for the homeostatic regulation of sleep drive. Adenosine receptor antagonists (caffeine) can therefore reduce the rebound of sleep that occurs following sleep deprivation, and also the potentiating effect of sleep deprivation on anaesthesia. Interestingly, sleep drive following propofol anaesthesia is also reduced due to alteration in extracellular adenosine concentration (see below).

Arousal from Sleep and Anaesthesia

Arousal from sleep is mediated through complex interactions of the brainstem and subcortical nuclei (see above). Of primary importance is the role of noradrenergic transmission and LC activity [20]. Similarly, emergence

Table 4.1 Neuronal system activity during anaesthesia and sleep

Neuronal system activity during anaesthesia and sleep					
Neurotransmitter system	Propofol	Barbiturates	Ketamine	NREM sleep	REM sleep
GABA	● Major Potentiation	● Major Potentiation	◉ Minor Potentiation	◉ Minor Potentiation	◉ Minor Potentiation
Acetylcholine	◉ Minor Potentiation	● Major inhibition	● Major inhibition	● Major inhibition	◉ Minor Potentiation
Serotonin	○ No change	◉ Minor Potentiation	◉ Minor Potentiation	◉ Minor Potentiation	◉ Minor Potentiation
NMDA	◉ Minor Potentiation	○ No change	● Major inhibition	◉ Minor Potentiation	◉ Minor Potentiation
Norepinephrine	◉ Minor Potentiation	◉ Minor Potentiation	◉ Minor Potentiation	● Major inhibition	● Major inhibition

● Major Potentiation   ◉ Minor Potentiation   ● Major inhibition   ◉ Minor inhibition   ○ No change

from general anaesthesia occurs through modulation of histaminergic, cholinergic, dopaminergic and orexinergic/hypocertinergic systems considered important in arousal networks [15]. Similar to sleep, evidence is growing for the central role of LC and noradrenergic transmission in regulating arousal from anaesthesia. For example, Vazey et al. demonstrated that increased noradrenergic transmission from the LC alone is sufficient to facilitate emergence from isoflurane anaesthesia [21]. This may be of importance during concomitant administration of alpha-adrenoceptor antagonists. The importance of noradrenergic transmission in arousal mechanisms is further highlighted by the finding that methylphenidate, a potent inhibitor of dopamine and NE transporters, induces emergence during isoflurane or propofol anaesthesia [22].

Electrophysiological Correlates of Brainstem Activity

Surface recordings of EEG reflect cortical neuronal activity, and altered states of consciousness are reflected in characteristic EEG changes. However, it is well recognised that the generation and maintenance of cortical activity is modulated by brainstem and basal forebrain structures. Although there is no direct neurophysiological correlate of REM sleep during anaesthesia, basal forebrain cholinergic neurons (receiving excitatory projections from the brainstem,and innervating the cerebral cortex) have been demonstrated to be active during REM sleep [23]. Electrical discharge from these basal forebrain neurons correlates positively with EEG power of gamma (30–60 Hz) and theta (4–8 Hz) frequency

bands. The EEG characteristics of the excitatory phase of general anaesthesia resemble those of REM sleep and may therefore be modulated by similar neural structures as those involved in REM sleep [24].

Neuroimaging studies have revealed that the transition from wakefulness to slow-wave sleep is associated with widespread deactivation in the upper brainstem, thalamus and basal forebrain, which is consistent with the earlier discussion [25]. Anaesthesia studies in human volunteers also establish a functional disconnection in the ascending reticular system between the brain stem nuclei and the thalamus and the cortex [26, 27]. Our current understanding of the neuropharmacology of brainstem sleep networks has focused research themes for treatment strategies in disorders of consciousness. Pharmacological modulation of neurotransmitter pathways described above (dopaminergic-amantadine, L-DOPA, methylphenidate, apomorphine; serotonergic-selective reuptake inhibitors; GABA agonists-zolpidem) can be employed to objectively assess neurological outcome following traumatic brain injury [28, 29].

Thalamic Networks, Sleep and Anaesthesia

The role of the thalamus in the conscious state is indisputable—it mediates organised behaviour and processes (through connections with basal ganglia and other subcortical nuclei) and transmits sensorimotor information (as a critical relay station in the ascending pathways) to the rest of the brain. The thalamocortical system plays a central role in information integration in the brain, and multiple animal and human volunteer studies have enabled the anatomical and functional delineation of the projection pathways between the various thalamic nuclei and cortical structures. In particular, the two major divisions of the thalamus, the specific relay nuclei and the more diffusely projecting 'nonspecific' nuclei, may collaborate to accomplish this task, with the specific system responsible for the transmission and encoding of sensory and motor information and the nonspecific system engaged in the control of cortical arousal and temporal conjunction of information across distributed cortical areas.

The location of the thalamus is also fundamentally important to the regulation of sleep and wakefulness, permitting top-down (corticothalamic) and bottom-up (spinothalamic) processing and integration of neuronal signalling [30]. The transition between sleep stages may disrupt information flow through the thalamic nuclei, and in that sense, the thalamus may serve as a consciousness switch [31]. The interaction between the thalamus and the cortex during the various stages of sleep has been studied in detail—for example, onset of sleep and awakening from sleep are both associated with changes in thalamic and cortical activity. However, sleep onset is characterised by thalamic deactivation preceding that of the cortex by several minutes [32]. In contrast, emergence from sleep is associated with synchronised reactivation of both structures [33]. The presence of a still active cortex during onset of sleep probably explains both the production of parasomnia hallucinations and over reported sleep latency (estimation of time needed to fall asleep). As will be discussed later, anaesthesia studies have demonstrated that induction of anaesthesia is associated with cortical deactivation preceding thalamic deactivation. Analysis of the activation-deactivation pattern at cortical and thalamic levels demonstrates that this asynchrony persists throughout the sleep cycle. Thalamocortical activity may alternate between periods of coupling and decoupling during REM sleep and stage 2 NREM sleep [34].

Given its location and critical functions related to arousal, damage to the thalamus often results in significant and life-threatening functional deficits and a reduced arousal state. The converse may be true—electrical stimulation of central thalamic nuclei in a patient in minimally conscious state (MCS) has been shown to temporarily reverse some of the behavioural deficits and improve cognitively mediated behaviour [35]. It is therefore unsurprising that such a vital subcortical structure has long been recognised to be fundamentally important to general anaesthetic mechanisms in the brain. The two major thalamic divisions, the specific versus nonspecific (medial and intralaminar nuclei) nuclei, show differential sensitivity to anaesthetic drugs. In the next section, recent evidence regarding anaesthetic drug action on the thalamus will be summarised.

Anaesthesia and Thalamic Activity

At doses sufficient to cause unconsciousness, anaesthetic drugs inhibit thalamic activity. Lighter stages of anaesthesia also influence thalamic connections with the rest of the brain. For example, complex interactions between the thalamus, the basal ganglia and the cerebral cortex that regulate behavioural arousal via the circuit mechanism (cortico-basal ganglia-thalamic circuit) are targeted by anaesthetic drugs acting via the GABA-A receptor. GABA-A activity at the basal ganglia suppresses the tonic inhibitory input to the thalamus that can result in paradoxical excitation. Iontophoretic injection of stimulants (nicotine) or antibodies (blocking a voltage-gated potassium channel) to anaesthetic agents into specific loci within the thalamus has demonstrated arousal when anaesthetised [36]. Early investigations characterising regional changes in brain metabolism and blood flow under different anaesthetics reported a decrease in thalamic activity under anaesthesia. This led to suggestions that unconsciousness under anaesthesia results from functional interruption of thalamocortical circuits at the level of the thalamus. Since reduced excitatory input to the thalamus from other sites may lead to the observation of reduced local blood flow and metabolism, this is perhaps a simplistic view of the mechanisms of thalamic underactivity under anaesthesia.

Failure of Information Transfer from Periphery to the Cortex

As a critical relay centre in the sensory pathways, the thalamus is an obvious focus for research into mechanisms of anaesthesia. In a recent human volunteer study, Liu et al. demonstrated that the specific thalamic nuclei involved in processing sensory information is unaltered under propofol anaesthesia, in contrast to the nonspecific thalamic nuclei that are significantly disrupted during anaesthesia [37]. Electrophysiological studies have revealed that anaesthetics can hyperpolarise thalamic neuronal resting membrane potential, thereby reducing synaptic transmission in response to somatosensory stimulation [38]. Ching et al. employed computational modelling to demonstrate that at a network level, alpha activity generated in the thalamus results in persistent and synchronous alpha activity in the cortex. The authors suggested that this thalamocortical synchrony may impede responsiveness to external stimuli [39]. Evidence that this may not be the primary mechanism of unconsciousness is offered by Boveroux et al. in a human volunteer study, where unconsciousness did not correlate with a reduction in thalamocortical connectivity in the sensory cortex [40]. Moreover, ketamine sedation is associated with reduced awareness despite preserved arousal behaviour, providing further opposition to the view that anaesthesia results primarily from the thalamus-mediated perpetual failure.

Suppression of Ascending Arousal Pathways: Thalamic Readout

The nonspecific thalamic nuclei serve as the main relay of information from one neocortical area to another and receive GABAergic input from other subcortical and pontine nuclei. Therefore the demonstration of impaired activity in the nonspecific thalamic nuclei under propofol and dexmedetomidine anaesthesia lends credence to the view that unconsciousness is mediated by suppressing the activity of the ascending arousal system [32, 37]. This is especially pronounced during transitions in level of consciousness—these are associated with greater changes in connectivity of nonspecific thalamic nuclei [37]. Electrophysiological studies afford excellent temporal resolution and thereby allow investigation of the temporal sequence surrounding the alteration in thalamocortical activity. For example, Baker et al. showed that during transition into both sleep and anaesthesia with propofol in rats, altered central medial thalamic activity preceded changes in the neocortex [32]. Velly et al. analysed data from cortical and implanted deep brain electrodes in patients with Parkinson's disease during induction of anaesthesia with propofol and sevoflurane. They reported that quantitative parameters derived from EEG but not from subcortical electrodes were able to predict consciousness and that those derived from subcortical electrodes were able to predict movement. The authors postulated that the cortex was the site mediating anaesthetic-induced unconsciousness with the subsequent thalamic depression reflecting a readout of diminished cortical activity [41]. Such inconsistency in findings may in part be related to the anatomical complexity of the thalamus. In a recent neuroimaging study by Mhuircheartaigh et al., propofol-induced unresponsiveness was associated with preserved thalamocortical connectivity while reducing functional disconnections from the putamen to the cortex [42]. Crucially, these basal ganglia circuits were impaired before thalamocortical connectivity was interrupted.

Thalamic Consciousness Switch

Loss of consciousness following administration of most anaesthetic drugs is associated with reduction in thalamic blood flow, activity and metabolism [43]. This occurs at doses that cause heavy sedation or at doses that are just beyond a loss of consciousness end point. More recent studies suggested a model of increased and coherent alpha frequency activity in the frontal cortex co-ordinated and driven by the thalamus during propofol-induced unconsciousness [39]. In addition, several positron emission tomography (PET) and functional magnetic resonance imaging (fMRI) studies have identified impaired thalamocortical connectivity during transition to loss of consciousness with various anaesthetic agents [40, 44]. This body of evidence from neuroimaging studies has led to the concept of a unitary consciousness switch at the level of the thalamus [45]. This model provides a convenient final common pathway for the plethora of effects that anaesthetic agents have at the receptor, neuronal and regional level. Early micro-infusion studies in animals established a direct anaesthetic effect on thalamic neurons. GABA agonist infusion in specific thalamic nuclei caused a loss of consciousness in rats, which was reversed by nicotine micro-infusions in the same nuclei [46]. This suggests a localised thalamic effect mediated by acetylcholine receptor antagonism. Hyperpolarisation of thalamic neurons by anaesthesia results in a switch from the tonic firing state of wakefulness to the burst firing state of unconsciousness. A loss of input from top-down (corticothalamic) and bottom-up (ascending arousal) circuits enhances this hyperpolarisation by inhibiting glutamatergic and cholinergic receptors, and increasing GABAergic transmission, respectively. Regardless of the underlying mechanisms, general anaesthesia ultimately follows the development of a hyperpolarisation block in thalamocortical neurons [45]. Experiments on mouse brain slices indicate that propofol acts on thalamocortical neurons through GABAergic pathways and via cyclic-nucleotide-gated channels [47].

Thalamocortical and Corticothalamic Loops

Thalamocortical connections exist not just during active brain states but also during periods of inactivity. These connections are closely correlated across distant brain regions, exhibiting strong temporal dynamics. These functional dynamics might constitute a signature of consciousness that is disrupted with the administration of anaesthesia. The resultant alterations in dominant functional configurations cause a loss of capacity to integrate information. There is now extensive evidence for functional disconnections in thalamocortical and corticothalamic pathways with anaesthesia (see above). In an elegant experiment involving multiple methodologies (PET and fMRI), Akeju et al. demonstrated a disruption of thalamic functional connectivity with unconsciousness induced by dexmedetomidine [48]. In a recent study, Barttfeld et al. examined the effect of propofol on functional thalamocortical networks and identified that the strength of connectivity within this network closely correlated with increasing depth of sedation [49]. The authors proposed that the thalamus acts as a key hub co-ordinating multiple functional networks into a 'network of networks'. With sedation, this hierarchy is disrupted, and the thalamus disengages from its role as a frontoparietal hub. Such dynamic reconfiguration results in increased local processing and decreased efficiency of information transfer, thus affecting effective information integration across the brain. Similar dynamic changes in thalamocortical functional connectivity are witnessed during the transition to sleep leading to a disruption in information transfer [50].

The role of the thalamus in the generation of unconsciousness remains contentious, with some suggestions that it may be a necessary but not sufficient component in maintaining unconsciousness. The mechanisms described above may all contribute to the thalamic effect. Whether the thalamus is responsible for unconsciousness by driving anaesthetic action or by working as part of thalamocortical and ascending arousal circuitry, it is highly unlikely that changes in thalamic activity are simply epiphenomenal to anaesthetic mechanisms [36].

Electrophysiological Correlates of Thalamic Activity

General anaesthesia is associated with changes in the brain's electrical activity. Many of these changes seen in the EEG are cortical in origin, but a significant proportion is generated in the thalamus. The pivotal role of higher-order thalamic nuclei is illustrated in the principal electrical signatures of sleep and anaesthesia (Table 4.2). For example, the thalamic reticular nucleus (TRN, a thin sheath of GABAergic neurons surrounding the thalamus) is key to the initiation of sleep spindles [51]. The TRN receives cholinergic input from the brainstem and has strong inhibitory input to the specific dorsal thalamic nuclei and thus is also essential for pain and sensory processing [52]. Optical stimulation of the cholinergic fibres innervating the TRN-initiated sleep in awake mice and promoted more NREM sleep in sleeping mice [53]. The GABAergic innervation of the TRN also makes it a potential target for anaesthetic drugs.

A key electrophysiological feature of NREM sleep and deep anaesthesia is slow-wave activity. These slow waves are the largest electrophysiological events of sleep [54] and are thought to be important for memory consolidation during natural sleep [55]. It is thought that the thalamic switch from

its tonic to its bursting mode (described above) is the source of this pattern [56]. The bursting mode favours a synchronised hyperpolarised slow oscillatory state in cortical neurons that are seen on the EEG as slow waves. These alterations in the firing mode of thalamic neurons are associated with a reduction in responsiveness to external stimuli. Evidence for its thalamic origin was recently published by Lewis et al. where local tonic activation of TRN rapidly induced slow-wave activity in a spatially restricted region of cortex [57]. Isoflurane anaesthesia in mice resulted in TRN activation and modulation of slow-wave dynamics and prolonged the duration of periodic suppressions. Given that cortical slow waves and arousal are often maintained in animals with thalamic lesions [58, 59], cortical slow waves may require co-ordinated cortical and thalamocortical neuronal activity that may be regulated at a local level by the TRN. Anaesthesia is associated with slow waves similar to the slow waves in NREM sleep [60, 61]. With increasing propofol anaesthesia, slow-wave activity was demonstrated to persist beyond loss of behavioural responsiveness with the thalamocortical system becoming isolated from sensory stimuli. Slow-wave saturation could therefore reflect loss of perception with increasing anaesthetic depth [62].

The second key electrophysiological feature of deep anaesthesia (but not sleep) is burst suppression. This pattern, characterised by alternating periods of synchronous high-voltage activity (bursts) and electrical silence (suppressions), is believed to represent a low-order dynamic mechanism that persists in the absence of higher-level brain activity [63]. Although the exact mechanism of this EEG pattern is uncertain, it is thought that both the cortex and the thalamus are involved in its generation [64]. The burst phase is associated with thalamic, brainstem and cortical sources, while the suppression phase is characterised by a 'cortical deafferentation', with coherent cortical sources and a silent thalamus. At a cellular level, evidence from rat slice

Table 4.2 Electrophysiological changes during anaesthesia and sleep

Electrophysiological changes during sleep and anaesthesia		
EEG signatures	Sleep	Anaesthesia
High-frequency, low-amplitude rthythms	Present (stage 1)	Present (stage 1)
Spindle activity	Present (stage 2)	Present
Slow waves	Present (NREM)	Present (stage 2)
Burst suppression	Absent	Present (stage 3)
Isoelectric EEG	Absent	Present (stage 4)

preparations indicates that anaesthetic effects at both gluta-mate and GABA synapses contribute to this pattern [65]. Since there is a parametric response of the proportion of time spent in suppression (burst suppression ratio) with depth of anaesthesia, this EEG signature is an important component of most 'depth of anaesthesia' monitors using spontaneous EEG.

Finally, Crick et al. proposed that consciousness is associated with phase-locked synchronous cortical regions oscillating in the 40 Hz γ-band [66]. This pattern is thought to be co-ordinated in the intralaminar thalamic nuclei, although thalamocortical circuits set up reverberating loops at this frequency with other networks thought to be neces-sary for arousal, perceptual integration and vigilance to occur [67]. Although there are some human studies indicating that this frequency band is suppressed under sleep and anaesthesia [68–70], the evidence for this remains patchy at best.

Cortical Networks, Sleep and Anaesthesia

The cerebral cortex has long been identified as a major site of anaesthetic action, and there is now irrefutable evidence for the role of the cortex in sleep and anaesthesia. Neverthe-less, there is less unanimity regarding the precise location of anaesthetic action in the cortex, or indeed whether the corti-cal changes seen are primary or as a result of influence on nuclei and networks further down the brain. The following section will attempt to briefly summarise the current evi-dence for cortical effects of sleep and anaesthesia.

Regional Changes in Response to Altered Conscious States

Sleep studies in human volunteer studies using PET have consistently demonstrated global and regional decreases in cerebral blood flow (CBF) [25, 71]. Some of the regions consistently highlighted in the studies include the posterior cingulate cortex (PCC) and the precuneus during deep sleep ([71]; Anderson et al. 1998). Similar findings have also been reported using functional MRI (fMRI). Higher-order cortical association areas are also more significantly affected during slow-wave sleep than primary sensory cortices [72]—a finding common to anaesthesia studies (see below). There-fore, deep sleep permits the processing of external sensory stimuli through the primary cortex, but higher-level sensory processing in polymodal association areas is prevented due to the functional dissociation between primary and higher-order cortex, thereby preventing arousal and conscious awareness of these stimuli. REM sleep, by contrast, is associated with significant activation in the pontine tegmen-tum and the thalamus and parts of the limbic cortex including the amygdala, hippocampus, orbitofrontal cortex and anterior cingulate cortex [25, 71, 73].

PET studies under anaesthesia have also demonstrated that whole-brain glucose metabolism is decreased by general anaesthetic drugs (including propofol, by up to 55 %), reflecting the reduced synaptic activity across the brain in the anaesthetised state. The cortex exhibits differential sen-sitivity to anaesthetic agents; in contrast to isoflurane and halothane, propofol caused a greater suppression of glucose metabolism in the temporal and occipital cortices and more regional changes in reduction of CMRGlu. These changes were more pronounced in the cortex (58 %) than in subcor-tical regions (48 %), and primary sensory cortical changes were less prominent than the higher sensory cortex. The largest and most consistent reductions in CBF were identified in the frontal cortex [74–76] and in the posterior parietal cortex [43]. This is a large multimodal association area consisting, in part, of the precuneus, the posterior cin-gulate cortex and the medial parietal cortex and is repeatedly mentioned in consciousness literature [77, 78]. These regions are also deactivated in unconscious states secondary to the vegetative state and in sleep [71, 79] (Fig. 4.2). They have also come under greater scrutiny over the past decade for their role in maintaining consciousness through func-tional connections with the rest of the cortex. This functional connectivity forms part of a much wider functional network (the DMN, see below) arguably representing baseline brain activity and global monitoring of the internal environment in conscious humans.

These changes are not restricted to the resting brain; there is now overwhelming evidence from functional imaging studies that propofol and other anaesthetic agents preferen-tially reduce activity in higher-order brain regions, but not in primary auditory areas in response to auditory stimulation, indicating a lack of higher-order integration in the cortex [37, 81–83].

The general assumption with most neuroimaging studies exploring regional changes to sleep and anaesthesia is that loss of functional activity reflects the neural correlates of consciousness. This is problematic on two counts—first, neuroimaging studies rely on the surrogate measure of altered CBF patterns to indicate altered neuronal activity, and second, the changes witnessed during loss of conscious-ness with anaesthetic drugs could be epiphenomenal and unrelated to the actual onset of unconsciousness.

Regional Interactions During Altered Conscious States

Brain regions don't act in isolation; instead they organise themselves into networks that display correlated and coher-ent activity both during rest (resting state networks) and cognitive activity. Alterations in brain networks with

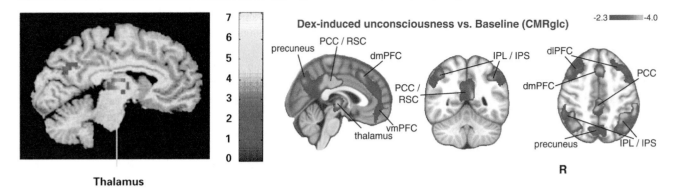

Fig. 4.2 Comparison of changes in brain activity and metabolism with NREM sleep (*left panel*) and dexmedetomidine-induced unconsciousness (*right panel*). Note the similarity in metabolic reduction in the thalamus and the precuneus in both conditions (Reproduced from Nofzinger et al. [80] with permission from Oxford University Press, and from Akeju et al. [48], with permission from eLife Sciences Publications, Ltd under a Creative Commons Attribution License)

anaesthesia would indicate correlated changes in anatomically distinct and distant brain regions that are not related to regional effects of drugs and may in fact represent large-scale changes in brain function. Such integrated functional brain networks are indeed altered in disorders of consciousness (see [84, 85] for some excellent reviews on this topic with description of typical methodology employed). Although early studies looking at functional connectivity between cortical regions identified no difference at various stages of sleep and anaesthesia, more recent studies utilising higher-resolution scanners and complex data analysis strategies have identified changes within and between cortical networks. The transition from wakefulness to slow-wave sleep has been studied in the context of altered functional connectivity; decreased thalamocortical connectivity and increased cortico-cortical connectivity associated with light sleep are replaced by a breakdown in cortico-cortical connectivity with slow-wave sleep [50], and also a decreased contribution of the PCC to the resting networks [86]. Early neuroimaging studies of anaesthesia studied task-related networks; connectivity in lower-order sensorimotor networks persists under deep anaesthesia, while higher-order association areas are more sensitive [40]. Resting state networks form part of 'intrinsic connectivity networks', a set of large-scale functionally connected brain networks identified in either resting state or task-based neuroimaging studies [87]. These networks include, among others, the medial frontoparietal default mode network (DMN), the dorsolateral frontoparietal executive control network (ECN) and the visual and auditory networks. Modulation of these brain networks is important, if not crucial, in processing cognitive stimuli in the conscious state [88–90], and it is thought that intact DMN connectivity is necessary for conscious awareness. The strength of the correlations within this network, and by implication, the integrity of the DMN, is dynamically modulated by the level of consciousness [40]. Human volunteer studies have revealed preferential modulation of higher-order functional connections with anaesthesia [91], although DMN effects are more variable, with some studies reporting no change [92], within network alterations [27], or across network decrease [40]. Some of these differences could be accounted for by the variations in the type and dosage of anaesthetic used and the methodology and analysis employed in the studies. Similar conflicting evidence is present for changes in the DMN during sleep stages [93–96] (Fig. 4.3). Many of the above studies have also demonstrated preserved connectivity between these networks and the thalamus [27, 40], indicating preservation of the corticothalamic circuits under anaesthesia. However, as has been described earlier, Liu et al. employed accurate delineation of the thalamic nuclei and identified altered cortical connectivity with the nonspecific thalamic nuclei [37].

Fragmentation of Neuronal Networks with Loss of Consciousness

Recent advances in signal processing and analyses techniques based on graph theoretical approaches have allowed the exploration of human fMRI and EEG datasets in unprecedented detail and the testing of specific hypotheses. Boly et al. and Spoormaker et al. showed in healthy volunteers that NREM sleep induces a reorganisation of large-scale resting networks into smaller independent modules [97, 98]. The authors postulate that the reported increase in modularity could reflect the failure of integration of information required to maintain consciousness. A similar reduction in whole-brain spatiotemporal integration associated with frontoparietal segregation and a pronounced breakdown of within and between network cortico-cortical connections have also been reported in anaesthesia studies [40, 60, 99, 100]. The importance of frontoparietal areas in the generation of conscious

Fig. 4.3 Changes in spatial configuration of the DMN with transitions in conscious level with sleep and sedation. (Panel **a**) Group statistical maps as obtained from 5-min epochs of wakefulness, stage 1 sleep, stage 2 sleep and slow-wave sleep. (Panel **b**) Illustrates the effect of mild and moderate sedation with propofol on the DMN (modified from Samann et al. [86], with permission from Oxford University Press and Stamatakis et al. [27] with permission from PLOS under a Creative Commons Attribution License)

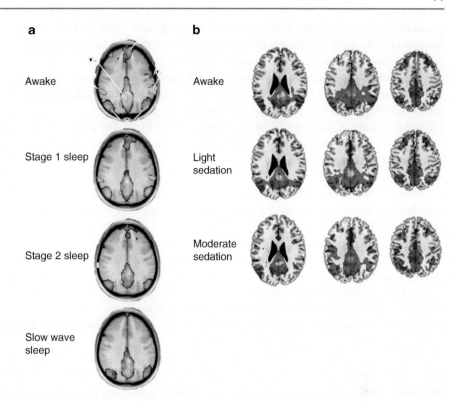

perception is illustrated in these studies, and disruption of their integration is probably a potent mechanism of unconsciousness following sleep and anaesthesia.

Cortical Information Transfer with Loss of Consciousness

Robust conclusions about the nature of brain connectivity changes with anaesthesia and sleep can be drawn with the investigation of strength and directionality of the change. Directional connectivity analyses have shown that information flow is impaired from the posterior (sensory and association) cortices to the anterior (executive prefrontal) areas in sleep [101] and anaesthesia [102–107], a finding that has also been demonstrated with simultaneous EEG/fMRI measurements [108] with propofol, sevoflurane and ketamine [109]. Change in cortical feedback connectivity in the presence of preserved feed-forward connectivity has therefore been proposed as a neurophysiological correlate of anaesthetic-induced unconsciousness.

Information Integration with Loss of Consciousness

Another approach to test the ability of the brain to integrate information is through transcranial magnetic stimulation (TMS) pulses applied to the conscious brain. This typically triggers widespread differentiated patterns of EEG

activation and is thought to reflect the ability of the brain to integrate information in the presence of an external stimulus. TMS activation during sleep and anaesthesia produces a more local and time-limited response [110, 111]. It is thought that the ability of cortical circuits to interact and to produce complex, integrated responses are diminished, resulting in a breakdown in effective connectivity between different cortical regions. Casali et al. further explored the complexity and distribution of this EEG response to TMS. They recorded TMS responses during wakefulness, sleep and anaesthesia with midazolam, xenon or propofol [112] and were able to identify a single measure that was bimodally distributed and separated all conscious from all unconscious individuals. It has therefore been proposed that anaesthesia-induced loss of consciousness is marked by deterioration in the quality and extent of information exchange.

Emergence from Anaesthesia

It is a common clinical knowledge that induction of anaesthesia occurs at higher anaesthetic concentrations than emergence from anaesthesia. Although the mechanisms behind this are currently unclear, mathematical modelling of transitions between consciousness states indicates the presence of a hysteresis loop, i.e. a switch from one state proceeds along a different concentration-response curve than led to entry into that state [113]. Contrary to common perception, this phenomenon cannot be fully explained by pharmacokinetic parameters. Freidman et al. have proposed the concept of neural inertia, an inherent tendency of the brain to resist transition between various conscious states [114], and one that must dissipate prior to anaesthetic emergence and normalisation of cognitive function. The clinical observation that sensitivity to induction of anaesthesia does not reliably predict recovery from anaesthesia may also result from similar mechanisms. Failure of resolution of neural inertia has been proposed to be responsible for coma and other pathological disorders of consciousness. Although the neural substrates for this phenomenon have not been elucidated, arousal-regulating pathways have been implicated [15, 115].

Neuroimaging studies have provided some evidence for anaesthetic hysteresis. As discussed extensively in the above sections, induction of anaesthesia results in widespread regional and global changes in cortical, subcortical and brainstem reactivity. Emergence from anaesthesia is however not a mirror image of induction. Evidence from an EEG study in rats indicates that during recovery from anaesthesia, the brain passes through several specific discrete activity states, and state transitions through an ordered sequence of states mediate recovery of consciousness [116]. A PET study in human volunteers showed that recovery from propofol and dexmedetomidine anaesthesia is associated with activation of the brainstem and thalamus before restoration of functional frontoparietal connectivity [117]. Common to many anaesthetic neuroimaging studies is the observation that regional brain activity and functional connectivity during emergence are increased well above the preanaesthetic baseline, for example [118, 119]. This may reflect the necessity for brain regions to function at supranormal levels to resolve neural inertia and restore a new behavioural state.

Sleep and Anaesthesia Interactions

The complementarity between sleep and anaesthesia permits the possibility that one could influence the other. Sleep deprivation potentiates the hypnotic effect of anaesthetics, probably mediated through adenosine [120]. Propofol anaesthesia also allows recovery from sleep deprivation in animals [121] with the hallmark features of recovery from natural sleep deprivation (increases in duration of NREM and REM). Anaesthesia alters sleep pattern in the postoperative period—the proportion of time spent in early NREM sleep is increased [122], and REM is initially suppressed with a subsequent rebound [123]. These findings are not replicated with opioid administration; opioids are associated with postoperative sleep impairment [124]. Further research into the relationship between anaesthesia and sleep homeostasis may contribute to the understanding of neurobiology of sleep disturbances in the postoperative period and ICU

and provide strategies to restore normal sleep patterns in a vulnerable population.

Consciousness: A Summary View

The above discussion has highlighted several recent studies of anaesthesia and sleep focusing on the mechanisms of onset of, transitions between and recovery from unconsciousness. The receptor, neuronal and network level effects of sleep and anaesthesia provide basis for some of the biological theories proposed for the mechanisms of consciousness. The reader is referred to Boly and Seth [125] for a concise review of the models of consciousness in the context of impaired conscious states. These concepts will be briefly discussed in the following section.

Biological Theories

This set of theories attempts to provide biologically plausible accounts of how brains generate conscious mental content posits that consciousness is a biological state of the brain with empirical correlations between the conscious experience and the brain. One key criterion underlying consciousness is the presence of specific patterns of activations. For example, synchronised neuronal electrical activity bringing together sensory modalities and thalamocortical circuits in the gamma range (75–100 Hz) [126–128] is said to facilitate cognitive binding by synchrony and synthesis of information content. Evidence from sleep and anaesthesia studies showing better correlation with loss of consciousness has allowed focus on these faster gamma frequencies than on Crick's 40 Hz theory (see above) [129, 130]. These frequencies may also be implicated in neural loops mediating recurrent processing; such loops in the visual system are claimed to be the source of visual experience [131–133] and are often absent during sleep and anaesthesia [104–107, 109, 134].

Conscious Access Hypothesis and the Global Neuronal Workspace Framework

In contrast to the above theories that emphasise synchronisation across neural circuits, Baars proposed that consciousness is related to the spread and reverberation of information across the brain [135]. According to this hypothesis, the brain consists predominantly of two types of neurons. The first type comprises functionally specialised neurons that communicate with similarly specialised neurons in a 'nonconscious' bottom-up manner and are activated even with stimuli that do not reach consciousness. This is exemplified in data from studies where primary sensory systems are active even during deep sleep or anaesthesia. The second type of neurons is a diffusely distributed set of neurons (the global workspace) that exchange information through long-range excitatory axons. These neurons include the cortical pyramidal cells (they enjoy long-range cortical connections with other cortical cells), with the prefrontal cortex as a major node of the global workspace due to its functional diversity and rich cortico-cortical connections [136]. This is supported by anaesthesia and sleep studies on fluctuations on resting state networks, especially the DMN. The hypothesis proposes that stimulation inhibits processing of concurrent stimuli and, with increasing salience, results in a sudden non-linear transition from a local to a global activity pattern (ignition). This is associated with several classic signatures of conscious access to a stimulus in the form of long-range phase synchrony and high-frequency oscillations [137].

Dynamic Core Hypothesis

In order to accommodate the concept of consciousness as a highly dynamic process, a highly specialised and differentiated group of thalamocortical neurons are said to constitute a 'dynamic core', characterised by high informability and allowing for the constant exchange of signals within the network [138]. A necessary feature of this dynamic system is that the composition of the core transcends traditional anatomical boundaries, varying significantly across individuals according to conscious states. Certain brain regions (such as the thalamocortical neurons) possess anatomical connectivity that is much more effective in generating coherent dynamic states than that of other regions.

The hypothesis also therefore embraces the concept of dynamic reentrant loops (above) within complex, widely dispersed, interconnected neural networks constituting a Global Workspace.

Integration of Information Hypothesis

This is closely related to the dynamic core hypothesis and proposes that conscious experience depends on rapid and effective integration of functionally diverse cognitive systems in the thalamocortical system. The highly integrated and indivisible nature and high information content of any conscious experience can be mathematically expressed as information integration, where the information generated is greater than the sum of the individual inbound contributions [133]. For consciousness to be present, the brain must be capable of selecting from a number of possibilities (highly differentiated) and presenting these selections as a unity (highly integrated) (Fig. 4.4). Such integration typically does not include neural circuits involving the basal ganglia and the cerebellum (brain regions are not considered critical for generating/maintaining consciousness; however, see [42] for an exception to this rule). A mathematical model of the capacity for information integration, denoted as Φ, has been described that is increased in systems maintaining consciousness and decreased in those that do not (e.g. basal ganglia, sleep and anaesthesia). Several indices have been calculated in studies to measure complexity of neural

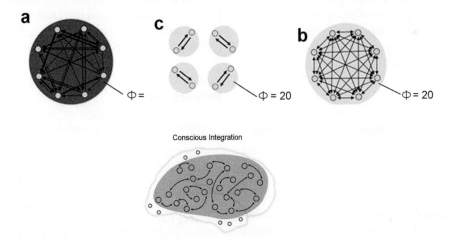

Fig. 4.4 A schematic of a system that is both functionally specialised and functionally integrated. *Top panel*: (*Left*, **a**) this network jointly maximises functional specialisation and functional integration among its elements, thereby resembling the anatomical organisation of the thalamocortical system. Note the heterogeneous arrangement of the incoming and outgoing connections: each element is connected to a different subset of elements, with different weights. (*Middle*, **c**) A loss of integration within the system to form four independent modules results in a net reduction of information integration. (*Right*, **b**) A loss of specialisation also results in reduction of information integration in the system. A homogenous distribution of the same amount of connectivity eliminates functional specialisation (Reproduced from Tononi [139] with permission from *BioMed Central*). *Bottom panel*: possible neural basis of conscious integration according to information integration theory. During conscious processing, the mechanisms integrating information above and beyond the union of their parts define a main complex (*dark orange*). This complex generates the subject's conscious experience (Reproduced from Mudrik et al. [140], with permission from Elsevier)

networks, and sleep and anaesthesia have been shown to reduce complexity, integration and differentiation [99, 141–143]. For example, Chennu et al. identified frontal shifts in alpha power and network topography with decreasing level of consciousness from propofol. Graph-theoretic network analysis found these frontal alpha networks to be characteristically compromised in terms of efficiency, indexing the loss of neural information integration that characterises consciousness [144].

In the following section, a brief summary of the other theoretical frameworks and models of consciousness is presented.

Other Theories

The basic premise of physical theories is that consciousness results from a change in the physical properties in the brain (global entropy [145], electromagnetic field changes [146], quantum effects [147], neural fields [148], to name a few). However, given the conventional methodology, such theories remain difficult to prove and do not provide answers to the fundamental question of why such physical changes should result in a subjective experience. The worldly discrimination theory relies on verbal report in response to environmental interactions and states that the ability to discriminate when presented with choice indicates the presence of conscious awareness, but only tests for the existence of first-order states or primary consciousness. In contrast, higher-order thought theories assume that consciousness is a mental state where one is aware of being aware and where conscious awareness crucially depends on higher-order representation. These theories do not explain the presence of conscious awareness in situations where objective assessment or behavioural reporting is difficult [149].

Consciousness and Anaesthesia: A Converging Paradigm?

The foregoing discussion suggests two themes. First, information transfer from the external environment does not follow a simple ascending pathway to the cortex to ensure conscious awareness, and consciousness is not mediated at any one brain region or network. It is probably best thought of as change in dynamic aspects in neuronal network communication. Although this process depends on intact function of brainstem-thalamocortical arousal circuits, the common denominator in the neural correlates of consciousness might rather be changes in distributed cortico-cortical processing. Second, a simple block of information transfer is inconsistent with unconsciousness under anaesthesia. General anaesthesia is probably a two-stage process targeting

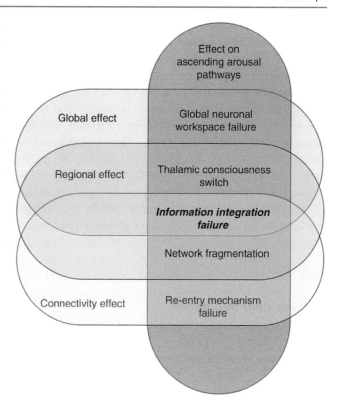

Fig. 4.5 Venn diagram illustrating the numerous mechanisms of anaesthetic unconsciousness. Common to all mechanisms is failure of integration of presented external information

sleep circuits at low doses and mechanisms across the entire brain at the higher doses required for surgery (Fig. 4.5). The basis of anaesthetic action is related more to specific changes in the connectivity patterns between regions, rather than changes in activity of isolated brain structures.

References

1. Saper CB, Chou TC, Scammell TE. The sleep switch: hypothalamic control of sleep and wakefulness. Trends Neurosci. 2001;24:726–31.
2. Saper CB, Fuller PM, Pedersen NP, Lu J, Scammell TE. Sleep state switching. Neuron. 2010;68:1023–42.
3. Moruzzi G, Magoun HW. Brain stem reticular formation and activation of the EEG. Electroencephalogr Clin Neurophysiol. 1949;1:455–73.
4. Lee SH, Dan Y. Neuromodulation of brain states. Neuron. 2012;76:209–22.
5. Leung LS, Luo T, Ma J, Herrick I. Brain areas that influence general anesthesia. Prog Neurobiol. 2014;122:24–44.
6. Lu J, Sherman D, Devor M, Saper CB. A putative flip-flop switch for control of REM sleep. Nature. 2006;441:589–94.
7. Nelson LE, Guo TZ, Lu J, Saper CB, Franks NP, Maze M. The sedative component of anesthesia is mediated by GABA (A) receptors in an endogenous sleep pathway. Nat Neurosci. 2002;5:979–84.
8. Luo T, Leung LS. Involvement of tuberomammillary histaminergic neurons in isoflurane anesthesia. Anesthesiology. 2011;115:36–43.

9. Correa-Sales C, Rabin BC, Maze M. A hypnotic response to dexmedetomidine, an alpha 2 agonist, is mediated in the locus coeruleus in rats. Anesthesiology. 1992;76:948–52.

10. Hu FY, Hanna GM, Han W, Mardini F, Thomas SA, Wyner AJ, et al. Hypnotic hypersensitivity to volatile anesthetics and dexmedetomidine in dopamine beta-hydroxylase knockout mice. Anesthesiology. 2012;117:1006–17.

11. Zhang Y, Yu T, Yuan J, Yu BW. The ventrolateral preoptic nucleus is required for propofol-induced inhibition of locus coeruleus neuronal activity. Neurol Sci. 2015;36:2177–84.

12. Mortazavi S, Thompson J, Baghdoyan HA, Lydic R. Fentanyl and morphine, but not remifentanil, inhibit acetylcholine release in pontine regions modulating arousal. Anesthesiology. 1999;90:1070–7.

13. Meuret P, Backman SB, Bonhomme V, Plourde G, Fiset P. Physostigmine reverses propofol-induced unconsciousness and attenuation of the auditory steady state response and bispectral index in human volunteers. Anesthesiology. 2000;93(3):708–17.

14. Plourde G, Chartrand D, Fiset P, Font S, Backman SB. Antagonism of sevoflurane anaesthesia by physostigmine: effects on the auditory steady-state response and bispectral index. Br J Anaesth. 2003;91(4):583–6.

15. Kelz MB, Sun Y, Chen J, Cheng Meng Q, Moore JT, Veasey SC, Dixon S, Thornton M, Funato H, Yanagisawa M. An essential role for orexins in emergence from general anesthesia. Proc Natl Acad Sci U S A. 2008;105:1309–14.

16. Kubota T, Hirota K, Yoshida H, Takahashi S, Ohkawa H, Anzawa N, Kushikata T, Matsuki A. Inhibitory effect of clonidine on ketamine-induced norepinephrine release from the medial prefrontal cortex in rats. Br J Anaesth. 1999;83:945–7.

17. Kushikata T, Hirota K, Yoshida H, Kudo M, Lambert DG, Smart D, Jerman JC, Matsuki A. Orexinergic neurons and barbiturate anesthesia. Neuroscience. 2003;121:855–63.

18. Porkka-Heiskanen T, Strecker RE, Thakkar M, Bjorkum AA, Greene RW, Mccarley RW. Adenosine: a mediator of the sleep-inducing effects of prolonged wakefulness. Science. 1997;276:1265–8.

19. Born J, Rasch B, Gais S. Sleep to remember. Neuroscientist. 2006;12:410–24.

20. Carter ME, Yizhar O, Chikahisa S, Nguyen H, Adamantidis A, Nishino S, Deisseroth K, de Lecea L. Tuning arousal with optogenetic modulation of locus coeruleus neurons. Nat Neurosci. 2010;13:1526–33.

21. Vazey EM, Aston-Jones G. Designer receptor manipulations reveal a role of the locus coeruleus noradrenergic system in isoflurane general anesthesia. Proc Natl Acad Sci U S A. 2014;111:3859–64.

22. Solt K, Cotten JF, Cimenser A, Wong KF, Chemali JJ, Brown EN. Methylphenidate actively induces emergence from general anesthesia. Anesthesiology. 2011;115:791–803.

23. Lee MG, Hassani OK, Alonso A, Jones BE. Cholinergic basal forebrain neurons burst with theta during waking and paradoxical sleep. J Neurosci. 2005;25:4365–9.

24. Brown EN, Lydic R, Schiff ND. General anesthesia, sleep, and coma. N Engl J Med. 2010;363:2638–50.

25. Braun AR, Balkin TJ, Wesenten NJ, Carson RE, Varga M, Baldwin P, Selbie S, Belenky G, Herscovitch P. Regional cerebral blood flow throughout the sleep-wake cycle. An H2(15)O PET study. Brain. 1997;120(Pt 7):1173–97.

26. Gili T, Saxena N, Diukova A, Murphy K, Hall JE, Wise RG. The thalamus and brainstem act as key hubs in alterations of human brain network connectivity induced by mild propofol sedation. J Neurosci. 2013;33:4024–31.

27. Stamatakis EA, Adapa RM, Absalom AR, Menon DK. Changes in resting neural connectivity during propofol sedation. PLoS One. 2010;5, e14224.

28. Gosseries O, Charland-Verville V, Thonnard M, Bodart O, Laureys S, Demertzi A. Amantadine, apomorphine and zolpidem in the treatment of disorders of consciousness. Curr Pharm Des. 2014;20:4167–84.

29. Thonnard M, Gosseries O, Demertzi A, Lugo Z, Vanhaudenhuyse A, Bruno MA, Chatelle C, Thibaut A, Charland-Verville V, Habbal D, Schnakers C, Laureys S. Effect of zolpidem in chronic disorders of consciousness: a prospective open-label study. Funct Neurol. 2013;28:259–64.

30. Tang L, Ge Y, Sodickson DK, Miles L, Zhou Y, Reaume J, Grossman RI. Thalamic resting-state functional networks: disruption in patients with mild traumatic brain injury. Radiology. 2011;260:831–40.

31. Alkire MT, Miller J. General anesthesia and the neural correlates of consciousness. Prog Brain Res. 2005;150:229–44.

32. Baker R, Gent TC, Yang Q, Parker S, Vyssotski AL, Wisden W, Brickley SG, Franks NP. Altered activity in the central medial thalamus precedes changes in the neocortex during transitions into both sleep and propofol anesthesia. J Neurosci. 2014;34:13326–35.

33. Magnin M, Rey M, Bastuji H, Guillemant P, Mauguiere F, Garcia-Larrea L. Thalamic deactivation at sleep onset precedes that of the cerebral cortex in humans. Proc Natl Acad Sci U S A. 2010;107:3829–33.

34. Rey M, Bastuji H, Garcia-Larrea L, Guillemant P, Mauguiere F, Magnin M. Human thalamic and cortical activities assessed by dimension of activation and spectral edge frequency during sleep wake cycles. Sleep. 2007;30:907–12.

35. Schiff ND, Giacino JT, Kalmar K, Victor JD, Baker K, Gerber M, Fritz B, Eisenberg B, Biondi T, O'Connor J, Kobylarz EJ, Farris S, Machado A, Mccagg C, Plum F, Fins JJ, Rezai AR. Behavioural improvements with thalamic stimulation after severe traumatic brain injury. Nature. 2007;448:600–3.

36. Mashour GA, Alkire MT. Consciousness, anesthesia, and the thalamocortical system. Anesthesiology. 2013;118:13–5.

37. Liu X, Lauer KK, Ward BD, Li SJ, Hudetz AG. Differential effects of deep sedation with propofol on the specific and nonspecific thalamocortical systems: a functional magnetic resonance imaging study. Anesthesiology. 2013;118:59–69.

38. Detsch O, Vahle-Hinz C, Kochs E, Siemers M, Bromm B. Isoflurane induces dose-dependent changes of thalamic somatosensory information transfer. Brain Res. 1999;829:77–89.

39. Ching S, Cimenser A, Purdon PL, Brown EN, Kopell NJ. Thalamocortical model for a propofol-induced alpha-rhythm associated with loss of consciousness. Proc Natl Acad Sci U S A. 2010;107:22665–70.

40. Boveroux P, Vanhaudenhuyse A, Bruno MA, Noirhomme Q, Lauwick S, Luxen A, Degueldre C, Plenevaux A, Schnakers C, Phillips C, Brichant JF, Bonhomme V, Maquet P, Greicius MD, Laureys S, Boly M. Breakdown of within- and between-network resting state functional magnetic resonance imaging connectivity during propofol-induced loss of consciousness. Anesthesiology. 2010;113:1038–53.

41. Velly LJ, Rey MF, Bruder NJ, Gouvitsos FA, Witjas T, Regis JM, Peragut JC, Gouin FM. Differential dynamic of action on cortical and subcortical structures of anesthetic agents during induction of anesthesia. Anesthesiology. 2007;107:202–12.

42. Mhuircheartaigh RN, Rosenorn-Lanng D, Wise R, Jbabdi S, Rogers R, Tracey I. Cortical and subcortical connectivity changes during decreasing levels of consciousness in humans: a functional magnetic resonance imaging study using propofol. J Neurosci. 2010;30:9095–102.

43. Fiset P, Paus T, Daloze T, Plourde G, Meuret P, Bonhomme V, Hajj-Ali N, Backman SB, Evans AC. Brain mechanisms of propofol-induced loss of consciousness in humans: a positron emission tomographic study. J Neurosci. 1999;19:5506–13.

44. White NS, Alkire MT. Impaired thalamocortical connectivity in humans during general-anesthetic-induced unconsciousness. Neuroimage. 2003;19:402–11.

45. Alkire MT, Haier RJ, Fallon JH. Toward a unified theory of narcosis: brain imaging evidence for a thalamocortical switch as the neurophysiologic basis of anesthetic-induced unconsciousness. Conscious Cogn. 2000;9:370–86.

46. Alkire MT, Mcreynolds JR, Hahn EL, Trivedi AN. Thalamic microinjection of nicotine reverses sevoflurane-induced loss of righting reflex in the rat. Anesthesiology. 2007;107:264–72.

47. Ying SW, Abbas SY, Harrison NL, Goldstein PA. Propofol block of I(h) contributes to the suppression of neuronal excitability and rhythmic burst firing in thalamocortical neurons. Eur J Neurosci. 2006;23:465–80.

48. Akeju O, Loggia ML, Catana C, Pavone KJ, Vazquez R, Rhee J, Contreras Ramirez V, Chonde DB, Izquierdo-Garcia D, Arabasz G, Hsu S, Habeeb K, Hooker JM, Napadow V, Brown EN, Purdon PL. Disruption of thalamic functional connectivity is a neural correlate of dexmedetomidine-induced unconsciousness. Elife. 2014;3, e04499.

49. Barttfeld P, Bekinschtein TA, Salles A, Stamatakis EA, Adapa R, Menon DK, Sigman M. Factoring the brain signatures of anesthesia concentration and level of arousal across individuals. Neuroimage Clin. 2015;9:385–91.

50. Spoormaker VI, Schroter MS, Gleiser PM, Andrade KC, Dresler M, Wehrle R, Samann PG, Czisch M. Development of a large-scale functional brain network during human non-rapid eye movement sleep. J Neurosci. 2010;30:11379–87.

51. Halassa MM, Siegle JH, Ritt JT, Ting JT, Feng G, Moore CI. Selective optical drive of thalamic reticular nucleus generates thalamic bursts and cortical spindles. Nat Neurosci. 2011;14:1118–20.

52. Hartings JA, Temereanca S, Simons DJ. State-dependent processing of sensory stimuli by thalamic reticular neurons. J Neurosci. 2003;23:5264–71.

53. Ni KM, Hou XJ, Yang CH, Dong P, Li Y, Zhang Y, Jiang P, Berg DK, Duan S, Li XM. Selectively driving cholinergic fibers optically in the thalamic reticular nucleus promotes sleep. Elife. 2016;5.

54. Achermann P, Borbely AA. Low-frequency (<1 Hz) oscillations in the human sleep electroencephalogram. Neuroscience. 1997;81:213–22.

55. Murphy M, Bruno MA, Riedner BA, Boveroux P, Noirhomme Q, Landsness EC, Brichant JF, Phillips C, Massimini M, Laureys S, Tononi G, Boly M. Propofol anesthesia and sleep: a high-density EEG study. Sleep. 2011;34:283–91A.

56. Steriade M, Timofeev I. Neuronal plasticity in thalamocortical networks during sleep and waking oscillations. Neuron. 2003;37:563–76.

57. Lewis LD, Voigts J, Flores FJ, Schmitt LI, Wilson MA, Halassa MM, Brown EN. Thalamic reticular nucleus induces fast and local modulation of arousal state. Elife. 2015;4, e08760.

58. Constantinople CM, Bruno RM. Effects and mechanisms of wakefulness on local cortical networks. Neuron. 2011;69:1061–8.

59. Steriade M, Nunez A, Amzica F. A novel slow (<1 Hz) oscillation of neocortical neurons in vivo: depolarizing and hyperpolarizing components. J Neurosci. 1993;13:3252–65.

60. Lewis LD, Weiner VS, Mukamel EA, Donoghue JA, Eskandar EN, Madsen JR, Anderson WS, Hochberg LR, Cash SS, Brown EN, Purdon PL. Rapid fragmentation of neuronal networks at the onset of propofol-induced unconsciousness. Proc Natl Acad Sci U S A. 2012;109:E3377–86.

61. Lukatch HS, Maciver MB. Synaptic mechanisms of thiopental-induced alterations in synchronized cortical activity. Anesthesiology. 1996;84:1425–34.

62. Ni Mhuircheartaigh R, Warnaby C, Rogers R, Jbabdi S, Tracey I. Slow-wave activity saturation and thalamocortical isolation during propofol anesthesia in humans. Sci Transl Med. 2013;5:208ra148.

63. Ching S, Purdon PL, Vijayan S, Kopell NJ, Brown EN. A neurophysiological-metabolic model for burst suppression. Proc Natl Acad Sci U S A. 2012;109:3095–100.

64. Japaridze N, Muthuraman M, Reinicke C, Moeller F, Anwar AR, Mideksa KG, Pressler R, Deuschl G, Stephani U, Siniatchkin M. Neuronal networks during burst suppression as revealed by source analysis. PLoS One. 2015;10, e0123807.

65. Lukatch HS, Kiddoo CE, Maciver MB. Anesthetic-induced burst suppression EEG activity requires glutamate-mediated excitatory synaptic transmission. Cereb Cortex. 2005;15:1322–31.

66. Crick F, Koch C. A framework for consciousness. Nat Neurosci. 2003;6:119–26.

67. Engel AK, Singer W. Temporal binding and the neural correlates of sensory awareness. Trends Cogn Sci. 2001;5:16–25.

68. Cantero JL, Atienza M, Madsen JR, Stickgold R. Gamma EEG dynamics in neocortex and hippocampus during human wakefulness and sleep. Neuroimage. 2004;22:1271–80.

69. John ER, Prichep LS, Kox W, Valdes-Sosa P, Bosch-Bayard J, Aubert E, Tom M, di Michele F, Gugino LD. Invariant reversible QEEG effects of anesthetics. Conscious Cogn. 2001;10:165–83.

70. Sleigh JW, Steyn-Ross DA, Steyn-Ross ML, Williams ML, Smith P. Comparison of changes in electroencephalographic measures during induction of general anaesthesia: influence of the gamma frequency band and electromyogram signal. Br J Anaesth. 2001;86:50–8.

71. Maquet P, Degueldre C, Delfiore G, Aerts J, Peters JM, Luxen A, Franck G. Functional neuroanatomy of human slow wave sleep. J Neurosci. 1997;17:2807–12.

72. Franks NP. General anaesthesia: from molecular targets to neuronal pathways of sleep and arousal. Nat Rev Neurosci. 2008;9:370–86.

73. Nofzinger EA, Mintun MA, Wiseman M, Kupfer DJ, Moore RY. Forebrain activation in REM sleep: an FDG PET study. Brain Res. 1997;770(1-2):192–201.

74. Kaisti KK, Langsjo JW, Aalto S, Oikonen V, Sipila H, Teras M, Hinkka S, Metsahonkala L, Scheinin H. Effects of sevoflurane, propofol, and adjunct nitrous oxide on regional cerebral blood flow, oxygen consumption, and blood volume in humans. Anesthesiology. 2003;99:603–13.

75. Kaisti KK, Metsahonkala L, Teras M, Oikonen V, Aalto S, Jaaskelainen S, Hinkka S, Scheinin H. Effects of surgical levels of propofol and sevoflurane anesthesia on cerebral blood flow in healthy subjects studied with positron emission tomography. Anesthesiology. 2002;96:1358–70.

76. Veselis RA, Feshchenko VA, Reinsel RA, Dnistrian AM, Beattie B, Akhurst TJ. Thiopental and propofol affect different regions of the brain at similar pharmacologic effects. Anesth Analg. 2004;99:399–408. table of contents.

77. Baars BJ, Ramsoy TZ, Laureys S. Brain, conscious experience and the observing self. Trends Neurosci. 2003;26:671–5.

78. Rees G, Kreiman G, Koch C. Neural correlates of consciousness in humans. Nat Rev Neurosci. 2002;3:261–70.

79. Laureys S, Goldman S, Phillips C, van Bogaert P, Aerts J, Luxen A, Franck G, Maquet P. Impaired effective cortical connectivity in vegetative state: preliminary investigation using PET. Neuroimage. 1999;9:377–82.

80. Nofzinger EA, Buysse DJ, Miewald JM, Meltzer CC, Price JC, Sembrat RC, Ombao H, Reynolds CF, Monk TH, Hall M, Kupfer DJ, Moore RY. Human regional cerebral glucose metabolism during non-rapid eye movement sleep in relation to waking. Brain. 2002;125:1105–15.

81. Adapa RM, Davis MH, Stamatakis EA, Absalom AR, Menon DK. Neural correlates of successful semantic processing during propofol sedation. Hum Brain Mapp. 2014;35:2935–49.

82. Kerssens C, Hamann S, Peltier S, Hu XP, Byas-Smith MG, Sebel PS. Attenuated brain response to auditory word stimulation with sevoflurane: a functional magnetic resonance imaging study in humans. Anesthesiology. 2005;103:11–9.

83. Ramani R, Qiu M, Constable RT. Sevoflurane 0.25 MAC preferentially affects higher order association areas: a functional magnetic resonance imaging study in volunteers. Anesth Analg. 2007;105:648–55.

84. Heine L, Soddu A, Gomez F, Vanhaudenhuyse A, Tshibanda L, Thonnard M, Charland-Verville V, Kirsch M, Laureys S, Demertzi A. Resting state networks and consciousness: alterations of multiple resting state network connectivity in physiological, pharmacological, and pathological consciousness states. Front Psychol. 2012;3:295.

85. Marino S, Bonanno L, Giorgio A. Functional connectivity in disorders of consciousness: methodological aspects and clinical relevance. Brain Imaging Behav. 2015;10:604–8.

86. Samann PG, Wehrle R, Hoehn D, Spoormaker VI, Peters H, Tully C, Holsboer F, Czisch M. Development of the brain's default mode network from wakefulness to slow wave sleep. Cereb Cortex. 2011;21:2082–93.

87. Seeley WW, Menon V, Schatzberg AF, Keller J, Glover GH, Kenna H, Reiss AL, Greicius MD. Dissociable intrinsic connectivity networks for salience processing and executive control. J Neurosci. 2007;27:2349–56.

88. Bressler SL. Large-scale cortical networks and cognition. Brain Res Brain Res Rev. 1995;20(3):288–304.

89. Goldman-Rakic PS. Topography of cognition: parallel distributed networks in primate association cortex. Annu Rev Neurosci. 1988;11:137–56.

90. Mesulam MM. Large-scale neurocognitive networks and distributed processing for attention, language, and memory. Ann Neurol. 1990;28(5):597–613.

91. Martuzzi R, Ramani R, Qiu M, Rajeevan N, Constable RT. Functional connectivity and alterations in baseline brain state in humans. Neuroimage. 2010;49:823–34.

92. Greicius MD, Kiviniemi V, Tervonen O, Vainionpaa V, Alahuhta S, Reiss AL, Menon V. Persistent default-mode network connectivity during light sedation. Hum Brain Mapp. 2008;29:839–47.

93. Horovitz SG, Braun AR, Carr WS, Picchioni D, Balkin TJ, Fukunaga M, Duyn JH. Decoupling of the brain's default mode network during deep sleep. Proc Natl Acad Sci U S A. 2009;106:11376–81.

94. Horovitz SG, Fukunaga M, de Zwart JA, van Gelderen P, Fulton SC, Balkin TJ, Duyn JH. Low frequency BOLD fluctuations during resting wakefulness and light sleep: a simultaneous EEG-fMRI study. Hum Brain Mapp. 2008;29:671–82.

95. Koike T, Kan S, Misaki M, Miyauchi S. Connectivity pattern changes in default-mode network with deep non-REM and REM sleep. Neurosci Res. 2011;69:322–30.

96. Larson-Prior LJ, Zempel JM, Nolan TS, Prior FW, Snyder AZ, Raichle ME. Cortical network functional connectivity in the descent to sleep. Proc Natl Acad Sci U S A. 2009;106:4489–94.

97. Boly M, Perlbarg V, Marrelec G, Schabus M, Laureys S, Doyon J, Pelegrini-Issac M, Maquet P, Benali H. Hierarchical clustering of brain activity during human nonrapid eye movement sleep. Proc Natl Acad Sci U S A. 2012;109:5856–61.

98. Spoormaker VI, Gleiser PM, Czisch M. Frontoparietal connectivity and hierarchical structure of the brain's functional network during sleep. Front Neurol. 2012;3:80.

99. Monti MM, Lutkenhoff ES, Rubinov M, Boveroux P, Vanhaudenhuyse A, Gosseries O, Bruno MA, Noirhomme Q, Boly M, Laureys S. Dynamic change of global and local information processing in propofol-induced loss and recovery of consciousness. PLoS Comput Biol. 2013;9, e1003271.

100. Schrouff J, Perlbarg V, Boly M, Marrelec G, Boveroux P, Vanhaudenhuyse A, Bruno MA, Laureys S, Phillips C, Pelegrini-Issac M, Maquet P, Benali H. Brain functional integration decreases during propofol-induced loss of consciousness. Neuroimage. 2011;57:198–205.

101. Massimini M, Ferrarelli F, Huber R, Esser SK, Singh H, Tononi G. Breakdown of cortical effective connectivity during sleep. Science. 2005;309:2228–32.

102. Blain-Moraes S, Tarnal V, Vanini G, Alexander A, Rosen D, Shortal B, Janke E, Mashour GA. Neurophysiological correlates of sevoflurane-induced unconsciousness. Anesthesiology. 2015;122:307–16.

103. Boly M, Moran R, Murphy M, Boveroux P, Bruno MA, Noirhomme Q, Ledoux D, Bonhomme V, Brichant JF, Tononi G, Laureys S, Friston K. Connectivity changes underlying spectral EEG changes during propofol-induced loss of consciousness. J Neurosci. 2012;32:7082–90.

104. Imas OA, Ropella KM, Ward BD, Wood JD, Hudetz AG. Volatile anesthetics disrupt frontal-posterior recurrent information transfer at gamma frequencies in rat. Neurosci Lett. 2005;387:145–50.

105. Ku SW, Lee U, Noh GJ, Jun IG, Mashour GA. Preferential inhibition of frontal-to-parietal feedback connectivity is a neurophysiologic correlate of general anesthesia in surgical patients. PLoS One. 2011;6, e25155.

106. Lee U, Kim S, Noh GJ, Choi BM, Hwang E, Mashour GA. The directionality and functional organization of frontoparietal connectivity during consciousness and anesthesia in humans. Conscious Cogn. 2009;18:1069–78.

107. Maksimow A, Silfverhuth M, Langsjo J, Kaskinoro K, Georgiadis S, Jaaskelainen S, Scheinin H. Directional connectivity between frontal and posterior brain regions is altered with increasing concentrations of propofol. PLoS One. 2014;9, e113616.

108. Jordan D, Ilg R, Riedl V, Schorer A, Grimberg S, Neufang S, Omerovic A, Berger S, Untergehrer G, Preibisch C, Schulz E, Schuster T, Schroter M, Spoormaker V, Zimmer C, Hemmer B, Wohlschlager A, Kochs EF, Schneider G. Simultaneous electroencephalographic and functional magnetic resonance imaging indicate impaired cortical top-down processing in association with anesthetic-induced unconsciousness. Anesthesiology. 2013;119:1031–42.

109. Lee U, Ku S, Noh G, Baek S, Choi B, Mashour GA. Disruption of frontal-parietal communication by ketamine, propofol, and sevoflurane. Anesthesiology. 2013;118:1264–75.

110. Ferrarelli F, Massimini M, Sarasso S, Casali A, Riedner BA, Angelini G, Tononi G, Pearce RA. Breakdown in cortical effective connectivity during midazolam-induced loss of consciousness. Proc Natl Acad Sci U S A. 2010;107:2681–6.

111. Massimini M, Ferrarelli F, Murphy M, Huber R, Riedner B, Casarotto S, Tononi G. Cortical reactivity and effective connectivity during REM sleep in humans. Cogn Neurosci. 2010;1:176–83.

112. Casali AG, Gosseries O, Rosanova M, Boly M, Sarasso S, Casali KR, Casarotto S, Bruno MA, Laureys S, Tononi G., Massimini M. A theoretically based index of consciousness independent of sensory processing and behavior. Sci Transl Med. 2013;5:198ra105.

113. Steyn-Ross ML, Steyn-Ross DA, Sleigh JW. Modelling general anaesthesia as a first-order phase transition in the cortex. Prog Biophys Mol Biol. 2004;85:369–85.

114. Friedman EB, Sun Y, Moore JT, Hung HT, Meng QC, Perera P, Joiner WJ, Thomas SA, Eckenhoff RG, Sehgal A, Kelz MB. A conserved behavioral state barrier impedes transitions between anesthetic-induced unconsciousness and wakefulness: evidence for neural inertia. PLoS One. 2010;5, e11903.

115. Joiner WJ, Friedman EB, Hung HT, Koh K, Sowcik M, Sehgal A, Kelz MB. Genetic and anatomical basis of the barrier separating wakefulness and anesthetic-induced unresponsiveness. PLoS Genet. 2013;9, e1003605.

116. Hudson AE, Calderon DP, Pfaff DW, Proekt A. Recovery of consciousness is mediated by a network of discrete metastable activity states. Proc Natl Acad Sci U S A. 2014;111:9283–8.

117. Langsjo JW, Alkire MT, Kaskinoro K, Hayama H, Maksimow A, Kaisti KK, Aalto S, Aantaa R, Jaaskelainen SK, Revonsuo A, Scheinin H. Returning from oblivion: imaging the neural core of consciousness. J Neurosci. 2012;32:4935–43.

118. Hudetz AG. General anesthesia and human brain connectivity. Brain Connect. 2012;2:291–302.

119. Plourde G, Belin P, Chartrand D, Fiset P, Backman SB, Xie G, Zatorre RJ. Cortical processing of complex auditory stimuli during alterations of consciousness with the general anesthetic propofol. Anesthesiology. 2006;104:448–57.

120. Tung A, Szafran MJ, Bluhm B, Mendelson WB. Sleep deprivation potentiates the onset and duration of loss of righting reflex induced by propofol and isoflurane. Anesthesiology. 2002;97:906–11.

121. Tung A, Bergmann BM, Herrera S, Cao D, Mendelson WB. Recovery from sleep deprivation occurs during propofol anesthesia. Anesthesiology. 2004;100:1419–26.

122. Moote CA, Knill RL. Isoflurane anesthesia causes a transient alteration in nocturnal sleep. Anesthesiology. 1988;69:327–31.

123. Gogenur I, Wildschiotz G, Rosenberg J. Circadian distribution of sleep phases after major abdominal surgery. Br J Anaesth. 2008;100:45–9.

124. Steinmetz J, Holm-Knudsen R, Eriksen K, Marxen D, Rasmussen LS. Quality differences in postoperative sleep between propofol-remifentanil and sevoflurane anesthesia in infants. Anesth Analg. 2007;104:779–83.

125. Boly M, Seth AK. Modes and models in disorders of consciousness science. Arch Ital Biol. 2012;150:172–84.

126. Seth AK, Baars BJ, Edelman DB. Criteria for consciousness in humans and other mammals. Conscious Cogn. 2005;14:119–39.

127. Tallon-Baudry C. The roles of gamma-band oscillatory synchrony in human visual cognition. Front Biosci (Landmark Ed). 2009;14:321–32.

128. Uhlhaas PJ, Pipa G, Neuenschwander S, Wibral M, Singer W. A new look at gamma? High- (>60 Hz) gamma-band activity in cortical networks: function, mechanisms and impairment. Prog Biophys Mol Biol. 2011;105:14–28.

129. Breshears JD, Roland JL, Sharma M, Gaona CM, Freudenburg ZV, Tempelhoff R, Avidan MS, Leuthardt EC. Stable and dynamic cortical electrophysiology of induction and emergence with propofol anesthesia. Proc Natl Acad Sci U S A. 2010;107:21170–5.

130. Hudetz AG, Vizuete JA, Pillay S. Differential effects of isoflurane on high-frequency and low-frequency gamma oscillations in the cerebral cortex and hippocampus in freely moving rats. Anesthesiology. 2011;114:588–95.

131. Dehaene S, Changeux JP. Ongoing spontaneous activity controls access to consciousness: a neuronal model for inattentional blindness. PLoS Biol. 2005;3, e141.

132. Lamme VA. Towards a true neural stance on consciousness. Trends Cogn Sci. 2006;10:494–501.

133. Tononi G. Consciousness as integrated information: a provisional manifesto. Biol Bull. 2008;215:216–42.

134. Lamme VA, Zipser K, Spekreijse H. Figure-ground activity in primary visual cortex is suppressed by anesthesia. Proc Natl Acad Sci U S A. 1998;95:3263–8.

135. Baars BJ. The conscious access hypothesis: origins and recent evidence. Trends Cogn Sci. 2002;6:47–52.

136. Gaillard R, Dehaene S, Adam C, Clemenceau S, Hasboun D, Baulac M, Cohen L, Naccache L. Converging intracranial markers of conscious access. PLoS Biol. 2009;7, e61.

137. Dehaene S, Sergent C, Changeux JP. A neuronal network model linking subjective reports and objective physiological data during conscious perception. Proc Natl Acad Sci U S A. 2003;100:8520–5.

138. Tononi G, Edelman GM. Consciousness and complexity. Science. 1998;282:1846–51.

139. Tononi G. An information integration theory of consciousness. BMC Neurosci. 2004;5:42.

140. Mudrik L, Faivre N, Koch C. Information integration without awareness. Trends Cogn Sci. 2014;18:488–96.

141. Hudetz AG, Liu X, Pillay S. Dynamic repertoire of intrinsic brain states is reduced in propofol-induced unconsciousness. Brain Connect. 2015;5:10–22.

142. Lee U, Mashour GA, Kim S, Noh GJ, Choi BM. Propofol induction reduces the capacity for neural information integration: implications for the mechanism of consciousness and general anesthesia. Conscious Cogn. 2009;18:56–64.

143. Schartner M, Seth A, Noirhomme Q, Boly M, Bruno MA, Laureys S, Barrett A. Complexity of multi-dimensional spontaneous EEG decreases during propofol induced general anaesthesia. PLoS One. 2015;10, e0133532.

144. Chennu S, O'Connor S, Adapa R, Menon DK, Bekinschtein TA. Brain connectivity dissociates responsiveness from drug exposure during propofol-induced transitions of consciousness. PLoS Comput Biol. 2016;12, e1004669.

145. John ER. A field theory of consciousness. Conscious Cogn. 2001;10:184–213.

146. Srinivasan R, Russell DP, Edelman GM, Tononi G. Increased synchronization of neuromagnetic responses during conscious perception. J Neurosci. 1999;19:5435–48.

147. Hameroff SR. The entwined mysteries of anesthesia and consciousness: is there a common underlying mechanism? Anesthesiology. 2006;105:400–12.

148. Libet B. Do the models offer testable proposals of brain functions for conscious experience? Adv Neurol. 1998;77:213–7.

149. Seth AK, Dienes Z, Cleeremans A, Overgaard M, Pessoa L. Measuring consciousness: relating behavioural and neurophysiological approaches. Trends Cogn Sci. 2008;12:314–21.

Mechanisms of Intravenous Anesthetic Action

5

Hugh C. Hemmings Jr. and Karl F. Herold

Summary

General anesthesia consists of key separable and independent neurobiological end points. Each of these involves distinct but possibly overlapping neuroanatomical and molecular mechanisms that converge to produce the characteristic behavioral end points of anesthesia: amnesia, unconsciousness, and immobility. The potency of various structurally dissimilar general anesthetics correlates with their solubilities in oil (lipophilicity), consistent with critical interactions with hydrophobic molecular targets. The pharmacologically relevant binding sites of general anesthetics are lipophilic cavities in proteins identified by a combination of site-directed mutagenesis and high-resolution structural analysis of anesthetic binding. Specific point mutations render putative target proteins insensitive to certain general anesthetics. Expression of these mutations in mice reduces anesthetic potency for specific end points.

The actions of various general anesthetics cannot be explained by a single molecular mechanism. Rather, multiple targets contribute to each component in an agent-specific manner. Major classes of general anesthetics include inhaled and intravenous anesthetics; the latter are more potent and possess more selective actions. Anesthetic-induced immobility involves primarily actions in the spinal cord, whereas sedation, unconsciousness, and amnesia involve supraspinal mechanisms, including endogenous memory, sleep, and consciousness networks.

H.C. Hemmings Jr., MD, PhD, FRCA (✉)
Department of Anesthesiology and Pharmacology, Weill Cornell Medical College, New York, NY, USA
e-mail: hchemmi@med.cornell.edu

K.F. Herold, MD, PhD
Department of Anesthesiology, Weill Cornell Medical College, New York, NY, USA
e-mail: kah2016@med.cornell.edu

Etomidate and propofol enhance inhibitory synaptic transmission postsynaptically and tonic inhibition extrasynaptically by potentiating ligand-gated ion channels activated by γ-aminobutyric acid (GABA). Ketamine suppresses excitatory synaptic transmission postsynaptically by inhibiting excitatory ionotropic NMDA-subtype glutamate receptors. Benzodiazepines and α_{2A} adrenergic receptor agonists (dexmedetomidine, clonidine) are not complete general anesthetics but are potent sedative agents that act by specific receptor-mediated mechanisms to produce sedation and anxiolysis.

Our understanding of the molecular, cellular, and network mechanisms of general anesthetics has made remarkable progress in the last 35 years. We now know that general anesthetics interact with membrane proteins critical to neuronal signaling in the central nervous system to produce the characteristic neurophysiological features that define general anesthesia: amnesia, sedation/unconsciousness, and immobility [1, 2]. Major progress in understanding the pharmacology of the intravenous anesthetics has been made using modern molecular genetic approaches that have identified critical actions at the molecular and cellular levels. Despite this progress, there are still gaps in our understanding of the sequence of events that leads from anesthetic-target interactions at the molecular level to the behavioral effects that characterize the composite state of clinical anesthesia. The focus of this chapter is on the mechanisms involved in the various actions of general anesthetics and sedatives most applicable to total intravenous anesthesia (TIVA), i.e., the intravenous anesthetics and their adjuvants. These agents are a chemically and pharmacologically diverse group (Fig. 5.1) that includes potent anesthetic/hypnotic agents (etomidate, propofol, ketamine) and sedatives (benzodiazepines, α_{2A} adrenergic receptor agonists).

A.R. Absalom, K.P. Mason (eds.), *Total Intravenous Anesthesia and Target Controlled Infusions*,
DOI 10.1007/978-3-319-47609-4_5

Fig. 5.1 Structures and primary molecular targets of representatives of the major classes of general anesthetics and anesthetic adjuvants used in total intravenous anesthesia. Individual elements displayed in the stick figures are represented by the following colors: hydrogen = *white*; carbon = *gray*; nitrogen = *dark blue*; oxygen = *red*; fluorine = *cyan*; chlorine = *green*

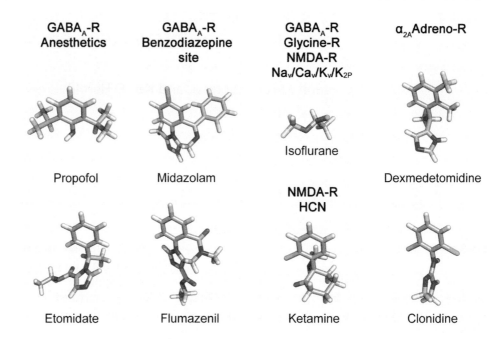

Overview of Molecular General Anesthetic Mechanisms

Ever since the first public demonstration of ether anesthesia in 1846, there has been intense scientific interest in the mechanisms for general anesthesia. The work of Meyer and Overton at the end of the nineteenth century produced the now famous correlation between anesthetic potency and solubility in olive oil, which indicated the hydrophobic (lipid-like) nature of the site(s) of action of a variety of structurally dissimilar anesthetic molecules [3, 4]. This correlation was the basis for early concepts of anesthetic action based on effects on cellular lipid bilayer membranes and led to an early focus of research on anesthetic effects on the physical properties of cell membranes. The appeal of this model of a single unified mechanism to explain anesthesia was its simplicity and ability to explain the actions of multiple structurally dissimilar anesthetics, which is difficult to accommodate using receptor-based pharmacological mechanisms. But research efforts to define how anesthetic interactions with lipid membranes might lead to the behavioral changes observed under anesthesia failed to identify plausible biophysical or neurophysiological mechanisms.

A shift from lipid-based to protein-based mechanisms occurred in the 1980s owing to the pioneering work of Franks and Lieb [5, 6]. They elegantly showed that general anesthetic potencies correlate equally well with both inhibition of firefly luciferase, a physiologically irrelevant soluble enzyme that serves as a lipid-free protein model for anesthetic binding and solubility in oil. This observation led to the paradigm-shifting concept that protein targets are also compatible with the Meyer-Overton correlation, which had a

profound impact on anesthesia research by directing efforts to identify the critical protein targets that underlie the various neurophysiological end points of anesthesia. Additional evidence against lipid-based theories of anesthetic action such as the stereoselectivity of several anesthetics has strengthened the case for specific binding sites on target proteins, in particular ion channels and neurotransmitter receptors [7]. Identification of the ion channels and receptors involved in the various anesthetic end points is a major aspect of current studies to define the pharmacological mechanisms of general anesthesia (Fig. 5.2).

The Composite Nature of the Anesthetic State

Progress in identifying the molecular mechanisms of anesthesia has occurred in parallel with efforts to understand the neurophysiology of the anesthetic state. General anesthetics induce a drug-induced coma-like state. General anesthesia consists of distinct but to some extent overlapping component states that involve separable mechanisms (e.g., amnesia, unconsciousness, immobility). These distinct neuropharmacological end points are mediated through effects on different anatomical regions of the central nervous system (CNS), involve different receptor mechanisms, and vary in relative potencies between specific agents [1]. Immobilization, which is mediated largely at the level of the spinal cord for inhaled anesthetics [8, 9], is supraspinally mediated for barbiturates and probably other intravenous anesthetics [10]. In contrast, amnesia, sedation, and unconsciousness involve supraspinal anesthetic effects on cerebrocortical function. Amnesia and sedation produced by intravenous

Fig. 5.2 Relationship between increasing anesthetic concentration and the observed pharmacological effects. With increasing doses and target-site anesthetic concentrations, desirable end points such as amnesia and loss of consciousness (hypnosis) are joined by various undesirable and off-target side effects, including cardiovascular and respiratory depression, the major cause of morbidity and mortality

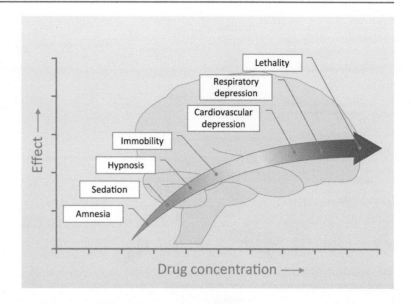

anesthetics can be functionally separated [11]. In patients, propofol and midazolam, for example, impair memory to similar extent when equisedative concentrations were maintained [12]. Yet, they affect memory differentially from effects on sedation, as measured by auditory event-related potentials in patients [11]. This indicates that their effects may be mediated by specific neuroanatomical areas that are not exclusive for one particular drug. Unconsciousness is itself heterogeneous, with distinct states of responsiveness and unconsciousness [13]. The composite pharmacology of general anesthesia consists of multiple distinct components that can be resolved both experimentally and clinically. Considerable evidence supports the notion that each component of anesthesia can be selectively induced in a dose- and agent-specific manner through distinct cellular, molecular, and network mechanisms in specific regions of the brain and spinal cord.

The regional specificity has been elegantly demonstrated for a number of intravenous anesthetics have been demonstrated using anatomically discrete brain microinjections of extremely small volumes of anesthetics and receptor antagonists. Microinjection of the anesthetic barbiturate pentobarbital into the mesopontine tegmentum induces a comatose state in rats very similar to general anesthesia, an example of the anatomical specificity of anesthetic actions that can result in generalized nervous system depression [14]. Microinjections of $GABA_A$ receptor antagonists into the tuberomammillary nucleus, a hypothalamic nucleus involved in the regulation of natural sleep, reverse the sedation produced by systemic administration of propofol [15]. In fact the α_{2A} adrenergic receptor agonist dexmedetomidine causes the two distinct states of sedation and loss of righting reflex (LORR) via two different brain regions, the preoptic hypothalamic area and the locus coeruleus (LC), respectively.

The effects of dexmedetomidine on loss of righting reflex were abolished upon selective α_{2A} adrenoreceptor knockdown in rodents, yet sedative effects were still observed [16]. These are examples of how intravenous anesthetics can produce certain substates of general anesthesia through agent-specific actions at discrete anatomic sites mediated by specific molecular targets. The implications of this anatomic and receptor specificity of anesthetic actions provide the scientific basis for the development of more specific drugs targeting the anesthetic substates.

The pharmacology of sedation is complex, with multiple drugs with distinct neuropharmacological profiles able to produce a state of sedation involving a number of distinct mechanisms (Chap. 4). In addition to lower doses of general anesthetics that produce sedation as part of their progressive dose-dependent effects, other drugs capable of producing sedation include α_{2A} adrenoceptor agonists, antimuscarinics, antihistamines, benzodiazepines, opioids, and ethanol, each with distinct pharmacokinetic and side effect profiles including respiratory and cardiovascular depression. Like general anesthesia, there is a continuum of sedation from anxiolysis to mild sedation, through deep sedation, to anesthesia, and eventually undesired toxicities, with distinct but overlapping agent-specific pharmacological mechanisms. In addition to their desired effects of amnesia, sedation, and hypnosis, all anesthetics have additional undesired side effects such as those summarized for the major drugs used for TIVA in Fig. 5.3. Individual drugs can even show opposing effects, which are thought to be mediated by distinct mechanisms. Dexmedetomidine, for example, causes hypotension at lower doses mainly due to inhibition of the sympathetic autonomic nervous system mediated by α_{2A} adrenoceptors, whereas at higher concentrations [17], activation of vascular α_{2B} adrenoceptors dominates resulting in a hypertensive response [18].

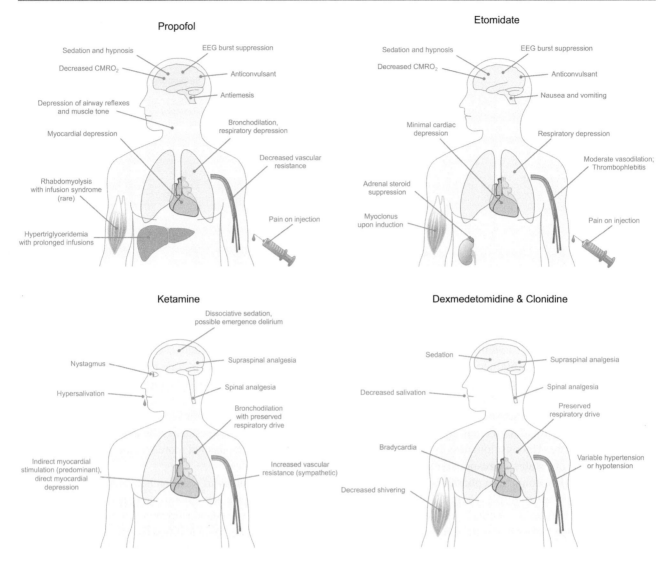

Fig. 5.3 Prominent effects and undesirable side effects of propofol, etomidate, ketamine, and the α_{2A} adrenoceptor agonists dexmedetomidine and clonidine. *CMRO$_2$* cerebral metabolic rate for oxygen, *EEG* electroencephalography

Integrated Effects on Central Nervous System Function

Immobility

Electroencephalography (EEG), a widely used monitor of brain activity, is used both in the study of anesthetic mechanisms and as a monitor of the depth of anesthesia (see Chap. 19). The lack of a correlation between electroencephalographic (cortical) activity and immobility (lack of movement in response to a noxious stimulus) is the basis for the current concept that immobility is mediated by anesthetic action primarily on the spinal cord rather than the cerebral cortex [19]. The finding that volatile anesthetics act on the spinal cord to suppress movement [8, 9] was important in the contemporary separation of anesthetic substates, of which immobility generally requires the highest drug concentrations (Fig. 5.2). Since the identification of the spinal cord as the principal site of anesthetic-induced immobility, attention has turned to the pharmacologic, genetic, and complex network mechanisms involved. A pharmacologic approach to investigate the receptors mediating anesthetic-induced immobility has led to the unanticipated finding that potentiation of GABA$_A$ receptors, an important target for many general anesthetics, is not involved in isoflurane-mediated immobility [20]. Propofol produces immobility through actions on the spinal cord as well. But unlike isoflurane, it does not depress dorsal horn activity upon noxious stimulation. Both anesthetics depress ventral horn neurons, though isoflurane to a larger extent than propofol. Interestingly the GABA$_A$ receptor inhibitor picrotoxin reverses the effects of propofol, but not isoflurane, to depress ventral horn neurons [21]. This apparent effect of propofol to produce immobility via GABAergic mechanisms in the ventral horn is in contrast to volatile anesthetics like isoflurane. The immobilizing effects of propofol are likely to be mediated by different regions of the nervous system than its sedative effects, due to actions in the tuberomammillary nucleus of the hypothalamus, for example [15]. However, a role for voltage-gated Na^+ channels was supported by the observations that intrathecal administration of the highly selective Na^+ channel inhibitor tetrodotoxin potentiates volatile anesthetic-induced immobility (reduces MAC), while the Na^+ channel activator veratridine does the opposite [22]. Transgenic mice engineered to express anesthetic-resistant $GABA_A$ receptor subunits showed that receptors containing α_1- or α_3-subunits do not contribute to the immobilizing action of isoflurane [23, 24]. While mice lacking the K^+ channels TASK-1, TASK-3, or TREK-1 K_{2P} channels are less sensitive to volatile anesthetics, their sensitivities to intravenous anesthetics is unaltered [25–27]. These findings suggest important roles for voltage-gated Na^+ and K^+ channels rather than $GABA_A$ receptors in spinally mediated immobility [28]. Anesthetic inhibition of afferent (noxious sensory) input to the spinal cord dorsal horn appears to play a subordinate role to the suppression of efferent (motor) output from the ventral horn, which is coordinated by neuronal networks organized in central pattern generators that control the activity of the cholinergic motoneurons [29].

Unconsciousness

Consciousness is easy to recognize but difficult to define neuroscientifically; it is a qualitative subjective state of sentience or awareness [30]. Loss of consciousness (or hypnosis) is a key feature of anesthesia. In addition to their clinical utility in ablating consciousness, anesthetic drugs provide essential tools for elucidating the central problem in neuroscience of scientifically defining consciousness by providing a pharmacological means to reversibly produce unconsciousness that can be used to facilitate identification of the neural correlates of consciousness [31]. The unconsciousness produced by anesthetics can be described as unresponsiveness to include states of awareness that lack explicit memory traces [13]. The study of consciousness has generated intense interest leading to a number of both testable and untestable hypotheses. One hypothesis of anesthesia proposes that somatosensory deafferentation in the thalamus is a mechanism for anesthetic-induced unconsciousness [32], which is supported by evidence that anesthetics can hyperpolarize and shunt thalamic neurons [33] and thereby impair thalamic transfer of sensory

information [34]. Functional brain imaging that shows preferential suppression of thalamic activity by some anesthetics has led to a thalamic switch hypothesis [32]. However, anesthetic-induced unconsciousness appears to involve more than a simple block of information transfer through the thalamus [35, 36].

Previous views of an anatomically discrete brain structure as the center of consciousness have given rise to the current concept that consciousness requires integration of information between multiple brain regions across large-scale neural networks [35, 37]. The rich connectivity of the cerebral cortex and its hierarchical organization enable extensive information integration in the brain. Highly connected nodes are preferentially interconnected, which is optimal for information integration [38, 39], and these pathways are promising targets for the hypnotic action of anesthetics. Recent evidence supports the view that anesthetics interfere with network synchronicity and coherence, and disruption of cortical functional and effective connectivity has been observed during midazolam-induced loss of responsiveness [40]. Thus breakdown of cortical connectivity rather than thalamic deafferentation might underlie loss of consciousness [41]. Unconsciousness would then be characterized by the fragmentation of cortical processing [35, 42]. Cortical electrical activity in the γ-band (40–90 Hz by EEG) has been proposed as a network-level target of general anesthetics [43–45].

Learning and Memory

Anterograde amnesia is a desirable anesthetic end point, particularly in the realm of preoperative and procedural sedation. It is produced at lower anesthetic concentrations than those required for unconsciousness and is a prominent action of benzodiazepines [46]. It can be measured in rodents using models of hippocampus-dependent spatial learning such as fear conditioning to place context or hippocampus-independent models such as fear conditioning to tone. Isoflurane disrupts hippocampus-dependent learning at about one-half the concentration necessary for disrupting hippocampus-independent learning [41]. Similarly, lower anesthetic concentrations inhibit explicit memory (memory that can be explicitly recalled) at lower doses than required to impair implicit memory (not subject to wilful recollection) [36]. These findings implicate the medial temporal lobe, including the hippocampus, as a target for the suppression of explicit memory by anesthetics, while effects on the amygdala are relevant to anesthetic impairment of implicit or other types of memory [47].

Evidence indicates that θ-rhythms (4–12 Hz by EEG) are important for hippocampus-dependent learning and memory [48]. Benzodiazepines [49] slow and suppress hippocampal θ-rhythms proportional to their impairment of hippocampus-dependent learning such that alterations in neuronal synchrony are a common network-level substrate for memory impairment. Synchronization between θ-rhythms in the amygdala and hippocampus during fear memory retrieval indicates that this mechanism also applies to impairment of other forms of memory by anesthetics [50]. The precise molecular and cellular mechanisms of memory impairment by general anesthetics and benzodiazepines, and of memory itself, remain to be elucidated, as with other components of anesthesia such as unconsciousness and sedation.

Sedation

Sedation is a decrease in activity, alertness, arousal, and/or vigilance on a behavioral continuum leading to hypnosis and can be achieved at anesthetic doses similar to those that produce amnesia. While there is no clear mechanistic or clinical separation between sedation and hypnosis, separate but overlapping substrates appear to separate sedation from amnesia [11, 51]. Genetic approaches have been particularly useful in dissecting the targets for benzodiazepine-induced sedation and amnesia and prove a paradigm for studying other more promiscuous drugs. A specific amino acid mutation (H101R) in the α_1 GABA$_A$ receptor subunit that eliminates sensitivity to modulation by benzodiazepines renders mice resistant to both the sedative and amnesic effects of benzodiazepines while maintaining other behavioral effects, among them anxiolysis [52]. The α_1-subunit is highly expressed in the CNS including the cerebrocortical areas and thalamus.

There is more than a superficial similarity between natural sleep and anesthetic-induced sedation and hypnosis, and the mechanisms of some anesthetics overlap natural sleep mechanisms through activation of known sleep-promoting nuclei in the hypothalamus [15]. The electroencephalographic patterns of natural slow-wave sleep resemble those of general anesthesia, consistent with similar effects on global cortical electrical activity [53]. Interestingly, recovery from sleep deprivation can occur during propofol anesthesia [54], providing further support for this concept. Anesthetic effects on other cortical [55] and subcortical structures [13] might also contribute to anesthetic-induced sedation and hypnosis. It is evident that sedative effects of intravenous anesthetics involve activation of GABA$_A$ receptors which results not necessarily in a general depression of the whole nervous system but rather actions on specific neuronal pathways in the hypothalamus (GABA$_A$ receptors in the tuberomammillary nucleus, TMN) that are associated with non-REM sleep as it has been shown for propofol and pentobarbital [15]. The TMN is of particular interest as animal experiments revealed that local injection of the GABA$_A$ receptor agonist muscimol into the TMN lead to a sedative state, but when injected into other brain regions such as the locus coeruleus or other sites in close proximity to the TMN, no such sedation was observed [15]. In addition, injection of the GABA$_A$ receptor antagonist gabazine attenuated the sedative effects of systemically administered GABAergic anesthetics.

Anesthetic Neurotoxicity

Early Postnatal Neurotoxicity

Extensive data from animal experiments indicate that multiple general anesthetics can cause persistent neurocognitive effects in neonatal animals of multiple species in addition to their desired effect of reversible anesthesia. This correlates with a discreet developmental sensitivity to both GABA$_A$ receptor potentiating and NMDA receptor-inhibiting anesthetics resulting in widespread programmed cell death known as apoptosis, which is probably due to a form of excitotoxicity (Chap. 45). This has generated significant concern among clinicians and parents, but its clinical significance remains unknown [56–63]. The landmark finding that postnatal exposure of the developing rodent brain to a cocktail of commonly used anesthetic drugs, either in combination or alone, for a period of several hours induced apoptotic cell death with long-term functional consequences identified this potentially harmful effect of general anesthesia in neonates [58]. Similar effects have been reproduced with all the commonly used general anesthetic drugs including propofol, ketamine, barbiturates, etomidate, and volatile anesthetics in species from rodents to nonhuman primates [64, 65]. Of interest, the α_{2A} adrenergic receptor agonist dexmedetomidine is not associated with neurotoxicity but rather can mitigate the toxic effects of other neurotoxic drugs such as propofol in animal experiments [66]. Translation of these findings, both quantitatively and qualitatively, from short-lived altricial (e.g., rodents) to long-lived precocial (e.g., *Homo sapiens*) species is difficult, but the convincing evidence for long-term neurocognitive deficits in nonhuman primates raises considerable concerns [67]. Environmental and pharmacological approaches to mitigating these effects provide strategies for minimizing the potential clinical impact of developmental neurotoxicity and are a current topic of active research [68].

Postoperative Cognitive Effects

Adverse postoperative cognitive effects following general anesthesia and surgery can result from predictable pharmacokinetic factors as well as unanticipated and poorly understood persistent pharmacological and toxic effects. Three recognized clinical entities occurring after anesthesia and surgery include delirium, dementia, and postoperative cognitive dysfunction (POCD). Delirium and dementia are defined clinical diagnoses, while POCD is not a clinical diagnosis but a phenomenon identified by comparing preoperative with postoperative neuropsychological test scores in surgical patients with matched control populations that did not undergo surgery. Based on these criteria, the incidence of POCD increases with age and underlying disease severity and frailty, but diagnosis is difficult and prone to artifacts. In contrast, delirium and dementia are more readily diagnosed by established criteria. Delirium is relatively common after anesthesia and is associated with a number of risk factors including age, preoperative cognitive impairment, use of volatile anesthetics in combination with other CNS-active drugs, as well as tracheal intubation [69, 70]. Recent clinical trials comparing the incidence of delirium in sedated ICU patients found a higher incidence of delirium with sedation achieved with propofol or benzodiazepines compared with dexmedetomidine [71].

Durable effects of inhaled anesthetics have been linked to memory deficits persisting for days in young adult mice through effects on the α_5-subunit of the $GABA_A$ receptor [72]. Moreover, immune and inflammation-mediated changes triggered by surgical trauma and anesthesia are potential mechanisms that underlie delirium and postoperative cognitive dysfunction [73, 74]. Experimental evidence from mice genetically susceptible to Alzheimer's disease-like neurodegeneration does not support a role of anesthetic agents in promoting such neurodegeneration [75]. These findings provide experimental support for clinical observations that cognitive decline after surgery is likely mediated by neuroinflammation rather than due to accelerated neurodegeneration or anesthetic neurotoxicity, although this is controversial and an active area of investigation [76]. The underlying disease trajectory rather than anesthesia or surgery is the major contributor to the long-term cognitive course of most patients [77].

Effects on the Cardiovascular and Respiratory Systems

Cardiovascular Effects

Cardiovascular function, like that of the CNS, depends on the integrated function of multiple ion channels, many of which are expressed in both of these excitable tissues. The cardiovascular effects of the general anesthetics are often deleterious side effects that limit the safety of these drugs, particularly in the critically ill, but there are also beneficial cardioprotective effects [78]. Most anesthetics produce agent- and dose-dependent reductions in myocardial contractility, systemic vascular resistance, and cardiac preload, with consequent reduction in mean arterial pressure, with agent-specific differences in relative potencies between cardiac and anesthetic effects [79]. Major targets for negative inotropic effects of anesthetics include blockade of cardiac Ca^{2+} channels (L-type; Ca_v1), sarcoplasmic Ca^{2+} handling, and the contractile protein apparatus. The resulting negative inotropic effect of reduced Ca^{2+} availability is enhanced by reduced Ca^{2+} sensitivity of myofibrils. Most anesthetics also produce vasodilation at clinical concentrations mediated both by direct endothelium-independent vasodilating effects on vascular smooth muscle cells (e.g., inhibition of smooth muscle Ca^{2+} influx via L-type Ca^{2+} channels, activation of hyperpolarizing K_{ATP} and K_{Ca} channels) and by indirect effects involving the sympathetic nervous system and the vascular endothelium (e.g., endothelium-dependent effects including nitric oxide production) [80].

General anesthetics also have agent-specific effects on heart rate and induction of arrhythmias due to actions on cardiac ion channels. Multiple ion channels are sensitive to anesthetics, many of which are potentially proarrhythmic. It is difficult to link anesthetic arrhythmogenicity to actions on specific channels [81]. Cardiac L-type Ca^{2+} channels are critical to the plateau phase of the cardiac action potential and electromechanical coupling and are inhibited by many anesthetics, leading to shortening of the refractory period. Multiple voltage-gated K^+ channels are also inhibited and can predispose to arrhythmias by delaying repolarization (see review by Thompson and Balser [82]).

Respiratory Effects

General anesthetics can cause significant respiratory depression at the concentrations used for surgical anesthesia, as well as potentially clinically significant effects at lower concentrations. These effects are significantly magnified when used concomitantly with other respiratory depressants such as opioids and benzodiazepines. The peripheral chemoreflexes and upper airway patency are particularly sensitive to subanesthetic concentrations of anesthetics [83–87]. These potentially serious effects involve depression of central respiratory networks mediated by depression of excitatory and facilitation of inhibitory transmission in the brainstem. The precise molecular targets responsible for the exquisite sensitivity of these networks to low concentrations of anesthetics remain to be elucidated. Ketamine and dexmedetomidine are unique in their lack of significant respiratory depression at clinically used concentrations [88, 89].

Molecular Sites of Anesthetic Action

Pharmacological Criteria for Identifying Sites Relevant to Anesthesia

As a result of the low potency and consequent promiscuity of most general anesthetics, specific criteria have been proposed to evaluate the relevance of the many potential molecular targets of anesthetics [90]. These criteria include inter alia reversibility, sensitivity (effects at clinically relevant concentrations), plausibility (target expression in relevant tissue or CNS region), cognate stereoselectivity for in vivo and in vitro effects of steroisomeric anesthetics (etomidate, pentobarbital, and neurosteroid anesthetics), appropriate sensitivity or insensitivity to model anesthetic and nonanesthetic compounds, and predictable responses to genetic manipulation of putative molecular targets. Targeted deletion (knockout mutation) of specific molecules implicated as anesthetic targets or genetic engineering to introduce specific mutations that modify anesthetic sensitivity (knock-in mutation) in experimental models is a powerful approach to test the involvement in anesthetic action. This approach has been particularly successful in analyzing the specific $GABA_A$ receptor subtypes involved in the effects of the GABAergic intravenous anesthetics propofol and etomidate and the sedative and amnesic effects of benzodiazepines where single amino acid substitutions in specific receptor subtypes eliminate specific drug actions both in vitro and in vivo [91] (see below).

From Model Proteins to Receptors

A variety of biophysical data derived from X-ray crystallography, molecular modeling, and structure function studies supports the concept that general anesthetics produce their cellular effects by binding in hydrophobic cavities formed in the three-dimensional structure of proteins, in particular membrane proteins [92, 93]. The lipophilic nature of these binding sites underlies the Meyer-Overton correlation between anesthetic potency and lipophilicity. The identification of anesthetic binding sites on plausible target proteins that meet the criteria outlined above is difficult due to the low affinity of most anesthetic-target protein interactions, the small number of high-resolution atomic structures of pharmacologically relevant target proteins, and the absence of potent and specific antagonists of anesthesia. Anesthetic binding sites identified in well-characterized model proteins for which three-dimensional atomic resolution structures are available but which are not themselves relevant to anesthesia, such as luciferase and albumin [92, 93], indicate that anesthetics bind in pockets with both nonpolar and polar noncovalent chemical interactions. Occupation of these cavities by anesthetics provides a mechanism for alteration of receptor and ion channel function by selective stabilization of particular confirmations. Convincing evidence supports the existence of anesthetic binding sites in critical neuronal signaling proteins including glycine, $GABA_A$, and NMDA receptors [93]. Amino acid residues critical for anesthetic actions and, by inference, binding have been identified in the α-subunit of the $GABA_A$ receptor [93] and NMDA receptor [94].

Structural studies using prokaryotic homologues of eukaryotic ion channels provide powerful models for identifying anesthetic binding sites in physiologically relevant proteins. Both propofol and desflurane have been co-crystalized with GLIC, a bacterial homologue of eukaryotic inhibitory ligand-gated ion channels (glycine and $GABA_A$ receptors). Both anesthetics bind in the upper part of the transmembrane segments of a single subunit (Fig. 5.4)

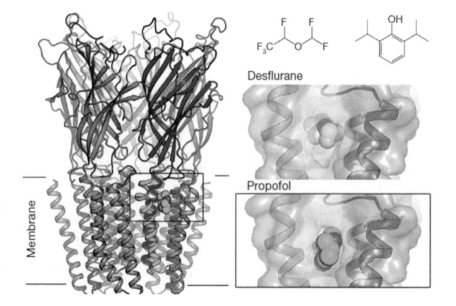

Fig. 5.4 X-ray crystal structures of propofol and desflurane bound to a pentameric ligand-gated ion channel. Membrane plane view of the bacterial homologue of mammalian pentameric ligand-gated ion channels (*Gloeobacter violaceus* or GLIC) with a bound general anesthetic molecule. From Nury H, et al., X-ray structure of general anesthetics bound to a pentameric ligand-gated ion channel (Reproduced from Nury et al. [95] with permission from Nature Publishing Group)

[95]. Molecular modeling has also been used to identify putative anesthetic binding sites in $GABA_A$ and glycine receptors, which suggests that different drugs can bind in different orientations within a single cavity or occupy different cavities within the protein to produce similar functional effects. Refinement of these molecular models will continue to provide new insights in the molecular basis for general anesthetic action that can be experimentally tested.

Molecular Targets of General Anesthetics

Ion channels have emerged as the most promising molecular targets for general anesthetics. The neurotransmitter-gated ion channels $GABA_A$, glycine, and NMDA-type glutamate receptors are leading candidates with appropriate CNS distributions, essential roles in inhibitory or excitatory synaptic transmission, and appropriate sensitivity to clinically relevant concentrations [1, 2]. Other ion channels that are sensitive to inhaled anesthetics include the HCN (hyperpolarization-activated cyclic nucleotide-gated) family of channels that give rise to pacemaker currents [2] and regulate neuronal excitability, two-pore domain (K_{2P}) K^+ channels that maintain resting membrane potential in many cells [96], and voltage-gated Na^+ and Ca^{2+} channels [2, 97].

General anesthetics can be divided into two broad classes based on their distinct pharmacologic properties. The first class exhibits positive modulation of $GABA_A$ receptors and includes both the potent inhaled (volatile) anesthetics, which also produce significant effects on a number of other plausible receptors/channels and intravenous anesthetics such as propofol and etomidate that represent more potent and specific positive modulators of $GABA_A$ receptors. The second class is inactive at $GABA_A$ receptors, but inhibits NMDA receptors, and includes the gaseous inhaled anesthetics cyclopropane, nitrous oxide, and xenon, as well as the intravenous anesthetic ketamine. These anesthetics also activate certain K_{2P} channels.

Ligand-Gated Ion Channels

Potentiation of Inhibitory $GABA_A$ and Glycine Receptors

Most intravenous anesthetics (including propofol, etomidate, barbiturates), all ether anesthetics (including isoflurane, sevoflurane, and desflurane), the alkane anesthetic halothane, and the neurosteroid anesthetics enhance the function of the inhibitory $GABA_A$ (Fig. 5.5) and glycine receptors (GlyRs). These belong to the Cys-loop ligand-gated ion channel superfamily that also includes the cation-permeable nicotinic acetylcholine and $5HT_3$ receptors. $GABA_A$ receptors are the principal transmitter-gated Cl^- channels in the brain and GlyRs in the spinal cord, with overlap in the diencephalon and brainstem. When activated

by ligand or drug binding, these ligand-gated ion channels conduct chloride which drives the membrane potential toward the Cl^- equilibrium potential, resulting in inhibition since the Cl^- equilibrium potential is usually more negative than the normal resting potential. Channel opening also reduces membrane resistance and "shunts" excitatory responses. Most $GABA_A$ and GlyRs are heteropentamers; the specific subunit composition of $GABA_A$ receptors determines their physiologic and pharmacologic properties and can vary between brain and neuronal compartments [98], for example, preferential expression of the α_5-subunit in the hippocampal CA1 area (a region important for memory formation) and extrasynaptic sites. The presence of a γ-subunit is required for benzodiazepine modulation of $GABA_A$ receptors. These receptors have been key to our understanding of anesthetic-receptor interactions. Using chimeric receptor constructs between anesthetic-sensitive $GABA_A$ and insensitive GlyR subunits, specific amino acid residues in transmembrane domains 2 and 3 critical to the action of inhaled anesthetics have been identified [99]. This laid the groundwork for the construction of anesthetic-resistant $GABA_A$ receptors and the generation of transgenic mice with altered anesthetic sensitivity (see below).

Inhibition of Excitatory Acetylcholine and Glutamate Receptors

Neuronal nicotinic acetylcholine receptors are cation selective heteropentameric ligand-gated ion channels that are also members of the Cys-loop family. Although usually heteropentamers composed of α- and β-subunits, functional homomeric receptors are formed by certain α-subunits. In the CNS, these receptors are localized primarily presynaptically [100], and homomeric α_7-receptors are highly permeable to Ca^{2+} [100]. Receptors consisting of $\alpha_4\beta_2$ subunits are very sensitive to inhibition by propofol and isoflurane [101, 102] which might contribute to amnesia.

The NMDA (N-methyl-D-aspartate) subtype of ionotropic glutamate receptors is a major postsynaptic receptor for glutamate, the principal excitatory neurotransmitter in the mammalian CNS [103]. NMDA receptors are defined pharmacologically by their selective activation by the agonist NMDA and exist as heteromers consisting of GluN1 and GluN2 subunits. Channel gating requires the agonist glutamate (or a synthetic agonist like NMDA) along with the endogenous co-agonist glycine; concomitant membrane depolarization is required to relieve voltage-dependent block by Mg^{2+}, which is typically provided by glutamate activation of non-NMDA glutamate receptors, which are subdivided into AMPA and kainate receptors based again on their sensitivities to selective exogenous agonists [103]. This requirement for both presynaptic glutamate release and postsynaptic depolarization allows NMDA receptors to

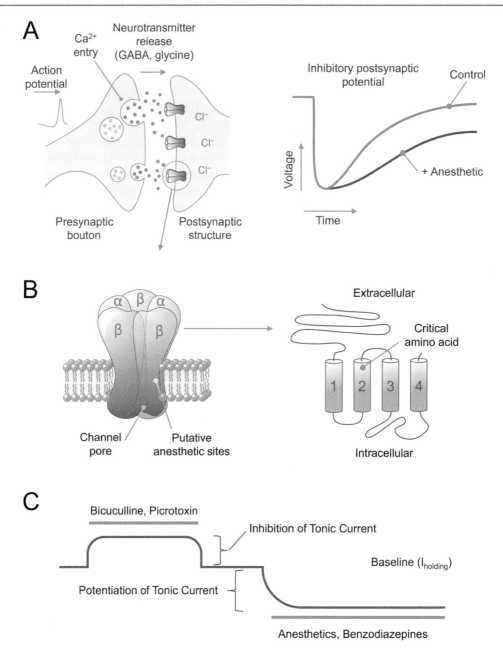

Fig. 5.5 Effects of intravenous anesthetics on inhibitory transmission. (a) A synapse in which an incoming action potential leads to Ca^{2+} influx and subsequent exocytosis of neurotransmitters (GABA, glycine, *blue dots*) into the synaptic cleft. Upon binding, pentameric postsynaptic GABA$_A$—or glycine receptors—are activated, and influx of Cl$^-$ through the channel pore leads to hyperpolarization of the postsynaptic neuron. *Right*: Intravenous anesthetics increase ionic current flowing through the pore enhancing postsynaptic inhibition. (b) A heteropentameric GABA$_A$ receptor complex with channel pore through which Cl$^-$ ions flow into the cell, with putative anesthetic binding sites in the transmembrane region. *Right*: Schematic of a single β-subunit

with four (1–4) transmembrane segments connected by extracellular and intracellular linkers. The critical anesthetic binding sites are thought to be located in transmembrane segment 2 (TM2). (c) Extrasynaptic GABA$_A$ receptors, in contrast to synaptic GABA$_A$ receptors, usually contain a δ-subunit and are highly sensitive to GABA, thus contributing to tonic inhibition from the low levels of ambient extrasynaptic GABA. They are highly sensitive to general anesthetics are candidate targets for intravenous anesthetics. Tonic inhibition is decreased (=depolarisation) by specific GABA$_A$ receptor inhibitors (bicuculline, picrotoxin) and increased (hyperpolarization) by intravenous anesthetics and benzodiazepines

function as coincidence detectors, which is thought to be critical to cellular mechanisms of synaptic plasticity in learning and memory. Given this role in synaptic plasticity, NMDA receptors are also involved in chronic

pain mechanisms. Ketamine, along with the inhaled anesthetics xenon, nitrous oxide, and cyclopropane, have minimal effects on GABA$_A$ receptors but depress excitatory glutamatergic synaptic transmission postsynaptically via NMDA glutamate receptor blockade, which is central to their neurodepressive effects (Fig. 5.3) [104, 105].

Voltage-Gated and Other Ion Channels

Voltage-gated Na$^+$ channels are critical to axonal conduction, synaptic integration, and neuronal excitability. Isoflurane and other volatile anesthetics, but not xenon or most intravenous anesthetics, inhibit the major mammalian Na$^+$ channel isoforms, including neuronal (Na$_v$1.2), skeletal muscle (Na$_v$1.4), cardiac (Na$_v$1.5), and peripheral (Na$_v$1.8) isoforms [106–110].

Multiple cellular functions depend on the tightly controlled concentration of intracellular-free Ca^{2+} ([Ca^{2+}]$_i$). This is determined largely by the activities of voltage-gated Ca^{2+} channels, plasma membrane and endoplasmic reticulum Ca^{2+}-ATPases (pumps), Na$^+$/Ca^{2+} exchangers, and mitochondrial Ca^{2+} uptake. Alteration of any of these mechanisms by anesthetics can affect the multiple processes regulated by Ca^{2+}, including synaptic transmission, gene expression, excitotoxicity, and muscle excitation-contraction coupling. Distinct Ca^{2+} channel subtypes are differentially expressed and are classified both pharmacologically and functionally as low voltage-activated (LVA; T-type) and high voltage-activated (HVA; L-, N-, R-, and P/Q-type) channels. The molecular identity of their pore-forming α-subunits is now widely used for classification [111]. Volatile anesthetics as well as higher concentrations of certain intravenous anesthetics inhibit certain Ca^{2+} channel isoforms but not others [112].

Ca^{2+} channel inhibition is an important contributor to the negative inotropic effects of volatile anesthetics and certain intravenous anesthetics prominent at higher doses. Negative inotropic effects of volatile anesthetics are mediated by reductions in Ca^{2+} availability, Ca^{2+} sensitivity of myofibril proteins, and cytosolic Ca^{2+} clearance. Volatile anesthetics reduce the Ca^{2+} transient and shorten action potential duration in cardiomyocytes by inhibiting L-type (Ca$_v$1.2) Ca^{2+} currents, resulting in a negative inotropic effect and arrhythmogenicity [81, 113, 114], in contrast to xenon which does not depress myocardial function or inhibit L-type Ca^{2+}, Na$^+$, or K$^+$ currents [115, 116]. Inhibition of Ca^{2+} currents in canine myocardial cells was greater with the intravenous anesthetic propofol as compared to etomidate, suggesting agent-specific effects of intravenous anesthetics on cardiac function [117].

Potassium (K$^+$) channels belong to a diverse ion channel family and regulate electrical excitability, muscle contractility, and neurotransmitter release. Given the large diversity in K$^+$ channel structure, function, and anesthetic sensitivity, there is considerable diversity in their sensitivity and response to anesthetics [118]: from relatively insensitive (voltage-gated K$^+$) [119] to sensitive (some members of the two-pore domain K$^+$ channels [K$_{2P}$] family), resulting in either inhibition, activation, or no effect on K$^+$ currents. Volatile anesthetic activation of certain "leak" K$^+$ channels was first observed in the snail Lymnaea [120], although the molecular identity of the affected ion channels was unknown. Activation of K$_{2P}$ channels by volatile and gaseous anesthetics, including xenon, nitrous oxide, and cyclopropane, was subsequently observed in mammals [121]. Increased K$^+$ conductance can hyperpolarize neurons, reducing responsiveness to excitatory synaptic input and possibly altering network synchrony. Targeted deletion of the TASK-1, TASK-3, and TREK-1 K$_{2P}$ channels in mice reduces sensitivity to immobilization by volatile anesthetics in an agent-specific manner, implicating these channels as contributory anesthetic targets in vivo [25–27]. Other members of this large family of K$^+$ channels are also sensitive volatile anesthetics [122].

Volatile anesthetics also inhibit HCN "pacemaker" channels, reducing the rate of rise of pacemaker potentials and the bursting frequency of certain neurons showing autorhythmicity. They decrease the I_h conductance in neurons [123] and modulate recombinant HCN1 and HCN2 channel isoforms at clinically relevant concentrations [124]. Because HCN channels contribute to resting membrane potential, control action potential firing, dendritic integration, neuronal automaticity, and temporal summation, and determine periodicity and synchronization of oscillations in many neuronal networks [125], the anesthetic modulation of these channels could play an important role in anesthetic effects on neuronal integrative functions.

Cellular Mechanisms

Neuronal Excitability

Neuronal excitability depends on a number of interrelated factors such as resting membrane potential, threshold for action potential initiation, and input resistance. These are determined by the regional, cellular, and subcellular expression and activity of various ion channels and receptors and thus can vary between compartments within a neuron. Neurons are very diverse, and thus anesthetic effects can vary not only between neuronal populations but also with the neurophysiological state of the neuron, such as its resting membrane potential and the activity of its synaptic inputs.

GABA$_A$ receptors located at extrasynaptic sites are particularly sensitive to the effects of both intravenous and volatile anesthetics (Fig. 5.5). Extrasynaptic GABA$_A$ receptors mediate tonic inhibition as opposed to phasic inhibition resulting from synaptic GABA release and activation of synaptic GABA$_A$ receptors. Extrasynaptic GABA$_A$ receptors have a high affinity for GABA and are tonically exposed to low ambient GABA concentrations in the extrasynaptic space [126]. Hippocampal neurons, which are critically involved in learning and memory, exhibit a large tonic current with activation of extrasynaptic α$_5$-subunit—containing GABA$_A$ receptors [127–130] that is highly sensitive to etomidate, propofol, midazolam, and isoflurane. These GABA$_A$ receptors are highly sensitive to low concentrations of propofol and isoflurane that produce amnesia but not unconsciousness. Receptors containing α$_5$-subunits also contribute to slow phasic (synaptic) currents that have been discovered in many brain regions [131]. These receptors provide a potential substrate for the amnesic properties of anesthetics.

Circuits and Networks

Rhythms and Simulations

The brain generates complex electrical rhythms through oscillations in field potentials with frequencies that range in from 10^{-1} to 10^2 Hz (cycles per second), as recorded at the scalp by electroencephalography as the electroencephalogram (EEG). These oscillations are state dependent, with characteristic multiple coexisting oscillations existing throughout the sleep-wake cycle. Lower frequency rhythms involve integration over longer time periods and engage larger areas of the brain, while higher frequency rhythms allow higher temporal resolution on local scales. Their physiologic roles are unclear, but rhythms of the brain reflect fundamental higher-order processing, and their modulation by anesthetics is a useful index of anesthetic action that is used in various EEG-based monitors of depth of anesthesia.

EEG frequencies from 1.5 to 4 Hz are referred to as δ-rhythms [132]. Slow rhythms are prominent during non-REM sleep (slow-wave sleep—SWS). δ-rhythms are commonly observed under general anesthesia and appear at loss of consciousness induced by propofol [133]. During natural SWS, δ-rhythms and sleep spindles are phase-related to a slower oscillation suggesting functional interaction [134]. Paroxysmal spindle-like waxing and waning oscillations overriding slower rhythms are also present in the cortical EEG under anesthesia, but the underlying physiology and functional significance are unknown.

θ-rhythms are most prominent in the hippocampus and are associated with sensorimotor and mnemonic functions during awake behavior [135]. A component of the θ-rhythm (type I) is affected by amnesic concentrations of isoflurane [136] and represents a potential network-level signature for anesthetic-induced amnesia. Type II θ-rhythm is slowed and potentiated under anesthesia [137].

γ-rhythms include an extremely broad and functionally heterogeneous spectrum of rhythms that can be subdivided into slow γ (30–50 Hz), γ (50–90 Hz), fast-γ, ultra-γ, or ε-rhythms (>90 Hz) [133]. GABAergic synaptic inhibition plays important roles in γ-physiology, which is reflected in their modulation by anesthetics. For example, isoflurane slows the frequency of evoked γ-oscillations (30–90 Hz, also known as 40 Hz rhythms) [138, 139].

A refinement of this strategy involves the anatomically discrete application of drugs to nuclei with known function. For example, the tuberomammillary nucleus (part of the endogenous sleep pathway) mediates the sedative component of anesthesia for some intravenous anesthetics (e.g., propofol) [15]. A discrete site of general anesthetic action for GABAergic drugs in the mesopontine tegmentum has also been proposed based on this strategy [14, 140].

Genetic Approaches

Genetic strategies to identifying drug targets usually focus on a particular gene, for example, one identified as potentially important to anesthesia. Targeted mutations that alter the sensitivity of specific neurotransmitter receptors or ion channels to anesthetics have been used to identify potential anesthetic binding sites [99]. The same mutations can be introduced into model organisms, usually mice, to create transgenic animals that are tested for their sensitivity to specific anesthetic end points to test the behavioral relevance of the altered gene product for the production of anesthesia.

GABA$_A$ Receptors

Results from transgenic animals illustrate both the utility and the difficulties of the genetic approach with respect to inhaled agents. The conditional forebrain-restricted GABA$_A$ receptor α$_1$-subunit knockout mouse was found to be less sensitive to isoflurane-induced amnesia than wild-type mice, and this led to the conclusion that action at these receptors contributes to its amnesic effects [141]. By contrast, a mouse harboring a mutation of the GABA$_A$ receptor α$_1$-subunit that renders the receptor insensitive to isoflurane in vitro did not show reduced sensitivity to either the amnesic or the immobilizing effects of isoflurane, leading to the conclusion that this subunit does not mediate the impairment of learning and memory by isoflurane [24]. Similar experiments indicate that action at the GABA$_A$ receptor β$_3$-subunit does not mediate immobility or amnesia by isoflurane [23]. This "bottom-up" genetic approach is a work intensive but powerful tool that has yielded clear results with the receptor-specific intravenous anesthetics [1], but it has proved more challenging to apply it to the more promiscuous inhaled agents (Fig. 5.6).

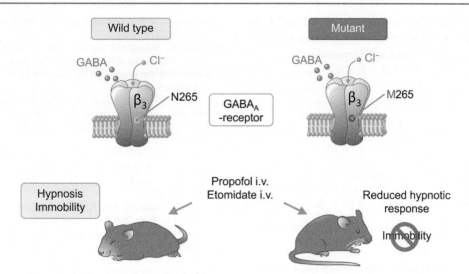

Fig. 5.6 Genetically engineered mice with mutations in the GABA$_A$ receptor serve as a model for identifying the molecular targets of general anesthetics. In a normal wild-type mouse, administration of propofol or etomidate leads to increased influx of chloride ions (Cl$^-$, *green*) through the channel pore after activation with the ligand GABA (*orange*). This produces the characteristic behavioral end point hypnosis and immobility. Mice carrying a knock-in mutation at amino acid residue 265 in the β3 subunit of the GABA$_A$ receptor (N265M), which eliminates anesthetic potentiation of the receptor in vitro, markedly attenuate the effects of propofol and etomidate in vivo by reducing hypnosis and eliminating immobilization. This provides strong support for this receptor as the principal anesthetic target for immobilization and an important contributor to unconsciousness induced by propofol or etomidate. (Reprinted from Jurd R, Arras M, Lambert S, et al. General anesthetic actions in vivo strongly attenuated by a point mutation in the GABA(A) receptor beta3 subunit. FASEB J. 2003;17:250–2. [142]. With permission from Federation of American Societies for Experimental Biology)

Glycine α$_1$-Containing Receptors Pharmacologic studies supported the notion that glycinergic neurotransmission might be the effector for the immobilizing action of inhaled anesthetics in the spinal cord, where glycine replaces GABA as the principal inhibitory transmitter. However, mice harboring mutations that render α$_1$-subunit-containing glycine receptors largely insensitive to alcohol and inhaled ether anesthetics do not demonstrate a concordant change in MAC values. As α$_1$ is the most widely expressed subunit in adult animals, it is unlikely that action at glycine receptors plays an important part in the immobilizing action of inhaled agents [143].

Two-Pore Domain K$^+$ Channels

The use of mice harboring knockout mutations of several two-pore domain K$^+$ channel (K$_{2P}$) family members (TASK-1, TASK-3, TREK-1) has demonstrated a role for these channels in volatile anesthesia [25–27]. TASK-1 and TASK-3 also show sensitivity toward etomidate (but not propofol), though the mechanisms by which etomidate impairs channel function seem to be distinct from volatile anesthetics [144]. Drugs with agonistic effects on GABA$_A$ receptors as well as propofol and benzodiazepines have a stronger effect on TASK-1 knockout mice as compared to wild type as they require a longer recovery time from anesthesia [26]. This effect was not observed in TREK-1 knockout mice, which showed no difference in recovery time after anesthesia

with pentobarbital [25]. One hypothesis for this increase in sensitivity is the upregulation of GABA$_A$ receptors in the knockout group [145].

For example, TREK-1 knockout mice are partially resistant to all volatile anesthetics tested with respect to both loss of righting reflex (a measure of consciousness) and immobility, but anesthesia can still be induced, albeit at higher anesthetic concentrations. Interestingly, responses to pentobarbital are unaffected, indicating that the mutation does not cause a generalized resistance to anesthesia.

Summary

Our understanding of the mechanisms of action of general anesthetics has advanced significantly over the last 30 years. The core component states of anesthesia (amnesia, sedation/unconsciousness, immobility) are separable behavioral states in vivo, the resolution of which at the molecular and cellular levels represents a major challenge for contemporary neuroscience. The paradigm has shifted from membrane lipids to hydrophobic cavities in proteins as the most likely targets for anesthetics [146]. Despite remarkable progress, a comprehensive understanding of general anesthetic action has not been achieved. Compared to inhaled anesthetics, the intravenous anesthetics exhibit more conventional receptor pharmacology. Accumulating evidence indicates that no universal target exists to explain all of the actions of every general anesthetic, or even of a single anesthetic agent, but an important role for GABA$_A$ receptors has been established for propofol, etomidate, and benzodiazepines.

References

1. Rudolph U, Antkowiak B. Molecular and neuronal substrates for general anaesthetics. Nat Rev Neurosci. 2004;5:709–20.
2. Hemmings Jr HC, Akabas MH, Goldstein PA, Trudell JR, Orser BA, Harrison NL. Emerging molecular mechanisms of general anesthetic action. Trends Pharmacol Sci. 2005;26:503–10.
3. Meyer H. Zur theorie der alkoholnarkose. Arch Exp Pathol Pharmakol. 1899;42:109–18.
4. Overton C. Studien über die Narkose zugleich ein Beitrag zur allgemeinen Pharmakologie. Jena: Verlag von Gustav Fischer; 1901.
5. Franks NP, Lieb WR. Do general anaesthetics act by competitive binding to specific receptors? Nature. 1984;310:599–601.
6. Franks NP, Lieb WR. Seeing the light: protein theories of general anesthesia. 1984. Anesthesiology. 2004;101:235–7.
7. Hall AC, Lieb WR, Franks NP. Stereoselective and non-stereoselective actions of isoflurane on the GABAA receptor. Br J Pharmacol. 1994;112:906–10.
8. Antognini JF, Schwartz K. Exaggerated anesthetic requirements in the preferentially anesthetized brain. Anesthesiology. 1993;79:1244–9.
9. Rampil IJ, Mason P, Singh H. Anesthetic potency (MAC) is independent of forebrain structures in the rat. Anesthesiology. 1993;78:707–12.
10. Stabernack C, Zhang Y, Sonner JM, Laster M, Eger 2nd EI. Thiopental produces immobility primarily by supraspinal actions in rats. Anesth Analg. 2005;100:128–36.
11. Veselis RA, Reinsel RA, Feshchenko VA. Drug-induced amnesia is a separate phenomenon from sedation: electrophysiologic evidence. Anesthesiology. 2001;95:896–907.
12. Veselis RA, Reinsel RA, Feshchenko VA, Wronski M. The comparative amnestic effects of midazolam, propofol, thiopental, and fentanyl at equisedative concentrations. Anesthesiology. 1997;87:749–64.
13. Sanders RD, Tononi G, Laureys S, Sleigh JW. Unresponsiveness not equal unconsciousness. Anesthesiology. 2012;116:946–59.
14. Devor M, Zalkind V. Reversible analgesia, atonia, and loss of consciousness on bilateral intracerebral microinjection of pentobarbital. Pain. 2001;94:101–12.
15. Nelson LE, Guo TZ, Lu J, Saper CB, Franks NP, Maze M. The sedative component of anesthesia is mediated by GABA(A) receptors in an endogenous sleep pathway. Nat Neurosci. 2002;5:979–84.
16. Zhang Z, Ferretti V, Guntan I, Moro A, Steinberg EA, Ye Z, Zecharia AY, Yu X, Vyssotski AL, Brickley SG, Yustos R, Pillidge ZE, Harding EC, Wisden W, Franks NP. Neuronal ensembles sufficient for recovery sleep and the sedative actions of alpha2 adrenergic agonists. Nat Neurosci. 2015;18:553–61.
17. Lakhlani PP, MacMillan LB, Guo TZ, McCool BA, Lovinger DM, Maze M, Limbird LE. Substitution of a mutant alpha2a-adrenergic receptor via "hit and run" gene targeting reveals the role of this subtype in sedative, analgesic, and anesthetic-sparing responses in vivo. Proc Natl Acad Sci U S A. 1997;94:9950–5.
18. Kamibayashi T, Maze M. Clinical uses of alpha2-adrenergic agonists. Anesthesiology. 2000;93:1345–9.
19. Rampil IJ, Laster MJ. No correlation between quantitative electroencephalographic measurements and movement response to noxious stimuli during isoflurane anesthesia in rats. Anesthesiology. 1992;77:920–5.
20. Zhang Y, Sonner JM, Eger 2nd EI, Stabernack CR, Laster MJ, Raines DE, Harris RA. Gamma-aminobutyric acidA receptors do not mediate the immobility produced by isoflurane. Anesth Analg. 2004;99:85–90.
21. Kungys G, Kim J, Jinks SL, Atherley RJ, Antognini JF. Propofol produces immobility via action in the ventral horn of the spinal cord by a GABAergic mechanism. Anesth Analg. 2009;108:1531–7.
22. Zhang Y, Guzinski M, Eger EI, Laster MJ, Sharma M, Harris RA, Hemmings HC. Bidirectional modulation of isoflurane potency by intrathecal tetrodotoxin and veratridine in rats. Br J Pharmacol. 2010;159:872–8.
23. Liao M, Sonner JM, Jurd R, Rudolph U, Borghese CM, Harris RA, Laster MJ, Eger 2nd EI. Beta3-containing gamma-aminobutyric acidA receptors are not major targets for the amnesic and immobilizing actions of isoflurane. Anesth Analg. 2005;101:412–8. Table of contents.
24. Sonner JM, Werner DF, Elsen FP, Xing Y, Liao M, Harris RA, Harrison NL, Fanselow MS, Eger 2nd EI, Homanics GE. Effect of isoflurane and other potent inhaled anesthetics on minimum alveolar concentration, learning, and the righting reflex in mice engineered to express alpha1 gamma-aminobutyric acid type A receptors unresponsive to isoflurane. Anesthesiology. 2007;106:107–13.
25. Heurteaux C, Guy N, Laigle C, Blondeau N, Duprat F, Mazzuca M, Lang-Lazdunski L, Widmann C, Zanzouri M, Romey G, Lazdunski M. TREK-1, a K+ channel involved in neuroprotection and general anesthesia. EMBO J. 2004;23:2684–95.
26. Linden AM, Aller MI, Leppa E, Vekovischeva O, Aitta-Aho T, Veale EL, Mathie A, Rosenberg P, Wisden W, Korpi ER. The in vivo contributions of TASK-1-containing channels to the actions of inhalation anesthetics, the alpha(2) adrenergic sedative dexmedetomidine, and cannabinoid agonists. J Pharmacol Exp Ther. 2006;317:615–26.
27. Linden AM, Sandu C, Aller MI, Vekovischeva OY, Rosenberg PH, Wisden W, Korpi ER. TASK-3 knockout mice exhibit exaggerated nocturnal activity, impairments in cognitive functions, and reduced sensitivity to inhalation anesthetics. J Pharmacol Exp Ther. 2007;323:924–34.
28. Westphalen R, Krivitski M, Amarosa A, Guy N, Hemmings H. Reduced inhibition of cortical glutamate and GABA release by halothane in mice lacking the K+ channel, TREK-1. Br J Pharmacol. 2007;152:939–45.
29. Jinks SL, Bravo M, Hayes SG. Volatile anesthetic effects on midbrain-elicited locomotion suggest that the locomotor network in the ventral spinal cord is the primary site for immobility. Anesthesiology. 2008;108:1016–24.
30. Searle JR. Consciousness. Annu Rev Neurosci. 2000;23:557–78.
31. Crick F, Koch C. A framework for consciousness. Nat Neurosci. 2003;6:119–26.
32. Alkire MT, Haier RJ, Fallon JH. Toward a unified theory of narcosis: brain imaging evidence for a thalamocortical switch as the neurophysiologic basis of anesthetic-induced unconsciousness. Conscious Cogn. 2000;9:370–86.
33. Ries CR, Puil E. Mechanism of anesthesia revealed by shunting actions of isoflurane on thalamocortical neurons. J Neurophysiol. 1999;81:1795–801.
34. Detsch O, Vahle-Hinz C, Kochs E, Siemers M, Bromm B. Isoflurane induces dose-dependent changes of thalamic somatosensory information transfer. Brain Res. 1999;829:77–89.
35. Alkire MT, Hudetz AG, Tononi G. Consciousness and anesthesia. Science. 2008;322:876–80.

36. Brown EN, Lydic R, Schiff ND. General anesthesia, sleep, and coma. N Engl J Med. 2010;363:2638–50.
37. Varela F, Lachaux JP, Rodriguez E, Martinerie J. The brainweb: phase synchronization and large-scale integration. Nat Rev Neurosci. 2001;2:229–39.
38. Bullmore E, Sporns O. The economy of brain network organization. Nat Rev Neurosci. 2012;13:336–49.
39. van den Heuvel MP, Sporns O. Rich-club organization of the human connectome. J Neurosci. 2011;31:15775–86.
40. Ferrarelli F, Massimini M, Sarasso S, Casali A, Riedner BA, Angelini G, Tononi G, Pearce RA. Breakdown in cortical effective connectivity during midazolam-induced loss of consciousness. Proc Natl Acad Sci U S A. 2010;107:2681–6.
41. Dutton RC, Maurer AJ, Sonner JM, Fanselow MS, Laster MJ, Eger 2nd EI. The concentration of isoflurane required to suppress learning depends on the type of learning. Anesthesiology. 2001;94:514–9.
42. Mashour GA. Fragmenting consciousness. Proc Natl Acad Sci U S A. 2012;109:19876–7.
43. Imas OA, Ropella KM, Ward BD, Wood JD, Hudetz AG. Volatile anesthetics enhance flash-induced gamma oscillations in rat visual cortex. Anesthesiology. 2005;102:937–47.
44. Imas OA, Ropella KM, Wood JD, Hudetz AG. Isoflurane disrupts anterio-posterior phase synchronization of flash-induced field potentials in the rat. Neurosci Lett. 2006;402:216–21.
45. John ER, Prichep LS, Kox W, Valdes-Sosa P, Bosch-Bayard J, Aubert E, Tom M, di Michele F, Gugino LD. Invariant reversible QEEG effects of anesthetics. Conscious Cogn. 2001;10:165–83.
46. Mohler H, Fritschy JM, Rudolph U. A new benzodiazepine pharmacology. J Pharmacol Exp Ther. 2002;300:2–8.
47. Alkire MT, Nathan SV. Does the amygdala mediate anesthetic-induced amnesia? Basolateral amygdala lesions block sevoflurane-induced amnesia. Anesthesiology. 2005;102:754–60.
48. Vertes RP. Hippocampal theta rhythm: a tag for short-term memory. Hippocampus. 2005;15:923–35.
49. Pan WX, McNaughton N. The medial supramammillary nucleus, spatial learning and the frequency of hippocampal theta activity. Brain Res. 1997;764:101–8.
50. Seidenbecher T, Laxmi TR, Stork O, Pape HC. Amygdalar and hippocampal theta rhythm synchronization during fear memory retrieval. Science. 2003;301:846–50.
51. Pryor KO, Murphy E, Reinsel RA, Mehta M, Veselis RA. Heterogeneous effects of intravenous anesthetics on modulatory memory systems in humans. Anesthesiology. 2007;107:A1218.
52. Rudolph U, Crestani F, Benke D, Brunig I, Benson JA, Fritschy JM, Martin JR, Bluethmann H, Mohler H. Benzodiazepine actions mediated by specific gamma-aminobutyric acid(A) receptor subtypes. Nature. 1999;401:796–800.
53. Murphy M, Bruno MA, Riedner BA, Boveroux P, Noirhomme Q, Landsness EC, Brichant JF, Phillips C, Massimini M, Laureys S, Tononi G, Boly M. Propofol anesthesia and sleep: a high-density EEG study. Sleep. 2011;34:283–91A.
54. Tung A, Bergmann BM, Herrera S, Cao D, Mendelson WB. Recovery from sleep deprivation occurs during propofol anesthesia. Anesthesiology. 2004;100:1419–26.
55. Hentschke H, Schwarz C, Antkowiak B. Neocortex is the major target of sedative concentrations of volatile anaesthetics: strong depression of firing rates and increase of GABAA receptor-mediated inhibition. Eur J Neurosci. 2005;21:93–102.
56. Perouansky M, Hemmings Jr HC. Neurotoxicity of general anesthetics: cause for concern? Anesthesiology. 2009;111:1365–71.
57. Durieux M, Davis PJ. The safety of key inhaled and intravenous drugs in pediatrics (SAFEKIDS): an update. Anesth Analg. 2010;110:1265–7.
58. Jevtovic-Todorovic V, Hartman RE, Izumi Y, Benshoff ND, Dikranian K, Zorumski CF, Olney JW, Wozniak DF. Early exposure to common anesthetic agents causes widespread neurodegeneration in the developing rat brain and persistent learning deficits. J Neurosci. 2003;23:876–82.
59. Young C, Jevtovic-Todorovic V, Qin YQ, Tenkova T, Wang H, Labruyere J, Olney JW. Potential of ketamine and midazolam, individually or in combination, to induce apoptotic neurodegeneration in the infant mouse brain. Br J Pharmacol. 2005;146:189–97.
60. Scallet AC, Schmued LC, Slikker Jr W, Grunberg N, Faustino PJ, Davis H, Lester D, Pine PS, Sistare F, Hanig JP. Developmental neurotoxicity of ketamine: morphometric confirmation, exposure parameters, and multiple fluorescent labeling of apoptotic neurons. Toxicol Sci. 2004;81:364–70.
61. Cattano D, Young C, Straiko MM, Olney JW. Subanesthetic doses of propofol induce neuroapoptosis in the infant mouse brain. Anesth Analg. 2008;106:1712–4.
62. Fredriksson A, Ponten E, Gordh T, Eriksson P. Neonatal exposure to a combination of N-methyl-D-aspartate and gamma-aminobutyric acid type A receptor anesthetic agents potentiates apoptotic neurodegeneration and persistent behavioral deficits. Anesthesiology. 2007;107:427–36.
63. Stratmann G. Review article: neurotoxicity of anesthetic drugs in the developing brain. Anesth Analg. 2011;113:1170–9.
64. Hudson AE, Hemmings Jr HC. Are anaesthetics toxic to the brain? Br J Anaesth. 2011;107:30–7.
65. Jevtovic-Todorovic V, Absalom AR, Blomgren K, Brambrink A, Crosby G, Culley DJ, Fiskum G, Giffard RG, Herold KF, Loepke AW, Ma D, Orser BA, Planel E, Slikker Jr W, Soriano SG, Stratmann G, Vutskits L, Xie Z, Hemmings Jr HC. Anaesthetic neurotoxicity and neuroplasticity: an expert group report and statement based on the BJA Salzburg Seminar. Br J Anaesth. 2013;111:143–51.
66. Li J, Xiong M, Nadavaluru PR, Zuo W, Ye JH, Eloy JD, Bekker A. Dexmedetomidine attenuates neurotoxicity induced by prenatal propofol exposure. J Neurosurg Anesthesiol. 2016;28:51–64.
67. Jevtovic-Todorovic V. Anesthesia and the developing brain: are we getting closer to understanding the truth? Curr Opin Anaesthesiol. 2011;24:395–9.
68. Shih J, May LD, Gonzalez HE, Lee EW, Alvi RS, Sall JW, Rau V, Bickler PE, Lalchandani GR, Yusupova M, Woodward E, Kang H, Wilk AJ, Carlston CM, Mendoza MV, Guggenheim JN, Schaefer M, Rowe AM, Stratmann G. Delayed environmental enrichment reverses sevoflurane-induced memory impairment in rats. Anesthesiology. 2012;116:586–602.
69. Munk L, Andersen G, Moller AM. Post-anaesthetic emergence delirium in adults: incidence, predictors and consequences. Acta Anaesthesiol Scand. 2016.
70. Guenther U, Riedel L, Radtke FM. Patients prone for postoperative delirium: preoperative assessment, perioperative prophylaxis, postoperative treatment. Curr Opin Anaesthesiol. 2016.
71. Djaiani G, Silverton N, Fedorko L, Carroll J, Styra R, Rao V, Katznelson R. Dexmedetomidine versus propofol sedation reduces delirium after cardiac surgery: a randomized controlled trial. Anesthesiology. 2016;124:362–8.
72. Zurek AA, Bridgwater EM, Orser BA. Inhibition of alpha5 gamma-aminobutyric acid type A receptors restores recognition memory after general anesthesia. Anesth Analg. 2012;114:845–55.
73. Wan Y, Xu J, Ma D, Zeng Y, Cibelli M, Maze M. Postoperative impairment of cognitive function in rats: a possible role for cytokine-mediated inflammation in the hippocampus. Anesthesiology. 2007;106:436–43.
74. Terrando N, Eriksson LI, Ryu JK, Yang T, Monaco C, Feldmann M, Jonsson Fagerlund M, Charo IF, Akassoglou K,

Maze M. Resolving postoperative neuroinflammation and cognitive decline. Ann Neurol. 2011;70:986–95.

75. Tang JX, Mardini F, Caltagarone BM, Garrity ST, Li RQ, Bianchi SL, Gomes O, Laferla FM, Eckenhoff RG, Eckenhoff MF. Anesthesia in presymptomatic Alzheimer's disease: a study using the triple-transgenic mouse model. Alzheimers Dement. 2011;7:521–31. e1.

76. Avidan MS, Searleman AC, Storandt M, Barnett K, Vannucci A, Saager L, Xiong C, Grant EA, Kaiser D, Morris JC, Evers AS. - Long-term cognitive decline in older subjects was not attributable to noncardiac surgery or major illness. Anesthesiology. 2009;111:964–70.

77. Avidan MS, Evers AS. Review of clinical evidence for persistent cognitive decline or incident dementia attributable to surgery or general anesthesia. J Alzheimers Dis. 2011;24:201–16.

78. Zaugg M, Lucchinetti E, Uecker M, Pasch T, Schaub MC. Anaesthetics and cardiac preconditioning. Part I. Signalling and cytoprotective mechanisms. Br J Anaesth. 2003;91:551–65.

79. Pagel PS, Hettrick DA, Lowe D, Gowrie PW, Kersten JR, Bosnjak ZJ, Warltier DC. Cardiovascular effects of verapamil enantiomer combinations in conscious dogs. Eur J Pharmacol. 1998;348:213–21.

80. Vulliemoz Y. The nitric oxide-cyclic 3',5'-guanosine monophosphate signal transduction pathway in the mechanism of action of general anesthetics. Toxicol Lett. 1998;100–101:103–8.

81. Huneke R, Fassl J, Rossaint R, Luckhoff A. Effects of volatile anesthetics on cardiac ion channels. Acta Anaesthesiol Scand. 2004;48:547–61.

82. Thompson A, Balser JR. Perioperative cardiac arrhythmias. Br J Anaesth. 2004;93:86–94.

83. Stuth EA, Krolo M, Tonkovic-Capin M, Hopp FA, Kampine JP, Zuperku EJ. Effects of halothane on synaptic neurotransmission to medullary expiratory neurons in the ventral respiratory group of dogs. Anesthesiology. 1999;91:804–14.

84. Nieuwenhuijs D, Sarton E, Teppema LJ, Kruyt E, Olievier I, van Kleef J, Dahan A. Respiratory sites of action of propofol: absence of depression of peripheral chemoreflex loop by low-dose propofol. Anesthesiology. 2001;95:889–95.

85. Hoshino Y, Ayuse T, Kurata S, Ayuse T, Schneider H, Kirkness JP, Patil SP, Schwartz AR, Oi K. The compensatory responses to upper airway obstruction in normal subjects under propofol anesthesia. Respir Physiol Neurobiol. 2009;166:24–31.

86. Nieuwenhuijs DJ, Olofsen E, Romberg RR, Sarton E, Ward D, Engbers F, Vuyk J, Mooren R, Teppema LJ, Dahan A. Response surface modeling of remifentanil-propofol interaction on cardiorespiratory control and bispectral index. Anesthesiology. 2003;98:312–22.

87. Gueye PN, Borron SW, Risede P, Monier C, Buneaux F, Debray M, Baud FJ. Buprenorphine and midazolam act in combination to depress respiration in rats. Toxicol Sci. 2002;65:107–14.

88. Venn RM, Hell J, Grounds RM. Respiratory effects of dexmedetomidine in the surgical patient requiring intensive care. Crit Care. 2000;4:302–8.

89. Hsu YW, Cortinez LI, Robertson KM, Keifer JC, Sum-Ping ST, Moretti EW, Young CC, Wright DR, Macleod DB, Somma J. Dexmedetomidine pharmacodynamics: Part I: Crossover comparison of the respiratory effects of dexmedetomidine and remifentanil in healthy volunteers. Anesthesiology. 2004;101:1066–76.

90. Franks NP, Lieb WR. Molecular and cellular mechanisms of general anaesthesia. Nature. 1994;367:607–14.

91. Zeller A, Jurd R, Lambert S, Arras M, Drexler B, Grashoff C, et al. Inhibitory ligand-gated ion channels as substrates for general anesthetic actions. In: Schüttler J, Schwilden H, editors. Modern anesthetics, Handbook of experimental pharmacology, vol. 182. Berlin Heidelberg: Springer; 2008. p. 31–51.

92. Bertaccini EJ, Trudell JR, Franks NP. The common chemical motifs within anesthetic binding sites. Anesth Analg. 2007;104:318–24.

93. Eckenhoff RG. Promiscuous ligands and attractive cavities: how do the inhaled anesthetics work? Mol Interv. 2001;1:258–68.

94. Dickinson R, Peterson BK, Banks P, Simillis C, Martin JC, Valenzuela CA, Maze M, Franks NP. Competitive inhibition at the glycine site of the N-methyl-D-aspartate receptor by the anesthetics xenon and isoflurane: evidence from molecular modeling and electrophysiology. Anesthesiology. 2007;107:756–67.

95. Nury H, Van Renterghem C, Weng Y, Tran A, Baaden M, Dufresne V, Changeux JP, Sonner JM, Delarue M, Corringer PJ. - X-ray structures of general anaesthetics bound to a pentameric ligand-gated ion channel. Nature. 2011;469:428–31.

96. Patel AJ, Honore E, Lesage F, Fink M, Romey G, Lazdunski M. Inhalational anesthetics activate two-pore-domain background K+ channels. Nat Neurosci. 1999;2:422–6.

97. Herold KF, Hemmings Jr HC. Sodium channels as targets for volatile anesthetics. Front Pharmacol. 2012;3:50.

98. Lynch JW. Molecular structure and function of the glycine receptor chloride channel. Physiol Rev. 2004;84:1051–95.

99. Mihic SJ, Ye Q, Wick MJ, Koltchine VV, Krasowski MD, Finn SE, Mascia MP, Valenzuela CF, Hanson KK, Greenblatt EP, Harris RA, Harrison NL. Sites of alcohol and volatile anaesthetic action on GABA(A) and glycine receptors. Nature. 1997;389:385–9.

100. Role LW, Berg DK. Nicotinic receptors in the development and modulation of CNS synapses. Neuron. 1996;16:1077–85.

101. Flood P, Ramirez-Latorre J, Role L. Alpha 4 beta 2 neuronal nicotinic acetylcholine receptors in the central nervous system are inhibited by isoflurane and propofol, but alpha 7-type nicotinic acetylcholine receptors are unaffected. Anesthesiology. 1997;86:859–65.

102. Violet JM, Downie DL, Nakisa RC, Lieb WR, Franks NP. Differential sensitivities of mammalian neuronal and muscle nicotinic acetylcholine receptors to general anesthetics. Anesthesiology. 1997;86:866–74.

103. Dingledine R, Borges K, Bowie D, Traynelis SF. The glutamate receptor ion channels. Pharmacol Rev. 1999;51:7–61.

104. Jevtovic-Todorovic V, Todorovic SM, Mennerick S, Powell S, Dikranian K, Benshoff N, Zorumski CF, Olney JW. Nitrous oxide (laughing gas) is an NMDA antagonist, neuroprotectant and neurotoxin. Nat Med. 1998;4:460–3.

105. Franks NP, Dickinson R, de Sousa SL, Hall AC, Lieb WR. How does xenon produce anaesthesia? Nature. 1998;396:324.

106. Herold KF, Nau C, Ouyang W, Hemmings HC. Isoflurane inhibits the tetrodotoxin-resistant voltage-gated sodium channel Nav1.8. Anesthesiology. 2009;111:591–9.

107. Ouyang W, Hemmings H. Depression by isoflurane of the action potential and underlying voltage-gated ion currents in isolated rat neurohypophysial nerve terminals. J Pharmacol Exp Ther. 2005;312:801–8.

108. Ouyang W, Hemmings H. Isoform-selective effects of isoflurane on voltage-gated Na + channels. Anesthesiology. 2007;107:91–8.

109. Ratnakumari L, Vysotskaya T, Duch D, Hemmings H. Differential effects of anesthetic and nonanesthetic cyclobutanes on neuronal voltage-gated sodium channels. Anesthesiology. 2000;92:529–41.

110. Shiraishi M, Harris R. Effects of alcohols and anesthetics on recombinant voltage-gated Na+ channels. J Pharmacol Exp Ther. 2004;309:987–94.

111. Catterall WA. Structure and regulation of voltage-gated Ca2+ channels. Annu Rev Cell Dev Biol. 2000;16:521–55.

112. Antognini J, Carstens E, Raines DE, Hemmings HC. Neural mechanisms of anesthesia. Totowa, NJ: Humana Press; 2003.

113. Hanley PJ, ter Keurs HE, Cannell MB. Excitation-contraction coupling in the heart and the negative inotropic action of volatile anesthetics. Anesthesiology. 2004;101:999–1014.

114. Rithalia A, Hopkins PM, Harrison SM. The effects of halothane, isoflurane, and sevoflurane on Ca2+ current and transient outward K + current in subendocardial and subepicardial myocytes from the rat left ventricle. Anesth Analg. 2004;99:1615–22. Table of contents.

115. Huneke R, Jungling E, Skasa M, Rossaint R, Luckhoff A. Effects of the anesthetic gases xenon, halothane, and isoflurane on calcium and potassium currents in human atrial cardiomyocytes. Anesthesiology. 2001;95:999–1006.

116. Stowe DF, Rehmert GC, Kwok WM, Weigt HU, Georgieff M, Bosnjak ZJ. Xenon does not alter cardiac function or major cation currents in isolated guinea pig hearts or myocytes. Anesthesiology. 2000;92:516–22.

117. Buljubasic N, Marijic J, Berczi V, Supan DF, Kampine JP, Bosnjak ZJ. Differential effects of etomidate, propofol, and midazolam on calcium and potassium channel currents in canine myocardial cells. Anesthesiology. 1996;85:1092–9.

118. Yost CS. Potassium channels: basic aspects, functional roles, and medical significance. Anesthesiology. 1999;90:1186–203.

119. Friederich P, Benzenberg D, Trellakis S, Urban BW. Interaction of volatile anesthetics with human Kv channels in relation to clinical concentrations. Anesthesiology. 2001;95:954–8.

120. Franks NP, Lieb WR. Volatile general anaesthetics activate a novel neuronal K+ current. Nature. 1988;333:662–4.

121. Franks NP, Honore E. The TREK K2P channels and their role in general anaesthesia and neuroprotection. Trends Pharmacol Sci. 2004;25:601–8.

122. Patel AJ, Honore E. Anesthetic-sensitive 2P domain K+ channels. Anesthesiology. 2001;95:1013–21.

123. Sirois JE, Lynch 3rd C, Bayliss DA. Convergent and reciprocal modulation of a leak K+ current and I(h) by an inhalational anaesthetic and neurotransmitters in rat brainstem motoneurones. J Physiol. 2002;541:717–29.

124. Chen X, Sirois JE, Lei Q, Talley EM, Lynch 3rd C, Bayliss DA. HCN subunit-specific and cAMP-modulated effects of anesthetics on neuronal pacemaker currents. J Neurosci. 2005;25:5803–14.

125. Robinson RB, Siegelbaum SA. Hyperpolarization-activated cation currents: from molecules to physiological function. Annu Rev Physiol. 2003;65:453–80.

126. Semyanov A, Walker MC, Kullmann DM, Silver RA. Tonically active GABA A receptors: modulating gain and maintaining the tone. Trends Neurosci. 2004;27:262–9.

127. Bai D, Zhu G, Pennefather P, Jackson MF, MacDonald JF, Orser BA. Distinct functional and pharmacological properties of tonic and quantal inhibitory postsynaptic currents mediated by gamma-aminobutyric acid(A) receptors in hippocampal neurons. Mol Pharmacol. 2001;59:814–24.

128. Bieda MC, MacIver MB. Major role for tonic GABAA conductances in anesthetic suppression of intrinsic neuronal excitability. J Neurophysiol. 2004;92:1658–67.

129. Caraiscos VB, Elliott EM, You-Ten KE, Cheng VY, Belelli D, Newell JG, Jackson MF, Lambert JJ, Rosahl TW, Wafford KA, MacDonald JF, Orser BA. Tonic inhibition in mouse hippocampal CA1 pyramidal neurons is mediated by alpha5 subunit-containing gamma-aminobutyric acid type A receptors. Proc Natl Acad Sci U S A. 2004;101:3662–7.

130. Caraiscos VB, Newell JG, You-Ten KE, Elliott EM, Rosahl TW, Wafford KA, MacDonald JF, Orser BA. Selective enhancement of tonic GABAergic inhibition in murine hippocampal neurons by low concentrations of the volatile anesthetic isoflurane. J Neurosci. 2004;24:8454–8.

131. Capogna M, Pearce RA. GABA A, slow: causes and consequences. Trends Neurosci. 2011;34:101–12.

132. Penttonen M, Buzsáki G. Natural logarithmic relationship between brain oscillators. Thalamus Relat Syst. 2003;2:145–52.

133. Lewis LD, Weiner VS, Mukamel EA, Donoghue JA, Eskandar EN, Madsen JR, Anderson WS, Hochberg LR, Cash SS, Brown EN, Purdon PL. Rapid fragmentation of neuronal networks at the onset of propofol-induced unconsciousness. Proc Natl Acad Sci U S A. 2012;109:E3377–86.

134. Steriade M, Nunez A, Amzica F. Intracellular analysis of relations between the slow (<1 Hz) neocortical oscillation and other sleep rhythms of the electroencephalogram. J Neurosci. 1993;13:3266–83.

135. Buzsaki G. Theta oscillations in the hippocampus. Neuron. 2002;33:325–40.

136. Perouansky M, Hentschke H, Perkins M, Pearce RA. Amnesic concentrations of the nonimmobilizer 1,2- dichlorohexafluorocyclobutane (F6, 2N) and isoflurane alter hippocampal theta oscillations in vivo. Anesthesiology. 2007;106:1168–76.

137. Bland BH, Bland CE, Colom LV, Roth SH, DeClerk S, Dypvik A, Bird J, Deliyannides A. Effect of halothane on type 2 immobility-related hippocampal theta field activity and theta-on/theta-off cell discharges. Hippocampus. 2003;13:38–47.

138. Madler C, Keller I, Schwender D, Poppel E. Sensory information processing during general anaesthesia: effect of isoflurane on auditory evoked neuronal oscillations. Br J Anaesth. 1991;66:81–7.

139. Munglani R, Andrade J, Sapsford DJ, Baddeley A, Jones JG. A measure of consciousness and memory during isoflurane administration: the coherent frequency. Br J Anaesth. 1993;71:633–41.

140. Sukhotinsky I, Zalkind V, Lu J, Hopkins DA, Saper CB, Devor M. Neural pathways associated with loss of consciousness caused by intracerebral microinjection of GABA A-active anesthetics. Eur J Neurosci. 2007;25:1417–36.

141. Sonner JM, Cascio M, Xing Y, Fanselow MS, Kralic JE, Morrow AL, Korpi ER, Hardy S, Sloat B, Eger 2nd EI, Homanics GE. Alpha 1 subunit-containing GABA type A receptors in forebrain contribute to the effect of inhaled anesthetics on conditioned fear. Mol Pharmacol. 2005;68:61–8.

142. Jurd R, Arras M, Lambert S, et al. General anesthetic actions in vivo strongly attenuated by a point mutation in the GABA (A) receptor beta3 subunit. FASEB J. 2003;17:250–2.

143. Borghese CM, Xiong W, Oh SI, Ho A, Mihic SJ, Zhang L, Lovinger DM, Homanics GE, Eger 2nd EI, Harris RA. Mutations M287L and Q266I in the glycine receptor alpha1 subunit change sensitivity to volatile anesthetics in oocytes and neurons, but not the minimal alveolar concentration in knockin mice. Anesthesiology. 2012;117:765–71.

144. Putzke C, Hanley PJ, Schlichthorl G, Preisig-Muller R, Rinne S, Anetseder M, Eckenhoff R, Berkowitz C, Vassiliou T, Wulf H, Eberhart L. Differential effects of volatile and intravenous anesthetics on the activity of human TASK-1. Am J Physiol Cell Physiol. 2007;293:C1319–26.

145. Steinberg EA, Wafford KA, Brickley SG, Franks NP, Wisden W. The role of K(2)p channels in anaesthesia and sleep. Pflugers Arch. 2015;467:907–16.

146. Herold KF, Sanford RL, Lee W, Schultz MF, Ingolfsson HI, Andersen OS, Hemmings Jr HC. Volatile anesthetics inhibit sodium channels without altering bulk lipid bilayer properties. J Gen Physiol. 2014;144:545–60.

Basic Pharmacology: Kinetics and Dynamics for Dummies

6

Johan Ræder

As anaesthesiologists, our drugs and their pharmacology are among our most important tools. Compared with most other physicians, we use high doses of very efficient and potent drugs with strong and actually intoxicating effects, for a very defined period of time. General anaesthesia may be said to be a "state of controlled drug intoxication", and for that reason the proper and thorough knowledge of pharmacology of the relatively few drugs we use is crucial.

In this chapter I will limit the discussion to general anaesthetic drugs (analgesics and hypnotics) given intravenously.

General Aspects

Basically the relation between a given dose and the observed effect may be split into two (Fig. 6.1):

1. Relation between dose and plasma level (pharmacokinetics)
2. Relation between plasma level and effect(s) (pharmacodynamics)

While we as clinical anaesthesiologists primarily are interested in the dose–effect relationship, it is still very useful to know the laws who dictate the plasma concentration. Better understanding of plasma concentration will help us in hitting the desired effect level more precisely.

As the mechanisms and target cells of strong hypnotic, analgesic and anti-nociceptive drugs are inside the central nervous system, the anaesthetic drugs have to be lipid soluble in order to penetrate the blood–brain barrier and be effective in the central nervous system. Lipid solubility creates two problems; the drugs are also distributed very extensively into all other cells and tissues, and they will not readily be excreted through the kidneys.

Fortunately, the brain and spinal cord is very well perfused so they will have access to a large number of drug molecules initially after a bolus dose or start of high-dose infusion, before other tissues "steal" a large number of drug molecules (Fig. 6.2). Then, the infusion has to be adjusted on an appropriate level to compensate for the ongoing loss of drug into tissues which are abundant in volume and not relevant for any anaesthetic effect, but some side effects. The speed and amount of drug diffusion into different organs is dependent upon blood flow to the organ, plasma concentration, concentration gradient between blood and tissue and drug solubility in the tissues.

The infusion has to compensate for both these mechanisms. The lipid-soluble IV drugs need to be transformed into water-soluble inactive metabolites, which subsequently are excreted renally (Fig. 6.3).

Whereas a lot of molecules have been tested and work for general anaesthesia, the present selection of common drugs have been through an almost evolutionary process with selection of the best drugs with some beneficial features in common: they have low toxicity, low potential of anaphylactic reactions, high speed of metabolism, inactive metabolites and metabolism by 1.order mechanism which ensure a constant fraction being metabolized all the time (see later). In contrast to zero-order metabolisms (a constant amount per time), the first-order mechanism will protect somewhat against unlimited accumulation with overdose. This is because with 1.order metabolism, potential accumulation of drug in plasma will also result in more drug molecules getting metabolized. By constant continuous dosing, the elimination will eventually (after three to five times the elimination half-life) increase until being equal to the supply of drugs per time, and the plasma will reach a stable ceiling level.

J. Ræder, MD, PhD (✉)
Department of Anaesthesiology—Ullevaal, Oslo University
Hospital and University of Oslo, Faculty of Medicine,
Kirkeveien, Oslo 0424, Norway
e-mail: johan.rader@medisin.uio.no

© Springer International Publishing AG 2017
A.R. Absalom, K.P. Mason (eds.), *Total Intravenous Anesthesia and Target Controlled Infusions*,
DOI 10.1007/978-3-319-47609-4_6

For most drugs, metabolism takes place in the liver. With a liver flow of 1.5 l per min in an adult, this will also be the maximum potential clearance of a liver-metabolized drug. *Clearance* is defined as the amount of blood which is fully cleaned of drug per time unit.

For some drugs, such as propofol, there is an extrahepatic metabolism (enzymes in lung, gut, etc.); thus, the clearance may be somewhat higher than liver blood flow. The even more efficient way of ensuring a rapid drug elimination is to construct drugs which are eliminated by enzymes being widespread in the body, and thus a more extensive and liver-independent degradation. This is the case with remifentanil, being degraded by tissue esterases very rapidly and extensively. There is also work in progress of having propofol-like or benzodiazepine drugs constructed this way in order to ensure an ultra-rapid metabolism.

With the neuromuscular blocking agents and reversal agents, there is no need to have lipid soluble drugs, because the effect site is on surface of the muscular membrane and accessible to water-soluble drugs. Although some of these also have a partly degradation in the liver, they do not diffuse so readily through membranes and into cells, thus their distribution volumes are lower.

A Good Model

A good model shall help us with describing what has happened and predict what is going to happen with a planned dose for a specific patient. Sometimes a model may also give some understanding as to what is happening and why, but this is not necessary for a model to be helpful. For instance, the commonly used three-compartment models may talk about distribution volumes of 2–300 l in a 70 kg adult, which has nothing to do with anatomy or physiology, but still the model may be very helpful in describing and predicting what is going on.

For intravenous drugs the plasma concentration will be determined by the dose given (in weight units of drug), the distribution to different tissues in the body and the elimination from the body. This is illustrated in Figs. 6.2 and 6.3, both being very rough anatomical models.

Such models may be developed further by listing every relevant organ in the body (including circulating blood) with

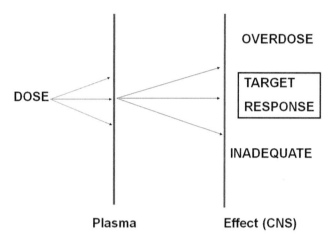

Fig. 6.1 A mg/kg dose will result in a spread of plasma concentrations of about ±30–50 % around an average, due to kinetic reasons. Even if we hit a specific plasma target, there will be a further and larger spread of effect, due to dynamic reasons

Fig. 6.2 Any injected drug will rapidly be distributed in artery blood to the central nervous system (brain in figure). However, on the way, much will be lost by uptake into the rest of the body (tissue) and by ongoing elimination (metabolism clearance)

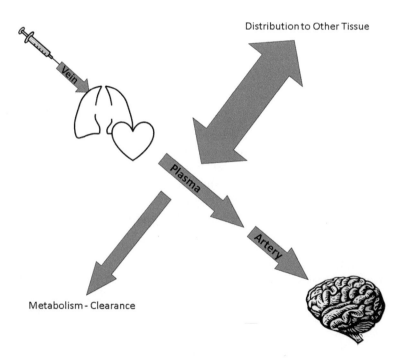

Fig. 6.3 Anatomical model of anaesthesia pharmacology: an anaesthetic drug is delivered to plasma from vaporizer (via lungs) or IV as bolus injections or infusions. From plasma the drug will diffuse into the CNS where the effects of sleep and anti-nociception (analgesia) are initiated. Simultaneously there will be a large amount of drug diffusing into the rest of the body. Also, a process of metabolism in the liver is starting by water soluble, inactive metabolite which is excreted in the urine

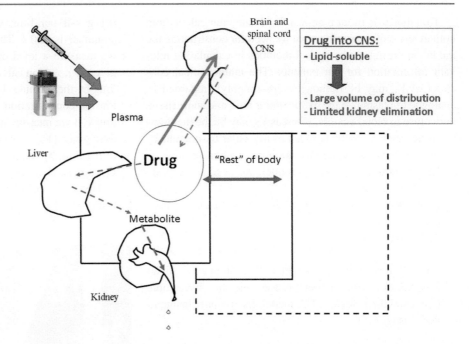

Fig. 6.4 This is a simplified model where all body are "pooled" into three compartments

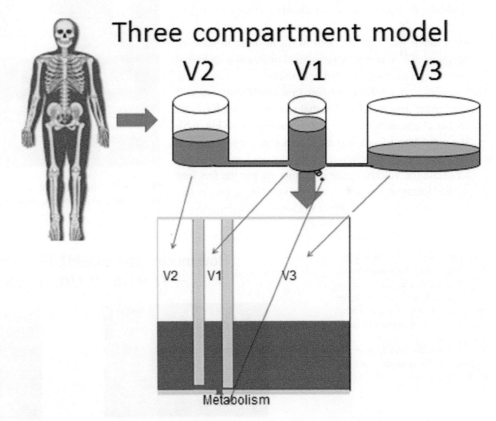

their volumes and weight and blood flow received). Then for each specific drug, we may add the solubility of the drug in the different organs and the diffusion speed of drug into or out of the organ and then construct a very accurate picture on how and where all drug molecules given IV will distribute at any given time in the total body.

Such an attempt of modelling is done. However, in order to construct such a model, we will need a vast amount of

measurements in all relevant tissues, and we do not actually need all this information in order to tell us the two major issues of interest: what is the concentration of drug in plasma? What is the anticipated effect in the target organs of brain and spinal cord?

Thus, we will do well by simplifying this model of ten organs into a construct of three compartments as we do in Fig. 6.4.

This model is more practical for dosing and calculation, both in terms of measuring what we need for constructing the model and using mathematical methods in calculating relevant information for our patients. The mathematical construct of V_1 may be (although very roughly!) regarded as analogue to plasma + the extracellular fluid and some tissue very close to blood vessels, whereas V_2 may be the medium-perfused parts of the body (such as muscular tissue) and V_3 the poorly perfused tissue, including fat and bone tissue.

But in order to use such a model, we need some basic terms and definitions.

Some pharmacokinetic terms, as defined by an everyday project:

The everyday project:

- The author will fill the sink with herbal salt in water for an adequate footbath, then empty the sink, then have some lunch and then (see the TCI model discussion) change to jeans! (Fig. 6.5).

Building the model for the steady-state situation:

1. How much water do we need to fill in order to have an adequate effect, that is, a water level of 10 cm with herbal salt at 1 g/l to cover the feet and ankle?
2. Obviously, if we have the feet in a small sink, we will need much less water and herbal salt than if we have the feet in a bathtub, nor to say in a swimming pool (Fig. 6.6). If we put 10 g of salt into the 10 cm water level bath and measure the concentration of salt to be 1 g/l, we may calculate the volume of the container we put the feet into by the formula: volume = dose given (10 g)/concentration of salt 1 g/l = 10 l. If we measure a concentration of

0.1 g salt per litre, we know that the volume of the container is 100 l. This is in parallel with IV drugs: if we measure a level of X in plasma and know the dose given (Y), we can calculate the distribution volume of the drug by the formula: Distribution volume = Dose given/Plasma concentration. This is in direct parallel with IV drugs: if we measure a level of X in plasma and know the dose given (Y), we can calculate the distribution volume of the drug by the formula: *Distribution volume* = Dose given/Plasma concentration.

However, in order to do more easy calculations, we want to have same concentrations in all three

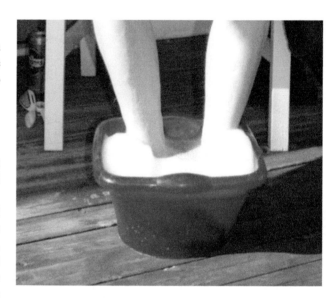

Fig. 6.5 The footbath analogy: an adequate amount of water to soak the feet with an appropriate concentration of salt (see text)

Fig. 6.6 The footbath analogy: how much water (=volume for distribution) do you need to fill in to have an adequate *level* of water to get your feet wet: not much in the sink—a huge amount in the pool. An adequate amount of water to soak the feet with an appropriate concentration of salt (see text)

How much water should be filled for adequate effect?
→ Foot bath !! (10 cm water)

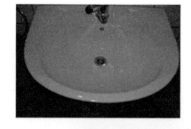

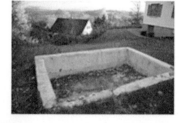

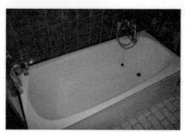

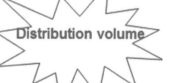

Distribution volume

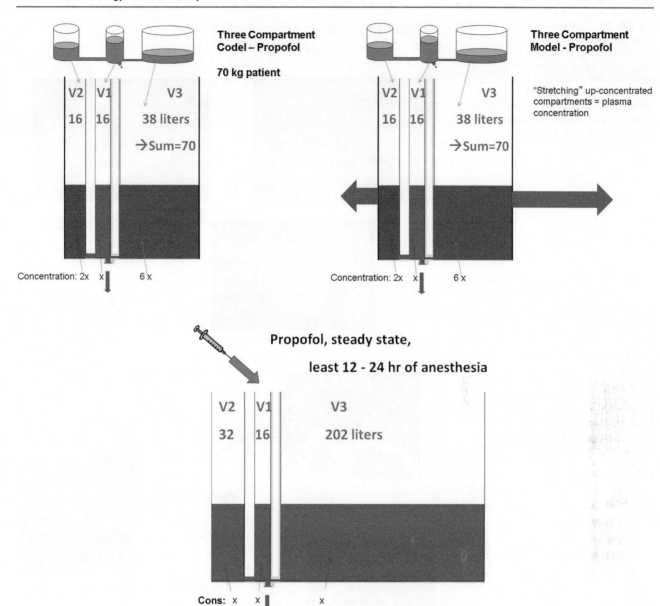

Fig. 6.7 (**a–c**) This is how a semi-anatomical model of compartments of total 70 l (**a**) in a 70 kg person may look like in terms of propofol concentrations (X-2X and 6X at steady state after a 12–24 h period of infusion). The higher concentration in V2 and V3 are due to the fact that much more drug binds in the tissue than V1 (which is mostly water), although the free fraction for diffusion equlibrium is the same in all compartments. In part (**b**) the two compartments, V_2 and V_3, are "stretched" in order to "dilute" the propofol to the same concentrations (part (**c**)) as V_1 has in part (**a**)

compartments; thus, we "stretch" the V_2 to twice the size, i.e. to 32 l, and V_3 to six times the size (Fig. 6.7c), i.e. 202 l, in order to have concentration of X everywhere (Fig. 6.7a).

Thus, we conclude that the total distribution volume of propofol at steady state in this model is 250 l in a 70 kg man, or 3.6 l per kg. If we extrapolate to a 60 kg woman, this will be $3.6 \times 60 = 216$ l.

3. Then we need to know how to empty the footbath when we are finished.

The rate of emptying will have to do with how much water we need to empty (i.e. the distribution volume, the higher the volume—the more to empty) and the size of the outlet (Fig. 6.8). The bigger the outlet, the higher rate of emptying. The speed of emptying through the outlet is called the *clearance* and should be measured in some amount (e.g. litres) per unit of time (e.g. min).

4. But we also need to know if the speed of water (ml/min) through the outlet is a constant amount irrespectively of

Fig. 6.8 This illustrates different clearances when you want to empty something, in the patient, a drug—in the figure a volume of water. The low clearance is from the sink, and the high clearance will be from the leaking swimming pool, whereas the lures in the bathroom floor have an intermediate clearance

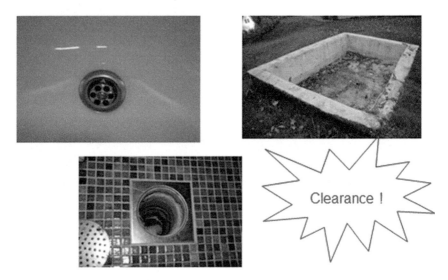

Fig. 6.9 The clearance of food by eating from a lunch table may have two approaches: either you want to taste a little of everything (the more food, the more you eat = 1.order process) or you just want to eat a preset amount, irrespective of how much you are offered (0-order process)

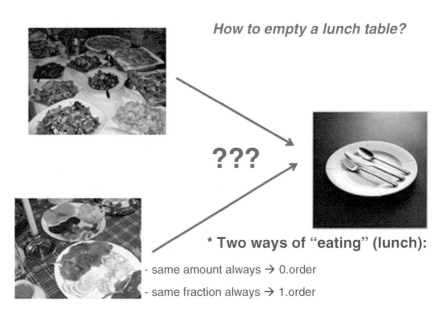

how much water there is in the sink or if there is some association of higher speed with higher amount. For that, we may look at the lunch table example:

Let's say there are two ways of eating from a lunch table (Fig. 6.9):

a. You take the same amount of food or calories, whether the table is huge with lots of dishes or small with just two to three dishes to choose from. This is 0-order way of eating and is the way the liver eats alcohol, about 0.15 units per hour, whether you have 4 units or 0.5 units per litre in your blood. It takes much more time to half empty the blood when you have 4 units at start.

b. You feel you like to taste a bite of everything on the table, that is, ten bites for ten dishes and three bites for three dishes. You will eat the same fraction of the table always, but the amount will be very different. This is the way the liver eats propofol; the liver will eat the same fraction whether the blood concentration is high or low (Fig. 6.10). This is the 1.order way of eating, which means it will take the same time to half empty the blood, irrespectively of the starting concentration.

Actually, the drugs we use in modern anaesthesia have a 1.order elimination, because 0.order elimination drugs are hard to dose, as they may accumulate to very high

Fig. 6.10 Liver clearance (i.e. metabolism) of lipid soluble drugs. The liver receives 1.5 L blood per min in an average adult. If every molecule in that delivery is metabolised to inactive substances, the clearance is 1.5 L per min. If only half of molecules is cleared (50 %), half of the 1.5 L are fully cleared (i.e. clearance is 0.75 l/min), whereas half is non-cleared. In the figure (from *top*) we see an illustration of 50, 75 and 100 % clearance

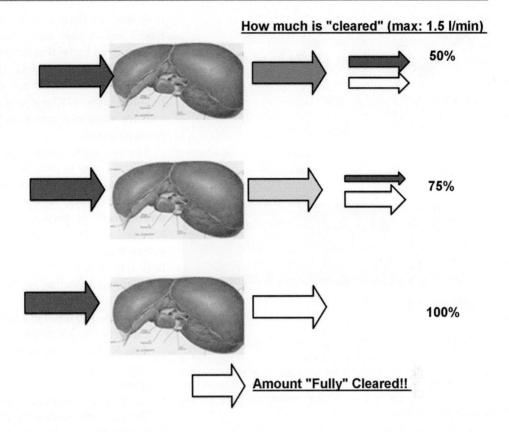

concentrations with dosing errors. With an infusion of a 1.order drug, the elimination (i.e. amount) will increase as the plasma concentration increase, until the amount eliminated is as high as the dose given per time unit, thus reaching an upper plateau or safe upper limit for plasma concentration after about three to five times the half-life of elimination.

5. But even though we have established our drug as a 1. order elimination drug, we need to know how big is the fraction eliminated every time or time unit. For the lunch example: do we take 1 bite of every dish or 2 bites? For the liver, which receives an "offer" of 1.5 l of blood every minute in the adult: how much does the liver eat from this offer? For propofol it is very simple and fortunate: the liver eats everything, that is, with a propofol concentration of 4 mg/l blood, the liver eats 6 mg propofol every minute (4 mg/l × 1.5 l per min). We may say that the liver clearance is 100 % of the flow, that is, 1.5 l is fully cleared every minute. If the liver instead is offered fentanyl, it only eats about 50 %, that is, for 1.5 l liver flow during a minute, there is only a 50 % clearance. Instead of saying "50 % clearance of 1.5 l", we instead divide the liver flow into volume of blood fully cleared and volume not cleared at all. For fentanyl: 1.5 l 50 % cleared will be the same as 0.75 l not cleared +0.75 l fully cleared. We will for simplicity always do this in our model, talk about

amount of blood fully cleared, that is, for fentanyl 0.75 l per minute.

Now, we have built a model for steady-state situation with distribution volume at steady state and clearance (Fig. 6.11). In this model the time to half the concentration when the dosing (or infusion) stops is given by the relation: $T\frac{1}{2} = k \times VD$/clearance. Also in this situation the dosing is very simple if we want to keep a steady plasma concentration; we simply replace the amount cleared every time unit; in our example of propofol of 4 mg/l blood concentration, we need to give 6 mg every minute. In this situation we do not actually need the three-compartment model; it is enough to know the clearance.

But very few anaesthetics last for 12–24 h, which is what we need to create a steady state. Thus we need to know more on two important situations:

a. How much drug do we need in the start?
b. How much drug do we need in the phase after start and until steady state is reached?

How Much Drug Do We Need in the Start?

In the very start, we do not need to pay much attention to elimination or distribution to slowly perfused tissues in V_2

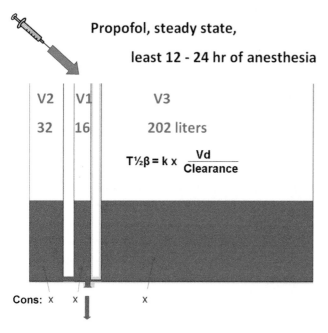

Fig. 6.11 Steady-state picture of propofol in a three-compartment model, 70 kg adult patient. Note that the V_2 and V_3 are upgraded in order to contain propofol at the same concentration as in plasma. In a pure anatomical model (total volume = 70 l), the V_2 would be 16 l and propofol concentration $2X$, whereas the V_3 would be 38 l and propofol concentration about $6X$

and V_3, but the focus is the size of V_1. Basically, we can do a blood sample just after a rapid bolus dose and calculate the immediate distribution volume, which is the same as V_1, by the formula:

$$\text{Drug concentration} = \text{Dose}/\text{volume of } V_1.$$

Here we may run into discussion about where to take our blood sample, and what will be the relevant concentration for the brain. If we, for instance, take a venous sample, as was done for the Marsh pharmacokinetic model, we may find that a 2 mg/kg dose in a 70 kg adult gave a venous plasma concentration of 4.4 mg/l, thus a volume of V_1 of 32 l.

However, if we do like the Schnider model and take an arterial sample, we may find a concentration of 25 mg/ml and calculate a V_1 of 5.5 l.

This discrepancy is some of the explanations for different models dosing quite differently in the start, but in a clinical situation, we also have to include the aspects of speed of infusion of drug into the CNS and the delay from plasma to onset of effect (see later).

How Much Drug Do We Need in the Phase After Start and Until Steady State Is Reached?

In this situation we have to compensate both for elimination of drug (clearance) and the distribution of drug into all tissues in the body. If we use the Marsh model and already have filled the V_1 with 4.4 mg/l of propofol, we know that during 12 h we shall fill another 234 l of body tissue (take 1030 mg/propofol), and we have to compensate for 6.6 mg eaten by the liver every minute, that is, 4752 mg propofol during 12 h to compensate for clearance and keep a steady concentration of 4.4 mg/l blood.

The question is how we adjust our infusion rate for such a project; we need to know the speed of diffusion into V_2 and V_3, or the time constants for such diffusion.

These data may be derived from plasma concentration measurements in volunteers or patients after defined dosing of drugs. The distribution and elimination of IV drugs after dosing, thanks to first-order elimination, follows logarithmic laws (Fig. 6.12) and may be well described in a three-compartment model, as we have used already.

A bolus dose will result in a very high initial plasma concentration (in V_1) which subsequently diffuses into V_2 and V_3 (Fig. 6.13). Because both V_2 and V_3 receives drug by a high concentration gradient initially, the decline in plasma concentration and decline in V_1 concentration is rapid, but then slower as V_2 comes in equilibrium with V_1. The third compartment (V_3) fills very slowly due to lower blood perfusion. Also, a constant (in terms of fraction of plasma drug metabolized per time) metabolism will go on, responsible for only a small fraction of total decline in plasma concentration initially.

Then all compartments (V_{1-3}) in the body are in diffusion equilibrium, and the drug amount metabolized is equal to the amount given per time unit if the concentration is steady.

With a model such as in Fig. 6.3 and data about V_1, V_2, V_3 and clearance and speed of equilibration between the compartments, computerized modelling may be used in order to predict the relevant plasma concentration in any patient at any time after a given setup for dosing (bolus (es) and/or infusion(s)). Examples of such modelling are presented in the Stanpump® (http://anesthesia.stanford.edu/pkpd), RUGLOOP® (http://users.skynet.be/fa491447/index.html) and Tivatrainer® (www.eurosiva.org) simulation programmes, which are very helpful for understanding intravenous dosing and predicting plasma levels.

The modelling of a fixed intravenous drug dose will surely depend on the patient weight; thus, the weight is always included in such models; basically quite simple: double weight means double dose in order to have same plasma concentration.

Taking other patient features into account may increase the precision of prediction, but they are often not included because they are difficult to calculate and interpret into mathematical models of drug pharmacokinetics. Examples

Fig. 6.12 Propofol plasma concentration (*red*) after a 2 mg/kg bolus dose in a 70 kg adult. The *green curve* is a qualitative estimation of strength of hypnotic effect. The peak effect is about 3–4 min after the start of bolus, and a result of the delay from plasma to CNS and the decay of the plasma curve

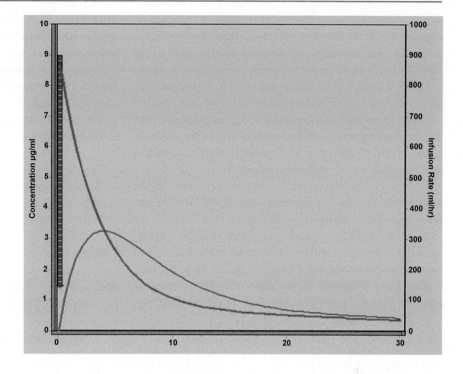

Fig. 6.13 Propofol is given for 1 h (*left panel*) or 6 h (*right panel*). Note that in both cases the V_2 is in equilibrium with the V_1, but the V_3 is "filled" less after 1 h than after 6 h. When the infusion stops the time to 50 %, drop in plasma concentration (=V_1) will be shorter after 1 h because the diffusion gradient to V_3 is larger

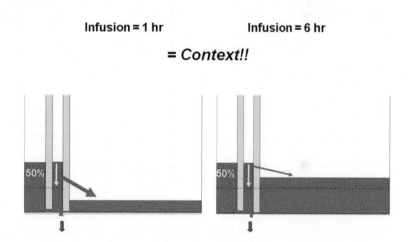

What About Stopping Dosing Before Steady State Is Reached?

One very important concept for the practical anaesthetist is to know what happens with the pharmacokinetics when we stop dosing before reaching steady state.

This concept is

The context-sensitive elimination time.

This is the time taken to achieve a predefined reduction of plasma concentration from the stop of dosing. The reduction is a net result of elimination (clearance) + distribution from plasma to nonequilibrated tissue. The term is usually used in conjunction with constant dosing (fixed dose per time unit) and looking for a reduction of 50 %, i.e. *the context-sensitive half-time*.

In Fig. 6.13, we have simulated the situation after 1 h of stable propofol infusion, compared with 6 h infusion. If we stop the infusion after 1 h, there is a large gradient of diffusion into V_3, "helping" us to half the concentration fairly quick, compared with the situation after 6 h, where the gradient is lower. In both situations the diffusion into V_3 adds to the contribution from the clearance, which is running all the time.

A 50 % reduction is usually the easiest to estimate and also fairly relevant for intermediate dosing of IV hypnotics for sleep and analgesics for stress response attenuation. With 50 % reduction in such doses, you may expect the patient to wake up (50 % reduction in hypnotic agent) and breathe spontaneously (50 % reduction in opioid).

Still, the context-sensitive concept may be used for any kind of dosing schedule and endpoints of 20, 80 % or any other degree of reduction may be applied.

With a carefully titrated and down-adjusted general anaesthetic combination for closing the wound at end of surgery, it may sometimes be relevant to check for only further 20 % reduction of analgesic or hypnotic drugs in order to have the patient breathing or awake, respectively.

With high dosing for, e.g. coronary surgery, it may be appropriate to look for 80 % reduction for the concentrations before breathing and verbal contact are achieved.

Figure 6.14 shows the context elimination half-life for propofol and some relevant opioids (see later for individual drug description).

Pharmacodynamics of intravenous drugs:
Pharmacodynamics has to do with both

a. Timing of effect onset/offset
b. Strength of effect
c. Type of effect

Timing

Basically a drug has to pass some steps from being in plasma into exerting effect (Fig. 6.15):

Fig. 6.14 This is a drawing of context-sensitive half-life of five relevant drugs as defined by duration of an infusion for constant plasma level

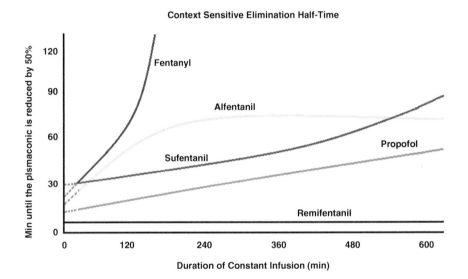

Fig. 6.15 The drug has a way to go from being in plasma until the relevant site for effect is reached (see text)

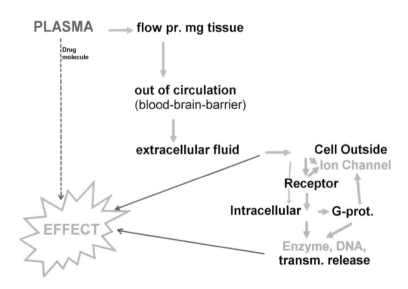

- Diffusion out of blood vessel (through blood–brain barrier)
- Diffusion in extracellular fluid
- Surface of effect or cell
- Binding to a receptor or cell surface or structure inside cell
- Biologic effect

The biologic effect may be fast, such as opening an ion channel, more slowly such as activating protein synthesis (e.g. NSAIDS) or even more slowly such as activating DNA and protein synthesis (e.g. corticosteroids). As the drugs differ both in their biological effect mechanism and how fast they get from plasma to the effect site, there is a difference in time to onset. This difference may be expressed by a constant, keO, a high constant means a rapid onset, or short $T\frac{1}{2}$ keO which is the time taken for 50 % equilibration from plasma to effect site. Both these terms are theoretical constructs based on assumption on stable plasma concentrations. In the three-compartment model, we may add an effect compartment, embedded in V_1 (since the CNS is very well perfused), as shown in Fig. 6.16.

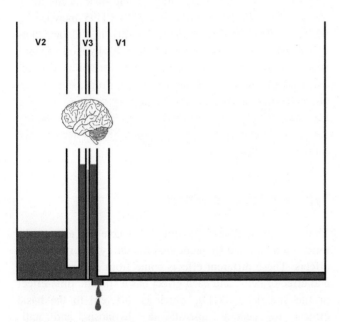

Fig. 6.16 Mathematically based three-compartment model with effect compartment embedded in V_1. In the middle is V_1, which receives drug and may be analogue to plasma and surrounding fluids. The level of *red* corresponds to drug concentration. From V_1 there is a good diffusion (*large opening*) of drug into V_2 which will get into equilibrium with V_1 within 10–30 min. A much slower diffusion takes place into V_3 (*narrow opening*) which is the larger part of the body, fairly poorly circulated. We may also note a constant "leakage" of drug from V_1, which represents the clearance, inactivation and/or excretion of drug. The small *green* compartment inside V_1 is the CNS or effect compartment. The level of drug (*red*; *green* in the brain) is an example of simulation 10 min after a bolus dose of propofol (from Tivatrainer®)

The time to peak effect after a bolus dose is the result of both the effect delay per se and the effects on plasma-to-brain gradient in dynamic change due to distribution of drug out of plasma. With infusion only, the time to peak effect will be prolonged, but this is due to the slow increase in plasma concentration more than delay from plasma to effect site (Fig. 6.17).

KeOs and time to peak effect are given for some drugs in Table 6.1.

Knowing the time to peak effect after bolus is useful in three important contexts:

1. Go for the maximum effect when the trauma is maximal, such as during intubation or start of surgery.
2. Titrate a drug until proper level. Titration is to give a dose and wait for full effect. If the full effect is insufficient, a new dose is given and then wait for effect and so on. With a short time to peak effect, the process of titration goes faster.
3. Anticipate risk of side effects. For instance, with a slow-acting drug such as morphine, the event of respiratory depression will evolve slowly, patients being gradually drowsy and then reduce the respiratory frequency before eventual apnoea by the time of the peak effect after 15–20 min. With alfentanil the maximal effect comes much more rapidly may be with a sudden apnoea 2 min after a bolus. Thus, with a slow-acting drug you have to watch longer in order to feel safe, and titration is slower. A positive aspect will be that you have more time to observe problems emerging and have some more time to call for help and find appropriate drugs and equipment needed. The negative effect of slow action is that you have to wait and observe the patient for longer in order to be sure to not miss the time of maximum side effect.

Strength of Effect

The computer programmes will usually simulate the time course and relative strength of effect changes, but not the actual level of clinical effect. For instance, with remifentanil the young and the elderly will have a fairly similar effect-site curve, but in the elderly the actual clinical effect may be twice as strong [1]. This is probably due to increased CNS sensitivity for opioids in the elderly and should be taken into account when choosing a dosing level or target of plasma or effect site in the elderly. It also seems that females need a little more hypnotic agent in order to be asleep than males; again the plasma or effect-site levels of drug may be similar, but the brain sensitivity may differ [2].

Fig. 6.17 Infusion is like rapidly repeated, with same interval, small, identical bolus doses over time. Time to peak effect is determined more by the slow rise in plasma, than delay in plasma-effect-site equilibration

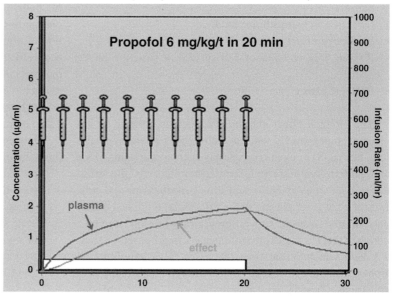

Infusion (= repeated small bolus doses)

Table 6.1 Delay (min) from drug being in plasma until effect

	$T\frac{1}{2}$ for equilibration	Time to maximal effect between plasma and effect site ($T\frac{1}{2}keO$) after a bolus dose
Barbiturates (thiopenthone)	1.2	1.0–2.0
Propofol	2.6	1.5–3.5
Midazolam	5.6	5–7
Diazepam	2	1–3
Opioids		
Remifentanil	1.2	1–2
Alfentanil	1.1	1.5–3
Fentanyl	5.8	4–5
Morphine	?	10–20
NSAID	?	15–30
Corticosteroid	?	60–120

The table shows in the middle column the half-life of equilibration from plasma to effect site for some relevant drugs (means that good data are not available), whereas the right column shows the time to maximal effect after a single bolus dose. The figures in both columns are average estimates from different sources and may vary considerably, whereas the *ranking* of speed between different drugs are better established

The strength of effect may be expressed in an intravenous analogue of MAC, the ED50 or EC50. Effective dose, ED50, is the dose needed in order to have the effect (e.g. sleep, no movement on incision) in 50 % of patients; the effective concentration, EC50, is the plasma concentration needed.

The variability in ED will always be larger than variability in EC, because a dose may result in a variety of plasma concentrations. With EC we anticipate a given plasma concentration and only compensate for variability in sensitivity.

In order to go from EC50 to EC95 (effective concentration for effect in 95 % of patients), the dose needs to be increased by 40–50 %; from ED50 to ED95 increase by 60–80 %. The interindividual variability in EC (and thus ED) is generally larger for opioids than for hypnotic agents, and we must be prepared for quite some variability in clinical need of opioids compared to other drugs, even in an otherwise normal patient. The range may be up to fivefold, i.e. the patient with minimal opioid need will require one-fifth of the dose in a patient with maximal need for the same standardized stimulus.

Type of Effect: Side Effect

The intravenous anaesthetic drugs also have side effects; the most important and frequent are circulatory and respiratory effects. These different effects come from different organs and effector cells, and each effect has a specific time-effect profile and delay (keO), which is different to the basic effects of general anaesthesia: hypnosis and anti-nociception.

Respiratory Effects

The opioids cause a dose-dependent reduction in respiration frequency, ending in apnoea. When the patients get drowsy and the respiratory rate is below 8–10 per minute, it may be a warning of apnoea potentially emerging. Inability to maintain free airway may be absent or present.

The ventilatory depression, being CNS driven, usually follows the analgesic and sedative effect fairly closely. Respiratory depression may be counteracted by stimulation, verbal or (more efficient) tactile and even painful. In a worst case, these effects may always be reversed by naloxone, which will also reverse the analgesia abruptly if not titrated very carefully.

The respiratory depression with hypnotics is usually regarded as less than with opioids, but it is difficult to sort out equipotency of these two drug classes, as the anaesthetic effects are quite different. Respiratory depression with hypnotics is clinically evident as inability to maintain free airway and shallow tidal volumes, whereas the ventilator frequency may be normal or low. Propofol will always result in apnoea with high doses, whereas the benzodiazepines are safer in terms of very high dose needed for respiratory arrest. Also, with the benzodiazepines, full reversal is possible with flumazenil.

Circulatory Effects

The circulatory effects will be a mixture of drug effects in the CNS and peripheral effects directly in the heart and vessel walls (vasodilatation), as well as the physiological effect of going to sleep with subsequent reduction in sympathetic nerve tone. A drop in blood pressure and heart rate during general anaesthetic induction is almost always seen (except with ketamine), unless the surgery or other stimulation starts concomitantly. Although elective patients also are slightly hypovolaemic (from fasting), they usually tolerate well a short-lasting drop in syst BP down to the 70–90 range, as organ flow is well maintained, and oxygen consumption low when being asleep. Kazama and co-workers have shown that the maximal drop in blood pressure is delayed for 2–3 min when compared to maximal hypnotic effect of propofol in the average adult. In the elderly, the delay after sleep is 5–6 min, and the drop is larger, probably due to stiffer myocardium and vessel walls in the elderly [2].

Intravenous Drug Interactions: Opioids and Hypnotics

Basically, general anaesthesia may be achieved with a very high dose of hypnotic drug alone. As a parallel, a patient with a severe benzodiazepine intoxication is unconscious and may not react to pain stimuli; thus surgery is possible. Propofol at a dose fivefold of being asleep will provide the same feature, but this is not very practical in terms of drug economy, cardiovascular depression and speed of recovery.

Opioids, on the other hand, may provide excellent abolishment of pain reaction when the dose is high enough but is not reliable as hypnotics. Although most patients will be asleep most of the time on a high-dose opioid, some may be fully awake in an unpredictable manner for periods. Thus, general anaesthesia with intravenous drugs only, total intravenous anaesthesia (TIVA), is usually achieved with a combination of opioid and hypnotic, most often propofol.

Opioids will reduce the dose need of propofol for sleep by 20–50 % at fairly low doses, such as alfentanil 1–2 mg in an adult, or remifentanil plasma level of 2.5–5.0 ng/ml. Increasing the opioid dose does not add much to further dose reduction of propofol for being asleep.

Thus a minimum dose of propofol at 3–4 mg/kg/h for maintenance or target of 1.5–1.8 µg/ml (Marsh model, see below) should be used for sleep, irrespectively if the opioid dose is high or low.

Propofol will reduce the need of opioids for antinociception in a dose-related manner, anything from 10 to 20 % reduction with a low sleeping dose (6 mg/kg/h or target 3 µg/ml) to almost 90–100 % if the dose is five to six times higher (target of 15–20 µg/ml).

The practical approach will depend on the type of opioid in use as demonstrated by Vuyk and colleagues in their important work on EC50 and EC95 values for propofol + opioid combination in open abdominal surgery (Table 6.2 [3]).

The major point with opioid + propofol combination is to use a high dose of the drug with shorter context-sensitive elimination half-life. With alfentanil or remifentanil that means to have a low and stable concentration of propofol to ensure sleep and then "play" with opioid adjustments in medium to high dose according to strength of nociceptive stimulation. This is also logical, because the variable stimulus during surgery is pain and nociception, whereas the need of being asleep is stable.

With short-lasting use of fentanyl (or low doses; i.e. 0.1–0.2 mg for a less than 30 min procedure, or less than 0.1 mg/h) the same strategy, i.e. low-dose propofol for sleep, may be used. However, if the use of fentanyl is more extensive, then a more rapid recovery will result by increasing the propofol dose with up to 100 % and subsequently reducing the dose of fentanyl.

As to respiratory depression, opioids are more potent than propofol, but the combination is synergistic.

Target Control Infusion (TCI) (See Chap. 8)

Target control infusion is no magic, but merely a device to help in dosing intravenous drugs more precisely and with less effort. As to the central nervous system and the clinical effector cells, they do not care for whether the drug is

Table 6.2 Recommended combinations of propofol + opioid

	Alfentanil EC$_{50}$–EC$_{95}$ (90–130 ng/ml)	Fentanyl EC$_{50}$–EC$_{95}$ (1.1–1.6 ng/ml)	Sufentanil EC$_{50}$–EC$_{95}$ (0.14–0.20 ng/ml)	Remifentanil EC$_{50}$–EC$_{95}$ (4.7–8.0 ng/ml)
Opioid				
Bolus	25–35 µg/kg in 30 s	3 µg/kg in 30 s	0.15–0.25 µg/kg in 30 s	1.5–2 µg/kg in 30 s
Infusion 1	50–75 µg kg^{-1} h^{-1} for 30 min	1.5–2.5 µg kg^{-1} h^{-1} for 30 min	0.15–0.22 µg kg^{-1} h^{-1}	13–22 µg kg^{-1} h^{-1} for 20 min
Infusion 2	30–42.5 µg kg^{-1} h^{-1} thereafter	1.3–2 µg kg^{-1} h^{-1} up to 150 min		11.5–19 µg kg^{-1} h^{-1} thereafter
Infusion 3		0.7–1.4 µg kg^{-1} h^{-1} thereafter		
	Propofol EC$_{50}$–EC$_{95}$ (3.2–4.4 µg/ml)	Propofol EC$_{50}$–EC$_{95}$ (3.4–5.4 µg/ml)	Propofol EC$_{50}$–EC$_{95}$ (3.3–4.5 µg/ml)	Propofol EC$_{50}$–EC$_{95}$ (2.5–2.8 µg/ml)
Propofol				
Bolus	2.0–2.8 mg/kg in 30 s	2.0–3.0 mg/kg in 30 s	2.0–2.8 mg/kg in 30 s	1.5 mg/kg in 30 s
Infusion 1	9–12 mg kg^{-1} h^{-1} for 40 min	9–15 mg kg^{-1} h^{-1} for 40 min	9–12 mg kg^{-1} h^{-1} for 40 min	7–8 mg kg^{-1} h^{-1} for 40 min
Infusion 2	7–10 mg kg^{-1} h^{-1} for 150 min	7–12 mg kg^{-1} h^{-1} for 150 min	7–10 mg kg^{-1} h^{-1} for 150 min	6–6.5 mg kg^{-1} h^{-1} for 150 min
Infusion 3	6.5–8 mg kg^{-1} h^{-1} thereafter	6.5–11 mg kg^{-1} h^{-1} thereafter	6.5–8 mg kg^{-1} h^{-1} thereafter	5–6 mg kg^{-1} h^{-1} thereafter

From Vuyk, Jaap; Mertens, Martijn J. Propofol Anesthesia and Rational Opioid Selection Determination of Optimal EC50EC95 Propofol Opioid Concentrations that Assure Adequate Anesthesia and a Rapid Return of Consciousness. Anesthesiology. Dec 1, 1997. Vo. 87. No 6. Reprinted with permission from Wolters Kluwer Health, Inc.

In the brackets are shown the appropriate target concentrations required, whereas the bolus + infusion figure show the relevant manual dosing for that target

The figures are based on measurements of plasma concentrations of different combinations of alfentanil and propofol during open abdominal surgery, and the optimal combination for most rapid emergence after 3 h anaesthesia. EC50 and EC95 are the dose combination needed to keep 50 % and 95 % of the patients nonmoving all the time, respectively. The figures for the other opioids are extrapolated from the alfentanil clinical tests

Generally in ambulatory patients, we will go even lower in propofol (1.8–2.2 µg/ml) unless the patient is paralyzed, then target of 2.5–2.8 may be appropriate during phases of deep relaxation (i.e. unable to move)

given by syringe, infusion or computer; the cells react upon the number of drug molecules present at the effect sites.

Still, with a TCI system, you may ensure a rapid onset, a stable effect when needed, a rapid offset or reduction in effect and less work with dosing and calculations.

The Logic of TCI

With a manual scheme for giving propofol, you may get to a good result in ensuring rapid and stable sleep in an adult by the following recipe: start with bolus 1.5 mg/kg together with an infusion of 10 mg/kg/h for 10 min, then adjust infusion to 8 mg/kg/h for another 10 min; then adjust to 6 mg/kg/h which is maintained for the rest of the case. If this seems to be too much, then adjust the infusion down by 2 mg/kg/min or if this seems to be too low dose, give another bolus of 0.5 mg/kg and adjust the infusion up with 2 mg/kg/h. Stop infusion by the end of the case (Fig. 6.18a).

This recipe is based on the weight of the patient and then simple calculations on bolus dose and pump rates. If we call this recipe for "Recipe X", we may programme a computerized pump to do this automatically. We programme the computer with patient weight and push the start button:

the computer will give the bolus dose and the infusion and automatically adjust rate after 10 and 20 min without any more actions from the anaesthetists. If the anaesthetist tells the computer to go "up", the computer will deliver the small bolus and adjust the infusion rate. If the anaesthetist tells the computer to go "down", the computer pump will stop for some minutes and then start the infusion at the lower level.

By programming this "Recipe X" into the computerized pump, we have made a simple TCI plasma system. If we run this programme in a series of patients and do measurements on stable propofol plasma concentrations 15 min after start of the programme, we may find that the average plasma concentration is about 3 µg/ml (Fig. 6.18b). Thus, we have programmed our pump to deliver a *plasma target concentration* of 3 µg/ml. If we test the plasma levels 15 min after doing the "up" and "down" adjustments, we may find a concentration of 4 and 2 µg/ml, respectively. Thus, we have made a programme for how the pump should work when we want to increase the target to four or reduce the target to two. By testing different ways of dosing, measuring plasma concentrations (in patients or volunteers) and fit into mathematical algorithms, we can make a programme for how to dose for any given target in any patient; the only thing we need to tell the computer in the OR is the weight of

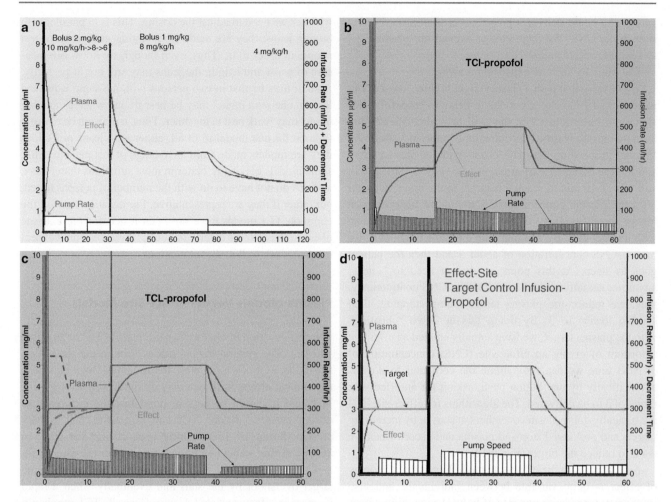

Fig. 6.18 (**a**) Plasma concentration (*red*) and relative strength of hypnotic effect (*green*) for a manual propofol regime of start bolus, then infusion adjusted at 10 and 20 min. Also shown is an increase in dosing at 30 min and decrease at 75 min (Marsh kinetic/dynamic model, Tivatrainer®). (**b**) Plasma target control infusion, TCI (pump rate are black columns) for target 3, then 5, then back to 3 again. Note that the pump gives a short-lasting bolus infusion at start and increasing the dose and stops temporarily by decreasing. Also note that the pump adjust far more frequently (=more accurately) than a manual regimen (as in Fig. 6.9). Also note the delay in effect, patient probably not being asleep until 5–7 min. (**c**) Same as in Fig. 4.11b, except for "cheating"

with a plasma target of 5.5 µg/min during induction, in order to get a more rapid effect (*green curve*); now patient will probably be asleep at 2–3 min. (**d**) Effect-site TCI for propofol. The pump is programmed to deliver an effect level corresponding to 3, then 5, then 3 again. Note the differences from Fig. 4.11 and plasma TCI: by start and increasing dose, there will be a plasma "overshoot" created by a more vigorous bolus infusion, then stopping for proper equilibration with the effect site. By decreasing effect level, the pump will stop and allow the plasma concentration to go below the new target, then giving a small bolus to "catch up" with the effect curve and keep stable at new level

the patient and the target we will like to have. This is the concept of the original Marsh *plasma target control infusion* algorithm, which was widely used with propofol-prefilled syringes for pumps programmed with the Diprifusor® software (www.eurosiva.org). When testing with blood samples, the Marsh algorithm gave quite different plasma levels in different patients (+/÷30–50 % around target) and also tended to give somewhat higher plasma levels than the preset target [4]. Still it was still very useful and gained high popularity in clinical everyday practice. It provided a stable level, and the clinicians soon learnt what a relevant proper starting target in their patients should be and how to easily adjust up or down according to clinical needs.

A limitation with the Marsh algorithm was that only weight was adjusted; there was no adjustment for the age of the patient and no adjustment for obese or slim body composition, only total weight. These limitations have been addressed in some of the other models, such as Schnider, Schuttler, Paedfusor, etc., where some of these covariates has been added to the weight for adjustment of dosing.

A major limitation with all models of plasma target and the plasma target concept is that they do not take into account the delay in drug equilibration between plasma and CNS. As the anaesthetic drug effect is not in plasma, but in the brain, we should rather like to have a computer pump who could deliver a preset concentration into effect sites in the CNS. We then have to expand our plasma TCI system into an *effect-site TCI system.*

The logic by such an expansion may be:

We observe that with a plasma target of three, most of our patients will go to sleep, but due to delay in propofol diffusion from plasma to CNS, this will take about 5–10 min, even though the plasma concentration is stable at 3 after 30 s. In order to speed up, we may "cheat" with the plasma target and tell the pump to start at target of 6 (Fig. 6.18b). It will still take 5–10 min to reach this target in the brain, but after 30 s the plasma concentration is 6 and we have a much higher speed (gradient) of diffusion of drug into CNS than with a target of 3. By 2–3 min with a plasma target of 6, we have a CNS concentration of about 3 and then the patient goes to sleep. At this point we do not need to "cheat" anymore; actually we will overdose the CNS continuously; thus, we reduce the plasma target (pump stopping, then starting lower) to 3. By doing this up-down "cheating" with the plasma target, we have actually created an effective algorithm of giving an effect-site (CNS) concentration of 3. Next time we can programme the computer to do this automatically by one button push, asking for an effect-site target of 3 to be delivered. The algorithms for effect-site TCI are basically doing plasma overshoot at start or by increasing targets and prolonged stop and plasma underscore when we want to reduce the target (Fig. 6.18c).

A problem with the effect-site modelling is that the delay of effect is quite variable between individuals, and also somewhat dependent upon rate of bolus/dosing, high versus low dose, state of circulation, etc. Also, the delay is hard to measure exactly and the relation may be both to arterial and venous drug concentration, which will differ during change in dosing. Still, the effect-site modelling gets closer to the clinical needs and is proven to be very useful in clinical work.

Exactly the same ways of making plasma TCI and effect-site TCI have been used with remifentanil, and also for other opioids, such as alfentanil, fentanil and sufentanil.

Different TCI Models

The TCI models are made from measurements of doses, plasma concentrations (venous or arterial) and effects in real patients or in volunteers. Even in a very standardized situation, volunteers or patients will differ in the values obtained; thus, ideally everyone should have their own Taylor-made model. However, as we use the models to make estimates on the average future patient, we need to use some average of the results from our test group and eventually adjust our dosing when starting our case and observe whether the patient seems to behave like average or

whether we need to adjust the dosing. This is in parallel with buying jeans; they are made from testing in a group of test people in order to fit. Thus, even though we know our measure of waist and length, the jeans may still not fit perfectly. Also, it may be that in two persons with the same waist and length, one jean model may be best in one whereas another model may work best in the other. Thus, it may not be realistic to hope for one model to fit all, either with jeans or TCI, as they are models made from an average of test persons. Still, some models may work better in most situations than others, and this do not have to do with the number of persons tested, but rather if they are representative. For instance, most of the common TCI modes have not been tested for the extreme obese or the extreme elderly or young; thus, we cannot expect them to work well in these situations.

Plasma Models Versus Effect-Site Models

The first question is whether to use a plasma TCI or an effect-site TCI. The general logical rule will be to use the effect-site mode, as this is more close to drug physiology including the clinical effect. Still, one may do quite well with plasma TCI, and it should be kept in mind that the difference in dosing between plasma TCI and effect-site TCI is only present during 10–15 min after each change (or start) in dosing; during stable conditions they deliver the same.

Using plasma TCI one should remember to do some target overshoot by the start and eventually when a rapid increase in effect is wanted. Using effect-site TCI one should remember that a higher bolus dose is given every time the dose is increased, and this may exert a stronger effect on respiration and haemodynamics. This stronger effect could be compensated by titrating the effect target in increments when needed for the fragile patient.

Remifentanil

For remifentanil there is only one model in major clinical use, the Minto model for both plasma and effect-site modus [1]. The Minto model hits on average well at the target, but a +/÷30–50 % deviation may be observed in the individual patient [4]. The model takes into consideration patient weight versus height ratio and also age for the plasma modelling. When used in the effect-site modus, it will only deliver a drug "concentration" in the CNS and not adjust as to how sensitive the patient will be for that concentration (dynamics). For instance, with no stimulation and effect-site infusion of 2 ng/ml, a 20-year-old patient may be breathing and awake, whereas an 80-year-old patient probably will be asleep and have apnoea. This is because the opioid sensitivity in the elderly is about twice that seen in the younger. The drug sensitivity is not built into the models, only the drug concentrations.

Propofol

With propofol there have been a number of groups who have made TCI models based on their measurements of plasma and effect delay in their series of patients or volunteers. Such measurements are not exact, and the results will also differ between individuals. For this reason, it is no surprise that different authors have come to different models. The basic differences between models are in their estimation of the size of V_1 and the delay of effect. Basically, if a model conclude that V_1 is large, then the initial dosing (in mg/kg) should be large, and if the delay is long (low keO, long $T\frac{1}{2}$ keO), the initial dose (overshoot) in effect-site modus should be large. Still, these differences are basically evident in the first 15 min of a case, after that the models will behave fairly similarly.

Also, it should be noted that some models compensate for weight/height ratio and/or age, whereas others only compensate for total weight. The common models do not compensate for differences in propofol sensitivity as may be decreased in children and slightly in females. For more detailed discussion on models, one is referred to Chap. XX, but some rough statements could be made.

- Marsh plasma TCI [5]: Generally delivers somewhat more than predicted, especially in the start (high V_1).
- Marsh effect—old: This model has a long delay in effect and will tend to overdose initially, compared with measurements in patients.
- Marsh effect—new [6]: This model has a short delay in effect, which will compensate somewhat for the overdosing done for the plasma part of the algorithm. Still it is a clinical impression that the delay is too short in this model, and a 25-50% overshoot in target for 1–2 min during the start of a case will work better in terms of getting asleep within 2–3 min.
- Schnider plasma: The Schnider model [7] is actually not developed for plasma modus and will (low V_1) underdose the patients initially. If used, the start target should be 50–100 % higher than with the Marsh model in order to have the same dose (mg/kg) delivered.
- Schnider effect: This has an intermediate delay in effect, which will compensate somewhat for the underdosing in plasma. It also compensate somewhat for thin/fat patients and elderly. Still, the target levels need to be a little higher than those for Marsh models. In the very obese, the formula for weight correction will be very wrong, and the model should not be used above 100–120 kg total weight.

- Kataria/Paedfusor: All models above do not compensate if the patient being is a child. Children have a higher V_1 and a higher clearance in relation to weight than adults. Both these children models will compensate for these features, resulting in a higher and more appropriate dose for a given target, both for start and maintenance in children. Paedfusor has an age dynamic change in clearance which is more precise for all children, whereas the kataria has a fixed rate for clearance which may result in overdose in children above 5-10 years of age.

Addendum

Interactions with inhalational agents

Dynamic interactions with intravenous agents:

Whereas the clinical effect and dose level in a population of intravenous drugs often is measured in plasma concentrations, e.g. EC_{50} which is the concentration needed to get 50 % of patients asleep, the corresponding effect of inhalational agents are usually measured with stable end-tidal concentrations. The minimum alveolar concentration (MAC) is defined as the concentration (i.e. dose level) needed to get 50 % of unconscious patients not moving when subjected to strong nociceptive or painful stimuli. Typically this will be 6 % for desflurane and 2 % for sevoflurane in an average adult. However, the inhalational agents are also potent sleeping agents, and the hypnotic effect is evident at doses about one-third of those needed to lay still upon pain. Thus, a term called MAC_{sleep} is defined as the stable end-tidal concentration needed to get 50 % of non-stimulated patients to sleep. Typically MAC_{sleep} is 2 % and 0.7 % for desflurane and sevoflurane, respectively.

The intravenous opioids and hypnotics will interact with inhalational agents, but somewhat differently according to class of IV drug and type of effect. The clinical interactions are logical; if you combine inhalational agent with a hypnotic, the combination is additive or supra-additive in terms of hypnotic effect. Still, the adding of an IV hypnotic does not add much to the anti-nociceptive or analgesic effect of the gas. On the other hand, if you add an opioid analgesic on top of the inhalational agent, the combination is additive or supra-additive in anti-nociceptive effect, whereas the opioid do not add much to the pure hypnotic effect [8–10]. However, for induction general anesthesia and deep unconsciousness for intubation or surgery, we need a combined anti-nociceptive and hypnotic effect for which the opioid-hypnotic combination is supra-additive.

The hypnotic potency measure, MAC_{sleep}, may be linearly and additively reduced by adding the hypnotic propofol or midazolam. With midazolam 0.1 mg/kg IV, MAC_{sleep} for a potent inhalational agent will be reduced by about 50 %, similarly with a propofol plasma level of 1.5 μg/ml.

1. The hypnotic potency measure, MAC_{sleep}, is reduced only by 10–20 % after a dose of fentanyl of 0.2 mg in the adult corresponding to a target of 7–8 ng/ml remifentanil or infusion of 0.3 μg/kg/min. Whereas some patients may be fully asleep on a high opioid dose alone, the individual variation is huge; thus, an average reduction in MAC_{sleep} of 50 % by adding opioid demands a very high dose of opioid (fentanyl 0.6 mg or other opioid in equipotent dose), and the effect is unpredictable.

2. The anaesthetic potency parameter, MAC, will be reduced by 60 % from a dose of fentanyl 0.2 mg and by 75 % by doubling this dose.

3. The anaesthetic potency parameter, MAC, will be reduced by hypnotics, by 30–40 % of adding midazolam 0.1 mg/kg bolus or propofol plasma level of 1.5 ng/ml. Still, the effect of further increased hypnotics IV is infra-additive. Still, very high (intoxicating) doses of hypnotics are actually also anti-nociceptive in clinical action.

References

1. Minto CF, Schnider TW, Egan TD, et al. Influence of age and gender on the pharmacokinetics and pharmacodynamics of remifentanil. I. Model development. Anesthesiology. 1997;86:10–23.
2. Hoymork SC, Raeder J. Why do women wake up faster than men from propofol anaesthesia? Br J Anaesth. 2005;95:627–33.
3. Vuyk J, Mertens MJ, Olofsen E, et al. Propofol anesthesia and rational opioid selection: determination of optimal EC50-EC95 propofol-opioid concentrations that assure adequate anesthesia and a rapid return of consciousness. Anesthesiology. 1997;87:1549–62.
4. Hoymork SC, Raeder J, Grimsmo B, Steen PA. Bispectral index, predicted and measured drug levels of target-controlled infusions of remifentanil and propofol during laparoscopic cholecystectomy and emergence. Acta Anaesthesiol Scand. 2000;44:1138–44.
5. Marsh B, White M, Morton N, Kenny GN. Pharmacokinetic model driven infusion of propofol in children. Br J Anaesth. 1991;67:41–8.
6. Vereecke HE, Vasquez PM, Jensen EW, et al. New composite index based on midlatency auditory evoked potential and electroencephalographic parameters to optimize correlation with propofol effect site concentration: comparison with bispectral index and solitary used fast extracting auditory evoked potential index. Anesthesiology. 2005;103:500–7.
7. Minto CF, Schnider TW, Gregg KM, et al. Using the time of maximum effect site concentration to combine pharmacokinetics and pharmacodynamics. Anesthesiology. 2003;99:324–33.
8. Katoh T, Ikeda K. The effects of fentanyl on sevoflurane requirements for loss of consciousness and skin incision. Anesthesiology. 1998;88:18–24.
9. Albertin A, Dedola E, Bergonzi PC, et al. The effect of adding two target-controlled concentrations (1-3 ng mL -1) of remifentanil on MAC BAR of desflurane. Eur J Anaesthesiol. 2006;23:510–6.
10. Inagaki Y, Sumikawa K, Yoshiya I. Anesthetic interaction between midazolam and halothane in humans. Anesth Analg. 1993;76:613–7.

Pharmacokinetic–Pharmacodynamic Modelling of Anesthetic Drugs

7

Johannes Hans Proost

Introduction

In a nutshell, the aim of pharmacokinetic–pharmacodynamic (PKPD) modelling is to be able to predict the time course of clinical effect resulting from different drug administration regimens and to predict the influence of various factors such as body weight, age, gender, underlying pathology and co-medication, on the clinical effect.

To enable this, the relationship between the administration of one or more drugs and the resulting time course of drug action is described quantitatively by mathematical models. Such PKPD models range from simple, purely empirical models to complex, mechanism-based, physiological models, which may include various related processes, such as drug interactions, disease progression, placebo effect, compliance and drop-out.

PKPD models are composite models consisting of a pharmacokinetic (PK) model and a pharmacodynamic (PD) model (Fig. 7.1). The PK model describes the relationship between drug administration and the resulting time course of drug concentration(s) in the body, usually the plasma concentration. The PD model describes the relationship between the drug concentration at the site of action (also denoted effect compartment, effect site or biophase) and the drug effect. Often a PKPD link model is required to describe the relationship between the plasma concentration and the concentration at the site of action, i.e. to account for time delays between both concentrations as a result of drug transport from plasma to the site of action.

The combination of a PK, PKPD link and PD model allows relating the drug dosing regimen to the time course of drug action. This relationship may be used to predict the time course of drug effect after a particular dose or dosing

regimen or to predict the dose or dosing regimen required to obtain a desired level of drug effect.

PKPD modelling can be performed using data from one individual subject (individual analysis) or from a group of individuals. Individual analysis is a valuable tool in therapeutic drug monitoring, allowing accurate individual dosing of, for example, immunosuppressive drug and antibiotics. However, population analysis has become the dominant approach over the last three decades, since it provides information about the PKPD behaviour of the 'typical subject' as well as about interindividual variability and the influence of covariates such as body weight, age, gender, underlying pathology and co-medication. The contribution of PKPD modelling to anaesthetic practice has been nicely illustrated in two review papers [1, 2] and two book chapters on interaction modelling in anaesthesia [3, 4]. A recommended general textbook on pharmacokinetics and pharmacodynamics is that by Rowland and Tozer [5], and for PKPD modelling and simulation, the book of Bonate [6] is recommended.

The aim of this chapter on PKPD modelling of anaesthetic drugs is to describe the general principles of PKPD modelling; to explain the principles of PKPD analysis; to provide an overview of PKPD modelling of drugs used in anaesthesia, including interactions of anaesthetic drugs; and to give some examples of the application of PKPD modelling in clinical anaesthetic practice. The focus of this chapter is on describing principles and methods, rather than a full review of literature on PKPD modelling of anaesthetic drugs.

Principles of Modelling

Pharmacokinetic Models

The pharmacokinetics of drugs are usually described by compartmental models (Fig. 7.2). Compartmental models are still considered as the basic PK models, despite their

J.H. Proost, PharmD PhD (✉)
Anesthesiology, University Medical Center Groningen, University of Groningen, Hanzeplein 1, Groningen 9713 GZ, The Netherlands
e-mail: j.h.proost@umcg.nl

© Springer International Publishing AG 2017
A.R. Absalom, K.P. Mason (eds.), *Total Intravenous Anesthesia and Target Controlled Infusions*,
DOI 10.1007/978-3-319-47609-4_7

pharmacokinetics   pharmacodynamics

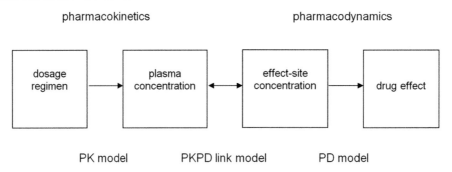

Fig. 7.1 Pharmacokinetics–pharmacodynamics concept. (i) The dosage regimen and the PK model determine the plasma concentration–time profile; (ii) the plasma concentration–time profile and the PKPD link model determine the effect-site concentration–time profile; and (iii) the effect-site concentration–time profile and the PD model determine the drug effect–time profile

Fig. 7.2 Pharmacokinetic two-compartment model. V_x is the apparent volume of compartment x, CL_{xy} is the intercompartmental clearance from compartment x to y, CL_{x0} is the elimination clearance from compartment x and R is the rate of drug entry in the system

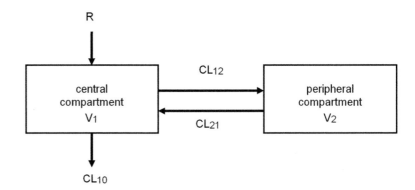

major limitations: they cannot describe the full complexity of pharmacokinetic process throughout the body, and they cannot be used for prediction of the pharmacokinetic behaviour of a drug based on in vitro data. The latter can be used in physiologically based pharmacokinetic (PBPK) models, which are mainly used in drug development for the prediction of PK based on physiological data (size and blood flow of various organs), physico-chemical data (partition coefficient, plasma protein binding) and data on enzymatic biotransformation. In anaesthesiology, PBPK models have been published for volatile anaesthetics (see below) and for propofol [7, 8]. More information on PBPK models can be found in the literature [9–11].

The usual approach in compartmental modelling is to start with the most simple, one-compartment model, with two model parameters: volume of distribution, which relates the amount of drug in the body to the plasma concentration, and clearance, which is defined as the rate of drug elimination divided by the plasma concentration. For many drugs used chronically in ambulant patients, the one-compartment model provides an adequate and robust description of the pharmacokinetic behaviour and can be used to guide dosing, e.g. in therapeutic drug monitoring.

In anaesthetic practice, the time frame of drug administration and drug action is often so short that the one-compartment model is insufficient to describe the pharmacokinetics adequately: drug mixing within the vascular space and drug distribution into tissues play a major role, and more complex models should be used. For the majority of drugs used in anaesthesia, a two-compartment or three-compartment model is able to describe the pharmacokinetics adequately (Fig. 7.2).

The principle of compartmental modelling is simple. The amount of drug in each compartment is assumed to be evenly distributed throughout the volume of the compartment, and the rates of drug elimination and drug transport to other compartments are assumed to be proportional to the drug concentration in the compartment (first-order kinetics, e.g. for enzymatic biotransformation, renal excretion and transport by blood flow and diffusion), where the apparent volume of the compartment is the amount in the compartment divided by the concentration in the compartment. Based on these principles, the model can be described in differential equations. As an example, consider a model with two compartments as depicted in Fig. 7.2. The change of the amount of drug in a compartment is the net result of the rate of entry of drug, that is, the sum of the amount drug administered to the compartment (e.g. an intravenous infusion or absorption rate after extravascular dosing) and the rate of transport from other compartments, diminished by the rate of exit, that is, the sum of the rates of removal from the compartment by elimination or by transport to other compartments. This leads to the following set of differential equations:

$$\frac{dA_1}{dt} = R + CL_{21} \cdot C_2 - CL_{12} \cdot C_1 - CL_{10} \cdot C_1 \qquad (7.1)$$

$$\frac{dA_2}{dt} = CL_{12} \cdot C_1 - CL_{21} \cdot C_2 \qquad (7.2)$$

where A_x and C_x are the amount and concentration of drug in compartment x, respectively, CL_{xy} is the intercompartmental clearance from compartment x to y, CL_{x0} is the elimination clearance from compartment x and R is the rate of drug entry in the system (if appropriate, as in the case of cisatracurium, elimination from the peripheral compartment can be added). A_x and C_x are related by

$$V_x = \frac{A_x}{C_x} \qquad (7.3)$$

where V_x is the apparent volume of compartment x.

For practical (as well as historical) reasons, Eq. (7.1) are often used in the following equivalent format:

$$\frac{dA_1}{dt} = R + k_{21} \cdot A_2 - k_{12} \cdot A_1 - k_{10} \cdot A_1 \qquad (7.4)$$

$$\frac{dA_2}{dt} = k_{12} \cdot A_1 - k_{21} \cdot A_2 \qquad (7.5)$$

where

$$k_{xy} = \frac{CL_{xy}}{V_x} \qquad (7.6)$$

Since only concentrations in the central compartment can be measured, it is not possible to estimate all five parameters (V_1, V_2, CL_{10}, CL_{12}, CL_{21}); only four parameters can be obtained from the bi-exponential plasma concentration decay profile (two slopes and two intercepts), implying that the model is over-parameterized. Usually this is solved by assuming that there is no net transport between two compartments if the concentrations in both compartments are equal; in this specific case $CL_{21} = CL_{12}$.

The same principles can be applied to any compartmental model, irrespective of its complexity. The differential equations can be solved mathematically in the case of a one-, two- or three-compartment model; in more complex cases, the differential equations can be solved numerically, irrespective of the complexity of the model.

However, it should be realized that the plasma concentration–time profile over the first few minutes after bolus injection cannot be described adequately using compartmental models and more advanced models for 'front-end kinetics' are required for a more accurate description of the plasma concentration [8, 12–14]. A shortcoming of compartmental models is the inherent assumption that the concentration within a compartment is homogeneous; mixing of a bolus administration over the entire vascular space takes a few minutes, and therefore the concentration in the various parts of the vascular bed is different and does not follow the time profile as described by a compartmental model, requiring a non-compartmental approach in PKPD modelling [15, 16].

Even after mixing within the vascular space is completed, there is still a concentration difference between the arterial and venous blood, which may persist for a prolonged period of time, due to a net transport to the perfused tissues. Theoretically, the concentration in venous blood is higher during the elimination phase. Several studies have shown that the choice between arterial and venous samples influences the results of PKPD modelling [17–21]. For PKPD modelling, the use of arterial concentrations is generally preferred, since this is the concentration entering the tissue where the effect site is located. On the other hand, it is likely that the concentration in venous blood is in equilibrium with the tissue concentration. More research on this topic seems necessary.

Pharmacokinetics is generally described in terms of plasma concentration, or serum concentration, which is equivalent for most drugs. However, for some drugs, blood concentrations may be measured, e.g. for propofol, both plasma concentration and blood concentrations are used in PKPD analysis. The blood-to-plasma concentration ratio of propofol was reported to be 1.1–1.3 [7, 22], and therefore blood concentrations and plasma concentration should not be assumed the same, but this topic does not get much attention in literature; in some papers the matrix blood or plasma is not even mentioned. As a result, propofol concentration data and PKPD models should be interpreted with care.

Finally, it should be realized that most drugs are partly bound to plasma proteins (albumin, alpha-1-acid glycoprotein, lipoproteins) and that the unbound concentration is the driving force for drug transport, including transport to the effect site, drug elimination and drug effect. However, since usually only the total drug concentration is measured, the term 'concentration' always refers to the total concentration, and as a result, PK analysis and parameters refer to the total concentration. However, the degree of plasma protein binding may change, either by displacement by other drugs or by changing protein concentrations. Fortunately, in most situations, such changes in free fraction do not have a clinical relevance, since the unbound drug concentration does not change significantly [23–25]. However, the exceptions to this rule are systemically administered drugs with high hepatic extraction and drugs with high active renal excretion. Propofol falls in the first category, and Hiraoka and co-workers [26] demonstrated that during cardiopulmonary bypass the unbound propofol concentration increased twofold, in accordance with the expected change [5]. In addition, the protein binding of propofol is still a matter of debate, e.g. with respect to the binding sites as well as methodological issues in the assay [27, 28]. More research on the binding of propofol and the clinical relevance of a change of the protein binding of propofol is still needed.

PKPD Link Models

Often a PKPD link model is required to describe the relationship between the plasma concentration and the concentration at the site of action, i.e. to account for time delays between both concentrations as a result of drug transport from plasma to the site of action. The concept of an effect compartment or effect site was introduced by Sheiner and colleagues to allow for the time delay between the plasma concentration of D-tubocurarine and the resulting muscle relaxation [29]. In a later paper, Holford and Sheiner [30] presented the PKPD link model in a more efficient description:

$$\frac{dC_e}{dt} = k_{e0} \cdot (C_{is} - C_e) \qquad (7.7)$$

where C and C_e are the drug concentrations in the central and effect compartments, respectively, and k_{e0} is a first-order equilibration rate constant, which may also be expressed as an equilibration half-life ($\ln(2)/k_{e0}$).

It should be noted that it is not possible to determine the effect-site concentration, since only plasma concentration is available for measurement. At equilibrium, the effect-site concentration may be different from the plasma concentration, due to various processes, including plasma protein binding, drug transporters (e.g. P-glycoprotein at the blood–brain barrier), convection and binding at the effect site. Therefore, the 'effect-site concentration' is actually a hypothetical concentration, defined as the concentration in plasma that is in equilibrium with the concentration at the effect site. Although this definition may sound complicated and hypothetical, it perfectly fits the need for a concentration at the effect site in terms of the plasma concentration.

Equation (7.7) should be considered as an approximation of the drug transport between plasma and effect site, which may be affected by the processes mentioned above. In some publications alternative models for linking plasma and effect compartment have been shown to be better suited, e.g., for mivacurium [31], where an interstitial compartment between plasma and effect compartment improved the fit significantly. However, the concept of effect-site concentration defined by Eq. (7.7) has been successfully applied for more than three decades, and still no generally applicable alternatives are available.

Pharmacodynamic Models

Continuous Responses

Many drug effects can be adequately described by the sigmoid E_{max} model or Hill equation:

$$E = E_{max} \cdot \left(\frac{C^\gamma}{C50^\gamma + C^\gamma}\right) \qquad (7.8)$$

where E is the drug effect; E_{max} is the maximal drug effect, i.e. the drug effect at very high concentration; C is the drug concentration at the site of action; $C50$ is the drug concentration at the site of action if E is 50 % of E_{max}; and γ is an exponent representing the steepness of the concentration–effect relationship. An example is shown in Fig. 7.3.

Equation (7.8) is also denoted as a logistic function, since it may be rewritten to the logistic function:

$$E = E_{max} \cdot \left(\frac{e^t}{1 + e^t}\right) \qquad (7.9)$$

where

$$t = -\gamma \cdot \ln(C50) + \gamma \cdot \ln(C) \qquad (7.10)$$

Note that Eqs. (7.9) and (7.10) are identical to Eq. (7.8). However, the traditional logistic function uses Eq. (7.11) instead of Eq. (7.10):

$$t = \beta_0 + \beta_1 \cdot C \qquad (7.11)$$

This logistic approach is flexible and can be extended to drug interactions [32]. However, this approach is not recommended, amongst others, because it does not describe the drug effect in the absence of the drug.

If the drug effect has a baseline value in the absence of drug, Eq. (7.8) may be expanded to

Fig. 7.3 Relationship between drug concentration and drug effect following the sigmoid E_{max} model (Eq. 7.8), for three hypothetical drugs (i) $C50 = 1$, $\gamma = 5$; (ii) $C50 = 0.5$, $\gamma = 5$, resulting in a shift to the *left*; (iii) $C50 = 1$, $\gamma = 10$, resulting in a steeper profile

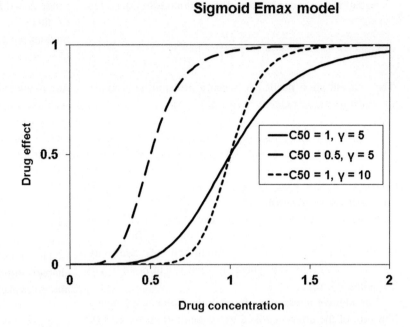

Equation (7.12) can be rewritten to

$$E = E_0 + (E_{max} - E_0) \cdot \left(\frac{U^\gamma}{1 + U^\gamma} \right) \qquad (7.13)$$

where U represents the normalized drug concentration, i.e. the drug concentration divided by $C50$

$$U = \frac{C}{C50} \qquad (7.14)$$

U is a dimensionless measure of potency, expressed in multiples of $C50$. The use of U instead of C is particularly useful in modelling of drug interactions (see below).

In spite of their widespread use in pharmacology and PKPD modelling, Eqs. (7.8) and (7.12) have a limited physiological and mechanistic basis. They reflect the relationship between drug concentration and effect in the case that the drug effect is proportional to the receptor occupancy, i.e. the fraction of receptors that is occupied by the drug. In this special case, $C50$ equals the equilibrium dissociation constant Kd and the slope of the concentration–effect relationship γ equals 1. In other cases, the sigmoid E_{max} model should be considered an empirical equation that often describes the concentration–effect relationship sufficiently accurately, as has been shown in numerous papers [33].

It should be noted that pharmacodynamic models such as those described by Eqs. (7.8) and (7.12) are expressed in terms of effect-site concentration (see above) or, in the case of a rapid equilibrium with plasma, in terms of plasma concentration. Including the dose in these equations, as has been done frequently in the past, is not logical in the concept of PKPD, where the dose determines the (effect-site) concentration via the PK model, and the concentration determines the drug effect via the PD model (Fig. 7.1).

Quantal Responses

Equations (7.8) and (7.12) describe the relationship between the drug concentration and the drug effect in the case that the drug effect is a continuous variable or graded response, e.g. mean arterial blood pressure. In the case of a binary response, also called all-or-none or quantal response or dichotomous variable, there are only two values for the response, 0 or 1, no or yes, responsive or nonresponsive (tolerant), etc. Modelling of this type of data is usually performed by logistic regression analysis. In the case of a single regressor, i.e. a single drug, logistic regression analysis is identical to Eq. (7.8), after rearrangement to

$$P = \frac{C^\gamma}{C50^\gamma + C^\gamma} \qquad (7.15)$$

where P is the probability of tolerance or non-responsiveness (within the range of 0–1).

$C50$ is the drug concentration associated with a probability of non-responsiveness of 0.5 (50 %).

Equation (7.15) can be rewritten, analogous to Eq. (7.13):

$$P = \frac{U^\gamma}{1 + U^\gamma} \qquad (7.16)$$

The concentration needed to reach a probability P can be obtained upon rearrangement of Eq. (7.15):

$$C = C50 \cdot \exp\left(\frac{\ln\left(\frac{P}{1-P}\right)}{\gamma}\right) \qquad (7.17)$$

Interaction Modelling

In the case of two or more drugs, several approaches can be used to describe the combined effect of the drug. Three types of drug interaction can be distinguished: (1) additivity, (2) supra-additivity (or synergism) and (3) infra-additivity (or antagonism).

For additive interaction of two drugs with equal potency, the sum of the effects evoked by concentrations (a) and (b) for drug A and drug B, respectively, is equal to the effect obtained with the administration of either drug A or B alone given in a concentration (a) + (b). If the potency of drug A and B is different (as is usually the case), the concentrations can be replaced by the values U, by dividing the concentrations by the corresponding $C50$.

For supra-additive interactions, the combination of drugs A and B will result in a more pronounced effect compared to additivity. For infra-additive interactions, the combination of drugs will result in a less pronounced effect compared to additivity conditions.

In general, additive interactions will occur in cases where the effect is elicited via a single pathway (e.g. an identical receptor), or a similar mechanism of action, as for inhalation anaesthetics and propofol, whereas supra-additive interaction may occur in the case of multiple pathways (e.g. N-methyl-D-aspartic acid and gamma-aminobutyric acid receptors), or a different action, as for general anaesthetics and opioids.

From a clinical point of view, supra-additive drug interactions have a clear advantage, because lower concentrations of the drugs are required, resulting in a lower drug exposure. On the other hand, additive drug interactions are easier to predict for the clinician in the absence of sophisticated tools (see below). In general, the occurrence of an infra-additive interaction is a disadvantage and should be avoided.

Interaction Models

In the case of two or more drugs, Eqs. (7.13) and (7.16) can be used if U represents the combined potency of the drugs. There are several options to relate U to the drug concentrations. For the easy of survey, only the case of two drugs A and B is shown, but the equations may be extended to three or more drugs [34]. More information about models, equations and mechanisms can be found in literature [35–39].

Additive Interaction Model

Additive interaction assumes that the effect of two drugs is equal to the sum of the effect of the two drugs taken separately. This is usually due to drugs acting via the same or similar mechanism. This is described by

$$U = U_A + U_B \qquad (7.18)$$

where U_A and U_B are the normalized concentrations of drugs A and B, normalized to $C50_A$ and $C50_B$, respectively.

This model, as well as the other models described in this chapter, implies that both drugs A and B are assumed to be able to evoke the maximal clinical effect.

Greco Model

The Greco model is a simplification of the original Greco model [36]:

$$U = U_A + U_B + \alpha \cdot U_A \cdot U_B \qquad (7.19)$$

where α is a dimensionless interaction parameter ($\alpha = 0$, additive; $\alpha < 0$, infra-additive; $\alpha > 0$, supra-additive).

The Greco model is the most simple and logical model that can be used for additive, supra-additive and infra-additive interactions. Although originally derived for continuous responses [36], it has also been applied successfully for binary responses [3, 40].

The single interaction parameter α is considered to be applicable for the total response surface and does not allow for adapting the shape of the interaction curve at different levels of drug effect. A limitation of the Greco model is the assumption that the steepness of the concentration–effect relationship is the same for both drugs. However, the Greco model has proven its suitability in many research papers.

Reduced Greco Model

In the case of the interaction, where drug B does not have a drug effect when given alone, or the effect is too small to accurately assess the $C50$ of that drug, the Greco model can be modified by leaving out the first term U_B from Eq. (7.19) and fixing α to 1, resulting in

$$U = U_A \cdot (1 + U_B) \qquad (7.20)$$

$C50_B$ may now be interpreted as the concentration of drug B that decreases $C50_A$ by 50 %. Since $U_B = C_B/C50_B$, when $C_B = C50_B$, $U_B = 1$ and $U = 2 \times U_A$, i.e. the concentration of the hypnotic required to achieve a certain potency U, and thus a certain drug effect, is reduced by a factor 2, compared to the concentration in the absence of drug B.

The reduced Greco model may be considered as a particular form of supra-additive interaction, i.e. where drug B does not elicit any effect when given alone.

Hierarchical Model

The original hierarchical model [41, 42], also denoted sequential model, was developed for the interaction of propofol (hypnotic, H) and remifentanil (opioid, O) and was based on observations that remifentanil potentiates the effect of propofol but does not affect the response when given alone. The model is defined by the following equations:

$$P = \frac{C_H{}^\gamma}{(C50_H \cdot \text{postopioid\_intensity})^\gamma + C_H{}^\gamma} \quad (7.21)$$

$$\text{postopioid\_intensity} = \text{preopioid\_intensity} \cdot \left(1 - \frac{C_O{}^{\gamma_O}}{(C50_O \cdot \text{prepioid\_intensity})^{\gamma_O} + C_O{}^{\gamma_O}}\right) \quad (7.22)$$

where postopioid_intensity is the stimulus intensity after attenuation by the opioid, and preopioid_intensity is the intensity of the stimulus in the absence of opioid.

It has been shown [37] that Eqs. (7.21) and (7.22) can be simplified to

$$U = U_A \cdot (1 + U_B{}^{\gamma_B}) \quad (7.23)$$

Comparing Eqs. (7.20) and (7.23), it follows that the hierarchical model is an extension of the reduced Greco model, i.e. by adding an exponent γ_B to U_B in Eq. (7.20), yielding Eq. (7.23), allowing more flexibility.

In the case of simultaneous analysis of two or more quantal responses, several constraints with respect to $C50_B$ can be applied, as described elsewhere in detail [37].

As for the reduced Greco model, the hierarchical model may be considered as a particular form of supra-additive interaction, i.e. where drug B does not elicit any effect when given alone.

Minto Model

The Minto model [34] may be described by the following equations:

$$\theta = \frac{U_A}{U_A + U_B} \quad (7.24)$$

where θ is the relative contribution of drug A to the total potency of both drugs, and its value is between 0 and 1

$$U_{50} = 1 - \beta_{U50} \cdot \theta \cdot (1 - \theta) \quad (7.25)$$

where U_{50} is the potency of two drugs in the combination θ yielding half-maximal effect and β_{U50} is a dimensionless interaction coefficient relating θ (fraction of drug A) and $1 - \theta$ (fraction of drug B) to U_{50} (higher-order functions of θ may be used to accommodate more complex shapes of interaction)

$$U = \frac{U_A + U_B}{U_{50}} \quad (7.26)$$

where U is the potency of the two drugs normalized to U_{50}.

The steepness parameter γ is a model parameter (similar as in other interaction models) or a function of the ratio of the drug concentrations (θ) and model parameters (γ_A, γ_B, β_γ). It may be written as a linear interpolation between γ_A and γ_B and an interaction term analogous to Eq. (7.25) (higher-order functions of θ may be used to accommodate more complex shapes of interaction):

$$\gamma = \gamma_A \cdot \theta + \gamma_B \cdot (1 - \theta) - \beta_\gamma \cdot \theta \cdot (1 - \theta) \quad (7.27)$$

Note that Eqs. (7.25) and (7.27) have been rearranged from the corresponding equations in the original paper of the Minto model [34] to clarify the interaction.

A particular property of the Minto model is its flexibility: any model parameter can be modelled as a function of its values for both compounds separately (e.g. $C50_A$ and $C50_B$) and one or more interaction parameters (e.g. β_{U50}). This flexibility may be an advantage, but it increases the risk of overparametrization (see below).

Two more approaches to response surface modelling with more than one interaction term have been presented in the literature. Fidler and Kern [43] called their approach the flexible interaction model, claiming a similar or slightly better fit for clinical interaction data. Kong and Lee [44] published a generalized interaction model for triple anaesthetic interactions [43]. These two approaches, as well as the Minto model, were reviewed [45] but were hardly used in anaesthetic literature. The logistic approach (Eq. 7.11) can be extended to drug interactions [32]. As was stated above, this approach is not recommended.

An extensive evaluation of the advantages and disadvantages of all available interaction models has not yet been performed.

Isoboles

Isoboles are used for a graphical representation of the interaction of two drugs. An isobole is a line in a graph of the concentration of drug A (X-axis) and drug B (Y-axis)

Fig. 7.4 Isoboles of 50 % effect for the interaction of two hypothetical drugs A and B. (i) Additive interaction ($\alpha = 0$); (ii) Supra-additive interaction ($\alpha = 3$); (iii) Infra-additive interaction ($\alpha = -0.75$)

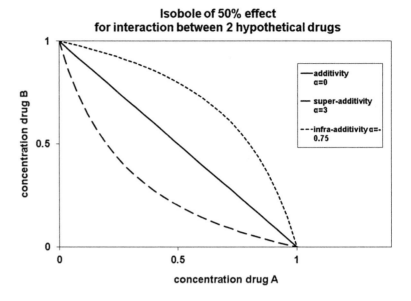

connecting all points where the effect is equal to a predefined value, e.g. 50 %.

An example of a 50 % isobole is shown in Fig. 7.4. For additive interaction, the isobole is a straight line, connecting the concentration of drug A producing 50 % effect and the concentration of drug B producing 50 % effect.

For a supra-additive interaction, the isobole is concave, i.e. the concentrations of drug A and/or drug B are lower than in the case of additive interaction. Similarly, in the case of an infra-additive interaction, the isobole is convex, i.e. the concentrations of drug A and/or drug B are higher than in the case of additive interaction.

So, an isobole provides a complete picture of the interaction of the two drugs, but only at the predefined drug effect level. For clinical practice, a wider range of response level should be available, for example, the 95 % isobole, representing the drug levels with a high probability of effect.

To obtain such an isobole requires a clinical study in many patients, in particular for binary responses, with at least three drug levels (drug A alone, drug B alone and a combination of A and B, e.g. in a ratio that $U_A = U_B$), aiming at the desired level of drug effect. If sufficient data are obtained at the desired level of drug effect, the isobole can be constructed. Data deviating from the desired level of drug effect cannot be used in this analysis.

Response Surface Modelling

A more rational approach is to perform a population pharmacokinetic–pharmacodynamic analysis (see below), using all available data. Each of the above-mentioned equations for drug interactions describes the combined drug response, either a continuous or a binary response, as a function of two (or more) drug concentrations and one or

more interaction parameters. These equations can be presented in the form of a three-dimensional graph, with typically the drug concentrations on the horizontal X- and Y-axes and the drug effect plotted on the vertical Z-axis. Therefore, this approach is denoted 'response surface modelling' and was introduced in anaesthesia by Minto and colleagues [34].

An example is shown in Fig. 7.5. Each horizontal cross-section of the response surface at a certain drug level represents an isobole, with two axes representing the drug concentrations.

Such pharmacodynamic response surface models have several distinct advantages over the 'classical' isobole approach:

- It integrates the information at any level of drug effect.
- It uses all data from (one or more) clinical studies.
- It can be applied to interactions of more than two drugs [34], although this has been applied rarely in literature until now.
- It allows predictions at any level of drug effect for any combination of drug concentrations.

Data Analysis

Nonlinear Regression Analysis

Once a clinical study has been performed and measurements of plasma concentration (PK) and/or drug effect (PD) are available, the question arises how these data can be analysed to obtain an appropriate model with reliable model parameter values. It is not the aim of this chapter to deal with data analysis extensively. For further reference, excellent papers and books are available [6].

Fig. 7.5 Response surface of the tolerance to laryngoscopy for the interaction between sevoflurane and remifentanil. The *contour lines* show the response surface calculated from the hierarchical interaction model (Eq. 7.23), the *open circles* represent the observations in patients responding to laryngoscopy and the *filled circles* represent the observations in patients tolerant to laryngoscopy

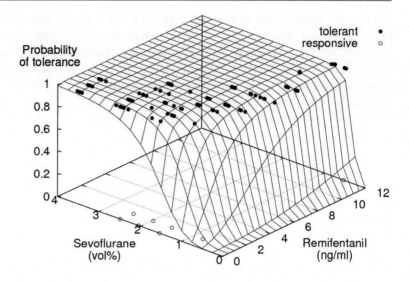

In short, this process is performed in the following steps:

1. Choose a model, in general, starting with the simplest model that may be appropriate to describe the available data. Often, this choice is based on the existing knowledge, e.g. a compartmental model for PK data or a sigmoid E_{max} model for PD data.
2. Assume 'reasonable' values for each of the model parameters. In general, the choice of these values is not critical, since all parameter values are estimated during the next steps.
3. Based on this model and parameter values, calculate the plasma concentration and drug effect at each time point where an observation is available. These calculated PK and/or PD values are usually denoted as 'predicted' values.
4. Define a measure for the difference between the observed and predicted PK and/or PD values. Usually, this measure is based on the likelihood principle, i.e. the likelihood that the actual observations have been obtained, given the model and its model parameter values. For practical reasons, −2 times the logarithm (base e) of the likelihood is calculated (minus 2 log likelihood or −2LL). This measure is often called 'objective function value' (OFV).
5. In the next step, all model parameters are adjusted until the 'best fit' is obtained, i.e. until the likelihood is maximal, corresponding to the minimum of −2LL. Now, we have obtained the parameter set describing the data 'best'.
6. The goodness-of-fit is tested by various diagnostic plots (see below).
7. Finally, various alternative models are analysed using the same procedure, and the results are statistically compared for selection of the most appropriate model.

To illustrate this process, we present here a simple, well-known example of a linear model:

$$Y = a + b \cdot X \qquad (7.28)$$

where a and b are model parameters, X is the independent variable (e.g. time or drug concentration) and Y is the dependent variable (e.g. plasma concentration or drug effect).

Suppose we have a set of observations Y_i ($i = 1,2,\ldots,n$) for the independent variable value X_i. These observations are expected to follow the trend of the linear model Eq. (7.28), with a certain deviation ε_i:

$$Y_i = a + b \cdot X_i + \varepsilon_i \qquad (7.29)$$

The predicted values, also called expected values, are calculated from the linear function:

$$\hat{Y}_i = a + b \cdot X_i \qquad (7.30)$$

The maximum likelihood, or the minimum of −2LL, corresponds to the following objective function value (omitting constant values):

$$\mathrm{OFV} = \sum_{i=1}^{n} \frac{\left(Y_i - \hat{Y}_i\right)^2}{\sigma_i^2} + \sum_{i=1}^{n} \ln\left(\sigma_i^2\right) \qquad (7.31)$$

where σ_i^2 is the variance of ε_i. For linear models, the parameters a and b can be calculated exactly, if the variance of the deviations ε_i is the same for each i and independent of the value of X or Y ($\sigma_i^2 = \sigma^2$). This method is known as linear regression analysis; details can be found in any textbook of statistics, and these are available in pocket calculators and spreadsheets.

However, in PKPD the relationship between Y and X is rarely linear, and often the variance of the deviations ε_i is dependent on the value of X or Y. In such cases, these equations are not valid, and the parameters cannot be calculated exactly (generally, even approximate solutions are not available). This implies that step 5 becomes much more complicated, and iterative procedures are required to adjust all parameters in such a way that the parameters corresponding to the minimum of the objective function value (OFV) are found in an efficient way. To this purpose of nonlinear regression analysis, several algorithms have been developed, e.g. the simplex, Gauss–Newton and Levenberg–Marquardt methods. These algorithms may be different in their most relevant properties:

1. Efficiency: how efficient the algorithm can find the best fitting parameter values is mainly relevant for the speed of execution. Although becoming less important with increasing computing power, the speed of execution may remain a relevant issue in the analysis of very large data sets with complex model structures.
2. Robustness: in some cases, the algorithm does not find the real, global minimum of the objective function values but converges to a local minimum, i.e. the lowest value around the parameter values, but not the lowest possible value (compare with the bottom of a lake in the mountains: it is the lowest point in the surrounding area of the lake, but not the lowest point of the country).

Both the speed of execution and risk of convergence to a local minimum are dependent on the set of starting values in the analysis (see item 1 above). To lower the risk of convergence to a local minimum, the analysis may be performed several times with different sets of starting values.

In general, commercially available software contains adequate implementations of suitable algorithms, and the user of these programmes does not need to know the details of such procedures.

Goodness-of-Fit

After fitting the parameters of a model to a set of observations, one needs criteria for the goodness-of-fit. The observations do not follow the model function exactly, for several reasons:

1. Measurement errors. For example, inevitable analytical errors implicit in plasma concentration or effect measurements. In general, such measurement errors are random errors, and their order of magnitude may be known from the precision of the assay, as assessed during the validation of the assay. If the magnitude of the residual errors is comparable to the precision of the assay, the goodness-of-fit is acceptable. In the case of measurements close to the lower limit of quantification, the relative errors in the analysis may be significantly larger than over the usual range.
2. Stochastic errors. Even if observations could be made without measurement error, and observations are made in the same subject, the plasma concentration or drug effect profiles will not be exactly reproducible, e.g. due to changes in heart rate and blood pressure, administration of other drugs, etc. These errors may be random or non-random.
3. Model misspecification. If an inappropriate model is chosen (e.g. a model with too few compartments or an incorrect model structure), the model will not be able to describe the observations adequately, resulting in systematic deviations between the observations and the model predicted values. Such systematic deviations can be detected by the visual methods described below.
4. Other errors in the procedure, such as dosing errors, deviations in the time of measurement, incorrect sampling procedure, etc. This type of error is most problematic, and no general solution can be given.

There are several methods for the assessment of the goodness-of-fit. However, exact and objective criteria for the evaluation of the goodness-of-fit do not exist. This is due to the following: (1) goodness-of-fit is not a single property and cannot be expressed in a single value, and (2) numerical measures of goodness-of-fit do not have an absolute meaning. Therefore, one must rely on somewhat subjective criteria. To ensure maximal objectivity, the criteria for accepting a set of model parameters obtained by the fitting procedure as a valid result should be defined explicitly before the analysis is started.

The following criteria could be used to ensure an acceptable goodness-of-fit:

– Visual inspection of the observed and calculated data should not reveal any significant lack of fit.
– Residuals (difference between observed and calculated data) or normalized residuals (residuals divided by the corresponding standard deviation) should be scattered randomly around zero, by visual inspection.
– Normalized residuals should be neither diverging nor converging when plotted against time or plotted against (logarithm of) observed values, by visual inspection.
– Residuals should not be serially correlated, as identified by visual inspection or by an appropriate statistical test (e.g. a Runs Test).
– Standard error of each relevant parameter should be lower than a predefined value (e.g. 50 % of the parameter value). High standard errors may reflect problems in the identifiability (see below).

– If any of the estimated parameter values is physiologically unfeasible or otherwise unlikely.
– Outlying data points should be dealt with explicitly and should not be discarded unless felt to be physiologically impossible. The impact of eliminating the outlier on the parameter estimates should be investigated.

Non-compliance with one or more of these criteria may indicate that an inappropriate structural model or an inappropriate residual error model (also called weighting scheme) was chosen.

Identifiability of Model Parameters

The procedure to obtain the best fitting set of model parameters can be performed only if each model parameter is uniquely identifiable from the observations [46, 47]. This implies that the same set of model parameters is obtained, irrespective of the initial set. In some cases one or more model parameters cannot be identified uniquely, because the measurement data do not contain enough 'information' on that particular parameter.

The problem of identifiability grows rapidly with increasing complexity of the model. In some cases the problem of identifiability can be solved by a proper experimental design. In most cases, problems of identifiability can be detected by inspection of the standard errors of the model parameters (the standard error of a model parameter is a measure of the credibility of the parameter value, which is provided by most fitting programmes). A high standard error (e.g. more than 50 % of the parameter value) indicates that the parameter value cannot be assessed from the data, most likely due to an identifiability problem. To solve this, the model should be simplified or modified.

Model Selection

Often the data may be described by more than one plausible model structure. In that case, each plausible model is analysed in a similar way. If the goodness-of-fit of more than one model is acceptable, we need a procedure for selecting the 'best' model.

It is a common practice to compare the results of different models, each yielding an acceptable goodness-of-fit, according to the following procedure. First, the models are classified hierarchically in a tree structure. The more complex models are considered as extensions of the simpler models, by adding extra parameters, for example, an extra compartment. One also may say that the simpler model is a special case of the more complex model, for example, because one or more parameters have a fixed value (in general a zero value). Then, starting with the simplest model, the models are compared in pairs according to their hierarchical relationship. Such a comparison can be based on

statistical criteria, such as the Akaike information criterion (AIC) [48]. For each model the AIC is calculated according to the following equation:

$$AIC = -2 \cdot loglikelihood + 2 \cdot P = OFV + 2 \cdot P \quad (7.32)$$

where P is the number of estimated parameters and OFV is the objective function value which equals -2 times the logarithm of the likelihood (Eq. 7.31).

The model with the lowest AIC value is accepted as the 'best' model. The addition of the term $2 \cdot P$ imposes a penalty on the addition of parameters, implying that adding a parameter must increase the likelihood sufficiently to be statistically justified.

A good model fits the data in a well-balanced manner. This can be difficult to achieve with unbalanced, real-world data sets when one relies solely on AIC for model development. Therefore, it seems logical to support decisions in model selection and evaluation on prediction performance metrics.

An interesting approach was used by Eleveld et al. in the development of a general purpose PK model for propofol [49]. Since the goal was good performance for all subgroups, they derived a predictive performance metric that is balanced between subgroups to guide model development. The predictive performance metric was defined as the percentage of observations with 'good' performance (absolute prediction error (APE) corresponding to APE ≤ 20 %) minus the percentage of observations with 'poor' performance (corresponding to APE > 60 %). The predictions used for this metric were obtained from twofold cross-validation as a guard against overfitting. With this method, the data set is split into two parts, D1 and D2. To evaluate a given model structure, its parameters are estimated using D1; the parameters are fixed and then used to predict D2. The process is repeated, exchanging D1 and D2. Predictions for D1 and D2 are combined to obtain a complete set of independent predictions. The predictive performance metric was calculated separately for five subgroups: young children (age <3 years), children (3 $\leq$ age < 18 years), adults (18 $\leq$ age < 70 years, BMI < 30), elderly (age $\geq$ 70 years) and high BMI individuals (BMI $\geq$ 30). For model development, the overall predictive performance metric was averaged over these five subgroups.

For quantal data, several metrics for prediction performance were proposed by Vereecke and colleagues [50]. From the prediction errors, i.e. the difference between the predicted probability of tolerance to a stimulus and the observed response (0 for responsive, 1 for tolerant), the mean prediction error (MPE) was calculated as a measure of bias, and mean absolute prediction error (MAPE) and root mean squared error (RMSE) were calculated as measures for precision. In addition, the prediction error score was calculated as the percentage of mispredicted responses, i.e. if tolerant, the probability of tolerance was less than 0.5, or if responsive, the probability of tolerance was more than 0.5.

An attractive feature of the above-mentioned metrics is that their value can be evaluated using 'common sense', e.g. by indicating the percentage of 'good predictions' or the typical percentage error in the predicted value. These values can then be evaluated with respect to the clinical acceptability.

Mechanistic vs. Empirical Models

In essence, all PK and PD models are empirical models, since they result mainly from experimental data, and are based on mechanistic information only to a very limited extend. For example, although the concept of clearance and volume of distribution has a mechanistic basis, e.g. the relationship between renal clearance and glomerular filtration rate, this only partly applies to the concept of peripheral compartments, since these are used without any mechanistic information about the anatomical and physiological structures associated with them. Also, as described above, the often used sigmoid E_{max} model (Eqs. 7.8 and 7.12) has some mechanistic basis for the case $\gamma = 1$, but not for other cases.

In practice, these (mainly) empirical models have been shown to be useful for the purpose of description and prediction. However, it may be expected that the use of more mechanistically based models (also denoted as semi-mechanistic models) may improve the predictive power of the model, and for that reason, the development of (more) mechanistic models should be encouraged.

Although anaesthesia is a complex situation, it should be realized that the PKPD of drugs used in anaesthesiology is not more complex than that in other areas of medicine, and perhaps even more simple, as a result of several factors that are usually more complex in other areas, as illustrated by the following examples, using the treatment of osteoporosis as an example of contrast [51, 52]:

1. In anaesthesiology the drug is given as a single dose or during a short period of time; in other areas drug dosing and drug effects are measured usually for a much longer period, with extreme cases over years, as in the case of osteoporosis.
2. As a result of the relative short time period, the influence of interindividual variability in hepatic and renal clearance is only moderate, where it may be a major cause of variability in treatment effects, in particular for genetic variability in the phenotypes of several cytochrome P450 enzymes (e.g. CYP2D6).

3. Drug effect is usually easily and often frequently or continuously measured.
4. Drug effect is usually a direct effect, whereas treatment effects are often indirect effects, with complicated relationships between effects on biomarkers and long-term effects, such as bone mineral density (BMD) and incidence of hip fractures in osteoporosis.
5. There is no underlying disease that may change during long-term treatment. For several diseases, disease progression models have been developed to separate the treatment effect from the disease progression [51, 52].
6. Placebo effect is unlikely to be interfering with the quantification of drug effect. For many drugs, in particular drugs used in psychiatry, placebo effect is large and quantification of drug effect requires special models [53].
7. Patient compliance is not an issue, in contrast to studies evaluating the effect of long-term treatment.

The change of the focus of PKPD models from purely descriptive to (more) mechanism-based models has attracted much interest over the past 10 years [54–58] and has resulted in the development of systems pharmacology, as an analogy to systems biology [59].

Population vs. Individual Approach

In 'classical' PK and PKPD analysis, the data from each individual subject is analysed separately. If a sufficient number of plasma concentration data and/or drug effect data are available for one individual (also called 'rich data'), model parameters for that individual can be estimated. This process can be applied to all subjects participating in a study. In a next step, the mean values and standard deviations of each parameter are calculated and presented and may be used in simulations for predictions. This approach is known as the standard two-stage (STS) approach.

Although the STS approach has been used in numerous papers on PK and PKPD modelling, it has some obvious limitations and disadvantages:

1. If the number of observations in each individual is small compared to the number of parameters to be estimated ('sparse data'), the parameters of that individual cannot be estimated with reasonable precision or cannot be estimated at all, e.g. if the number of observations is less than the number of parameters.
2. In some cases, the parameters of each individual cannot be estimated reliably, for example, in a PK analysis without data during the elimination phase or with increasing concentrations during the elimination phase, or in the case of binary data, if all observations are identical, i.e. either responsive or tolerant. This does not allow an

estimation of $C50$ for that individual. As a result, STS cannot be applied in these cases.

3. STS overestimates the interindividual variability of model parameters.
4. STS is sensitive to outlier data. Outlier data may result in estimated parameters that are far from the mean value or expected value. As a result, mean and standard deviation may be biased.

For these reasons, the STS approach has been largely abandoned in favour of various methods for population analysis, where all data are analysed simultaneously. The population approach has become the dominant approach over the last decades, since it has distinct advantages over the individual approach:

1. Population analysis is more efficient and more accurate than individual analysis with respect to the PKPD behaviour of the 'typical subject'.
2. Population analysis is more accurate and more precise with respect to the estimation of interindividual variability. It has been shown that interindividual variability is overestimated in individual analysis [60].
3. Population analysis is more flexible in model assumptions with respect to interindividual and residual variability. For example, in PD analysis, it is likely that there is interindividual variability in $C50$, but not (necessarily) in the steepness of the concentration–effect relationship (γ). Interindividual variability in clearance and $C50$ is usually assumed to be log-normally distributed, whereas other parameters may be assumed to be normally distributed. Also, residual variability is usually assumed to be the same in all subjects. Such choices can be made in population modelling.
4. Population analysis is more efficient in the estimation of the influence of covariates like body weight, age, gender, underlying pathology and co-medication. Covariates can be included in the structural PK or PKPD model and are essential in population analysis since they allow a more precise prediction of PK or PKPD in individuals.

The number of methods for population analysis has grown over the last decades. Each method has its own advantages, disadvantages and limitations, both with respect to the underlying statistical basis and to the flexibility of the available software.

The oldest and still by far the most used software package for population analysis is NONMEM (Icon Development Solutions, Hanover, MD), an acronym for nonlinear mixed effects modelling. NONMEM was developed in the late 1970s of the previous century by Lewis B. Sheiner and Stuart L. Beal of the NONMEM Project Group, University of California at San Francisco.

For NONMEM, several 'front-end' packages are available to create an environment to create the control file (a list of instructions for the NONMEM programme), to display the results in tables and graphics and to perform additional analysis, such as bootstrap analysis and log-likelihood profiling for the assessment of confidence intervals, for visual predictive checks (VPC) and for archiving. Such packages include PsN (http://psn.sourceforge.net), PLT Tools (www.pltsoft.com) and Pirana (www.pirana-software.com).

Since the introduction of NONMEM in 1979, other methods and software for population analysis have been developed, e.g. nonparametric methods, parametric expectation-maximum methods and iterative two-stage Bayesian methods, WinBugs and Monolix. A description of software for PK and PKPD falls outside the scope of this chapter. A regularly updated list of PKPD software can be found at www.boomer.org/pkin/soft.html.

Basic Aspects of NONMEM

In short, the procedure in NONMEM is as follows. The assumed model structure is described in a so-called control file, including information of PK models (most common models are provided in a built-in library) and specific commands.

The observed values are collected in a data file, together with the time of observation, dosing information and covariate information (e.g. weight, age, gender, study group).

After running the results are provided in an output file and user-defined tables. The original NONMEM output is rather user-unfriendly: limited information is provided, presented in an inconveniently arranged text file, without any graphics. Therefore, the above-mentioned front-end packages are very useful for a clear and well-organized presentation of the results.

In general, the following parameter values are estimated:

1. Structural model parameters, also called 'typical values', denoted θ (THETA, numbered 1, 2, etc.). These θ's are the same for each subject.
2. Interindividual variability in the structural model parameters denoted ω (OMEGA). Each individual deviates from the typical value θ with a deviation η (ETA, one value for each subject). The mean values of all η's are assumed to be zero, and their variance is ω.
3. Residual variability, also called residual error or intra-individual variability. Each individual observation deviated from the model-predicted value with a deviation ε (EPS). The mean values of all ε's are assumed to be zero, and their variance is σ (SIGMA).

The user must provide initial values for each of the values θ, ω and σ. As for individual analysis, the choice of these initial values is, generally speaking, not critical, although values far from the 'optimal' value may increase the risk of convergence to a local minimum (see above) and thus not the optimal solution and may increase the computation time.

During the NONMEM run, all values θ, ω and σ are estimated; alternatively, these values can be kept constant by adding the word FIX to the initial value. From a statistical point of view, θ is a fixed effect (with a fixed, albeit yet unknown value), and ω and σ are random effects (each subject is assumed to be randomly assigned to the study, and each observation is assumed to be statistically independent); this type of analysis is called mixed effects modelling. For nonlinear functions, the process can be described by nonlinear mixed effects modelling.

Simultaneous vs. Sequential PKPD Analysis

In a PKPD analysis, there are usually two sets of observed data, i.e. plasma concentrations (also called PK data) and drug effect observations (PD data), and two models, the PK and the PD model (which may include the PKPD link model). All the data can be analysed by different procedures, which will be described here shortly. A more detailed description of these procedures and comparison of them can be found in the literature [61, 62]. For convenience, we adopted the acronym from those papers:

1. SIM: simultaneous analysis of PK and PD models in a single run. From a statistical point, this is the best and most logical way to perform the analysis, provided that the data are 'ideal', i.e. that the data are equally informative with respect to the PK and PD model. If this is not the case, the simultaneous analysis may result in biased estimates of the PK and/or PD parameters, as has been demonstrated in literature [62–64]. Other limitations of this approach are the increased risk of convergence to local minima and long execution times.

   For these reasons, one of the following sequential procedures may be used. First, the PK analysis is performed, estimating only the PK parameters (θ, ω, σ), using only the PK model and PK data. In the next step, the PD analysis is performed, estimating the PD parameters (θ, ω, σ).

2. IPP (individual PK parameters): After the PK step, Bayesian (also called 'post hoc') parameter estimates are provided by NONMEM, and these parameters are used as fixed values in the PD analysis, estimating only the PD parameters (θ, ω, σ), using only the PD data. Although two different runs have to be performed, the total execution time is usually much shorter than for the simultaneous analysis [61–64]. However, this method

suffers from a statistical 'sin': the PK parameters are considered as exactly known values without any error, since only the point estimates are used. Actually, the PK parameters are not exactly known; only point estimates and their standard error (and/or confidence interval) are known. Therefore, the results are 'too optimistic', and the standard errors and confidence intervals of the PD parameters are underestimated significantly and population values may be biased [61–64].

3. IPPSE (individual PK parameters with standard errors): To avoid the above-mentioned problem of the sequential analysis, the standard error of the individual PK parameters may be included in the analysis to account for the uncertainty of the individual PK parameters, as was proposed by Lacroix et al. [61]. This method combines good accuracy and precision with reasonable execution times.

4. PPP&D (population PK parameters and dynamics): Alternatively, the individual PK parameters may be estimated in the PD run, but with fixed values of the typical PK parameter values and their variances as obtained from the PK analysis; this procedure is similar to the simultaneous approach, except for the fixed values of the typical PK parameter values and their variances, thus avoiding the limitations of the simultaneous analysis. In general, this approach may be considered the 'ideal' solution for the earlier mentioned problems with the other methods, at the cost of a limited increase of the execution time.

5. Nonparametric PK model: Unadkat and colleagues described an alternative to the IPP method, by replacing the compartmental PK model by a nonparametric PK model, i.e. assuming that the plasma concentration can be described by connecting the observed concentrations with straight line, either on a linear scale or a logarithmic scale [65]. This method requires some adaptations of the usual software. The advantage of this approach is that the PD analysis is completely independent of the PK analysis and that bias in the PK model is not transferred to the PD model; for this reason this approach was applied in several studies [31, 63, 66, 67]. In addition, this approach can be applied also in cases where a compartmental PK model does not seem to be appropriate, e.g. in the case of secondary plasma concentration peaks as a result of enterohepatic circulation. However, the method has the same disadvantages as approach IPP and requires sufficiently frequent sampling in each individual for an accurate description of the plasma concentration profile. Proost and colleagues compared the nonparametric PK, SIM and IPP methods and concluded that the nonparametric PK approach performed similarly to IPP [63].

Optimal Study Design

The study design is a key factor to obtain accurate and precise parameter estimates. Although this is quite obvious, it may be questioned whether the design of the study is evaluated thoroughly in the typical clinical study. Data to support this are lacking, but it seems likely that more accurate and precise results can be obtained in well-designed studies.

A problem inherent to 'optimal study design' is that such a design can be assessed only if the results of the study are known. For example, the well-known power analysis to determine the number of subjects in a study requires information on the expected variability, which must be estimated based on earlier information or pilot studies.

In general, the following factors determine the optimal design of PKPD studies:

– The primary and secondary objectives of the study
– The required accuracy and precision of the PKPD parameters and/or the required prediction performance
– The underlying PKPD model, its parameters and their interindividual and residual variability

The procedure for the assessment of the optimal study design should provide optimal values for, amongst others, the number of subjects, the number of observations per subject and the time points of observations.

The importance of time points of observations in PK studies was demonstrated by D'Argenio in 1981 [68], introducing various methods to assess the optimal time points of sampling for individual pharmacokinetic analysis, known as D-optimality and several more. More recently, this work was extended by several authors [69–71].

The optimal design of 'classical' clinical studies is nowadays performed by clinical trial simulation (CTS), allowing selection of the optimal design parameters for a study. The principle of CTS is to generate a large number of study results, based on the assumed clinical parameters, using a process called Monte Carlo simulations, where study parameters are simulated from the assumed mean, standard deviation and statistical distribution. Similar procedures can be used in PKPD studies. A major limitation of these Monte Carlo-based methods is the enormous computational burden; even in the present time with very fast computers, this still is an issue.

A critical point in optimal study design of PKPD studies is the fact that the optimal conditions are often in conflict with the 'classical' design of clinical studies. Two examples to clarify this point will be given here.

The first example refers to the optimal time point of the observations. In particular in cases where the number of observations per subject is small ('sparse data'), it is important that the time points are well spread over the relevant time period of the study, implying that the times of observations, for PK and/or PD, are not the same for each subject; the optimal sampling strategy may even have different time points for each subject. Such a study design will not be acceptable from a 'classical' clinical study point of view, since one cannot summarize the data in a table, such as 'drug effect was an increase of 5.0 (SD 0.7) units after 1 hour and 2.5 (SD 0.5) units after 4 hours', and a statistical analysis of these data is not possible. Actually, a population PKPD analysis is the only way to analyse this type of data.

The second example is the dose (or concentration, in the case of inhaled anaesthetics or TCI infusion) in relation to the (expected) drug effect. If the observed effects are well spread over the entire range, parameter estimation is likely to be precise and accurate, as shown in Fig. 7.6a. However, in a 'classical' clinical study, all patients would receive the same dose or a few different doses. In general, these doses are chosen to be effective, in order to avoid insufficient drug effect. As a result, at most time points, the observed drug effect is large, and small drug effects are lacking. So, the data are not well spread over the range from zero to full drug effect (Fig. 7.6b). As a result, the estimates of $C50$, γ and E_0 will be imprecise, even in cases where the total number of observations is large. For other drugs, where doses are relatively low to avoid adverse effects at higher concentrations, the drug concentrations are too low to estimate $C50$, γ and E_{max} precisely (Fig. 7.6c).

These examples show that the optimal design of PKPD studies may be hampered by the requirements posed by the 'classical' clinical study design or by ethical reasons that do not allow choice of the optimal doses.

The optimal design for interaction studies may be much more complex than that for a single drug, and, in spite of its importance, this topic seems to be largely neglected in literature. Short and colleagues [72] compared several designs for interaction studies based on response surface methodology in a simulation study, to select the most satisfactory study design and to estimate the number of patients needed to adequately describe the entire response surface. They concluded that the 'crisscross' design was most appropriate: in half of the patients, drug A is kept constant at one of a series of predefined levels and drug B is tested at various levels, and in the other half of the patients, drug B is kept constant at one of a series of predefined level and drug A is tested at various levels. For details we refer to the original publication [72].

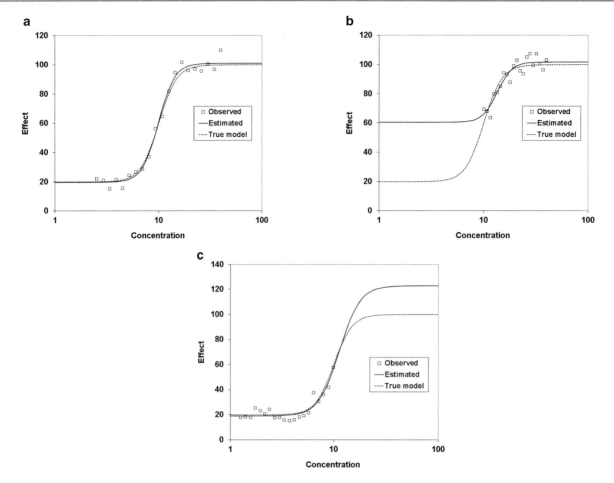

Fig. 7.6 Fitting drug effect data to the sigmoid E_{max} model. The *dashed line* shows the relationship according to the sigmoid E_{max} model with the true values of the parameters, the *open squares* show 20 simulated data points with added random error in the drug effect ('observed') and the *solid line* shows the best fitting sigmoid E_{max} model with baseline E_0 (Eq. 7.12). (**a**) Observations are well spread over the relevant range, resulting in accurate parameter estimates. (**b**) Observations are located in the upper range of effect, resulting in poor parameter estimates for $C50$, γ and E_0. (**c**) Observations are located in the lower range of effect, resulting in poor parameter estimates for $C50$, γ and E_{max}

Reporting PKPD Studies

A clear and consistent presentation of the results of PKPD studies is essential for a good understanding and in subsequent use of these results in patient care, drug development or research. Unfortunately, a survey of publications of PKPD studies shows that much can be improved, since many publications lack relevant information (e.g. with respect to calculations, units, residual error, model assumptions, model selection, diagnostic plots) or use uncommon or confusing symbols; it is recommended to use the generally accepted symbols as published [73, 74], and the use of software- or model-specific symbols should be avoided (e.g. denoting the volume of the central compartment as V_2 instead of V_c (or V_1), since it is used in the NONMEM code reflecting the volume of compartment 2, in cases where compartment 1 is used for the absorption compartment).

The statistical and technical aspects of PKPD modelling may be difficult to explain to readers not or less familiar with PKPD and pharmacometric concepts. However, this should be a challenge to clarify the aims, methods, results and discussion of PKPD studies for a wide audience, rather than hiding the message by unnecessarily technical writing, and still provide all essential details in the report or article. The possibility to provide part of such information as supplementary data on a website linked to the journal allows keeping the main article clear and succinct without lack of essential information.

Both the FDA and EMA published guidelines for population pharmacokinetic studies [75, 76].

Recently, a paper entitled 'Reporting a population pharmacokinetic-pharmacodynamic study: a journal's perspective' was published [77], followed by 'Reporting

Guidelines for Clinical Pharmacokinetic Studies: The ClinPK Statement' [78].

Earlier, Viby-Mogensen and colleagues published a paper on good clinical research practice (GCRP) of pharmacokinetic studies of neuromuscular blocking agents, including design, analysis and reporting of such studies [79], as a companion to papers on GCRP of pharmacodynamic studies of neuromuscular blocking agents [80]. Both papers were the result of consensus conferences of a large group of experts in the field.

PKPD Modelling of Drugs Used in Anaesthesia

Neuromuscular Blocking Agents

In 1979, Sheiner and colleagues published their classical paper on PKPD modelling of neuromuscular blocking agents (NMBA), introducing the concept of the 'effect compartment' to describe the relationship between the plasma concentration and the concentration at the site of action, i.e. to account for time delays between both concentrations as a result of drug transport from plasma to the site of action [29]. This idea, described above, solved the problem of the observed time delay between the plasma concentration of the NMBA and the resulting muscle relaxation, without the need of an extra pharmacokinetic compartment describing the plasma concentration profile, as was used in the model of Hull et al. [81].

The concept of the effect compartment has given an enormous impetus to PKPD modelling of almost all classes of drugs, within and outside anaesthesiology, and even today, Sheiner's PKPD link model is still by far the most commonly used approach in describing time delays of effect due to pharmacokinetics. It is obvious that the proof of principle of the effect compartment concept could be demonstrated only with a data set with sufficient PK and PD data and well-defined PK and PD models. To this purpose, NMBAs are most appropriate: the effect, i.e. the degree of muscle relaxation, can be quantified accurately by measuring muscle contraction force upon electrical stimulation, and the PD model can be used in its most simple form, since in Eq. (7.12) E_0 (pre-dose muscle contraction force, usually expressed as 100 % of control) and E_{max} are zero (complete relaxation or complete neuromuscular blockade), thus leaving only three parameters to be estimated (k_{e0}, $C50$ and γ).

This simple model has been described successfully for almost all NMBAs used in clinical practice. As described above, Viby-Mogensen and colleagues published a paper on good clinical research practice (GCRP) of pharmacokinetic studies of neuromuscular blocking agents, including design, analysis and reporting of such studies [79].

In most published studies, and for most compounds, the value of γ was in the range of 3–8, and the question arises whether this range reflects real differences between compounds or is due to methodological issues or inter-study variability. From a pharmacological point of view, it seems likely that the relationship between receptor occupancy of a nondepolarizing NMBA and the degree of neuromuscular block is independent of the chemical structure of the NMBA, and thus γ is a property of the neuromuscular system, and the same for all nondepolarizing NMBAs [82], but different for different muscles. Unfortunately, this hypothesis has never been tested thoroughly.

Donati and Meistelman [83] proposed a PKPD model for NMBAs, taking into account the binding of the NMBA to the acetylcholine receptors in the synaptic cleft, instead of the 'inert' effect compartment of the Sheiner model. This binding to receptors, also called the 'buffering hypothesis' as observed in in vitro experiments [84], has profound effects on the potency and time course of NMBAs, since binding to receptor lowers the unbound concentration in the effect compartment, thus increasing the onset time and increasing the dose needed to reach a certain degree of block [83, 85]. This model may explain the observed relationship between onset time and potency [86–88], but it is still unclear whether this 'buffering hypothesis' plays a dominant role in the observed relationship between onset time and potency, since conflicting observations have been reported [89, 90].

Beaufort and co-workers [91] showed that inhibition of the enzymatic degradation of suxamethonium and mivacurium increases the onset time of submaximal neuromuscular block, as predicted by PKPD modelling [85, 92].

The models described above have a common feature that they assume that the drug effect (neuromuscular block) is dependent on the (unbound) NMBA concentration in the effect compartment. From a mechanistic point of view, this is cumbersome, since the drug effect is the result of interaction of the drug molecules with the acetylcholine receptors, and thus it seems logical to relate the drug effect to the receptor occupancy. This concept has been used by D'Hollander and Delcroix [93], but this approach has not been explored further. Actually, as a result of the very fast binding and release of the NMBA and acetylcholine receptor, there is a fixed relationship between unbound drug concentration and receptor occupancy, and therefore both approaches are essentially identical.

A modification of this approach was applied to explain the increased sensitivity to NMBAs and the prolonged time course in myasthenic patients [67]. Using the classical approach (Sheiner model, using Eqs. (7.7) and (7.12)), $C50$ and γ were significantly decreased in myasthenic patients compared to controls. Using the unbound receptor model (URM), which relates the drug effect to the number of unbound acetylcholine receptors (i.e. the number of receptors available for neurotransmission by acetylcholine), explained the increased sensitivity to NMBAs and the prolonged time course in myasthenic patients as a result of a decreased number of acetylcholine receptors, in accordance with the known mechanism of myasthenia gravis, illustrating the advantage of a (more) mechanistic model over a merely empirical model. The results of this clinical PKPD study were confirmed in a study with pigs [66] and in an experimental setting with an antegrade perfused rat peroneal nerve anterior tibialis muscle model [94], in which experimental autoimmune myasthenia gravis was evoked by injection of alpha-bungarotoxin or by injecting monoclonal antibodies against rat acetylcholine receptors.

Several studies have been performed describing the different effects of NMBAs on different muscles [95, 96]. Vecuronium and rocuronium showed an earlier, but less deep, neuromuscular block at the adductor laryngeal muscle compared to the adductor pollicis, resulting in a larger value of k_{e0} (shorter equilibrium time) and a larger $C50$ (lower potency) as shown by PKPD modelling [96].

In the case of (cis)atracurium, the PK model should take into account both central and peripheral Hofmann elimination, a chemical degradation process independent of enzyme activity [97]. For mivacurium the classical PKPD link model did not result in acceptable model fitting, and an additional interstitial compartment was postulated to describe the PKPD of mivacurium adequately [31].

As described earlier, the plasma concentration–time profile cannot be accurately described by a compartmental model during the first minutes after administration due to the processes of mixing over the vascular space, and consequently, a PKPD model cannot describe the drug effect accurately over this time period. Beaufort and colleagues [15] and Ducharme and colleagues [16] investigated the influence of the compartmental approach in experiments with frequent arterial blood sampling, with intervals of 10 s and 1.2 s, respectively, and using a non-compartmental PK model. Their results showed that model parameters with frequent sampling were significantly different from that obtained from conventional compartmental modelling.

Only a few PKPD studies on the depolarizing NMBA suxamethonium (succinylcholine) have been published, partly as a result of the methodological issue of the rapid breakdown by plasma cholinesterase [98–100].

An alternative approach was introduced by Verotta and Sheiner [101–103] by performing PKPD modelling without plasma concentration measurements. In this approach, a one- or two-compartment PK model is assumed, and the parameters of this PK model together with the PD parameters are estimated from the PD measurements. Since

no concentrations are measured, $C50$ cannot be estimated, but instead of $C50$ the drug potency is modelled as an infusion rate associated with 50 % effect. For compounds following one-compartment kinetics, and for comparisons between compounds or between muscles, this approach may be attractive, but in other cases the value of this approach seems limited.

Nigrovic and colleagues published some extended PKPD models, e.g. to explain the competition of NMBAs and acetylcholine [104] and the phenomenon of twitch fade [105]. Such models may be helpful in a quantitative understanding of the processes involved, but their clinical relevance seems limited.

Interaction of Neuromuscular Blocking Agents

Several studies on the interaction of different NMBAs have been published in literature [106–108]. These studies were analysed using isobolographic analysis. Nigrovic and Amann [109] published a theoretical model describing the additive or supra-additive interaction of NMBAs. However, no PKPD models supported by full PKPD analysis describing the interaction of different NMBAs could be found in literature.

The overall pattern of these studies is that interactions of NMBAs of the same chemical group (aminosteroids such as rocuronium, vecuronium, pipecuronium and pancuronium or benzylisoquinolinium compounds such as cisatracurium, atracurium, mivacurium, metocurine and D-tubocurarine) are additive or mildly synergistic and that interactions of NMBAs of a different chemical group are synergistic. The clinical relevance of these findings remains to be demonstrated.

Reversal of Neuromuscular Block

The reversal of neuromuscular block by acetylcholinesterase inhibitors such as neostigmine and edrophonium has been modelled as an extension of the PKPD model of NMBAs [110–113].

The development of sugammadex introduced a novel concept to reverse neuromuscular block by forming a stable complex with rocuronium [114–118]. Due to the very high affinity of sugammadex for rocuronium, and to a lesser extend for vecuronium, unbound plasma concentrations of these NMBAs are rapidly reduced after injection of sugammadex.

The pharmacokinetics of sugammadex was investigated by non-compartmental analysis [116]. The PKPD of rocuronium and vecuronium, sugammadex and their interaction was successfully modelled, allowing investigation of the characteristics of the reversal of neuromuscular block of rocuronium and vecuronium by sugammadex in a quantitative manner [57].

In a case report in which a temporary decrease in train-of-four response was observed after reversal of muscle relaxation with a small dose (0.5 mg/kg) of sugammadex administered 42 min after 0.9 mg/kg of rocuronium, it was hypothesized that this muscle relaxation rebound occurs when the dose of sugammadex is sufficient for complex formation with rocuronium in the central compartment, but insufficient for redistribution of rocuronium from peripheral to central compartments, rather than dissociation of the sugammadex–rocuronium complex [119]. This hypothesis was supported by a PKPD modelling approach, and simulations indicated that muscle relaxation rebound can occur for doses of sugammadex in a limited critical range.

Volatile Anaesthetics

The classical measure of potency of volatile anaesthetics is the minimum alveolar concentration (MAC), defined as the concentration in the alveoli at which 50 % of the patients do not react to a standardized skin incision. Comparing this definition with Eq. (7.15), it follows that the MAC equals $C50$ for the stimulus skin incision. In this approach, the steepness γ is not explicitly determined; instead, anaesthesiologists use practical rules, e.g. that a concentration of 1.3 times the MAC results in adequate suppression of response after skin incision. Assuming that this coincides with a level of $P = 0.9$, it follows from Eq. (7.15) that γ of volatile anaesthetics is about 8. In addition, in the case of two or more anaesthetics, their MAC values may be added, implying that the assumed interaction is additive.

The concept of MAC as well as full PKPD models assumes equilibrium conditions of the concentrations in the alveoli, blood and brain. The time course of the concentrations in these areas can be described by pharmacokinetic models [120].

Several pharmacokinetic models for volatile anaesthetics were published [121–129]. Such models may be helpful for a better understanding of the time course of action of volatile anaesthetics as well as the influence of physico-chemical properties of the anaesthetic drug (e.g. blood–gas partition coefficient) and patient characteristics (e.g. cardiac output); their practical benefit remains to be demonstrated.

An overview of the clinical pharmacokinetics of sevoflurane can be found in the literature [130].

Intravenous Anaesthetics

Numerous PK models for intravenous anaesthetics have been published, in particular for propofol. The models for propofol derived by Marsh [131] and by Schnider [132, 133] are widely used and have been evaluated in TCI settings [8, 134–137]. In addition, PK and PKPD models have been developed for special patient groups, in particular in obesity [138, 139], children [140–142], infants [143] and obese children [144].

Eleveld and colleagues [49] developed a 'general purpose pharmacokinetic model' for propofol, using data from 21 previously published propofol data sets containing data from young children, children, adults, elderly and obese individuals, including data sets available from the Open TCI Initiative website (www.opentci.org). In total, 10,927 drug concentration observations from 660 individuals (age range 0.25–88 years, weight range 5.2–160 kg) were analysed. The goal was to determine a PK model with robust predictive performance for a wide range of patient groups and clinical conditions. A three-compartment allometric model was estimated with NONMEM using weight, age, sex and patient status as covariates. A predictive performance metric focused on intraoperative conditions was devised and used along with the AIC to guide model development. The predictive performance of the final model was better than or similar to that of specialized models, even for the subpopulations on which those models were derived. This general purpose model seems promising for the application of TCI in a wide range of patient groups and clinical conditions, although further prospective evaluation of the model is needed.

For several other intravenous anaesthetics, population PK models have been published, e.g. for midazolam in adults [145], infants [146] and obesity [147] and for dexmedetomidine in children [148] and adults [149].

Interaction of Anaesthetics

Harris and co-workers [150] found an additive interaction of sevoflurane and propofol for loss of consciousness and response to skin incision, using the Dixon up-and-down method and isobolographic techniques.

This interaction was also investigated by Schumacher et al. [151]. Using the response surface modelling approach, they showed that the interaction was additive for all investigated end points: BIS suppression, state and response entropy, tolerance of shake and shout, tetanic stimulation, laryngeal mask airway insertion and laryngoscopy. This implies that, for these end points, sevoflurane and propofol can be interchanged, with 1 mg/l propofol corresponding to 0.42 vol.% sevoflurane.

A similar study by Diz et al., using midazolam premedication and low doses of opioids, confirmed the additive interaction between propofol and sevoflurane on BIS [152]. The findings of these three studies are in line with the above-mentioned assumption of additivity of volatile anaesthetics.

The interaction of sevoflurane and nitrous oxide was modelled by Vereecke and colleagues [50]. Since this study also included the interaction with opioids, it is described below.

The interaction between midazolam and propofol has been studied by several researchers, with varying results. It has been shown that midazolam and propofol influence each others' kinetics [153–155], complicating the analysis of the interaction, although the observed PD interaction appeared not to be attributed to PK changes of the unbound concentrations of the drugs [156]. Some publications reported a synergistic interaction for sedation and loss of responsiveness [157–159], but others reported an additive interaction [43, 160]. A synergistic interaction was also found in a triple interaction study on midazolam, propofol and alfentanil by Minto and co-workers, as described below.

Opioids

The PK of the opioids used in anaesthesia has been investigated in several studies, which were reviewed about 20 years ago [161, 162]. More recent pharmacokinetic studies with opioids commonly used in anaesthesia seem to be absent in literature, except for remifentanil.

The PK of remifentanil was investigated by Egan and co-workers [163–165], by Minto and co-workers [166, 167] and by Drover and Lemmens [168]. The PK model of Minto et al. has been and is still widely used for TCI application. The performance of this model was validated in obese patients [169]. However, Mertens and colleagues [170] compared the predictive performance of remifentanil TCI using the above-mentioned five models and concluded that the three models by Egan and co-workers performed better than the Minto and Drover models.

The PD of opioids has been studied in many publications, using different end points of opioid effect. The oldest papers studied the MAC reduction of isoflurane by fentanyl [171, 172], alfentanil [172], sufentanil [173] and remifentanil [174]. Katoh and co-workers investigated the MAC reduction of sevoflurane by fentanyl [175]. It should be noted that MAC reduction studies are actually interaction studies (see below); they are mentioned here because these studies were aiming at measurement of the potency of the opioids.

Bouillon performed two studies comparing the respiratory depressant potency of remifentanil, alfentanil and piritramide [176, 177].

Gambus and co-workers [178] investigated the EEG-derived canonical univariate parameter (CUP) and the spectral edge ($SE_{95\%}$) as effect parameters of fentanyl, alfentanil, sufentanil, trefentanil and remifentanil. The potency of these compounds was expressed in their $C50$ (denoted IC50 in that paper). These $C50$ values are 5- to 20-fold the $C50$ values obtained in the MAC reduction studies, questioning whether these values can be used to compare the potency of opioids to provide the antinociceptive component of a balanced anaesthesia technique.

An overview of $C50$ values of alfentanil, fentanyl, sufentanil and remifentanil for the above-mentioned end points, as well as for the minimum effective plasma concentration providing postoperative analgesia (MEAC), can be found in *Miller's Anesthesia* [179].

Interaction of Opioids

The opioids most commonly used in anaesthesia (fentanyl, alfentanil, sufentanil and remifentanil) are pure μ-receptor opioid agonists [180]. Therefore, it may be assumed that their interaction is additive, implying that they can be interchanged, provided that (1) their different pharmacokinetics are considered; these differences may be exploited by changing the opioids towards the end of the surgical procedure to maintain the optimal analgesic treatment, and (2) the equipotent doses, or in TCI, equipotent concentrations are known. Unfortunately, as mentioned above, the equipotent doses and concentrations are dependent on the observed end point of opioid effect. Therefore, there is still a need for comparative studies determining the equipotent concentrations of the opioids used in anaesthesia on the clinically relevant end points such as reduction of $C50$ of propofol and analgesic effect. The latter would be measured as experimental pain, either attenuation of a standard stimulus or increasing pain tolerance.

Interaction of Volatile Anaesthetics and Opioids

The interaction studies on the MAC reduction of volatile anaesthetics by opioids have been described above, because these studies were aiming at measurement of the potency of the opioids.

The interaction between sevoflurane and remifentanil was studied by Manyam et al. [32], measuring sedation and responsiveness using the Observer's Assessment of Alertness and Sedation Scale (OAAS) and several painful stimuli: electrical titanic stimulus, pressure algometry (reproducible pressure on the anterior tibia) and 50 °C hot temperature sensation in volunteers. In this study, end-tidal vapour pressure was used as input for the PD model, although there was no equilibrium with effect-site concentrations. Therefore, the results of this study are of limited validity. The same group published a reanalysis of these data [181].

The interaction between sevoflurane and remifentanil was also investigated by Heyse and colleagues [37], measuring responsiveness using the OAAS scale and several painful stimuli: electrical tetanic stimulus, laryngeal mask airway insertion and laryngoscopy. They applied several available mathematical approaches in modelling the concentration–effect data to identify which approach works best. The hierarchical model was found to fit best to the data, the same model that was developed by Bouillon et al. [41] to describe the interaction between propofol and remifentanil.

In the study of Heyse and colleagues, also several continuous measures of hypnotic and analgesic effect were obtained before and after the above-mentioned series of noxious and non-noxious stimulations [182]. Using a response surface methodology, an additive interaction between sevoflurane and remifentanil was found for the EEG-derived measures bispectral index (BIS), state entropy (SE) and response entropy (RE).

For the composite variability index (CVI), a moderate synergism was found. The comparison of pre- and poststimulation data revealed a shift of $C50$ of sevoflurane for BIS, SE and RE, with a consistent increase of 0.3 vol.% sevoflurane. The surgical pleth index (SPI) data did not result in plausible parameter estimates, neither before nor after stimulation.

These modelling results confirm the reduction of the MAC of volatile anaesthetics as a result of a synergistic interaction, as has been shown in several MAC reduction studies Once the interaction between sevoflurane and remifentanil is established using response surface modelling, it is tempting to predict the interactions of other volatile anaesthetics using MAC equivalencies and/or other opioids, using remifentanil equivalents, i.e. remifentanil concentrations equipotent to the other opioid. Although it is likely that such predictions are valid, their clinical validity and safety need to be established in prospective studies.

Vereecke and colleagues [50] expanded the hierarchical model for sevoflurane and opioids for the combined administration of sevoflurane, opioids and nitrous oxide (N_2O), using historical data on the somatic (motor) and autonomic (hemodynamic) responsiveness to incision, the MAC and MAC-BAR, respectively [175]. Four potential actions of N_2O were postulated: (1) N_2O is equivalent to A ng/ml of fentanyl (additive); (2) N_2O reduces $C50$ of fentanyl by a factor B; (3) N_2O is equivalent to X vol.% of sevoflurane

(additive); and (4) N_2O reduces $C50$ of sevoflurane by a factor Y. They found that 66 vol.% N_2O combines an additive effect corresponding to 0.27 ng/ml fentanyl (A) with an additive effect corresponding to 0.54 vol.% sevoflurane (X). This allows incorporation of the effect of N_2O into the hierarchical interaction model.

Interaction of Intravenous Anaesthetics and Opioids

The interaction of propofol with opioids has been investigated in many papers, for a variety of PD end points and for various opioids, e.g. for fentanyl [183, 184], alfentanil [154, 185, 186] and remifentanil. The latter have been extensively studied for a variety of effects, including EEG-derived indices [41, 187–189], cardiorespiratory end points [190–193] and sedation and responsiveness using OAAS [41].

Response surface modelling of the propofol—remifentanil interaction was performed in several studies using the Greco interaction model [194–196]. This resulted in very high $C50$ values for remifentanil as a result of the low sensitivity of the end points (amongst others, OAAS and laryngoscopy). Bouillon and co-workers [41] performed a study in volunteers using the same end points. They introduced the hierarchical model and found that the hierarchical model performed better than the Minto model. For the EEG-derived measures BIS and approximate entropy (AE), the interaction between propofol and remifentanil was additive. The results of Bouillon et al. for propofol are in excellent agreement with that for sevoflurane of Heyse et al. [37, 182] for all reported end points, confirming the similarity of the PKPD properties of sevoflurane and propofol.

Vereecke and co-workers [197] reanalysed the pooled data of three studies on the interaction of propofol–remifentanil [41], sevoflurane–propofol [151] and sevoflurane–remifentanil [37] to develop a triple interaction model for the probability to tolerate laryngoscopy (P_{TOL}), combining Eqs. (7.18) and (7.23) to

$$U = \left(\frac{C_{SEVO}}{C50_{SEVO}} + \frac{C_{PROP}}{C50_{PROP}} \right) \cdot \left(1 + \left(\frac{C_{REMI}}{C50_{REMI}} \right)^{\gamma_o} \right)$$

(7.33)

The pooled analysis resulted in unique $C50$ values for each compound and a common value for γ, whereas γ_O was not significantly different from 1. Based on P_{TOL}, a given combination of propofol and remifentanil can be converted to an equipotent combination of sevoflurane and remifentanil and vice versa.

This model was used to extend the noxious stimulation response index (NSRI), an anaesthetic depth indicator related to P_{TOL}, presented for propofol and remifentanil [42]. The NSRI was extended for sevoflurane by modification of the original definition of NSRI [197]. NSRI is scaled between 100 (when no anaesthetic drugs are administered) and 0 (indicating very profound anaesthesia), in addition, for $P_{TOL} = 0.5$, NSRI is 50, and for $P_{TOL} = 0.9$, NSRI is 20, leading to the following equation:

$$NSRI = \frac{100}{1 + \left(\frac{P_{TOL}}{1-P_{TOL}}\right)^{s}} \quad (7.34)$$

where $S =$ slope factor $= 0.63093$. P_{TOL} was estimated from the end-tidal concentration of sevoflurane and effect-site concentrations of propofol and remifentanil [197].

NSRI was found to be a better predictor of P_{TOL} compared to bispectral index (BIS), state and response entropy (SE, RE), composite variability index (CVI) and surgical pleth index (SPI), as well as end-tidal concentration of sevoflurane and effect-site concentrations of propofol and remifentanil [197]. These data suggest that NSRI may be of interest as a universal pharmacology-based anaesthesia indicator reflecting the total potency of any combination of sevoflurane, propofol and remifentanil.

Zanderigo and colleagues [198] modelled the relationship between desired and undesired effects simultaneously by defining a new parameter called 'well-being', defined as a superposition of desired and undesired effects. The synergistic response for both desired and adverse effects was used to identify a preferred range of propofol and remifentanil concentrations that provide adequate anaesthesia, associated with the lowest risk of side effects. This approach has not resulted in more publications, in spite of its attractive characteristics.

In a triple interaction study on midazolam, propofol and alfentanil, Vinik and co-workers [160] used isobolographic techniques to determine whether combinations of midazolam–propofol, propofol–alfentanil, midazolam–alfentanil and midazolam–propofol–alfentanil interacted in a synergistic or additive way. Only the midazolam–propofol interaction was not significantly different from additivity.

Using data from an earlier study [159] with midazolam, propofol and alfentanil, Minto and co-workers found significant synergistic interactions of each pair of these compounds, but no additional triple interaction when three drugs were combined [34]. A weak point of this study is that observations were made at fixed time points after administration of known doses, but the actual concentrations were not known. This implies that this study does not provide a full surface response model allowing estimating the effect of any combination of midazolam, propofol and alfentanil. Therefore, a well-designed study of the midazolam–propofol–opioid interaction assessed at near steady state, using standardized end points of hypnotic drug effect, is still missing.

Applications of PKPD Models

PKPD models offer a wide range of applications in anaesthesiology, for example:

1. Drug administration by TCI, as is nowadays routinely applied for propofol and opioids such as remifentanil, throughout Europe and Asia. The clinical value of TCI has been demonstrated in validation studies [8, 134, 135, 137]. Due to regulatory differences, TCI pumps are not yet allowed in the United States [136].
2. Drug advisory displays, such as SmartPilot View (Dräger, Lübeck, Germany) and Navigator Suite (GE Healthcare, Madison, WI), have a large potential to help the anaesthesiologist. Such displays provide real-time individualized predictions of anaesthetic drug effects, accounting for administered doses, drug interactions and patient characteristics, allowing rational, timely and reproducible drug titration. These predictions are presented either as isoboles (SmartPilot View) or coloured zones of desired effect on the effect-site concentration graphs (Navigator Suite). In order to guarantee optimal performance, adequate PKPD models must be available and prospectively validated.

The application of drug advisory displays in clinical practice has several potential advantages. They allow a titration of the drug dose to, for example, the 95 % isobole, i.e. a near-maximal effect while minimizing overdose, a process called 'surfing the waves' [136]. Also in cases where the individual patient behaves differently from the expected typical patient, the isoboles can still be used to guide dosing, taking into account the clinical observations in that patient.

The anaesthesiologist should be aware of the limitations to these drug displays. The predictions of drug concentration and effects are based on population models. This means that the concentrations and effects individual patients may deviate from the predictions shown on the display. From a clinical point of view, it may diminish the user's confidence in the system, but from a statistical point of view, the prediction is not 'wrong'. In addition, even for the typical patient, PKPD predictions are not perfect and are based on models obtained from studies in a limited number of patients with possibly a suboptimal study design, e.g. with respect to co-medication affecting drug effect or insufficient time to reach steady-state conditions.

3. Prediction of the time course of drug action, e.g. to confirm the anaesthesiologist's knowledge and expertise, in particular in complex or unusual circumstances, but also in daily practice, e.g. to determine the optimal dosing of anaesthetics and opioids during anaesthesia. Quantitative PKPD knowledge of their combined effects (either 'at hand' or in a drug advisory displays) allows exploitation of the synergistic interaction, aiming at drug concentrations close to the 95 % isobole ('surfing the waves'), i.e. sufficient to elicit the desired level of anaesthesia in a large majority of patients, but avoid prolonged drug effect and increased risk of adverse effects, while keeping the optimal balance between depth of anaesthesia and cardiovascular stability and, at the same time, ensuring a rapid recovery.

Conclusions

The development of PKPD modelling techniques and models over the last decades has undoubtedly increased our knowledge and understanding of the relationship between dose administration profile and clinical effect, enabling prediction of time course of the clinical effects of drugs routinely used in clinical anaesthetic practice. Great progress has been made in understanding pharmacodynamic interactions. This knowledge has recently been implemented in drug advisory displays, allowing the anaesthesiologists to better understand interactions between different drugs and to better predict the future time courses of clinical effects of combinations of drugs, thus contributing to more adequate and safer anaesthesia.

References

1. Minto CF, Schnider TW. Contributions of PK/PD modeling to intravenous anesthesia. Clin Pharmacol Ther. 2008;84:27–38.
2. Sadean MR, Glass PSA. Pharmacokinetic–pharmacodynamic modeling in anesthesia, intensive care and pain medicine. Curr Opin Anaesthesiol. 2009;22:463–8.
3. Bouillon TW. Hypnotic and opioid anesthetic drug interactions on the CNS, focus on response surface modelling, modern anesthetics. In: Schuttler J, Schwilden H, editors. Handbook of experimental pharmacology, vol. 182. Berlin Heidelberg: Springer; 2008. p. 471–875.
4. Vereecke HEM, Proost JH, Eleveld DJ, Struys MMRF. Drug interactions in anesthesia. In: Johnson K, editor. Clinical pharmacology for anesthesiology. McGraw-Hill Education; 2015. ISBN-13: 978-0071736169 ISBN-10: 0071736166.
5. Rowland M, Tozer T. Clinical pharmacokinetics and pharmacodynamics: concepts and applications. 4th ed. Philadelphia: Lippincott Williams and Wilkins; 2010.
6. Bonate PL. Pharmacokinetic-pharmacodynamic modeling and simulation. 2nd ed. New York: Springer; 2011. ISBN 978-1-4419-9484-4.
7. Levitt DG, Schnider TW. Human physiologically based pharmacokinetic model for propofol. BMC Anesthesiol. 2005;5:4. doi:10.1186/1471-2253-5-4.
8. Masui K, Upton RN, Doufas AG, Coutzee JF, Kazama T, Mortier EP, Struys MMRF. The performance of compartmental and physiologically based recirculatory pharmacokinetic models for propofol: a comparison using bolus, continuous, and target-controlled infusion data. Anesth Analg. 2010;111(2):368–79.
9. Edginton AN, Theil FP, Schmitt W, Willmann S. Whole body physiologically-based pharmacokinetic models: their use in clinical drug development. Expert Opin Drug Metab Toxicol. 2008;4(9):1143–52.
10. Nestorov I. Whole-body physiologically based pharmacokinetic models. Expert Opin Drug Metab Toxicol. 2007;3(2):235–49.
11. Rostami-Hodjegan A. Physiologically based pharmacokinetics joined with in vitro–in vivo extrapolation of ADME: a marriage under the arch of systems pharmacology. Clin Pharmacol Ther. 2012;92(1):50–61.
12. Avram MJ, Krejcie TC. Using front-end kinetics to optimize target-controlled drug infusions. Anesthesiology. 2003;99:1078–86.
13. Krejcie TC, Henthorn TK, Niemann CU, Klein C, Gupta DK, Gentry WB, Shanks CA, Avram MJ. Recirculatory pharmacokinetic models of blood, extracellular fluid and total body water administered concomitantly. J Pharmacol Exp Ther. 1996;278:1050–7.
14. Struys MMRF, Coppens MJ, De Neve N, Mortier EP, Doufas AG, Van Bocxlaer JFP, Shafer SL. Influence of administration rate on propofol plasma-effect site equilibration. Anesthesiology. 2007;107(3):386–96.
15. Beaufort TM, Proost JH, Kuizenga K, Houwertjes MC, Kleef UW, Wierda JMKH. Do plasma concentrations obtained from *early* arterial blood sampling improve pharmacokinetic/pharmacodynamic modeling? J Pharmacokinet Biopharm. 1999;27(2):173–90.
16. Ducharme J, Varin F, Bevan DR, Donati F. Importance of early blood sampling on vecuronium pharmacokinetic and pharmacodynamic parameters. Clin Pharmacokinet. 2003;24(6):507–18.
17. Chiou WL. The phenomenon and rationale of marked dependence of drug concentration on blood sampling site. Implications in pharmacokinetics, pharmacodynamics, toxicology and therapeutics (Part I). Clin Pharmacokinet. 1989;17(3):175–99.
18. Donati F, Varin F, Ducharme J, Gill SS, Théorêt Y, Bevan DR. Pharmacokinetics and pharmacodynamics of atracurium obtained with arterial and venous blood samples. Clin Pharmacol Ther. 1991;49(5):515–22.
19. Hermann DJ, Egan TD, Muir KT. Influence of arteriovenous sampling on remifentanil pharmacokinetics and pharmacodynamics. Clin Pharmacol Ther. 1999;65(5):511–8.
20. Levitt DG. Physiologically based pharmacokinetic modeling of arterial—antecubital vein concentration difference. BMC Clin Pharmacol. 2004;4:2.
21. Olofsen E, Mooren R, van Dorp E, Aarts L, Smith T, den Hartigh J, Dahan A, Sarton E. Arterial and venous pharmacokinetics of morphine-6-glucuronide and impact of sample site on pharmacodynamic parameter estimates. Anesth Analg. 2010;111(3):626–32.
22. Weaver BMQ, Staddon GE, Raptopoulos D, Mapleson WW. Partitioning of propofol between blood cells, plasma and deproteinised plasma in sheep. J Vet Anaesth. 1998;25(1):19–23.

23. Benet LZ, Hoener B. Changes in plasma protein binding have little clinical relevance. Clin Pharmacol Ther. 2002;71(3):115–21.

24. Heuberger J, Schmidt S, Derendorf H. When is protein binding important? J Pharm Sci. 2013;102(9):3458–67.

25. Roberts JA, Pea F, Lipman J. The clinical relevance of plasma protein binding changes. Clin Pharmacokinet. 2013;52:1–8.

26. Hiraoka H, Yamamoto K, Okano N, Morita T, Goto F, Horiuchi R. Changes in drug plasma concentrations of an extensively bound and highly extracted drug, propofol, in response to altered plasma binding. Clin Pharmacol Ther. 2004;75(4):324–30.

27. Mazoit JX, Samii K. Binding of propofol to blood components: implications for pharmacokinetics and for pharmacodynamics. Br J Clin Pharmacol. 1999;47(1):35–42.

28. Suarez E, Calvo R, Zamacona MK, Lukas J. Binding of propofol to blood components. Br J Clin Pharmacol. 2000;49(4):380–1.

29. Sheiner LB, Stanski DR, Vozeh S, Miller RD, Ham J. Simultaneous modeling of pharmacokinetics and pharmacodynamics: application to d tubocurarine. Clin Pharmacol Ther. 1979;25:358–71.

30. Holford NHG, Sheiner LB. Understanding the dose effect relationship: clinical application of pharmacokinetic-pharmacodynamic models. Clin Pharmacokinet. 1981;6:429–53.

31. Schiere S, Proost JH, Roggeveld J, Wierda JMKH. An interstitial compartment is necessary to link the pharmacokinetics and pharmacodynamics of mivacurium. Eur J Anaesthesiol. 2004;21(11):882–91.

32. Manyam SC, Gupta DK, Johnson KB, White JL, Pace NL, Westenskow DR, Egan TD. Opioid-volatile anesthetic synergy: a response surface model with remifentanil and sevoflurane as prototypes. Anesthesiology. 2006;105(2):267–78.

33. Goutelle S, Maurin M, Rougier F, Barbaut X, Bourguignon L, Ducher M, Maire P. The Hill equation: a review of its capabilities in pharmacological modelling. Fundam Clin Pharmacol. 2008;22(6):633–48.

34. Minto CF, Schnider TW, Short TG, Gregg KM, Gentilini A, Shafer SL. Response surface model for anesthetic drug interactions. Anesthesiology. 2000;92:1603–16.

35. Greco WR, Bravo GO, Parsons JC. The search for synergy: a critical review from a response surface perspective. Pharmacol Rev. 1995;47(2):331–85.

36. Greco WR, Park HS, Rustum YM. Application of a new approach for the quantitation of drug synergism to the combination of cis-diamminedichloroplatinum and 1-beta-D-arabinofuranosyl-cytosine. Cancer Res. 1990;50:5318–27.

37. Heyse B, Proost JH, Schumacher PM, Bouillon TW, Vereecke HEM, Eleveld DJ, Luginbühl M, Struys MMRF. Sevoflurane remifentanil interaction: Comparison of different response surface models. Anesthesiology. 2012;116(2):311–23.

38. Jonker DM, Visser SAG, van der Graaf PH, Voskuyl RA, Danhof M. Towards a mechanism-based analysis of pharmacodynamic drug–drug interactions in vivo. Pharmacol Ther. 2005;106:1–18.

39. Tallarida RJ. Drug synergism: its detection and applications. J Pharmacol Exp Ther. 2001;298(3):865–72.

40. Bol CJ, Vogelaar JP, Tang JP, Mandema JW. Quantification of pharmacodynamic interactions between dexmedetomidine and midazolam in the rat. J Pharmacol Exp Ther. 2000;294:347–55.

41. Bouillon TW, Bruhn J, Radulescu L, Andresen C, Shafer TJ, Cohane C, Shafer SL. Pharmacodynamic interaction between propofol and remifentanil regarding hypnosis, tolerance of laryngoscopy, bispectral index, and electroencephalographic approximate entropy. Anesthesiology. 2004;100:1353–72.

42. Luginbuhl M, Schumacher PM, Vuilleumier P, Vereecke H, Heyse B, Bouillon TW, Struys MM. Noxious stimulation response index: a novel anesthetic state index based on hypnotic-opioid interaction. Anesthesiology. 2010;112:872–80.

43. Fidler M, Kern SE. Flexible interaction model for complex interactions of multiple anesthetics. Anesthesiology. 2006;105(2):286–96.

44. Kong M, Lee JJ. A generalized response surface model with varying relative potency for assessing drug interaction. Biometrics. 2006;62:986–95.

45. Lee S. Drug interactions: focussing on response surface models. Korean J Anesthesiol. 2010;58(5):421–34.

46. Godfrey KR, Chapman MJ, Vajda S. Identifiability and indistinguishability of nonlinear pharmacokinetic models. J Pharmacokinet Biopharm. 1994;22:229–51.

47. Jacquez JA, Perry T. Parameter estimation—local identifiability of parameters. Am J Physiol. 1990;258:E727–36.

48. Ludden TM, Beal SL, Sheiner LB. Comparison of the Akaike Information Criterion, the Schwarz Criterion and the F test as guides to model selection. J Pharmacokinet Biopharm. 1994;22:431–45.

49. Eleveld DJ, Proost JH, Cortinez LI, Absalom AR, Struys MMRF. A general purpose pharmacokinetic model for propofol. Anesth Analg. 2014;118(6):1221–37.

50. Vereecke HEM, Proost JH, Heyse B, Eleveld DJ, Katoh T, Luginbühl M, Struys MMRF. Interaction between nitrous oxide, sevoflurane and opioids: a response surface approach. Anesthesiology. 2013;118(4):894–902.

51. Post TM, Cremers SC, Kerbusch T, Danhof M. Bone physiology, disease and treatment: towards disease system analysis in osteoporosis. Clin Pharmacokinet. 2010;49(2):89–118.

52. Post TM, Schmidt S, Peletier LA, de Greef R, Kerbusch T, Danhof M. Application of a mechanism-based disease systems model for osteoporosis to clinical data. J Pharmacokinet Pharmacodyn. 2013;40(2):143–56.

53. Pilla Reddy V, Kozielska M, Johnson M, Vermeulen A, de Greef R, Liu J, Groothuis GMM, Danhof M, Proost JH. Structural models describing placebo treatment effects in schizophrenia and other neuropsychiatric disorders. Clin Pharmacokinet. 2011;50(7):429–50.

54. Danhof M, de Jongh J, De Lange ECM, Della Pasqua O, Ploeger BA, Voskuyl RA. Mechanism-based pharmacokinetic-pharmacodynamic modeling: biophase distribution, receptor theory, and dynamical systems analysis. Annu Rev Pharmacol Toxicol. 2007;47:357–400.

55. Danhof M, De Lange ECM, Della Pasqua O, Ploeger BA, Voskuyl RA. Mechanism-based pharmacokinetic-pharmacodynamic (PK-PD) modeling in translational drug research. Trends Pharmacol Sci. 2008;29(4):186–91.

56. Mager DE, Jusko WJ. Development of translational pharmacokinetic–pharmacodynamic models. Clin Pharmacol Ther. 2008;83(6):909–12.

57. Ploeger BA, Smeets J, Strougo A, Drenth HJ, Ruigt G, Houwing N, Danhof M. Pharmacokinetic-pharmacodynamic model for the reversal of neuromuscular blockade by sugammadex. Anesthesiology. 2009;110(1):95–105.

58. Ploeger BA, van der Graaf PH, Danhof M. Incorporating receptor theory in mechanism-based pharmacokinetic-pharmacodynamic (PK-PD) modeling. Drug Metab Pharmacokinet. 2009;24(1):3–15.

59. Van der Graaf PH. Pharmacometrics and systems pharmacology. CPT Pharmacometrics Syst Pharmacol. 2012;1, e8. doi:10.1038/psp.2012.8.

60. Proost JH, Eleveld DJ. Performance of an iterative two-stage Bayesian technique for population pharmacokinetic analysis of rich data sets. Pharm Res. 2006;23(12):2748–59. Erratum in Pharm Res 2007;24(8):1599.

61. Lacroix BD, Friberg LE, Karlsson MO. Evaluation of IPPSE, an alternative method for sequential population PKPD analysis. J Pharmacokinet Pharmacodyn. 2012;39(2):177–93.

62. Zhang L, Beal SL, Sheiner LB. Simultaneous vs. sequential analysis for population PK/PD data I: best-case performance. J Pharmacokinet Pharmacodyn. 2003;30:387–404.

63. Proost JH, Schiere S, Eleveld DJ, Wierda JMKH. Simultaneous versus sequential pharmacokinetic-pharmacodynamic population analysis using an Iterative two-stage Bayesian technique. Biopharm Drug Dispos. 2007;28(8):455–73.

64. Zhang L, Beal SL, Sheiner LB. Simultaneous vs. sequential analysis for population PK/PD data II: robustness of methods. J Pharmacokinet Pharmacodyn. 2003;30:405–16.

65. Unadkat JD, Bartha F, Sheiner LB. Simultaneous modeling of pharmacokinetics and pharmacodynamics with nonparametric kinetic and dynamic models. Clin Pharmacol Ther. 1986;40:86–93.

66. De Haes A, Proost JH, De Baets MH, Stassen MHW, Houwertjes MC, Wierda JMKH. Pharmacokinetic-pharmacodynamic modeling of rocuronium in case of a decreased number of acetylcholine receptors: a study in myasthenic pigs. Anesthesiology. 2003;98(1):133–42.

67. De Haes A, Proost JH, Kuks JBM, van den Tol DC, Wierda JMKH. Pharmacokinetic-pharmacodynamic modeling of rocuronium in myasthenic patients is improved by taking into account the number of unbound acetylcholine receptors. Anesth Analg. 2002;95(3):588–96.

68. D'Argenio DZ. Optimal sampling times for pharmacokinetic experiments. J Pharmacokinet Biopharm. 1981;9(6):739–56.

69. Bazzoli C, Retouta S, Mentré F. Design evaluation and optimisation in multiple response nonlinear mixed effect models: PFIM 3.0. Comput Methods Programs Biomed. 2010;98:55–65.

70. Dokoumetzidis A, Aarons L. Bayesian optimal designs for pharmacokinetic models: sensitivity to uncertainty. J Biopharm Stat. 2007;17(5):851–67.

71. Hooker AC, Foracchia M, Dodds MG, Vicini P. An evaluation of population D-optimal designs via pharmacokinetic simulations. Ann Biomed Eng. 2003;31:98–111.

72. Short TG, Ho TY, Minto CF, Schnider TW, Shafer SL. Efficient trial design for eliciting a pharmacokinetic-pharmacodynamic model-based response surface describing the interaction between two intravenous anesthetic drugs. Anesthesiology. 2002;96:400–8.

73. Adis Data Information. Clinical pharmacokinetics preferred symbols. 2006. http://static.springer.com/sgw/documents/1372030/application/pdf/40262_CPK_symbols.pdf. Accessed 21 Aug 2015.

74. Rowland M, Tucker G. Symbols in pharmacokinetics. J Pharmacokinet Biopharm. 1980;8(5):497–507.

75. Food and Drug Administration. Guidance for industry—population pharmacokinetics. 1999. http://www.fda.gov/downloads/Drugs/.../Guidances/UCM072137.pdf. Accessed 21 Aug 2015.

76. Committee for medicinal products for human use (CHMP) and European Medicines Agency. Guideline on reporting the results of population pharmacokinetic analyses. 2007. http://www.ema.europa.eu/docs/en_GB/document_library/Scientific_guideline/2009/09/WC500003067.pdf. Accessed 21 Aug 2015.

77. Jamsen KM, McLeay SC, Barras MA, Green B. Reporting a population pharmacokinetic-pharmacodynamic study: a journal's perspective. Clin Pharmacokinet. 2014;53:111–22.

78. Kanji S, Hayes M, Ling A, Shamseer L, Chant C, Edwards DJ, Edwards S, Ensom MH, Foster DR, Hardy B, Kiser TH, la Porte C, Roberts JA, Shulman R, Walker S, Zelenitsky S, Moher D. Reporting guidelines for clinical pharmacokinetic studies: the ClinPK statement. Clin Pharmacokinet. 2015;54(7):783–95.

79. Viby-Mogensen J, Østergaard D, Donati F, Fisher D, Hunter J, Kampmann JP, Kopman A, Proost JH, Rasmussen SN, Skovgaard LT, Varin F, Wright PMC. Pharmacokinetic studies of neuromuscular blocking agents: Good Clinical Research Practice (GCRP). Acta Anaesthesiol Scand. 2000;44(10):1169–90.

80. Fuchs-Buder T, Claudius C, Skovgaard LT, Eriksson LI, Mirakhur RK, Viby-Mogensen J. Good clinical research practice in pharmacodynamic studies of neuromuscular blocking agents II: the Stockholm revision. Acta Anaesthesiol Scand. 2007;51:789–808.

81. Hull CJ, Van Beem HBH, McLeod K, Sibbald A, Watson MJ. A pharmacokinetic model for pancuronium. Br J Anaesth. 1978;50:1113–23.

82. Nigrovic V, Amann A. Physiologic-pharmacologic interpretation of the constants in the Hill equation for neuromuscular block: a hypothesis. J Pharmacokinet Pharmacodyn. 2002;29(2):189–206.

83. Donati F, Meistelman C. A kinetic-dynamic model to explain the relationship between high potency and slow onset time for neuromuscular blocking drugs. J Pharmacokinet Biopharm. 1991;19:537–52.

84. Glavinovic MI, Law Min JC, Kapural L, Donati F, Bevan DR. Speed of action of various muscle relaxants at the neuromuscular junction binding vs buffering hypothesis. J Pharmacol Exp Ther. 1993;265:1181–6.

85. Proost JH, Wierda JMKH, Meijer DKF. An extended pharmacokinetic/pharmacodynamic (PK/PD) model describing quantitatively the influence of plasma protein binding, tissue binding, and receptor binding on the potency and time course of action of drugs. J Pharmacokinet Biopharm. 1996;24(1):45–77.

86. Bowman WC, Rodger IW, Houston J, Marshall IG, McIndewar I. Structure-action relationships among some desacetoxy analogues of pancuronium and vecuronium in the anesthetized cat. Anesthesiology. 1988;89:57–62.

87. Kopman AF. Molar potency and the onset of action of rocuronium [Letter]. Anesth Analg. 1994;78:815.

88. Kopman AF. Pancuronium, gallamine, and d-tubocurarine compared: Is speed of onset inversely related to drug potency? Anesthesiology. 1989;70:915–20.

89. Proost JH, Houwertjes MC, Wierda JMKH. Is time to peak effect of neuromuscular blocking agents dependent on dose? Testing the concept of buffered diffusion. Eur J Anaesthesiol. 2008;25(7):572–80.

90. Proost JH, Wright PMC. A pharmacokinetic-dynamic explanation of the rapid onset/offset of rapacuronium. Eur J Anaesthesiol. 2001;18 Suppl 23:83–9.

91. Beaufort TM, Nigrovic V, Proost JH, Houwertjes MC, Wierda JMKH. Inhibition of the enzymic degradation of suxamethonium and mivacurium increases the onset time of submaximal neuromuscular block. Anesthesiology. 1998;89(3):707–14.

92. Proost JH, Wierda JMKH. Pharmacokinetic aspects of the onset of action of neuromuscular blocking agents. Anasthesiol Intensivmed Notfallmed Schmerzther. 2000;35(2):98–100.

93. D'Hollander AA, Delcroix C. An analytical pharmacodynamic model for non-depolarizing neuromuscular blocking agents. J Pharmacokinet Biopharm. 1981;9:27–40.

94. De Haes A, Proost JH, De Baets MH, Stassen MHW, Houwertjes MC, Wierda JMKH. Decreased number of acetylcholine receptors is the mechanism that alters the time course of muscle relaxants in myasthenia gravis: a study in a rat model. Eur J Anaesthesiol. 2005;22(8):591–6.

95. Donati F, Meistelman C, Plaud B. Vecuronium neuromuscular blockade at the vocal cords and adductor pollicis in humans. Anesthesiology. 1991;74:833–7.

96. Plaud B, Proost JH, Wierda JMKH, Barre J, Debaene B, Meistelman C. Pharmacokinetics and pharmacodynamics of rocuronium at the vocal cords and the adductor pollicis in humans. Clin Pharmacol Ther. 1995;58:185–91.

97. Laurin J, Nekka F, Donati F, Varin F. Assuming peripheral elimination: its impact on the estimation of pharmacokinetic parameters of muscle relaxants. J Pharmacokinet Biopharm. 1999;27(5):491–512.

98. Kato M, Shiratori T, Yamamuro M, Haga S, Hoshi K, Matsukawa S, Jalal IM, Hashimoto Y. Comparison between in vivo and in vitro pharmacokinetics of succinylcholine in humans. J Anesth. 1999;13(4):189–92.

99. Roy JJ, Donati F, Boismenu D, Varin F. Concentration-effect relation of succinylcholine chloride during propofol anesthesia. Anesthesiology. 2002;97(5):1082–92.

100. Torda TA, Graham GG, Warwick NR, Donohue P. Pharmacokinetics and pharmacodynamics of suxamethonium. Anaesth Intensive Care. 1997;25(3):272–8.

101. Bragg P, Fisher DM, Shi J, Donati F, Meistelman C, Lau M, Sheiner LB. Comparison of twitch depression of the adductor pollicis and the respiratory muscles. Pharmacodynamic modeling without plasma concentrations. Anesthesiology. 1994;80(2):310–9.

102. Fisher DM, Wright PM. Are plasma concentration values necessary for pharmacodynamic modeling of muscle relaxants? Anesthesiology. 1997;86(3):567–75.

103. Verotta D, Sheiner LB. Semiparametric analysis of non-steady-state pharmacodynamic data. J Pharmacokinet Biopharm. 1991;19 (6):691–712.

104. Nigrovic V, Amann A. Competition between acetylcholine and a nondepolarizing muscle relaxant for binding to the postsynaptic receptors at the motor end plate: simulation of twitch strength and neuromuscular block. J Pharmacokinet Pharmacodyn. 2003;30 (1):23–51.

105. Bhatt SB, Kohl J, Amann A, Nigrovic V. The relationship between twitch depression and twitch fade during neuromuscular block produced by vecuronium: correlation with the release of acetylcholine. Theor Biol Med Model. 2007;4:24.

106. Breslin DS, Jiao K, Habib AS, Schultz J, Gan TJ. Pharmacodynamic interactions between cisatracurium and rocuronium. Anesth Analg. 2004;98(1):107–10.

107. Kim KS, Chun YS, Chon SU, Suh JK. Neuromuscular interaction between cisatracurium and mivacurium, atracurium, vecuronium or rocuronium administered in combination. Anaesthesia. 1998;53 (9):872–8.

108. Naguib M, Samarkandi AH, Ammar A, Elfaqih SR, Al-Zahrani S, Turkistani A. Comparative clinical pharmacology of rocuronium, cisatracurium, and their combination. Anesthesiology. 1998;89 (5):1116–24. Erratum in: Anesthesiology 1999; 90(4):1241.

109. Nigrovic V, Amann A. Simulation of interaction between two non-depolarizing muscle relaxants: generation of an additive or a supra-additive neuromuscular block. J Pharmacokinet Pharmacodyn. 2004;31(2):157–79.

110. Unadkat JD, Sheiner LB, Hennis PJ, Cronelly R, Miller RD, Sharma M. An integrated model for the interaction of muscle relaxants with their antagonists. J Appl Physiol. 1986;61:1593–8.

111. Van den Broek L, Proost JH, Wierda JMKH, Njoo MD, Hennis PJ. Neuromuscular and cardiovascular effects of neostigmine and methyl-atropine administered at different degrees of rocuronium-induced neuromuscular block. Eur J Anaesthesiol. 1994;11:481–7.

112. Van den Broek L, Proost JH, Wierda JMKH. Early and late reversibility of rocuronium bromide. Eur J Anaesthesiol. 1994;11 Suppl 9:128–32.

113. Verotta D, Kitts J, Rodriguez R, Caldwell J, Miller RD, Sheiner LB. Reversal of neuromuscular blockade in humans by neostigmine and edrophonium: a mathematical model. J Pharmacokinet Biopharm. 1991;19:713–29.

114. Bom A, Epemolu O, Hope F, Rutherford S, Thomson K. Selective relaxant binding agents for reversal of neuromuscular blockade. Curr Opin Pharmacol. 2007;7:298–302.

115. Epemolu O, Bom A, Hope F, Mason R, Cert HN. Reversal of neuromuscular blockade and simultaneous increase in plasma rocuronium concentration after the intravenous infusion of the novel reversal agent Org 25969. Anesthesiology. 2003;99:632–7.

116. Gijsenbergh F, Ramael S, Houwing N, van Iersel T. First human exposure of Org 25969, a novel agent to reverse the action of rocuronium bromide. Anesthesiology. 2005;103:695–703.

117. Sorgenfrei IF, Norrild K, Bo Larsen P, Stensballe J, Østergaard D, Prins ME, Viby-Mogensen J. Reversal of rocuronium-induced neuromuscular block by the selective relaxant binding agent sugammadex a dose-finding and safety study. Anesthesiology. 2006;104:667–74.

118. Sparr HJ, Vermeyen KM, Beaufort AM, Rietbergen H, Proost JH, Saldien V, Velik-Salchner C, Wierda JMKH. Early reversal of profound rocuronium-induced neuromuscular blockade by sugammadex in a randomized multicenter study: efficacy, safety, and pharmacokinetics. Anesthesiology. 2007;106 (5):935–43.

119. Eleveld DJ, Kuizenga K, Proost JH, Wierda JMKH. A temporary decrease in twitch response during reversal of rocuronium-induced muscle relaxation with a small dose of sugammadex. Anesth Analg. 2007;104(3):582–4.

120. Kennedy R, McKellow M, French R, Sleigh J. Sevoflurane end-tidal to effect-site equilibration in women determined by response to laryngeal mask airway insertion. Anesth Analg. 2013;117:786–91.

121. Bailey JM. The pharmacokinetics of volatile anesthetic agent elimination: a theoretical study. J Pharmacokinet Biopharm. 1989;17(1):109–23.

122. Enlund M, Kietzmann D, Bouillon T, Züchner K, Meineke I. Population pharmacokinetics of sevoflurane in conjunction with the AnaConDa: toward target-controlled infusion of volatiles into the breathing system. Acta Anaesthesiol Scand. 2008;52 (4):553–60.

123. Lerou JGC, Booij LHDJ. Model-based administration of inhalation anaesthesia. 1. Developing a system model. Br J Anaesth. 2001;86(1):12–28.

124. Lerou JGC, Booij LHDJ. Model-based administration of inhalation anaesthesia. 2. Exploring the system model. Br J Anaesth. 2001;86(1):29–37.

125. Lerou JGC, Booij LHDJ. Model-based administration of inhalation anaesthesia. 3. Validating the system model. Br J Anaesth. 2002;88(1):24–37.

126. Lerou JGC, Booij LHDJ. Model-based administration of inhalation anaesthesia. 4. Applying the system model. Br J Anaesth. 2002;88(2):175–83.

127. Lu CC, Tsai CS, Hu OY, Chen RM, Chen TL, Ho ST. Pharmacokinetics of isoflurane in human blood. Pharmacology. 2008;81(4):344–9.

128. Yasuda N, Lockhart SH, Eger EI, Weiskopf RB, Johnson BH, Freire BS, Fassoulaki A. Kinetics of desflurane, isoflurane, and halothane in humans. Anesthesiology. 1991;74:489–98.

129. Yasuda N, Lockhart SH, Eger EI, Weiskopf RB, Liu J, Laster M, Taheri S, Peterson NA. Comparison of kinetics of sevoflurane and isoflurane in humans. Anesth Analg. 1991;72(3):316–24.

130. Beline M, Wilke HJ, Harder S. Clinical pharmacokinetics of sevoflurane. Clin Pharmacokinet. 1999;36(1):13–26.

131. Marsh B, White M, Morton N, Kenny GN. Pharmacokinetic model driven infusion of propofol in children. Br J Anaesth. 1991;67:41–8.

132. Schnider TW, Minto CF, Gambus PL, Andresen C, Goodale DB, Shafer SL, Youngs EJ. The influence of method of administration and covariates on the pharmacokinetics of propofol in adult volunteers. Anesthesiology. 1998;88(5):1170–82.

133. Schnider TW, Minto CF, Shafer SL, Gambus PL, Andresen C, Goodale DB, Youngs EJ. The influence of age on propofol pharmacodynamics. Anesthesiology. 1999;90(6):1502–16.

134. Absalom AR, Mani V, De Smet T, Struys MMRF. Pharmacokinetic models for propofol—defining and illuminating the devil in the detail. Br J Anaesth. 2009;103(1):26–37.

135. Coppens M, Van Limmen JG, Schnider T, Wyler B, Bonte S, Dewaele F, Struys MM, Vereecke HE. Study of the time course of the clinical effect of propofol compared with the time course of the predicted effect-site concentration: performance of three pharmacokinetic-dynamic models. Br J Anaesth. 2010;104 (4):452–8.

136. Egan TD, Shafer SL. Target-controlled infusions for intravenous anesthetics: surfing USA not! Anesthesiology. 2003;99 (5):1039–41.

137. Struys M, Versichelen L, Thas O, Herregods L, Rolly G. Comparison of computer-controlled administration of propofol with two manually controlled infusion techniques. Anaesthesia. 1997;52(1):41–50.

138. Cortinez LI, Anderson BJ, Penna A, Olivares L, Munoz HR, Holford NHG, Struys MMRF, Sepulveda P. Influence of obesity on propofol pharmacokinetics: derivation of a pharmacokinetic model. Br J Anaesth. 2010;105(4):448–56.

139. La Colla L, Albertin A, La Colla G, Ceriani V, Lodi T, Porta A, Aldegheri G, Mangano A, Khairallah I, Fermo I. No adjustment vs. adjustment formula as input weight for propofol target-controlled infusion in morbidly obese patients. Eur J Anaesthesiol. 2009;26:362–9.

140. Choi BM, Lee HG, Byon HJ, Lee SH, Lee EK, Kim HS, Noh GJ. Population pharmacokinetic and pharmacodynamic model of propofol externally validated in children. J Pharmacokinet Pharmacodyn. 2015;42(2):163–77.

141. Coppens MJ, Eleveld DJ, Proost JH, Marks LA, Van Bocxlaer JF, Vereecke H, Absalom AR, Struys MMRF. An evaluation of using population pharmacokinetic models to estimate pharmacodynamic parameters for propofol and bispectral index in children. Anesthesiology. 2011;115(1):83–93.

142. Peeters MYM, Allegaert K, Blusse van Oud-Alblas HJ, Cella M, Tibboel D, Danhof M, Knibbe CAJ. Prediction of propofol clearance in children from an allometric model developed in rats, children and adults versus a 0.75 fixed-exponent allometric model. Clin Pharmacokinet. 2010;49(4):269–75.

143. Peeters MY, Prins SA, Knibbe CA, DeJongh J, van Schaik RH, van Dijk M, van der Heiden IP, Tibboel D, Danhof M. Propofol pharmacokinetics and pharmacodynamics for depth of sedation in nonventilated infants after major craniofacial surgery. Anesthesiology. 2006;104(3):466–74.

144. Diepstraten J, Chidambaran V, Sadhasivam S, Esslinger HR, Cox SL, Inge TH, Knibbe CAJ, Vinks AA. Propofol clearance in morbidly obese children and adolescents: influence of age and body size. Clin Pharmacokinet. 2012;51(8):543–51.

145. Somma J, Donner A, Zomorodi K, Sladen R, Ramsay J, Geller E, Shafer SL. Population pharmacodynamics of midazolam administered by target controlled infusion in SICU patients after CABG surgery. Anesthesiology. 1998;89(6):1430–43.

146. Peeters MY, Prins SA, Knibbe CA, Dejongh J, Mathôt RA, Warris C, van Schaik RH, Tibboel D, Danhof M. Pharmacokinetics and pharmacodynamics of midazolam and metabolites in nonventilated infants after craniofacial surgery. Anesthesiology. 2006;105(6):1135–46.

147. van Rongen A, Vaughns JD, Moorthy G, Barrett JS, Knibbe CA, van den Anker JN. Population pharmacokinetics of midazolam and its metabolites in overweight and obese adolescents. Br J Clin Pharmacol. 2015. doi:10.1111/bcp.12693. Epub ahead of print.

148. Potts AL, Anderson BJ, Warman GR, Lerman J, Diaz SM, Vilo S. Dexmedetomidine pharmacokinetics in pediatric intensive care—a pooled analysis. Pediatr Anesth. 2009;19(11):1119–29.

149. Hannivoort LN, Eleveld DJ, Proost JH, Reyntjens KMEM, Absalom AR, Vereecke HEM, Struys MMRF. Development of an optimized pharmacokinetic model of dexmedetomidine using target controlled infusion in healthy volunteers. Anesthesiology. 2015;123:357–67.

150. Harris RS, Lazar O, Johansen JW, Sebel PS. Interaction of propofol and sevoflurane on loss of consciousness and movement to skin incision during general anesthesia. Anesthesiology. 2006;104(6):1170–5.

151. Schumacher PM, Dossche J, Mortier EP, Luginbuehl M, Bouillon TW, Struys MM. Response surface modeling of the interaction between propofol and sevoflurane. Anesthesiology. 2009;111 (4):790–804.

152. Diz JC, Del Rio R, Lamas A, Mendoza M, Duran M, Ferreira LM. Analysis of pharmacodynamic interaction of sevoflurane and propofol on Bispectral Index during general anaesthesia using a response surface model. Br J Anaesth. 2009;104(6):733–9.

153. Lichtenbelt BJ, Olofsen E, Dahan A, van Kleef JW, Struys MM, Vuyk J. Propofol reduces the distribution and clearance of midazolam. Anesth Analg. 2010;110(6):1597–606.

154. Vuyk J, Hennis PJ, Burm AG, de Voogt JW, Spierdijk J. Comparison of midazolam and propofol in combination with alfentanil for total intravenous anesthesia. Anesth Analg. 1990;71 (6):645–50.

155. Vuyk J, Lichtenbelt BJ, Olofsen E, van Kleef JW, Dahan A. Mixed-effects modeling of the influence of midazolam on propofol pharmacokinetics. Anesth Analg. 2009;108(5):1522–30.

156. Teh J, Short TG, Wong J, Tan P. Pharmacokinetic interactions between midazolam and propofol: an infusion study. Br J Anaesth. 1994;72(1):62–5.

157. McClune S, McKay AC, Wright PM, Patterson CC, Clarke RS. Synergistic interaction between midazolam and propofol. Br J Anaesth. 1992;69(3):240–5.

158. Short TG, Chui PT. Propofol and midazolam act synergistically in combination. Br J Anaesth. 1991;67(5):539–45.

159. Short TG, Plummer JL, Chui PT. Hypnotic and anaesthetic interactions between midazolam, propofol and alfentanil. Br J Anaesth. 1992;69(2):162–7.

160. Vinik HR, Bradley Jr EL, Kissin I. Triple anesthetic combination: propofol-midazolam-alfentanil. Anesth Analg. 1994;78(2):354–8.

161. Lemmens HJM. Pharmacokinetic-pharmacodynamic relationships for opioids in balanced anaesthesia. Clin Pharmacokinet. 1995;29(4):231–42.

162. Scholz J, Steinfath M, Schulz M. Clinical pharmacokinetics of alfentanil, fentanyl and sufentanil: an update. Clin Pharmacokinet. 1996;31(4):275–92.

163. Egan TD, Huizinga B, Gupta SK, Jaarsma RL, Sperry RJ, Yee JB, Muir KT. Remifentanil pharmacokinetics in obese versus lean patients. Anesthesiology. 1998;89(3):562–73.

164. Egan TD, Lemmens HJ, Fiset P, Hermann DJ, Muir KT, Stanski DR, Shafer SL. The pharmacokinetics of the new short-acting opioid remifentanil (GI87084B) in healthy adult male volunteers. Anesthesiology. 1993;79(5):881–92.

165. Egan TD, Minto CF, Hermann DJ, Barr J, Muir KT, Shafer SL. Remifentanil versus alfentanil: comparative pharmacokinetics and pharmacodynamics in healthy adult male volunteers. Anesthesiology. 1996;84(4):821–33. Erratum in: Anesthesiology 1996;85(3):695.

166. Minto CF, Schnider TW, Egan TD, Youngs E, Lemmens HJ, Gambus PL, Billard V, Hoke JF, Moore KH, Hermann DJ, Muir KT, Mandema JW, Shafer SL. Influence of age and gender on the pharmacokinetics and pharmacodynamics of remifentanil. I Model development. Anesthesiology. 1997;86:10–23.

167. Minto CF, Schnider TW, Shafer SL. Pharmacokinetics and pharmacodynamics of remifentanil. II Model application. Anesthesiology. 1997;86:24–33.

168. Drover DR, Lemmens HJ. Population pharmacodynamics and pharmacokinetics of remifentanil as a supplement to nitrous oxide anesthesia for elective abdominal surgery. Anesthesiology. 1998;89(4):869–77.

169. La Colla L, Albertin A, La Colla G, Porta A, Aldegheri G, Di Candia D, Gigli F. Predictive performance of the 'Minto' remifentanil pharmacokinetic parameter set in morbidly obese patients ensuing from a new method for calculating lean body mass. Clin Pharmacokinet. 2010;49(2):131–9.

170. Mertens MJ, Engbers FH, Burm AG, Vuyk J. Predictive performance of computer-controlled infusion of remifentanil during propofol/remifentanil anaesthesia. Br J Anaesth. 2003;90(2):132–41.

171. McEwan AI, Smith C, Dyar O, Goodman D, Smith LR, Glass PS. Isoflurane minimum alveolar concentration reduction by fentanyl. Anesthesiology. 1993;78(5):864–9.

172. Westmoreland CL, Sebel PS, Gropper A. Fentanyl or alfentanil decreases the minimum alveolar anesthetic concentration of isoflurane in surgical patients. Anesth Analg. 1994;78:23–8.

173. Brunner MD, Braithwaite P, Jhaveri R, McEwan AI, Goodman DK, Smith LR, Glass PSA. MAC reduction of isoflurane by sufentanil. Br J Anaesth. 1994;72:42–6.

174. Lang E, Kapila A, Shlugman D, Hoke JF, Sebel PS, Glass PS. Reduction of isoflurane minimal alveolar concentration by remifentanil. Anesthesiology. 1996;85(4):721–8.

175. Katoh T, Kobayashi S, Suzuki A, Iwamoto T, Bito H, Ikeda K. The effect of fentanyl on sevoflurane requirements for somatic and sympathetic responses to surgical incision. Anesthesiology. 1999;90:398–405.

176. Bouillon T, Bruhn J, Radulescu L, Andresen C, Cohane C, Shafer SL. A model of the ventilatory depressant potency of remifentanil in the non-steady state. Anesthesiology. 2003;99(4):779–87.

177. Bouillon T, Garstka G, Stafforst D, Shafer S, Schwilden H, Hoeft A. Piritramide and alfentanil display similar respiratory depressant potency. Acta Anaesthesiol Scand. 2003;47(10):1231–41.

178. Gambus PL, Gregg KM, Shafer SL. Validation of the alfentanil canonical univariate parameter as a measure of opioid effect on the electroencephalogram. Anesthesiology. 1995;83:747–56.

179. Struys MMRF, Absalom AR, Shafer SL. Intravenous drug delivery systems. In: Miller RD, Cohen NH, Eriksson LI, Fleisher LA, Wiener-Kronisch JP, Young WL, editors. Miller's anesthesia. 8th ed. St. Louis: Saunders; 2014. p. 929.

180. Glass PS, Gan TJ, Howell S. A review of the pharmacokinetics and pharmacodynamics of remifentanil. Anesth Analg. 1999;89 Suppl 4:S7–14.

181. Johnson KB, Syroid ND, Gupta DK, Manyam SC, Pace NL, LaPierre CD, Egan TD, White JL, Tyler D, Westenskow DR. An evaluation of remifentanil-sevoflurane response surface models in patients emerging from anesthesia: model improvement using

effect-site sevoflurane concentrations. Anesth Analg. 2010;111(2):387–94.

182. Heyse B, Proost JH, Hannivoort LN, Eleveld DJ, Luginbühl M, Struys MMRF, Vereecke HEM. A response surface model approach for continuous measures of hypnotic and analgesic effect during sevoflurane-remifentanil interaction: quantifying the pharmacodynamic shift evoked by stimulation. Anesthesiology. 2014;120(6):1390–9.

183. Kazama T, Ikeda K, Morita K. The pharmacodynamic interaction between propofol and fentanyl with respect to the suppression of somatic or hemodynamic responses to skin incision, peritoneum incision, and abdominal wall retraction. Anesthesiology. 1998;89(4):894–906.

184. Smith C, McEwan AI, Jhaveri R, Wilkinson M, Goodman D, Smith LR, Canada AT, Glass PS. The interaction of fentanyl on the Cp50 of propofol for loss of consciousness and skin incision. Anesthesiology. 1994;81(4):820–8.

185. Schwilden H, Fechner J, Albrecht S, Hering W, Ihmsen H, Schuttler J. Testing and modelling the interaction of alfentanil and propofol on the EEG. Eur J Anaesthesiol. 2003;20(5):363–72.

186. Vuyk J, Lim T, Engbers FH, Burm AG, Vletter AA, Bovill JG. The pharmacodynamic interaction of propofol and alfentanil during lower abdominal surgery in women. Anesthesiology. 1995;83(1):8–22.

187. Bruhn J, Bouillon TW, Radulescu L, Hoeft A, Bertaccini E, Shafer SL. Correlation of approximate entropy, bispectral index, and spectral edge frequency 95 (SEF95) with clinical signs of "anesthetic depth" during coadministration of propofol and remifentanil. Anesthesiology. 2003;98(3):621–7.

188. Ropcke H, Konen-Bergmann M, Cuhls M, Bouillon T, Hoeft A. Propofol and remifentanil pharmacodynamic interaction during orthopedic surgical procedures as measured by effects on bispectral index. J Clin Anesth. 2001;13(3):198–207.

189. Vanluchene AL, Vereecke H, Thas O, Mortier EP, Shafer SL, Struys MM. Spectral entropy as an electroencephalographic measure of anesthetic drug effect: a comparison with bispectral index and processed midlatency auditory evoked response. Anesthesiology. 2004;101(1):34–42.

190. Bouillon T, Schmidt C, Garstka G, Heimbach D, Stafforst D, Schwilden H, Hoeft A. Pharmacokinetic-pharmacodynamic modeling of the respiratory depressant effect of alfentanil. Anesthesiology. 1999;91(1):144–55.

191. LaPierre CD, Johnson KB, Randall BR, Egan TD. A simulation study of common propofol and propofol-opioid dosing regimens for upper endoscopy: implications on the time course of recovery. Anesthesiology. 2012;117(2):252–62.

192. LaPierre CD, Johnson KB, Randall BR, White JL, Egan TD. An exploration of remifentanil-propofol combinations that lead to a loss of response to esophageal instrumentation, a loss of responsiveness, and/or onset of intolerable ventilatory depression. Anesth Analg. 2011;113(3):490–9.

193. Nieuwenhuijs DJ, Olofsen E, Romberg RR, Sarton E, Ward D, Engbers F, Vuyk J, Mooren R, Teppema LJ, Dahan A. Response surface modeling of remifentanil-propofol interaction on cardio-respiratory control and bispectral index. Anesthesiology. 2003;98(2):312–22.

194. Johnson KB, Syroid ND, Gupta DK, Manyam SC, Egan TD, Huntington J, White JL, Tyler D, Westenskow DR. An evaluation of remifentanil propofol response surfaces for loss of responsiveness, loss of response to surrogates of painful stimuli and laryngoscopy in patients undergoing elective surgery. Anesth Analg. 2008;106(2):471–9.

195. Kern SE, Xie G, White JL, Egan TD. Opioid-hypnotic synergy: a response surface analysis of propofol-remifentanil pharmacodynamic interaction in volunteers. Anesthesiology. 2004;100(6):1373–81.

196. Mertens MJ, Olofsen E, Engbers FH, Burm AG, Bovill JG, Vuyk J. Propofol reduces perioperative remifentanil requirements in a synergistic manner: response surface modeling of perioperative remifentanil-propofol interactions. Anesthesiology. 2003;99 (2):347–59.
197. Hannivoort LN, Vereecke HEM, Proost JH, Heyse BEK, Eleveld DJ, Bouillon TW, et al. Probability to tolerate laryngoscopy and noxious stimulation response index as general indicators of the anaesthetic potency of sevoflurane, propofol, and remifentanil. Br J Anaesth. 2016;116(5):624–31.
198. Zanderigo E, Sartori V, Sveticic G, Bouillon T, Schumacher P, Morari M, Curatolo M. The well-being model: a new drug interaction model for positive and negative effects. Anesthesiology. 2006;104(4):742–53.

Principles of Target-Controlled Infusions

Steven L. Shafer

Pharmacokinetics

Volume and clearance are the basic physiological concepts underlying target-controlled infusions (TCI) of intravenous anesthetic drugs. Following intravenous injection, drug is distributed within the body's volume of distribution, as shown in Fig. 8.1. The volume of distribution is the volume of the blood or plasma, along with whatever other tissues contribute to the initial dilution of the drug (e.g., the lungs). Volume usually has units of liters. Clearance describes the physiological process by which drug is removed from the blood, plasma, or tissue. The arrows in Fig. 8.2 show the flow of blood in and out of the clearing organ, typically the liver for most anesthetic drugs. The clearance is the rate of flow times the fraction removed by the liver. If the liver removes all of the drug, as is the case for propofol, then clearance equals liver blood flow. The liver removes about half of the fentanyl that flows in. The clearance of fentanyl is thus about half of liver blood flow. Clearance has units of flow, typically liters per hour or milliliters per minute.

Figure 8.3 combines the basic principles of Figs. 8.1 and 8.2. This is the simple "one-compartment model." Drug is administered into the "central" (and only) compartment. This is the volume of distribution and is typically designated in equations as V. Drug is removed from the central compartment by the process of clearance. Clearance is typically designated in equations as Cl. When a bolus of drug is injected into a system represented by a one-compartment model, as shown in Fig. 8.3, the drug concentration decreases over time in a log-linear manner.

Most intravenous drugs used in anesthesia practice are very soluble in fat. This is particularly the case with

propofol. As a result, the simple one-compartment model shown in Fig. 8.3 can't describe the drug concentrations observed after bolus drug delivery. To accommodate the movement of drug into body fat requires the addition of a second compartment, as shown in Fig. 8.4. In the two-compartment model, the peripheral compartment is substantially larger than the central compartment, because most anesthetic drugs preferentially partition into body tissues (e.g., fat, muscle) rather than remain in the central compartment (i.e., the blood or plasma).

The two-compartment model shown in Fig. 8.4 is not satisfactory to describe the behavior of intravenous anesthetic drugs [1]. Figure 8.5 shows the time course of drug concentration following intravenous injection of a typical intravenous anesthetic drug. The simulation is based on fentanyl pharmacokinetics, but the choice of drug and drug dose doesn't matter. The general behavior which is shown in Fig. 8.5 is shared among the intravenous opioids, hypnotics, and muscle relaxants used in anesthesia. In Fig. 8.5 the Y axis has the units "percent of initial concentration." That is why it starts at 100 (%).

The first observation about Fig. 8.5 is that the curve is not straight, even though it is plotted on a log Y axis. That means that the drug cannot be described by a one-compartment model. The second observation is that there are three distinct curve segments. In the first segment, shown in dark red, the drug concentration decreases almost an order of magnitude over a few minutes. In the second segment, shown in blue, the rate of decrease in concentration is initially rapid. However, over an hour or two the rate of decline gradually slows. The third segment, in green, is log-linear.

Figure 8.6 shows the usual interpretation of the three curve segments shown in Fig. 8.5. We can envision the body as being composed of three tanks. There is a central tank, which is where we inject the bolus. There are two peripheral tanks, representing peripheral volumes of distribution. The bigger peripheral tank might represent body fat, while the smaller peripheral tank might represent muscle and

S.L. Shafer, MD(✉)
Department of Anesthesiology, Perioperative and Pain Medicine, Stanford University School of Medicine, 300 Pasteur Drive, MC-5640, Stanford, CA 94305-5640, USA
e-mail: steven.shafer@stanford.edu

© Springer International Publishing AG 2017
A.R. Absalom, K.P. Mason (eds.), *Total Intravenous Anesthesia and Target Controlled Infusions*,
DOI 10.1007/978-3-319-47609-4_8

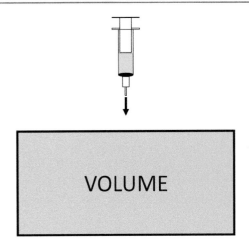

Fig. 8.1 The volume of distribution accounts for the dilution of drug when it is first injected into the body

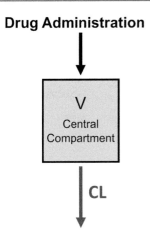

Fig. 8.3 The one-compartment model integrates the concepts of volume and clearance shown in Figs. 8.1 and 8.2

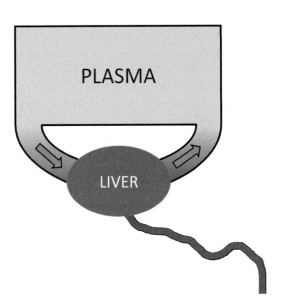

Fig. 8.2 Clearance is the flow of blood or plasma from which the drug is completely removed. If the drug is cleared by the liver, then clearance is liver blood flow times the fraction extracted by the liver

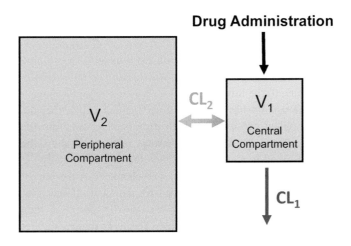

Fig. 8.4 The two-compartment model adds a second compartment to account for preferential uptake by peripheral tissues

rapidly equilibrating tissues. The central tank is connected to two peripheral tanks by pipes at the base. There is also a pipe that drains the central tank. Initially, all of the drug appears in the central tank. The height of fluid in the tank corresponds to drug concentration in each tank.

Initially, during the red segment phase, there are three places for the drug to go. Drug can flow to the tanks on either side of the central tank or can flow out of the system through the pipe draining the central tank. Because there are three pipes that initially drain the tank, the drug concentration falls quickly.

With the transition from the red segment to the blue segment, the drug concentration in the central tank falls below the drug concentration in the tank to the right.

Because drug flows down its concentration gradient, when the concentration in the central tank is less than that in the small peripheral tank, drug flow reverses. Drug now returns to the central tank from the peripheral tank. This acts as a brake on how quickly drug concentration can fall in the central tank. It is this reversal of flow that accounts for the gradual slowing of the rate of descent in the blue segment. By the end of the blue segment, the drug concentration in the central tank has fallen below the drug concentration in both peripheral tanks. Drug then returns to the central tank from both peripheral tanks, which greatly slows the rate of drug decrease.

The final, log-linear green segment is characterized as the "terminal slope" of the concentration curve. During this phase, there is only one way for drug to leave the central tank: the drainage pipe. However, as soon as drug leaves the central tank, it is almost (but not quite) replaced by drug that flows in from the peripheral tanks. The result is that the little

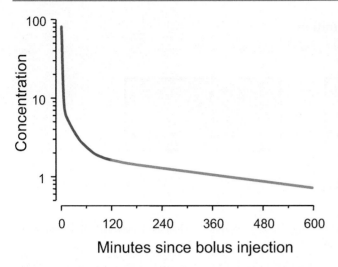

Fig. 8.5 For most intravenous anesthetic drugs, there are three distinct phases following bolus injection. As shown by the *dark red segment*, initially the concentrations fall by an order of magnitude over a few minutes. In the second phase, shown in *blue*, the rate at which the concentrations fall diminishes over an hour or so. In the final phase, shown in *green*, the concentrations decrease in a log-linear manner

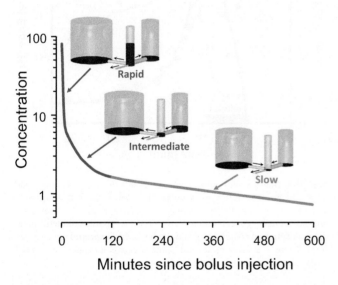

Fig. 8.6 The behavior shown in Fig. 8.5 is explained by a hydraulic model. In this model, there are three tanks, connected by pipes at the base. The drug concentration in each tank is represented by the height of the liquid in the tank. Initially all of the drug is placed in the central tank. Over time, drug flows into the peripheral tanks through the pipes at the base and then returns to the central tank once the concentration is low enough to reverse net drug flow. Drug leaves the system through the small pipe draining the center tank

drain pipe on the central tank is draining all three tanks, not just the central tank. Because it is draining all three tanks, they drain slowly. The log-linear behavior appears because the relative fraction of drug in each tank remains constant once this final equilibration has been reached. It is not a one-compartment model, but because the fraction in each tank remains constant, it behaves like a one-compartment model.

Figure 8.7 shows the three-compartment model corresponding to the three-tank model in Fig. 8.6. Drug is administered into V_1, the central compartment. As mentioned previously, the central compartment is thought of as consisting of the blood (or plasma) and tissues (e.g., the lungs) that equilibrate almost instantly with the blood. Drug equilibrates with two peripheral compartments. V_3, the larger peripheral compartment, is thought to be the fat compartment. V_2, the smaller peripheral compartment, is thought to represent muscle and rapidly equilibrating tissues. CL_1 is the clearance from the central compartment, which often represents hepatic clearance (although remifentanil is cleared by nonspecific plasma and tissue esterases). CL_2 is the clearance between the central compartment and compartment 2. CL_3 is the clearance between the central compartment and compartment 3.

For the purposes of explaining the principles of TCI, I will represent the three-compartment model as being "true." However, the model is "true" only to the extent that the three-compartment model accurately predicts drug concentration following any arbitrary dose. Compartment models are merely mathematical relationships expressed as volumes and clearances. The only component of these models that matches real physiology is central clearance, CL_L. All three volumes, and both peripheral clearances, are just empirically derived terms that describe the pharmacokinetics. They only vaguely relate to true anatomic structures and physiological processes.

Figure 8.8 shows the mathematics that is embodied in the three-compartment model. The blood (or plasma) concentration over time following bolus injection (black dots) is described by the sum of three exponential terms, $C(t) = Ae^{-\alpha t} + Be^{-\beta t} + Ce^{-\gamma t}$. The three individual exponential components appear as color-matched lines. The terms A, B, C, α, β, and γ in the triexponential equation can be mathematically converted into V_1, V_2, V_3, CL_1, CL_2, and CL_3 in the compartmental representation through a complex calculation.

Pharmacodynamics

Anesthetic drugs work in tissues, not in the blood or plasma. Understanding the behavior of anesthetic drugs in the blood (or plasma) is necessary to understanding target-controlled drug delivery, but it is not enough. We also need to understand the process by which the blood (or plasma) concentration equilibrates with the concentration of drug at the site of drug effect. Equilibration models were originally proposed by Sheiner [2], and independently by Hull [3], to describe the onset of neuromuscular relaxation following administration of D-tubocurarine and pancuronium, respectively. Equilibration models have been created for nearly all intravenous anesthetic drugs, including opioids and propofol. Because nearly all of these have measured plasma concentration,

Drug Administration

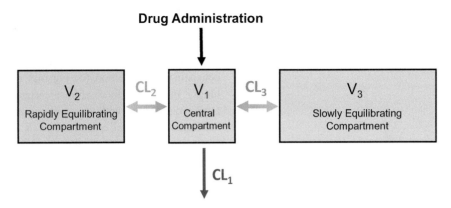

Fig. 8.7 This is the three-compartment model that is both necessary and sufficient, to describe the pharmacokinetics of most intravenous anesthetic drugs. It is a compartmental representation of the hydraulic model in Fig. 8.6

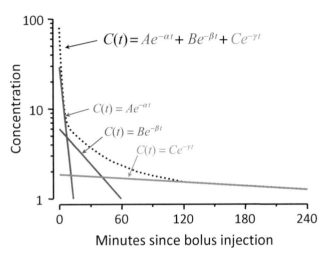

$$C(t) = Ae^{-\alpha t} + Be^{-\beta t} + Ce^{-\gamma t}$$

$$C(t) = Ae^{-\alpha t}$$

$$C(t) = Be^{-\beta t}$$

$$C(t) = Ce^{-\gamma t}$$

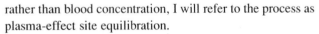

Minutes since bolus injection

Fig. 8.8 The three-compartment model shown in Fig. 8.7 captures the same mathematical relationship as the sum of exponentials shown here following bolus injection. The overall shape of the *curve* is the sum of three separate mono-exponential equations, which are color-matched here. The models in Figs. 8.7 and 8.8 can be interconverted mathematically

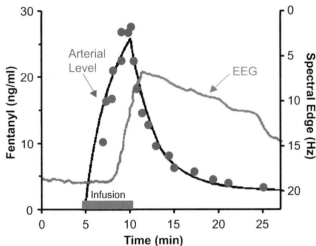

Fig. 8.9 Stanski and colleagues used infusions of fentanyl and alfentanil to characterize the equilibration delay between the plasma and the brain. This figure, adapted from Scott et al. [4], shows the arterial fentanyl concentration (*red dots*), the pharmacokinetic fit to the concentration (*black line*), and the 95 % EEG spectral edge (*green line*). There is a delay of several minutes between changes in arterial fentanyl concentration and the brain response

rather than blood concentration, I will refer to the process as plasma-effect site equilibration.

Figure 8.9 shows the rise and fall in arterial drug concentration during a brief infusion of fentanyl [4]. The blue bar shows the duration of the fentanyl infusion. During the infusion, the arterial fentanyl concentrations (red dots) rise rapidly, reaching a peak by the end of the infusion. Once the infusion is turned off, the plasma fentanyl concentrations fall very quickly, consistent with the red segment of Figs. 8.5 and 8.6. The black line is the fit of a three-compartment pharmacokinetic model to the arterial fentanyl concentrations. The green line is fentanyl drug effect on the brain, as determined using 95 % EEG spectral edge frequency (shown on the Y axis to the right of the data). The spectral edge is about 18 Hz at baseline. During the

fentanyl infusion there is initially no change in spectral edge, reflecting the delay caused by plasma-effect site equilibration. About 2–3 min after starting the fentanyl infusion, the spectral edge starts to respond. It then rises quickly, as drug continues to cross from the plasma into the brain. Because of this equilibration delay, the spectral edge continues to rise for 1–2 min after turning off the infusion, simply because it takes a few minutes for the fentanyl concentration in the plasma to drop below the fentanyl concentration in the brain. The brain recovers much more slowly than the plasma, again reflecting the delay in plasma-brain equilibration.

Figure 8.10 shows the same experiment repeated for alfentanil [4]. The rise and fall in arterial alfentanil concentrations in Fig. 8.6 is not very different from the rise and fall in fentanyl concentrations in Fig. 8.5. However, the brain response is very different. The EEG starts to respond within a minute to the rising alfentanil concentration. After the alfentanil infusion is turned off, the EEG begins to fall almost immediately, again reflecting the rapid plasma-brain equilibration of alfentanil. The plasma-brain equilibration delay for remifentanil is very similar to that of alfentanil, shown in Fig. 8.6.

The plasma-brain brain equilibration delay shown in Figs. 8.9 and 8.10 can be incorporated into a pharmacokinetic model by adding an "effect site" to the model, as shown in Fig. 8.11. The effect site is connected to the plasma by a pipe, shown as the red arrow from the plasma to the effect site. In the model, the effect site is assumed to have trivial (nearly 0) volume, and so very little drug actually flows to the effect site. Drug is removed from the effect site by a clearance process that is defined by a single rate constant: k_{e0}. Because the effect site is arbitrarily small, the rate of plasma-effect site equilibration is completely determined by the value of k_{e0}. As will be demonstrated below, it is important to know the value of k_{e0} for drugs given by TCI, because this information allows you to titrate the drug concentration in the brain, where the drugs actually work, rather than the concentration in the plasma.

How TCI Pumps Work

TCI devices consist of three components, a computer, an infusion pump, and the interface between them. The computer is responsible for interacting with the user. Based on this interaction, the computer selects the pharmacokinetic model and calculates the infusion rate required to rapidly achieve and maintain desired drug concentration. The infusion pump gives drugs at a constant rate, based on instructions from the computer. While this may seem like a simple task, the pump has many sensors to measure how much drug was given every moment and detect any problems (e.g., air-in-line, occluded tubing). These must be communicated quickly to the computer. The interface provides a two-way link between the computer and the pump. At regular intervals (e.g., every 10 s), the communication link transmits a status update from the pump to the computer. The computer determines the infusion rate necessary to rapidly achieve and maintain the desired concentration and transmits the necessary instructions to the pump. The computer also updates the pharmacokinetic model (e.g.,

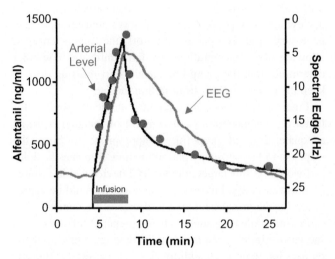

Fig. 8.10 As shown here, the brain responds much more quickly to changes in plasma alfentanil concentration than to changes in plasma fentanyl concentration (Fig. 8.9). This figure is also adapted from Scott et al. [4]

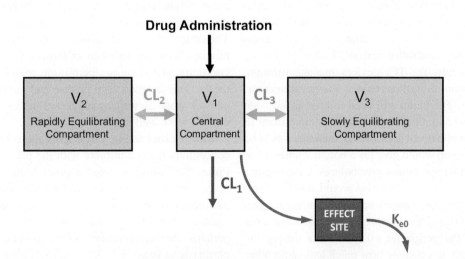

Fig. 8.11 For intravenous anesthetics, it is possible to fully account for the equilibration delay between the plasma and the site of drug effect by adding an effect site to the model. The equilibration delay requires only one additional parameter, k_{e0}

Fig. 8.11) and the real-time display of the patient status to the clinician. These three components are integrated into a single device in commercial TCI systems.

When the pharmacokinetics of drugs are described by a one-compartment model, as shown in Fig. 8.3, then it is easy to rapidly achieve and maintain a steady drug concentration. Let's say you want a drug concentration of 2 units/ml. You first give a bolus of drug that is $2 \times V$, the volume of distribution. That will immediately achieve the desired concentration of 2 units/ml. You then start an infusion, set to $2 \times$ clearance. That will maintain a concentration of 2 units/ml. If anesthetic drugs were described by one-compartment models, there would be very little for a TCI computer to calculate. Unfortunately, an initial bolus followed by a constant-rate infusion is unable to rapidly achieve and maintain a stable drug concentration for any of the intravenous anesthetics, because none of them are described by one-compartment models.

In 1968 Kruger-Thiemer [5] published the equations needed to rapidly achieve and maintain a steady-state concentration for drugs described by a two-compartment model. This was extended to an arbitrary number of compartments in 1981 by Schwilden [6]. As noted by both authors, the infusion rates must decrease exponentially to maintain a steady concentration, reflecting the accumulation of drug in peripheral compartments.

To understand TCI it is not necessary to understand exponentially decreasing infusion rates. While these are required to maintain steady concentrations, that is not the goal during anesthesia. The goal is to rapidly achieve, maintain, and *titrate* the anesthetic drug effect. If everything is stable, then a steady concentration is fine. However, in anesthesia very little is "stable." Surgical stimulation varies throughout the case. The patient's tolerance for hemodynamic depression may change over the course of anesthesia. Coadministration of other drugs may alter anesthetic requirements. The goal is not to maintain a single steady concentration. The goal is to titrate the intravenous anesthetic in a highly controlled manner [7, 8].

To understand how the TCI devices manage titration, let's say that we want to start our case at a target concentration of 2 units/ml. The pump will need to give an infusion that raises the concentration in the central compartment to 2 units/ml. If the pump could give a bolus, then this would be very simple: the pump would give (as a bolus) 2 units/ml $\times$ V_1. Since infusion pumps cannot give boluses, the computer has to compute the infusion rate that would quickly (e.g., within 10 s) produce the desired drug concentration. This will be a bit more than 2 units/ml $\times V_1$, because some drug will "leak" into the peripheral compartments during the infusion. It's simple to calculate how much leaks into other compartments, or is removed by systemic (e.g., hepatic) clearance, over the 10 s. The pump gives this extra amount,

so that 10 s into the case the concentration in the central compartment is *exactly* 2 units/ml.

Over the next 10 s, the pump computes how much drug will leave the central compartment. This is a simple calculation, requiring nothing more than multiplication [9, 10]. The pump gives this amount of drug. As before, it has to give a little extra to precisely account for the additional "leak" from the central to peripheral compartments over 10 s and for systemic clearance from the central compartment.

If higher concentrations are necessary, the user increases the target concentration. The computer repeats the above steps, raising the concentration in the central compartment to the desired target as quickly as possible—typically about 10 s. However, it is basically the same calculation: how much drug must be infused into the central compartment in 10 s to achieve the new concentration? If lower concentrations are necessary, the computer turns off the pump entirely, allowing the concentrations to fall, until the computer determines that the pump must again start infusing drug to keep the concentrations from falling too far.

Figure 8.12 shows what is pharmacologically possible for fentanyl. A concentration of 6 ng/ml of fentanyl, with an adequate dose of propofol, is appropriate to blunt the response to laryngoscopy and intubation. The anesthesiologist would set this target, and the TCI device would achieve it almost instantly. Following intubation, it would be appropriate for the anesthesiologist to decrease the fentanyl concentration while the patient is being prepared for surgery, as shown in Fig. 8.12. In this hypothetical example, after the preparation there is an additional delay waiting for the surgeon. The anesthesiologist chooses an additional decrease in fentanyl concentration, since the patient is unstimulated. In a few minutes the surgeon arrives, and the anesthesiologist raises the target fentanyl concentration in anticipation of incision. The concentration is then gradually lowered, until a concentration is found at which the patient has exactly the right fentanyl concentration for stable maintenance. The concentrations are again raised for skin closure. A few minutes later, the infusion is turned off, and the fentanyl concentrations decrease, permitting awakening from anesthesia. This appears very precise and elegant. However, it doesn't work as well as suggested in Fig. 8.12. In fact, it doesn't work well at all.

Turning back to Fig. 8.9, it takes about 3 min for the brain concentration to equilibrate with the plasma concentration. Figure 8.12 shows us what is possible in the plasma, but it ignores plasma-effect site equilibration. Since intubation is performed in the first few minutes, and it takes 3 min for the brain to respond to the increase in fentanyl concentration, perhaps the equilibration delay between the blood and plasma is an issue.

It is. We can calculate the concentration of fentanyl in the effect site, as shown by the dashed red line in Fig. 8.13.

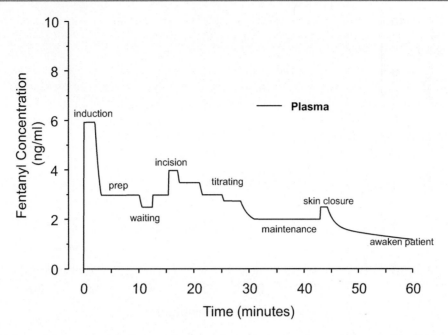

Fig. 8.12 Using TCI it is possible to very precisely titrate the plasma fentanyl concentration, as demonstrated in this figure

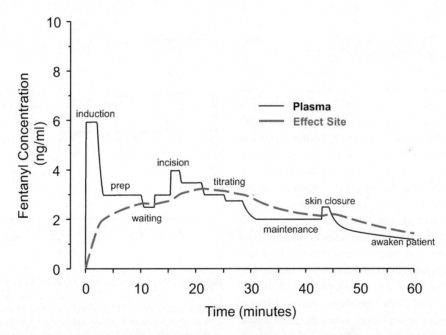

Fig. 8.13 The *dashed red line* shows the effect site fentanyl concentration expected with the titration described in Fig. 8.12. Although it is possible to very precisely titrate the plasma concentration, this is of little value because the plasma is not the site of fentanyl drug effect. Indeed, the slurred onset and offset of fentanyl implied by the *red dashed line* suggest that titrating the plasma, rather than the site of drug effect, could result in inadequate fentanyl concentrations in the effect site at critical moments of the case

Because of the plasma-brain equilibration delay, at the time of intubation the fentanyl concentration at the site of drug effect is inadequate to blunt the noxious stimulation. The precise titration described for Fig. 8.12 is possible for the plasma, but that is irrelevant. What matters is the brain concentration. As shown in Fig. 8.12, the concentrations of fentanyl in the effect site are very poorly titrated. Effect site fentanyl concentrations rise gradually, and fall gradually, with little evidence of titration.

Shafer and Gregg developed an algorithm to control the drug concentration in the effect site (e.g., the brain) rather than the plasma [11]. There is no way around the equilibration delay, but understanding that delay permits control of effect site concentration and provides the anesthesiologist

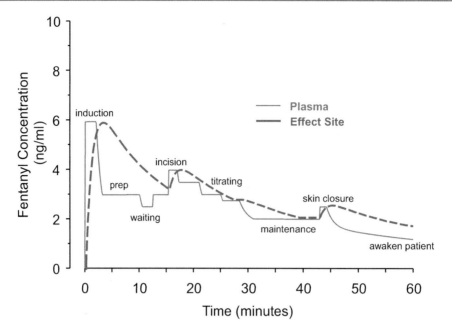

Fig. 8.14 TCI devices can target the site of drug effect, rather than the plasma, as shown by the *dashed red line*. In the case of fentanyl, the equilibration delay results in titration that is far less precise than implied (inappropriately) by the ability to rapidly titrate the plasma concentration

with information on the equilibration delay during the onset and offset of drug effect. The dashed red line in Fig. 8.14 shows the fentanyl concentration in the effect site, when the pump targets effect site concentration rather than plasma concentration. As shown in Fig. 8.14, intubation must be delayed for a few minutes to account for plasma-brain equilibration delay (matching what you already know). Additionally, the precise decreases in plasma fentanyl concentration possible in the plasma aren't possible in the effect site. Figure 8.14 illustrates how the fentanyl concentration can be titrated in the effect site as precise as possible, given the biology of plasma-effect site equilibration.

Figure 8.15 shows the same anesthetic as described above for fentanyl, but using remifentanil rather than fentanyl. The remifentanil concentrations must be about 50 % higher than the fentanyl concentrations, because remifentanil is less potent than fentanyl. The black line shows precise titration of plasma remifentanil concentration. When the anesthesiologist lowers the concentrations of remifentanil, they decrease a little faster than they did for fentanyl (Fig. 8.12), reflecting the rapid esterase metabolism of remifentanil. As mentioned above, remifentanil rapidly equilibrates with the brain. This rapid plasma-effect site equilibration results in the effect site levels coming reasonably close to the plasma levels during titration (dashed red line).

Figure 8.16 shows the effect site remifentanil concentration when the anesthesiologist chooses to titrate the concentration of remifentanil in the effect site (dashed red line). The target concentrations are quickly achieved in the effect site and can be titrated precisely, because the

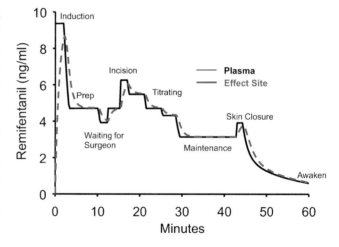

Fig. 8.15 This figure shows the titration of remifentanil, rescaled from Figs. 8.12, 8.13, and 8.14 to reflect the decreased potency of remifentanil compared to fentanyl. Because the plasma-brain equilibration of remifentanil is much faster than for fentanyl, the effect site concentrations (*dashed red line*) more closely follow the plasma concentrations

pharmacokinetic model includes plasma-effect site equilibration (Fig. 8.11).

Propofol also equilibrates quickly with the brain. Figure 8.17 shows the plasma concentration for the same hypothetical anesthetic. The anesthesiologist selects a target concentration of 5 mcg/ml for intubation and 2 mcg/ml for maintenance of anesthesia. Although a TCI device can accomplish this, the delay required for equilibration with the brain results in the effect site propofol concentrations

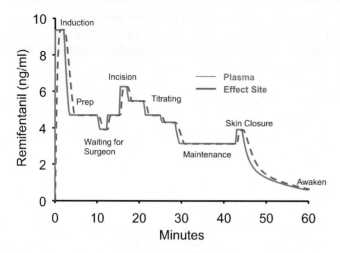

Fig. 8.16 Even though the plasma-effect site equilibration is fast for remifentanil, titration is still more accurate if the TCI device targets the concentration at the site of remifentanil drug effect (*dashed red line*)

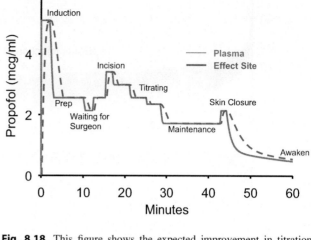

Fig. 8.18 This figure shows the expected improvement in titration when the TCI device targets the propofol concentration in the effect site (*dashed red line*)

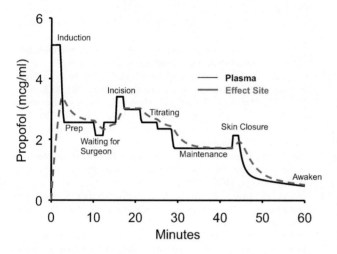

Fig. 8.17 This figure shows titration of propofol for the same anesthetic shown in Figs. 8.12, 8.13, 8.14, 8.15, and 8.16. Although plasma-brain equilibration of propofol is rapid, there is a risk of inadequate propofol concentrations in the effect site (*dashed red line*) at critical moments in the case because of the equilibration delay

well below the target concentration at critical points during the case (dashed red line).

Figure 8.18 shows the effect site concentration (dashed red line) when the effect site is specifically targeted by the TCI device. Because the TCI device understands plasma-effect site equilibration, the effect site propofol concentrations should be adequate at intubation, incision, and skin closure.

The first generation of TCI devices were only able to target the plasma drug concentration, limiting utility. All currently available TCI devices permit targeting the concentration at the site of drug effect. This should always be selected, because the effect site accounts for the physiologically imposed delay in concentration between the plasma and the site of drug effect.

Variability

The discussion so far has ignored pharmacokinetic variability. Pharmacokinetic variability represents biology, just as the plasma-brain equilibration delay represents biology. While we cannot eliminate pharmacokinetic variability, we can characterize it and incorporate this knowledge into our models, just as we do for the plasma-brain equilibration delay.

Based on concerns expressed by the US Food and Drug Administration on the effects of TCI on biological variability [12], Hu et al. developed a theoretical framework comparing the variability of TCI drug delivery with the variability of drugs administered by bolus injection [13]. They noted that "the accuracy of TCI delivery for many intravenous anesthetic drugs, including fentanyl [14–17], alfentanil [18–21], sufentanil [22, 23], remifentanil [24, 25], propofol [26–35], etomidate [36], thiopental [37] and midazolam [38, 39], dexmedetomidine [40], and lidocaine [41] resembles the accuracy observed after simple infusions or bolus drug delivery." Based on the pharmacokinetics of propofol [42], the authors documented using simulation that the expected variability from TCI is similar to conventional infusions and less than expected following bolus injection (Fig. 8.19). The authors also proved mathematically that the coefficient of variation in concentration following *any* drug input (e.g., TCI) *cannot exceed the coefficient of variation in concentration following bolus injection*. Most anesthetic drugs that might be given using TCI are approved by the FDA for administration by bolus injection, including fentanyl, alfentanil, sufentanil, remifentanil, morphine, hydromorphone, propofol, etomidate, thiopental, ketamine, vecuronium, atracurium, cisatracurium, dexmedetomidine, midazolam,

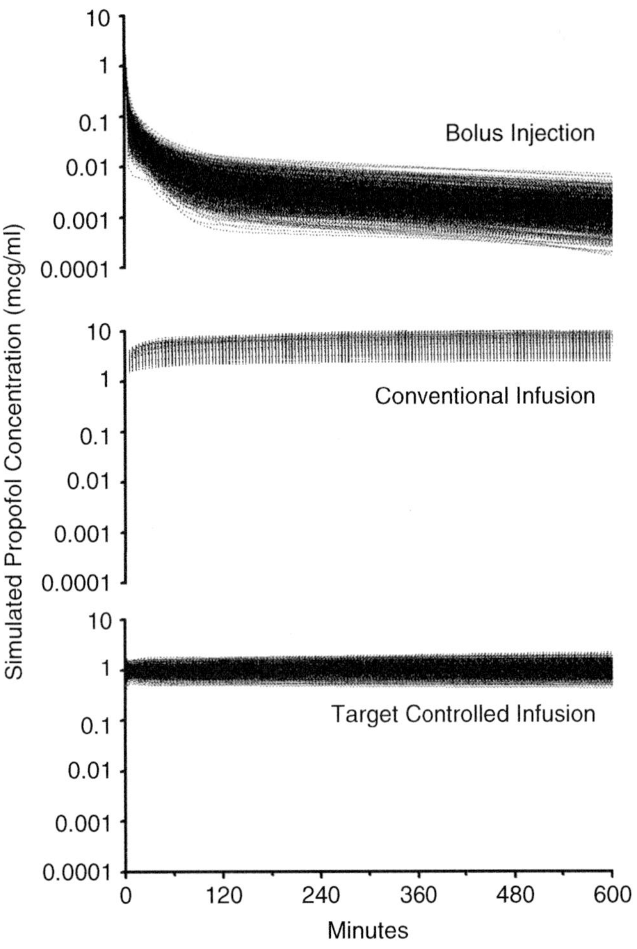

Fig. 8.19 This figure shows propofol simulations in 1000 patients, based on the pharmacokinetics reported by Schnider [42], for bolus injection, single-rate continuous infusion, and TCI. The variability with TCI will be similar to the variability with a single-rate continuous infusion and less than the variability following bolus injection. The figure is from Struys et al. [43] (used with permission of the author)

and lorazepam. Variability with bolus injection of these drugs necessarily exceeds the variability following TCI delivery.

Conclusion

Volume and clearance are the fundamental processes that govern pharmacokinetics. Because intravenous anesthetics require multicompartmental models, rapidly achieving, maintaining, and precisely titrating the concentration of intravenous anesthetics are only possible using TCI. Additionally, TCI systems are able to rapidly achieve, maintain, and titrate the drug concentration at the site of drug effect, which is the clinically relevant target (e.g., the brain). Although biological variability exists, the variability with TCI is similar to the variability seen with conventional infusions and less than expected following bolus injection.

These concepts are covered in greater detail in a recent set of review papers on the history [43], safety [44], and current status [45] of target controlled anesthetic drug delivery.

Conflict of Interest Dr. Shafer is the author of the computer program STANPUMP. STANPUMP is in the public domain, and Dr. Shafer has no financial ties to the use of the program.

References

* Stanski DR, Watkins WD. Drug disposition in anesthesia. New York: Grune and Stratton; 1982. p. 12–8.
* Sheiner LB, Stanski DR, Vozeh S, Miller RD, Ham J. Simultaneous modeling of pharmacokinetics and pharmacodynamics: application to d-tubocurarine. Clin Pharmacol Ther. 1979;25:358–71.
* 3. Hull CJ, Van Beem HB, McLeod K, Sibbald A, Watson MJ. A pharmacodynamic model for pancuronium. Br J Anaesth. 1978:50:1113–23.
* 4. Scott J, Ponganis KV, Stanski DR. Anesthesiology. 1985;62:234–41.
* Kruger-Thiemer E. Continuous intravenous infusion and multicompartment accumulation. Eur J Pharmacol. 1968;4:317–24.
* Schwilden H. A general method for calculating the dosage scheme in linear pharmacokinetics. Eur J Clin Pharmacol. 1981;20:379
  –86.
* Egan TD, Shafer SL. Target-controlled infusions for intravenous anesthetics: surfing USA not! Anesthesiology. 2003;99:1039–41.
* 8. Shafer SL, Egan T. Target-controlled infusions: surfing USA Redux. Anesth Analg. 2016;122:1–3.
* Maitre PO, Shafer SL. A simple pocket calculator approach to predict anesthetic drug concentrations from pharmacokinetic data. Anesthesiology. 1990;73:332–6.
* Bailey JM, Shafer SL. A simple analytical solution to the threecompartment pharmacokinetic model suitable for computercontrolled infusion pumps. IEEE Trans Biomed Eng. 1991;38:522–5.
* Shafer SL, Gregg KM. Algorithms to rapidly achieve and maintain stable drug concentrations at the site of drug effect with a computercontrolled infusion pump. J Pharmacokinet Biopharm. 1992;20:147–69.
* Bazaral MG, Ciarkowski A. Food and drug administration regulations and computer-controlled infusion pumps. Int Anesthesiol Clin. 1995;33:45–63.
* Hu C, Horstman DJ, Shafer SL. Variability of target-controlled infusion is less than the variability after bolus injection. Anesthesiology. 2005;102:639–45.
* Alvis JM, Reves JG, Govier AV, Menkhaus PG, Henling CE, Spain JA, Bradley E. Computer-assisted continuous infusions of fentanyl during cardiac anesthesia: comparison with a manual method. Anesthesiology. 1985;63:41–9.
* Glass PS, Jacobs JR, Smith LR, Ginsberg B, Quill TJ, Bai SA, Reves JG. Pharmacokinetic model-driven infusion of fentanyl: assessment of accuracy. Anesthesiology. 1990;73:1082–90.
* Ginsberg B, Howell S, Glass PS, Margolis JO, Ross AK, Dear GL, Shafer SL. Pharmacokinetic model-driven infusion of fentanyl in children. Anesthesiology. 1996;85:1268–75.
* Shafer SL, Varvel JR, Aziz N, Scott JC. Pharmacokinetics of fentanyl administered by computer-controlled infusion pump. Anesthesiology. 1990;73:1091–102.
* Ausems ME, Stanski DR, Hug CC. An evaluation of the accuracy of pharmacokinetic data for the computer assisted infusion of alfentanil. Br J Anaesth. 1985;57:1217–25.

19. Schuttler J, Kloos S, Schwilden H, Stoeckel H. Total intravenous anaesthesia with propofol and alfentanil by computer-assisted infusion. Anaesthesia. 1988;43(Suppl):2–7.

20. Raemer DB, Buschman A, Varvel JR, Philip BK, Johnson MD, Stein DA, Shafer SL. The prospective use of population pharmacokinetics in a computer-driven infusion system for alfentanil. Anesthesiology. 1990;73:66–72.

21. Fiset P, Mathers L, Engstrom R, Fitzgerald D, Brand SC, Hsu F, Shafer SL. Pharmacokinetics of computer-controlled alfentanil administration in children undergoing cardiac surgery. Anesthesiology. 1995;83(5):944–55.

22. Hudson RJ, Henderson BT, Thomson IR, Moon M, Peterson MD. Pharmacokinetics of sufentanil in patients undergoing coronary artery bypass graft surgery. J Cardiothorac Vasc Anesth. 2001;15:693–9.

23. Schraag S, Mohl U, Hirsch M, Stolberg E, Georgieff M. Recovery from opioid anesthesia: the clinical implication of context-sensitive half-times. Anesth Analg. 1998;86:184–90.

24. Hoymork SC, Raeder J, Grimsmo B, Steen PA. Bispectral index, predicted and measured drug levels of target-controlled infusions of remifentanil and propofol during laparoscopic cholecystectomy and emergence. Acta Anaesthesiol Scand. 2000;44:1138–44.

25. Mertens MJ, Engbers FH, Burm AG, Vuyk J. Predictive performance of computer-controlled infusion of remifentanil during propofol/remifentanil anaesthesia. Br J Anaesth. 2003;90:132–41.

26. Coetzee JF, Glen JB, Wium CA, Boshoff L. Pharmacokinetic model selection for target controlled infusions of propofol. Assessment of three parameter sets. Anesthesiology. 1995;82:1328–45.

27. Vuyk J, Engbers FH, Burm AG, Vletter AA, Bovill JG. Performance of computer-controlled infusion of propofol: an evaluation of five pharmacokinetic parameter sets. Anesth Analg. 1995;81:1275–82.

28. Bailey JM, Mora CT, Shafer SL. Pharmacokinetics of propofol in adult patients undergoing coronary revascularization. The multicenter study of Perioperative Ischemia Research Group. Anesthesiology. 1996;84:1288–97.

29. Struys MM, De Smet T, Depoorter B, Versichelen LF, Mortier EP, Dumortier FJ, Shafer SL, Rolly G. Comparison of plasma compartment versus two methods for effect compartment–controlled target-controlled infusion for propofol. Anesthesiology. 2000;92:399–406.

30. Swinhoe CF, Peacock JE, Glen JB, Reilly CS. Evaluation of the predictive performance of a 'Diprifusor' TCI system. Anaesthesia. 1998;53 Suppl 1:61–7.

31. Doufas AG, Bakhshandeh M, Bjorksten AR, Shafer SL, Sessler DI. Induction speed is not a determinant of propofol pharmacodynamics. Anesthesiology. 2004;101:1112–21.

32. Fechner J, Albrecht S, Ihmsen H, Knoll R, Schwilden H, Schuttler J. Predictability and precision of "target-controlled infusion" (TCI) of propofol with the "Disoprifusor TCI" system. Anaesthesist. 1998;47:663–8.

33. Barr J, Egan TD, Sandoval NF, Zomorodi K, Cohane C, Gambus PL, Shafer SL. Propofol dosing regimens for ICU sedation based upon an integrated pharmacokinetic-pharmacodynamic model. Anesthesiology. 2001;95:324–33.

34. Absalom A, Amutike D, Lal A, White M, Kenny GN. Accuracy of the 'Paedfusor' in children undergoing cardiac surgery or catheterization. Br J Anaesth. 2003;91:507–13.

35. Li YH, Zhao X, Xu JG. Assessment of predictive performance of a Diprifusor TCI system in Chinese patients. Anaesth Intensive Care. 2004;32:141–2.

36. Schuttler J, Schwilden H, Stoekel H. Pharmacokinetics as applied to total intravenous anaesthesia. Practical implications. Anaesthesia. 1983;38(Suppl):53–6.

37. Buhrer M, Maitre PO, Hung OR, Ebling WF, Shafer SL, Stanski DR. Thiopental pharmacodynamics. I. Defining the pseudo-steady-state serum concentration-EEG effect relationship. Anesthesiology. 1992;77:226–36.

38. Zomorodi K, Donner A, Somma J, Barr J, Sladen R, Ramsay J, Geller E, Shafer SL. Population pharmacokinetics of midazolam administered by target controlled infusion for sedation following coronary artery bypass grafting. Anesthesiology. 1998;89:1418–29.

39. Barr J, Zomorodi K, Bertaccini EJ, Shafer SL, Geller E. A double-blind, randomized comparison of i.v. lorazepam versus midazolam for sedation of ICU patients via a pharmacologic model. Anesthesiology. 2001;95:286–98.

40. Dyck JB, Maze M, Haack C, Azarnoff DL, Vuorilehto L, Shafer SL. Computer-controlled infusion of intravenous dexmedetomidine hydrochloride in adult human volunteers. Anesthesiology. 1993;78:821–8.

41. Schnider TW, Gaeta R, Brose W, Minto CF, Gregg KM, Shafer SL. Derivation and cross-validation of pharmacokinetic parameters for computer-controlled infusion of lidocaine in pain therapy. Anesthesiology. 1996;84:1043–50.

42. Schnider TW, Minto CF, Gambus PL, Andresen C, Goodale DB, Shafer SL, Youngs EJ. The influence of method of administration and covariates on the pharmacokinetics of propofol in adult volunteers. Anesthesiology. 1998;88:1170–82.

43. Struys MMRF, De Smet T, Glen JB, Vereecke HEM, Absalom AR, Schnider TW. The history of target-controlled infusion. Anesth Analg. 2016;122:56–69.

44. Schnider TW, Minto CF, Struys MMRF, Absalom AR. The safety of target-controlled infusions. Anesth Analg. 2016;122:79–85.

45. Absalom AR, Glen JB, Zwart GJC, Schnider TW, Struys MMRF. Target-controlled infusion—a mature technology. Anesth Analg. 2016;122:70–8.

Performance of Target-Controlled Infusion Systems

9

Matthew T.V. Chan

The purpose of a target-controlled infusion (TCI) system is to calculate and administer the drug infusion profile required to achieve and maintain a user-defined target plasma or effect-site concentration of the drug. Such a system involves hardware that includes a syringe driver, user interface, power supply, and a microprocessor. The microprocessor is loaded with one or more pharmacokinetic models (or even combined pharmacokinetic and pharmacodynamic models) and software to control the interface. It asks the user to select the desired drug and model, who thereafter enters the values of any model covariates (patient characteristics such as age, height, weight and gender), and select the initial target concentration. The microprocessor is therefore programmed with an infusion algorithm that can use the pharmacokinetic parameters of the user-selected model, scaled according to the values of the covariates, to calculate the infusion rate profiles necessary to achieve the user-selected target concentrations.

For the same target concentration, different pharmacokinetic models will produce important differences in the amount of drug required to be infused and may influence the accuracy of the TCI device [1]. It is therefore important to understand the predictive performance of different models in order to choose the appropriate one for any individual patient. This chapter outlines the methodology for assessing the performance of TCI systems, evaluates the common sources of error, and reports on the accuracy of various TCI protocols.

Measurements of Performance

The performance of TCI systems is evaluated by comparing the predicted and measured values of the blood or plasma concentration [2]. It should be noted that plasma drug

concentration, in many circumstances, cannot be measured in real time. Therefore, the ability of TCI systems to target plasma concentrations is generally reported after post hoc measurements and analyses. Although online measurement of end-tidal propofol concentration has been reported [3–5], routine clinical use is still limited by current technological development. In contrast, drug effect assessed by, for example, changes in the processed electroencephalogram for hypnotics and train-of-four ratio for neuromuscular blockers, may be monitored online. In these scenarios, performance measures can be computed in real time. This has been shown to facilitate fine-tuning of TCI systems, such as closed-loop infusion systems designed to target drug effect during anesthesia (Fig. 9.1) [6–10].

Varvel and others have recommended five indices to quantify TCI performance [11].

1. Percentage performance error (PE)
   This is the weighted residual of the target value at any given time point. It indicates the deviation of observed value from its predicted value [11]. Mathematically, for the i-th subject, the PE at j-th time point is given by

$$\text{PE}_{ij} = \frac{\text{Observed value}_{ij} - \text{Predicted value}_{ij}}{\text{Predicted value}_{ij}} \times 100\%.$$

2. Median performance error (MDPE)
   This is a measure of bias and indicates whether drug delivery with the TCI system is systematically above or below the target value.

$$\text{MDPE}_i = \text{Median} \left\{ \text{PE}_{ij}, j = 1, \ldots, N_i \right\}$$

where N_i is the number of observations obtained in the i-th patient.

Alternatively, bias can be expressed as the ratio between observed and predicted values. Logarithmic transformation of the ratio is commonly presented.

M.T.V. Chan, MBBS, PhD, FANZCA, FHKCA, FHKAM(✉)
Department of Anaesthesia and Intensive Care, The Chinese University of Hong Kong, Prince of Wales Hospital, Shatin, Hong Kong
e-mail: mtvchan@cuhk.edu.hk

© Springer International Publishing AG 2017
A.R. Absalom, K.P. Mason (eds.), *Total Intravenous Anesthesia and Target Controlled Infusions*,
DOI 10.1007/978-3-319-47609-4_9

Fig. 9.1 Closed-loop control of propofol infusion aiming to maintain a bispectral value of 80 in a patient receiving sedation for gastrointestinal endoscopy. The infusion was controlled by an automated proportional-integral-differential control algorithm. The initial period showed a big variation in BIS producing a large performance error. The control algorithm was changed with a 20 % increase in the control of "proportional" value (*arrow*), and this resulted in a lower performance error

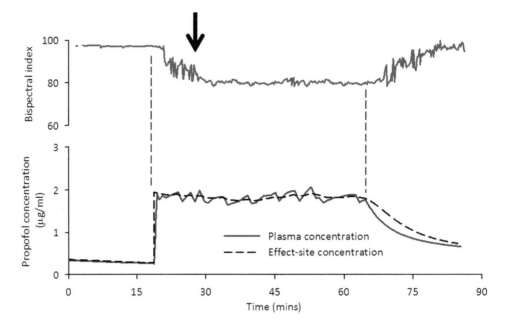

3. Median absolute performance error (MDAPE)

This measure indicates the inaccuracy of the TCI system and is a quantitative measure of how far the observed value deviates from the target:

$$MDAPE_i = Median\left\{\left|PE_{ij}\right|, j = 1, \ldots, N_i\right\}$$

4. Wobble

This index indicates the within-subject variability of the TCI system and is calculated as the median absolute deviation of PE from the bias of the system (MDPE):

$$Wobble_i = Median\left\{\left|PE_{ij} - MDPE_{ij}\right|, j = 1, \ldots, N_i\right\}$$

5. Divergence

This is the slope of linear regression between the $MDAPE_i$ and time. Divergence shows whether inaccuracy of the TCI system changes over time.

An ideal TCI system would produce an observation that matches perfectly with the predicted value. Therefore, the performance error (MDAPE) and bias (MDPE) should approach zero, and the ratio between the observed and predicted value would be of unity. The TCI system should also be stable over time, so that wobble and divergence should be as low as possible.

A useful way to display the performance of a TCI system is to plot the observed and predicted target values over time. Figure 9.2a shows the typical deviations of observed propofol concentration from its predicted value in a patient who was enrolled in a randomized trial evaluating the effect of hyperventilation in patients having craniotomy for removal of brain tumor [12]. Anesthesia was induced and maintained with effect-site-targeted propofol infusion using an open TCI system—computer control infusion pump [13] (CCIP), based on the Schnider pharmacokinetic and pharmacodynamic datasets [14, 15]. Since effect-site concentration cannot be measured, comparisons were made between observed and predicted propofol concentrations in the plasma. Figures 9.2b, c illustrates the bias of the TCI system over time in the same patient. The TCI system produced a lower plasma concentration than predicted during the initial 2 h of infusion. This negative performance error was however offset by the overshoots in the remaining period of anesthesia when the observed plasma concentrations were 14–29 % higher than that of predicted. Consequently, the overall mean ratio of observed-to-predicted concentration (0.99) and MDPE (1.2 %) were small. Inaccuracy (MDAPE) of the TCI system in the patient was 13.8 (95 % confidence intervals (CI): 1.2–27.2 %), Fig. 9.2d.

Analyses can also be performed with population data. Figure 9.3 shows the changes of performance error, absolute performance error, and ratio of observed-to-predicted concentrations over time in 30 patients enrolled in our craniotomy hyperventilation trial [12]. By pooling data from all patients, the MDPE was −2.6 % (95% CI: −25.7 to 24.8 %), Fig. 9.3a, and the mean ratio of observed-to-predicted concentration was 0.97 (95% CI: 0.74–1.25), Fig. 9.3b. It should be noted that confidence intervals were wide, suggesting that a large proportion of performance errors were higher or lower than the average values. The MDAPE indicates the overall inaccuracy of the TCI system and was 16.4 % (95% CI: 1.9–27.0 %) in our dataset, Fig. 9.3c. Interestingly, the absolute performance errors tended to become smaller with time, and this indicated convergence of performance with the TCI system

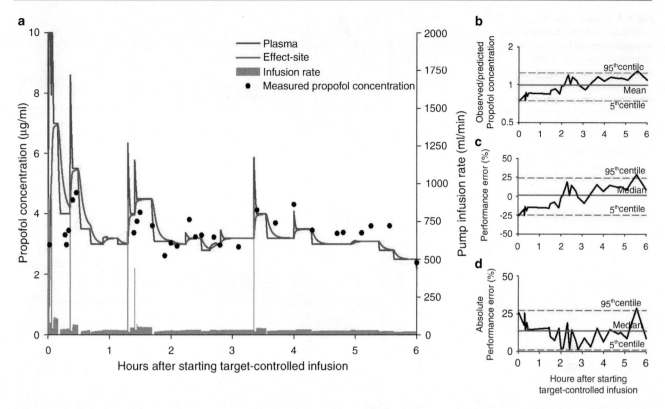

Fig. 9.2 (**a**) Target-controlled propofol infusion delivered to a 62-year-old man undergoing excision of frontal tumor. The *blue and red lines* indicate predicted plasma and effect-site concentrations, respectively. The *gray bar* shows the pump infusion rate. Measured (observed) propofol concentrations are shown by *black circles*. (**b**) Time course of observed-to-predicted propofol concentrations, (**c**) performance errors, and (**d**) absolute performance errors. Median (or mean as indicated), 5th, and 95th centile values are also shown

(Fig. 9.3d). Finally, in our sample dataset, the median wobble was 15.0 % (95% CI: 3.8–21.0 %), indicating the variability of performance error in each of the subjects.

These analyses illustrate how the performance indices may be used to quantify the accuracy of TCI system. However, clinical interpretation is more complex. Currently, there is no consensus on the maximum performance error that could be considered acceptable in routine clinical practice. Empirically, Eleveld and colleagues suggested that an absolute performance error <20 % represents good performance, whereas an error >60 % is considered to indicate a poorly performing TCI system [16]. Others have recommended that an absolute performance error <20 to 40 % and a MDPE <10 to 20 % would be clinically acceptable [17, 18]. Although a 20–40 % error seems excessive, this has not been shown to increase the rate of adverse events during TCI [19]. Interestingly, in a systematic study evaluating the discrepancy between end-tidal (predicted) and arterial (observed) isoflurane concentrations, Zbinden and co-workers showed that an ordinary vaporizer produced a negative bias with an arterial isoflurane concentration that was 17.0 % (95% CI: 5.9–27 %) lower than that predicted by end-tidal gas monitoring [20, 21].

Sources of Errors

Table 9.1 summarizes the potential factors that may influence the performance of TCI systems. This includes hardware problems, where inaccuracy of infusion devices may result in a failure to deliver the exact amount of drug intended. In practice, though, hardware problems are rare, and regulatory approval requires that pumps actually administer the intended concentration with high precision. If inaccuracies arise from mechanical problems, then they are more likely to be caused by mechanical failure of one or more components, including problems with the syringe and/or plunger [22–27]. There are also potential software errors, such as incorrect implementation of models or infusion algorithms that might produce large errors in the prediction of drug infusion rates required, or programming errors that might shut down the system unexpectedly. Again, with stringent testing, software errors are rare. Finally, and probably most importantly, there are human errors in drug delivery. This could be due to incorrect pump programming, syringe swap [28], disconnection of venous cannula, or incorrect drug dilution.

Fig. 9.3 Time course of (**a**) performance errors, (**b**) observed-to-predicted propofol concentrations, (**c**) absolute performance errors, and (**d**) regression of absolute performance errors with time in 30 patients having craniotomy for brain tumor excision. *Solid line* indicates the median (or mean) value. The 5th and 95th centile values are shown as *dotted line*

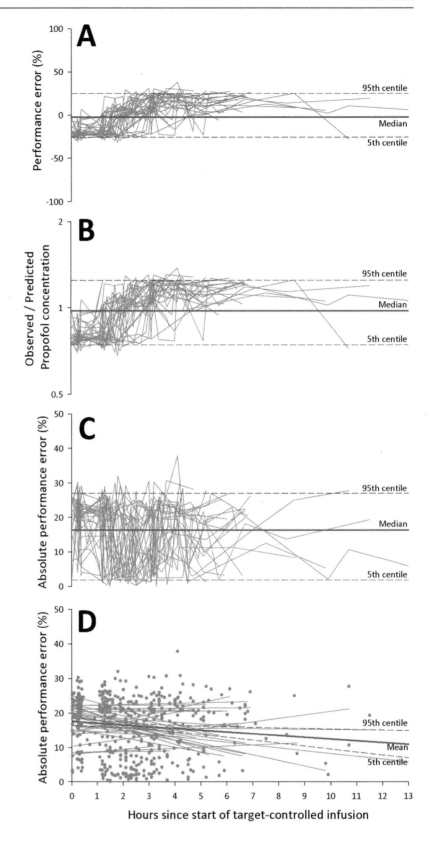

Hardware

Before the mid-1990s, limitations in processing power limited technological developments. However, with the advances of computing technology, smaller and faster microprocessors have been developed and incorporated into ordinary syringe pumps to enable implementation of the infusion algorithms required for TCI [29, 30]. Some groups have even developed software programs that are capable of driving syringe pumps from mobile devices through wireless networks without observable delay [31].

Downstream drug delivery could however affect TCI performance. It should be noted that modern syringe pumps are infusion control devices that are capable of delivering a wide range of flow rates from 0.1 to >1000 ml/h. In general, these devices produce an inaccuracy of $<\pm5$ % of expected volume infused [32, 33]. Nevertheless, several factors may delay infusion start-up and affect flow stability (Table 9.2). In this respect, a misplaced or loose plunger of a large syringe can delay the onset of infusion [34–39]. This is particularly important when a compliant syringe plunger stopper is used or when compliant infusion delivery lines [40, 41] and antisiphon or anti-reflux devices are used [42–44]. This may contribute to a lower amount of drug being delivered than programmed, resulting in a negative performance error, particularly during the early phase of an infusion. Other factors such as concurrent infusions using multi-access devices [45, 46] and small air bubbles in the infusion line will also contribute to flow irregularity and affect infusion accuracy [47, 48]. There are also extreme conditions, such as strong magnetic fields [49], radio frequency, and hyperbaric conditions [50, 51], that may affect pump performance to different extents. Nevertheless, when hardware problems are carefully prevented by priming of the infusion system (with the flush or purge function) before starting the infusion, the performance error for remifentanil TCI was reduced by 1.6–7.9 % during induction of anesthesia and 0–0.3 % in the maintenance phase [36]. The current data suggest that hardware factors do not contribute substantially to the inaccuracy of TCI systems.

Software

In contrast to hardware performance, the accuracy of TCI is heavily influenced by software factors. In this respect, the prediction performance of TCI systems is heavily dependent on the validity and relevance of the pharmacokinetic model chosen by the user to the patient receiving the infusion. Table 9.3 shows seven sets of pharmacokinetic models for propofol that have been implemented in commercially available and open TCI systems (open systems provide the user with a choice of drugs and models, as opposed to the first generation of pumps, which only enabled TCI of propofol using the Marsh model) [14, 52–60]. It should be noted that the rate constants differ significantly among the different models. Consequently, there is a large variation in the predicted plasma propofol concentration with any given amount of drug infused according to the specific models applied, or conversely that for a given target concentration, the infusion rates necessary, as estimated by the models, will differ significantly. Using computer simulations, Absalom and co-workers found that the Marsh model required at least 20 % more propofol to maintain the same target plasma concentration compared with the Schnider model in middle-aged adults of normal proportions [1]. This finding highlights the importance for specification of appropriate pharmacokinetic model.

Table 9.1 Sources of errors in drug delivery during target-controlled infusion

Hardware
• Delayed communication or disconnection between the infusion pump and computer
• Inaccuracy of the infusion pump
• Syringe, venous infusion line disconnection
Software
• Inappropriate pharmacokinetic and pharmacodynamic models
• Incorrect infusion rate control algorithms
Human errors
• Syringe swap
• Incorrect drug dilution
• Venous cannula disconnection

Table 9.2 Factors contributing to drug delivery error in target-controlled infusion

Factors	Potential mechanisms	Counter measures
Start-up delay	• Loose fitting of syringe plunger • Large dead space volume in the infusion delivery line • Large compliant syringe • Use of antisiphon or anti-reflux devices	• Priming of infusion devices • Use syringe with smaller diameter • Tight fit between thumb rest and syringe drive
Flow stability	• Concurrent use of multi-access infusion devices • Use of antisiphon or anti-reflux devices • Air bubbles in the infusion delivery line	• Use of dedicated venous line • Eliminate bubbles in the infusion delivery line

Table 9.3 Reported propofol pharmacokinetic models for target-controlled infusion

	V_1	V_2	V_3	k_{10} (min^{-1})	k_{12} (min^{-1})	k_{13} (min^{-1})	k_{14} (min^{-1})	k_{21} (min^{-1})	k_{31} (min^{-1})	k_{e0} (min^{-1})
Dyck [52]	$9.64 - (0.051 \times \text{age})$, L/kg	–	$571 - (1.66 \times \text{age})$	$(0.652 + 0.015 \times \text{weight})/V_1$	$1.68/V_1$	$(2.670 - 0.015 \times \text{age})/V_1$	–	$V_1 \times k_{12}/19.4$	$V_1 \times k_{13}/(571 - 1.66 \times \text{age})$	–
Gepts [53]	0.228, L/kg	0.476, L/kg	2.895, L/kg	0.119	0.114	0.042	0.00002	0.055	0.003	0.239
Kataria [54]	0.41, L/kg	$0.78 \times \text{weight} + 3.1 \times \text{age} - 16$, L	6.9, L/kg	0.085	$k_{21} \times V_2/V_1$	0.063	–	$0.077 \times \text{weight}/(0.78 \times \text{weight} + 3.1 \times \text{age} - 16)$	0.004	–
Marsh [55]	0.227, L/kg	0.463, L/kg	2.886, L/kg	0.119	0.112	0.042	0.00002	0.055	0.003	0.26
Paedfusor [56–59]	0.458, L/Kg	0.95, L/Kg	5.82, L/Kg	$(70 \times \text{weight}^{-0.3})/458.3$	0.114	0.042	0.00002	0.055	0.003	0.26
Schnider [14]	4.27, L	$18.9 - 0.391 \times (\text{age}, 53)$, L	238	C_1/V_1	$k_{21} \times V_2/V_1$	$k_{31} \times V_3/V_1$	$k_{41}/10{,}000$	C_2/V_2	C_3/V_3	0.456
		where		$C_1 = 1.89 + [(\text{weight} - 77) \times 0.046] + [(\text{LBM} - 59) \times (-0.068)] + [(\text{height} - 177) \times 0.026]$ $C_2 = 1.29 - 0.024 \times (\text{age} - 53)$ $C_3 = 0.836$ $\text{LBM} = 1.1 \times \text{weight} - 128 \times (\text{weight}/\text{height})^2$ for male or $1.07 \times \text{weight} - 148 \times (\text{weight}/\text{height})^2$ for female						
Tackley [60]	0.32, L/kg	0.525, L/kg	2.071, L/kg	0.087	0.105	0.022	–	0.064	0.003	–

LBM lean body mass

Performance of Target-Controlled Infusions

In order to select the best pharmacokinetic model, one needs to understand the underlying processes in deriving these datasets. Table 9.4 summarizes the patient characteristics of studies producing the various pharmacokinetic models for opioids [61–72], etomidate [73], ketamine [74], midazolam [75], thiopental [76, 77], propofol [14, 16, 52–60, 78, 79], and muscle relaxants [80]. Earlier studies recruited a small number of volunteers or healthy patients having trivial elective surgery, and their pharmacokinetic parameters may not represent those patients at extreme age with multiple

Table 9.4 Patient characteristics of commonly used pharmacokinetic dataset in target-controlled infusion

Author[Reference]	Patient characteristics	No. of patients	Male sex, no. (%)	Covariates
Alfentanil				
Lemmens [61]	Adults (24–79 years), ASA 1–2	36	15 (41.7)	Weight ($\leq$50 vs. >50 years), gender
Maitre [62]	Adults with various risks (24–91 years), ASA 1–3	45	–	Weight, age, gender
Scott [63]	Adults (20–89 years), ASA 1–2	17	17 (100)	Weight
Fentanyl				
Hudson [64]	Adults (67.2 $\pm$ 8.7 years)[b], ASA 2–3	10	9 (90)	Weight
McClain [65]	Healthy volunteers (22–29 years)	7	7 (100)	Weight
Scott [63]	Adults (20–89 years), ASA 1–2	17	17 (100)	Weight
Shafer [66]	Adults (58 $\pm$ 11 years)[b], ASA 1–4	21	7 (33.3)	Weight
Varvel [67]	Adults (33–57 years), ASA 1–2	8	3 (37.5)	Weight
Remifentanil				
Egan [68]	Healthy volunteers (22–38 years)	10	10 (100)	Weight
Minto [69, 70]	Healthy volunteers (60–65 years)	65	38 (58.5)	Age, gender, lean body mass (weight and height)
Sufentanil				
Bovill [71]	Adults (22–64 years), ASA 1–2	10	7 (70)	Weight
Gepts [72]	Adults (14–68 years), ASA 1–2	25	14 (56)	Weight
Etomidate				
Arden [73]	Adults (22–82 years), ASA 1–2	21	20 (95.2)	Weight
Ketamine				
Domino [74]	Healthy volunteers (26–41 years)	8	8 (100)	Weight
Midazolam				
Greenblatt [75]	Healthy volunteers (24–37 years)	20	10 (50)	Weight
	Elderly volunteers (60–79 years)	20	9 (45)	Weight
Propofol				
Dyck [52]	Adults (20 $\geq$ 65 years)	60	60 (100)	Weight, age
Eleveld [16]	Patients/volunteers from 21 datasets (0–88 years)	660	433 (72.2)	Weight, age, gender, healthy (*vs.* patient)
Gepts [53]	Adults, ASA 1	18	13 (72.2)	Weight
Kataria [54]	Children (3–11 years), ASA 1	53	28 (52.8)	Weight, age
Kirkpatrick [78]	Adults (65–80 years), ASA 1–2	12	–	Weight
	Adults (18–35 years), ASA 1	12	–	Weight
Marsh[a] [55]	Children (1–10 years), ASA 1	30	–	Weight
Paedfusor [56–59]	–	–	–	Weight
Shafer [79]	Adults (43 $\pm$ 14 years), ASA 1–3	50	22 (44)	Weight
Schnider [14]	Adults (26–81 years)	24	13 (54.2)	Age, gender, lean body mass (weight and height)
Tackley [60]	Adults (24–65 years), ASA 1–2	16	–	Weight
Thiopental				
Stanski [76]	Healthy volunteers (20–40 years)	6	–	Weight, age
	Adult patients (20–61), ASA 1–3	58	–	
Sorbo [77]	Children (5 months–13 years), ASA 1–2	16	9 (56.3)	Weight
Rocuronium				
van den Broek [80]	Adult patients (18–65), ASA 1–3	36	–	Weight

ASA American Society of Anesthesiologists
[a]Modified and incorporated in Diprifusor [29]
[b]Values are mean $\pm$ standard deviation

comorbidities. There are also important differences in the study methodology, such as the use of venous sampling in the Marsh model [55] which might have underestimated the plasma propofol concentration, because venous sampling produced lower concentrations than arterial measurements.

There is a major impact on TCI performance when patient characteristics are different from those of the subjects involved in the study from which the pharmacokinetic parameters were derived. Table 9.5 lists the studies that evaluated the bias (MDPE) and accuracy (MDAPE) of TCI

Table 9.5 Performance of target-controlled infusion for propofol using different pharmacokinetic models

Study[Reference]	Year	Patient characteristics	No. of patients	MDAPE (%)	MDPE (%)
Dyck model					
Coetzee [81]	1995	Adult (21–50 year), nonobese, ASA 1–2, having orthopedic or gynecologic surgery	10	47.1	43.1
Eleveld model					
Cortínez [94]	2014	Adult (2–60 years), BMI > 35 kg/m^2, elective laparoscopic bariatric surgery	20	27.5	18.2
Gepts model					
Short [82]	1996	Adult (20–60 years) patients, ASA 1–2, Asian, elective surgery >2 h	40	19.2–33.8	19.5–25.3
Oei-Lim [83]	1998	Adult (18–60 years) patients, ASA 1–2, sedation for dental procedure	53	16–25	−0.02 to −5
Marsh model					
Coetzee [81]	1995	Adult (21–50 year), nonobese, ASA 1–2, having orthopedic or gynecologic surgery	10	28.6	−0.9
Barvais [84]	1996	Adult (40–75 years) patients, ASA 2–4, having elective coronary artery bypass graft surgery	21	9.6–212	23–185
Swinhoe [17]	1998	Adult (29–68 years), ASA 1–3, elective surgery >2 h	46	22.6–25.0	13.8–17.7
Pandin [85]	2000	Adult (36–69 years), ASA 1–2, nonobese elective surgery >12 h	10	22.1	−12.1
Sabate Tenas [86]	2003	Adult (18–54 years), ASA 2–3, end-stage renal failure having kidney transplant	40	16.3–21.2	−1.1 to 3.45
Cavaliere [87]	2005	Adult (37–70 years) critically ill patients with and without hypoalbuminemia (<24 g/L) receiving propofol sedation	20	22–27	−5 to −6
Li [88]	2005	Adult (17–68 years), ASA 1–2, elective abdominal surgery >2–5 h	27	23.3	14.9
Wu [89]	2005	Adult (29–53 years), ASA 2–4, liver transplantation	10	339–588	339–588
Wietasch [90]	2006	Adult (58 ± 13 years)[a], ASA 1–3, elective surgery >1 h with concurrent remifentanil infusion	54	60.7	58.6
Albertin [91]	2007	Adult (32–64 years), ASA 2–3, morbid obesity with BMI > 45 kg/m^2, elective intestinal bypass	20	33.1	−32.9
La Colla [92]	2009	Adult (25–62 years), ASA 2–3, morbid obesity with BMI > 45 kg/m^2, elective intestinal bypass	24	20.6–31.7	−16.3 to −31.7
Cowley [93]	2013	Adult (53 ± 15 years)[a], ASA 1–3, elective craniotomy	50	29.4	27.6
Cortínez [94]	2014	Adult (20–60 years), BMI > 35 kg/m^2, elective laparoscopic bariatric surgery	20	39.9	36.6
Tachibana [95]	2014	Adult (47.8 ± 10 years)[a], Japanese, ASA 1–2, elective surgery	75	20–40	20–40
Sitsen [96]	2015	Adult (44.9 ± 15.1 years)[a], ASA 1–2, elective surgery requiring 20-segment epidural block	28	37	32
Mathew [97]	2016	Adult (18–65 years), Indian, ASA 2–3, elective open heart surgery	23	8	−6.4
Paedfusor					
Absalom [101]	2007	Children (1–15 years), ASA 2–3, elective cardiac surgery or catheterization	29	9.7	4.1
Panchatsharam [102]	2014	Children (9–17 years), ASA 1–2, scoliosis surgery with blood loss of 6.6 ml/kg	13	46.3	46.3
Schnider model					
Doufas [10]	2003	Adult (18–50 years) healthy volunteers	20	17–22	−13 to −18
Cortínez [94]	2014	Adult (20–60 years), BMI > 35 kg/m^2, elective laparoscopic bariatric surgery	20	79.7	79.7
Shafer model					
Lim [98]	1997	Adult (41 ± 8 years)[a] patients, ASA 1–2, elective craniotomy	15	20.6	−5.3
Tackley Model					
Coetzee [81]	1995	Adult (21–50 year), nonobese, ASA 1–2, having orthopedic or gynecologic surgery	10	24.4	−2.8

ASA American Society of Anesthesiologists, *BMI* body mass index, *MDPE* median performance error, *MDAPE* median absolute performance error
[a]Values are mean ± standard deviation

Table 9.6 Performance of target-controlled infusion for remifentanil using Minto or Egan pharmacokinetic model

Study[Reference]	Year	Patient characteristics	No. of patients	MDAPE (%)	MDPE (%)
Minto model					
La Colla [99]	2010	Adults (34–49 years), all females, ASA 2–3, BMI > 65 kg/m^2, elective Roux-en-Y bypass surgery	15	20.5–53.4	−18.9 to −53.4
Mertens [100]	2003	Adults (20–65 years), all females, ASA 1–2, elective lower abdominal surgery	30	20	−15
Egan model					
Mertens [100]	2003	Adults (20–65 years), all females, ASA 1–2, elective lower abdominal surgery	30	19–30	1 to −6

ASA American Society of Anesthesiologists, *BMI* body mass index, *MDPE* median performance error, *MDAPE* median absolute performance error

systems for propofol based on the Dyck [81], Gepts [82, 83], Marsh [17, 81, 84–97], Schnider [11, 94], Shafer [98], and Tackley models [81]. Among adult patients undergoing elective noncardiac surgery, the average bias for the majority of TCI systems was about 15 % with an absolute performance error in the range of 20–30 %. Similar data are observed with remifentanil (Table 9.6) [99, 100]. The Paedfusor uses pediatric pharmacokinetic model for propofol that was developed specifically for children, and when used to control TCI propofol administration for children undergoing cardiac surgery or cardiac catheterization, it performed very well [101]. In contrast, pharmacokinetic models based on nonobese patients performed poorly when used in morbidly obese patients undergoing bariatric surgery [94].

Eleveld and colleagues have produced a general pharmacokinetic model that can be used for TCI propofol administration to a wide range of patients, by analyzing 21 published datasets that included data from 660 volunteers or patients, including obese patients, patients from different age groups, and those with liver diseases [16]. When this "universal" model was internally validated on subsets (data from pediatric, elderly, and obese patients) of the combined dataset, it performed either as well as or even better than the predictions of specialist models for those subsets. The model incorporates four covariates (age, gender, weight, and patient *vs.* volunteer). Cortinez et al. recently used their own model designed for use in obese patients, to control TCI propofol administration to 20 obese patients, and took blood for propofol assays. They then tested the predicted performance of their model, as well as the ability of several other models, to predict the measured propofol concentrations. The Eleveld allometric pharmacokinetic model showed the best overall predictive performance [94].

Apart from preoperative patient characteristics, intraoperative events may also affect the pharmacokinetic profile of a drug. With regard to propofol, pharmacokinetic parameters vary with changes in liver perfusion and function. In patients undergoing liver transplantation, the Marsh model underestimated the plasma propofol concentration by fourfold, primarily due to a reduction in drug clearance [89]. Interestingly, extensive epidural block and significant intraoperative blood loss have also been shown to impair the predictive performance of pharmacokinetic models for propofol [96, 102]. Similar changes are reported for remifentanil [103]. Theoretically, the use of physiological models may account for acute changes in perfusion and be able to adjust for the alterations in volumes and clearances among different organs [104]. However, this type of model is complex to implement and has not been widely adopted in TCI systems, and its performance has not been prospectively evaluated. Moreover, the additional complexity of making real-time adaptations to the model parameters will be challenging.

In circumstances where intraoperative events appear to be causing a significant change in the pharmacokinetics of one or more drugs, likely leading to underestimation of plasma concentrations, it is wise to decrease the target concentrations to avoid drug overdose.

Conclusions

In summary, current TCI systems generally tend to underestimate plasma concentrations with a performance error of about 20–40 %. In extreme conditions, such as morbid obesity, predictive performance of pharmacokinetic models can be severely impaired, resulting in a potentially dangerous infusion profile, with risks of either drug overdose or inadvertent under dosage [1]. This is mainly due to misspecification of pharmacokinetic models or the use of pharmacokinetic models not designed for use in that population of patients. Safe and efficient use of TCI will therefore require sound knowledge of pharmacokinetics and of the methodology used during development of the available models, to inform the choice of an appropriate model with appropriate scaling of model parameters according to the model covariates.

References

1. Absalom AR, Mani V, De Smet T, Struys MM. Pharmacokinetic models for propofol-defining and illuminating the devil in the detail. Br J Anaesth. 2009;103:26–37.

2. Sheiner LB, Beal SL. Some suggestions for measuring predictive performance. J Pharmacokinet Biopharm. 1981;9:503–12.

3. Grossherr M, Hengstenberg A, Meier T, Dibbelt L, Igl BW, Ziegler A, Schmucker P, Gehring H. Propofol concentration in exhaled air and arterial plasma in mechanically ventilated patients undergoing cardiac surgery. Br J Anaesth. 2009;102:608–13.

4. Takita A, Masui K, Kazama T. On-line monitoring of end-tidal propofol concentration in anesthetized patients. Anesthesiology. 2007;106:659–64.

5. Colin P, Eleveld DJ, van den Berg JP, Vereecke HE, Struys MM, Schelling G, Apfel CC, Hornuss C. Propofol breath monitoring as a potential tool to improve the prediction of intraoperative plasma concentrations. Clin Pharmacokinet. 2015.

6. Ngan Kee WD, Khaw KS, Ng FF, Tam YH. Randomized comparison of closed-loop feedback computer-controlled with manual-controlled infusion of phenylephrine for maintaining arterial pressure during spinal anaesthesia for caesarean delivery. Br J Anaesth. 2013;110:59–65.

7. Morley A, Derrick J, Mainland P, Lee BB, Short TG. Closed loop control of anaesthesia: an assessment of the bispectral index as the target of control. Anaesthesia. 2000;55:953–9.

8. Ionescu CM, De Keyser R, Torrico BC, De Smet T, Struys MM, Normey-Rico JE. Robust predictive control strategy applied for propofol dosing using BIS as a controlled variable during anesthesia. IEEE Trans Biomed Eng. 2008;55:2161–70.

9. Absalom AR, Sutcliffe N, Kenny GN. Closed-loop control of anesthesia using Bispectral index: performance assessment in patients undergoing major orthopedic surgery under combined general and regional anesthesia. Anesthesiology. 2002;96:67–73.

10. Doufas AG, Bakhshandeh M, Bjorksten AR, Greif R, Sessler DI. A new system to target the effect-site during propofol sedation. Acta Anaesthesiol Scand. 2003;47:944–50.

11. Varvel JR, Donoho DL, Shafer SL. Measuring the predictive performance of computer-controlled infusion pumps. J Pharmacokinet Biopharm. 1992;20:63–94.

12. Gelb AW, Craen RA, Rao GS, Reddy KR, Megyesi J, Mohanty B, Dash HH, Choi KC, Chan MT. Does hyperventilation improve operating condition during supratentorial craniotomy? A multicenter randomized crossover trial. Anesth Analg. 2008;106:585–94.

13. Tam YH. Computer control infusion pump (CCIP) version 2.4; released in December, 2010. Available at www.cuhk.edu.hk/med/ans/softwares.htm.

14. Schnider TW, Minto CF, Gambus PL, Andresen C, Goodale DB, Shafer SL, Youngs EJ. The influence of method of administration and covariates on the pharmacokinetics of propofol in adult volunteers. Anesthesiology. 1998;88:1170–82.

15. Schnider TW, Minto CF, Shafer SL, Gambus PL, Andresen C, Goodale DB, Youngs EJ. The influence of age on propofol pharmacodynamics. Anesthesiology. 1999;90:1502–16.

16. Eleveld DJ, Proost JH, Cortinez LI, Absalom AR, Struys MM. A general purpose pharmacokinetic model for propofol. Anesth Analg. 2014;118:1221–37.

17. Swinhoe CF, Peacock JE, Glen JB, Reilly CS. Evaluation of the predictive performance of a 'Diprifusor' TCI system. Anaesthesia. 1998;53 Suppl 1:61–7.

18. Schuttler J, Kloos S, Schwilden H, Stoeckel H. Total intravenous anaesthesia with propofol and alfentanil by computer-assisted infusion. Anaesthesia. 1988;43(Suppl):2–7.

19. Schnider TW, Minto CF, Struys MM, Absalom AR. The safety of target-controlled infusions. Anesth Analg. 2016;122:79–85.

20. Zbinden AM, Petersenfelix S, Thomson DA. Anesthetic depth defined using multiple noxious stimuli during isoflurane/oxygen anesthesia. II. hemodynamic responses. Anesthesiology. 1994;80:261–7.

21. Zbinden AM, Maggiorini M, Petersenfelix S, Lauber R, Thomson DA, Minder CE. Anesthetic depth defined using multiple noxious stimuli during isoflurane/oxygen anesthesia. I. Motor reactions. Anesthesiology. 1994;80:253–60.

22. Smith JH, Karthikeyan G. Foreign body occlusion of syringe driver mechanism. Eur J Anaesthesiol. 2007;24:1063–4.

23. Maruyama K, Hara K. Accidental propofol infusion from a pre-filled propofol syringe. Br J Anaesth. 2004;93:479–80.

24. Laurent S, Fry R, Nixon C. Serial failure of Diprifuser infusion pumps. Anaesthesia. 2001;56:596–7.

25. Cox IR. Target controlled infusion pump failure due to worn drive nut. Anaesth Intensive Care. 2012;40:186–7.

26. Corcoran EL, Riley RH. Occlusion of a syringe pump by plastic cap. Anaesth Intensive Care. 2003;31:234.

27. Breslin D. Failure of a 'Diprivan 1%' prefilled propofol syringe. Anaesthesia. 2000;55:1030–1.

28. Sistema Espanol de Notificacion en Seguridad en Anestesia y R. Incorrect programming of a target controlled infusion pump. Case SENSAR of the trimester. Rev Esp Anestesiol Reanim 2014;61:e27-30.

29. Glen JB. The development of 'Diprifusor': a TCI system for propofol. Anaesthesia. 1998;53 Suppl 1:13–21.

30. Absalom AR, Glen JI, Zwart GJ, Schnider TW, Struys MM. -Target-controlled infusion: a mature technology. Anesth Analg. 2016;122:70–8.

31. Wijnen B, Hunt EJ, Anzalone GC, Pearce JM. Open-source syringe pump library. PLoS One. 2014;9, e107216.

32. Connor SB, Quill TJ, Jacobs JR. Accuracy of drug infusion pumps under computer control. IEEE Trans Biomed Eng. 1992;39:980–2.

33. Schraag S, Flaschar J. Delivery performance of commercial target-controlled infusion devices with Diprifusor module. Eur J Anaesthesiol. 2002;19:357–60.

34. Weiss M, Fischer J, Neff T, Baenziger O. The effects of syringe plunger design on drug delivery during vertical displacement of syringe pumps. Anaesthesia. 2000;55:1094–8.

35. Neff T, Fischer J, Fehr S, Baenziger O, Weiss M. Start-up delays of infusion syringe pumps. Paediatr Anaesth. 2001;11:561–5.

36. Kim JY, Moon BK, Lee JH, Jo YY, Min SK. Impact of priming the infusion system on the performance of target-controlled infusion of remifentanil. Korean J Anesthesiol. 2013;64:407–13.

37. Neff T, Fischer J, Fehr S, Baenziger O, Weiss M. Evaluation of the FASTSTART mode for reducing start-up delay in syringe pump infusion systems. Swiss Med Wkly. 2001;131:219–22.

38. Chae YJ, Kim JY, Kim DW, Moon BK, Min SK. False selection of syringe-brand compatibility and the method of correction during target-controlled infusion of propofol. Korean J Anesthesiol. 2013;64:251–6.

39. Schmidt N, Saez C, Seri I, Maturana A. Impact of syringe size on the performance of infusion pumps at low flow rates. Pediatr Crit Care Med. 2010;11:282–6.

40. Weiss M, Banziger O, Neff T, Fanconi S. Influence of infusion line compliance on drug delivery rate during acute line loop formation. Intensive Care Med. 2000;26:776–9.

41. Neff SB, Neff TA, Gerber S, Weiss MM. Flow rate, syringe size and architecture are critical to start-up performance of syringe pumps. Eur J Anaesthesiol. 2007;24:602–8.

42. Weiss M, Fischer J, Neff T, Schulz G, Banziger O. Do antisiphon valves reduce flow irregularities during vertical displacement of infusion pump systems? Anaesth Intensive Care. 2000;28:680–3.

43. Lannoy D, Decaudin B, Dewulf S, Simon N, Secq A, Barthelemy C, Debaene B, Odou P. Infusion set characteristics such as antireflux valve and dead-space volume affect drug delivery: an experimental study designed to enhance infusion sets. Anesth Analg. 2010;111:1427–31.

44. McCarroll C, McAtamney D, Taylor R. Alteration in flow delivery with antisyphon devices. Anaesthesia. 2000;55:355–7.

45. Decaudin B, Dewulf S, Lannoy D, Simon N, Secq A, Barthelemy C, Debaene B, Odou P. Impact of multiaccess infusion devices on in vitro drug delivery during multi-infusion therapy. Anesth Analg. 2009;109:1147–55.
46. Timmerman AM, Snijder RA, Lucas P, Lagerweij MC, Radermacher JH, Konings MK. How physical infusion system parameters cause clinically relevant dose deviations after setpoint changes. Biomed Tech (Berl). 2015;60:365–76.
47. Schulz G, Fischer J, Neff T, Banziger O, Weiss M. The effect of air within the infusion syringe on drug delivery of syringe pump infusion systems. Anaesthesist. 2000;49:1018–23.
48. Davey C, Stather-Dunn T. Very small air bubbles (10 - 70 microl) cause clinically significant variability in syringe pump fluid delivery. J Med Eng Technol. 2005;29:130–6.
49. Adapa RM, Axell RG, Mangat JS, Carpenter TA, Absalom AR. Safety and performance of TCI pumps in a magnetic resonance imaging environment. Anaesthesia. 2012;67:33–9.
50. Bell J, Weaver LK, Deru K. Performance of the Hospira Plum A plus (HB) hyperbaric infusion pump. Undersea Hyperb Med. 2014;41:235–43.
51. Lavon H, Shupak A, Tal D, Ziser A, Abramovich A, Yanir Y, Shoshani O, Gil A, Leiba R, Nachum Z. Performance of infusion pumps during hyperbaric conditions. Anesthesiology. 2002;96:849–54.
52. Dyck JB, Shafer SL. Effects of age on propofol pharmacokinetics. Semin Anesth. 1992;11:2–4.
53. Gepts E, Camu F, Cockshott ID, Douglas EJ. Disposition of propofol administered as constant rate intravenous infusions in humans. Anesth Analg. 1987;66:1256–63.
54. Kataria BK, Ved SA, Nicodemus HF, Hoy GR, Lea D, Dubois MY, Mandema JW, Shafer SL. The pharmacokinetics of propofol in children using three different data analysis approaches. Anesthesiology. 1994;80:104–22.
55. Marsh B, White M, Morton N, Kenny GN. Pharmacokinetic model driven infusion of propofol in children. Br J Anaesth. 1991;67:41–8.
56. Schuttler J, Stoeckel H, Schwilden H. Pharmacokinetic and pharmacodynamic modelling of propofol ('Diprivan') in volunteers and surgical patients. Postgrad Med J. 1985;61 Suppl 3:53–4.
57. Schuttler J, Ihmsen H. Population pharmacokinetics of propofol: a multicenter study. Anesthesiology. 2000;92:727–38.
58. Absalom A, Kenny G. 'Paedfusor' pharmacokinetic data set. Br J Anaesth. 2005;95:110.
59. Absalom A, Amutike D, Lal A, White M, Kenny GN. Accuracy of the 'Paedfusor' in children undergoing cardiac surgery or catheterization. Br J Anaesth. 2003;91:507–13.
60. Tackley RM, Lewis GT, Prys-Roberts C, Boaden RW, Dixon J, Harvey JT. Computer controlled infusion of propofol. Br J Anaesth. 1989;62:46–53.
61. Lemmens HJ, Burm AG, Hennis PJ, Gladines MP, Bovill JG. Influence of age on the pharmacokinetics of alfentanil. Gender dependence. Clin Pharmacokinet. 1990;19:416–22.
62. Maitre PO, Vozeh S, Heykants J, Thomson DA, Stanski DR. Population pharmacokinetics of alfentanil: the average dose-plasma concentration relationship and interindividual variability in patients. Anesthesiology. 1987;66:3–12.
63. Scott JC, Stanski DR. Decreased fentanyl and alfentanil dose requirements with age. A simultaneous pharmacokinetic and pharmacodynamic evaluation. J Pharmacol Exp Ther. 1987;240:159–66.
64. Hudson RJ, Thomson IR, Cannon JE, Friesen RM, Meatherall RC. Pharmacokinetics of fentanyl in patients undergoing abdominal aortic surgery. Anesthesiology. 1986;64:334–8.
65. McClain DA, Hug Jr CC. Intravenous fentanyl kinetics. Clin Pharmacol Ther. 1980;28:106–14.
66. Shafer SL, Varvel JR, Aziz N, Scott JC. Pharmacokinetics of fentanyl administered by computer-controlled infusion pump. Anesthesiology. 1990;73:1091–102.
67. Varvel JR, Shafer SL, Hwang SS, Coen PA, Stanski DR. Absorption characteristics of transdermally administered fentanyl. Anesthesiology. 1989;70:928–34.
68. Egan TD, Lemmens HJ, Fiset P, Hermann DJ, Muir KT, Stanski DR, Shafer SL. The pharmacokinetics of the new short-acting opioid remifentanil (GI87084B) in healthy adult male volunteers. Anesthesiology. 1993;79:881–92.
69. Minto CF, Schnider TW, Egan TD, Youngs E, Lemmens HJM, Gambus PL, Billard V, Hoke JF, Moore KHP, Hermann DJ, Muir KT, Mandema JW, Shafer SL. Influence of age and gender on the pharmacokinetics and pharmacodynamics of remifentanil. I. Model development. Anesthesiology. 1997;86:10–23.
70. Minto CF, Schnider TW, Shafer SL. Pharmacokinetics and pharmacodynamics of remifentanil. II. Model application. Anesthesiology. 1997;86:24–33.
71. Bovill JG, Sebel PS, Blackburn CL, Oei-Lim V, Heykants JJ. The pharmacokinetics of sufentanil in surgical patients. Anesthesiology. 1984;61:502–6.
72. Gepts E, Shafer SL, Camu F, Stanski DR, Woestenborghs R, Van Peer A, Heykants JJ. Linearity of pharmacokinetics and model estimation of sufentanil. Anesthesiology. 1995;83:1194–204.
73. Arden JR, Holley FO, Stanski DR. Increased sensitivity to etomidate in the elderly: initial distribution versus altered brain response. Anesthesiology. 1986;65:19–27.
74. Domino EF, Domino SE, Smith RE, Domino LE, Goulet JR, Domino KE, Zsigmond EK. Ketamine kinetics in unmedicated and diazepam-premedicated subjects. Clin Pharmacol Ther. 1984;36:645–53.
75. Greenblatt DJ, Abernethy DR, Locniskar A, Harmatz JS, Limjuco RA, Shader RI. Effect of age, gender, and obesity on midazolam kinetics. Anesthesiology. 1984;61:27–35.
76. Stanski DR, Maitre PO. Population pharmacokinetics and pharmacodynamics of thiopental: the effect of age revisited. Anesthesiology. 1990;72:412–22.
77. Sorbo S, Hudson RJ, Loomis JC. The pharmacokinetics of thiopental in pediatric surgical patients. Anesthesiology. 1984;61:666–70.
78. Kirkpatrick T, Cockshott ID, Douglas EJ, Nimmo WS. Pharmacokinetics of propofol (diprivan) in elderly patients. Br J Anaesth. 1988;60:146–50.
79. Shafer A, Doze VA, Shafer SL, White PF. Pharmacokinetics and pharmacodynamics of propofol infusions during general anesthesia. Anesthesiology. 1988;69:348–56.
80. van den Broek L, Wierda JM, Smeulers NJ, van Santen GJ, Leclercq MG, Hennis PJ. Clinical pharmacology of rocuronium (Org 9426): study of the time course of action, dose requirement, reversibility, and pharmacokinetics. J Clin Anesth. 1994;6:288–96.
81. Coetzee JF, Glen JB, Wium CA, Boshoff L. Pharmacokinetic model selection for target controlled infusions of propofol. Assessment of three parameter sets. Anesthesiology. 1995;82:1328–45.
82. Short TG, Lim TA, Tam YH. Prospective evaluation of pharmacokinetic model-controlled infusion of propofol in adult patients. Br J Anaesth. 1996;76:313–5.
83. Oei-Lim VL, White M, Kalkman CJ, Engbers FH, Makkes PC, Ooms WG. Pharmacokinetics of propofol during conscious sedation using target-controlled infusion in anxious patients undergoing dental treatment. Br J Anaesth. 1998;80:324–31.
84. Barvais L, Rausin I, Glen JB, Hunter SC, D'Hulster D, Cantraine F, d'Hollander A. Administration of propofol by target-controlled infusion in patients undergoing coronary artery surgery. J Cardiothorac Vasc Anesth. 1996;10:877–83.

85. Pandin PC, Cantraine F, Ewalenko P, Deneu SC, Coussaert E, d'Hollander AA. Predictive accuracy of target-controlled propofol and sufentanil coinfusion in long-lasting surgery. Anesthesiology. 2000;93:653–61.

86. Sabate Tenas S, Soler Corbera J, Queralto Companyo JM, Baxarias Gascon P. Predictive capability of the TCI Diprifusor system in patients with terminal chronic renal insufficiency. Rev Esp Anestesiol Reanim. 2003;50:381–7.

87. Cavaliere F, Conti G, Moscato U, Meo F, Pennisi MA, Costa R, Proietti R. Hypoalbuminaemia does not impair Diprifusor performance during sedation with propofol. Br J Anaesth. 2005;94:453–8.

88. Li YH, Xu JH, Yang JJ, Tian J, Xu JG. Predictive performance of 'Diprifusor' TCI system in patients during upper abdominal surgery under propofol/fentanyl anesthesia. J Zhejiang Univ Sci B. 2005;6:43–8.

89. Wu J, Zhu SM, He HL, Weng XC, Huang SQ, Chen YZ. Plasma propofol concentrations during orthotopic liver transplantation. Acta Anaesthesiol Scand. 2005;49:804–10.

90. Wietasch JK, Scholz M, Zinserling J, Kiefer N, Frenkel C, Knufermann P, Brauer U, Hoeft A. The performance of a target-controlled infusion of propofol in combination with remifentanil: a clinical investigation with two propofol formulations. Anesth Analg. 2006;102:430–7.

91. Albertin A, Poli D, La Colla L, Gonfalini M, Turi S, Pasculli N, La Colla G, Bergonzi PC, Dedola E, Fermo I. Predictive performance of 'Servin's formula' during BIS-guided propofol-remifentanil target-controlled infusion in morbidly obese patients. Br J Anaesth. 2007;98:66–75.

92. La Colla L, Albertin A, La Colla G, Ceriani V, Lodi T, Porta A, Aldegheri G, Mangano A, Khairallah I, Fermo I. No adjustment vs. adjustment formula as input weight for propofol target-controlled infusion in morbidly obese patients. Eur J Anaesthesiol. 2009;26:362–9.

93. Cowley NJ, Hutton P, Clutton-Brock TH. Assessment of the performance of the Marsh model in effect site mode for target controlled infusion of propofol during the maintenance phase of general anaesthesia in an unselected population of neurosurgical patients. Eur J Anaesthesiol. 2013;30:627–32.

94. Cortinez LI, De la Fuente N, Eleveld DJ, Oliveros A, Crovari F, Sepulveda P, Ibacache M, Solari S. Performance of propofol target-controlled infusion models in the obese: pharmacokinetic and pharmacodynamic analysis. Anesth Analg. 2014;119:302–10.

95. Tachibana N, Niiyama Y, Yamakage M. Evaluation of bias in predicted and measured propofol concentrations during target-controlled infusions in obese Japanese patients: an open-label comparative study. Eur J Anaesthesiol. 2014;31:701–7.

96. Sitsen E, Olofsen E, Lesman A, Dahan A, Vuyk J. Epidural blockade affects the pharmacokinetics of propofol in surgical patients. Anesth Analg. 2015;122:1341–9. doi:10.1213/ANE.0000000000001090.

97. Mathew PJ, Sailam S, Sivasailam R, Thingnum SK, Puri GD. Performance of target-controlled infusion of propofol using two different pharmacokinetic models in open heart surgery - a randomised controlled study. Perfusion. 2016;31:45–53.

98. Lim TA, Gin T, Tam YH, Aun CS, Short TG. Computer-controlled infusion of propofol for long neurosurgical procedures. J Neurosurg Anesthesiol. 1997;9:242–9.

99. La Colla L, Albertin A, La Colla G, Porta A, Aldegheri G, Di Candia D, Gigli F. Predictive performance of the 'Minto' remifentanil pharmacokinetic parameter set in morbidly obese patients ensuing from a new method for calculating lean body mass. Clin Pharmacokinet. 2010;49:131–9.

100. Mertens MJ, Engbers FH, Burm AG, Vuyk J. Predictive performance of computer-controlled infusion of remifentanil during propofol/remifentanil anaesthesia. Br J Anaesth. 2003;90:132–41.

101. Absalom AR, Lee M, Menon DK, Sharar SR, De Smet T, Halliday J, Ogden M, Corlett P, Honey GD, Fletcher PC. Predictive performance of the Domino, Hijazi, and Clements models during low-dose target-controlled ketamine infusions in healthy volunteers. Br J Anaesth. 2007;98:615–23.

102. Panchatsharam S. Callaghan M, Day R. Measured versus predicted blood propofol concentrations in children during scoliosis surgery. Anesth Analg: Sury MR; 2014.

103. Johnson KB, Kern SE, Hamber EA, McJames SW, Kohnstamm KM, Egan TD. Influence of hemorrhagic shock on remifentanil: a pharmacokinetic and pharmacodynamic analysis. Anesthesiology. 2001;94:322–32.

104. Masui K, Upton RN, Doufas AG, Coetzee JF, Kazama T, Mortier EP, Struys MM. The performance of compartmental and physiologically based recirculatory pharmacokinetic models for propofol: a comparison using bolus, continuous, and target-controlled infusion data. Anesth Analg. 2010;111:368–79.

How to Select a PK/PD Model

10

Kenichi Masui

PK Model and Predicted Plasma Concentration

To control the drug effect, not the infusion rate but the drug concentration should be titrated. For volatile anesthetics, inhaled and exhaled concentration can be measured in real time using a commercial device. For propofol, exhaled concentration can also be measured in real time under experimental settings [1], and blood concentration can be measured intermittently [2]. However, the measurement of the real concentration of intravenous drugs is not general in daily anesthesia practice.

When the drug is administered by a bolus and/or infusion, estimation of the achieved drug concentrations is not easy without the use of a computer. Figure 10.1 shows three time courses of propofol plasma concentration at 8 mg/kg/h for 60 min without or with an initial bolus (1 or 2 mg/kg), given to a 70 kg adult patient, calculated using the pharmacokinetic model developed by Marsh et al. [3].

During a constant rate infusion, the propofol plasma concentration may increase or decrease. A simulation of the time course of propofol plasma concentration after a 2 mg/kg bolus followed by an infusion at 8 mg/kg/h (bold line in Fig. 10.1) shows that the propofol plasma concentration decreases monotonically after it has reached a peak (after the end of bolus infusion) and then increases monotonically 15 min after the start of propofol administration.

Dose regimen also influences the plasma concentration during a constant rate infusion. In Fig. 10.1, the propofol plasma concentrations are different among three dose regimens, especially during the first 10 min. For example, at 8 min after the start of propofol administration, the plasma concentrations are 2.0 μg/ml if no bolus was given (thin solid line in Fig. 10.1), 2.7 μg/ml with a 1 mg/kg bolus (bold

dashed line in Fig. 10.1), and 3.4 μg/ml with a 2 mg/kg bolus (bold solid line in Fig. 10.1). These examples illustrate that the context of the dosing influences the relationship between the infusion rate and plasma drug concentration.

Pharmacokinetic parameters are used to estimate plasma concentration of a drug. The following simple calculation estimates the drug concentration at steady state (C_{ss}):

$$C_{ss} = \text{infusion rate} / CL_{tot} \qquad (10.1)$$

where infusion rate is the infusion rate of the drug and CL_{tot} is the total body clearance of the drug. In anesthetic practice, this equation can be used to give a rough estimation of drug concentration. However, it is difficult to know when steady state is established.

Pharmacokinetic model parameters can be used to estimate the time course of drug concentration as shown in the above examples (Fig. 10.1). The following differential equations describe a three-compartment pharmacokinetic model (Fig. 10.2):

$$\frac{dA_1}{dt} = \text{Dose} - (k_{10} + k_{12} + k_{13}) \cdot A_1 + k_{21} \cdot A_2 + k_{31} \cdot A_3$$

$$\frac{dA_2}{dt} = k_{12} \cdot A_1 - k_{21} \cdot A_2$$

$$\frac{dA_3}{dt} = k_{13} \cdot A_1 - k_{31} \cdot A_3$$

$$k_{10} = \frac{CL_1}{V_1}, k_{12} = \frac{CL_2}{V_1}, k_{13} = \frac{CL_3}{V_1}, k_{21} = \frac{CL_2}{V_2}, k_{31} = \frac{CL_3}{V_3}$$

$$(10.2)$$

where A_i is the drug amount in the ith compartment, t is the time, dose is the infusion rate of the drug at time t, k_{10} is the elimination rate constant, k_{ij} is the equilibration rate constant between the ith and jth compartments, CL_i is the clearance for the ith compartment, and V_i is the distribution volume of the ith compartment. Predicted concentration of a drug can be easily obtained using simulation software incorporating

K. Masui, MD, PhD (✉)
Anesthesiology Department, National Defense Medical College Hospital, Namiki 3-2, Tokorozawa, Saitama 359-8513, Japan
e-mail: kenichi@masuinet.com

A.R. Absalom, K.P. Mason (eds.), *Total Intravenous Anesthesia and Target Controlled Infusions*, DOI 10.1007/978-3-319-47609-4_10

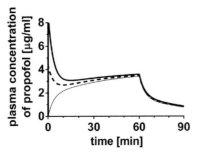

Fig. 10.1 Time course of plasma propofol concentrations arising from three different dosing schemes. All three time courses show the predicted plasma concentration of propofol administered at 8 mg/kg/h for 60 min without (*thin solid line*) or with an initial bolus of 1 mg/kg (*bold dashed line*) or 2 mg/kg (*bold solid line*). Predicted concentrations were calculated using the pharmacokinetic model developed by Marsh et al. [3]

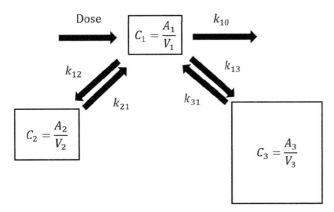

Fig. 10.2 Three-compartment model. A simple mathematical three-compartment pharmacokinetic model. When a drug is infused intravenously, the drug is infused into the central (the first) compartment (dose). In this compartment model, A_i is the drug amount in the ith compartment, and V_i is the distribution volume of the ith compartment. C_i is the drug concentration in the ith compartment, calculated as A_i/V_i. K_{10} is the elimination rate constant, and k_{ij} is the equilibration rate constant between the ith and jth compartments. Generally, C_1 is the plasma or blood concentration of the drug. The differential equations of a three-compartment model are shown in Eq. 10.2

these equations with pharmacokinetic parameter values (pharmacokinetic model).

Predicted concentration is a good alternative to measured concentration of intravenous drug to see the drug concentration. The prediction of drug concentrations using pharmacokinetic models offers not only an estimation of the present concentration but also the time course of the concentration throughout the past, present, and future. Accordingly, predicted concentration helps to assess and control the drug effect in clinical practice. After assessing the concentration–clinical effect relationship of the drug using the past and present drug concentrations, the anesthesiologist can make a dosing plan using the predicted future drug concentrations.

However, there are two problems with the use of predicted plasma concentrations to control the drug effect. One is that the plasma is not the effect site for the main indications for the

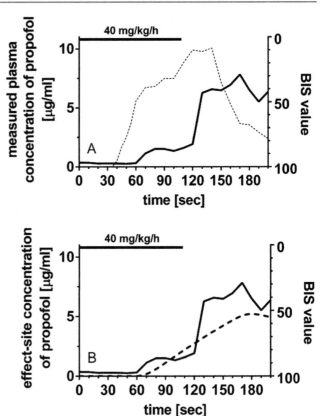

Fig. 10.3 The relationship between propofol concentration and propofol effect against time. (**a**) Time courses of measured plasma concentration of propofol and estimated propofol effect using a BIS monitor from a patient in our previous study [30]. Propofol was infused at 40 mg/kg/h for 108 s. A time delay is observed between the measured plasma concentration of propofol and estimated BIS value. (**b**) Time courses of effect-site concentration of propofol and estimated propofol effect using a BIS monitor in the same patient as in Fig. 10.3a. There is no time delay between the effect-site concentration and BIS value. The effect-site concentration was estimated with the raw data of measured plasma propofol concentrations and BIS values from the same patients using an effect-site pharmacodynamic model (Fig. 10.4 and Eq. 10.3) and sigmoid E_{max} model (Eq. 10.4) [30]. In this case, an appropriate k_{e0} value is applied to calculate the effect-site concentration because the k_{e0} value was estimated for the specific individual. When a population k_{e0} value is used to estimate effect-site concentration, there may be a discrepancy between effect-site concentration and clinical effect because the population k_{e0} value may be different from individual k_{e0} value

anesthetics or opioids (see section "PD Model and Effect-Site Concentration"). The other is that the pharmacokinetic model may not appropriately estimate the plasma concentration of the drug over time (see section "Consideration of Model Applicability").

PD Model and Effect-Site Concentration

The effect site for the main effects of the anesthetics and opioids is the brain or spinal cord. Therefore, a time delay is observed in the relationship between the plasma concentration and clinical effect. Figure 10.3a clearly shows the time

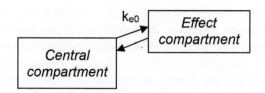

Fig. 10.4 Effect-compartment model. This is a simple scheme of the effect-compartment model. k_{e0} is the equilibration rate constant between the central compartment and the effect compartment, i.e., between the plasma concentration and the effect-site concentration of the drug. The predicted plasma concentration of the central compartment concentration is estimated by a compartment model (Fig. 10.2). Equilibration half-time may be a more intuitive concept than k_{e0} value, in describing the relationship between the plasma and effect-site concentrations. Equilibration half-time ($t_{1/2}k_{e0}$) is calculated as ln $2/k_{e0}$

delay between the measured plasma concentrations of propofol and estimated BIS values [4, 5].

To take this time delay into account, an effect-site pharmacodynamic model [6] (Fig. 10.4) can be applied using the following equation:

$$\frac{dC_e}{dt} = k_{e0}(C_1 - C_e) \qquad (10.3)$$

where C_e is the effect-site concentration, t is the time, k_{e0} is the equilibration rate constant between the plasma and effect site, and C_1 is the drug concentration in the central compartment of the compartment model. If the pharmacokinetic parameters for the compartment model (all k values in Eq. 10.2) and for the effect-site model (k_{e0} in Eq. 10.3) are obtained, effect-site concentration can be calculated. These parameters may be found in published literature.

To determine the k_{e0} value using Eq. 10.3, the observed plasma concentrations (C_1) and effect-site concentration (C_e) are necessary. However, effect-site concentration cannot be measured. Instead, the effect of the drug is observed, and an additional pharmacodynamic model such as a sigmoid E_{max} model is applied to determine the k_{e0}. The sigmoid E_{max} model is described using the following equation:

$$E = E_0 + (E_{max} - E_0) \cdot \frac{C_e^{\gamma}}{C_e^{\gamma} + EC_{50}^{\gamma}} \qquad (10.4)$$

where E is the observed drug effect, E_0 is the baseline measurement of the observed effect when no drug is present, E_{max} is the maximum possible drug effect, C_e is the estimated effect-site concentration, EC_{50} is the effect-site concentration associated with 50 % maximum drug effect, and γ is the steepness of the effect-site concentration versus effect relationship. When applying Eqs. 10.3 and 10.4 simultaneously with the observed effect of the drug and

the data of plasma concentrations, all the pharmacodynamic parameters including E_0, E_{max}, EC_{50}, γ, and k_{e0} will be estimated.

The estimated k_{e0} value enables calculation of the time course of the effect-site concentration. There is no time delay between the effect-site concentration and the drug effect when using the appropriate k_{e0} value (Fig. 10.3b). In experimental settings, estimation of the k_{e0} value is useful for pharmacodynamic analysis. In clinical practice, an estimate of the effect-site concentration is also useful because the effect-site concentration is expected to reflect the clinical effect. However, there are limitations of the use of k_{e0} values for predicting effect-site concentration. One important limitation is the significant interindividual variability of the k_{e0} value (see section "Consideration of Effect-Site Model Application").

Consideration of Model Applicability

The applicability of a pharmacokinetic/pharmacodynamic model should be considered carefully when using the model for prediction. The use of an inappropriate model may cause incorrect estimations of the relationship between the drug concentration and its effect, which may increase the risk of complications such as anesthetic awareness caused by inadequate doses and concentration-related drugs side effect arising from excessive doses.

In pharmacokinetic studies, a pharmacokinetic model is developed for either prediction or description. With prediction, the model is developed to predict the drug concentration for subjects other than the subjects from whom the model was developed. With description, the model is developed to describe the measured concentrations of collected samples in a group of subjects, for a pharmacokinetic analysis, which is not intended to be used for the prediction. A model developed for description may not be suitable for prediction of drug concentrations in other subjects.

To develop an appropriate population pharmacokinetic model, model validation is generally performed to evaluate the predictability of the developed final model using a validation data set not used for building the model and parameter estimation [7]. Two types of statistically robust validations are external and internal validation. To quantify the predictability of the developed model, some metrics are applied. Visual inspection of graphical displays is also applied to evaluate the predictability.

A validated pharmacokinetic model is one with evidence for prediction of the drug concentration. However, this may still be applicable to conditions that are applied during drug administration in the subjects of the validation data set.

External Validation

External validation is the most stringent type of validation [7]. For this type of validation, two data sets are needed. One is used for the model development, and the other is for testing the external validation of the model. It is possible to apply a data set from another experiment. For the validation, metrics and/or visual inspection is applied.

There are two types of external validation. For the first type, an example might be validation of a pharmacokinetic model that has been developed from data from subjects aged 30–60 years. For this model, the predictability (external validity) may be tested using a new data set from other subjects aged 30–60 years, or subjects aged 25–65 years, or something similar to the original age range. This is a standard external validation.

The other external validation procedure is extrapolation. The validation data set should include data from subjects with focused demographics (such as age and weight) involved in a study with specific methodology condition (sampling interval or duration) which is different from the demographics or methodology involved in the model development study. This external validation of the pharmacokinetic model may expand the applicability of the model to a different population. Short et al. developed a population pharmacokinetic model of propofol using the data set obtained from 3- to 10-year-old children [8]. Sepúlveda et al. evaluated the performance of the Short pharmacokinetic model using a data set obtained from children aged 3–26 months and found that the Short model had acceptable performance [9]. This external validation study has shown that the applicability of the Short model can be expanded from the age group of the original subjects (3–10 years) to a wide age group (3 months–10 years).

Internal Validation

External validation is the most robust but needs two data sets, i.e., more subjects and samples, requiring more resources, such as man power, time, and cost, during the model development procedure. Internal validation is a method of using all the data collected data for the model development itself. Internal validation is always considered when external validation is not applied. Resampling techniques such as bootstrapping [10] and cross validation [10] and prediction-corrected visual predictive check [11] are used.

An internally validated pharmacokinetic model may be used to predict drug concentrations in patients whose age is within the range of the study population used for the model development. However, it is possible that this method of validation also involves extrapolation, because age is not the only factor that might have influenced the results of the pharmacokinetic model. Before an internally validated model is used to predict drug concentrations in a patient, it should be considered whether the patient characteristics and other dosing conditions and methods are similar to (strictly, within the range of) those used in the subjects from whom the original model was developed. The types of the factors that must be considered are explained below (see section "Subject Characteristics and Methods Used for Development of a PK Model to be Applied for Prediction").

"Validation" or "Evaluation"

"Validation" is a strong term. A "validated" pharmacokinetic model should be suitable for prediction of drug concentrations in samples taken from subjects with different characteristics and using different dosing and study methods.

To confirm the model's validity for various conditions, the data set for the external validation should include those conditions. However, it is common for the external validation data set to only include a limited number of the subjects under limited conditions. In other words, an external validation procedure generally only confirms a limited range of external validity.

Yano, Beal, and Sheiner proposed the use of the term of "evaluation": "We use the weaker term 'evaluation' rather than the stronger one 'validation', as we believe one cannot truly validate a model, except perhaps in the very special case that one can both specify the complete set of alternative models that must be excluded and one has sufficient data to attain a preset degree of certainty with which these alternatives would be excluded. We believe that such cases are rare at best" [12].

Performance Error Derivatives: Metrics

Quantitative indices (metrics) are used to evaluate the population model. In the study of anesthetic pharmacology, performance error derivatives proposed by Varvel et al. [13] are frequently used. The original aim to develop the derivatives is measuring the predictive performance of computer-control infusion pumps [14–16], which is a predecessor of target-controlled infusion pumps [17].

Performance Error (PE)

The performance error (PE, generally calculated as percentage performance error) of a model with regard to one blood sample is calculated using the following equation:

$$PE_{ij} = \frac{Cm_{ij} - Cp_{ij}}{Cp_{ij}} \times 100 \qquad (10.5)$$

where PE_{ij} is the performance error of jth sample in ith individual, Cm_{ij} is the measured (observed) drug concentration of jth sample in ith individual, and Cp_{ij} is the predicted drug concentration (using pharmacokinetic model) of jth sample in ith individual. This equation is standardized by predicted concentration. A PE value of zero means that the pharmacokinetic model predicted the concentration perfectly.

This standardization has several merits. When the difference between a Cm_{ij} and a Cp_{ij} is 1, the difference can be evaluated as small at a Cm_{ij} of 10, whereas the difference can be evaluated as large at a Cm_{ij} of 2. In this case, PE_{ij} is calculated to be 11 % ($Cm_{ij} = 10$ and $Cp_{ij} = 9$) or 100 % ($Cm_{ij} = 2$ and $Cp_{ij} = 1$). The standardization quantifies the difference in a similar manner to the idea of coefficient of variation, which shows the relative variability calculated as standard deviation divided by the mean. This standardization of PE_{ij} would be similar to the point of view of an anesthesiologist considering the drug concentration. Additionally, constant coefficient of variation models or lognormal models (similar to coefficient of variation models) as random effects is used to describe interindividual and intraindividual variability in population models [18]. This is one advantage of using PE_{ij}.

Another further strength is that predicted concentrations, and not measured concentrations, are used as standard. In clinical and research work, clinicians and researchers are almost always dealing with predicted concentrations instead of measured concentration. Therefore, the use of predicted concentration as standard is reasonable.

During model evaluation, the term "prediction error" may be used instead of "performance error." With respect to this term, the equations of PE and PE derivatives are the same.

In standard pharmacometrics, the performance error is calculated as ODV minus PDV, where ODV is the value of the observed dependent variable, e.g., observed drug concentration, and PDV is the value of the predicted dependent variable. This is the same concept as used in an additive error model for interindividual and intraindividual variability in population models [18].

Performance Error Derivatives and Visual Inspection of the Model

There are four original performance error derivatives, namely, median absolute performance error (MDAPE), median performance error (MDPE), divergence, and wobble.

MDAPE indicates the inaccuracy of the prediction. In the ith subject,

$$MDAPE_i = median\{|PE_{ij}|, j = 1, 2, \cdots, N_i\} \qquad (10.6)$$

where $MDAPE_i$ is MDAPE of the ith subject, PE_{ij} is the performance error of the jth sample in the ith subject (Eq. 10.5), and N_i is the number of |PE| values obtained from the ith subject. The closer to zero the $MDAPE_i$, the more accurate the model for prediction of concentrations in the ith individual.

MDPE reflects the bias of the prediction. In the ith subject:

$$MDPE_i = median\{PE_{ij}, j = 1, 2, \cdots, N_i\} \qquad (10.7)$$

where $MDPE_i$ is MDPE of the ith subject, PE_{ij} is the performance error of the jth sample in the ith subject (Eq. 10.5), and N_i is the number of PE values obtained from the ith subject. An $MDPE_i$ of zero means that the model has no bias in its prediction of concentrations in the ith subject. An MDPE larger or smaller than zero indicates underprediction (i.e., measured concentration > predicted concentration) or overprediction (i.e., predicted concentration > measured concentration), respectively.

Divergence shows the rate of change of absolute performance error against time. $Divergence_i$ (generally expressed in %/h) is calculated as the slope of the linear regression of absolute performance error versus time. A negative value of divergence indicates that the predicted concentration comes closer to measured concentration over time.

Wobble quantifies the intraindividual variability of the prediction error. In the ith subject:

$$Wobble_i = median\{|PE_{ij}\text{-}MDPE_i|, j = 1, 2, \cdots, N_i\} \qquad (10.8)$$

where $Wobble_i$ is wobble of the ith subject, PE_{ij} is the performance error of the jth sample in the ith subject (Eq. 10.5), $MDPE_i$ is the median performance error in the ith subject (Eq. 10.7), and N_i is the number of PE values obtained from the ith subject. The smaller value of the wobble, the more stable the predictions of the pharmacokinetic model.

The population estimate for each of these performance error derivatives is generally calculated as the mean of the individual estimates. For example, population MDPE is calculated using the following equation:

$$MDPE = mean\{MDPE_i, i = 1, 2, \cdots, N\} \qquad (10.9)$$

where $MDPE_i$ is MDPE of the ith subject and N is the number of the subjects in the population.

Two Types of Divergence

As mentioned above, the original divergence parameter proposed by Varvel was the measure of divergence of APE, calculated as the slope of the linear regression of absolute performance error over time. Since then another divergence parameter has been proposed, which is divergence in PE, calculated as the slope of the linear regression of performance error over time [19]. Glen et al. proposed the use of both divergence parameters to evaluate the predictive performance of pharmacokinetic models [19]. Divergence APE and divergence PE reveal different information and may result in seemingly contradictory evaluations of a model as shown and explained in Fig. 10.5.

Acceptable Ranges of PE Derivatives

An MDPE between −20 and 20 % and an MDAPE <30 % during target-controlled infusion are regarded as acceptable [20, 21]. These can be used as criteria for external evaluation of a model. In many studies evaluating the accuracy of model prediction [9, 22, 23], expected performance of drug delivery devices such as target-controlled infusion pumps tends to be an MDPE of around 20–30 % [24].

There are no published criteria for acceptable values of divergence and wobble. A divergence APE <3–5 %/h and divergence PE between −5 and −3 %/h and between 3 and 5 %/h may be acceptable. A divergence APE of 3–5 %/h means absolute performance error increases 30–50 % over 10 h. A larger than 50 % increase of APE seems to be unacceptable. For target-controlled infusions of propofol, positive divergence PE is more preferable than negative one. As a negative divergence PE means that PE decreases against time, implying that the measured concentration is decreasing relative to the predicted concentration, there is a risk of awareness in this case.

It is difficult to define an acceptable value of wobble because not only will the accuracy and relevance of the prediction model parameters influence performance, but wobble may also be influenced by physiological factors

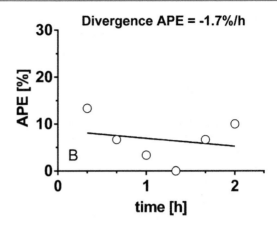

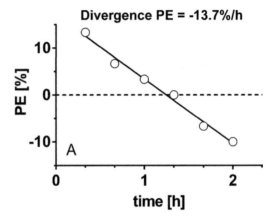

Fig. 10.5 Two types of divergence. Six absolute performance errors (APE) and performance errors (PE) obtained from six pairs of measured and predicted drug concentrations during 2 h are depicted in **a** and **b**, respectively. For this data set, original divergence (divergence APE) is −1.7 %/h, which indicates that the APE decreases to zero versus time, i.e., predicted concentration is getting closer to measured concentration as time progresses. On the other hand, divergence PE is −13.7 %/h, which indicates PE decreases 13.7 %/h over time. The decrement of PE means that measured concentration decreases against predicted concentration over time. When the drug is administered using target-controlled infusion, measured concentration gradually decreases. Therefore, a pharmacokinetic model with large negative divergence PE is associated with an increased risk of insufficient drug effect. The two types of divergence, original divergence (divergence APE) and divergence PE, provide different information

such as cardiac output or uncompensated bleeding [25–27] that may increase the intraindividual variability of the prediction. By definition the wobble value will be less than MDAPE (Eq. 10.8).

Limitation of Performance Error Standardized by Predicted Concentration

As explained above, there are both advantages and disadvantages of using performance error standardized by predicted concentration (Eq. 10.5).

Performance error has a minimum value of -100% when the measured concentration is zero but can theoretically be infinitely large (e.g., when a measured value is high, while the predicted value is close to zero). This means that the evaluation using this PE is asymmetric with respect to overprediction and underprediction. For example, consider the two combinations of measured and predicted concentrations, respectively, "2 µg/ml and 3 µg/ml" (overprediction) versus "3 µg/ml and 2 µg/ml" (underprediction). For the overprediction combination, the prediction error is -33.3%, whereas for the underprediction combination the prediction error is 50%. When using performance error standardized by predicted concentration (Eq. 10.5), a model overestimating the concentration tends to be assessed as better than a model underestimating the concentration. This estimation tendency is preferable to avoid higher (but not lower) measured concentrations.

Possible Alternatives of Performance Error

To obtain symmetry in the performance error, a modification of performance error, or another index, is necessary.

We previously developed another index as an alternative to performance error defined using the Eq. 10.5. During the evaluation of a pharmacokinetic model, plots are often made of Cm/Cp (the ratio of measured to predicted concentrations) displayed against a variable such as time or predicted concentration. These plots are often described as goodness of fit plots (explained in the next section) [22, 28, 29]. For these plots, a logarithmic y-axis is used for Cm/Cp. On any logarithmic axis, by definition Y and 1/Y are symmetrical because y = Y and y = 1/Y are equidistant from y = 1. Accordingly, we proposed the log-transformed value of Cm/Cp as a new index [22]. To calculate this index, the following equation is applied:

$$ \mathrm{PE}_{ij} = \log\left(\frac{Cm_{ij}}{Cp_{ij}}\right) \quad (10.10) $$

where PE_{ij} is the performance error of jth sample in ith individual, Cm_{ij} is the measured (observed) drug concentration of jth sample in ith individual, and Cp_{ij} is the predicted drug concentration of jth sample in ith individual. When a pharmacokinetic model predicts a single sample perfectly (i.e., $Cm_{ij} = Cp_{ij}$), prediction error is 0, which is the same value for perfect prediction using Eq. 10.5. For all imperfect predictions, the performance errors calculated by Eqs. 10.5 and 10.10 are different.

Equation 10.10 can be rearranged to:

$$ Cm_{ij} = 10^{PE_{ij}} \cdot Cp_{ij} \quad (10.11) $$

A value of 1 for PE_{ij} means that Cm_{ij} is ten times Cp_{ij}, and a value of -1 means that Cm_{ij} is one-tenth of Cp_{ij}. The PE values calculated using Eq. 10.10 are distributed symmetrically on a linearly scaled axis (not logarithmic axis). Using this logarithmic transformation, we can calculate PE derivatives of MDAPE (Eq. 10.6), MDPE (Eq. 10.7), divergences (divergence APE and divergence PE), and wobble (Eq. 10.8).

The meaning of the ratio Cm/Cp is intuitive. However, the values of PE calculated using either Eqs. 10.5 or 10.10 are quite different, e.g., when Cm is 4.5 and Cp is 3, PE is calculated to be 50% by Eq. 10.5 or to be 0.18 by Eq. 10.10 (Fig. 10.6). Therefore, it is difficult to compare PE derivatives from Eq. 10.10 with ones calculated from Eq. 10.5 [22].

Another PE definition can be considered:

$$ \mathrm{PE}_{ij} = \begin{cases} \dfrac{Cm_{ij} - Cp_{ij}}{Cp_{ij}} \times 100 & \left[\text{if } Cm_{ij} \geq Cp_{ij}\right] \\[2ex] \dfrac{Cm_{ij} - Cp_{ij}}{Cm_{ij}} \times 100 & \left[\text{if } Cm_{ij} < Cp_{ij}\right] \end{cases} \quad (10.12) $$

where PE_{ij} is the performance error of jth sample in ith individual, Cm_{ij} is the measured (observed) drug concentration of jth sample in ith individual, and Cp_{ij} is the predicted drug concentration of jth sample in ith individual. The first equation is the same as Eq. 10.5. The second equation is added for the symmetry. For example, with this approach, the two combinations of measured and predicted concentrations, "2 and 3" (over prediction) and "3 and 2" (underprediction), are symmetric. For these concentration combinations, the prediction errors are -33.3% and 33.3%, respectively, using Eq. 10.12 (the latter prediction error is calculated to be 50% using Eq. 10.5).

Figure 10.6 shows the performance error distribution of different concentration combinations. With the PE defined by Eq. 10.5 (Fig. 10.6, Type A), the distribution of the PE is asymmetric with respect to the zero value of PE. On the other hand, the distribution of PEs is symmetric, when PE is defined according to Eq. 10.12 (Fig. 10.6, Type B) or Eq. 10.10 (Fig. 10.6, Type C). Only the PE values defined by Eq. 10.5 have a lower boundary (as mentioned the minimum value is -100%).

For PEs calculated using Eq. 10.5 (Fig. 10.6, Type A) and Eq. 10.12 (Fig. 10.6, Type B), the PE values are completely the same for any combination of Cm and Cp resulting in $PE \geq 0$. For example in Fig. 10.6, the circle or square for the

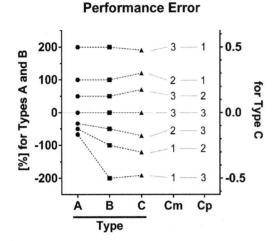

Fig. 10.6 Three types of performance error. The following are three different equations for calculation of the performance error (PE): A (Eq. 10.5) $PE = \frac{Cm-Cp}{Cp} \times 100$, B (Eq. 10.12)

$$PE = \begin{cases} \dfrac{Cm-Cp}{Cp} \times 100 \; [\text{if } Cm \geq Cp] \\ \dfrac{Cm-Cp}{Cm} \times 100 \; [\text{if } Cm < Cp] \end{cases}, \; C \; (\text{Eq. 10.10}) \; PE = \log\left(\frac{Cm}{Cp}\right),$$

where Cm is the measured (observed) concentration and Cp is the predicted concentration estimated using a pharmacokinetic model. Each *circle*, *square*, and *triangle* indicates each PE value

combination of "$Cm = 2$" and "$Cp = 1$" resulting in PE of 100 % has the same distance from the gray line for PE of zero (meaning perfect prediction). On the other hand, the PE value is different for any combination of Cm and Cp resulting in PE < 0. For example in Fig. 10.6, the PE values for the combination of "$Cm = 1$" and "$Cp = 2$" are −50 % with Eq. 10.5 (Fig. 10.6, Type A) and −100 % with Eq. 10.12 (Fig. 10.6, Type B) resulting in different distances from the gray line for PE of zero.

As mentioned above, the distribution of PE values is different when PE is calculated by Eq. 10.12 (Fig. 10.6, Type B) and Eq. 10.10 (Fig. 10.6, Type C). For example in Fig. 10.6, the concentration combination of "$Cm = 2$" and "$Cp = 1$" results in PE values of 200 % by Eq. 10.12 (Fig. 10.6, Type B) and 0.48 by Eq. 10.10 (Fig. 10.6, Type C).

All three PE definitions, by Eqs. 10.5, 10.10, and 10.12, have similar limitations. Firstly, when predicted concentration is zero, a PE value cannot be determined. If one use a simple compartment model such as two- or three-compartment model, predicted concentration is never zero except at the time before drug administration and at a long enough time (depending on total body clearance and accumulation of the drug) after the end of drug administration. However, it is possible that predicted concentrations reach zero a short period of time after the end of an infusion of an ultra-short-acting (rapidly cleared) drug. A predicted concentration of zero is also possible when using a complicated pharmacokinetic model, such as a simple compartment

model, with a lag time, a transit delay function [30], or an absorption model. In these cases, extra assumptions or different mathematical approaches are necessary to be able to calculate PE values for samples taken when the predicted concentration of zero [22].

Goodness of Fit Plots

To evaluate a pharmacokinetic model, different types of goodness of fit plots can be used to facilitate visual inspection of the data.

Observed Versus Predicted Variables

This goodness of fit plot shows the relationship between observed and predicted concentration in every sample on a two-dimensional graph (Fig. 10.7a). The predicted variable is displayed on a horizontal axis, logarithmically scaled. A vertical logarithmic axis indicates the observed variable. The axes should not be switched each other because the plot should describe the predictive ability of the model.

Each of the samples is commonly shown as independent point. In some cases, all the sample points from each individual are connected sequentially using lines. A line for identity (the line of y = x) is usually shown. A point on this line indicates that the prediction is perfect for that concentration.

A regression line or curve is usually fitted to the data using Friedman's supersmoother, a highly automated variable span smoother [31], and superimposed on the goodness of fit plot. The line or curve helps assessors evaluate the model prediction. When the model prediction is acceptable, the regression line or the Friedman's supersmoother curve lies near the line of identity.

Observed/Predicted Variables Versus Time

This variation of a goodness of fit plot shows the time course of Cm (measured or observed concentrations) divided by Cp (predicted concentrations) (Fig. 10.7b). The vertical (logarithmic) axis indicates the Cm/Cp ratio and the horizontal axis indicates time. A Friedman's supersmoother curve shown on this plot shows the prediction stability versus time. When a model has an excellent predictability, the smoother is depicted near the line of y = 1 over time.

When the regression line on this plot is estimated, the slope of this line is numerically the same as divergence PE calculated using Eq. 10.10. Thus, divergence PE is a quantitative (or summarized) index of this goodness of fit plot.

Observed/Predicted Variables Versus Predicted Variable

This goodness of fit plot shows the relation between Cm/Cp versus Cp (Fig. 10.7c). The vertical logarithmic axis

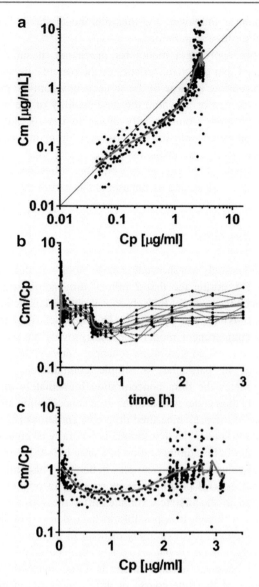

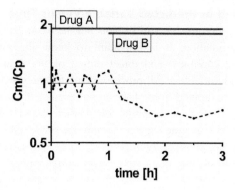

Fig. 10.8 Example of model performance during administration of two drugs. Each *filled circle* indicates the *Cm/Cp* ratio for a single blood sample for drug A in an individual. Drug A is infused for 3 h. Drug B is infused for 2 h, starting at 1 h after the start of drug A. A pharmacokinetic model for drug A predicts plasma concentrations well during the first hour but overestimates during the next 2 h. This overestimation may be caused by time effects and/or by the coadministration of drug B

Other Goodness of Fit Plots

Some investigators display goodness of fit plots using performance error instead of *Cm/Cp* ratio, e.g., performance error versus time or performance error versus *Cp*.

A plot with PE − $MDPE_i$ on the vertical normal axis, with time on the horizontal access, was used in a previous article to show two other types of goodness of fit plot [28]. One type shows one point per sample, and the other shows all individual regression lines whose slopes depict the individual divergence PE.

Interpreting Goodness of Fit Plots

When considering the interpretation of the plots, at least two steps are necessary.

At the first step, visual inspection of the plots should be performed without taking into account other factors, e.g., characteristics of the subjects or drug dosing methodology. When inspecting the plot of *Cm/Cp* versus time, the influence of time on the predictability should be assessed.

For the second step, the plots should be carefully inspected, this time taking into account other factors. An illustration involving another important factor follows (see also Fig. 10.8). Assume that drug A was infused for 3 hours. A 2 h infusion of drug B was started 1 h after the start of administration of the drug A. Figure 10.8 shows a hypothetical time course of *Cm/Cp* for drug A, showing overestimation of the concentration during the last 2 h. Is the cause of the underestimation just time? Without taking into account the administration of drug B, time seems to influence the predictions of the concentration of the drug A. However, it may be that the infusion of drug B inhibits the metabolism of drug A.

Fig. 10.7 Goodness of fit plots. These two-dimensional graphs show predictive performance of the pharmacokinetic model. Each *filled circle* indicates a sample in all figures. The *solid line* in (**a**) is the line of identity between measured concentration (*Cm*) and predicted concentration (*Cp*). *Dashed lines* connect all samples from each individual in (**b**). *Gray bold lines* indicate the Friedman's supersmoother curve

indicates the *Cm/Cp* ratio, and on the horizontal axis, the predicted variable is indicated on either a normal or a logarithmic scale. A Friedman's supersmoother added to this plot shows the prediction stability versus predicted variable. When a model has excellent predictability, the smoother will remain near the line of *y* = 1 over time.

Although this plot provides similar information to a plot of *Cm* versus *Cp* (in both plots horizontal axes indicate *Cp*, the predicted variable), this plot helps to focus attention on the predictive performance with respect to the magnitude of the predicted variable.

Observed or Predicted Variable Versus Time

These are not goodness of fit plots but the basic data for the model evaluation. It is important to know the raw data (observed variables) and direct output of the final model (predicted variables). All processed data for the goodness of fit plots are derived from observed and predicted variables.

Simultaneous presentation of predicted and observed variables versus time (instead of only the predicted variable versus time) may be preferable in some cases, as visual inspection of the plots may yield further insights into the data.

Subject Characteristics and Methods Used for Development of a PK Model to Be Applied for Prediction

In the previous section, the performance error derivatives such as MDPE and MDAPE, used for model evaluation, were explained. These metrics give an objective value of the overall model performance.

When the model is applied to a patient in clinical practice, the patient will a set of patient characteristics such as age and weight, and these may or may not be outside of the range of these characteristics of the subjects from whom the model was developed. However, the methodology used during drug administration and blood sampling in the development study is also very relevant and may influence the predictive performance of the model. Particularly relevant and important issues include method of dosing, sampling interval, and modeling approach.

Patient Characteristics

Age influences drug disposition [32–34]. For example, hepatic and renal clearances are lower in elderly subjects than in young adults. The ratios of body water, extracellular water, and fat in neonates are different from adults. Sex [35–37] and obesity [38–40] also influence drug disposition. The influence of these covariates depends on the drug characteristics. A population pharmacokinetic model often includes covariates in the calculation of pharmacokinetic parameters.

The parameter set of the Short model [8] only includes total body weight as a covariate. Therefore, predicted plasma propofol concentration can easily be calculated mathematically using the Short model in any patient. However, this model was developed using a blood concentration data set obtained from children from 3 to 10 years old and later evaluated using a data set from patients younger than 3 years. As there was no evaluation in adolescents and adults, the applicability of the Short model to adolescents

and adults is unknown, and thus this model should not be applied to these populations.

Before applying a model for prediction, it should be confirmed that the characteristics of the patients are similar and appropriate to those of the subjects in whom the model was developed or in whom the predictability of the model was confirmed. Commercially available devices such as target-controlled infusion pumps and drug information displays [41] automatically check that the patient characteristics are appropriate, but this relies on correct input of the patient data by the user at the start of the device.

Sampling Time

A previous study has shown that early blood samples (taken every 10 s during the first 2 min of drug administration) influenced the result of the subsequent pharmacokinetic and pharmacodynamic analysis [42]. This study clarified that a simple compartment model does not provide an accurate description of concentration changes shortly following injection. In particular, a simple compartment model overestimates the drug concentration immediately after a bolus and then underestimates the drug concentration around the time of the peak measured drug concentrations [22, 42].

In many studies the first sample is generally taken at least 1 min after bolus administration of a drug [43–45] to reduce the total volume of blood samples in human. This limits the ability of general pharmacokinetic models to predict concentration in the first few minutes after the start of drug infusion. Although it is possible to have dense samples in the early phase, it is extremely difficult to improve predictive ability in the early phase to predict drug concentration in the first minutes because there is large interindividual variability of the time course of drug concentration in the first minute [30].

Unless samples are taken long after the end of a drug infusion, predictive ability will tend to be weak for the period after an infusion has stopped. To develop a pharmacokinetic model capable of long-duration predictions, later samples are needed to adequately characterize the elimination phase. If a model is developed using blood samples collected during a continuous infusion and for only 30 min after the end of the infusion, it may not have predictability at 30 min or later after the end of infusion.

Sampling Site

Both arterial and venous samples are used for pharmacokinetic modeling. Theoretically, arterial and venous drug concentrations are the same at steady state. When the transit rate of the drug from the intravascular to the extravascular space is faster than that from the extravascular to the intravascular space, then arterial concentration will be higher than venous concentrations.

A previous study investigated the time course arterial and venous plasma concentrations of midazolam [46] during a 15 min infusion and up to 200 min afterward. Arterial concentrations of midazolam were higher during the infusion and lower after the infusion than venous concentrations of midazolam.

For pharmacodynamic modeling, whose aim is to describe continuous changes of clinical drug effect, arterial blood sampling has some distinct advantages [47]. When the effect-site concentration is calculated, a pharmacokinetic model developed using arterial samples may be better as input function to the pharmacodynamic model.

Method of Dosing

Infusion rate may influence the predictive performance of a pharmacokinetic model.

Our previous study clarified higher infusion rates were associated with more overprediction, when using the Marsh pharmacokinetic model, but not the Schnider, Schüttler, and Upton models for prediction of propofol concentrations [22]. Another study showed that the Gepts model [48] (the prototype model of the Marsh model) predicted propofol concentration appropriately during infusion and underestimated concentrations from 90 s and onward after the end of the infusion. A pharmacokinetic model developed from samples obtained after a bolus but without any continuous infusion may underestimate propofol plasma concentrations from subjects in subsequent study who receive an infusion [49].

Another factor that may influence predictability is the first-pass arterial concentration of the drug. The concept of a two-compartment recirculatory pharmacokinetic model is useful to understand the first-pass concentration [50]. In this concept, the total arterial drug concentration at any time is calculated as the sum of the first-pass concentration and the recirculated concentration. After the end of a drug infusion (except immediately after stopping the infusion), the first-pass concentration is zero. If a data set used for pharmacokinetic model development has a little or no information on drug concentrations during a continuous infusion, the model may underestimate the drug concentration, i.e., the model predictions of drug concentration may be lower than the measured concentrations. Commonly pharmacokinetic model analyses are performed with blood samples obtained after a bolus infusion. Most samples obtained with this procedure are thus taken during a period when no infusion of the drug was occurring.

Again, dosing regimen may influence the predictive performance of the pharmacokinetic model. Before the pharmacokinetic model is applied for prediction, it is better to confirm the details of the dosing regimen at the stages of model development and external evaluation.

Modeling Approach

Pharmacokinetic modeling approach is also thought to influence the predictive performance [44, 51, 52]. In a standard two-stage analysis [53], each of the population parameters is calculated as the mean of the individual parameters. If the sample size is small, or if the data set is unbalanced, this will result in several biased individual parameter estimates. Thus, the averaged parameters of the two-stage analysis may be inappropriate.

Dense sampling data is necessary for the standard two-stage approach. Modeling approaches such as nonlinear mixed effect modeling techniques are generally preferable for the more typical population modeling studies these days that only have available sparse sampling data.

Consideration of Effect-Site Model Application

To estimate the effect-site concentration of a drug, a pharmacodynamic parameter, k_{e0}, is necessary along with a pharmacokinetic parameter set.

For some drugs, many pharmacokinetic parameter sets have been published. An example is propofol for which more than 20 models have been published [9, 29, 54]. In some pharmacokinetic/pharmacodynamic studies, the k_{e0} value was simultaneously estimated with the pharmacokinetic parameters. In this case, one can apply the combination of the pharmacokinetic parameter sets and corresponding k_{e0} value to calculate the effect-site concentration if the model has acceptable predictive performance.

However, in standard pharmacokinetic studies, k_{e0} is not estimated because of a lack of pharmacodynamic data. As the k_{e0} value also depends on the associated pharmacokinetic model, it is necessary to integrate a pharmacokinetic parameter set from one study with a k_{e0} value from another study. For a k_{e0} value calculation, an alternative approach is to use "time-to-peak effect" with a pharmacokinetic parameter set [55]. With this method, numerical calculation of k_{e0} is performed based on time-to-peak effect data, using one equation along with pharmacokinetic parameter values.

Another approach to determine k_{e0} of propofol has been reported [56]. In this study, patients were randomized to an effect-site target-controlled infusion with 1 of 6 k_{e0} values. Once a desired level of sedation was reached, the target plasma concentration was locked at the effect-site concentration estimated at that time. The stability of objective measures of sedation/anesthesia was then recorded and examined. If there was a change over time in the measure of clinical effect, then the k_{e0} value was assumed to have been inaccurate. For sedative drugs, this approach enables calculation of a k_{e0} value for a population pharmacokinetic model without blood sampling. This approach relies heavily on the (unlikely) assumption that the pharmacodynamics of propofol do not change over time (i.e., that the relationship between effect-site concentration and depth of sedation or anesthesia is constant).

In some cases, several k_{e0} values have been linked with one pharmacokinetic model. For example, the Marsh pharmacokinetic model for adults [3] has two different k_{e0} values of 0.26 and 1.21 [57] incorporated into commercial target-controlled infusion devices. This difference is large (see section "Tips to Apply PK/PD Simulation"). The performance characteristics of the pharmacokinetic model with a k_{e0} may help to select one of the different k_{e0} values.

At pseudo-steady state, the change of the effect-site concentration over time is small and almost the same as the change in plasma concentration of the drug. In this situation, the existence and use of different k_{e0} values are not really relevant. The choice of k_{e0} is much more relevant when blood concentrations are changing, and the k_{e0} is used to estimate an effect-site concentration for clinical advisory purposes and for effect-site targeting, when the k_{e0} determines the level of plasma overshoot/undershoot with target concentration increases or decreases, respectively.

Fundamentally, the k_{e0} value is derived from population pharmacokinetic and pharmacodynamic estimates. Although a population k_{e0} is applied to an individual in anesthetic practice, discrepancy may exist between the true k_{e0} value in the individual and the population k_{e0} value.

Calculation of effect-site concentration is challenging. When using any k_{e0} value, one should be always aware that the applied k_{e0} may be inappropriate. When using the effect-site concentration target-controlled infusions, especially during and after target concentration changes, it is better to also use a monitor of pharmacodynamic effect, such as electroencephalogram-based monitoring.

Compartment Model Versus Physiological Model

A simple compartment model performs poorly in estimating drug concentrations in early phase after a bolus dose [42]. Physiological models seem to predict drug concentrations better than simple compartment models because they take into account hemodynamic factors such as cardiac output and blood flow to organs such as the liver and kidney.

Previously, we compared the predictive performance of three compartment models for propofol [22], developed by Marsh et al. [3], Schnider et al. [43], and Schüttler et al. [58], and one physiological model for propofol developed by Upton et al. [59]. The data sets for the evaluation were taken under four different conditions. Briefly, the "bolus" data set was taken after a 2.5 mg/kg bolus administered within 10 s with samples at 0.5, 1, 2, 3, 4, and 5 min after the start of administration. The "short infusion" data set was from subjects receiving an infusion of 1.2 mg/kg over 27–432 s at an infusion rate of 10–160 mg/kg/h, with samples taken every 5 s during the first 1 min, every 10 s during the second minute, and then at regular intervals of between 10 and 60 s until up to 530 s after the start of infusion. The "TCI" data set was taken during target-controlled infusion using the Marsh [3], Dyck [28], or Tackley [60] models over 33–206 min, with samples at 10–20 min after the start of propofol administration, at 2, 5, and 10 min after each adjustment of the targeted concentration, and every 15–20 min subsequently or just before adjusting the targeted concentration. The "long infusion" data set was taken during target-controlled drug delivery by the Schnider model over 110–245 min, with samples collected 1–7 times over the first 10 min after each 0.5 or 1.0 increment of effect-site concentration. The total number of the blood samples was 2155.

The former two data sets required the four evaluated pharmacokinetic models to predict propofol concentration in challenging circumstances. By definition subjects in the "bolus" data set had a sudden increase of the plasma concentration at around 30 sec and sudden decrease afterward. The "short infusion" data set includes dense samples especially in the first 2 min. The latter two data sets included samples at relatively stable conditions compared with those in opposite the other sets.

Contrary to expectation, the physiological model did not improve the predictive performance compared with the compartment models. For the overall prediction of concentrations achieved with the "bolus" and "short infusion" types of infusions, it is difficult for simple compartment models to predict the higher concentrations in the first minutes after the start of drug administration, whereas physiological model theoretically should perform better with these higher concentrations. However, there were discrepancies between the peak times of measured and predicted concentrations in most cases. For the prediction of the "TCI" and "long infusion" data sets, overall predictive ability was similar between the Schnider and Upton models with the exception of predictions of the higher concentrations.

An advantage of physiological models is that the model has a parameter for cardiac output. If the real-time change of cardiac output is used for the model prediction, the predictive ability may be improved. However, it is not common to estimate the cardiac output in clinical practice. If completely noninvasive cardiac output monitors are available in the future, the situation for predicting the drug concentration may evolve.

Compartment models are not perfect but can predict drug concentrations in clinical practice with reasonable accuracy. At the moment, no physiological models are available on drug delivery devices or drug information displays. Naturally, this does not mean that physiologically based model has value. Physiologically based model remains useful for detailed analysis of drug disposition [61, 62].

Selection of PK/PD Model

For Commercial Target-Controlled Infusion Pump

Current commercial TCI pumps contain two propofol pharmacokinetic models, the Marsh and Schnider model for adults [3, 43]. Unless one model is deactivated, users are then forced to make a choice of model. Some pumps also offer two pediatric pharmacokinetic models, the Kataria and the Paedfusor models [51, 63]. Additionally, different commercial pumps may have two different k_{e0} values for the Marsh model (0.26 or 1.21) [64].

Marsh or Schnider Model for Propofol in Adults

TCI systems implementing these models can administer very different bolus sizes after an increase in target concentration, despite the user inputting the same target concentration.

With target-controlled infusions in plasma concentration targeting mode, the initial bolus dose of propofol only depends on the distribution volume of the central compartment of the pharmacokinetic model. The Schnider model has a smaller central compartment volume (4.27 L) than the Marsh model (0.228 L/kg) in the standard size adult. The smaller the central compartment, the smaller the bolus dose size after an increment of the targeted concentration. During effect-site target-controlled infusion, not only the distribution volume of the central compartment but also k_{e0} value influences the bolus dose. The smaller k_{e0} value, the larger the bolus dose, since the system will estimate that a larger plasma concentration overshoot is required to drive or drag down the concentration gradient into the effect site. To avoid hemodynamic instability during effect-site concentration targeting, the Schnider model or alternatively the Marsh model with a larger (faster) k_{e0} value should be used,

because in this way a smaller bolus volume will be administered on starting the infusion or increasing the target.

Models for Obese Adult Patients: Propofol and Remifentanil

Specific pharmacokinetic models of propofol for obese patients have been published, such as the Cortinez and van Kralingen models [65, 66]. However, these models have not been incorporated into the commercial pumps. Cortinez et al. reported that the Marsh or Schnider model with adjusted body weight instead of total body weight achieved the acceptable performance error (MDPE of −3.5 % and MDAPE of 21.7 % for the Marsh model with adjusted body weight and MDPE of 8.6 % and MDAPE of 20.1 % for the Schnider model with adjusted body weight) among the examined pharmacokinetic models including the Cortinez and van Kralingen models [40]. The evaluation data set included 3 males and 17 females, age between 21 and 53, and body mass index between 35 and 52. The adjusted body weight (ABW) is calculated as

$$\begin{cases} \text{ABW} = \text{IBW} + 0.4 \times (\text{TBW} - \text{IBW}) \\ \text{IBW} = 45.4 + 0.89 \times (\text{HT} - 152.4) + 4.5 \times \text{Male} \end{cases}$$

$$(10.13)$$

where IBW is the ideal body weight calculated using the second equation, TBW (kg) is the total body weight, HT is the height (cm), and male is the dichotomous variable (1 for male and 0 for female) [38]. These results have indicated that both Marsh and Schnider models can be applied to obese patients with adjusted body weight.

For remifentanil, the Minto model [37] is only the choice in commercial target-controlled infusion pumps. However, this model (and also the Schnider model) includes a problematic lean body mass calculated using the James equations [67]:

$$\text{LBM} = \begin{cases} 1.1 \times \text{TBW} - 128 \times \left(\frac{\text{TBW}}{\text{HT}}\right)^2 [\text{for male}] \\ 1.07 \times \text{TBW} - 148 \times \left(\frac{\text{TBW}}{\text{HT}}\right)^2 [\text{for female}] \end{cases}$$

$$(10.14)$$

where TBW is total body weight (kg) and HT is height (cm). This calculation yields a maximum value of lean body mass, for any height, at a body mass index (calculated as $\text{TBW}/(\text{HT}/100)^2$) of 43.0 for male and 36.1 for female subjects, i.e., a patient with a BMI value >43 has a lower calculated LBM than a patient with a BMI = 43. Therefore, when used to control a target-controlled infusion, the Minto model will result in lower infusion rates for a given target concentration in a subject with BMI > 43 than a patient with BMI = 43. To fix this problem, commercial pumps have programmed in upper limits of BMI or body weight depending on height and sex and cannot operate in target-controlled infusion mode above these limits.

La Colla et al. [68] confirmed that fat-free mass, calculated using the Janmahasatian equations [69] instead of the James equations, greatly improved the predictive performance of the Minto model in 15 female subjects. The Janmahasatian equations for the fat-free mass (FFM) are:

$$FFM = \begin{cases} \dfrac{9.27 \times 10^3 \times TBW}{6.68 \times 10^3 + 216 \times BMI} & \text{[for male]} \\[3ex] \dfrac{9.27 \times 10^3 \times TBW}{8.78 \times 10^3 + 244 \times BMI} & \text{[for female]} \end{cases}$$

(10.15)

where TBW is total body weight (kg) and BMI is body mass index. Since the equations for LBM cannot be changed in current commercial pumps, La Colla et al. proposed to use a "fictitious height" for obese patients receiving target-controlled infusions of propofol with commercial pumps [70]. The calculation result of the LBM equation with the fictitious height and total body weight is the same as the calculation result of the FFM equation with the real height and total body weight. The Minto model can also be used with FFM equations in the commercial pumps when the "fictitious height" is entered on start-up. Fictitious height (FH) is calculated as:

$$FH = \begin{cases} \sqrt{\dfrac{128 \times TBW \times (6.68 \times 10^3 + 216 \times BMI)}{-1922 + 1.1 \times 216 \times BMI}} & \text{[for male]} \\[3ex] \sqrt{\dfrac{148 \times TBW \times (8.78 \times 10^3 + 244 \times BMI)}{124.6 + 1.07 \times 244 \times BMI}} & \text{[for female]} \end{cases}$$

(10.16)

where TBW is total body weight and BMI is body mass index.

The user can select to use either total body weight or adjusted body weight with a propofol pharmacokinetic model or either lean body mass or fat-free mass with the remifentanil models on the commercial target-controlled infusion pumps. This is also, so to speak, a form of model selection.

For Simulation Software

When using the commercial target-controlled infusion devices, one selects a model from a limited list of choices as mentioned above. On the other hand, when using simulation software (see also the next section), one can select a model freely from the list of prepared models in the simulation software or all published models.

There are several methods for model selection available to the user:

(a) Select a model that is used in the commercial devices.
(b) Select a model recommended in a published study.
(c) Select a model recommended by experts.
(d) Select a model according to the discretion of the software user.

The first one, (a), is a sure choice to have an appropriate model but may be conservative. There may be another better model for your patient. The second one, (b), may be a good choice but the derivation or evaluation study may have been biased or limited by specific methodological techniques. For example, La Colla et al. [68] confirmed that the fat-free mass instead of the lean body mass improved predictive performance of the Minto model in only female subjects. Therefore, the applicability in male subjects is unknown. The third one, (c), would be a nice choice. Experts are aware of various information about the models such as the background, methodology used, results of external evaluations, merits, and limitations. Note that different experts may recommend different models for the same drug because each model has different merits. The fourth one, (4), is an excellent but tough choice. Appropriate model selection needs specialized knowledge of pharmacometrics. For this choice, it is necessary to know the details of background of published models and the results of the model evaluations and to confirm whether the model development and evaluation are appropriate.

Environment for PK/PD Simulation

Pharmacokinetic/pharmacodynamic simulation is feasible using either commercial environment or specialized simulation software.

Target-controlled infusion pumps and drug information displays [41] are available in clinical practice. These are safe to use but often include a model developed in patients with a limited range of patient characteristics, and the pumps offer a restricted choice of models.

Simulation software products designed to calculate drug concentration profiles associated with drug administration regimens have far fewer limitations because the software allows the use of any pharmacokinetic/pharmacodynamic model for which the parameter sets are available. STANPUMP [71], RUGLOOP II [72], and TIVA Trainer [73] are very well-known programs and have been used in many published studies. Many other software products have also been developed on Windows OS, Mac OS, iOS, or Android OS platforms, including our software [74].

Tips to Apply PK/PD Simulation

Predicted Concentration Depends on Applied PK/PD Model

The predicted plasma concentrations associated with a given drug administration regimen are different between two different models [22]. The effect-site concentrations are also different between different combinations of pharmacokinetic and pharmacodynamic models, e.g., between "the Marsh pharmacokinetic model with k_{e0} of 0.26" and "the Schnider pharmacokinetic model with k_{e0} of 0.456" or between "the Marsh pharmacokinetic model with k_{e0} of 0.26" and "the Marsh pharmacokinetic model with k_{e0} of 1.21."

Figure 10.9 shows the difference in the time course of propofol plasma and effect-site concentration during the same dosing (1.5 mg/kg bolus followed by 8 mg/kg/h until 20 min) simulated by the Marsh model with k_{e0} of 0.26 or 1.21 and the Schnider model with k_{e0} of 0.456. The predictive performances are similar among the different models during pseudo-steady-state conditions, whereas the time courses of predicted concentration simulation are different during the periods when concentrations are changing, including the early phase after the start of drug administration.

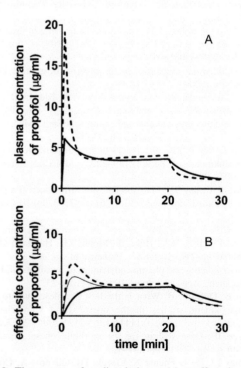

Fig. 10.9 Time course of predicted plasma (**a**) or effect-site concentration (**b**) of propofol. Propofol is given as a 1.5 mg/kg bolus (at 12,000 mg/h) followed by an infusion at 8 mg/kg/h for 20 min to a subject (30 years old, male, weight 70 kg, and height 170 cm). The *solid lines* indicate the time course predicted by the Marsh model, and *dashed lines* indicate the time course predicted by the Schnider model. For the calculation of the effect-site concentration (in **b**), the applied k_{e0} values are 0.26 (*bold solid line*) and 1.21 (*thin solid line*) for the Marsh model and 0.456 (*dashed line*) for the Schnider model

A Model Name Means Sole Model Parameter Sets?

Different anesthesiologists may use the same model name to refer to different model parameter sets.

As mentioned above, the Marsh model is integrated with two different k_{e0} values—0.26 or 1.21 min^{-1} in commercial devices. The former may be called "original Marsh model" and the latter "modified Marsh model." However, some may simply refer to both of these as the "Marsh model." The Marsh model with another k_{e0} value could also be called a "Marsh model" [57, 75].

The Schnider model is also integrated with different k_{e0}s in different commercial devices—a fixed value of 0.456 or a k_{e0} value derived from a time-to-peak effect of 1.6 min [76]. In this case, both models are generally referred to as a "Schnider model."

Other examples are the Kataria and Murat models for propofol in children [44, 51]. In these articles describing the model development, multiple model parameter sets are shown. It is thus also possible that a model referred to as a "Kataria model" is different between two different studies.

Only Using One Model May Be Better for One Drug

In clinical practice, the availability of different models for one drug may pose dangers for patients. Unwary anesthesiologists may be unaware of the differences between the models, and the differences may confound attempts to understand interindividual variability in relationships between target concentration and drug effect. It may be better for departments to only activate or allow one combination of pharmacokinetic and pharmacodynamic models for one drug. If more than one model is available to use in one hospital, the name of the model should be written in the anesthetic record. In addition, the anesthesiologists should recognize that a predicted concentration value has different meanings with different models.

References

1. Takita A, Masui K, Kazama T. On-line monitoring of end-tidal propofol concentration in anesthetized patients. Anesthesiology. 2007;106(4):659–64. doi:10.1097/01.anes.0000264745.63275.59. 00000542-200704000-00006 [pii].
2. Liu B, Pettigrew DM, Bates S, Laitenberger PG, Troughton G. Performance evaluation of a whole blood propofol analyser. J Clin Monit Comput. 2012;26(1):29–36. doi:10.1007/s10877-011-9330-0.
3. Marsh B, White M, Morton N, Kenny GN. Pharmacokinetic model driven infusion of propofol in children. Br J Anaesth. 1991;67 (1):41–8.

4. Sigl JC, Chamoun NG. An introduction to bispectral analysis for the electroencephalogram. J Clin Monit. 1994;10(6):392–404.

5. Flaishon R, Windsor A, Sigl J, Sebel PS. Recovery of consciousness after thiopental or propofol. Bispectral index and isolated forearm technique. Anesthesiology. 1997;86(3):613–9.

6. Derendorf H, Meibohm B. Modeling of pharmacokinetic/pharmacodynamic (PK/PD) relationships: concepts and perspectives. Pharm Res. 1999;16(2):176–85.

7. Williams PJ, Kim YH, Ette EI. The epistemology of pharmacometrics. In: Ette EI, Williams PJ, editors. Pharmacometrics: the science of quantitative pharmacology. Hoboken: Wiley; 2007. p. 223–44.

8. Short TG, Aun CS, Tan P, Wong J, Tam YH, Oh TE. A prospective evaluation of pharmacokinetic model controlled infusion of propofol in paediatric patients. Br J Anaesth. 1994;72(3):302–6.

9. Sepulveda P, Cortinez LI, Saez C, Penna A, Solari S, Guerra I, Absalom AR. Performance evaluation of paediatric propofol pharmacokinetic models in healthy young children. Br J Anaesth. 2011;107(4):593–600. doi:10.1093/bja/aer198.

10. Williams PJ, Kim YH. Resampling techniques and their application to pharmacometrics. In: Ette EI, Williams PJ, editors. Pharmacometrics: the science of quantitative pharmacology. Hoboken: Wiley; 2007. p. 401–19.

11. Bergstrand M, Hooker AC, Wallin JE, Karlsson MO. Prediction-corrected visual predictive checks for diagnosing nonlinear mixed-effects models. AAPS J. 2011;13(2):143–51. doi:10.1208/s12248-011-9255-z.

12. Yano Y, Beal SL, Sheiner LB. Evaluating pharmacokinetic/pharmacodynamic models using the posterior predictive check. J Pharmacokinet Pharmacodyn. 2001;28(2):171–92.

13. Varvel JR, Donoho DL, Shafer SL. Measuring the predictive performance of computer-controlled infusion pumps. J Pharmacokinet Biopharm. 1992;20(1):63–94.

14. Alvis JM, Reves JG, Govier AV, Menkhaus PG, Henling CE, Spain JA, Bradley E. Computer-assisted continuous infusions of fentanyl during cardiac anesthesia: comparison with a manual method. Anesthesiology. 1985;63(1):41–9.

15. Ausems ME, Stanski DR, Hug CC. An evaluation of the accuracy of pharmacokinetic data for the computer assisted infusion of alfentanil. Br J Anaesth. 1985;57(12):1217–25.

16. Schwilden H. A general method for calculating the dosage scheme in linear pharmacokinetics. Eur J Clin Pharmacol. 1981;20(5):379–86.

17. Glen JB. The development of 'Diprifusor': a TCI system for propofol. Anaesthesia. 1998;53 Suppl 1:13–21.

18. Owen JS, Fiedler-Kelly J. Population model concepts and terminology. In: Introduction to population pharmacokinetic/pharmacokinetic analysis with nonlinear mixed effects models. Hoboken: Wiley; 2014. p. 9–27.

19. Glen JB, Servin F. Evaluation of the predictive performance of four pharmacokinetic models for propofol. Br J Anaesth. 2009;102 (5):626–32. doi:10.1093/bja/aep043.

20. Glass PS, Shafer S, Reves JG. Intravenous drug delivery systems. In: Miller RD, editor. Miller's anesthesia. 6th ed. Philadelphia: Elsevier (Churchill Livinstone); 2004, p. 439–80.

21. Schuttler J, Kloos S, Schwilden H, Stoeckel H. Total intravenous anaesthesia with propofol and alfentanil by computer-assisted infusion. Anaesthesia. 1988;43(Suppl):2–7.

22. Masui K, Upton RN, Doufas AG, Coetzee JF, Kazama T, Mortier EP, Struys MM. The performance of compartmental and physiologically based recirculatory pharmacokinetic models for propofol: a comparison using bolus, continuous, and target-controlled infusion data. Anesth Analg. 2010;111(2):368–79. doi:10.1213/ANE.0b013e3181bdcf5b.

23. Coppens M, Van Limmen JG, Schnider T, Wyler B, Bonte S, Dewaele F, Struys MM, Vereecke HE. Study of the time course of the clinical effect of propofol compared with the time course of

the predicted effect-site concentration: performance of three pharmacokinetic-dynamic models. Br J Anaesth. 2010;104 (4):452–8. doi:10.1093/bja/aeq028.

24. Struys MMRF, Absalom AR, Shafer SL. Intravenous drug delivery system. In: Miller RD, editor. Miller's anesthesia, vol. 1. Philadelphia: Elsevier Saunders; 2015. p. 919–57.

25. Kurita T, Kazama T, Morita K, Fujii S, Uraoka M, Takata K, Sato S. Influence of fluid infusion associated with high-volume blood loss on plasma propofol concentrations. Anesthesiology. 2004;100 (4):871–8. discussion 875A-876A.

26. Kurita T, Morita K, Kazama T, Sato S. Influence of cardiac output on plasma propofol concentrations during constant infusion in swine. Anesthesiology. 2002;96(6):1498–503.

27. Kurita T, Uraoka M, Jiang Q, Suzuki M, Morishima Y, Morita K, Sato S. Influence of cardiac output on the pseudo-steady state remifentanil and propofol concentrations in swine. Acta Anaesthesiol Scand. 2013;57(6):754–60. doi:10.1111/aas.12076.

28. Coetzee JF, Glen JB, Wium CA, Boshoff L. Pharmacokinetic model selection for target controlled infusions of propofol. Assessment of three parameter sets. Anesthesiology. 1995;82(6):1328–45.

29. Coppens MJ, Eleveld DJ, Proost JH, Marks LA, Van Bocxlaer JF, Vereecke H, Absalom AR, Struys MM. An evaluation of using population pharmacokinetic models to estimate pharmacodynamic parameters for propofol and bispectral index in children. Anesthesiology. 2011;115(1):83–93. doi:10.1097/ALN.0b013e31821a8d80.

30. Masui K, Kira M, Kazama T, Hagihira S, Mortier EP, Struys MM. Early phase pharmacokinetics but not pharmacodynamics are influenced by propofol infusion rate. Anesthesiology. 2009;111(4):805–17. doi:10.1097/ALN.0b013e3181b799c1.

31. Friedman JH. A variable span scatterplot smoother. Laboratory for Computational Statistics, Stanford University Technical Report No. 5; 1984.

32. Greenblatt DJ, Sellers EM, Shader RI. Drug therapy: drug disposition in old age. N Engl J Med. 1982;306(18):1081–8. doi:10.1056/NEJM198205063061804.

33. Vuyk J. Pharmacodynamics in the elderly. Best Pract Res Clin Anaesthesiol. 2003;17(2):207–18.

34. Kearns GL, Abdel-Rahman SM, Alander SW, Blowey DL, Leeder JS, Kauffman RE. Developmental pharmacology--drug disposition, action, and therapy in infants and children. N Engl J Med. 2003;349 (12):1157–67. doi:10.1056/NEJMra035092.

35. Wilson K. Sex-related differences in drug disposition in man. Clin Pharmacokinet. 1984;9(3):189–202. doi:10.2165/00003088-198409030-00001.

36. Soldin OP, Chung SH, Mattison DR. Sex differences in drug disposition. J Biomed Biotechnol. 2011;2011:187103. doi:10.1155/2011/187103.

37. Minto CF, Schnider TW, Egan TD, Youngs E, Lemmens HJ, Gambus PL, Billard V, Hoke JF, Moore KH, Hermann DJ, Muir KT, Mandema JW, Shafer SL. Influence of age and gender on the pharmacokinetics and pharmacodynamics of remifentanil. I. Model development. Anesthesiology. 1997;86(1):10–23.

38. Green B, Duffull SB. What is the best size descriptor to use for pharmacokinetic studies in the obese? Br J Clin Pharmacol. 2004;58(2):119–33. doi:10.1111/j.1365-2125.2004.02157.x.

39. Coetzee JF. Dose scaling for the morbidly obese. South Afr J Anaesth Analg. 2011;20(1):67–72.

40. Cortinez LI, De la Fuente N, Eleveld DJ, Oliveros A, Crovari F, Sepulveda P, Ibacache M, Solari S. Performance of propofol target-controlled infusion models in the obese: pharmacokinetic and pharmacodynamic analysis. Anesth Analg. 2014;119(2):302–10. doi:10.1213/ANE.0000000000000317.

41. Struys MM, De Smet T, Mortier EP. Simulated drug administration: an emerging tool for teaching clinical pharmacology during anesthesiology training. Clin Pharmacol Ther. 2008;84(1):170–4. doi:10.1038/clpt.2008.76.

42. Ducharme J, Varin F, Bevan DR, Donati F. Importance of early blood sampling on vecuronium pharmacokinetic and pharmacodynamic parameters. Clin Pharmacokinet. 1993;24(6):507–18. doi:10.2165/00003088-199324060-00006.

43. Schnider TW, Minto CF, Gambus PL, Andresen C, Goodale DB, Shafer SL, Youngs EJ. The influence of method of administration and covariates on the pharmacokinetics of propofol in adult volunteers. Anesthesiology. 1998;88(5):1170–82.

44. Murat I, Billard V, Vernois J, Zaouter M, Marsol P, Souron R, Farinotti R. Pharmacokinetics of propofol after a single dose in children aged 1-3 years with minor burns. Comparison of three data analysis approaches. Anesthesiology. 1996;84 (3):526–32.

45. Saint-Maurice C, Cockshott ID, Douglas EJ, Richard MO, Harmey JL. Pharmacokinetics of propofol in young children after a single dose. Br J Anaesth. 1989;63(6):667–70.

46. Tuk B, Herben VM, Mandema JW, Danhof M. Relevance of arteriovenous concentration differences in pharmacokinetic-pharmacodynamic modeling of midazolam. J Pharmacol Exp Ther. 1998;284(1):202–7.

47. Stanski DR, Hudson RJ, Homer TD, Saidman LJ, Meathe E. Pharmacodynamic modeling of thiopental anesthesia. J Pharmacokinet Biopharm. 1984;12(2):223–40.

48. Gepts E, Camu F, Cockshott ID, Douglas EJ. Disposition of propofol administered as constant rate intravenous infusions in humans. Anesth Analg. 1987;66(12):1256–63.

49. Miyabe-Nishiwaki T, Masui K, Kaneko A, Nishiwaki K, Nishio T, Kanazawa H. Evaluation of the predictive performance of a pharmacokinetic model for propofol in Japanese macaques (Macaca fuscata fuscata). J Veterinary Pharmacol Ther. 2013;36 (2):169–73. doi:10.1111/j.1365-2885.2012.01404.x.

50. Upton RN. The two-compartment recirculatory pharmacokinetic model--an introduction to recirculatory pharmacokinetic concepts. Br J Anaesth. 2004;92(4):475–84.

51. Kataria BK, Ved SA, Nicodemus HF, Hoy GR, Lea D, Dubois MY, Mandema JW, Shafer SL. The pharmacokinetics of propofol in children using three different data analysis approaches. Anesthesiology. 1994;80(1):104–22.

52. Fisher DM. Propofol in pediatrics. Lessons in pharmacokinetic modeling. Anesthesiology. 1994;80(1):2–5.

53. Ette EI, Williams PJ, Ahmad A. Population pharmacokinetic estimation methods. In: Ette EI, Williams PJ, editors. Pharmacometrics: the science of quantitative pharmacology. Hoboken: Wiley; 2007. p. 265–85.

54. Eleveld DJ, Proost JH, Cortinez LI, Absalom AR, Struys MM. A general purpose pharmacokinetic model for propofol. Anesth Analg. 2014;118(6):1221–37. doi:10.1213/ANE.0000000000000165.

55. Minto CF, Schnider TW, Gregg KM, Henthorn TK, Shafer SL. Using the time of maximum effect site concentration to combine pharmacokinetics and pharmacodynamics. Anesthesiology. 2003;99(2):324–33.

56. Thomson AJ, Nimmo AF, Engbers FH, Glen JB. A novel technique to determine an 'apparent ke0' value for use with the Marsh pharmacokinetic model for propofol. Anaesthesia. 2014;69(5):420–8. doi:10.1111/anae.12596.

57. Absalom AR, Mani V, De Smet T, Struys MM. Pharmacokinetic models for propofol--defining and illuminating the devil in the detail. Br J Anaesth. 2009;103(1):26–37. doi:10.1093/bja/aep143.

58. Schuttler J, Ihmsen H. Population pharmacokinetics of propofol: a multicenter study. Anesthesiology. 2000;92(3):727–38.

59. Upton RN, Ludbrook G. A physiologically based, recirculatory model of the kinetics and dynamics of propofol in man. Anesthesiology. 2005;103(2):344–52.

60. Tackley RM, Lewis GT, Prys-Roberts C, Boaden RW, Dixon J, Harvey JT. Computer controlled infusion of propofol. Br J Anaesth. 1989;62(1):46–53.

61. Avram MJ, Sanghvi R, Henthorn TK, Krejcie TC, Shanks CA, Fragen RJ, Howard KA, Kaczynski DA. Determinants of thiopental induction dose requirements [see comments]. Anesth Analg. 1993;76(1):10–7.

62. Avram MJ, Krejcie TC, Niemann CU, Klein C, Gentry WB, Shanks CA, Henthorn TK. The effect of halothane on the recirculatory pharmacokinetics of physiologic markers [see comments]. Anesthesiology. 1997;87(6):1381–93.

63. Absalom A, Kenny G. 'Paedfusor' pharmacokinetic data set. Br J Anaesth. 2005;95(1):110. doi:10.1093/bja/aei567.

64. Seo JH, Goo EK, Song IA, Park SH, Park HP, Jeon YT, Hwang JW. Influence of a modified propofol equilibration rate constant (k (e0)) on the effect-site concentration at loss and recovery of consciousness with the Marsh model. Anaesthesia. 2013;68 (12):1232–8. doi:10.1111/anae.12419.

65. Cortinez LI, Anderson BJ, Penna A, Olivares L, Munoz HR, Holford NH, Struys MM, Sepulveda P. Influence of obesity on propofol pharmacokinetics: derivation of a pharmacokinetic model. Br J Anaesth. 2010;105(4):448–56. doi:10.1093/bja/aeq195.

66. van Kralingen S, Diepstraten J, Peeters MY, Deneer VH, van Ramshorst B, Wiezer RJ, van Dongen EP, Danhof M, Knibbe CA. Population pharmacokinetics and pharmacodynamics of propofol in morbidly obese patients. Clin Pharmacokinet. 2011;50 (11):739–50. doi:10.2165/11592890-000000000-00000.

67. Research DMGoO, Waterlow JC, James WPT, Security GBDoHaS, Council MR. Research on obesity: a report of the DHSS/MRC group. London; 1976.

68. La Colla L, Albertin A, La Colla G, Porta A, Aldegheri G, Di Candia D, Gigli F. Predictive performance of the 'Minto' remifentanil pharmacokinetic parameter set in morbidly obese patients ensuing from a new method for calculating lean body mass. Clin Pharmacokinet. 2010;49(2):131–9. doi:10.2165/11317690-000000000-00000.

69. Janmahasatian S, Duffull SB, Ash S, Ward LC, Byrne NM, Green B. Quantification of lean bodyweight. Clin Pharmacokinet. 2005;44 (10):1051–65. doi:10.2165/00003088-200544100-00004.

70. La Colla L, Albertin A, La Colla G. Pharmacokinetic model-driven remifentanil administration in the morbidly obese: the 'critical weight' and the 'fictitious height', a possible solution to an unsolved problem? Clin Pharmacokinet. 2009;48(6):397–8. doi:10.2165/00003088-200948060-00005.

71. Shafer SL, Gregg KM. Algorithms to rapidly achieve and maintain stable drug concentrations at the site of drug effect with a computer-controlled infusion pump. J Pharmacokinet Biopharm. 1992;20 (2):147–69.

72. Struys MM, Coppens MJ, De Neve N, Mortier EP, Doufas AG, Van Bocxlaer JF, Shafer SL. Influence of administration rate on propofol plasma-effect site equilibration. Anesthesiology. 2007;107(3):386–96.

73. Engbers F. Basic pharmacokinetic principles for intravenous anaesthesia. In: Vuyk J, Schraag S, editors. Advances in modelling and clinical application of intravenous anaesthesia. New York: Springer; 2003.

74. Masui K. http://www.masuinet.com.

75. Lim TA. A novel method of deriving the effect compartment equilibrium rate constant for propofol. Br J Anaesth. 2003;91 (5):730–2.

76. Schnider T, Minto C. Pharmacokinetic models of propofol for TCI. Anaesthesia. 2008;63(2):206. doi:10.1111/j.1365-2044.2007. 05419_1.x. author reply 206–207.

Part III

Pharmacology of the Intravenous Anesthetic Agents

Propofol PK-PD

Douglas J. Eleveld

Introduction

Propofol is an intravenous anesthetic in very wide use in modern medical practice. In the literature, propofol is referred to by a number of names: Diprivan, Disoprivan, ICI-35868, 2,6-bis(1-methylethyl)phenol, Rapinovet, 2,6-diisopropylphenol, and disoprofol. Propofol is flexible in application and has a good profile of side effects. Rapid injection allows for a rapid onset and a short duration of action while continuous infusion allows for longer periods of stable anesthesia or sedation. The continuous infusion rate can be varied to meet patient needs and achieve varying levels of anesthetic depth.

Propofol originally appeared on the market in 1977; however, it was later removed due to undesirable side effects related to the formulation using Cremophor EL, a polyethoxylated castor oil. The drug was reformulated using emulsion of soya oil and propofol in water and again brought to the market in 1986 as Diprivan. Diprivan has been extremely successful and is even considered by the World Health Organization as one of the most important injectable anesthetics in medicine [1].

Propofol Pharmacokinetics and Pharmacodynamics

Propofol is administered intravenously. With regard to pharmacokinetics (PK), its primary route of elimination is hepatic, and the inactive metabolites are excreted by the kidney (http://www.drugbank.ca/drugs/DB00818). Like many intravenous drugs, propofol is highly protein bound

with a free fraction of about 1.2–1.7 %. The bound fraction is evenly distributed between erythrocytes and human serum albumin [2]. The rate at which propofol blood concentration decreases after administration depends on the preceding time course of administration. This is known as the context-sensitive decrement time, and it increases for longer duration infusions. The typical context-sensitive 80 % decrement times are predicted to be less than 50 min for infusions up to about 2 h, but it increases to 120–480 min for very long infusions of more than 12 h [3]. Individuals will not necessarily exhibit these values exactly; the degree of interindividual variability is not negligible.

Propofol pharmacodynamic (PD) effects are achieved by interacting with the GABA neurotransmitter system by increasing membrane accumulation of GABAARβ3 subunits [2]. This results in enhanced evoked and miniature synaptic GABA receptor currents. The complex mechanism of action of propofol is not well known and seems to involve many different physiological systems. Hypnosis and general anesthesia are consequences of propofol causing the disruption of processes needed to integrate information in the gamma frequency band [4]. Loss of consciousness occurs when the synchronization needed between different areas in the brain to support information processing is altered. Propofol appears to disrupt these processes in a dose-dependent manner.

The Role of PK and PD Models

Propofol PK and PD models are useful mathematical descriptions of the distribution, metabolism, excretion, and drug effect of propofol in the body. They are designed to characterize the interaction of the drug with the body and enable the prediction of propofol distribution, metabolism, excretion, and degree of drug effect in different circumstances than those in which the data was obtained. Extrapolation to different drug-dosing regimens and to

D.J. Eleveld, PhD(✉)
Department of Anesthesiology, University Medical Center Groningen, University of Groningen, Hanzeplein 1, Groningen 9713GZ, The Netherlands
e-mail: d.j.eleveld@umcg.nl

© Springer International Publishing AG 2017
A.R. Absalom, K.P. Mason (eds.), *Total Intravenous Anesthesia and Target Controlled Infusions*,
DOI 10.1007/978-3-319-47609-4_11

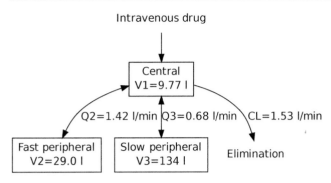

Intravenous drug

Fig. 11.1 Compartmental model for propofol using the Eleveld PK model for a 70-kg, 35-year-old male patient

different populations is one of the most fundamental and important applications of PK and PD models. They also enable insight into underlying physiological processes by allowing examination of the characteristics of various structures in the model and thus enabling comparisons of information about the underlying physiological processes obtained by other means.

For propofol, the majority of PK models in the literature are three-compartment mammillary models. These models consist of three virtual or simulated volumes intended to represent tissues in the body which have differing physico-chemical properties. Mammillary models consist of a central compartment connected to peripheral compartments, without connections between the peripheral compartments. These three structures each represent tissues with similar physicochemical properties. They are lumped together to represent the characteristics and behavior of the collected tissue types. In this sense, they are greatly simplified versions of the understood physiological processes underlying drug absorption, distribution, and elimination. Figure 11.1 shows a schematic diagram of a compartmental model for propofol. The particular values for volumes and clearances given are those from a population typical reference individual from the Eleveld PK model for propofol [5] representing a 70-kg, 35-year-old male patient (as opposed to healthy volunteer).

The three compartments in the above PK model represent the volumes for the initial or central drug distribution volume ($V1$), the intermediate or fast-peripheral drug distribution ($V2$), and the slow-peripheral drug distribution ($V3$). When an intravenous dose of propofol is administered, it is assumed to be immediately and completely distributed throughout the central compartment volume. This is of course not true; however, for the vast majority of applications of the PK model, this captures the behavior of drug administration to a satisfactory degree. When drug appears in the central compartment, it immediately begins transporting to the fast-peripheral and slow-peripheral compartments, as well as being eliminated from the body

(or otherwise rendered inactive). The rates of drug transport are represented by $Q2$, $Q3$, and CL, respectively. The distinction between $V2$ and $V3$ as fast or slow is essentially arbitrary; $V2$ is taken to represent the compartment with the faster equilibration time compared to $V3$. Sometimes a total volume of distribution parameter is described, Vss, which is the sum of $V1$, $V2$, and $V3$. The behavior of the three-compartment model can be fully described by a set of linear differential equations. For the standard three-compartment PK model, these are:

$$\partial A1/\partial t = A2 \cdot k21 + A3 \cdot k31 + A1 \cdot (k10 + k12 + k13) + \text{dosing}$$

$$\partial A2/\partial t = A1 \cdot k12 + A2 \cdot k21$$

$$\partial A3/\partial t = A1 \cdot k13 + A3 \cdot k31$$

where $\partial A1/\partial t$ represents the derivative of $A1$, the amount of drug in the central compartment, with respect to time, i.e., the rate of change in $A1$. Likewise $\partial A2/\partial t$ and $\partial A3/\partial t$ represent the derivatives of drug amounts in the fast- and slow-peripheral compartments, respectively. The values for $A1$, $A2$, and $A3$ represent the amount of drug accumulated in the central, fast-peripheral, and slow-peripheral compartments, respectively. The predicted concentration of drug in a compartment is the amount of the drug divided by the corresponding volume; thus, the predicted concentration in the central compartment is $A1/V1$. Usually for propofol, before initial dosing, these variables are assumed zero. In contrast, for endogenous compounds, the amounts in the compartments may have some steady-state values. Intravenous drug dosing is applied to the central compartment, and thus following a bolus dose, the amount of drug in the central compartment, $A1$, is stepwise increased at the moment of dosing. For a continuous infusion, the derivative of the amount of drug in the central compartment is increased by the rate of continuous infusion per unit time. The rate constant $k10$ represents the rate of drug transport out of the body (or otherwise rendered inactive), and $k21$, $k12$, $k31$, and $k13$ represent the rate of drug transport between the peripheral compartments and the central compartment. Calculation of these rate constants from more meaningful compartmental volumes and clearances is:

$$k10 = CL/V1$$
$$k12 = Q2/V1$$
$$k21 = Q2/V2$$
$$k13 = Q3/V1$$
$$k31 = Q3/V3$$

The differential equations can be used to obtain a predicted time course of drug distribution and elimination by finding an approximate solution using an ordinary-differential-equation (ODE) solver algorithm. If the infusion profile consists of simple bolus administrations or as continuous infusions of fixed rate and duration, then analytical solutions are available for three-compartment models which can predict drug distribution profiles directly from the model compartmental characteristics using the model parameters and the timing and amounts of the bolus doses and continuous infusions. The analytical solutions have the benefit of being exact and not requiring approximation. These analytical solutions can also be used to find approximate solutions for more complex infusion profiles. The arbitrary infusion profile can be approximated by a summation of bolus doses and continuous infusions, and then the superposition principle of linear systems is applied using the results of the separate individual components of the infusion profile. When these are summed, they predict the time course of drug distribution from the more complex infusion profile. While this can be computationally complex for complex dosing profiles, in many realistic cases, it is considerably more efficient than using an ODE solver.

Sigmoidal E_{max} Pharmacodynamic Models

While the PK of propofol receives considerable attention in modern anesthetic medicine and research, it is in reality a secondary issue. Drugs are primarily administered to achieve some desired drug effect. It is the desired drug PD effect which determines rational drug therapy, not the time course of drug concentrations in the body needed to achieve the desired effect. While the PK of anesthetic is indeed important to understand and consider, it is not the raison d'être of anesthetic drug dosing. For propofol, in nearly all cases, this is some degree of anesthesia or sedation.

Propofol central compartment concentrations show considerable hysteresis with the majority of PD effects, and thus a theoretical effect compartment is often used to introduce a delay between propofol central compartment concentrations and the PD effects. This "collapses" the hysteresis loop and establishes a fixed relationship between a hypothetical effect-site concentration and the concordant EEG effects. In addition, there are often upper and lower limits for PD effects, and there may only be a limited range of propofol concentrations between which the drug effect varies between these limits. Thus, for the majority of PD effects of propofol, a sigmoidal E_{max} model is used where the effect-site concentrations follow the central compartment concentration by a first-order time constant, typically referred to as k_{e0}. The differential equations for the effect compartment are:

$$\partial Ce/\partial t = k_{e0} \cdot (A(1)/V1 - Ce)$$

where $A(1)$ and $V1$ maintain the same meaning as in the PK differential equations as the amount of propofol in the central compartment and the volume of the central compartment. The equation $\partial Ce/\partial t$ represents the rate of change in concentration of propofol in a hypothetical effect compartment over time. Note that the differential equations do not consider the amount or mass of drug transfer between the central and effect compartments. The amount is assumed small enough to be negligible. This approach allows the PK model estimation to be performed separately from the PD model estimation.

The equation for transforming the predicted propofol effect-site concentration to a scaled drug effect is:

$$\text{Effect} = E_0 - (E_0 - E_{max}) \cdot \frac{Ce^{\gamma}}{Ce50^{\gamma} + Ce^{\gamma}}$$

where Ce represents the predicted effect-site concentration at some time point, E_0 is the drug effect in the absence of propofol, E_{max} is the theoretical maximal drug effect in the presence of arbitrarily high concentrations of propofol, $Ce50$ represents the predicted effect-site concentration when drug effect is halfway between E_0 and E_{max}, and γ describes the steepness of the relationship between effect-site concentration and drug effect.

Interindividual Variability

While Fig. 11.1 shows the compartmental volumes and clearances for a particular population typical individual, all of the PK parameters show considerable interindividual variability. This is expressed as variability in model parameters across individuals but manifests itself as a variability in time course of drug concentrations for a given drug administration regimen. To provide an impression of the degree of variability of propofol distribution and elimination, Fig. 11.2 shows the time course for 100 hypothetical individuals, all of which are 70-kg, 35-year-old male patients, but who have randomly generated PK parameters, based on the variability of the different PK parameters in real datasets. The left panel shows the time course of propofol central compartment concentration following a bolus dose of 2 mg/kg. The right panel shows the propofol central compartment concentration for an infusion of 0.2 mg/kg/min for a duration of 30 min. This figure gives the reader an impression of the degree of variability across the population.

Fig. 11.2 The time course of propofol central compartment concentration for 100 simulated individuals who are 70-kg, 35-year-old male patients. Model parameters calculated using the Eleveld PK model

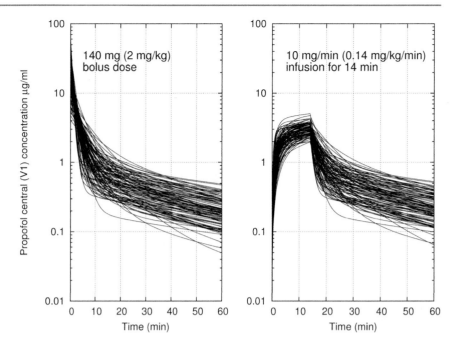

A Short History of Compartmental PK-PD Models for Propofol

A considerable number of PK models for propofol can be found in the literature. For the most part, these have been focused on some specific subpopulation such as children, adults, or the obese. More recently, PK models have been published which attempt to provide unified models for multiple subpopulations. An exhaustive historical review would be too lengthy for this chapter, so we will focus on a selection of the models which are particularly relevant to the scientific progress of propofol PK models and TCI applications.

One of the first investigations of the PK of Diprivan appeared in the literature in 1985 and was performed by Kay [6] who obtained propofol concentration data from 12 patients and estimated a three-compartment PK model to capture the distribution and elimination characteristics. The estimated CL was about 1.8 l/min, and the volume of distribution was quite large, about 755 l. This verified the idea that the very high lipid solubility of propofol would lead to large a volume of distribution.

The first important development toward the possibility of administration of propofol using target-controlled infusion (TCI) was the development of the Diprifusor TCI system. This system was based on PK parameters proposed by Gepts [7] and later modified by Marsh in 1991 (the Marsh parameters were published in passing in an article on the performance of an adapted model in children) [8]. The TCI system allows drug infusion profiles to be calculated which would achieve some desired concentration profile in a population typical individual. When applied to an individual selected from a population, the exact desired concentration profile would not be exactly replicated. However, the approach does enable TCI system users to modulate anesthetic depth with greater ease and accuracy compared to the more straightforward direct determination and manual implementation of infusion rates. Although the equations of the Diprifusor PK model are typically presented as rate constants, here they are presented as volumes and clearances referenced to 70 kg:

$$V1(l) = 15.96 \cdot (\text{WGT}/70)$$

$$V2(l) = 33.08 \cdot (\text{WGT}/70)$$

$$V3(l) = 202.6 \cdot (\text{WGT}/70)$$

$$CL(l/\text{min}) = 1.90 \cdot (\text{WGT}/70)$$

$$Q2(l/\text{min}) = 1.82 \cdot (\text{WGT}/70)$$

$$Q3(l/\text{min}) = 0.67 \cdot (\text{WGT}/70)$$

In 1994, the Kataria PK model [8] was published. It focused not only on the development of a PK model for propofol for children but also on some appropriate numerical methods for PK model estimation and evaluating PK model predictive performance. The focus was on comparing the performance of PK models developed from a population approach and those developed using a naive-pooled approach. The conclusion was that, although the naive-pooled approach may provide good model fits to data, the resulting model is not optimal for predictions under conditions differing from the experiment itself. Thus, predictions from a population PK model are expected to be superior than those developed using a naive-pooled approach. The equations for the Kataria PK model are:

$$V1(l) = 0.41 \cdot \text{WGT}$$

$$V2(l) = 0.78 \cdot \text{WGT} + 3.1 \cdot \text{AGE} - 16$$

$$V3(l) = 6.9 \cdot \text{WGT}$$

$$CL(l/\text{min}) = 0.035 \cdot \text{WGT}$$

$$Q2(l/\text{min}) = 0.077 \cdot \text{WGT}$$

$$Q3(l/\text{min}) = 0.026 \cdot \text{WGT}$$

where WGT is the individual's weight in kg and AGE is the individual's age in years. Note that the Kataria model parameters do not have good extrapolation properties. A 12-kg, 2-year-old child is predicted to have a V2 less than zero. As such the slope of the age relationship is likely overestimated.

In 1998 Schnider published a PK model [9] intended to investigate the influence of methods of administration—bolus versus continuous infusions—on the estimated PK parameters. Patient covariates such as lean body mass and weight were found to play a role in parameter scaling for some, but not all parameters. A year later Schnider followed up the PK model with the corresponding PD analysis [10] which found an influence of age on both the k_{e0} (plasma-effect-site equilibration rate constant) and the steady-state sensitivity EC50 of individuals to propofol. The PD measure was the CUP (canonical univariate parameter) which is an encephalographic (EEG) measure intended to describe drug effect (hypnosis). For the same dose, older individuals were found to be more sensitive than younger individuals but achieved these drug effects more slowly than younger individuals. The Schnider model has found considerable success as a PK-PD model for TCI applications and is programmed into a number of commercially available infusion pumps. The equations for the Schnider PK and models are:

$$V1(l) = 4.27$$

$$V2(l) = 18.9 - 0.391 \cdot (\text{AGE} - 53)$$

$$V3(l) = 238$$

$$CL(l/\text{min}) = 1.89 + 0.0456 \cdot (\text{WGT} - 77) - 0.0681 \cdot (\text{LBM} - 59) + 0.0246 \cdot (\text{HGT} - 177)$$

$$Q2(l/\text{min}) = 1.29 - 0.024 \cdot (\text{AGE} - 53)$$

$$Q3(l/\text{min}) = 0.836$$

where HGT is the individual's height in cm, AGE is the individual's age in years, and LBM is the individual's estimated lean body mass. Schnider used the James equation [11] to estimate LBM as follows:

$$\text{LBM} = \begin{cases} 1.1 \cdot \text{WGT} - 128 \cdot (\text{WGT}/\text{HGT})^2, & \text{male} \\ 1.07 \cdot \text{WGT} - 148 \cdot (\text{WGT}/\text{HGT})^2, & \text{female} \end{cases}$$

When applied to large, obese individuals, the Schnider model exhibits paradoxical behavior, predicting very small values for lean body mass (LBM) for very large individuals [12]. This is a result of the quadratic form of the James equation, having a convex parabolic shape. Some commercial applications of the Schnider PK-PD model avoid the paradoxical behavior by refusing to accept some ranges of patient weights as inputs.

In 2000, Schuttler published a large multicenter PK analysis [13] by using data from seven different datasets from five different research groups. This was the first attempt to produce a unified PK model for both children and adult populations. It was the largest PK analysis to date by a considerable margin involving 4112 propofol concentrations from 270 individuals over a wide age range of 3–88 years. The final model used total body weight, age, method of administration (bolus vs. infusion), and sampling site (arterial vs. venous sampling) as covariates. The final model showed that PK model compartmental volumes and clearances (with the exception of V3) could be scaled to normalized total body weight to power exponents between 0.55 and 0.75. The equations of the Schuttler model are:

$$V1(l) = 9.3 \cdot (\text{WGT}/70)^{0.71} \cdot (\text{AGE}/30)^{-0.39} \cdot \left\{ \begin{array}{ll} 1, & \text{infusion} \\ 2.61, & \text{bolus} \end{array} \right\}$$

$$V2(l) = 44.2 \cdot (\text{WGT}/70)^{0.61} \cdot \left\{ \begin{array}{ll} 1, & \text{infusion} \\ 1.73, & \text{bolus} \end{array} \right\}$$

$$V3(l) = 266$$

$$CL(l/\text{min}) = 1.44 \cdot (\text{WGT}/70)^{0.75} - \left\{ \begin{array}{ll} 0, & \text{AGE} \leq 60 \\ 0.045 \cdot (\text{AGE} - 60), & \text{AGE} > 60 \end{array} \right\}$$

$$Q2(l/\text{min}) = 2.25 \cdot (\text{WGT}/70)^{0.62} \cdot \left\{ \begin{array}{ll} 1, & \text{arterial} \\ 0.6, & \text{venous} \end{array} \right\} \cdot \left\{ \begin{array}{ll} 1, & \text{infusion} \\ 3.02, & \text{bolus} \end{array} \right\}$$

$$Q3(l/\text{min}) = 0.92 \cdot (\text{WGT}/70)^{0.55} \cdot \left\{ \begin{array}{ll} 1, & \text{infusion} \\ 0.52, & \text{bolus} \end{array} \right\}$$

Despite being the most well-supported PK model at the time, it did not find widespread clinical application. A possible reason for the lack of acceptance is that the Schuttler PK model proposes different values for *V1, V2, Q2,* and *Q3* depending on the method of administration, bolus, or continuous infusions. In clinical applications, drug doses are often in the form of both boluses and continuous infusions. Those considering the applying of the Schuttler model for clinical application may be uncertain which of the predicted parameter values should be used for a proposed drug infusion regimen containing both boluses and continuous infusions. In reality, this is not an insurmountable technical problem if separate compartmental state variables can be maintained, one for each method of administration. The principle of superposition, a property of all linear systems, allows the predicted concentrations for the separate state variables to be additively combined. This is possible because the PK for an individual is linear with respect to dose and drug concentrations. Unfortunately, the superposition principle does not help solve the problem of whether the rate of infusion is an important criterion for discerning whether some drug administration should be considered a bolus or an infusion. Overall, perhaps the additional numerical complexity of this approach and the uncertainty of the precise distinction between a bolus dose and a continuous infusion were a barrier to more widespread application of the Schuttler PK model compared to other PK models.

In 2001 and 2003, the Paedfusor PK model was investigated in two studies [14, 15] although the specific PK parameter set used was only published in 2005 in a separate publication [16]. The notable aspect of this model was nonlinear scaling of *k10,* which was scaled to weight to a power exponent of −0.3. This corresponds to a scaling of CL to a power exponent of 0.7 to total body weight. This is interestingly close to the power exponent of 0.75 found by Schuttler. This same power exponent of 0.75 is predicted by allometric scaling

theory which has been supported by subsequently developed PK models. The Paedfusor PK model has been programmed into in commercially available TCI infusion pumps. The equations of the Paedfusor model were published as rate constants and unwieldy to express as volumes and clearances. The equations of the Paedfusor model are:

$$V1(l) = \left\{ \begin{array}{ll} 0.4584 \cdot \text{WGT}, & 1 < \text{AGE} \leq 12 \\ 0.4000 * \text{WGT}, & \text{AGE} = 13 \\ 0.3420 * \text{WGT}, & \text{AGE} = 14 \\ 0.2480 * \text{WGT}, & \text{AGE} = 15 \\ 0.22857 * \text{WGT}, & \text{AGE} = 16 \end{array} \right\}$$

$$k10(\text{min}^{-1}) = \left\{ \begin{array}{ll} 0.1527 \cdot \text{WGT}^{-3}, & 1 < \text{AGE} \leq 12 \\ 0.0678, & \text{AGE} = 13 \\ 0.0792, & \text{AGE} = 14 \\ 0.0954, & \text{AGE} = 15 \\ 0.1190, & \text{AGE} = 16 \end{array} \right\}$$

$$k12(\text{min}^{-1}) = 0.114$$
$$k21(\text{min}^{-1}) = 0.055$$
$$k13(\text{min}^{-1}) = 0.0419$$
$$k31(\text{min}^{-1}) = 0.0033$$
$$ke0(\text{min}^{-1}) = 0.26$$

In 2005, Knibbe et al. published an interspecies two-compartment PK model [17] using data from rats, children, and adults. This impressive feat was made possible with the use of allometric scaling, a mathematical technique to scale models for body size. While allometric scaling has been a topic of interest in the biological sciences, it only came to the forefront in PK modeling in propofol in 1999 in a publication in the pediatric anesthesia sciences [18]. Allometric scaling has since found widespread application in PK models, especially those concerning patient groups with a wide range of sizes. The equations for the Knibbe PK model are:

$$V1(l) = 20.6 \cdot (WGT/70)^{0.98}$$
$$V2(l) = 71.9 \cdot (WGT/70)^{1.1}$$
$$CL(l/\text{min}) = 1.63 \cdot (WGT/70)^{0.78}$$
$$Q2(l/\text{min}) = 1.45 \cdot (WGT/70)^{0.73}$$

Also in 2005, Upton published a physiologically based PK model [19] which utilized considerable physiological information as model structural elements. The model structure was rather complex and required a considerable number of assumptions to make the model estimable from PK observations while avoiding issues of numerical stability and identifiability. Because of the complexity of the model equations, we do not repeat them here.

In 2010 Cortínez published a PK model [20] targeted to obese and lean individuals, applying concepts from allometric scaling to data collected from three different studies. They investigated whether other methods of parameter scaling such as linear scaling and the application of fat-free-mass (FFM) concepts could lead to an improved model but found that scaling the PK model parameters to total body weight using the theoretical allometric scaling power exponents provided the best model. The equations of the Cortínez PK model are:

$$V1(l) = 4.48 \cdot (WGT/70)$$
$$V2(l) = 18.9 \cdot (WGT/70) \cdot e^{-0.0164 \cdot (AGE-50)}$$
$$V3(l) = 237 \cdot (WGT/70)$$
$$CL(l/\text{min}) = 1.92 \cdot (WGT/70)^{0.75}$$
$$Q2(l/\text{min}) = 1.45 \cdot (WGT/70)^{0.75} \cdot e^{-0.0153 \cdot (AGE-50)}$$
$$Q3(l/\text{min}) = 0.86 \cdot (WGT/70)^{0.75}$$

Currently, the most well-supported PK model for propofol is the general purpose PK model published by Eleveld [5] in 2014. This model was based on propofol data from several studies publicly available via the Open TCI website (http://www.opentci.org/) as well as other studies. The analyzed data contains 10,927 drug concentration observations from 660 individuals over an age range of 0.25–88 years and a weight range of 5.2–160 kg. The patient covariates used were weight, age, gender, and patient status (healthy volunteer vs. patient). The final model uses concepts from allometric scaling where volumes are assumed to scale linearly with normalized weight and clearances to the ¾ power exponent. Predictive performance of the model has been evaluated in the obese [21] and in cancer patients [22] and was found to be clinically acceptable. Further prospective evaluation of this model is needed to establish whether it can replace specialized PK models for children and adults and the obese. The equations of the Eleveld general purpose PK model for propofol are:

$$f_{\text{sigmoid}}(x, E50, \lambda) = x^\lambda / (x^\lambda + E50^\lambda)$$

$$ADLT = f_{\text{sigmoid}}(WGT, 16.6, 2.75)$$

$$f_{\text{aging}}(x) = e^{-0.001 \cdot (AGE-35) \cdot x}$$

$$CLAG = 1 - f_{\text{sigmoid}}(PMA, 69.2, 8)$$

$$PMAL = \begin{cases} f_{\text{sigmoid}}(PMA, 22.2, 8), & \text{male} \\ 0, & \text{female} \end{cases}$$

$$KGEN = e^{0.225 \cdot (CLAG \cdot (1-PMAL) + (1-CLAG) \cdot PMAL) \cdot ADLT}$$

$$V1(l) = \begin{cases} 5.74, & \text{healthy} \\ 9.77, & \text{patient} \end{cases} \cdot \frac{ADLT}{ADLT_{\text{ref}}} \cdot \begin{cases} 1, & \text{male} \\ 0.830, & \text{female} \end{cases} \cdot f_{\text{aging}}(3.55) \cdot e^{\begin{cases} \eta1, & \text{healthy} \\ \eta2, & \text{patient} \end{cases}}$$

$$V2(l) = \begin{cases} 11.8, & \text{healthy} \\ 29.0, & \text{patient} \end{cases} \cdot \left(\frac{WGT}{70}\right) \cdot f_{\text{aging}}(8.91) \cdot e^{\eta3}$$

$$V3(l) = \begin{cases} 222, & \text{healthy} \\ 134, & \text{patient} \end{cases} \cdot \left(\frac{WGT}{70}\right)^{0.35} \cdot \frac{ADLT}{ADLT_{\text{ref}}} \cdot e^{\eta4}$$

$$CL(l/\text{min}) = \begin{cases} 1.83, & \text{healthy} \\ 1.53, & \text{patient} \end{cases} \cdot \left(\frac{WGT}{70}\right)^{0.75} \cdot \frac{KGEN}{KGEN_{\text{ref}}} \cdot f_{\text{aging}}(3.55) \cdot e^{\eta5}$$

$$Q2(l/\text{min}) = \begin{cases} 3.10, & \text{healthy} \\ 1.42, & \text{patient} \end{cases} \cdot \left(\frac{V2}{29.0}\right)^{0.75} \cdot f_{\text{aging}}((1-ADLT) \cdot 27.6 + ADLT \cdot 6.34) \cdot e^{\eta6}$$

$$Q3(l/\text{min}) = \begin{cases} 1.08, & \text{healthy} \\ 0.608, & \text{patient} \end{cases} \cdot \left(\frac{V3}{134}\right)^{0.75} \cdot f_{\text{aging}}(6.34) \cdot e^{\begin{cases} \eta7, & \text{healthy} \\ 0, & \text{patient} \end{cases}}$$

Perspective

If one considers the development of propofol PK models in the literature over the years, it is interesting to note that the individual models have not changed significantly since the 1985 when Kay showed that the individual time course of propofol concentration could be characterized by a mammillary three-compartment PK model. More than 25 years later, the same basic model is still in use. It is an interesting coincidence to note the predicted rate of clearance established by Kay in 1985 was 1.8 l/min while the rate predicted in 2014 by Eleveld was 1.53 l/min for patients and 1.83 l/min for healthy volunteers. Over the course of almost 30 years, the estimate of propofol clearance for adults has hardly changed.

There has been a lack of widespread applications of individual models more complex than the three-compartment mammillary model. This suggests that the quality and quantity of the individual PK data gathered in these investigations are not sufficiently informative to construct more detailed models on an individual level. This should put some perspective on efforts to develop PK models with a better connection to physiology, i.e., models with more detailed representation of physiological process as structures. If this approach is to become viable, PK modeling studies would likely need significantly more detailed and diverse kinds of observations than the 5–25 PK samples combined with on the order of ten covariate observations per individual.

What has changed significantly over the years is the breadth of demographic groups on which the PK models focus. The earliest models were targeted to healthy adult volunteers or adults undergoing some specific surgical intervention. Since 2005, these demographic groups have broadened significantly, and this has created more challenging conditions under which models can be developed and evaluated. The end result is improved models and more confidence in users that a chosen model is appropriate for some desired application. This broadening of demographic groups applied to propofol PK models has been the result of the application of allometric scaling.

Another aspect that has changed over the years is the choice a priori model structure. Earlier developed PK models tended to utilize (estimated) constants for parameter values in their a priori models. No covariates at all were assumed, not even weight. If the data was not very informative for those parameters, then hierarchical model building would not result in the addition of any covariates at all. For those parameters, the final model would simply be a constant value. While this approach can be numerically justified from the point of view of maintaining simplicity in the final structural model, the final models are less useful than they could be. Constant parameters are in general poor when good extrapolation properties are desired. One example of this is V1 in the Schnider model, which is a constant with no covariates at all. Extrapolation of the Schnider model to children is probably not sensible because it is very unlikely that children would have the same value for V1 as adults. If that were indeed true, then children and adults would require the same total dose amount (e.g., in mg) to achieve the same initial concentration. Anesthesiologists with clinical experience are likely to understand that children require smaller doses to achieve the same drug levels as an adult. If, on the other hand, Schnider had chosen a different a priori function for V1, then it is possible that the final model would have shown more reasonable extrapolation behavior and a smaller V1 for children than for adults. This model would then propose more reasonable initial doses and concentrations and thus likely be more useful for extrapolation. Most of the recently developed PK models incorporate allometric scaling in the a priori model. This approach has the positive property of ensuring more reasonable, but of course not necessarily perfect, extrapolation properties and making the final models more useful in general.

A Very Short Introduction to Allometric Scaling Theory

The term allometry was first coined by Huxley and Tessier [23] in 1936. Allometry is the study of the relationship of the size of an organism to diverse characteristics of that organism. The motivation for this study is the realization that many natural phenomena appear to have a predictable relationship with the size or scale of the organism in which the phenomena is observed. For example, in the biological sciences, considerable research over the years has been devoted to the study of metabolic rate. This was assumed to scale to the $2/3$ power exponent since this is the scaling ratio for surface area in relation to volume for many geometrical shapes. The reasoning was based on the idea that metabolic rate was related to energy generation which is related to heat generation. Energy loss must have a clear relationship with surface area since the surface is the only pathway for energy transfer out of the organism and into the environment. The balance between energy generation and loss in an organism determines the rate of change of temperature in the organism. If energy generation is greater than loss, then temperature must go up. Conversely, temperature can decrease if surface area is increased and energy generation held constant provided the starting temperature of the organism is higher than its immediate environment.

Fig. 11.3 In 1947 Kleiber showed data supporting the 3/4 power scaling exponent for metabolic rate. The 2/3 power scaling exponent was at the time widely believed to be correct. Source: https://commons.wikimedia.org/wiki/File:Kleiber1947.jpg [24]. Reproduced under Creative Commons Attribution-Share Alike 3.0 Unported license. Accessed 5/16/2016

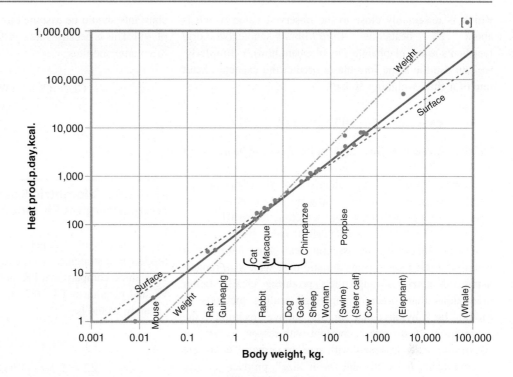

The work of Kleiber [24] suggested that experimental data of metabolic rate do not support the claim that it scaled to the ⅔ power as does surface area, but to the ¾ power (see Fig. 11.3). Kleiber did not provide a sound theoretical basis for this observation, and for many years, this issue was not resolved. It was not clear whether the reasoning supporting scaling with surface area was wrong or that the data selection or interpretation of Kleiber was incorrect. Considerable debate occurred in the following years.

Many of these issues of allometric scaling exponents were resolved with the seminal work by West [25] which modeled organisms as space-filling hierarchical branching networks. Their assumptions were reasonable and generic: (1) area-preserving branching for the transmission of energy containing substance utilized by the organism, (2) invariance of the terminal branching networks, and (3) the system as a whole would be energy efficient to minimize transmission losses. The conclusion was that power functions are reasonable scaling functions and that the appropriate exponent depends on the units of the characteristic of interest. Characteristics with units related to size, such as mass or volume, are associated with scaling exponents of 1; these would be expected to scale linearly with the size of the organism. Characteristics with units related to time intervals are associated with scaling exponents of ¼, and when the characteristic is inverted to have the units per unit time, then the exponent is also inverted to −¼. As a consequence of these rules, characteristics with combined units, for example, mass or volume per unit time, would be expected to scale to the ¾ power exponent.

Thus, the value of characteristic A would be expected to equal to some constant multiplied by body size to some exponent b. Thus, when body size is equated to total body weight (WGT), then:

$$A = k \cdot (\mathrm{WGT}/\mathrm{WGT}_{\mathrm{ref}})^b$$

where A is the characteristic of interest and $\mathrm{WGT}_{\mathrm{ref}}$ is a reference weight which determines the interpretation of the constant scaling factor k.

An Example: Allometric Scaling of Heart Rate

An introductory example is the relationship between heart rate and body size. It is well known that heart rates of large animals are slower than that of humans which are correspondingly slower to those of smaller animals. Allometric scaling theory suggests that rates expressed on a per minute basis scale to the power exponent of −¼. We can thus fill in this scaling equation for adult humans assuming a total body weight of 70 kg and an assumed resting heart rate of 60 beats/min as:

$$\mathrm{beats/min} = 60 \cdot (70\mathrm{kg}/70\mathrm{kg})^{-1/4} = 60$$

Using this equation to predict the heart rate of an Asian elephant weighing 3000 kg would be:

$$\mathrm{beats/min} = 60 \cdot (3000\mathrm{kg}/70\mathrm{kg})^{-1/4} = 23.5$$

which is reasonably close to the observed value which is about 28 beats/min (http://library.sandiegozoo.org/factsheets/asian_elephant/asian_elephant.htm). Similarly, we can use the same formula to predict the expected heart rate of a child weighing 10 kg:

$$\text{beats/min} = 60 \cdot (10\text{kg}/70\text{kg})^{-1/4} = 97.6$$

which is reasonably close to the normal resting heart rate of 80–130 for children 1–2 years old. Boys reach 10 kg at about 11 months (http://library.sandiegozoo.org/factsheets/asian_elephant/asian_elephant.htm) and girls at 14 months (http://www.cdc.gov/growthcharts/data/set1clinical/cj41l017.pdf). Of course, the prediction is not perfect, and it would be naive to expect otherwise. The essential realization here is that when predicting some characteristic over wide size ranges, using allometric scaling often produces clearly better predictions than other "competing" scaling methods. It should be obvious that in the above example, the assumptions "heart rate is constant with respect to size" or "heart rate scales inversely with size" or perhaps "heart rate is completely unpredictable with size" produce clearly poorer predictions compared to allometric scaling. When one considers some characteristic over a wide demographic range, then the difference in predictive performance is often so large that it becomes hard to consider these truly "competing" hypotheses. These alternative scaling methods could be better described as simply mathematically convenient assumptions rather than well-founded methods for size scaling.

Applying Allometric Scaling Simple PK Models

The usual way to apply allometric scaling to PK studies is to scale volumes to the power exponent of 1 and clearances to the power exponent of 0.75; thus:

$$\text{Volume} = V_{\text{ref}} \cdot (\text{WGT}/\text{WGT}_{\text{ref}})$$

$$\text{Clearance} = \text{CL}_{\text{ref}} \cdot (\text{WGT}/\text{WGT}_{\text{ref}})^{0.75}$$

where V_{ref} and CL_{ref} are the volume and clearance associated with the reference individual of total body weight 70 kg. Here we use WGT as the size descriptor.

In the above example, the scaling occurs relative to WGT of 70 kg. Technically a different reference value could be used without changing the functional relationship between volume and clearance and WGT. The only difference is the interpretation of the reference values V_{ref} and CL_{ref}.

Some researchers prefer to construct PK models using rate constant $k10$ to describe the rate of eliminations of drug from the body instead of clearances. Note that in this case rate

constants should be assumed to scale to the power exponent of $-\frac{1}{4}$. This is because rate constants are the ratio of clearance to volume and thus:

$$k = \frac{\text{CL}}{V} = \frac{\text{CL}_{\text{ref}} \cdot (\text{WGT}/\text{WGT}_{\text{ref}})^{0.75}}{V_{\text{ref}} \cdot (\text{WGT}/\text{WGT}_{\text{ref}})}$$

$$= k_{\text{ref}} \cdot (\text{WGT}/\text{WGT}_{\text{ref}})^{-0.25}$$

Applying Allometric Scaling to Multi-compartmental PK Models

Most studies apply allometric scaling to multi-compartmental models in a straightforward extension to simple PK models. For a three-compartment PK model with volumes $V1$, $V2$, and $V3$ and clearances CL, $Q2$, and $Q3$, the allometric scaling equation would be:

$$V1 = V1_{\text{ref}} \cdot (\text{WGT}/\text{WGT}_{\text{ref}})$$

$$V2 = V2_{\text{ref}} \cdot (\text{WGT}/\text{WGT}_{\text{ref}})$$

$$V3 = V3_{\text{ref}} \cdot (\text{WGT}/\text{WGT}_{\text{ref}})$$

$$\text{CL} = \text{CL}_{\text{ref}} \cdot (\text{WGT}/\text{WGT}_{\text{ref}})^{0.75}$$

$$Q2 = Q2_{\text{ref}} \cdot (\text{WGT}/\text{WGT}_{\text{ref}})^{0.75}$$

$$Q3 = Q3_{\text{ref}} \cdot (\text{WGT}/\text{WGT}_{\text{ref}})^{0.75}$$

The underlying assumption with this approach is that the volumes and clearances scale linearly to WGT.

Compartmental Allometry in Multi-compartmental PK Models

The study by Eleveld developing a general-purpose PK model for propofol suggested that there is some advantage in scaling the inter-compartmental clearance $Q2$ and $Q3$ relative to the estimated size of the corresponding compartment instead of total body weight. Thus:

$$Q2 = Q2_{\text{ref}} \cdot (V2/V2_{\text{ref}})^{0.75}$$

$$Q3 = Q3_{\text{ref}} \cdot (V3/V3_{\text{ref}})^{0.75}$$

Note that in the absence of interindividual variability in $V2$ and $V3$, this is exactly the same as the usual approach to scaling $Q2$ and $Q3$ to WGT. However, when interindividual variability does occur and is factored into the calculations of $Q2$ and $Q3$, then the ratios are not equal, and $V2$ and $V3$ may be higher or lower depending on the individual. Essentially, compartmental allometry assumes that $Q2$ will be correlated with *V2* and *Q3* correlated with *V3*. The precise degree of correlation is not fixed; it depends on the relative unknown variabilities of the volumes and clearances.

The reasoning behind compartmental allometry is that the volume of a compartment scales linearly with its size, and thus the reverse is also true that the size of the compartment scales linearly with its volume. In multi-compartmental models where there is interindividual variability, we explicitly estimate the compartmental volumes in each particular individual. These volume estimates can be used as estimates of the size of the compartment in the particular individual.

The Initial Distribution of Propofol

The initial distribution of intravenously injected propofol, sometimes referred to as the front-end kinetics, occurs in the following manner: Once injected in a vein, propofol is transported via blood flow toward the heart. If administered at the wrist, it arrives in the right atrium via the superior vena cava, and the action of the heart pumps the propofol and blood to the pulmonary artery via the right ventricle. After circulation through the lungs, the propofol and blood return to the left atrium, and subsequently the left ventricle pumps the blood through the aortic valve to the aorta. Once the blood is in the systemic circulation, it is transported throughout the body tissues including the brain. Here propofol exerts its primary influence on various structures in the brain to produce the well-known hypnotic and amnestic effects so essential to its application in anesthesia.

Intravenous injection of propofol does not immediately result in an evenly and homogenous distribution of propofol throughout the blood. There is a peak of high concentration that passes through the circulation and which gradually dissipates as well-mixed steady state is approached. As the venous blood flow transports the dose of propofol toward the heart, there is likely a degree of mixing and greater, more even distribution of propofol. In the right ventricle, the blood-borne propofol is likely further mixed due to the turbulence of flow through the tricuspid and pulmonary valves. In the capillaries of the lung, it seems likely that little additional mixing occurs due to the tendency for laminar flow in fluid transmission when cross-sectional area is small as in the small capillaries of the lung. Upon returning from the heart, again further mixing likely occurs due to turbulence from the mitral and aortic valves and blood flow to the aorta for distribution throughout the body. Overall, the result of the first pass of propofol through the heart and lungs is considerable mixing and even distribution of an intravenous dose throughout the blood. Each time the propofol is circulated, its distribution throughout the circulating blood becomes more and more well mixed and homogenous.

There is scientific debate whether the lungs play a significant role in the distribution or elimination of propofol. Some studies support this claim (http://www.cdc.gov/growthcharts/data/set1clinical/cj41l018.pdf) while others refute it [27]. Thus, propofol injection rate and amount, cardiac output, and myocardial blood flow play a role in the immediate mixing and distribution of a bolus dose of propofol.

It is fairly well established that the speed of administration of the initial dose influences the PK of propofol and not the PD [28, 29].

For current compartmental PK models for propofol, the initial distribution volume is assumed to be represented by the central compartment volume, *V1*. Many PK models differ considerably in how *V1* is handled. The Marsh and Diprifusor models predict that *V1* increases linearly with total body weight. In contrast, the Schnider PK model uses a constant value for *V1*, i.e., *V1* is independent of weight. Obviously, the use of a constant value *V1* does not extrapolate well to small body sizes, and the Schnider PK model should not be used in children. Allometric scaling theory suggests that volumes scale linearly with body size, and Cortinez used this property in a propofol PK model for obese individuals. In the investigation by Eleveld, the many PK datasets were combined, and a single PK model was estimated. In this investigation, Eleveld found that *V1* increases approximately linearly for small body sizes but reaches a plateau for total body weights greater than about 40 kg. The reason for this deviation of *V1* scaling from allometric scaling theory may be that *V1* represents an apparent distribution volume and other variables such as incomplete mixing and limited cardiac output may dominate the apparent *V1* for large body sizes but have less obvious influence for smaller individuals.

In their investigation, Eleveld et al. found a difference between initial distribution volumes for patients compared to volunteers, even though that investigation considered both arterial and venous samples. They found that initial distribution volume was primarily determined by the patient vs. healthy volunteer covariate and that no further difference could be detected between arterial and venous samples. Indeed, other studies have found that only in samples taken soon after propofol administration—earlier than 60 s from drug administration—do arterial and venous propofol blood concentrations differ [30].

The Elimination of Propofol

Elimination of propofol occurs predominantly in the liver via cytochrome P450 (CYP) isoforms which are involved in the oxidation of propofol by human liver microsomes. Of the isoforms, only CYP2B6 is strongly related to propofol clearance suggesting that it is part of the essential pathway for propofol elimination in the liver [31]. It is oxidized to 1,4-di-isopropylquinol which is subsequently subjected to glucuronidation. The total clearance of propofol is greater than hepatic blood flow, supporting the existence of additional pathways of propofol elimination. It is well supported that the kidneys play an important role in propofol clearance [32].

There is scientific debate of the role of the lungs, whether it is a pathway for elimination or rather that propofol is only temporarily distributed to the lungs and subsequently released back into the blood. Propofol can be measured in exhaled breath and thus technically is a pathway for elimination. However, the measured propofol concentrations in breath are extremely small, on the order of parts per billion [33], and thus the total amount of propofol eliminated in this manner is likely negligible compared to other pathways.

Examination of some PK models from the literature of propofol suggests that propofol clearance is not proportional to total body weight but scales more rapidly than linearly for smaller individuals and more slowly than linear for larger individuals. The Marsh and Diprifusor models scale clearance linearly with total body weight, and there have been concerns that the model is biased for large, obese individuals [34]. This would be consistent with an overprediction of clearance in this group due to the model performing linear extrapolation of clearance from nonobese to large obese individuals. The Schnider model showed a more complex covariate relationship where clearance increased with total body weight, decreased with lean body mass as predicted by the James equation, and increased with height. More recently, PK models based on allometric theory such as those by Cortinez and Eleveld found that propofol clearance scales to the ¾ power of total body weight. Eleveld additionally found that clearance decreases slightly with age and that there appear to be gender differences with females showing slightly increased clearance for adolescents and young adults.

For very young individuals, the physiological and biochemical mechanisms involved in elimination of propofol are not fully developed, and consequently propofol clearance is much lower in this group. Post-menstrual age, an indicator of the time since conception, seems to be the strongest indicator of propofol clearance toward adult values; however, events near birth likely also play a role since clearance increases markedly about 10 days after birth [35].

Intermediate Distribution

Essentially all of the propofol PK models from the literature show an intermediate-rate distribution, faster than the initial rate but slower than the terminal rate. For three-compartment PK models, this property is characterized by the so-called fast-peripheral compartment often denoted as $V2$ with an associated inter-compartmental clearance of $Q2$.

Most propofol PK models show increased $V2$ and $Q2$ with increasing weight, and this agreement with allometric scaling theory suggests that volumes scale linearly and clearances scale to the ¾ power of body size. This property is found for the Cortinez and Eleveld PK models. The exception to this is the Schnider model in which $V2$ and $Q2$ both decrease with age.

Slow Distribution

Propofol is highly soluble in lipids. Even in nonobese individuals, this results in very large volumes of distribution, and this is evident by the quite large volumes of distribution for all of the published PK models for propofol. Typically, $V3$ has the largest volume often on the order of at least 200 l for a 70 kg individual; this is considerably larger than the blood volume.

The large volume of distribution for propofol probably contributes to its favorable clinical profile for short procedures. Recovery from a single sedative dose of propofol can be rather rapid due to immediate redistribution of drug from the blood into deep compartments. After the initial drug effects have worn off, drug returning to the blood from deep compartments arrives sufficiently slowly that the mechanisms of elimination clearance are able to maintain low enough blood concentration that substantial drug effect does not reoccur.

Obesity

Obesity is the accumulation of excess body fat to an extent that it has a negative impact on health, well-being, and life expectancy. The prevalence of obesity across the world has increased considerably in the last decades, and this trend appears to continue or possibly even accelerate. The causes of obesity from a medical point of view can be relatively simple; it can be as simple as excessive food intake. However, determining effective treatments can be very complex because of the interwoven aspects of the role of food and exercise in modern societies. Regardless of the causes and treatments of obesity, all medical practitioners are likely to be increasingly often presented with an obese patient. Thus, they should have procedures to treat patients with this condition.

A confounding factor in the discussion of the relationship between obesity and the PK and PD of propofol (or any other drug) is that, although obesity is well defined as a concept, the precise quantification of obesity in routine clinical practice is not currently possible. Even though technology exists

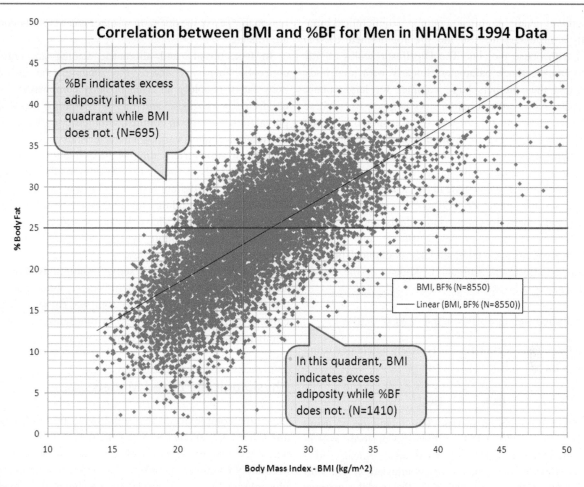

Fig. 11.4 The correlation between body mass index (BMI) and percentage body fat (%) for 8550 men in the NCHS NHANES 199 data. Clearly BMI does not have a strong relationship with body fat. Source: Mark Warren. 11-30-2010 https://commons.wikimedia.org/wiki/File: Correlation_between_BMI_and_Percent_Body_Fat_for_Men_in_ NCHS%27_NHANES_1994_Data.PNG. Reproduced under Creative Commons Attribution-Share Alike 3.0 Unported license. Accessed 5/16/2016

to estimate the body composition of patients reasonably accurately and inexpensively, anesthesiologists are nearly never provided with this information in clinical practice. Obtaining accurate information about an individual's body composition is even beyond the realm of current PK and PD studies; there are no published propofol PK or PD studies which consider accurate individualized body composition measures as covariates to PK or PD model parameters. Many studies do consider BMI and predicted LBM and FFM formulas. The formulas for LBM and FFM are simple predictors based on weight and height, and no further individualization is performed. It is also known that BMI has a tenuous relationship with the percentage of body fat [36]; this can be seen in Fig. 11.4. Despite this well-known problem, there is still the tendency of some to define obesity as being present if a patient has a BMI greater than 30. This can greatly impede scientific discussion when different parties use different definitions of obesity.

As a result of the high lipid solubility, propofol might be expected to exhibit an increasingly large volume of distribution in obese individuals. If we consider the propofol PK models from the literature, we do not see a clear indication of this, and the values for $V3$ are not strongly different when obese individuals are considered. For example, for a nonobese 35-year-old, 70-kg male patient, the predicted $V3$ for the Diprifusor, Schnider, and Schuttler PK models are 202, 238, 266 l, respectively. Interestingly, the PK models which specifically included data obtained from obese individuals were the Cortinez and Eleveld PK models which predict values for $V3$ of 237 l and 134 l, respectively. So it does not appear to be the case that $V3$ is increased in obese individuals. Thus, there is no clear relationship between $V3$ and body fat.

Although obese individuals are routinely treated in clinical practice, none of the PK-PD models specifically targeted toward obese individuals are preprogrammed in commercially available infusion pumps. So in clinical practice, it is necessary to use the preprogrammed PK-PD models with obese patients. The Diprifusor scales all PK volume and clearance parameters linearly with total body weight and thus predicts large volumes for large, obese individuals. As a result, it administers large doses to obese individuals, and clinically these have been shown to be too large. At the same time, the Schnider model exhibits paradoxical behavior for very large obese individuals due to poor extrapolation properties of the James equation used to estimate lean body mass, a covariate in the Schnider model. One technique to use these PK-PD models is to determine adjusted body sizes for obese individuals and use these adjusted sizes as inputs to the Diprifusor and Schnider PK-PD models currently commercially available. The most well-known adjustment formula is known as the Servin formula [37]:

$$\text{Adjusted weight} = \text{IBW} + 0.4 \cdot (\text{WGT} - \text{IBW})$$

where ideal body weight (IBW) is typically calculated using Lemmens formula [38]:

$$\text{IBW} = 22 \cdot \text{HGT}^2$$

where HGT is height in meters. This technique of using adjusted body weights has been found to perform well in obese individuals [21, 34], but this is most logically done with the Marsh model. The use of an adjusted weight with the Schnider model is less logical as the model equations will generate an inappropriately low estimations of lean body mass, and thus of metabolic clearance, potentially resulting in administration of inadequate doses.

The (Non-)connection Between Obesity and Allometric Scaling

Obese individuals are often physically large individuals with high body weights. It is the clinical experience of many anesthesiologists that obese individuals typically require lower amounts of propofol administration (on a per kg basis) to achieve the same drug effect as a nonobese individual. At the same time, allometric scaling suggests that, for example, elimination clearance scales (in theory) to the ¾ power exponent of size, which in most cases is assumed to be total body weight. Thus, allometric scaling also suggests that propofol clearance in large individuals is lower than less large individuals (on a per kg basis); and thus when allometric scaling is used to calculate model parameters to be used for TCI, maintenance infusion rates will be lower (on a per kg basis) than those administered to smaller nonobese individuals, for the same target concentration. It is thus

reasonable to ask the question whether these two phenomena are related.

In fact, obesity and allometric scaling are unrelated concepts. Obesity concerns the accumulation of excess body fat; it is solely an issue of body composition. Small children can be obese and this is becoming increasingly prevalent in society. In contrast, allometric scaling concerns the relationship of various characteristics with size. One could view allometric scaling as the correction for different sized individuals of "normal" body composition and mature development. In the context of this discussion, this would relate to nonobese adults and children where the relevant physiological processes have developed sufficiently to reach (allometry scaled) adult levels. Allometric scaling is intended to characterize a law of nature, to describe how things scale with size given some assumptions about their structure. The fact that in modern society obese individuals are often large individuals has complex causes related to cultural and sociological issues. In this sense, obesity and allometric scaling are unrelated phenomena.

Physiologically Based Models

Given the complexity of the initial distribution of propofol and other intravenous drugs, it should be obvious that two- and three-compartment models are too simplistic to very accurately characterize early-phase drug distribution. More physiologically based models have been described by Upton; however, these kinds of models have found considerably less clinical application compared to simple two- and three-compartment models. The reason for this is likely the increased numerical complexity of the physiologically based models. The number of components rises rapidly as physiological systems are added to the model and the amount of relevant data available is typically not sufficient to characterize these systems in their full, complex descriptions. Ultimately, a considerable number of assumptions and/or simplifications to the model must be made to make the models numerically tractable. For example, the fraction of blood flow through organs involved in elimination, such as the liver and the kidneys, must be differentiated from blood flow through other organs. However, this fraction is not well known, and it likely varies in a complex manner with anesthetic state and other factors influencing cardiac output and vascular resistance.

Some attempts have been made at a hybrid approach, combining physiologically based concepts with compartmental modeling concepts; however, these models have had considerably less development for clinical applications compared to three-compartment models. In clinical practice, one simply accepts that the simple compartmental models are not necessarily accurate over short time scales but may be expected to be reasonably well optimized over longer time scales.

Electroencephalographic (EEG) Effects

The favorable hypnotic effects of propofol are its primary reason for use in very large numbers of general anesthetics across the world. This PD effect is reflected in the individual's EEG patterns which are generated by electrical activity in the brain. Monitoring EEG during general anesthesia has been technically possible for more that half a century. The rapid advance in technology and in particular semiconductor technology and computing over the last century has driven parallel advancements in EEG monitoring technology as well.

Propofol profoundly influences EEG responses during general anesthesia. Overall, the influence of propofol on the power of various EEG frequency bands is complex, showing a biphasic response, comprising an initial increase from baseline in power at low propofol concentrations and a subsequent decrease from baseline for higher concentrations and deeper planes of anesthesia [40]. Under general anesthesia, propofol causes a reduction in the ability of the brain to process information in the gamma wave band frequencies [4]. Low-frequency signals increase in amplitude at loss of consciousness along with a shift of spatially coherent alpha oscillations from the occipital to the frontal regions [41]. Deeper levels of anesthesia are indicated by burst suppression. This complexity, coupled with the considerable interindividual variation in the PK and PD across individuals, has made the unambiguous classification of EEG signals according to anesthetic state more difficult compared to other fields of research. This has likely hindered technological advancements in EEG monitoring.

Despite, or perhaps because of, these difficulties, a number of very different algorithmic and methodological approaches have been developed, and a number of devices have become commercially available which monitor a patient's EEG during general anesthesia. Many of these devices can often also store and analyze EEG information and interface with hospital data management systems.

The effect-site equilibration time constant for EEG effects is typically estimated to be around 1.6 and 3 min [42, 43]. Some studies suggest that a fixed time constant is not appropriate and that the effect-site time constant may vary with different propofol concentrations since propofol shows dose-dependent decreases in cerebral blood flow velocity to about 40 % of its baseline value [44]. The time to equilibration of the effect site is likely inversely related to cerebral blood flow velocity since slower blood flow would increase equilibration times in a mixed system.

Bispectral Index (BIS)

The bispectral index (BIS) is an EEG monitor introduced in 1994 by Aspect Medical Systems Inc (now part of Medtronic, Dublin, Ireland) as a monitor of hypnosis or anesthetic depth during general anesthesia [45]. It has found considerable clinical application, and BIS monitors are used to titrate anesthetic dosing and to reduce the likelihood of awareness with recall. Propofol has a predictable influence on the BIS, and studies have shown that 50 % of maximal BIS depression is achieved with propofol concentrations of slightly higher than 3 µg/ml and the steepness of the concentration-effect relationship is not extreme [46]. When described using a sigmoidal Emax PD model, the gamma parameter is in general close to 1.5.

Hemodynamics

Like most general anesthetics, propofol has hemodynamic side effects. With maintained blood pressure, it causes matched reductions in cerebral blood flow and cerebral metabolic oxygen consumption [47]. An induction dose can lead to hypotension and thereby also cerebral ischemia. In data from over 25,000 patients receiving propofol [47], the overall incidence of hypotension (systolic blood pressure <90 mmHg) was 15.7 % with most of these occurring within 10 min of induction with propofol. Bradycardia (heart rate <50 beats/min) occurred in 4.8 % of patients with nearly half occurring in the first 10 min. Hypotension occurred more frequently in the elderly, females, Caucasians, and patients undergoing abdominal and integumentary procedures. The risk of hypotension is increased in the presence of opioids and long-term administration of beta-adrenergic receptor-blocking drugs. Simultaneous bradycardia and hypotension had a low rate of incidence. Although clearly recognizable, the hemodynamic effects were frequently of sufficiently low intensity and short duration so as not to require additional supportive pharmacological intervention.

The mechanism for decreased blood pressure is thought to be mostly due to decreased peripheral resistance as a result of a decreased sympathetic vasoconstrictor nerve activity as there seems to be no significant direct vascular responses at therapeutic concentrations of propofol [48]. Propofol appears to also cause mild reductions in myocardial contractility. The degree of hypotension is related to dose and rate of propofol administration, with larger and more rapid dosing showing greater effects.

During induction of anesthesia, a rapid onset of anesthesia is often desirable, and thus a larger dose is administered, at a faster rate than during maintenance of anesthesia. The result is higher peak concentrations of propofol during induction which dissipate with propofol distribution and stabilize toward constant levels during maintenance provided continuous infusion is administered for maintenance. These transient higher concentrations probably contribute to the observed higher rates of undesirable hemodynamic side effects. Thus, it seems reasonable that this hemodynamic depression can be related to drug concentrations at some hypothetical effect site related to the vascular system. However, related time constants and EC50 values and sigmoidicity values are not known.

Respiration

Propofol is a respiratory depressant and can cause apnea especially at the high concentrations associated with induction due to the relatively large doses and rapid administration intended to achieve a fast onset of effect. It is known to cause bronchodilation [49] and is thought to decrease airway resistance by causing central airway dilation [50]. It is thought to have an effect on the smooth musculature of the airway [51]. It reduces central respiratory drive and is associated with significant decreases in respiratory rate, minute volume, tidal volume, mean inspiratory flow rate, and functional residual capacity [52].

Propofol is sometimes used for conscious sedation and has been shown to increase blood carbon dioxide tension and decrease the ventilatory response to hypoxia [53]. When patients are given propofol TCI using the Schnider PK-PD model, then respiratory depression begins to occur (5 % threshold) at 3.09 μg/ml, and the EC50 is 3.99 μg/ml. Since this is close to the EC50 values thought to cause depression in the BIS, the onset of respiratory depression is likely to occur for doses intended to cause sedation or low levels of anesthesia. This underlines the risks associated with propofol for conscious sedation without adequate care for respiratory support if needed.

Injection Pain

An undesirable pharmacodynamic effect of intravenous propofol injection is a cold sensation or a feeling of intense burning in the arm directly after injection. The experience can be so severe that at the induction of anesthesia patients can have the strong desire to physically remove the infusions and leave the operating theater. Importantly, the painful experience from injection of propofol appears to occur before the amnesic effects have started. Thus, the very negative experience can often be clearly remembered, and some patients view pain on injection from propofol as the most painful part of the entire perioperative process. Given the very wide application of induction of general anesthesia using propofol, it should be clear that a large numbers of people undergo this, stated mildly, very unpleasant experience.

The underlying physiological mechanism of the propofol injection pain is not fully understood. The pain appears to be most severe when propofol is injected in smaller veins and rapidly. The original propofol formulation using polyethoxylated castor oil also showed pain on injection, but the change in formation to soya oil emulsion did not appear to strongly reduce this effect [54]. The conclusion that the solvent is not the primary cause seems reasonable, although a subsequent study has shown that a newer propofol formulation, in a different lipid emulsion, is associated with less pain, suggesting that the vehicle may well play a role [55]. The site of effect is thought to be local where propofol interacts with specific types of nociceptive receptors and the pain is transmitted by thinly myelinated A delta fibers [56].

Since the painful effect is localized to the arm of injection, a logical approach would be to change the localized conditions to reduce or eliminate the effect. However, because the underlying mechanism is not well understood, a considerable variety of different approaches have been tried such as warming and cooling of the propofol before injection, the use of different injection sites, and injection of additional analgesics such as lidocaine and opioids such as fentanyl, alfentanil, meperidine, and metoclopramide. The analgesics have been given before propofol injection or as a mixture with the propofol, and sometimes a tourniquet technique is used at injection. A systematic review of clinical trials investigating measures to prevent pain on propofol injection was performed by Picard [57]. It was found that changing the temperature of the injected propofol did not significantly reduce pain on propofol injection. The most effective technique was found to be intravenous lidocaine administered as a Bier's block 30–120 s before injection of propofol. This allows the lidocaine to most effectively influence the local conditions before the propofol is injected and thus block the mechanisms by which the propofol causes the burning sensation.

While the effectiveness of lidocaine pretreatment superficially suggests that it is the local anesthetic effects of lidocaine which reduce pain on injection, other mechanisms may be relevant. For instance, binding of lidocaine to the vascular smooth muscle [58] may be responsible for the blocking of interaction with propofol with the vascular smooth muscle thereby reducing pain on injection of propofol. This mechanism is supported by the observation that metoclopramide also reduces pain on propofol injection [59] despite its very low levels of direct local anesthetic effect [60].

Propofol Infusion Syndrome

Propofol infusion syndrome is a rare but often fatal syndrome that can occur in patients who receive long-term administration of propofol (more than 24 h) at doses greater than 4 mg/kg/h. It is thus most relevant to intensive care situation over several days. The underlying mechanism is related to impaired fatty acid oxidation and dysfunction of mitochondrial respiration that cause raised levels of intermediaries in the metabolism of long-chain, medium-chain, and short-chain fatty acids [61]. Early recognition and stopping of the propofol infusion are essential. Some research suggests that hemofiltration is also a helpful treatment [62].

Current approaches to PK and PD modeling of propofol are not likely to be useful for elucidating the mechanism of propofol infusion syndrome. Current PK models reach steady state within a few hours and, after steady state has been reached, do not predict any changes in propofol concentrations. The relevant systems regarding fatty acid oxidation are not considered in any propofol PK or PD models in current literature, even in physiological-based models. Current PK and PK models would need to become considerably improved before they are likely to be found useful to understanding propofol infusion syndrome.

Summary

The widespread use of propofol in routine clinical practice makes it essential that clinicians appreciate its unique PK and PD characteristics. It is, after all, these characteristics which make it so suitable for widespread clinical use. An open, scientific process allows all patients and clinicians to benefit from the recent advancements in research in propofol in particular and in PK and PD in general.

References

1. World Health Organization. "WHO Model List of Essential Medicines" (PDF). October 2013, p 6. Retrieved 8 Sept 2015.
2. Mazoit JX, Samii K. Binding of propofol to blood components: implications for pharmacokinetics and for pharmacodynamics. Br J Clin Pharmacol. 1999;47(1):35–42.
3. Hannivoort LN, Eleveld DJ, Proost JH, Reyntjens KM, Absalom AR, Vereecke HE, Struys MM. Development of an optimized pharmacokinetic model of dexmedetomidine using target-controlled infusion in healthy volunteers. J Am Soc Anesthesiol. 2015;123(2):357–67.
4. Lee U, Mashour GA, Kim S, Noh GJ, Choi BM. Propofol induction reduces the capacity for neural information integration: implications for the mechanism of consciousness and general anesthesia. Conscious Cogn. 2009;18(1):56–64.
5. Eleveld DJ, Proost JH, Cortínez LI, Absalom AR, Struys MM. A general purpose pharmacokinetic model for propofol. Anesth Analg. 2014;118(6):1221–37.
6. Kay NH, Uppington J, Sear JW, Douglas EJ, Cockshott ID. Pharmacokinetics of propofol ('Diprivan') as an induction agent. Postgrad Med J. 1984;61:55–7.
7. Gepts E, Camu F, Cockshott ID, Douglas EJ. Disposition of propofol administered as constant rate intravenous infusions in humans. Anesth Analg. 1987;66(12):1256–63.
8. Kataria BK, Ved SA, Nicodemus HF, Hoy GR, Lea D, Dubois MY, et al. The pharmacokinetics of propofol in children using three different data analysis approaches. Anesthesiology. 1994;80(1):104–22.
9. Schnider TW, Minto CF, Cambus PL, Andresen C, Goodale DB, Shafer SL, Youngs EJ. The influence of method of administration and covariates on the pharmacokinetics of propofol in adult volunteers. Anesthesiology. 1998;88:1170–82.
10. Schnider TW, Minto CF, Shafer SL, Gambus PL, Andresen C, Goodale DB, Youngs EJ. The influence of age on propofol pharmacodynamics. Anesthesiology. 1999;90(6):1502–16.
11. DHSS/MRC Group on Obesity Research, and John Conrad Waterlow. Research on obesity: a report of the DHSS/MRC group. HM Stationery Office; 1976.
12. Absalom AR, Mani V, De Smet T, Struys MMRF. Pharmacokinetic models for propofol—defining and illuminating the devil in the detail. Br J Anaesth. 2009;103(1):26–37.
13. Schüttler J, Ihmsen H. Population pharmacokinetics of propofol: a multicenter study. Anesthesiology. 2000;92(3):727–38.
14. Amutike D, Lal A, Absalom A, Kenny GNC. Accuracy of the Paedfusor-a new propofol target-controlled infusion system for children. Br J Anaesth. 2001;87(1):175P–6.
15. Absalom A, Amutike D, Lal A, White M, Kenny GNC. Accuracy of the 'Paedfusor' in children undergoing cardiac surgery or catheterization. Br J Anaesth. 2003;91(4):507–13.
16. Absalom A, Kenny G. 'Paedfusor' pharmacokinetic data set. Br J Anaesth. 2005;95(1):110.
17. Knibbe CA, Zuideveld KP, Aarts LP, Kuks PF, Danhof M. Allometric relationships between the pharmacokinetics of propofol in rats, children and adults. Br J Clin Pharmacol. 2005;59(6):705–11.
18. McFarlan CS, Anderson BJ, Short TG. The use of propofol infusions in paediatric anaesthesia: a practical guide. Pediatr Anesth. 1999;9(3):209–16.
19. Upton RN, Ludbrook G. A physiologically based, recirculatory model of the kinetics and dynamics of propofol in man. Anesthesiology. 2005;103(2):344–52.
20. Cortinez LI, Anderson BJ, Penna A, Olivares L, Munoz HR, Holford NHG, et al. Influence of obesity on propofol pharmacokinetics: derivation of a pharmacokinetic model. Br J Anaesth. 2010;105(4):448–56.
21. Cortínez LI, De la Fuente N, Eleveld DJ, Oliveros A, Crovari F, Sepulveda P, et al. Performance of propofol target-controlled infusion models in the obese: pharmacokinetic and pharmacodynamic analysis. Anesth Analg. 2014;119(2):302–10.
22. Przybyłowski K, Tyczka J, Szczesny D, Bienert A, Wiczling P, Kut K, et al. Pharmacokinetics and pharmacodynamics of propofol in cancer patients undergoing major lung surgery. J Pharmacokinet Pharmacodyn. 2015;42(2):111–22.
23. Huxley JS, Teissier G. Terminology of relative growth. Nature. 1936;137(3471):780–1.
24. Kleiber M. Body size and metabolic rate. Physiol Rev. 1947;27(4):511–41.
25. West GB, Brown JH, Enquist BJ. A general model for the origin of allometric scaling laws in biology. Science. 1997;276(5309):122–6.

26. Dawidowicz AL, Fornal E, Mardarowicz M, Fijalkowska A. The role of human lungs in the biotransformation of propofol. Anesthesiology. 2000;93(4):992–7.

27. Hiraoka H, Yamamoto K, Miyoshi S, Morita T, Nakamura K, Kadoi Y, et al. Kidneys contribute to the extrahepatic clearance of propofol in humans, but not lungs and brain. Br J Clin Pharmacol. 2005;60(2):176–82.

28. Doufas AG, Bakhshandeh M, Bjorksten AR, Shafer SL, Sessler DI. Induction speed is not a determinant of propofol pharmacodynamics. Anesthesiology. 2004;101(5):1112.

29. Masui K, Kira M, Kazama T, Hagihira S, Mortier EP, Struys MM. Early phase pharmacokinetics but not pharmacodynamics are influenced by propofol infusion rate. Anesthesiology. 2009;111(4):805–17.

30. Major E, Aun C, Yate PM, Savege TM, Verniquet AJW, Adam H, Douglas EJ. Influence of sample site on blood concentrations of ICI 35 868. Br J Anaesth. 1983;55(5):371–5.

31. Oda Y, Hamaoka N, Hiroi T, Imaoka S, Hase I, Tanaka K, et al. Involvement of human liver cytochrome P4502B6 in the metabolism of propofol. Br J Clin Pharmacol. 2001;51(3):281–5.

32. Takizawa D, Hiraoka H, Goto F, Yamamoto K, Horiuchi R. Human kidneys play an important role in the elimination of propofol. J Am Soc Anesthesiol. 2005;102(2):327–30.

33. Colin P, Eleveld DJ, van den Berg JP, Vereecke HE, Struys MM, Schelling G, et al. Propofol breath monitoring as a potential tool to improve the prediction of intraoperative plasma concentrations. Clin Pharmacokinet. 2016;55:849.

34. Albertin A, Poli D, La Colla L, Gonfalini M, Turi S, Pasculli N, et al. Predictive performance of 'Servin's formula' during BIS®-guided propofol-remifentanil target-controlled infusion in morbidly obese patients. Br J Anaesth. 2007;98(1):66–75.

35. Allegaert K, Peeters MY, Verbesselt R, Tibboel D, Naulaers G, De Hoon JN, Knibbe CA. Inter-individual variability in propofol pharmacokinetics in preterm and term neonates. Br J Anaesth. 2007;99(6):864–70.

36. Corral AR, Somers VK, Sierra-Johnson J, Thomas RJ, Collazo-Clavell ML, Korinek J, et al. Accuracy of body mass index to diagnose obesity in the USA adult population. Int J Obes. 2008;32(6):959–66.

37. Servin F, Farinotti R, Haberer JP, Desmonts JM. Propofol infusion for maintenance of anesthesia in morbidly obese patients receiving nitrous oxide. A clinical and pharmacokinetic study. Anesthesiology. 1993;78(4):657–65.

38. Lemmens HJ, Brodsky JB, Bernstein DP. Estimating ideal body weight–a new formula. Obes Surg. 2005;15(7):1082–3.

39. Niedermeyer E, da Silva FL, editors. Electroencephalography: basic principles, clinical applications, and related fields. Philadelphia: Lippincott Williams & Wilkins; 2005.

40. Kuizenga K, Wierda JMKH, Kalkman CJ. Biphasic EEG changes in relation to loss of consciousness during induction with thiopental, propofol, etomidate, midazolam or sevoflurane. Br J Anaesth. 2001;86(3):354–60.

41. Purdon PL, Pierce ET, Mukamel EA, Prerau MJ, Walsh JL, Wong KFK, et al. Electroencephalogram signatures of loss and recovery of consciousness from propofol. Proc Natl Acad Sci. 2013;110(12):E1142–51.

42. Struys MM, De Smet T, Depoorter B, Versichelen LF, Mortier EP, Dumortier F, et al. Comparison of plasma compartment versus two methods for effect compartment--controlled target-controlled infusion for propofol. Anesthesiology. 2000;92(2):399–406.

43. Wakeling HG, Zimmerman JB, Howell S, Glass PS. Targeting effect compartment or central compartment concentration of propofol: what predicts loss of consciousness? Anesthesiology. 1999;90(1):92–7.

44. Ludbrook GL, Visco E, Lam AM. Propofol: relation between brain concentrations, electroencephalogram, middle cerebral artery blood flow velocity, and cerebral oxygen extraction during induction of anesthesia. Anesthesiology. 2002;97(6):1363–70.

45. Sigl JC, Chamoun NG. An introduction to bispectral analysis for the electroencephalogram. J Clin Monit. 1994;10(6):392–404.

46. Rigouzzo A, Girault L, Louvet N, Servin F, De-Smet T, Piat V, et al. The relationship between bispectral index and propofol during target-controlled infusion anesthesia: a comparative study between children and young adults. Anesth Analg. 2008;106(4):1109–16.

47. Hug Jr CC, McLeskey CH, Nahrwold ML, Roizen MF, Stanley TH, Thisted RA, et al. Hemodynamic effects of propofol: data from over 25,000 patients. Anesth Analg. 1993;77 Suppl 4:S21–9.

48. Robinson BJ, Ebert TJ, O'brien TJ, Colinco MD, Muzi M. Mechanisms whereby propofol mediates peripheral vasodilation in humans. Sympathoinhibition or direct vascular relaxation? Anesthesiology. 1997;86(1):64–72.

49. Conti G, Dell'Utri D, Vilardi V, De Blasi RA, Pelaia P, Antonelli M, et al. Propofol induces bronchodilation in mechanically ventilated chronic obstructive pulmonary disease (COPD) patients. Acta Anaesthesiol Scand. 1993;37(1):105–9.

50. Peratoner A, Nascimento CS, Santana MCE, Cadete RA, Negri EM, Gullo A, et al. Effects of propofol on respiratory mechanic and lung histology in normal rats. Br J Anaesth. 2004;92(5):737–40.

51. Ouedraogo N, Roux E, Forestier F, Rossetti M, Savineau JP, Marthan R. Effects of intravenous anesthetics on normal and passively sensitized human isolated airway smooth muscle. Anesthesiology. 1998;88(2):317–26.

52. Sebel PS, Lowdon JD. Propofol: a new intravenous anesthetic. Anesthesiology. 1989;71(2):260.

53. Blouin RT, Seifert HA, Babenco HD, Conard PF, Gross JB. Propofol depresses the hypoxic ventilatory response during conscious sedation and isohypercapnia. Anesthesiology. 1993;79(6):1177–82.

54. Kay B, Rolly GICI. ICI 35868-The effect of a change of formulation on the incidence of pain after intravenous injection. Acta Anaesthesiol Belg. 1976;28(4):317–22.

55. Sun NC, Wong AY, Irwin MG. A comparison of pain on intravenous injection between two preparations of propofol. Anesth Analg. 2005;101(3):675–8.

56. Klement W, Arndt JO. Pain on injection of propofol: effects of concentration and diluent. Br J Anaesth. 1991;67(3):281–4.

57. Picard P, Tramer MR. Prevention of pain on injection with propofol: a quantitative systematic review. Anesth Analg. 2000;90(4):963–9.

58. Nicol ME, Moriarty J, Edwards J, Robbie DS, A'Hern RP. Modification of pain on injection of propofol—a comparison between lignocaine and procaine. Anaesthesia. 1991;46(1):67–9.

59. Liaw WJ, Pang WW, Chang DP, Hwang MH. Pain on injection of propofol: the mitigating influence of metoclopramide using different techniques. Acta Anaesthesiol Scand. 1999;43(1):24–7.

60. Ganta R, Fee JPH. Pain on injection of propofol: comparison of lignocaine with metoclopramide. Br J Anaesth. 1992;69(3):316–7.

61. Wolf A, Weir P, Segar P, Stone J, Shield J. Impaired fatty acid oxidation in propofol infusion syndrome. Lancet. 2001;357(9256):606–7.

62. Karakitsos D, Poularas J, Kalogeromitros A, Karabinis A. The propofol infusion syndrome treated with haemofiltration. Is there a time for genetic screening? Acta Anaesthesiol Scand. 2007;51(5):644–5.

Douglas E. Raines

Etomidate

Clinical Development and Therapeutic Actions of Etomidate

Etomidate is a highly potent and efficacious sedative-hypnotic agent that is commonly used to induce anesthesia (Fig. 12.1). It was one of several dozen imidazole-based compounds synthesized by Janssen Pharmaceuticals in the early 1960s as part of a program to develop new antifungal drugs [1]; imidazole-based drugs have antifungal properties because they suppress the biosynthesis of the steroid ergosterol, which is a critical component of the fungal cytoplasmic membrane [2, 3].Upon testing these compounds for safety in rats, ten were unexpectedly found to possess hypnotic activity. Studies using a wide range of doses revealed that etomidate's therapeutic index in rats (12) was higher than those of the other hypnotic imidazole compounds (range, 5.0–9.1) or existing intravenous hypnotic agents such as pentobarbital (5.0) and phenobarbital (2.0), suggesting that it might have unique value as an anesthetic agent.

The initial characterization of etomidate by Janssen Pharmaceuticals utilized a racemic mixture of the drug. Upon synthesis and study of its two enantiomers, it became evident that essentially all of etomidate's hypnotic activity is mediated by the R enantiomer and that the therapeutic index of that enantiomer is approximately twice as high as that of the racemic mixture [4]. Consequently, it was etomidate's R enantiomer that was ultimately developed for clinical use.

Etomidate's comparatively high therapeutic index (defined in unventilated animals) is almost certainly attributable to its relatively modest effects on respiratory function. Studies of etomidate in humans show that it produces little or no change in respiratory parameters when given alone at clinically relevant doses [5, 6]. When given along with remifentanil, etomidate produces less respiratory depression than propofol [7]. Studies utilizing steady-state end-tidal carbon dioxide concentrations revealed that although an induction dose of etomidate (0.3 mg/kg) decreases the ventilatory drive in response to changing levels of carbon dioxide (i.e., reduces the slope of the carbon dioxide concentration—ventilatory response curve), it doubles minute ventilation when end-tidal carbon dioxide is held constant at 46 mmHg [8]. For these reasons, etomidate may be preferable to other hypnotic agents when spontaneous ventilation is desired [9–11].

Cardiovascular function is similarly preserved after etomidate administration. Etomidate does not release histamine and maintains hemodynamic stability even in patients with valvular and coronary artery disease [12–14]. As a consequence, its greatest value may be as an anesthetic induction agent for patients with significant cardiac disease. Etomidate also maintains cerebral perfusion pressure while reducing cerebral metabolic requirements and blood flow, features that are desirable in patients with space-occupying intracranial lesions [15]. In dogs, hepatic arterial and portal blood flow is reduced by etomidate [16]. Nevertheless in humans, etomidate minimally affects the metabolism of coadministered drugs [17].

It has been reported that etomidate can enhance focal epileptogenic activity in patients with epilepsy and produce generalized epileptiform electroencephalographic activity in patients without a history of seizure disorders [18]. As a sedative-hypnotic agent for electroconvulsive therapy, etomidate induces seizures that are longer in duration and with fewer side effects than methohexital [19]. For this reason, etomidate has often been advocated for patients undergoing electroconvulsive therapy and, in particular, those who are seizure resistant [20–22]. Bispectral (BIS)

D.E. Raines, MD(✉)
Department of Anesthesia, Critical Care, and Pain Medicine,
Massachusetts General Hospital, 55 Fruit Street, GRB444,
Boston, MA 02114, USA
e-mail: draines@partners.org

© Springer International Publishing AG 2017
A.R. Absalom, K.P. Mason (eds.), *Total Intravenous Anesthesia and Target Controlled Infusions*,
DOI 10.1007/978-3-319-47609-4_12

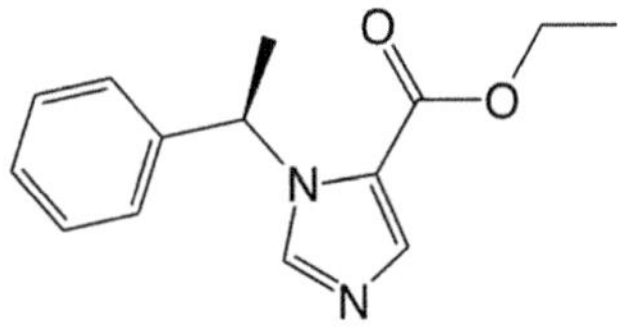

Fig. 12.1 The molecular structure of etomidate. Etomidate has a single chiral carbon. The R enantiomer (shown) is the more potent form and the one used clinically

index values of patients who have received etomidate correlate with predicted blood concentrations. However, with etomidate, loss of consciousness tends to occur at BIS values that are lower than those seen with other anesthetic agents including propofol and sevoflurane [23].

Etomidate Pharmacokinetics and Pharmacodynamics

Anesthetic induction upon administering a typical bolus dose of etomidate (0.3 mg/kg) occurs within seconds and lasts 3–5 min [24]. With such bolus dosing, plasma etomidate concentrations reach a peak value of approximately 300 ng/ml before falling in a triexponential manner. Analysis using a three-compartment open pharmacokinetic model yields an initial half-life after bolus administration of 2.6 ± 1.3 min, an intermediate half-life of 28.7 ± 14 min, and an apparent elimination half-life of 4.6 ± 2.6 h. The two early exponential phases are consistent with etomidate's rapid distribution into the brain with resultant anesthetic induction followed by its extensive redistribution into other tissues leading to anesthetic emergence. The late exponential phase, which defines etomidate's elimination half-life, reflects the slow, rate-limiting return of the drug from the deep peripheral compartment and hepatic elimination. Although compartmental models do not define each compartment in terms of an actual biological organ or tissue, it seems likely that fat contributes significantly to that deep compartment [4]. Etomidate is metabolized in the liver by hepatic esterases to a carboxylic acid metabolite that has no known pharmacological activity and is excreted primarily in the urine [25].

With prolonged continuous etomidate infusion, hypnotic recovery is significantly slower than after single bolus administration. When infused for 30 ± 26 min as the hypnotic component of a total intravenous anesthetic regimen for gynecological surgery, emergence occurred (on average) 20 ± 9 min after terminating the etomidate infusion, and patients remained drowsy for 4–6 h after leaving the recovery room [26]. Hebron et al. reported that awakening from

even moderate levels of sedation and steady-state plasma concentrations averaging only 158 ± 36 ng/ml occurred approximately 40 min after discontinuing etomidate infusions lasting 2 days [27, 28]. As expected from its several hour terminal elimination half-life, etomidate concentrations in the plasma remained measurable (as high as 150 ng/ml in one patient) for 24 h after terminating such prolonged infusions.

Studies in humans and animals have sought to define how pathological states modify etomidate pharmacokinetics. Human studies have shown that etomidate's clearance rate is unaffected by hepatic cirrhosis. However, etomidate's terminal elimination half-life is prolonged (to 9 h) because its volume of distribution is increased [29]. Elderly patients or those with hepatic or renal failure may require lower dosing because plasma protein binding is reduced [30, 31]. Studies in pigs have shown that hemorrhagic shock only minimally affects etomidate pharmacokinetics. The only notable change was a reduction in the volume of the two peripheral compartments, which likely reflected redistribution of blood flow away from these compartments as cardiac output was reduced.

Suppression of Adrenocortical by Etomidate

The most notable and potentially serious side effect of etomidate administration is the suppression of adrenocortical steroid synthesis. The ability of etomidate to suppress stress-induced steroid synthesis was first reported in 1982 by Preziosi and Vacca, but its clinical significance at the time was unclear [32]. However in their seminal letter to Lancet the following year, Ledingham and Watt reported that critically ill multiple trauma patients in their intensive care unit who received prolonged etomidate infusions for sedation had a mortality that was almost threefold higher than those who received benzodiazepines (69 % versus 25 %, $p < 0.0005$) [33]. They postulated that this increased death rate was attributable to etomidate's suppression of adrenocortical function. In vitro studies using adrenocortical cells and in vivo studies in both surgical and nonsurgical patients showed that etomidate inhibited the adrenocortical cytochrome P450 enzyme 11α-hydroxylase and blocked the conversion of 11-deoxycortisol to cortisol [34–37]. After a single bolus dose of etomidate, this adrenocortical suppression lasts approximately 6 h in healthy individuals [38, 39]. However in the critically ill, such suppression can last for days [40–42].

Prior to the publication of the Ledingham and Watt letter and the subsequent full report of the study, etomidate was enthusiastically recommended as a continuously infusible sedative because it maintained respiratory drive and hemodynamic stability [33, 43–46]. Since that time, the use of prolonged etomidate infusions has been almost completely abandoned out of concerns that it increases morbidity and mortality. An interesting exception is in patients with Cushing's syndrome where low-dose etomidate infusions continue to be used to reduce cortisol synthesis and ameliorate the symptoms of hypercortisolemia [47–51]

Etomidate continues to be used as a single bolus to induce anesthesia at the start of surgery, particularly in the elderly and critically ill. However, even this limited use is controversial as it is known to suppress adrenocortical function for many hours or even days [52–56]. Clinical studies and meta-analyses aiming to evaluate the impact of a single dose of etomidate on morbidity and mortality in the critically ill have yielded apparently conflicting results with some suggesting significant deleterious effects [57–62] and others suggesting no affect at all [63–66]. Thus, we are in a state of clinical equipoise with respect to the use of single-dose etomidate in the critically ill.

Other Adverse Effects of Etomidate

Involuntary movements (myoclonus) are commonly observed after etomidate administration, with some studies reporting an incidence as high as 80 % in unpremedicated patients [67–70]. Such movements may resemble myoclonic seizures, but are physiologically distinct. Although the mechanism of etomidate-induced myoclonus is not clear, it has been suggested that it occurs because etomidate depresses inhibitory neural circuits in the central nervous system sooner and at lower concentrations than excitatory circuits [70]. Regardless of the mechanism, myoclonus can be significantly reduced or completely prevented by administering a variety of drugs with central nervous system depressant effects including opiates [71, 72], benzodiazepines [73], dexmedetomidine [74], thiopental [74], lidocaine [75], and magnesium [76].

Pain at the injection site is another common side effect of etomidate administration, although its incidence is highly dependent upon the size of the vein into which it is injected [77] and the formulation that is used. When etomidate is formulated in either cyclodextrin [78] or a lipid emulsion of medium- and long-chain triglycerides [79, 80], the incidence of injection pain is significantly less than when dissolved in a 35 % propylene glycol/water mixture. The underlying mechanism for such pain may be etomidate's ability to activate transient receptor potential (TRP) ion channels present in sensory neurons [81]. By lowering the free-aqueous etomidate concentration and/or reducing solution osmolality, lipid emulsion and cyclodextrin formulations may reduce TRP channel activation, leading to less pain on injection.

Finally, postoperative nausea and vomiting have long been associated with etomidate administration with reported incidences as high as 40 % [77, 82, 83]. However, a prospective study using etomidate formulated in a lipid emulsion found an incidence of nausea that was no greater than that produced by propofol perhaps suggesting that the emetogenic trigger in etomidate is the propylene glycol solvent and not the anesthetic itself. [84]

Molecular Mechanisms of Etomidate Action

Etomidate produces sedation and hypnosis by binding to and enhancing the function of $GABA_A$ receptors. This conclusion is strongly supported by numerous studies including those demonstrating high correlations between the in vivo hypnotic potencies of etomidate and etomidate analogues and their in vitro $GABA_A$ receptor enhancing activities [85–87]. They are further supported by studies showing that an amino acid mutation that reduces etomidate's ability to enhance $GABA_A$ receptor function also reduces the sensitivity of transgenic mice containing that mutation to etomidate's hypnotic and immobilizing actions [88]. In electrophysiological experiments, $GABA_A$ receptor enhancement may be detected at low etomidate concentrations as an increase in the receptor's sensitivity to GABA (i.e., a leftward shift in the GABA concentration-response curve), a phenomenon commonly termed agonist potentiation. At high concentrations, etomidate can also directly activate $GABA_A$ receptors even in the absence of GABA. Site-directed mutagenesis and modeling studies by Forman et al. suggest that both agonist potentiation and direct activation result from etomidate binding to the same class of sites on the $GABA_A$ receptor's open channel state [89, 90].

The etomidate-binding sites on $GABA_A$ receptors responsible for enhancement are thought to be located within the receptor's transmembrane domain at the interfaces between the α- and β-subunits. $GABA_A$ receptors containing α_2- or α_3-subunits are more sensitive to etomidate's enhancing actions than those containing the α_1-subunit [86, 91]. This subunit selectivity may be contrasted with that exhibited by propofol, which modulates $GABA_A$ receptors containing α_1-, α_2-, or α_3-subunits with equal potency [86]. It is, therefore, tempting to speculate that at least some of the pharmacodynamic differences between etomidate and propofol (e.g., incidence of myoclonus) are due to their differing selectivities for the various $GABA_A$ receptor subtypes present in the central nervous system. In addition to the enhancing sites, there is also a distinct site(s) that causes channel inhibition. This inhibitory site lacks the enantiomeric selectivity exhibited by the enhancing site and almost certainly binds etomidate with much lower affinity [86]. Therefore, it is unlikely that this site contributes to etomidate's pharmacology when the drug is given at clinically relevant doses.

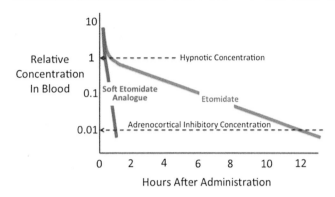

Fig. 12.2 Time-dependent change in hypnotic drug concentrations after single intravenous bolus administration. After administering a hypnotic dose of etomidate, the concentration of etomidate in the blood must fall by two orders of magnitude before adrenocortical function recovers. Because etomidate is relatively slowly metabolized, such recovery requires many hours (12 h in this figure). Soft etomidate analogues are designed to be rapidly metabolized to accelerate both hypnotic and adrenocortical recoveries

Rapidly Metabolized Etomidate Analogues

The prolonged adrenocortical suppression produced by etomidate results from two important aspects of etomidate's pharmacology. First, etomidate is approximately 100-fold more potent a suppressor of adrenocortical function than it is a sedative-hypnotic [24, 92, 93]. Consequently, an anesthetic induction dose of etomidate represents a massive overdose with respect to its ability to suppress adrenocortical function. Second, etomidate's terminal elimination half-life is rather long: 3–5 h [24, 29]. Thus, after just a single anesthetic induction dose of etomidate, many hours must pass before etomidate's concentration in the blood falls below that which suppresses adrenocortical steroid synthesis. It is within this mechanistic context that the strategy emerged to design rapidly metabolized analogues of etomidate [94]. The premise was that because these "soft" analogues would be metabolized much more rapidly than the "hard" drug (i.e., etomidate) upon which they are based, recovery from adrenocortical suppression would occur significantly more quickly (Fig. 12.2). In addition, it was hypothesized that hypnotic recovery would similarly occur more quickly—particularly after prolonged infusion—because of this more rapid elimination.

Methoxycarbonyl Etomidate (MOC-Etomidate): The Prototypical Soft Etomidate Analogue

MOC-etomidate was the first soft etomidate analogue to be synthesized and studied (Fig. 12.3a) [94]. Similar to remifentanil and esmolol, it contains a metabolically labile

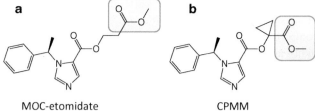

Fig. 12.3 The molecular structures of (**a**) methoxycarbonyl etomidate (MOC-etomidate) and (**b**) cyclopropyl-methoxycarbonyl metomidate (CPMM). The metabolically labile ester moiety in each etomidate analogue is highlighted by the *blue box*

ester moiety that is attached to the pharmacophore via a two-carbon spacer. Thus, it was anticipated that MOC-etomidate would be rapidly hydrolyzed by nonspecific esterases to a carboxylic acid metabolite that possessed significantly less pharmacological activity than the parent compound, MOC-etomidate.

Initial studies of MOC-etomidate in both tadpoles and rats demonstrated that similar to etomidate, MOC-etomidate rapidly induces hypnosis (albeit with potency that is 1/5 to 1/10 that of etomidate), has a high therapeutic index, and enhances $GABA_A$ receptor function. However, compared to etomidate, it is much more rapidly metabolized. For example, in pooled human liver s9 fraction, MOC-etomidate was hydrolyzed with a half-life of 4.4 min, whereas etomidate was not measurably hydrolyzed even after 40 min. Therefore, after single bolus administration, MOC-etomidate is ultrashort acting as a hypnotic and does not produce prolonged adrenocortical suppression.

In the soft analogue strategy of drug design, the pharmacological activity of the metabolite is a critical determinant of drug pharmacology. Ideally, the metabolite would have no activity at all, but in practice this is rarely the case. In the case of MOC-etomidate, the carboxylic acid metabolite that forms upon hydrolysis has potencies for activating $GABA_A$ receptors, producing hypnosis, and inhibiting cortisol synthesis that are ~300-fold less than those of MOC-etomidate [95]. Although this potency difference between metabolite and parent drug is sufficiently large to achieve the goal of rapid recovery after bolus administration and similar to that of esmolol (also 300-fold), it is less than those reported for both remifentanil (4600-fold) and remimazolam (1600-fold) [96–98].

Subsequent studies focused on assessing the potential value of MOC-etomidate as a hypnotic maintenance agent [99]. MOC-etomidate was infused into rats for periods of time ranging from 5 to 30 min. After the infusion ended, the time required for rats to recover was measured using electro-encephalographic (burst suppression ratio) and behavioral (loss of righting reflexes) endpoints. After 5-minute infusions, the electroencephalogram recovered to near baseline values and righting reflexes returned in 1–2 min. However, with longer MOC-etomidate infusion times, recovery times were dramatically longer. Such marked context sensitivity was unexpected because it had not been observed with other commonly used soft drugs. Chemical analysis of the blood and cerebrospinal fluid revealed that during MOC-etomidate infusions, MOC-etomidate metabolite concentrations reached levels sufficient to cause hypnosis. After MOC-etomidate infusions ended, metabolite concentrations decreased on the timescale of hours, paralleling the time required for electroencephalographic and behavioral recoveries. This strongly suggested that the delayed recovery after prolonged MOC-etomidate infusions was caused by a large accumulation of the weakly active metabolite in the central nervous system. Thus, MOC-etomidate provided a proof of principle that soft etomidate analogues could be produced. However, its relatively low potency and very rapid metabolism required the administration of extremely large doses to maintain hypnosis and resulted in sufficient metabolite accumulation to markedly delay recovery. This made the drug unsuitable for clinical development as a continuously infused hypnotic maintenance agent.

Cyclopropyl-Methoxycarbonyl Metomidate (CPMM): A Second-Generation Soft Etomidate Analogue

To ameliorate the problem of metabolite accumulation during prolonged infusion, work was begun to develop second-generation soft etomidate analogues with optimized pharmacokinetic and pharmacodynamic properties [100]. These efforts focused on modifying the structure of the spacer that links the metabolically labile ester moiety to the etomidate pharmacophore. It was hypothesized that the hydrolysis rate could be beneficially slowed (thus reducing infusion requirements and metabolite accumulation) by adding substituent groups onto that spacer to modestly increase steric hindrance. At the same time, it was hoped that such structural modifications would increase hypnotic potency. Thirteen new soft etomidate analogues were produced whose spacers were either one or two carbons in length and contained various aliphatic-protecting groups to slow hydrolysis. In vitro and in vivo studies revealed that the metabolic half-lives in rat blood and hypnotic potencies in rats ranged by more than an order of magnitude. The most promising of these compounds was cyclopropyl-methoxycarbonyl metomidate (CPMM). It differs from MOC-etomidate in that its spacer is only one carbon in length and contains a cyclopropyl substituent group (Fig. 12.3b). Compared to MOC-etomidate, its hypnotic potency in rats is eightfold higher, and it is metabolized by

esterases slightly more slowly. Because of these pharmacodynamic and pharmacokinetic differences, infusion dosing of CPMM is one to two orders of magnitude lower than that of MOC-etomidate.

Studies in both rats and dogs showed that hypnotic recovery after terminating a continuous infusion of CPMM occurs within several minutes regardless of the infusion duration [101, 102]. Such context-insensitive recovery is distinct from that exhibited by either etomidate or propofol. Adrenocortical function similarly recovers rapidly after infusion termination. In rats, adrenocorticotropic hormone-stimulated plasma corticosterone concentrations returned to baseline values within 30 min after terminating a 2-h CPMM infusion. In dogs, adrenocortical responsiveness 90 min after terminating a 2-h CPMM infusion was equivalent to that observed after terminating a 2-h propofol infusion, suggesting that with CPMM infusions lasting only a few hours, any adrenocortical suppression was likely to be clinically unimportant.

Pharmacokinetic studies in dogs confirmed that CPMM is rapidly hydrolyzed to the expected carboxylic acid metabolite in vivo [102]. After a single CPMM bolus dose, venous plasma concentrations rapidly increased and then fell by nearly three orders of magnitude over the subsequent hour. CPMM's terminal elimination half-life was 16.1 ± 2.99 min, which was significantly faster than that of etomidate (60.1 ± 10.4 min). The clearance of CPMM was not only significantly faster than that of etomidate (211 ± 26 versus 14.7 ± 2.78 ml $\cdot$ kg^{-1} min^{-1}, respectively); it was also more than an order of magnitude greater than the total hepatic blood flow. This implied that the primary site of CPMM metabolism in these dogs was extrahepatic. After 2-h infusions, CPMM's terminal elimination half-life was sixfold longer (96.8 ± 38.5 min) than that observed after single bolus administration and essentially identical to that of etomidate (88.1 ± 14.1 min). The similar terminal elimination half-lives of CPMM and etomidate after 2-h infusions suggest a common rate-controlling step. Previous pharmacokinetic modeling studies of etomidate indicate that this step is the slow return of drug into the central compartment from a poorly perfused deep compartment (e.g., fat) into which the drug had accumulated during the infusion period [24].

So how does CPMM compare with propofol? Both anesthetics enhance the function of GABA$_A$ receptors [103]. However, CPMM retains etomidate's ß-subunit selectivity. This suggests that CPMM and etomidate act on the same GABA$_A$ receptor subtypes. In tadpoles, an animal common model system for quantifying the hypnotic potencies of anesthetic agents, CPMM was found to be approximately half as potent as propofol with median hypnotic concentrations of 2.6 ± 0.19 μM and 1.3 ± 0.04 μM, respectively [103]. However, CPMM's median hypnotic

a

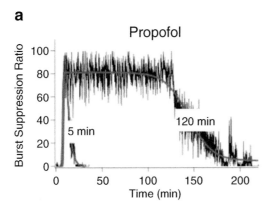

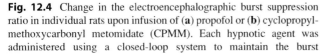

b

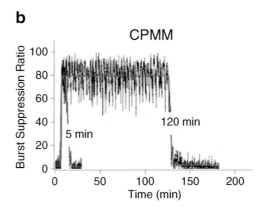

Fig. 12.4 Change in the electroencephalographic burst suppression ratio in individual rats upon infusion of (**a**) propofol or (**b**) cyclopropyl-methoxycarbonyl metomidate (CPMM). Each hypnotic agent was administered using a closed-loop system to maintain the burst suppression ratio at 80 % for either 5 or 120 min (in the presence of 1 % isoflurane). The *red curves* are fits of each data set to a biphasic sigmoidal equation

dose in rats is approximately 1/6 that of propofol. This apparent discrepancy likely relates to the different extents to which CPMM and propofol bind to plasma proteins; protein binding is expected to be ~75 % for CPMM (i.e., similar to etomidate) compared to 98 % for propofol. Encephalographic recovery times in rats following propofol infusion are highly dependent upon the infusion duration (Fig. 12.4). For example, the time required for the burst suppression ratio to recover to within 10 % of baseline was 9.7 ± 2.3 min after a 5-min propofol infusion but 45 ± 11 min after a 120-min infusion. In contrast and as noted above, recovery after CPMM infusion is short and independent of infusion duration (Fig. 12.5). Such infusion duration-independent recovery is similar to that seen with remifentanil, which is also rapidly metabolized by nonspecific esterases to an essentially inactive carboxylic metabolite.

Studies in rats suggest that CPMM may offer important advantages over etomidate in the setting of sepsis. In a lipopolysaccharide inflammatory model of sepsis, plasma corticosterone concentrations in rats were up to ninefold higher during 1-h infusions of CPMM as compared to etomidate suggesting that CPMM's intrinsic ability to inhibit 11β-hydroxylase is significantly lower than that of etomidate [104]. In addition, plasma cytokine concentrations were lower, metabolic derangement was less, and survival was higher in rats that received CPMM as compared to those that received etomidate.

Under the name ABP-700, CPMM has recently completed phase 1 clinical studies in healthy human volunteers. Although the results have not been formally reported, public comments made by The Medicines Company indicate that ABP-700's pharmacology in humans mirrors that seen in animals with an onset and offset of hypnotic action that are fast and effects on adrenocortical steroid synthesis that are similar to that seen with propofol.

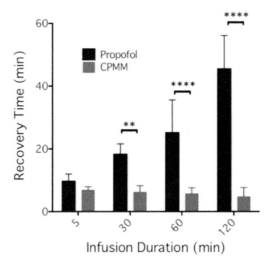

Fig. 12.5 90 % electroencephalographic burst suppression ratio recovery time in the rat as a function of propofol or CPMM infusion duration. This recovery time is defined as the time when the infusion ended until the time that the burst suppression returned to within 10 % of the post-infusion baseline value. The data shows that recovery times increased with infusion duration with propofol but not with CPMM. For infusion times of 30 min and longer, recovery times were significantly shorter after infusion of CPMM versus propofol. Each bar is the mean ($\pm$SD) obtained using five rats. Studies were performed in a background of 1 % isoflurane. ****$p < 0.0001$; **$p < 0.001$

Pyrrole Etomidate Analogues

X-ray crystallographic studies of binding of imidazole-containing molecules to cytochrome P450 enzymes indicate that high-affinity binding requires a coordination bond between the basic nitrogen in the imidazole ring and the heme iron located at the enzyme's active site [105–107]. Because 11β-hydroxylase is a cytochrome P450 enzyme, it was hypothesized that etomidate's high binding affinity to

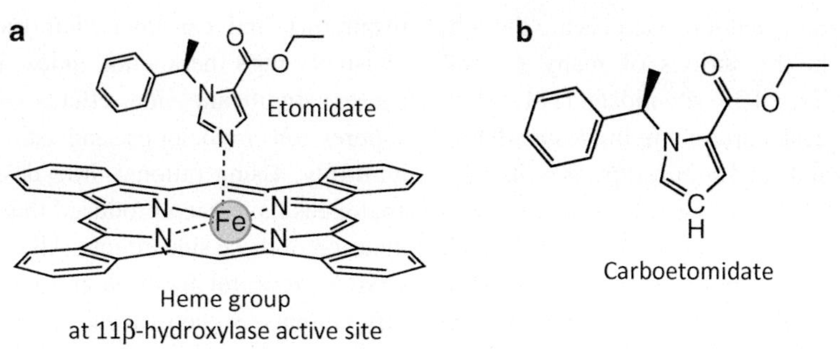

Fig. 12.6 Carboetomidate is a pyrrole etomidate analogue in which the basic nitrogen in etomidate's imidazole ring has been replaced with a —CH moiety. (**a**) Computer docking studies using homology a model of 11α-hydroxylase indicate that etomidate binds with high affinity to the enzyme (and potently inhibits its function) because the basic nitrogen in etomidate's imidazole ring forms a coordination bond with the enzyme's heme iron. (**b**) Molecular structure of carboetomidate. The basic nitrogen in etomidate's imidazole ring has been replaced by a —CH moiety

this enzyme similarly resulted from analogous coordination bonding (Fig. 12.6a). Thus, it was predicted that binding affinity could be substantially reduced (and adrenocortical suppression eliminated) by replacing this nitrogen with other atoms that are incapable of forming coordination bonds. At the same time, it was hoped that such a molecular change would not greatly impact GABA$_A$ receptor potency (and thus hypnotic activity) and preserve etomidate's beneficial properties such as its minimal affects on cardiovascular and respiratory function and its high therapeutic index.

Carboetomidate

Carboetomidate is a pyrrole analogue of etomidate in which the basic nitrogen has been replaced with a —CH group (Fig. 12.6b) [108]. Studies in GABA$_A$ receptors demonstrated that carboetomidate retains etomidate's ability to enhance GABA$_A$ receptor function. It produces loss of righting reflexes (an animal surrogate for hypnosis) in both tadpoles and rats. However, its potency is nearly an order of magnitude lower than that of etomidate. This was a surprising observation because carboetomidate is significantly more hydrophobic than etomidate and, therefore, predicted by the Meyer-Overton correlation to be a more potent hypnotic. This suggests that etomidate's imidazole nitrogen also contributes to etomidate binding to the GABA$_A$ receptor, a conclusion supported by quantitative structure-activity analyses (unpublished data). At equihypnotic doses, carboetomidate produces even less hypotension than etomidate in rats and does not suppress adrenocortical steroid synthesis. Studies in human adrenocortical carcinoma cells demonstrated that the reason that carboetomidate does not suppress adrenocortical function is that it is three orders of magnitude less potent an inhibitor of cortisol synthesis than is etomidate.

Carboetomidate's relatively low affinity for 11-β-hydroxylase has also been demonstrated directly using binding and spectroscopic techniques. [109] In contrast to etomidate, carboetomidate is unable to reduce the irreversible photoincorporation of an etomidate photoaffinity label or produce a type 2 difference spectrum. Such a spectrum is indicative of a complexation with the enzyme's heme iron. Computer docking studies utilizing homology models of 11β-hydroxylase provided further support for a critical interaction between the basic nitrogen in etomidate's imidazole ring. In addition, these studies indicate that etomidate's carbonyl carbon and its phenyl ring interact with discrete regions within the enzyme's active site. This suggests that alterations to these parts of etomidate's molecular scaffold might similarly reduce binding to 11β-hydroxylase.

Carboetomidate's lack of significant adrenocortical inhibitory activity suggests that it might be a safer alternative to etomidate in patients with sepsis. To test this hypothesis, etomidate and carboetomidate were administered to endotoxemic rats as either a single bolus induction dose or as multiple doses to maintain hypnosis over 3.5 h [110]. A control group of rats were also studied that received endotoxin (lipopolysaccharide) and given dimethyl sulfoxide vehicle only. Measurements of plasma adrenocorticotropic hormone, corticosterone, and cytokine concentrations demonstrated that carboetomidate had no effect on the inflammatory response to endotoxin administration as carboetomidate group rats and vehicle group rats had plasma adrenocorticotropic hormone, corticosterone, and cytokine concentrations that were not significantly different at any time point of the study. In contrast, corticosterone concentrations were significantly and persistently lower, and pro-inflammatory cytokine levels were higher in rats that received etomidate.

Carboetomidate's pharmacology was further explored by assessing its ability to modulate the function of neuronal nicotinic acetylcholine, serotonin, and N-methyl-D-aspartate receptors. These three ligand-gated ion channels are thought to play important roles in the actions of many general anesthetics but are not affected by etomidate [111, 112]. Carboetomidate inhibited peak current amplitudes mediated by both the acetylcholine and serotonin receptors with half-inhibitory concentrations of 13 µM and 1.93 µM, respectively. In addition, carboetomidate increased the rate with which it induced serotonin receptors to isomerize to an inactivatable desensitized state. Given the important role that serotonin receptors play in mediating nausea and vomiting, these results showing that carboetomidate inhibits the function of serotonin receptors suggest that carboetomidate might be less emetogenic than etomidate. However, similar to etomidate, carboetomidate does not affect the function of N-methyl-D-aspartate receptors.

Methoxycarbonyl Carboetomidate (MOC-Carboetomidate)

The molecular modifications made to etomidate to shorten its duration of action (to produce MOC-etomidate or CPMM) or reduce its adrenocortical inhibitory potency (to produce carboetomidate) involve distinct regions of the etomidate molecular scaffold. This suggested that it might be possible to incorporate both modifications into a single molecular entity to produce an etomidate analogue that is both ultrashort acting and completely devoid of adrenocortical side effects. MOC-carboetomidate is the prototype of such an analogue. Similar to MOC-etomidate, it contains a metabolically labile ester moiety attached to the etomidate scaffold via a two-carbon spacer. In common with carboetomidate, the basic nitrogen in the imidazole ring has been replaced with a −CH moiety.

As predicted by its structure, MOC-carboetomidate's pharmacodynamic profile closely parallels that of carboetomidate, whereas its pharmacodynamic behavior is similar to MOC-etomidate [113]. It enhances the function of GABA$_A$ receptors and produces loss of righting reflexes in tadpoles and rats. However, MOC-carboetomidate's potency was only half those of either MOC-etomidate or carboetomidate. This has important negative implications for a rapidly metabolized hypnotic agent because it means that extremely large doses would need to be administered to maintain anesthesia for any significant length of time.

Summary and Conclusion

It has been more than 50 years since etomidate was first synthesized and found to be a potent hypnotic agent. Among currently available clinical general anesthetics, it remains a popular choice because it offers unparalleled preservation of respiratory and cardiovascular function and possesses an unusually high therapeutic index. Unfortunately, etomidate causes significant side effects—including adrenocortical suppression, myoclonus, and pain on injection—that limit its utility. Using rational drug design strategies, etomidate analogues have been produced that reduce the magnitude or duration of these side effects. All of these analogues enhance GABA$_A$ receptor function and produce hypnosis in laboratory animals. Some of these analogues may be best considered to be lead compounds that establish a proof of principle and provide pharmacological insights. Other analogues (e.g., CPMM) are obvious clinical candidates that have reached or will soon reach clinical trials.

Conflicts of Interest

Dr. Raines is an inventor of intellectual property related to the design of etomidate analogues. His interests were reviewed by the Massachusetts General Hospital and Partners HealthCare in accordance with their conflict of interest policies.

Acknowledgment This is supported by grant R01-GM087316 from the National Institutes of Health, Bethesda, MD, and the Department of Anesthesia, Critical Care, and Pain Medicine, Massachusetts General Hospital, Boston, Massachusetts.

References

1. Godefroi EF, Janssen PA, Vandereycken CA, Vanheertum AH, Niemegeers CJ. Dl-1-(1-arylalkyl)imidazole-5-carboxylate esters. A novel type of hypnotic agents. J Med Chem. 1965;8:220–3.
2. Lepesheva GI, Waterman MR. Sterol 14alpha-demethylase cytochrome P450 (CYP51), a P450 in all biological kingdoms. Biochim Biophys Acta. 2007;1770:467–77.
3. Lepesheva GI, Hargrove TY, Kleshchenko Y, Nes WD, Villalta F, Waterman MR. CYP51: a major drug target in the cytochrome P450 superfamily. Lipids. 2008;43:1117–25.
4. Heykants JJ, Meuldermans WE, Michiels LJ, Lewi PJ, Janssen PA. Distribution, metabolism and excretion of etomidate, a short-acting hypnotic drug, in the rat. Comparative study of (R)-(+)-(−−)-Etomidate. Arch Int Pharmacodyn Ther. 1975;216:113–29.
5. Criado A, Maseda J, Garcia Carmona MT, Dominguez E, Avello F. Pulmonary function and tissue oxygenation studies during anesthetic induction with etomidate. Acta Anaesthesiol Belg. 1983;34:5–13.
6. Rifat K, Gamulin Z, Gemperle M. Effects of Etomidate on ventilation and blood gases. Ann Anesthesiol Fr. 1976;17:1217–22.
7. Toklu S, Iyilikci L, Gonen C, Ciftci L, Gunenc F, Sahin E, Gokel E. Comparison of etomidate-remifentanil and propofol-remifentanil sedation in patients scheduled for colonoscopy. Eur J Anaesthesiol. 2009;26:370–6.
8. Choi SD, Spaulding BC, Gross JB, Apfelbaum JL. Comparison of the ventilatory effects of etomidate and methohexital. Anesthesiology. 1985;62:442–7.
9. Falk J, Zed PJ. Etomidate for procedural sedation in the emergency department. Ann Pharmacother. 2004;38:1272–7.
10. Mandt MJ, Roback MG, Bajaj L, Galinkin JL, Gao D, Wathen JE. Etomidate for short pediatric procedures in the emergency department. Pediatr Emerg Care. 2012;28:898–904.

11. Cicero M, Graneto J. Etomidate for procedural sedation in the elderly: a retrospective comparison between age groups. Am J Emerg Med. 2011;29:1111–6.

12. Doenicke A. Etomidate, a new intravenous hypnotic. Acta Anaesthesiol Belg. 1974;25:307–15.

13. Gooding JM, Weng JT, Smith RA, Berninger GT, Kirby RR. Cardiovascular and pulmonary responses following etomidate induction of anesthesia in patients with demonstrated cardiac disease. Anesth Analg. 1979;58:40–1.

14. Gooding JM, Corssen G. Effect of etomidate on the cardiovascular system. Anesth Analg. 1977;56:717–9.

15. Moss E, Powell D, Gibson RM, McDowall DG. Effect of etomidate on intracranial pressure and cerebral perfusion pressure. Br J Anaesth. 1979;51:347–52.

16. Thomson IA, Fitch W, Hughes RL, Campbell D, Watson R. Effects of certain i.v. anaesthetics on liver blood flow and hepatic oxygen consumption in the greyhound. Br J Anaesth. 1986;58:69–80.

17. Atiba JO, Horai Y, White PF, Trevor AJ, Blaschke TF, Sung ML. Effect of etomidate on hepatic drug metabolism in humans. Anesthesiology. 1988;68:920–4.

18. Gancher S, Laxer KD, Krieger W. Activation of epileptogenic activity by etomidate. Anesthesiology. 1984;61:616–8.

19. Janouschek H, Nickl-Jockschat T, Haeck M, Gillmann B, Grozinger M. Comparison of methohexital and etomidate as anesthetic agents for electroconvulsive therapy in affective and psychotic disorders. J Psychiatr Res. 2013;47:686–93.

20. Khalid N, Atkins M, Kirov G. The effects of etomidate on seizure duration and electrical stimulus dose in seizure-resistant patients during electroconvulsive therapy. J ECT. 2006;22:184–8.

21. Tan HL, Lee CY. Comparison between the effects of propofol and etomidate on motor and electroencephalogram seizure duration during electroconvulsive therapy. Anaesth Intensive Care. 2009;37:807–14.

22. Ayhan Y, Akbulut BB, Karahan S, Gecmez G, Oz G, Gurel SC, Basar K. Etomidate is Associated With Longer Seizure Duration, Lower Stimulus Intensity, and Lower Number of Failed Trials in Electroconvulsive Therapy Compared With Thiopental. J ECT. 2014.

23. Kuizenga K, Wierda JM, Kalkman CJ. Biphasic EEG changes in relation to loss of consciousness during induction with thiopental, propofol, etomidate, midazolam or sevoflurane. Br J Anaesth. 2001;86:354–60.

24. Van Hamme MJ, Ghoneim MM, Ambre JJ. Pharmacokinetics of etomidate, a new intravenous anesthetic. Anesthesiology. 1978;49:274–7.

25. Ghoneim MM, Van Hamme MJ. Hydrolysis of etomidate. Anesthesiology. 1979;50:227–9.

26. Avram MJ, Fragen RJ, Linde HW. High-performance liquid chromatographic assay for etomidate in human plasma: results of preliminary clinical studies using etomidate for hypnosis in total intravenous anesthesia. J Pharm Sci. 1983;72:1424–6.

27. Hebron BS, Edbrooke DL, Newby DM, Mather SJ. Pharmacokinetics of etomidate associated with prolonged i.v. infusion. Br J Anaesth. 1983;55:281–7.

28. Hebron BS. Plasma concentrations of etomidate during an intravenous infusion over 48 hours. Anaesthesia. 1983;38(Suppl):39–43.

29. van Beem H, Manger FW, van Boxtel C, van Bentem N. Etomidate anaesthesia in patients with cirrhosis of the liver: pharmacokinetic data. Anaesthesia. 1983;38(Suppl):61–2.

30. Carlos R, Calvo R, Erill S. Plasma protein binding of etomidate in patients with renal failure or hepatic cirrhosis. Clin Pharmacokinet. 1979;4:144–8.

31. Arden JR, Holley FO, Stanski DR. Increased sensitivity to etomidate in the elderly: initial distribution versus altered brain response. Anesthesiology. 1986;65:19–27.

32. Preziosi P, Vacca M. Etomidate and corticotrophic axis. Arch Int Pharmacodyn Ther. 1982;256:308–10.

33. Ledingham IM, Watt I. Influence of sedation on mortality in critically ill multiple trauma patients. Lancet. 1983;1:1270.

34. de Jong FH, Mallios C, Jansen C, Scheck PA, Lamberts SW. Etomidate suppresses adrenocortical function by inhibition of 11 beta-hydroxylation. J Clin Endocrinol Metab. 1984;59:1143–7.

35. Wagner RL, White PF, Kan PB, Rosenthal MH, Feldman D. Inhibition of adrenal steroidogenesis by the anesthetic etomidate. N Engl J Med. 1984;310:1415–21.

36. Fellows IW, Bastow MD, Byrne AJ, Allison SP. Adrenocortical suppression in multiply injured patients: a complication of etomidate treatment. Br Med J (Clin Res Ed). 1983;287:1835–7.

37. Fragen RJ, Shanks CA, Molteni A, Avram MJ. Effects of etomidate on hormonal responses to surgical stress. Anesthesiology. 1984;61:652–6.

38. De Coster R, Helmers JH, Noorduin H. Effect of etomidate on cortisol biosynthesis: site of action after induction of anaesthesia. Acta Endocrinol (Copenh). 1985;110:526–31.

39. Schenarts CL, Burton JH, Riker RR. Adrenocortical dysfunction following etomidate induction in emergency department patients. Acad Emerg Med. 2001;8:1–7.

40. Absalom A, Pledger D, Kong A. Adrenocortical function in critically ill patients 24 h after a single dose of etomidate. Anaesthesia. 1999;54:861–7.

41. Vinclair M, Broux C, Faure P, Brun J, Genty C, Jacquot C, Chabre O, Payen JF. Duration of adrenal inhibition following a single dose of etomidate in critically ill patients. Intensive Care Med. 2008;34:714–9.

42. den Brinker M, Hokken-Koelega AC, Hazelzet JA, de Jong FH, Hop WC, Joosten KF. One single dose of etomidate negatively influences adrenocortical performance for at least 24h in children with meningococcal sepsis. Intensive Care Med. 2008;34:163–8.

43. Watt I, Ledingham IM. Mortality amongst multiple trauma patients admitted to an intensive therapy unit. Anaesthesia. 1984;39:973–81.

44. Newby DM, Edbrooke DL, Mather SJ, Bird TM, Hebron BS. Etomidate as a sedative agent in intensive care: observations on its cardiovascular effects. Acta Anaesthesiol Scand. 1983;27:218–21.

45. Edbrooke DL, Newby DM, Mather SJ, Dixon AM, Hebron BS. Safer sedation for ventilated patients. A new application for etomidate. Anaesthesia. 1982;37:765–71.

46. Edbrooke DM, Hebron BS, Mather SJ, Dixon AM. Etomidate infusion: a method of sedation for the intensive care unit. Anaesthesia. 1981;36:65.

47. Schulte HM, Benker G, Reinwein D, Sippell WG, Allolio B. Infusion of low dose etomidate: correction of hypercortisolemia in patients with Cushing's syndrome and dose–response relationship in normal subjects. J Clin Endocrinol Metab. 1990;70:1426–30.

48. Greening JE, Brain CE, Perry LA, Mushtaq I, Sales Marques J, Grossman AB, Savage MO. Efficient short-term control of hypercortisolaemia by low-dose etomidate in severe paediatric Cushing's disease. Horm Res. 2005;64:140–3.

49. Bilgin YM, van der Wiel HE, Fischer HR, De Herder WW. Treatment of severe psychosis due to ectopic Cushing's syndrome. J Endocrinol Invest. 2007;30:776–9.

50. Diez JJ, Iglesias P. Pharmacological therapy of Cushing's syndrome: drugs and indications. Mini Rev Med Chem. 2007;7:467–80.

51. Molitch ME. Current approaches to the pharmacological management of Cushing's disease. Mol Cell Endocrinol. 2014.

52. Jackson Jr WL. Should we use etomidate as an induction agent for endotracheal intubation in patients with septic shock?: a critical appraisal. Chest. 2005;127:1031–8.

53. den Brinker M, Joosten KF, Liem O, de Jong FH, Hop WC, Hazelzet JA, van Dijk M, Hokken-Koelega AC. Adrenal insufficiency in meningococcal sepsis: bioavailable cortisol levels and impact of interleukin-6 levels and intubation with etomidate on adrenal function and mortality. J Clin Endocrinol Metab. 2005;90:5110–7.

54. Kulstad EB, Kalimullah EA, Tekwani KL, Courtney DM. Etomidate as an induction agent in septic patients: red flags or false alarms? West J Emerg Med. 2010;11:161–72.

55. de la Grandville B, Arroyo D, Walder B. Etomidate for critically ill patients. Con: do you really want to weaken the frail? Eur J Anaesthesiol. 2012;29:511–4.

56. Pearl RG. Review: etomidate increased mortality and adrenal insufficiency in adults with sepsis. Ann Intern Med. 2013;158: JC2–10.

57. Lipiner-Friedman D, Sprung CL, Laterre PF, Weiss Y, Goodman SV, Vogeser M, Briegel J, Keh D, Singer M, Moreno R, Bellissant E, Annane D. Adrenal function in sepsis: the retrospective Corticus cohort study. Crit Care Med. 2007;35:1012–8.

58. Hildreth AN, Mejia VA, Maxwell RA, Smith PW, Dart BW, Barker DE. Adrenal suppression following a single dose of etomidate for rapid sequence induction: a prospective randomized study. J Trauma. 2008;65:573–9.

59. Warner KJ, Cuschieri J, Jurkovich GJ, Bulger EM. Single-dose etomidate for rapid sequence intubation may impact outcome after severe injury. J Trauma. 2009;67:45–50.

60. Chan CM, Mitchell AL, Shorr AF. Etomidate is associated with mortality and adrenal insufficiency in sepsis: a meta-analysis*. Crit Care Med. 2012;40:2945–53.

61. Komatsu R, You J, Mascha EJ, Sessler DI, Kasuya Y, Turan A. Anesthetic induction with etomidate, rather than propofol, is associated with increased 30-day mortality and cardiovascular morbidity after noncardiac surgery. Anesth Analg. 2013;117:1329–37.

62. Haddad JJ, Saade NE, Safieh-Garabedian B. Cytokines and neuro-immune-endocrine interactions: a role for the hypothalamic-pituitary-adrenal revolving axis. J Neuroimmunol. 2002;133:1–19.

63. Jung B, Clavieras N, Nougaret S, Molinari N, Roquilly A, Cisse M, Carr J, Chanques G, Asehnoune K, Jaber S. Effects of etomidate on complications related to intubation and on mortality in septic shock patients treated with hydrocortisone: a propensity score analysis. Crit Care. 2012;16:R224.

64. McPhee LC, Badawi O, Fraser GL, Lerwick PA, Riker RR, Zuckerman IH, Franey C, Seder DB. Single-dose etomidate is not associated with increased mortality in ICU patients with sepsis: analysis of a large electronic ICU database. Crit Care Med. 2013;41:774–83.

65. Wagner CE, Bick JS, Johnson D, Ahmad R, Han X, Ehrenfeld JM, Schildcrout JS, Pretorius M. Etomidate use and postoperative outcomes among cardiac surgery patients. Anesthesiology. 2014;120:579–89.

66. Gu WJ, Wang F, Tang L, Liu JC. Single-Dose Etomidate Does Not Increase Mortality in Patients with Sepsis: A Systematic Review and Meta-Analysis of Randomized Controlled Trials and Observational Studies. Chest. 2014.

67. He L, Ding Y, Chen H, Qian Y, Li Z. BuButorphanol pre-treatment prevents myoclonus induced by etomidate: a randomised, double-blind, controlled clinical trial. Swiss Med Wkly. 2014;144:w14042.

68. Yates AM, Wolfson AB, Shum L, Kehrl T. A descriptive study of myoclonus associated with etomidate procedural sedation in the ED. Am J Emerg Med. 2013;31:852–4.

69. Reddy RV, Moorthy SS, Dierdorf SF, Deitch Jr RD, Link L. Excitatory effects and electroencephalographic correlation of

etomidate, thiopental, methohexital, and propofol. Anesth Analg. 1993;77:1008–11.

70. Doenicke AW, Roizen MF, Kugler J, Kroll H, Foss J, Ostwald P. Reducing myoclonus after etomidate. Anesthesiology. 1999;90:113–9.

71. Stockham RJ, Stanley TH, Pace NL, Gillmor S, Groen F, Hilkens P. Fentanyl pretreatment modifies anaesthetic induction with etomidate. Anaesth Intensive Care. 1988;16:171–6.

72. Hueter L, Schwarzkopf K, Simon M, Bredle D, Fritz H. Pretreatment with sufentanil reduces myoclonus after etomidate. Acta Anaesthesiol Scand. 2003;47:482–4.

73. Schwarzkopf KR, Hueter L, Simon M, Fritz HG. Midazolam pretreatment reduces etomidate-induced myoclonic movements. Anaesth Intensive Care. 2003;31:18–20.

74. Mizrak A, Koruk S, Bilgi M, Kocamer B, Erkutlu I, Ganidagli S, Oner U. Pretreatment with dexmedetomidine or thiopental decreases myoclonus after etomidate: a randomized, double-blind controlled trial. J Surg Res. 2010;159:e11–6.

75. Gultop F, Akkaya T, Bedirli N, Gumus H. Lidocaine pretreatment reduces the frequency and severity of myoclonus induced by etomidate. J Anesth. 2010;24:300–2.

76. Un B, Ceyhan D, Yelken B. Prevention of etomidate-related myoclonus in anesthetic induction by pretreatment with magnesium. J Res Med Sci. 2011;16:1490–4.

77. Holdcroft A, Morgan M, Whitwam JG, Lumley J. Effect of dose and premedication on induction complications with etomidate. Br J Anaesth. 1976;48:199–205.

78. Doenicke A, Roizen MF, Nebauer AE, Kugler A, Hoernecke R, Beger-Hintzen H. A comparison of two formulations for etomidate, 2-hydroxypropyl-beta-cyclodextrin (HPCD) and propylene glycol. Anesth Analg. 1994;79:933–9.

79. Doenicke AW, Roizen MF, Hoernecke R, Lorenz W, Ostwald P. Solvent for etomidate may cause pain and adverse effects. Br J Anaesth. 1999;83:464–6.

80. Nyman Y, Von Hofsten K, Palm C, Eksborg S, Lonnqvist PA. -Etomidate-Lipuro is associated with considerably less injection pain in children compared with propofol with added lidocaine. Br J Anaesth. 2006;97:536–9.

81. Matta JA, Cornett PM, Miyares RL, Abe K, Sahibzada N, Ahern GP. General anesthetics activate a nociceptive ion channel to enhance pain and inflammation. Proc Natl Acad Sci U S A. 2008;105:8784–9.

82. Yelavich PM, Holmes CM. Etomidate: a foreshortened clinical trial. Anaesth Intensive Care. 1980;8:479–83.

83. Fruergaard K, Jenstrup M, Schierbeck J, Wiberg-Jorgensen F. Total intravenous anaesthesia with propofol or etomidate. Eur J Anaesthesiol. 1991;8:385–91.

84. St Pierre M, Dunkel M, Rutherford A, Hering W. Does etomidate increase postoperative nausea? A double-blind controlled comparison of etomidate in lipid emulsion with propofol for balanced anaesthesia. Eur J Anaesthesiol. 2000;17:634–41.

85. Tomlin SL, Jenkins A, Lieb WR, Franks NP. Stereoselective effects of etomidate optical isomers on gamma-aminobutyric acid type A receptors and animals. Anesthesiology. 1998;88:708–17.

86. Pejo E, Santer P, Jeffrey S, Gallin H, Husain SS, Raines DE. Analogues of etomidate: modifications around etomidate's chiral carbon and the impact on in vitro and in vivo pharmacology. Anesthesiology. 2014;121:290–301.

87. Belelli D, Muntoni AL, Merrywest SD, Gentet LJ, Casula A, Callachan H, Madau P, Gemmell DK, Hamilton NM, Lambert JJ, Sillar KT, Peters JA. The in vitro and in vivo enantioselectivity of etomidate implicates the GABAA receptor in general anaesthesia. Neuropharmacology. 2003;45:57–71.

88. Jurd R, Arras M, Lambert S, Drexler B, Siegwart R, Crestani F, Zaugg M, Vogt KE, Ledermann B, Antkowiak B, Rudolph U.

General anesthetic actions in vivo strongly attenuated by a point mutation in the GABA(A) receptor beta3 subunit. FASEB J. 2003;17:250–2.

89. Rusch D, Zhong H, Forman SA. Gating allosterism at a single class of etomidate sites on alpha1beta2gamma2L GABA A receptors accounts for both direct activation and agonist modulation. J Biol Chem. 2004;279:20982–92.

90. Forman SA. Monod-Wyman-Changeux allosteric mechanisms of action and the pharmacology of etomidate. Curr Opin Anaesthesiol. 2012;25:411–8.

91. Belelli D, Lambert JJ, Peters JA, Wafford K, Whiting PJ. The interaction of the general anesthetic etomidate with the gamma-aminobutyric acid type A receptor is influenced by a single amino acid. Proc Natl Acad Sci U S A. 1997;94:11031–6.

92. Crozier TA, Beck D, Wuttke W, Kettler D. Relation of the inhibition of cortisol synthesis in vivo to plasma etomidate concentrations. Anaesthesist. 1988;37:337–9.

93. Lambert A, Mitchell R, Robertson WR. Effect of propofol, thiopentone and etomidate on adrenal steroidogenesis in vitro. Br J Anaesth. 1985;57:505–8.

94. Cotten JF, Husain SS, Forman SA, Miller KW, Kelly EW, Nguyen HH, Raines DE. Methoxycarbonyl-etomidate: a novel rapidly metabolized and ultra-short-acting etomidate analogue that does not produce prolonged adrenocortical suppression. Anesthesiology. 2009;111:240–9.

95. Ge RL, Pejo E, Haburcak M, Husain SS, Forman SA, Raines DE. Pharmacological studies of methoxycarbonyl etomidate's carboxylic acid metabolite. Anesth Analg. 2012;115:305–8.

96. Shaffer JE, Quon CY, Gorczynski RJ. Beta-adrenoreceptor antagonist potency and pharmacodynamics of ASL-8123, the primary acid metabolite of esmolol. J Cardiovasc Pharmacol. 1988;11:187–92.

97. Hoke JF, Cunningham F, James MK, Muir KT, Hoffman WE. Comparative pharmacokinetics and pharmacodynamics of remifentanil, its principle metabolite (GR90291) and alfentanil in dogs. J Pharmacol Exp Ther. 1997;281:226–32.

98. Kilpatrick GJ, McIntyre MS, Cox RF, Stafford JA, Pacofsky GJ, Lovell GG, Wiard RP, Feldman PL, Collins H, Waszczak BL, Tilbrook GS. CNS 7056: a novel ultra-short-acting Benzodiazepine. Anesthesiology. 2007;107:60–6.

99. Pejo E, Ge R, Banacos N, Cotten JF, Husain SS, Raines DE. Electroencephalographic recovery, hypnotic emergence, and the effects of metabolite following continuous infusions of a rapidly metabolized etomidate analog in rats. Anesthesiology. 2012;116:1057–65.

100. Husain SS, Pejo E, Ge R, Raines DE. Modifying methoxycarbonyl etomidate inter-ester spacer optimizes in vitro metabolic stability and in vivo hypnotic potency and duration of action. Anesthesiology. 2012;117:1027–36.

101. Ge R, Pejo E, Husain SS, Cotten JF, Raines DE. Electroencephalographic and hypnotic recoveries after brief and prolonged infusions of etomidate and optimized soft etomidate analogs. Anesthesiology. 2012;117:1037–43.

102. Campagna JA, Pojasek K, Grayzel D, Randle J, Raines DE. Advancing novel anesthetics: pharmacodynamic and pharmacokinetic studies of cyclopropyl-methoxycarbonyl metomidate in dogs. Anesthesiology. 2014;121:1203–16.

103. Ge R, Pejo E, Gallin H, Jeffrey S, Cotten JF, Raines DE. The pharmacology of cyclopropyl-methoxycarbonyl metomidate: a comparison with propofol. Anesth Analg. 2014;118:563–7.

104. Santer P, Pejo E, Feng Y, Chao W, Raines DE. Cyclopropyl-methoxycarbonyl metomidate: studies in a lipopolysaccharide inflammatory model of sepsis. Anesthesiology. 2015;123:368–76.

105. Scott EE, White MA, He YA, Johnson EF, Stout CD, Halpert JR. Structure of mammalian cytochrome P450 2B4 complexed with 4-(4-chlorophenyl)imidazole at 1.9-A resolution: insight into the range of P450 conformations and the coordination of redox partner binding. J Biol Chem. 2004;279:27294–301.

106. Ouellet H, Podust LM, de Montellano PR. Mycobacterium tuberculosis CYP130: crystal structure, biophysical characterization, and interactions with antifungal azole drugs. J Biol Chem. 2008;283:5069–80.

107. Seward HE, Roujeinikova A, McLean KJ, Munro AW, Leys D. Crystal structure of the Mycobacterium tuberculosis P450 CYP121-fluconazole complex reveals new azole drug-P450 binding mode. J Biol Chem. 2006;281:39437–43.

108. Cotten JF, Forman SA, Laha JK, Cuny GD, Husain SS, Miller KW, Nguyen HH, Kelly EW, Stewart D, Liu A, Raines DE. Carboetomidate: a pyrrole analog of etomidate designed not to suppress adrenocortical function. Anesthesiology. 2010;112:637–44.

109. Shanmugasundararaj S, Zhou X, Neunzig J, Bernhardt R, Cotten JF, Ge R, Miller KW, Raines DE. Carboetomidate: an analog of etomidate that interacts weakly with 11beta-hydroxylase. Anesth Analg. 2013;116:1249–56.

110. Pejo E, Feng Y, Chao W, Cotten JF, Le Ge R, Raines DE. Differential effects of etomidate and its pyrrole analogue carboetomidate on the adrenocortical and cytokine responses to endotoxemia. Crit Care Med. 2012;40:187–92.

111. Pierce DW, Pejo E, Raines DE, Forman SA. Carboetomidate inhibits alpha4/beta2 neuronal nicotinic acetylcholine receptors at concentrations affecting animals. Anesth Analg. 2012;115:70–2.

112. Desai R, Miller KW, Raines DE. The pyrrole etomidate analog carboetomidate potently inhibits human 5-HT3A receptor function: comparisons with etomidate and potential implications for emetogenesis. Anesth Analg. 2013;116:573–9.

113. Pejo E, Cotten JF, Kelly EW, Le Ge R, Cuny GD, Laha JK, Liu J, Lin XJ, Raines DE. In vivo and in vitro pharmacological studies of methoxycarbonyl-carboetomidate. Anesth Analg. 2012;115:297–304.

Dexmedetomidine: The Science and Clinical Aspects in Adults and Children

13

Mohamed Mahmoud

Introduction

Choosing the appropriate sedative/anesthetic agent is an integral part of providing patient comfort and safety. The adverse respiratory profile of the traditional sedative agents, along with the stress response to the procedure, creates the need for a novel sedative agent that can be used safely in both healthy and high-risk patients. Ideally this agent should provide adequate level of anesthesia/sedation required for successful and timely completion of the procedure and attenuate the stress response to procedure, while minimizing the risk of adverse events.

Dexmedetomidine (DEX) (Precedex®, Hospira, Lake Forest, IL, USA, and Dexdor, Orion Corporation, Espoo, Finland) possesses many desirable properties of an ideal sedative/anesthetic agent. The enthusiasm for this novel agent stems from several factors including the unique mechanism of action, lack of an ideal agent for procedural sedation, and adverse effects associated with the traditional sedative/anesthetic agents. The Mechanism of action and physiological effects of DEX are distinct from those of traditional drugs used in procedural sedation, such as benzodiazepines, opioids, and propofol. It provides sedative properties paralleling natural sleep (patients appear to be asleep, but are readily roused) and attenuates the stress response to the procedure, anxiolysis, and analgesic-sparing effect with minimal respiratory depression through action on alpha-2 adrenoceptor in the locus ceruleus sleep [1–7]. In addition, DEX may also provide some neuroprotective activity against ischemic and hypoxic injury [8–11].

The use of DEX is associated with predictable hemodynamic variations related to cardiovascular system depression including bradycardia; hypotension, resulting from its sympatholytic activity; as well as hypertension. The extent of these hemodynamic variations is related to the age of the patient, to the dose and the rate of titration of the drug, as well as to concomitant sources of hemodynamic instability such as volume depletion, severe myocardial dysfunction, heart block, and high vagal tone.

This chapter provides an evidence-based review of the literature regarding the current clinical uses of DEX in adults and children. We will provide a descriptive account of the end-organ effects, the mechanism of action, pharmacology, pharmacokinetics, the side effects, and precautions before its administration.

History and Approval

The use of alpha-2 adrenoceptor agonists as sedative/anesthetics is not new. The veterinary experience has proved for years that alpha-2 adrenoceptor agonists are safe agents for analgesia and sedation [12], and much of current knowledge was gained from this application. Alpha-2 adrenoceptor agonists have been used since 1970 to treat patients with hypertension and patients withdrawing from long-term abuse of drugs or alcohol.

Despite the lack of respiratory depression, DEX was initially approved in the United States by the Food and Drug Administration (FDA) in 1999 for sedation in adults whose airways were intubated in the intensive care unit (ICU). In October 2008, DEX received FDA approval for monitored anesthesia care in adults. Currently FDA approved for the provision sedation of adult patients via bolus and continuous infusion for up to 24 h on intubated adults as well as for adult procedural sedation in areas outside the ICU and operating room setting. It was approved in Europe in 2011 for light to moderate ICU sedation for adults (intubated or non-intubated) in the ICU via continuous infusion, at higher doses than approved for in the United

M. Mahmoud, MD(✉)
Department of Anesthesia and Pediatrics, Cincinnati Children's Hospital Medical Center, University of Cincinnati, 3333 burnet Avenue, Cincinnati, OH 45229, USA
e-mail: mohamed.mahmoud@cchmc.org

A.R. Absalom, K.P. Mason (eds.), *Total Intravenous Anesthesia and Target Controlled Infusions*,
DOI 10.1007/978-3-319-47609-4_13

States, and without a restriction on duration of administration.

To date, there are no FDA-approved indications for its use in pediatric population [13, 14]. Although not yet approved by the FDA for use in the pediatric population, given its beneficial physiological effects and favorable adverse effect profile, there is an ever-growing experience with its use for pediatric procedural sedation and critical care medicine particularly as concerns of neurotoxicity from other anesthetic agents have arisen recently [13, 14].

Pharmacology and Pharmacokinetics

DEX incorporates an imidazoline structure. It is the pharmacologically active dextro-isomer of medetomidine [15]. The physiological effects of alpha-2 agonists are mediated by the different alpha-2 adrenoceptors subtypes [16, 17] (Fig. 13.1). It is a proximately eight times more specific for $\alpha 2$ adrenoceptors with $\alpha 2:\alpha 1$ selectivity ratio of 1620:1, compared with 200:1 for clonidine making it a complete agonist at the alpha-2 adrenoceptor [18]. It is available in a water-soluble solution without the addition of lipid or propylene glycol and is not associated with pain following intravenous administration. The pharmacological actions of DEX result from interactions with all three

subtypes (alpha-2A, alpha-2B, and alpha-2C). The effects of DEX are dose dependent and can be reversed by administration of a selective $\alpha 2$ antagonist, such as atipamezole [19].

The physiological effects of DEX are mediated via postsynaptic alpha-2 adrenoceptor and activation of a pertussis toxin-sensitive guanine nucleotide regulatory protein (G protein) resulting in decreased adenyl cyclase activity [20]. A reduction of intracellular cyclic adenosine monophosphate (cAMP) and cAMP-dependent protein kinase activity results in the dephosphorylation of ion channels [21]. Alterations in ion channel function, ion translocation, and membrane conductance lead to decreased neuronal activation and the clinical effects of sedation and anxiolysis. The hypnotic effect of DEX is mediated by the change in membrane ion conductance which leads to a hyperpolarization of the membrane, which suppresses neuronal firing in the locus ceruleus as well as activity in the ascending noradrenergic pathway. Decreased noradrenergic output from the locus coeruleus allows for increased firing of inhibitory neurons including gamma aminobutyric acid (GABA) which further inhibited the locus ceruleus and tuberomamillary nucleus. This inhibitory response also causes a decrease in the release of histamine which results in a hypnotic response. There is some evidence that sedation induced with DEX resembles normal sleep [4, 22]; in rats, the pattern of c-Fos expression (a marker of activation of

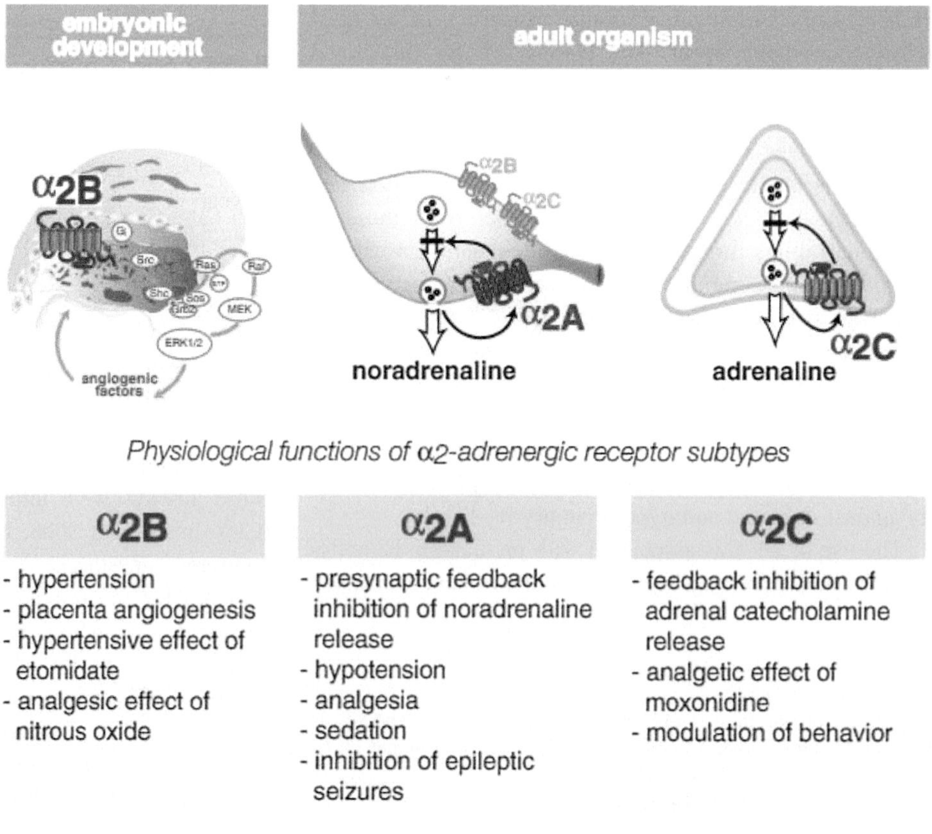

Fig. 13.1 Physiological functions of a2 adrenoceptor subtypes derived from gene-targeted mouse models. Endogenous catecholamines stimulate a2 adrenoceptors to mediate essential physiological functions (*upper panels*): The a-2B adrenoceptor subtype is required for vascular development of the placenta in mice, and a-2A and a-2C adrenoceptor subtypes regulate catecholamine release from sympathetic nerves and the adrenal gland, respectively. Pharmacological stimulation of a2 adrenoceptors results in a variety of biological effects (*lower panels*). From Brede M, Philipp M, Knaus A, et al. Alpha-2 adrenoceptor subtypes—novel functions uncovered in gene-targeted mouse models. Biol Cell. 2004; 96:343–48. Used with permission from John Wiley and Sons

Physiological functions of α2-adrenergic receptor subtypes

α2B	α2A	α2C
- hypertension - placenta angiogenesis - hypertensive effect of etomidate - analgesic effect of nitrous oxide	- presynaptic feedback inhibition of noradrenaline release - hypotension - analgesia - sedation - inhibition of epileptic seizures	- feedback inhibition of adrenal catecholamine release - analgetic effect of moxonidine - modulation of behavior

neurons) is qualitatively similar to that seen during normal NREM sleep, suggesting that endogenous sleep pathways are causally involved in DEX-induced sedation [4].

Centrally acting alpha-2 adrenergic agonists also activate receptors in the medullary vasomotor center reducing norepinephrine with a resultant central sympatholytic effect leading to decreased heart rate (HR) and blood pressure (BP). The sedative and anxiolytic effects of DEX result primarily from stimulation of parasympathetic outflow and inhibition of sympathetic outflow from the locus coeruleus in the brainstem.

The precise mechanisms and pathways by which DEX induces analgesia have not been fully elucidated. The brain, spinal cord, and peripheral mechanisms all seem operant. The most important of these sites may be the spinal cord, where the analgesic effects are believed to be related with the activation of both α2-C and α2-A, situated in the neurons of the superficial dorsal horn especially in the lamina II [23–25], which directly decreases pain transmission by reducing the release of pro-nociceptive transmitter, substance P, and glutamate from primary afferent terminals and by hyperpolarizing spinal interneurons via G-protein-mediated activation of potassium channels. Suppression of activity in the descending noradrenergic pathway may also modulate nociceptive neurotransmission and terminate propagation of pain signals leading to analgesia [26]. One should be aware that the analgesic potential of DEX, however, does not approximate the potency of opioids.

The pharmacokinetic profile of DEX includes a rapid distribution phase (6 min), a terminal elimination half-life of approximately 2 h [3, 27, 28], and a steady-state volume of distribution of 118 l. DEX exhibits linear kinetics over the recommended dosage range of 0.2–0.7 mcg/kg/h delivered via continuous intravenous infusion for up to 24 h. DEX is 93 % protein bound [3] and is extensively metabolized through both the cytochrome P450 enzyme system, primarily by CYP2A6, and direct glucuronidation in the liver to inactive metabolites [29]. A very small fraction of DEX is excreted unchanged in urine and feces. DEX administration has been described by intravenous, intramuscular, intranasal (IN) [30], and buccal route [31]. Via the nasal and buccal route, DEX bioavailability approximates 65 % (35–93 %) and 81.8 % (72.6–92.1 %), respectively [32, 33]. The bioavailability of DEX by the oral route is very poor (16 %) and administration by such a route is unwarranted [32].

Information on the pharmacokinetics of DEX in the pediatric population is limited, especially in children younger than 2 year of age. Infants appear to require larger doses of DEX compared with older children [34]. A recent study that examined pharmacokinetics of intravenous DEX in children under 11 years of age showed that total plasma clearance is similar in younger and older children, but the volume of distribution and the terminal elimination half-life were greater in children younger than 2 years of age compared with older children [28]. A recent study that examined the pharmacokinetics of DEX in 23 neonates (age, 1 day–1 month) and 36 infants (age, 1 month–24 months) after open heart surgery showed that continuous infusions of up to 0.3 mcg/kg/h in neonates and 0.75 mcg/kg/h in infants were well tolerated. The study concluded that DEX clearance is significantly diminished in full-term newborns and increases rapidly in the first few weeks of life. The dependence of clearance on age during the first few weeks of life most likely reflects the relative immaturity of metabolic processes during the newborn period [35].

A recent study examined the pharmacokinetics of prolonged infusion (maximum duration of 14 days) of high dose of DEX in critically ill patients [36]. The authors quantified for the first time in humans the concentrations of the previously poorly characterized H3 metabolite of DEX. The result of their study suggests that DEX obeys linear pharmacokinetics up to the dose of 2.5 mcg/kg/h. They could not establish any new safety findings despite the high dosing regimen and prolonged infusions. Abrupt cessation of DEX may produce withdrawal symptoms similar to those seen with clonidine withdrawal (i.e., agitation, irritability, headache, and rebound hypertension). In clinical practice DEX has been used for more than 24 h. However, the manufacturer recommends that DEX not be used for more than 24 h [29].

End-Organ Effects of Dexmedetomidine

Effect of Dexmedetomidine on Respiration

The recent enthusiasm for DEX use for variety of pediatric and adult procedures stems from the ability to maintain ventilation and airway patency in the presence of increasing level of sedation especially in patients with obstructive sleep apnea (OSA). The administration of anesthetic/sedative agents increases airway collapsibility due to increase closing pressure [37], loss of pharyngeal muscular tone [38], and failure of coordination of phasic activation of upper airway muscles with diaphragmatic activity [39]. These agents depress upper airway dilator muscle activity and diaphragm muscles to varying degrees. One possible explanation for the difference between the anesthetic/sedative agents on airway collapsibility can be attributed to the impact of pharmacologic mechanisms of the sedative or sleep-inducing actions on processes that control motor efferents to pharyngeal musculature as well as afferents from airway mechanoreceptors. In contrast to traditional sedative agents, DEX produces a state closely resembling physiological sleep [4, 5], which gives further support to earlier experimental evidence for activation of normal NREM pathways. A recent study compared the respiratory effect of DEX to that of remifentanil in six healthy male volunteers and reported similarity between the hypercapnic arousal phenomenon during DEX infusions and natural sleep [22].

The ability to maintain spontaneous ventilation and upper airway tone makes DEX an attractive choice for sleep endoscopy and dynamic airway imaging [40–42] [43]. Providing anesthesia that mimics physiological sleep and the need to avoid the use of airway interventions in these procedures is a challenge but is critical for accurate interpretation of the airway evaluation [44, 45]. A recent retrospective study reviewed the records of 52 children receiving DEX and 30 children receiving propofol for anesthesia during MRI sleep studies and showed that the total number of airway interventions was significantly less in the DEX group than in the propofol group [40]. The same authors examined the effects of increasing depth of DEX anesthesia on upper airway morphology in 23 children with normal airway. Images of the upper airway were obtained during low (1 mcg/kg/h) and high (3 mcg/kg/h) dose of DEX anesthesia. The authors concluded that increasing doses of DEX in children with normal airway are associated with statistically significant reductions in airway dimensions at the level of the posterior nasopharynx and retroglossal airway; these changes were small in magnitude and do not appear to be associated with clinical signs of airway obstruction in [41].

Recently a prospective, single-blinded controlled comparative study examined the dose–response effects of DEX and propofol on airway morphology in children and adolescents with OSA. MRI images of the upper airway measurements were obtained during low (1 mcg/kg/h) and high (3 mcg/kg/h) doses of DEX or low (100 mcg/kg/min) and high (200 mcg/kg/min) doses of propofol. Most airway measurements demonstrated statistically nonsignificant associations with increasing doses of propofol and DEX. As dosage increased, average airway dimensions were typically unchanged or slightly increased with DEX compared to unchanged or slightly decreased with propofol. An airway intervention was required for oxygen desaturation in three children (11 %) in the DEX group versus seven children (23 %) in the propofol group. The authors concluded that both agents provided an acceptable level of anesthesia for sleep cine MRI studies in patients with OSA with statistically nonsignificant changes in airway dimensions [42].

Cardiovascular and Hemodynamic Effects

The hemodynamic effects of DEX result from peripheral and central mechanisms. DEX displays a biphasic, dose-dependent BP response. The initial response to rapid DEX infusion may be a transient hypertension related to stimulation of peripheral postsynaptic alpha-2B adrenergic receptors which results in vasoconstriction, whereas the eventual decrease in BP and HR results from central presynaptic alpha-2A adrenergic receptor stimulated sympatholysis. Hypotension and bradycardia associated with DEX administration have been reported in adults and children, especially in the presence of comorbid cardiac disease, when administered with other medications that possess negative chronotropic effects or following large [3] or rapid bolus doses. DEX can mediate a significant increase in BP when the plasma concentration of DEX increases from 0.5 to 3.2 ng/ml. The pressor effect of DEX has been shown to correlate with the rate of IV infusion and plasma concentration of the drug [46]. In general, at serum concentrations greater than 1 mcg/l, the BP changes from a mild decrease from baseline to an elevation (Fig. 13.2) [47]. Although decreases in HR and a biphasic effect on BP are observed with increasing doses of DEX, the literature supports that concurrent hemodynamic collapse or need for pharmacologic resuscitation does not occur. Rather, a recent publication suggests that the bradycardia associated with alpha-2 adrenergic agonists in children may not require treatment nor for adverse hemodynamic consequence [48]. Although bradycardia and hypotension have been described in patients receiving DEX, to date, there are only rare reports of clinically significant bradycardia with the use of DEX in infants and children. This exaggerated physiological effect seems to be related to the use of a loading dose and/or preexisting hypovolemia, and the occurrence of hypotension can be attenuated by pretreatment with balanced salt solution boluses [49].

A recent study that utilized a continuous noninvasive cardiac output to measure the hemodynamic effects of DEX sedation in healthy children undergoing radiological imaging studies found a significant decrease in HR within 5–10 min of initiating a DEX bolus (2 mcg/kg bolus over 10 min). HR and cardiac index (CI) decreased after a single bolus and recovered to baseline within 60 min after a brief exposure (completed the procedure within 10 min). No changes in stroke index (SI) or systemic vascular resistance index were observed after a brief exposure, but prolonged exposure (procedures lasting longer than 10 min) leads to decreases in HR, CI, and SI that did not recover back to baseline.

A common concern with this novel sedative agent is bradycardia. Bradycardia or a decrease in resting HR (up to a 30 % decrease from baseline) is expected and should be considered as a predictable physiologic response anticipated with DEX. The HR responses are rarely of clinical significance, as they do not usually require intervention [3, 48, 50] [51]. An accidental overdose with the administration of DEX up to 0.5 mcg/kg/min and an infusion up to 10 mcg/kg/h did not result in hypotension or severe bradycardia [52, 53]. Extreme bradycardia can occur if

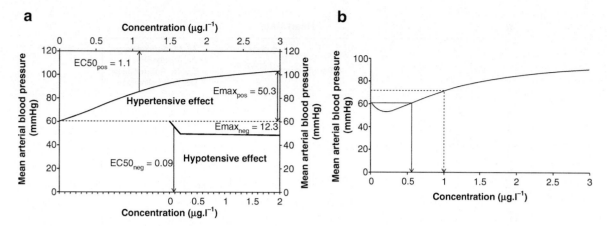

Fig. 13.2 Hyper- and hypotensive effect of dexmedetomidine on mean arterial blood pressure. (**a**) Composite Emax model, showing hyper- and hypotensive effect of dexmedetomidine on mean arterial blood pressure (MAP). (**b**) Combined hyper- and hypotensive effect of dexmedetomidine on MAP. The *solid arrow* indicates the concentration at which the hypertensive effect begins; the *dashed arrow* indicates the concentration producing a 20 % increase in MAP from baseline. From Potts AL, Anderson BJ, Holford NH, Vu TC, Warman GR. Dexmedetomidine hemodynamics in children after cardiac surgery. Pediatric anesthesia. 2010;20(5):425–33. Used with permission from John Wiley and Sons

administered to a patient receiving digoxin and syncope, likely from a vasovagal response, and has been cited in the literature as well as in the package insert [29, 54, 55]. A recent study examined the effect of DEX on sinus node, atrioventricular node, and conduction pathways and found a decrease in HR with significant depression of sinus and atrioventricular nodal function in a clinical study in pediatric patients undergoing electrophysiological study [56]. However, a prospective observational controlled study in pediatric patients with congenital heart disease showed DEX does not have direct effect on cardiac conduction [57]. In healthy women undergoing elective hysterectomy, a 6.2 % prevalence of intraoperative and 14.1 % prevalence of postoperative bradycardia (HR less than 40 beats/min) were noted in patients premedicated with intramuscular DEX (2.5 mg/kg) when administered with or without fentanyl [58]. Severe bradycardia (HR, 27 beats/min) and transient sinus arrest (20–30 s) have been reported in two healthy subjects who had received intramuscular DEX [59].

Although there are no absolute contraindications to DEX in the literature or package insert, it is recommended that DEX be avoided in patients with depressed left ventricular function, recent high-degree AV block, and volume depletion and in children receiving digoxin, beta adrenergic blockers, calcium channel blockers, or other agents which predispose to bradycardia or hypotension.

Caution should be exercised when administering anticholinergics to treat isolated DEX-associated bradycardia in children, as intravenous glycopyrrolate has been shown to elicit immediate, significant hypertension [60]. In dogs, administration of intramuscular atropine with intramuscular DEX reversed HR changes and hypotension, but

arrhythmias (atrioventricular block, premature ventricular contractions, and bigeminy) were observed [61]. A recent retrospective study showed that the administration of prophylactic anticholinergic (atropine or glycopyrrolate) administration prior to DEX in pediatric imaging studies did not show any advantage other than a transient clinically insignificant increase in HR and systolic blood pressure (SBP) (Fig. 13.3a, b). In fact transient exaggerated SBP was noted in a greater number of patients who received anticholinergics as compared to not using prophylactic anticholinergic [62].

ECG abnormalities as noted by RR prolongation and junctional escape rhythms at 2 mcg/kg, administered as a single dose, have been reported with DEX use [6]. The concomitant administration of DEX with medications that have negative chronotropic effects (propofol, pyridostigmine, succinylcholine, and remifentanil) may potentiate vagotonic or negative chronotropic effects [63]. Asystole following 0.5 mg atropine to treat a HR in the 1930s was reported in a 52-year-old woman receiving a DEX infusion during general anesthesia (fentanyl, propofol, sevoflurane) [64].

The DEX package insert recommends administering the drug (1 mcg/kg) over a 10-min infusion to attenuate dose-dependent, biphasic, hemodynamic response caused by peripheral α2 adrenoreceptor stimulation and subsequent central α2 adrenoreceptor-mediated sympatholysis. However, rapid infusion of 0.25, 0.5, 1.0, or 2.0 mcg/kg DEX over 2 min was well tolerated in healthy volunteers with a biphasic hemodynamic effect observed initially and eventual decrease from baseline of the mean arterial pressure (MAP) at 60 min of 14, 16, 23, and 27 % [6]. Rapid boluses in small

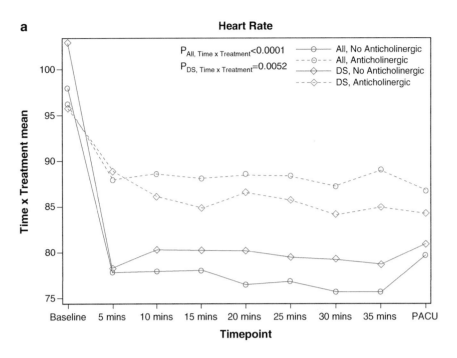

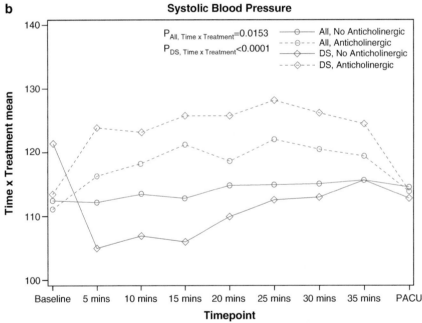

Fig. 13.3 (**a**) Changes in heart rate after DEX sedation attributed to receiving or not receiving an anticholinergic pretreatment. In this retrospective descriptive study, we reviewed the records of 163 children receiving dexmedetomidine anesthesia during MRI studies. The heart rate between the patients receiving an anticholinergic and not receiving an anticholinergic at baseline, during the scan period, and in the post-anesthesia care unit (PACU) is shown and compared. The *x*-axis represents the heart rate at baseline (before the start of the scan), during the scan at 5-min intervals (5 min through 35 min), and in the PACU. The *y*-axis indicates the least squares estimates of time and treatment interaction mean effect. There was a significant reduction in the heart rates during scan period when an anticholinergic was not used compared with using a prophylactic anticholinergic in all patients ($P < 0.0001$) and in patients with Down syndrome (DS) ($P = 0.0052$). The *solid line and the broken line with the round dot* indicate the heart rate for all patients. The *solid line and the broken line with the diamond dot* indicate the heart rate for patients with DS. (**b**) Changes in systolic blood pressure after DEX sedation attributed to receiving or not receiving an anticholinergic pretreatment. In this retrospective descriptive study, we reviewed the records of 163 children receiving dexmedetomidine anesthesia during MRI studies. The systolic blood pressure between the patients receiving an anticholinergic and not receiving an anticholinergic at baseline, during the scan period, and in the post-anesthesia care unit (PACU) is shown and compared. The *x*-axis represents the systolic blood pressure at baseline (before the start of the scan), during the scan at 5-min intervals (5 min through 35 min), and in the PACU. The *y*-axis indicates the least squares estimates of time and treatment interaction mean effect. There was a significant reduction in systolic blood pressure during scan period when an anticholinergic was not used compared with when a prophylactic anticholinergic was used in all patients ($P = 0.0153$) and in patients with Down syndrome (DS) ($P < 0.0001$). The *solid line and the broken line with the round dot* indicate the systolic blood pressure for all patients. The *solid line and the broken line with the diamond dot* indicate the systolic blood pressure for patients with DS

doses (0.25 and 0.5 mcg/kg) have been shown to be well tolerated in 12 pediatric heart transplant patients undergoing cardiac catheterization. The denervation of the sinoatrial node, however, should be considered as a potential factor for the minimal observed response [46]. A recent study examined the dose–response DEX bolus over 5 s administered to healthy children. The maximum elevation in MAP was a 33 % increase from baseline and the maximum decrease in HR was 36 % from baseline (Fig. 13.3). An ED50 (no hemodynamic response in half of the subjects) of 0.49 mcg/kg was extrapolated to avoid hemodynamic responses in half of the subjects [65].

In addition to its potential to cause hypotension, hypertension, and bradycardia, a significant area of concern is DEX's effect on pulmonary vascular resistance (PVR). The results of studies on the effect of DEX on pulmonary hemodynamics vary along with the doses and study conditions that were used. At present, there is limited information regarding the effect of DEX on the pulmonary vasculature and PVR in adults and children with varying degrees of pulmonary hypertension (PH). The perioperative infusion of DEX without a loading dose is not associated with any increase in the mean pulmonary artery pressure (MPAP) [66, 67]. In the animal model, DEX (2 mcg/kg over 1 min) transiently increased MPAP and PVR [68]. Similar transient pulmonary hemodynamic changes have been shown in healthy adult volunteers subjected to increasing DEX infusions to a plasma concentration of 1.9 ng/ml [6]. Post cardiac surgery, DEX doses as permitted by labeling had minimal effect on the pulmonary artery pressure, leaving ventricular function unchanged [69].

The effect of DEX on infants and children with pulmonary hypertension can be variable. Children with pulmonary hypertension as compared to those without both demonstrated no significant change in pulmonary vascular resistance, pulmonary artery pressure, and cardiac index in response to up to 1 mcg/kg DEX bolus followed by a continuous infusion of 0.7 mcg/kg/h [70]. In contrast, a recent FDA-monitored study evaluating the effect of DEX on PVR in children with pulmonary hypertension was terminated due to increased PVR in addition to premature ventricular complexes, bradycardia (<60 bpm), and hypotension in one of the subjects [71]. Another prospective observational pilot study demonstrated that DEX after congenital cardiac surgery did not have a demonstrable effect on pulmonary artery pressure of children who did not have pulmonary hypertension [69]. Given the potential impact of these findings on infants and children with preexisting pulmonary hypertension, future studies are needed before advocating routine DEX in this patient population.

Endocrine, Renal, and Hepatic Effects of Dexmedetomidine

Because DEX contains an imidazole ring, there are theoretical concerns regarding its effects on steroidogenesis. In the concentrations that are used clinically, there is no evidence to suggest that can depress adrenocortical function to the extent that occurs with etomidate [72]. DEX administration for up to 7 days in dogs failed to suggest any adrenal shock or severe impairment of the hypothalamic–pituitary axis [73].

There seems to be no evidence of significant accumulation of any metabolic products that would limit the prolonged use of DEX. DEX has been used more than 2 months on a 9-month-old infant with liver cirrhosis, who underwent liver transplantation. The respiratory conditions improved when DEX was added to midazolam and fentanyl. The infant was then successfully extubated 10 weeks later. No serious adverse effects or disturbance of liver function was found when DEX was used as a prolonged infusion up to 1.4 mcg/kg/h [74]. DEX was also used in six patients with severe renal impairment. The authors showed that there was no difference between renal disease and control groups. However, DEX resulted in a more prolonged sedation in subjects with renal disease [75]. A recent study showed that a metabolite called H3 was quantified, but seemed to have no relevant pharmacologic activity [36].

The α2 adrenoreceptors are widely distributed in the renal proximal and distal tubules, peritubular vasculature, as well as in systemic tissues. DEX seems to induce diuresis by inhibiting the antidiuretic action of vasopressin (AVP), enhance renal blood flow and glomerular filtration, and increase urine output [76, 77]. Recent animal studies showed that it can also protect against radiocontrast nephropathy by preserving outer medullary renal blood flow [78]. Anesthesia/sedation providers should also be aware of the potential development of polyuric syndrome when DEX is used. A recent case report in adult patient who underwent posterior spinal fusion under general anesthesia with isoflurane, sufentanil, DEX, and lidocaine infusions showed that urine output increased from 150 to 950 ml/h. An increasing serum sodium, low urine specific gravity, and increased serum osmolarity occurred simultaneously with the polyuria. Within 2 h of discontinuing the DEX infusion, urine output greatly decreased and all signs of the polyuric syndrome resolved spontaneously in 24 h [79]. Despite the diuretic effect of DEX, in adults, the 74 % increase in urinary output that has been seen for up to 4 h post cardiac surgery does not affect renal function when compared to placebo in a double-blind design [80]. There is some data to support a renoprotective effect of DEX. A retrospective review of cardiac and thoracic surgeries in adults who received a DEX infusion of up to 0.6 mcg/kg/h for up to 24 h postoperatively revealed a decrease in a 30-day mortality and decrease in serum markers for acute kidney injury [81]. Similar results were found in children who received intravenous iodine contrast for cardiac angiography. Compared to the control group, children 6 months–6 years of age had decreased elevation in plasma endothelin, renin, and markers of acute renal injury [82]. Future studies are warranted to delineate the patient population, surgical procedures, and resultant effect of DEX on renal function.

Effect of Dexmedetomidine on the Central Nervous System

Because of the complexity associated with normal brain development, the developing nervous system has been hypothesized to be more susceptible than the mature brain to certain neurotoxic insults. The issue of anesthetic-induced neurotoxicity is a topic of ongoing interest and has continued to gain attention and research support over the past decade, as some studies have suggested that inhalational and intravenous anesthetics may both cause neurotoxicity [83–86] and may contribute to neuronal apoptosis in neonates. One of the most interesting directions of DEX research involves its potential for neuroprotection particularly in children. To date, only DEX and possibly xenon have been proposed to be neuroprotective in animal studies [87].

The precise mechanism of the neuroprotective effect of alpha-2 adrenergic agonists is not clear. DEX's neuroprotective effects may be mediated by a reduction in caspase-3 expression (a proapoptotic factor); increased expression of active (autophosphorylated) focal adhesion kinase (FAK), a nonreceptor tyrosine kinase which plays a role in cellular plasticity and survival; and upregulation of antiapoptotic proteins [88, 89].

Catecholaminergic neurotransmission is also considered to possibly be related to the neuroprotective effect of DEX. Cerebral ischemia is associated with an increase in circulating and extracellular brain catecholamine concentrations. The treatment with agents that are capable of reducing the release of norepinephrine in the brain (e.g., alpha-2 agonists) may provide protection against the damaging effect of cerebral ischemia. Various animal models with complete and incomplete as well as transient and permanent ischemic injury have attempted to define DEX's protective effects during central nervous system injury [90–92] and attenuated hypoxic-ischemic brain injury in developing brains, highly susceptible to neuronal damage [93, 94]. Moreover, improvement in functional neurological outcomes was

shown after brain injury [95]. As mentioned before, the exact mechanisms of neuroprotection are not clear, but catecholamine pathways play an important role, and a positive correlation between circulating norepinephrine and neurological outcome was revealed after cerebral ischemia [96]. Several studies demonstrate that DEX reduces excitatory neurotransmitter (e.g., glutamate) and may protect against excitotoxic injury to the developing brain [93, 97].

It is possible that an opioid-based technique with DEX may be a better alternative than current volatile anesthetic techniques in neonates. Large, multicenter studies designed to assess the effect of DEX on neurocognitive development are required to confirm the neuroprotective beneficial effect in humans.

The effects on memory formation of $\alpha 2$ adrenoceptor agonists in both animals and man remain controversial in the literature. These contradictory findings can be ascribed to the dose used, the type of memory involved, and the timing of drug administration [98]. Several animal studies report disruption of memory formation induced by $\alpha 2$ adrenoceptor agonists. In ten healthy adult male volunteers, sequential 40-min infusions of DEX were administered to achieve plasma concentrations of 0.5, 0.8, 1.2, 2.0, 3.2, 5.0, and 8.0 ng/ml [45]. The two volunteers who received the highest incremental dose (calculated to achieve a plasma concentration of 8.0 ng/ml) were not arousable even with vigorous shaking. Picture recall and recognition were preserved during the lowest incremental infusion (0.5 ng/ml) but were 0 % (0 of 10) and 20 % (2 of 10), respectively, with the second and third infusion levels (0.8 and 1.2 ng/ml). Another study examined recall with DEX confirmed that with increasing serum concentrations of DEX, there is a decrease in the Observer Assessment of Alertness/Sedation (OASS) scale and visual analog scale [99]. With increasing plasma concentrations of DEX administered to healthy adult volunteers, the correct recall or recognition of a picture decreased [99]. There is no literature to date which describes the effect of DEX on memory acquisition, recall, and amnesia in children.

In adults, it has been suggested that on continuous recognition tasks using photograph recognition to differentiate working from long-term memory, DEX impairs familiarity more than recognition [100]. Whether a similar response is seen in children is yet to be determined. Thus, until the effect of DEX on amnesia has been clarified, the authors suggest that synergistic administration of amnestic medications be administered if recall is unwanted.

The available information indicates that DEX causes a reduction of cerebral blood flow (CBF) in humans [101, 102]. A recent study showed that CBF was not associated with reduction without a parallel reduction in cerebral metabolic rate [103].

Periprocedural Applications of Dexmedetomidine

A summary of the current adult and pediatric periprocedural applications of DEX is provided in Table 13.1.

Pre-procedural Applications: Anxiolysis

Premedication with DEX not only offers anxiolysis, sedation, and analgesia but also helps in attenuating the stress responses to tracheal intubation/extubation and emergence from anesthesia. DEX administration has been described as a premedication by intramuscular, IN [30], and buccal route [31]. The buccal route ensures more compliance and better absorption, while the intranasal technique causes no

discomfort during administration and is relatively quick and simple. The nasal route is effective and well tolerated for sedation and postoperative analgesia in adults in the dose of 1 mcg/kg given 45 min before surgery [104].

When used as a premedication in pediatric patients, IN DEX has been shown to produce more satisfactory effect of sedation than buccal DEX (1 mcg/kg) or oral midazolam (0.5 mg/kg) [31, 105, 106]. Compared to IN dose of DEX (1 mcg/kg), higher IN doses of DEX (2 mcg/kg over 1 mcg/kg) are more efficacious at producing sedation, anxiolysis, better acceptance to a mask inhalation induction, and less cardiovascular variability [30].

A recent study that examined the onset time of IN DEX premedication (1 mcg/kg) in 100 healthy children aged 1–12 years undergoing elective surgery showed that the median onset time of sedation was 25 min and the median duration

Table 13.1 Current common periprocedural applications of dexmedetomidine in adults and children

Pre-procedural applications	Advantage
Anxiolysis	Easy and quick arousal from sedation Minimal respiratory depression Attenuates sympathetic hemodynamic response
Periprocedural applications	
Airway procedures Rigid bronchoscopy Drug-induced sleep endoscopy MRI sleep studies Open thyroplasty Anterior mediastinal mass biopsy	Obtunds airway reflexes while maintaining stable hemodynamic and respiratory profiles in spontaneously ventilating children and provides sedative properties paralleling natural sleep
Neurosurgical procedures	
Posterior spine fusions	Lowers propofol and inhalational agent requirements and facilitates intraoperative wake-up tests
Brain tumor and epileptic seizure foci resection	Preserves epileptiform activity and allows comfortable and cooperative sedation
Cardiac surgery	Blunts sympathetic response, provides analgesia and sedation postoperatively, and expedites extubation
Invasive procedures	
Extracorporeal shock wave lithotripsy Burn dressing change Lumbar puncture Bone marrow biopsy Central venous line placement Chest tube insertion	Combining ketamine and dexmedetomidine in these procedures provides sedation, analgesia, amnesia, and hemodynamic stability
Vascular surgery Carotid endarterectomy Carotid angioplasty and stenting	Provides excellent hemodynamics due to its sympatholytic effects
Bariatric surgery	Potentiates opioid analgesia with minimal additional respiratory depression
Post-procedural applications	
Adenotonsillectomy Postoperative shivering Postoperative emergence agitation	May reduce the incidence of severe emergence agitation, opioid requirements, and episodes of oxygen desaturation in children with obstructive sleep apnea
Sedation in the pediatric intensive care	Produces a state of cooperative sedation associated with minimal respiratory depression and facilitates withdrawal from benzodiazepines or opioids
Miscellaneous applications	
Palliative care Treatment of cyclic vomiting syndrome	May provide a bridge to wean the patients' dependency on opioids

was 85 min [107]. At a higher dose, 2 mcg/kg IN DEX (compared to 0.5 mg oral midazolam) produced shorter onset of sedation without a demonstrable difference in conditions at induction, emergence, and recovery [108]. In a prospective, randomized, open-label clinical trial, children were enrolled into one of the three groups of premedication: midazolam 0.5 mg/kg PO, clonidine 4 mcg/kg PO, or transmucosal DEX 1 mcg/kg. All groups produced similar anxiolysis, ease of separation from parents, recovery, and discharge time. DEX had advantages (compared to midazolam) with respect to analgesia and attenuation of sympathetic hemodynamic response [109].

A recent meta-analysis of 13 randomized controlled trials (RCTs) on non-intravenous (IN, sublingual, or oral) DEX versus midazolam was performed to examine the efficacy in improving perioperative sedation and analgesia and in reducing postoperative agitation when used as a preanesthetic medication in 1033 children. The authors concluded that DEX as a premedication is superior to midazolam in ensuring satisfactory levels of sedation in children undergoing surgery, both at separation from parents and at emergence [110].

DEX that is characterized by an easy and quick arousal from sedation resembling natural sleep makes it theoretically a promising premedication. On the other hand its slow onset of anxiolysis makes it an unsuitable substitute for oral midazolam [111]. The current major limitations of studies examining efficacy of DEX in improving perioperative sedation are the significant heterogeneity between studies in the scales and measures used for sedation and children's anxiety evaluation, differences in the anesthesia protocols, and differences in the doses. More studies are needed to evaluate the effect of premedication routes on various outcome measures like preoperative anxiety levels, induction time, emergence excitation, postoperative analgesic requirements, and postoperative behavior disturbances. Randomized clinical trials are also required to identify optimal doses and appropriate monitoring of DEX use for premedication.

Intra-procedural Applications

Airway Procedures

Tracheal intubation without the use of muscle relaxants is commonly used in pediatric anesthesia. A single dose of DEX (1 mcg/kg) has been shown to improve intubation conditions in children after induction with propofol (3 mg/kg) and remifentanil (2 mcg/kg) without muscle relaxants in 60 ASA physical status I children aged 5–10 years [112]. DEX did not affect the hemodynamic response to intubation.

IV administration of DEX (1 mcg/kg) has also been found to decrease the target effect-site concentration of propofol and remifentanil that is required for suspension laryngoscopy by 1.29 μg/ml and 0.64 ng/ml, respectively. Single-dose bolus injection of DEX (0.5 mcg/kg) before tracheal extubation has been shown to attenuate airway-circulatory reflexes during extubation [113].

Airway procedures such as rigid bronchoscopy are challenging and require meticulous anesthesia management including airway access for the surgeons, adequate oxygenation and gas exchange to avoid hypoxemia, and stabilized hemodynamics. Total intravenous propofol anesthesia, with or without remifentanil, is a common technique used in these procedures. Challenges with this technique include the ability to maintain spontaneous respiration, protect the airway, and prevent laryngospasm. Comparatively, DEX offers some advantages: In contrast to other agents, DEX converges on sleep pathways at the locus ceruleus and is associated with changes in neuronal activity similar to those seen in deeper stages of NREM sleep, without significant respiratory depression [114, 115]. The ability to maintain spontaneous ventilation and upper airway tone makes DEX an attractive choice for this scenario, particularly for children with severe preoperative airway impairment [40, 45]. Previous reports have demonstrated that for rigid bronchoscopy, DEX offers advantages of obtunding airway reflexes while maintaining stable hemodynamic and respiratory profiles in spontaneously ventilating children [116–118].

Open thyroplasty with vocal cord medialization is another challenging airway surgery performed to treat dysphonia. To optimize surgical repair, the patients need to be awake or lightly sedated during the procedure. The anesthesia challenges require that the non-intubated patient has adequate anxiolysis, sedation, and analgesia while maintaining the ability to phonate on command. In combination with local anesthetic, DEX has been described for this case scenario to maintain spontaneous ventilation and patient cooperation during laryngoplasty [119]. The favorable physiological effects of DEX on airway in addition to the antisialagogic [120] effect make it a useful anesthetic choice in adults and children who have a potential for airway catastrophe such as those with history of known difficult airway. Incorporating and expanding the applications of DEX into appropriate airway surgeries will be invaluable, as it has already been successfully implemented for patients at risk of airway collapse or a difficult airway [121–123]. By maintaining spontaneous ventilation and avoiding respiratory depression, DEX has been useful for those at risk of suffering fatal cardiopulmonary, respiratory, and cardiovascular complications [124].

Dexmedetomidine Use During Neurosurgical Procedures

The addition of DEX to anesthetic regimen is desirable in neurosurgical procedures and may contribute significantly to patient comfort and safety. A recent randomized trial evaluated the opioid-sparing effect of an intraoperative DEX infusion (0.2–0.5 mcg/kg/h) after craniotomy and demonstrated the opioid-sparing effect of DEX as evidenced by (1) a reduced verbal numerical pain rating scale, (2) a prolonged time before an analgesic request, (3) a reduced opioid requirement to control postoperative pain, and (4) fewer opioid-related side effects [125]. DEX has been used a as an adjunct to total intravenous anesthesia (TIVA) in the perioperative regimen used in the care of patients undergoing posterior spine fusion due to the anesthetic-sparing effects by lowering the propofol and inhalational agent requirements and facilitating emergence from anesthesia for the intraoperative wake-up test (when requested) and at the completion of surgery [63, 126]. It is also often continued into the postoperative period because of its ability to provide sedation and potentiate opioid analgesia with minimal additional respiratory depression. One should know that the potential risks of adding high doses of DEX to the anesthesia regimen in neurosurgical procedures require motor evoked potentials (MEP) monitoring

(Fig. 13.4). A target plasma concentration of 0.4 ng/ml DEX and 2.5 mcg/ml propofol seems to have minimal effect on MEP. Higher plasma serum DEX concentrations, however, may attenuate the amplitude of MEP [127]. DEX (0.2–0.7 mcg/kg/h) can also be used as an adjunct to establish and maintain controlled hypotension (mean arterial BP of 55–65 mmHg) during anterior spinal fusion [128]. Its concomitant effect, when used for controlled hypotension, on cardiac function, cerebral blood flow, and cerebral perfusion pressure has not been carefully evaluated.

Brain mapping and neurophysiologic testing have recently become an integral part of many neurosurgical techniques, brain tumor and epileptic seizure foci resection in particular. The anesthetic regimen for these tests should aim for a deep plane of anesthesia during the highly stimulating craniotomy and then a fully awake, comfortable, and cooperative patient during lesion resection in order to provide instant neurological feedback [129, 130]. Clinicians should also carefully balance the anesthetic depth in order to avoid untoward incidents such as airway obstruction, respiratory depression, hypercarbia, coughing, and hypotension. A key advantage of using DEX in these procedures is maintaining ventilation and airway patency in the presence of increasing level of sedation. Another critical advantage is ability to easily awaken patients by verbal stimulation. DEX 0.1–0.3 mcg/kg/h has been shown to maintain respiratory

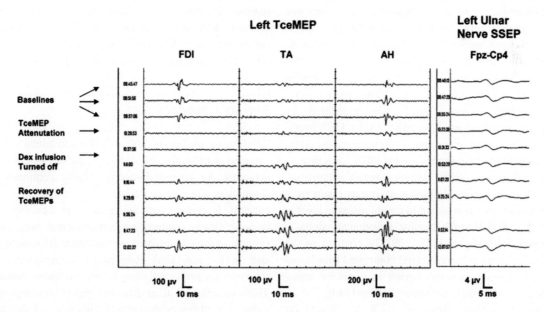

Fig. 13.4 Significant attenuation of transcranial electrical motor evoked potential amplitude after infusion of dexmedetomidine. Samples of transcranial electrical motor evoked potentials (TceMEP) recorded in a 13-year-old, 90-kg female patient with kyphoscoliosis presented for posterior spinal fusion with instrumentation of T2 to L3. Total intravenous anesthesia (TIVA) was initiated immediately after intubation with propofol 200 mcg/kg/min, remifentanil 0.5 mcg/kg/min, and dexmedetomidine 0.5 mcg/kg/h. Samples from left first dorsal interosseous (FDI), tibialis anterior (TA), and abductor hallucis (AH) muscles 1 h after starting TIVA (baselines), 1.5 h after acquisition of baselines (TceMEP attenuation), and during a 2-h period after the infusion of dexmedetomidine (DEX) were stopped (recovery of TceMEPs). Cortical somatosensory evoked potentials (SSEP) to stimulation of the left ulnar nerve recorded during the same time period as the TceMEPs are shown

drive and airway patency while still enabling the patient to be awakened and responsive to verbal stimulation for functional brain mapping [131].

Common anesthetic agents (both inhalational and intravenous) that are used for general anesthesia are known to suppress brain electrical activity by stimulating the GABA-A receptors in the cerebral cortex. DEX acts on subcortical areas of the brain and does not bind to the GABA receptors. It preserves epileptiform activity in children with seizure disorders, facilitating localization and identification of seizure foci [115, 132]. In a recent prospective study, electrocardiogram was monitored during DEX infusion in 34 adult patients undergoing anterior temporal lobe resection with amygdalohippocampectomy for drug-resistant mesial temporal lobe epilepsy. The authors concluded the DEX is useful during intraoperative electrocorticogram recording in epilepsy surgery as it enhances or does not alter spike rate in most of the cases, without any major adverse effects [133].

Cardiac Procedures

Adult and pediatric cardiac surgery is associated with a high risk of cardiovascular and other complications that may lead to increased morbidity and mortality and prolonged hospital stays. Alpha-2 agonists have many desirable effects, including analgesia, anxiolysis, inhibition of central sympathetic outflow, and blunting of the sympathetic response, that improve hemodynamic stability, positively affect myocardial oxygen supply and demand, may provide myocardial protection, and maximize neurocognitive function and expedite extubation [134–136]. Administration of DEX prior to global ischemia/reperfusion resulted in a reduction in infarct size, which was abrogated by pretreatment with yohimbine. This indicates that DEX exerts a cardioprotective effect against ischemia/reperfusion injury [137]. Several studies also suggested that DEX has a protective effect against myocardial ischemia injury in animals. These effects are not centrally mediated; it may result from preventing an increase in myocardial norepinephrine level in the ischemic region through cardiac presynaptic alpha-2-adrenoreceptor stimulation [138, 139]. In contrast to the previous studies, a recent randomized controlled trial found DEX did not provide cardioprotection in coronary artery bypass grafting with cardiopulmonary bypass [140].

The cardioprotective effects of DEX are based on blunting hemodynamic responses to perioperative stress, i.e., controlling HR through centrally mediated sympatholysis [141]. Under conditions of regional ischemia, DEX has been shown to exhibit cardioprotective effects: it optimized the blood flow of coronary arteries [142] and decreased lactate release during emergence from general anesthesia [143]. As an adjunct to anesthetic induction, DEX blunts the hemodynamic response to endotracheal intubation in patients undergoing cardiac surgery [144, 145]. A retrospective study in adults showed that perioperative DEX use was associated with a decrease in postoperative mortality up to 1 year and reduced the risk of overall complications and delirium in patients undergoing cardiac surgery [146]. In children (1–6 years) undergoing cardiac surgery, DEX 0.5 mcg/kg IV followed by an infusion of 0.5 mcg/kg/h attenuates the hemodynamic and neuroendocrine (epinephrine, norepinephrine, blood glucose, plasma cortisol) responses at time of incision, time of sternotomy, and after bypass [147]. Whether there is a long-term benefit on reducing delirium and mortality in the pediatric population is yet to be determined.

Although the negative chronotropic effect of DEX is considered as an adverse event, it has been used as a therapeutic maneuver in various clinical scenarios. In a retrospective study, 13 (93 %) of 14 children who received DEX for atrial and junctional tachyarrhythmias were converted to normal sinus rhythm [148]. Another prospective cohort study of pediatric patients undergoing cardiothoracic surgery [149] found that perioperative use of DEX may reduce the incidence of both ventricular (0 % vs. 25 %) and supraventricular (6 % vs. 25 %) tachyarrhythmias without significant adverse effects. The same authors examined the potential efficacy of DEX in the acute treatment of AV nodal-dependent reentrant tachyarrhythmias in pediatric patients compared with adenosine. The authors showed that the administration of DEX (0.7 ± 0.3 mcg/kg) successfully terminated 26 episodes of supraventricular tachycardia (96 %) at a median time of 30 s (20–35 s) [31].

Bariatric Surgery

Worldwide, obesity in both children and adults continues to increase in most countries and to a greater extent in modern societies. As a result bariatric surgery continues to grow throughout the world. Perioperative management of these patients is more challenging than in nonobese patients because airway anatomy is often abnormal with excess pharyngeal tissue and tongue size making it difficult to ventilate and to intubate [150]. Respiratory comorbidities in these patients may profoundly impact the anesthetic management. These patients are at an increased risk of developing opioid-induced ventilatory depression. Because of the increased risks with the conventional opioid-based anesthesia, DEX was recently added as an adjunct to anesthetic regimen to potentiate opioid analgesia with minimal additional respiratory depression. A recent study showed that using DEX infusion (0.2–0.8 mcg/kg/h) during laparoscopic bariatric surgery decreased fentanyl use, antiemetic therapy, and the length of stay in the recovery room. However, it failed to facilitate late recovery (e.g., bowel function) or improve the patients' overall quality of recovery [151]. Although the study did not facilitate late recovery, rapid turnover of these procedure and early recovery of these patients can be extremely important in busy practices.

Dexmedetomidine Applications During Vascular Surgeries

Perioperative management of hypertension is very important in patients who undergo carotid endarterectomy (CEA). If not managed appropriately, the patients can have intracerebral bleed, left ventricular failure, myocardial infarction, or fatal arrhythmias. The sympatholytic effect and the hemodynamic stability provided by DEX make it an attractive choice in these procedures [152]. A recent study recruited 54 patients for CEA under regional anesthesia and enrolled 25 patients in the DEX group and 29 patients in the standard group (midazolam and fentanyl). Patients in the DEX group received 0.5 mcg/kg bolus over 10 min followed by infusion of 0.2 mcg/kg/h. DEX provided less intraoperative and postoperative hypertension and tachycardia. But the incidence of bradycardia and hypotension was also more in the DEX group [153]. In conjunction with local anesthesia, DEX provided adequate sedation for a patient for axillofemoral bypass graft in a patient with history of difficult airway [154].

Dexmedetomidine for Dental Procedures

DEX appears to provide the desirable properties for successful dental sedation than traditional sedatives because of its analgesic property, antisalivatory properties, anxiolytic and sympatholytic effects, and less cognitive impairment and respiratory depression. It has been trialed for adult and pediatric dental sedation via different routes [155–161]. Along with its beneficial effects, DEX was reported to exert potential anti-inflammatory and antioxidant effects. Previous studies revealed that DEX significantly decreased the levels of inflammatory cytokines [162]. Compared to midazolam, DEX appears to provide better sedation and postoperative analgesia via anti-inflammatory and antioxidation pathway during office-based artificial tooth implantation [163]. A recent study that compared the efficacy (sedation, anxiolysis, analgesia, operating conditions, and patients' satisfaction) and safety of DEX and midazolam as sedatives for dental outpatient procedures showed that DEX works, as well as midazolam, for outpatient dental procedures and can be used as an alternative to midazolam [164]. Conversely, a Japanese study compared intravenous

sedation with DEX and propofol for minor oral surgery and reported hypotension and bradycardia with DEX but no difference in respiratory depression with propofol [165].

Although the bioavailability of DEX is poor via the oral route, a prospective, triple-blind, randomized study compared the efficacy and safety of one of the three doses of oral DEX (3, 4, and 5 mcg/kg) combined with ketamine (8 mg/kg) for pediatric dental sedation. The study showed that ketamine and DEX at 5 mcg/kg provided faster onset of sedation, higher intra- and postoperative analgesia and anterograde amnesia, and delayed recovery from sedation when compared with lower dose of DEX groups [166].

Regional Anesthesia

Clonidine has been employed clinically to achieve the desired effects in regional anesthesia (epidural, intrathecal, peripheral nerve block) for decades [167]. The successful use of epidural clonidine in adults led to its evaluation in pediatric caudal block, and so far there is reasonable extensive clinical experience and published literature to dispel any concern regarding its neurotoxicity. DEX has been described with regional blocks in both adults and children. In adults, a meta-analysis of 16 RCTs included 1092 adults and compared outcomes between DEX (intrathecal, epidural, or caudal) and bupivacaine or ropivicaine. DEX was found to decrease the pain and prolong the analgesia. Although there was an increased incidence of bradycardia in the DEX group, it was not associated with hypotension and did not warrant treatment [168]. Similarly, the combination of caudal DEX and bupivacaine (1 mcg/kg and 2.5 mg/kg, respectively) in children has been shown to decrease the sevoflurane requirements, incidence of emergence agitation, adjuvant postoperative analgesics, and duration of postoperative pain relief, to a greater degree as compared to bupivacaine alone. The addition of caudal DEX to bupivacaine did not affect the hemodynamic response [169]. Epidural DEX and clonidine produced similar analgesia, duration of action, and hemodynamic profile when used with bupivacaine (2.5 mg/kg) for lower abdominal surgery in children [170]. A recent meta-analysis concluded that the addition of DEX to a caudal anesthetic provided extended duration of postoperative pain relief in 328 pediatric patients. There was no statistically significant effect on hemodynamics and adverse events with the addition of DEX to the local anesthetic. Subgroup analysis showed no advantage of the 2 mcg/kg of caudal DEX over the 1 mcg/kg in terms of analgesia [171]. Currently there are still some concerns regarding neuraxial DEX safety. DEX via the neuraxial route is off label and the safety has not been established in humans. In animal models, perineural administration of DEX attenuated inflammation in the sciatic nerve via reducing inflammatory cytokine levels [172]. However, in rabbits, epidural DEX elicited what appeared to be a demyelination of oligodendrocytes in the white matter of the spinal cord [173]. Future studies are warranted in order to support or dispel the concerns of neurotoxicity from DEX.

Caution should be exercised when DEX sedation is used in infants and neonates receiving epidural analgesia, without support from external warming devices. Infants depend more on non-shivering thermogenesis than on shivering and vasoconstriction. In mice, DEX causes hypothermia [174]. The effect is attenuated in animals that are genetically deficient in alpha-2 adrenoceptor. The hypothermic response is postulated to interference with non-shivering thermogenesis and reduction of metabolic heat production [175]. Recently a 2-day-old neonate receiving epidural analgesia, without using external warming devices, developed hypothermia (33 °C axillary) and bradycardia (HR 75 beats/min). There was no change in the HR following the administration of atropine and naloxone that was unresponsive to atropine [176]. The epidural infusion was discontinued and the infant was placed under a radiant warmer. Over the next 2–3 h, the temperature was improved.

Dexmedetomidine Applications for Ambulatory Procedures

Clear understanding of the pharmacokinetic effects of the chosen anesthetic agent is critical for brief procedures in the operating room. An important factor influencing the anesthetic regimen in ambulatory practice is rapid home discharge. There are few studies that examined the use of DEX for ambulatory procedures, perhaps because its half-life and analgesic properties do not lend themselves to the fast pace (induction, emergence, and recovery) of most short procedures. The undesirable prolongation of recovery length of stay associated with administering high dose of DEX for brief procedure makes it a poor choice that does not appear to offer advantages over current standard of practices.

Pressure equalizing tubes procedure is a very common brief (10–15 min) surgical procedure in the pediatric population. Some form of analgesia is required in most children despite the brief nature of the procedure with limited tissue trauma. Management of pain can be a challenge because this procedure is often performed without intravenous access; the options for providing analgesia may be limited. Choosing nasal DEX administration for this procedure is theoretically reasonable because it has been shown to have analgesic effects without significant respiratory depression. DEX administration has been described for this procedure, but without an advantage over intranasal fentanyl or acetaminophen [177]. Early experience with this agent demonstrated it to be ineffective during upper gastrointestinal endoscopy in

children; it was not found to offer any advantages either alone or in combination with propofol [178].

A recent study examined the use of DEX as a sole sedative agent (1 mcg/kg infused over 10 min followed by a maintenance dose of 0.2–0.8 mcg/kg/h) in office-based oral and maxillofacial surgery procedures [179]. The authors showed that the prolonged recovery time makes DEX undesirable for busy office-based practices. They recommended using DEX for patients with a high risk of respiratory complications (e.g., obese patients or those with a history of sleep apnea). Findings in other adult studies also clearly demonstrate that DEX significantly prolongs length of stay in the PACU for brief procedure such as colonoscopy [180].

Several studies found that the perioperative use of DEX can help to reduce opioid requirements and to potentiate analgesia in various surgical procedures. This opioid-sparing analgesic effect of DEX may be advantageous for short procedures. In a double-blind controlled trial, children who received high doses of IV DEX (2 and 4 mcg/kg) immediately following endotracheal intubation had a lower opiate requirement and longer opiate-free interval in recovery than the group that received a single IV dose of fentanyl (1 or 2 mcg/kg) [181]. DEX may be an option to minimize intraoperative narcotic use, particularly for tonsillectomies. 1 mcg/kg and morphine IV 100 mcg/kg have exhibited comparable morphine-sparing effects and time to discharge readiness post-tonsillectomy and adenoidectomy [182]. This opioid-sparing analgesic and recovery profile of DEX in children following tonsillectomy and adenoidectomies may be particularly advantageous in those at risk of postoperative apnea or respiratory compromise.

Dexmedetomidine Use for Procedural Sedation

DEX has been successfully used as a sole sedative agent for diagnostic radiologic procedures, like MRI, CT scans, and nuclear medicine studies [183, 184]. A bolus of 2 mcg/kg followed by an infusion of 1 mcg/kg has been shown to provide successful sedation for CT imaging [50, 185]. At these doses, a decrease in HR and mean arterial BP was observed, still within normal range for age, along with a 16 % incidence of sinus arrhythmia. When used as a sole agent within the dosing guidelines of the FDA, DEX does not provide consistent success for sedation in MRI [186]. The literature reveals that higher doses of DEX (bolus of 3 mcg/kg^{-1} and infusion of 2 mcg/kg/h) were successful for 97.6 % of 747 children undergoing MRI [51]. In 16 %, the HR decreased below 20 % of age-adjusted clinical normal values, with mean arterial BPs remaining within 20 % of age-adjusted norms.

Although DEX has been shown to provide effective sedation for noninvasive procedures, it has been largely unsuccessful in providing adequate analgesia when used alone for painful procedures [13, 51, 180, 187, 188]. Using high doses of DEX to overcome this problem in order to provide adequate depth of sedation in these procedures may lead to significant hemodynamic instability specifically bradycardia which eventually can limit DEX use in infants and children. IV DEX in combination with IV ketamine may be a successful combination, with relatively fast onset and amnesia, sedation, analgesia, and hemodynamic stability [189, 190]. Combining the two agents has been described in adults and children for extracorporeal shock wave lithotripsy [191], lumbar puncture [192], bone marrow biopsy, burn dressing changes [193, 194], chest tube insertion, and femoral cutdown for tunneled central venous catheter placement [195]. This combination can also be useful for patients with history of mitochondrial disorders and malignant hyperthermia (MH). Although this combination in one patient is rare, it poses a unique challenging situation for anesthesia providers. In the animal model, DEX has been shown to have beneficial effects on the mitochondrial membrane in ischemic rats [196]. If this quality extends to humans, DEX could offer advantages for use within this challenging scenario. The most effective regimen for combing DEX and ketamine appears to be the use of a bolus dose of both agents, DEX (1 mcg/kg) and ketamine (1–2 mg/kg), to initiate sedation. This can then be followed by a DEX infusion (1–2 mcg/kg/h) with supplemental bolus doses of ketamine (0.5–1 mg/kg) as needed.

Post-procedural Applications

The saying "an ounce of prevention is worth a pound of cure" should encapsulate the mindset of dealing with emergence agitation (EA). Prevention is definitely better than treatment. A restless recovery from anesthesia may not only cause injury to the child or to the surgical site, but it may also lead to the accidental removal of surgical dressings, IV catheters, and drains. Emergence delirium and agitation (ED and EA), described as early as 1961, are relatively common, particularly after volatile anesthetics in the pediatric population [197, 198]. It is associated with prolonged recovery time and the potential for maladaptive behavior for up to 2 weeks [198–200]. It is relatively common for pediatric ambulatory procedures and can be associated with morbidity in the recovery period [201, 202]. A recent meta-analysis showed that alpha-2-agonists (clonidine or DEX), given by oral, intravenous, or caudal route, had a prophylactic effect in preventing EA in children anesthetized with sevoflurane or desflurane [88]. DEX 0.25–1 mcg/kg has been shown to prevent and treat postoperative agitation in pediatric population [116, 203–205]. The perioperative infusion of 0.2 mcg/kg/

h decreases the incidence and frequency of postoperative agitation in children after sevoflurane without prolonging the time to extubate or discharge [206]. Compared to placebo, DEX (0.5 and 1 mcg/kg) decreases the incidence of EA from 47.6 to 4.8 %, albeit a slightly prolonged emergence and time to extubation [204, 205]. In comparison with fentanyl (1 mcg/kg), intraoperative DEX (2 mcg/kg bolus followed by 0.7 mcg/kg/h) reduced the incidence of severe EA, the postoperative opioid requirements, and the episodes of desaturation in children with OSA following tonsillectomy and adenoidectomy [207].

The use of the DEX as an infusion over 10 min to treat agitation in a delirious child is impractical, although some practitioners administer DEX as a rapid (less than 5 s) IV bolus to treat EA. Rapid IV administration (<5 s) of 0.25–0.5 mcg/kg DEX has been described in children undergoing cardiac catheterization without hemodynamic consequence [46]. A recent prospective, double-blind, randomized study examined the effect of rapid (2–3-second) IV bolus injection of DEX on emergence agitation and the hemodynamic response in 400 patients, aged 4–10 years, undergoing tonsillectomy with or without adenoidectomy, with or without myringotomy, and/or tympanostomy tube insertion. The study concluded that rapid IV bolus administration of DEX in children improved the recovery profile by reducing the incidence of EA. A statistically significant change in hemodynamics was noticed, but none of these patients required any intervention for hemodynamic changes. One concern with using small doses of DEX for prophylaxis or treatment of agitation is cost. Collaboration with the pharmacy to reduce the cost of DEX per patient is advised for this scenario. Preparing a sterilely 10-ml syringes of DEX in 4 mcg ml^{-1} solutions can significantly reduce the cost and waste of DEX.

Many adult studies demonstrated the efficacy of DEX in the setting of postoperative shivering [208–211]. DEX decreases vasoconstriction and may have a role in altering thermoregulatory shivering. In a prospective, nonrandomized open-label study in 24 children ranging in age from 7 to 16 years who shivered after general anesthesia, 0.5 mcg/kg IV DEX over 3–5 min stopped the shivering in all of the children within 5 min, without recurrence. No adverse effects were observed with the rapid bolus [212].

Although intraoperative DEX has been reported to reduce opioid consumption in children, the opioid-sparing effects of DEX are still not completely understood in children. DEX has been shown in adults to alter the pain perception, specifically to decrease the perception of pain inducted by cold and ischemia [213]. In adults, intraoperative DEX has been shown in a recent meta-analysis to decrease postoperative pain scores and morphine consumption [214]. A recent meta-analysis of 11 RCTs examined intraoperative DEX versus placebo or opioids on postoperative pain, analgesic consumption, and adverse events in 434 children undergoing surgery. The study demonstrated that intraoperative use of DEX provided similar postoperative analgesia compared to intraoperative opioid use and better postoperative analgesia compared to placebo use [215].

Sedation in Critical Care Unit

Choosing the appropriate sedative agent is an integral part of optimizing outcomes and preventing complications in ICU. The ideal sedative agent should aim for improve tolerance with mechanical ventilation , preventing accidental device removal, reducing myocardial oxygen demands, increasing patient comfort and safety and finally does not have significant accumulation of any metabolic products that would limit the prolonged use. Shortening the time to extubation and the duration of mechanical ventilation are also among key factors in reducing ICU costs and resource utilization. γ-Aminobutyric acid receptor agonist medications are the most commonly used sedatives for ICU patients, yet recent evidence indicates that DEX may have distinct advantages in these critically ill patients. This novel sedative agent is an attractive choice in the ICU environment because it maintains respiratory drive and airway patency while still enabling the patient to be awakened and responsive to verbal stimulation upon demand. Another advantage is ongoing sedation can be maintained with the use of DEX during and following extubation. DEX seems to gain a place in the ICU as a safer sedative agent, deftly replacing traditional sedatives like propofol and benzodiazepines.

The use of DEX has been associated with lower risk of delirium and coma compared with propofol, lorazepam, and midazolam [216, 217]. A recent meta-analysis which included a total of 24 trials involving 2419 critically ill patients from over 11 countries concluded that DEX reduced the length of ICU stay. The risk of bradycardia was, however, higher when both a loading dose and high maintenance doses of DEX were used [218]. DEX has been shown to reduce the time to extubation compared with traditional sedative agents [216, 219, 220].

A recent study of two-phase three multicenter, randomized, double-blind trials carried out from 2007 to 2010 examined the efficacy of DEX vs. midazolam or propofol in maintaining sedation, reducing duration of mechanical ventilation, and improving patients' interaction with nursing care. The authors of this trial showed that among ICU patients receiving prolonged mechanical ventilation, DEX was not inferior to midazolam and propofol in maintaining light to moderate sedation. DEX reduced duration of mechanical ventilation compared with midazolam and improved patients' ability to communicate pain compared with midazolam and propofol (Fig. 13.5). Patients who received DEX did experience higher incidences of hypotension and bradycardia compared to the midazolam group, but there was no difference in these adverse effects between the propofol and DEX groups. The authors concluded that DEX is a feasible agent for long-term sedation [219].

A recent meta-analysis study examined all randomized controlled trials exploring the clinical benefits of DEX versus propofol for sedating adult in 1202 ICU patients. The primary outcomes of this study were length of ICU stay, duration of mechanical ventilation, and risk of ICU mortality. Secondary outcomes included risk of delirium, hypotension, bradycardia, and hypertension. The authors concluded that DEX may offer advantages over propofol in terms of decrease in the length of ICU stay and the risk of delirium. However, transient hypertension may occur when DEX is administered with a loading dose or at high infusion rates [221].

From the cost-minimization prospective, DEX appears to be a preferable option compared with standard sedative agents (propofol or midazolam) used to provide light to moderate ICU sedation exceeding 24 h. The saving potential results primarily from shorter time to extubation [222].

The use of DEX for a period greater than 24 h has been studied [223, 224]. In a Phase IV study, DEX was safe in dosages up to 1.4 mcg/kg/h for greater than 24 h and did not produce rebound tachycardia or hypertension when abruptly discontinued [223, 225]. In an observational study of 136 patients at ten institutions, a third of these patients received DEX for a period greater than 24 h. The average length of treatment was 54 h, with a range of 24.5–123.5 h [226]. There were no reports of rebound symptoms.

Limited data are available regarding prolonged administration to children. Several studies have evaluated the usefulness of DEX in the pediatric ICU and showed that it is effective in sedating infants and children up to 3 days [27, 227, 228]. In these studies, DEX spared the doses of benzodiazepines and opioids, although bradycardia and hypotension were notable in 27 % of children. The successful use of DEX for 4 days in a child after tracheal reconstruction for subglottic stenosis has been recently reported [229]. A recent retrospective study of 38 spontaneously breathing and mechanically ventilated children undergoing cardiothoracic surgery showed that DEX provided adequate sedation 93 % of the time and adequate analgesia 83 % of the time. Side effects included hypotension (15 %) and transient bradycardia in one patient [34].

In conclusion, evidence continues to accumulate through several studies targeting the use of DEX in ICU and shows that it is a valuable agent for providing sedation and anxiolysis in this setting. Data are promising, but are still limited, and further prospective studies of both short-term and long-term DEX infusions in infants and children are needed to support its use as a safe and effective agent for

a MIDEX trial

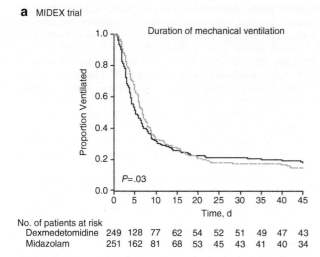

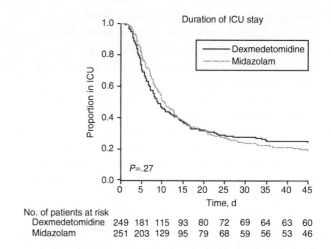

No. of patients at risk

Dexmedetomidine	249	128	77	62	54	52	51	49	47	43
Midazolam	251	162	81	68	53	45	43	41	40	34

No. of patients at risk

Dexmedetomidine	249	181	115	93	80	72	69	64	63	60
Midazolam	251	203	129	95	79	68	59	56	53	46

b PRODEX trial

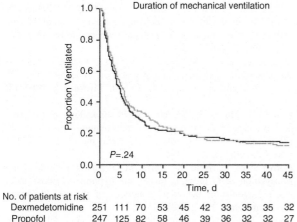

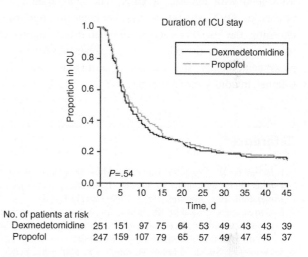

No. of patients at risk

Dexmedetomidine	251	111	70	53	45	42	33	35	35	32
Propofol	247	125	82	58	46	39	36	32	32	27

No. of patients at risk

Dexmedetomidine	251	151	97	75	64	53	49	43	43	39
Propofol	247	159	107	79	65	57	49	47	45	37

Fig. 13.5 Duration of mechanical ventilation and intensive care unit stay. In the MIDEX trial (midazolam vs. dexmedetomidine), the median duration of mechanical ventilation was, for dexmedetomidine, 123 h (interquartile range [IQR], 67–337 h) and, for midazolam, 164 h (IQR, 92–380 h) (Gehan-Wilcoxon $P = 0.03$). The median length of stay in the intensive care unit (ICU) from randomization until the patient was medically fit for discharge was, for dexmedetomidine, 211 h (IQR, 115–831 h) and, for midazolam, 243 h (IQR, 140–630 h; Gehan-Wilcoxon $P = 0.27$). In the PRODEX trial (propofol vs. dexmedetomidine), the median duration of mechanical ventilation was, for dexmedetomidine, 97 h (IQR, 45–257 h) and, for propofol, 118 h (IQR, 48–327 h) (Gehan-Wilcoxon $P = 0.24$). The median length of stay in the ICU from randomization until the patient was medically fit for discharge was, for dexmedetomidine, 164 h (IQR, 90–480 h) and, for propofol, 185 h (93–520 h; Cox's proportional hazards test $P = 0.54$). Study drugs were given for a maximum of 336 h in both trials

maintaining sedation in critically ill patients requiring mechanical ventilation.

Conclusion

Are there more unanswered questions about the use of DEX in the management of anesthesia/sedation in children and adults? Evidence continues to accumulate through many studies targeting the use of this novel sedative agent for a variety of procedures in pediatric and adult population. The enthusiasm for the growing interest in the use of DEX over the past few years stems from its unique mechanism of action and the favorable sedative and anxiolytic properties together with its limited effects on hemodynamic and respiratory function. We still have many unanswered questions, and further studies are required to examine organoprotective effects in humans, long-term evaluation, impact of age on side effects, the effect of prolonged administration, and interactions with other anesthetic/sedative agents to support its use as a safe and effective agent for maintaining sedation in healthy and critically ill patients. These issues are likely to be sorted out as experience with DEX use grows.

DEX has organoprotective effects, reducing cerebral, cardiac, intestinal, and renal injury. There is substantial in vivo and in vitro evidence that DEX has neuroprotective properties. It is time to investigate its value as a neuroprotectant in clinical practice. There is an urgent need to confirm the neuroprotective beneficial effects in more experimental and clinical studies to examine existence of associations between early anesthetic exposure of DEX and long-term neurocognitive function.

In conclusion, data regarding the use of DEX in adults and children are promising, but are still limited. The benign effect of DEX on ventilatory drive is one of the major advantages of DEX over other traditional sedative agents. For patients with respiratory compromise for whom the preservation of spontaneous ventilation and airway tone is preferable or those for whom the preservation of neuromonitoring with or without patient responsiveness is the goal, DEX should be strongly considered. As is the case with any novel agent, there is a significant learning curve associated with the use of DEX. The few predicted side effects of DEX should always be kept in mind before choosing the patients for its administration. An in-depth understanding of the pharmacologic, pharmacokinetic, and pharmacodynamic effects of DEX is critical to maximize its safe use in adults and children.

References

1. Belleville JP, Ward DS, Bloor BC, Maze M. Effects of intravenous dexmedetomidine in humans. I. Sedation, ventilation, and metabolic rate. Anesthesiology. 1992;77(6):1125–33.
2. Correa-Sales C, Rabin BC, Maze M. A hypnotic response to dexmedetomidine, an alpha 2 agonist, is mediated in the locus coeruleus in rats. Anesthesiology. 1992;76(6):948–52.
3. Petroz GC, Sikich N, James M, van Dyk H, Shafer SL, Schily M, et al. A phase I, two-center study of the pharmacokinetics and pharmacodynamics of dexmedetomidine in children. Anesthesiology. 2006;105(6):1098–110.
4. Nelson LE, Lu J, Guo T, Saper CB, Franks NP, Maze M. The alpha2-adrenoceptor agonist dexmedetomidine converges on an endogenous sleep-promoting pathway to exert its sedative effects. Anesthesiology. 2003;98(2):428–36.
5. Doze VA, Chen BX, Maze M. Dexmedetomidine produces a hypnotic-anesthetic action in rats via activation of central alpha-2 adrenoceptors. Anesthesiology. 1989;71(1):75–9.
6. Bloor BC, Ward DS, Belleville JP, Maze M. Effects of intravenous dexmedetomidine in humans. II. Hemodynamic changes. Anesthesiology. 1992;77(6):1134–42.
7. Akeju O, Pavone KJ, Westover MB, Vazquez R, Prerau MJ, Harrell PG, et al. A comparison of propofol- and dexmedetomidine-induced electroencephalogram dynamics using spectral and coherence analysis. Anesthesiology. 2014;121 (5):978–89.
8. Sanders RD, Sun P, Patel S, Li M, Maze M, Ma D. Dexmedetomidine provides cortical neuroprotection: impact on anaesthetic-induced neuroapoptosis in the rat developing brain. Acta Anaesthesiol Scand. 2010;54(6):710–6.
9. Li Y, Zeng M, Chen W, Liu C, Wang F, Han X, et al. Dexmedetomidine reduces isoflurane-induced neuroapoptosis partly by preserving PI3K/Akt pathway in the hippocampus of neonatal rats. PLoS One. 2014;9(4), e93639.
10. Tachibana K, Hashimoto T, Kato R, Uchida Y, Ito R, Takita K, et al. Neonatal administration with dexmedetomidine does not impair the rat hippocampal synaptic plasticity later in adulthood. Paediatr Anaesth. 2012;22(7):713–9.
11. Sanders RD, Xu J, Shu Y, Januszewski A, Halder S, Fidalgo A, et al. Dexmedetomidine attenuates isoflurane-induced neurocognitive impairment in neonatal rats. Anesthesiology. 2009;110(5):1077–85.
12. Clarke KW, Hall LW. "Xylazine"--a new sedative for horses and cattle. Vet Rec. 1969;85(19):512–7.
13. Mason KP, Lerman J. Review article: Dexmedetomidine in children: current knowledge and future applications. Anesth Analg. 2011;113(5):1129–42.
14. Mahmoud M, Mason KP. Dexmedetomidine: review, update, and future considerations of paediatric perioperative and periprocedural applications and limitations. Br J Anaesth. 2015;115(2):171–82.
15. Bhana N, Goa KL, McClellan KJ. Dexmedetomidine. Drugs. 2000;59(2):263–8. discussion 9–70.
16. Brede M, Philipp M, Knaus A, Muthig V, Hein L. alpha2-adrenergic receptor subtypes - novel functions uncovered in gene-targeted mouse models. Biol Cell. 2004;96(5):343–8.
17. Kobilka BK, Matsui H, Kobilka TS, Yang-Feng TL, Francke U, Caron MG, et al. Cloning, sequencing, and expression of the gene coding for the human platelet alpha 2-adrenergic receptor. Science. 1987;238(4827):650–6.
18. Virtanen R, Savola JM, Saano V, Nyman L. Characterization of the selectivity, specificity and potency of medetomidine as an alpha 2-adrenoceptor agonist. Eur J Pharmacol. 1988;150 (1–2):9–14.
19. Panzer O, Moitra V, Sladen RN. Pharmacology of sedative-analgesic agents: dexmedetomidine, remifentanil, ketamine, volatile anesthetics, and the role of peripheral mu antagonists. Crit Care Clin. 2009;25(3):451–69.
20. Correa-Sales C, Reid K, Maze M. Pertussis toxin-mediated ribosylation of G proteins blocks the hypnotic response to an alpha 2-agonist in the locus coeruleus of the rat. Pharmacol Biochem Behav. 1992;43(3):723–7.
21. Nacif-Coelho C, Correa-Sales C, Chang LL, Maze M. Perturbation of ion channel conductance alters the hypnotic response to the alpha 2-adrenergic agonist dexmedetomidine in the locus coeruleus of the rat. Anesthesiology. 1994;81 (6):1527–34.
22. Hsu YW, Cortinez LI, Robertson KM, Keifer JC, Sum-Ping ST, Moretti EW, et al. Dexmedetomidine pharmacodynamics: part I: crossover comparison of the respiratory effects of dexmedetomidine and remifentanil in healthy volunteers. Anesthesiology. 2004;101(5):1066–76.
23. Ishii H, Kohno T, Yamakura T, Ikoma M, Baba H. Action of dexmedetomidine on the substantia gelatinosa neurons of the rat spinal cord. Eur J Neurosci. 2008;27(12):3182–90.
24. Roudet C, Mouchet P, Feuerstein C, Savasta M. Normal distribution of alpha 2-adrenoceptors in the rat spinal cord and its modification after noradrenergic denervation: a quantitative autoradiographic study. J Neurosci Res. 1994;39(3):319–29.
25. Stone LS, Broberger C, Vulchanova L, Wilcox GL, Hokfelt T, Riedl MS, et al. Differential distribution of alpha2A and alpha2C adrenergic receptor immunoreactivity in the rat spinal cord. J Neurosci. 1998;18(15):5928–37.
26. Guo TZ, Jiang JY, Buttermann AE, Maze M. Dexmedetomidine injection into the locus ceruleus produces antinociception. Anesthesiology. 1996;84(4):873–81.
27. Diaz SM, Rodarte A, Foley J, Capparelli EV. Pharmacokinetics of dexmedetomidine in postsurgical pediatric intensive care unit patients: preliminary study. Pediatr Crit Care Med. 2007;8 (5):419–24.

28. Vilo S, Rautiainen P, Kaisti K, Aantaa R, Scheinin M, Manner T, et al. Pharmacokinetics of intravenous dexmedetomidine in children under 11 yr of age. Br J Anaesth. 2008;100(5):697–700.

29. Dextor (dexmedetomidine) package insert. Espo, Finland: Orion Corporation; 2014.

30. Wang SS, Zhang MZ, Sun Y, Wu C, Xu WY, Bai J, et al. The sedative effects and the attenuation of cardiovascular and arousal responses during anesthesia induction and intubation in pediatric patients: a randomized comparison between two different doses of preoperative intranasal dexmedetomidine. Paediatr Anaesth. 2014;24(3):275–81.

31. Cimen ZS, Hanci A, Sivrikaya GU, Kilinc LT, Erol MK. Comparison of buccal and nasal dexmedetomidine premedication for pediatric patients. Paediatr Anaesth. 2013;23(2):134–8.

32. Anttila M, Penttila J, Helminen A, Vuorilehto L, Scheinin H. Bioavailability of dexmedetomidine after extravascular doses in healthy subjects. Br J Clin Pharmacol. 2003;56(6):691–3.

33. Iirola T, Vilo S, Manner T, Aantaa R, Lahtinen M, Scheinin M, et al. Bioavailability of dexmedetomidine after intranasal administration. Eur J Clin Pharmacol. 2011;67(8):825–31.

34. Chrysostomou C, Di Filippo S, Manrique AM, Schmitt CG, Orr RA, Casta A, et al. Use of dexmedetomidine in children after cardiac and thoracic surgery. Pediatr Crit Care Med. 2006;7(2):126–31.

35. Su F, Gastonguay MR, Nicolson SC, DiLiberto M, Ocampo-Pelland A, Zuppa AF. Dexmedetomidine pharmacology in neonates and infants after open heart surgery. Anesth Analg. 2016;122:1556–66.

36. Iirola T, Aantaa R, Laitio R, Kentala E, Lahtinen M, Wighton A, et al. Pharmacokinetics of prolonged infusion of high-dose dexmedetomidine in critically ill patients. Crit Care. 2011;15(5):R257.

37. Eastwood PR, Platt PR, Shepherd K, Maddison K, Hillman DR. Collapsibility of the upper airway at different concentrations of propofol anesthesia. Anesthesiology. 2005;103(3):470–7.

38. Dhonneur G, Combes X, Leroux B, Duvaldestin P. Postoperative obstructive apnea. Anesth Analg. 1999;89(3):762–7.

39. Brouillette RT, Thach BT. A neuromuscular mechanism maintaining extrathoracic airway patency. J Appl Physiol. 1979;46(4):772–9.

40. Mahmoud M, Gunter J, Donnelly LF, Wang Y, Nick TG, Sadhasivam S. A comparison of dexmedetomidine with propofol for magnetic resonance imaging sleep studies in children. Anesth Analg. 2009;109(3):745–53.

41. Mahmoud M, Radhakrishman R, Gunter J, Sadhasivam S, Schapiro A, McAuliffe J, et al. Effect of increasing depth of dexmedetomidine anesthesia on upper airway morphology in children. Paediatr Anaesth. 2010;20(6):506–15.

42. Mahmoud M, Jung D, Salisbury S, McAuliffe J, Gunter J, Patio M, et al. Effect of increasing depth of dexmedetomidine and propofol anesthesia on upper airway morphology in children and adolescents with obstructive sleep apnea. J Clin Anesth. 2013;25:529–41.

43. Truong MT, Woo VG, Koltai PJ. Sleep endoscopy as a diagnostic tool in pediatric obstructive sleep apnea. Int J Pediatr Otorhinolaryngol. 2012;76(5):722–7.

44. Chatterjee D, Friedman N, Shott S, Mahmoud M. Anesthetic dilemmas for dynamic evaluation of the pediatric upper airway. Semin Cardiothorac Vasc Anesth. 2014;18(4):371–8.

45. Mahmoud M, Gunter J, Sadhasivam S. Cine MRI airway studies in children with sleep apnea: optimal images and anesthetic challenges. Pediatr Radiol. 2009;39(10):1034–7.

46. Jooste EH, Muhly WT, Ibinson JW, Suresh T, Damian D, Phadke A, et al. Acute hemodynamic changes after rapid intravenous bolus dosing of dexmedetomidine in pediatric heart transplant patients undergoing routine cardiac catheterization. Anesth Analg. 2010;111(6):1490–6.

47. Potts AL, Anderson BJ, Holford NH, Vu TC, Warman GR. Dexmedetomidine hemodynamics in children after cardiac surgery. Paediatr Anaesth. 2010;20(5):425–33.

48. Mason KP, Lonnqvist PA. Bradycardia in perspective-not all reductions in heart rate need immediate intervention. Paediatr Anaesth. 2015;25(1):44–51.

49. Mason KP, Turner DP, Houle TT, Fontaine PJ, Lerman J. Hemodynamic response to fluid management in children undergoing dexmedetomidine sedation for MRI. AJR Am J Roentgenol. 2014;202(6):W574–9.

50. Mason KP, Zgleszewski SE, Prescilla R, Fontaine PJ, Zurakowski D. Hemodynamic effects of dexmedetomidine sedation for CT imaging studies. Paediatr Anaesth. 2008;18(5):393–402.

51. Mason KP, Zurakowski D, Zgleszewski SE, Robson CD, Carrier M, Hickey PR, et al. High dose dexmedetomidine as the sole sedative for pediatric MRI. Paediatr Anaesth. 2008;18(5):403–11.

52. Jorden VS, Pousman RM, Sanford MM, Thorborg PA, Hutchens MP. Dexmedetomidine overdose in the perioperative setting. Ann Pharmacother. 2004;38(5):803–7.

53. Ramsay MA, Luterman DL. Dexmedetomidine as a total intravenous anesthetic agent. Anesthesiology. 2004;101(3):787–90.

54. Patel VJ, Ahmed SS, Nitu ME, Rigby MR. Vasovagal syncope and severe bradycardia following intranasal dexmedetomidine for pediatric procedural sedation. Paediatr Anaesth. 2014;24(4):446–8.

55. Berkenbosch JW, Tobias JD. Development of bradycardia during sedation with dexmedetomidine in an infant concurrently receiving digoxin. Pediatr Crit Care Med. 2003;4(2):203–5.

56. Hammer GB, Drover DR, Cao H, Jackson E, Williams GD, Ramamoorthy C, et al. The effects of dexmedetomidine on cardiac electrophysiology in children. Anesth Analg. 2008;106(1):79–83.

57. Chrysostomou C, Komarlu R, Lichtenstein S, Shiderly D, Arora G, Orr R, et al. Electrocardiographic effects of dexmedetomidine in patients with congenital heart disease. Intensive Care Med. 2010;36(5):836–42.

58. Aantaa R, Kanto J, Scheinin M, Kallio A, Scheinin H. Dexmedetomidine, an alpha 2-adrenoceptor agonist, reduces anesthetic requirements for patients undergoing minor gynecologic surgery. Anesthesiology. 1990;73(2):230–5.

59. Scheinin H, Aantaa R, Anttila M, Hakola P, Helminen A, Karhuvaara S. Reversal of the sedative and sympatholytic effects of dexmedetomidine with a specific alpha2-adrenoceptor antagonist atipamezole: a pharmacodynamic and kinetic study in healthy volunteers. Anesthesiology. 1998;89(3):574–84.

60. Mason KP, Zgleszewski S, Forman RE, Stark C, DiNardo JA. An exaggerated hypertensive response to glycopyrrolate therapy for bradycardia associated with high-dose dexmedetomidine. Anesth Analg. 2009;108(3):906–8.

61. Congdon JM, Marquez M, Niyom S, Boscan P. Evaluation of the sedative and cardiovascular effects of intramuscular administration of dexmedetomidine with and without concurrent atropine administration in dogs. J Am Vet Med Assoc. 2011;239(1):81–9.

62. Subramanyam R, Cudilo EM, Hossain MM, McAuliffe J, Wu J, Patino M, et al. To pretreat or not to pretreat: prophylactic anticholinergic administration before dexmedetomidine in pediatric imaging. Anesth Analg. 2015;121(2):479–85.

63. Peden CJ, Cloote AH, Stratford N, Prys-Roberts C. The effect of intravenous dexmedetomidine premedication on the dose requirement of propofol to induce loss of consciousness in patients receiving alfentanil. Anaesthesia. 2001;56(5):408–13.

64. Ingersoll-Weng E, Manecke Jr GR, Thistlethwaite PA. Dexmedetomidine and cardiac arrest. Anesthesiology. 2004;100(3):738–9.

65. Dawes J, Myers D, Gorges M, Zhou G, Ansermino JM, Montgomery CJ. Identifying a rapid bolus dose of dexmedetomidine (ED50) with acceptable hemodynamic outcomes in children. Paediatr Anaesth. 2014;24(12):1260–7.

66. Ickeringill M, Shehabi Y, Adamson H, Ruettimann U. Dexmedetomidine infusion without loading dose in surgical patients requiring mechanical ventilation: haemodynamic effects and efficacy. Anaesth Intensive Care. 2004;32(6):741–5.

67. Nishibe S, Imanishi H, Mieda T, Tsujita M. The effects of dexmedetomidine administration on the pulmonary artery pressure and the transpulmonary pressure gradient after the bidirectional superior cavopulmonary shunt. Pediatr Cardiol. 2015;36(1):151–7.

68. Kastner SB, Kull S, Kutter AP, Boller J, Bettschart-Wolfensberger R, Huhtinen MK. Cardiopulmonary effects of dexmedetomidine in sevoflurane-anesthetized sheep with and without nitric oxide inhalation. Am J Vet Res. 2005;66(9):1496–502.

69. Lazol JP, Lichtenstein SE, Jooste EH, Shiderly D, Kudchadker NA, Tatum GH, et al. Effect of dexmedetomidine on pulmonary artery pressure after congenital cardiac surgery: a pilot study. Pediatr Crit Care Med. 2010;11(5):589–92.

70. Friesen RH, Nichols CS, Twite MD, Cardwell KA, Pan Z, Pietra B, et al. The hemodynamic response to dexmedetomidine loading dose in children with and without pulmonary hypertension. Anesth Analg. 2013;117(4):953–9.

71. Nathan AT, Nicolson SC, McGowan FX. A word of caution: dexmedetomidine and pulmonary hypertension. Anesth Analg. 2014;119(1):216–7.

72. Venn RM, Bryant A, Hall GM, Grounds RM. Effects of dexmedetomidine on adrenocortical function, and the cardiovascular, endocrine and inflammatory responses in post-operative patients needing sedation in the intensive care unit. Br J Anaesth. 2001;86(5):650–6.

73. Maze M, Virtanen R, Daunt D, Banks SJ, Stover EP, Feldman D. Effects of dexmedetomidine, a novel imidazole sedative-anesthetic agent, on adrenal steroidogenesis: in vivo and in vitro studies. Anesth Analg. 1991;73(2):204–8.

74. Enomoto Y, Kudo T, Saito T, Hori T, Kaneko M, Matsui A, et al. Prolonged use of dexmedetomidine in an infant with respiratory failure following living donor liver transplantation. Paediatr Anaesth. 2006;16(12):1285–8.

75. De Wolf AM, Fragen RJ, Avram MJ, Fitzgerald PC, Rahimi-Danesh F. The pharmacokinetics of dexmedetomidine in volunteers with severe renal impairment. Anesth Analg. 2001;93(5):1205–9.

76. Villela NR, do Nascimento Junior P, de Carvalho LR, Teixeira A. Effects of dexmedetomidine on renal system and on vasopressin plasma levels. Experimental study in dogs. Rev Bras Anestesiol. 2005;55(4):429–40.

77. Frumento RJ, Logginidou HG, Wahlander S, Wagener G, Playford HR, Sladen RN. Dexmedetomidine infusion is associated with enhanced renal function after thoracic surgery. J Clin Anesth. 2006;18(6):422–6.

78. Billings FT, Chen SW, Kim M, Park SW, Song JH, Wang S, et al. alpha2-Adrenergic agonists protect against radiocontrast-induced nephropathy in mice. Am J Physiol Renal Physiol. 2008;295(3):F741–8.

79. Greening A, Mathews L, Blair J. Apparent dexmedetomidine-induced polyuric syndrome in an achondroplastic patient undergoing posterior spinal fusion. Anesth Analg. 2011;113(6):1381–3.

80. Leino K, Hynynen M, Jalonen J, Salmenpera M, Scheinin H, Aantaa R, et al. Renal effects of dexmedetomidine during coronary artery bypass surgery: a randomized placebo-controlled study. BMC Anesthesiol. 2011;11:9.

81. Ji F, Li Z, Young JN, Yeranossian A, Liu H. Post-bypass dexmedetomidine use and postoperative acute kidney injury in patients undergoing cardiac surgery with cardiopulmonary bypass. PLoS One. 2013;8(10), e77446.

82. Bayram A, Ulgey A, Baykan A, Narin N, Narin F, Esmaoglu A, et al. The effects of dexmedetomidine on early stage renal functions in pediatric patients undergoing cardiac angiography using non-ionic contrast media: a double-blind, randomized clinical trial. Paediatr Anaesth. 2014;24(4):426–32.

83. Wilder RT, Flick RP, Sprung J, Katusic SK, Barbaresi WJ, Mickelson C, et al. Early exposure to anesthesia and learning disabilities in a population-based birth cohort. Anesthesiology. 2009;110(4):796–804.

84. Brambrink AM, Evers AS, Avidan MS, Farber NB, Smith DJ, Zhang X, et al. Isoflurane-induced neuroapoptosis in the neonatal rhesus macaque brain. Anesthesiology. 2010;112(4):834–41.

85. Slikker Jr W, Zou X, Hotchkiss CE, Divine RL, Sadovova N, Twaddle NC, et al. Ketamine-induced neuronal cell death in the perinatal rhesus monkey. Toxicol Sci. 2007;98(1):145–58.

86. Satomoto M, Satoh Y, Terui K, Miyao H, Takishima K, Ito M, et al. Neonatal exposure to sevoflurane induces abnormal social behaviors and deficits in fear conditioning in mice. Anesthesiology. 2009;110(3):628–37.

87. Cattano D, Williamson P, Fukui K, Avidan M, Evers AS, Olney JW, et al. Potential of xenon to induce or to protect against neuroapoptosis in the developing mouse brain. Can J Anaesth. 2008;55(7):429–36.

88. Dahmani S, Stany I, Brasher C, Lejeune C, Bruneau B, Wood C, et al. Pharmacological prevention of sevoflurane- and desflurane-related emergence agitation in children: a meta-analysis of published studies. Br J Anaesth. 2010;104(2):216–23.

89. Engelhard K, Werner C, Eberspacher E, Bachl M, Blobner M, Hildt E, et al. The effect of the alpha 2-agonist dexmedetomidine and the N-methyl-D-aspartate antagonist S(+)-ketamine on the expression of apoptosis-regulating proteins after incomplete cerebral ischemia and reperfusion in rats. Anesth Analg. 2003;96(2):524–31.

90. Kuhmonen J, Pokorny J, Miettinen R, Haapalinna A, Jolkkonen J, Riekkinen Sr P, et al. Neuroprotective effects of dexmedetomidine in the gerbil hippocampus after transient global ischemia. Anesthesiology. 1997;87(2):371–7.

91. Jolkkonen J, Puurunen K, Koistinaho J, Kauppinen R, Haapalinna A, Nieminen L, et al. Neuroprotection by the alpha2-adrenoceptor agonist, dexmedetomidine, in rat focal cerebral ischemia. Eur J Pharmacol. 1999;372(1):31–6.

92. Degos V, Charpentier TL, Chhor V, Brissaud O, Lebon S, Schwendimann L, et al. Neuroprotective effects of dexmedetomidine against glutamate agonist-induced neuronal cell death are related to increased astrocyte brain-derived neurotrophic factor expression. Anesthesiology. 2013;118(5):1123–32.

93. Laudenbach V, Mantz J, Lagercrantz H, Desmonts JM, Evrard P, Gressens P. Effects of alpha(2)-adrenoceptor agonists on perinatal excitotoxic brain injury: comparison of clonidine and dexmedetomidine. Anesthesiology. 2002;96(1):134–41.

94. Ma D, Hossain M, Rajakumaraswamy N, Arshad M, Sanders RD, Franks NP, et al. Dexmedetomidine produces its neuroprotective effect via the alpha 2A-adrenoceptor subtype. Eur J Pharmacol. 2004;502(1–2):87–97.

95. Hoffman WE, Kochs E, Werner C, Thomas C, Albrecht RF. Dexmedetomidine improves neurologic outcome from incomplete ischemia in the rat. Reversal by the alpha 2-adrenergic antagonist atipamezole. Anesthesiology. 1991;75(2):328–32.

96. Altman JD, Trendelenburg AU, MacMillan L, Bernstein D, Limbird L, Starke K, et al. Abnormal regulation of the

sympathetic nervous system in alpha2A-adrenergic receptor knockout mice. Mol Pharmacol. 1999;56(1):154–61.

97. Huang R, Chen Y, Yu AC, Hertz L. Dexmedetomidine-induced stimulation of glutamine oxidation in astrocytes: a possible mechanism for its neuroprotective activity. J Cereb Blood Flow Metab. 2000;20(6):895–8.

98. van Oostrom H, Stienen PJ, Doornenbal A, Hellebrekers LJ. The alpha(2)-adrenoceptor agonist dexmedetomidine suppresses memory formation only at doses attenuating the perception of sensory input. Eur J Pharmacol. 2010;629(1–3):58–62.

99. Ebert TJ, Hall JE, Barney JA, Uhrich TD, Colinco MD. The effects of increasing plasma concentrations of dexmedetomidine in humans. Anesthesiology. 2000;93(2):382–94.

100. Veselis RA, Pryor KO, Reinsel RA, Li Y, Mehta M, Johnson Jr R. Propofol and midazolam inhibit conscious memory processes very soon after encoding: an event-related potential study of familiarity and recollection in volunteers. Anesthesiology. 2009;110(2):295–312.

101. Prielipp RC, Wall MH, Tobin JR, Groban L, Cannon MA, Fahey FH, et al. Dexmedetomidine-induced sedation in volunteers decreases regional and global cerebral blood flow. Anesth Analg. 2002;95(4):1052–9.

102. Zornow MH, Maze M, Dyck JB, Shafer SL. Dexmedetomidine decreases cerebral blood flow velocity in humans. J Cereb Blood Flow Metab. 1993;13(2):350–3.

103. Drummond JC, Dao AV, Roth DM, Cheng CR, Atwater BI, Minokadeh A, et al. Effect of dexmedetomidine on cerebral blood flow velocity, cerebral metabolic rate, and carbon dioxide response in normal humans. Anesthesiology. 2008;108(2):225–32.

104. Cheung CW, Ng KF, Liu J, Yuen MY, Ho MH, Irwin MG. Analgesic and sedative effects of intranasal dexmedetomidine in third molar surgery under local anaesthesia. Br J Anaesth. 2011;107(3):430–7.

105. Yuen VM, Hui TW, Irwin MG, Yuen MK. A comparison of intranasal dexmedetomidine and oral midazolam for premedication in pediatric anesthesia: a double-blinded randomized controlled trial. Anesth Analg. 2008;106(6):1715–21.

106. Ghali AM, Mahfouz AK, Al-Bahrani M. Preanesthetic medication in children: a comparison of intranasal dexmedetomidine versus oral midazolam. Saudi J Anaesth. 2011;5(4):387–91.

107. Yuen VM, Hui TW, Irwin MG, Yao TJ, Wong GL, Yuen MK. Optimal timing for the administration of intranasal dexmedetomidine for premedication in children. Anaesthesia. 2010;65(9):922–9.

108. Talon MD, Woodson LC, Sherwood ER, Aarsland A, McRae L, Benham T. Intranasal dexmedetomidine premedication is comparable with midazolam in burn children undergoing reconstructive surgery. J Burn Care Res. 2009;30(4):599–605.

109. Schmidt AP, Valinetti EA, Bandeira D, Bertacchi MF, Simoes CM, Auler Jr JO. Effects of preanesthetic administration of midazolam, clonidine, or dexmedetomidine on postoperative pain and anxiety in children. Paediatr Anaesth. 2007;17(7):667–74.

110. Pasin L, Febres D, Testa V, Frati E, Borghi G, Landoni G, et al. Dexmedetomidine vs midazolam as preanesthetic medication in children: a meta-analysis of randomized controlled trials. Paediatr Anaesth. 2016;25:468–76.

111. Sun Y, Lu Y, Huang Y, Jiang H. Is dexmedetomidine superior to midazolam as a premedication in children? A meta-analysis of randomized controlled trials. Paediatr Anaesth. 2014;24(8):863–74.

112. Hauber JA, Davis PJ, Bendel LP, Martyn SV, McCarthy DL, Evans MC, et al. Dexmedetomidine as a rapid bolus for treatment and prophylactic prevention of emergence agitation in anesthetized children. Anesth Analg. 2015;121(5):1308–15.

113. Guler G, Akin A, Tosun Z, Eskitascoglu E, Mizrak A, Boyaci A. Single-dose dexmedetomidine attenuates airway and circulatory reflexes during extubation. Acta Anaesthesiol Scand. 2005;49(8):1088–91.

114. Huupponen E, Maksimow A, Lapinlampi P, Sarkela M, Saastamoinen A, Snapir A, et al. Electroencephalogram spindle activity during dexmedetomidine sedation and physiological sleep. Acta Anaesthesiol Scand. 2008;52(2):289–94.

115. Mason KP, O'Mahony E, Zurakowski D, Libenson MH. Effects of dexmedetomidine sedation on the EEG in children. Paediatr Anaesth. 2009;19(12):1175–83.

116. Shukry M, Kennedy K. Dexmedetomidine as a total intravenous anesthetic in infants. Paediatr Anaesth. 2007;17(6):581–3.

117. Seybold JL, Ramamurthi RJ, Hammer GB. The use of dexmedetomidine during laryngoscopy, bronchoscopy, and tracheal extubation following tracheal reconstruction. Paediatr Anaesth. 2007;17(12):1212–4.

118. Chen KZ, Ye M, Hu CB, Shen X. Dexmedetomidine vs remifentanil intravenous anaesthesia and spontaneous ventilation for airway foreign body removal in children. Br J Anaesth. 2014;112(5):892–7.

119. Abdelmalak B, Gutenberg L, Lorenz RR, Smith M, Farag E, Doyle DJ. Dexmedetomidine supplemented with local anesthesia for awake laryngoplasty. J Clin Anesth. 2009;21(6):442–3.

120. Penttila J, Helminen A, Anttila M, Hinkka S, Scheinin H. Cardiovascular and parasympathetic effects of dexmedetomidine in healthy subjects. Can J Physiol Pharmacol. 2004;82(5):359–62.

121. Tsai CJ, Chu KS, Chen TI, Lu DV, Wang HM, Lu IC. A comparison of the effectiveness of dexmedetomidine versus propofol target-controlled infusion for sedation during fibreoptic nasotracheal intubation. Anaesthesia. 2010;65(3):254–9.

122. Stricker P, Fiadjoe JE, McGinnis S. Intubation of an infant with Pierre Robin sequence under dexmedetomidine sedation using the Shikani Optical Stylet. Acta Anaesthesiol Scand. 2008;52(6):866–7.

123. Iravani M, Wald SH. Dexmedetomidine and ketamine for fiberoptic intubation in a child with severe mandibular hypoplasia. J Clin Anesth. 2008;20(6):455–7.

124. Mahmoud M, Tyler T, Sadhasivam S. Dexmedetomidine and ketamine for large anterior mediastinal mass biopsy. Paediatr Anaesth. 2008;18(10):1011–3.

125. Song J, Ji Q, Sun Q, Gao T, Liu K, Li L. The opioid-sparing effect of intraoperative dexmedetomidine infusion after craniotomy. J Neurosurg Anesthesiol. 2016;28:14–20.

126. Tobias JD. Dexmedetomidine: applications in pediatric critical care and pediatric anesthesiology. Pediatr Crit Care Med. 2007;8(2):115–31.

127. Mahmoud M, Sadhasivam S, Salisbury S, Nick TG, Schnell B, Sestokas AK, et al. Susceptibility of transcranial electric motor-evoked potentials to varying targeted blood levels of dexmedetomidine during spine surgery. Anesthesiology. 2010;112(6):1364–73.

128. Tobias JD, Berkenbosch JW. Initial experience with dexmedetomidine in paediatric-aged patients. Paediatr Anaesth. 2002;12(2):171–5.

129. Frost EA, Booij LH. Anesthesia in the patient for awake craniotomy. Curr Opin Anaesthesiol. 2007;20(4):331–5.

130. Rozet I. Anesthesia for functional neurosurgery: the role of dexmedetomidine. Curr Opin Anaesthesiol. 2008;21(5):537–43.

131. Ard J, Doyle W, Bekker A. Awake craniotomy with dexmedetomidine in pediatric patients. J Neurosurg Anesthesiol. 2003;15(3):263–6.

132. Souter MJ, Rozet I, Ojemann JG, Souter KJ, Holmes MD, Lee L, et al. Dexmedetomidine sedation during awake craniotomy for

seizure resection: effects on electrocorticography. J Neurosurg Anesthesiol. 2007;19(1):38–44.

133. Chaitanya G, Arivazhagan A, Sinha S, Reddy KR, Thennarasu K, Bharath RD, et al. Dexmedetomidine anesthesia enhances spike generation during intra-operative electrocorticography: a promising adjunct for epilepsy surgery. Epilepsy Res. 2015;109:65–71.

134. Ellis JE, Drijvers G, Pedlow S, Laff SP, Sorrentino MJ, Foss JF, et al. Premedication with oral and transdermal clonidine provides safe and efficacious postoperative sympatholysis. Anesth Analg. 1994;79(6):1133–40.

135. Muzi M, Goff DR, Kampine JP, Roerig DL, Ebert TJ. Clonidine reduces sympathetic activity but maintains baroreflex responses in normotensive humans. Anesthesiology. 1992;77(5):864–71.

136. Curtis JA, Hollinger MK, Jain HB. Propofol-based versus dexmedetomidine-based sedation in cardiac surgery patients. J Cardiothorac Vasc Anesth. 2013;27(6):1289–94.

137. Okada H, Kurita T, Mochizuki T, Morita K, Sato S. The cardioprotective effect of dexmedetomidine on global ischaemia in isolated rat hearts. Resuscitation. 2007;74(3):538–45.

138. Riha H, Kotulak T, Brezina A, Hess L, Kramar P, Szarszoi O, et al. Comparison of the effects of ketamine-dexmedetomidine and sevoflurane-sufentanil anesthesia on cardiac biomarkers after cardiac surgery: an observational study. Physiol Res. 2012;61 (1):63–72.

139. Yoshitomi O, Cho S, Hara T, Shibata I, Maekawa T, Ureshino H, et al. Direct protective effects of dexmedetomidine against myocardial ischemia-reperfusion injury in anesthetized pigs. Shock. 2012;38(1):92–7.

140. Tosun Z, Baktir M, Kahraman HC, Baskol G, Guler G, Boyaci A. Does dexmedetomidine provide cardioprotection in coronary artery bypass grafting with cardiopulmonary bypass? A pilot study. J Cardiothorac Vasc Anesth. 2013;27(4):710–5.

141. Talke P, Li J, Jain U, Leung J, Drasner K, Hollenberg M, et al. Effects of perioperative dexmedetomidine infusion in patients undergoing vascular surgery. The Study of Perioperative Ischemia Research Group. Anesthesiology. 1995;82(3):620–33.

142. Roekaerts PM, Prinzen FW, De Lange S. Beneficial effects of dexmedetomidine on ischaemic myocardium of anaesthetized dogs. Br J Anaesth. 1996;77(3):427–9.

143. Willigers HM, Prinzen FW, Roekaerts PM, de Lange S, Durieux ME. Dexmedetomidine decreases perioperative myocardial lactate release in dogs. Anesth Analg. 2003;96(3):657–64.

144. Menda F, Koner O, Sayin M, Ture H, Imer P, Aykac B. Dexmedetomidine as an adjunct to anesthetic induction to attenuate hemodynamic response to endotracheal intubation in patients undergoing fast-track CABG. Ann Card Anaesth. 2010;13(1):16–21.

145. Kunisawa T, Nagata O, Nagashima M, Mitamura S, Ueno M, Suzuki A, et al. Dexmedetomidine suppresses the decrease in blood pressure during anesthetic induction and blunts the cardiovascular response to tracheal intubation. J Clin Anesth. 2009;21 (3):194–9.

146. Ji F, Li Z, Nguyen H, Young N, Shi P, Fleming N, et al. Perioperative dexmedetomidine improves outcomes of cardiac surgery. Circulation. 2013;127(15):1576–84.

147. Mukhtar AM, Obayah EM, Hassona AM. The use of dexmedetomidine in pediatric cardiac surgery. Anesth Analg. 2006;103(1):52–6.

148. Chrysostomou C, Beerman L, Shiderly D, Berry D, Morell VO, Munoz R. Dexmedetomidine: a novel drug for the treatment of atrial and junctional tachyarrhythmias during the perioperative period for congenital cardiac surgery: a preliminary study. Anesth Analg. 2008;107(5):1514–22.

149. Chrysostomou C, Sanchez-de-Toledo J, Wearden P, Jooste EH, Lichtenstein SE, Callahan PM, et al. Perioperative use of

dexmedetomidine is associated with decreased incidence of ventricular and supraventricular tachyarrhythmias after congenital cardiac operations. Ann Thorac Surg. 2011;92(3):964–72.

150. Ramsay MA, Saha D, Hebeler RF. Tracheal resection in the morbidly obese patient: the role of dexmedetomidine. J Clin Anesth. 2006;18(6):452–4.

151. Tufanogullari B, White PF, Peixoto MP, Kianpour D, Lacour T, Griffin J, et al. Dexmedetomidine infusion during laparoscopic bariatric surgery: the effect on recovery outcome variables. Anesth Analg. 2008;106(6):1741–8.

152. Sidorowicz M, Owczuk R, Kwiecinska B, Wujtewicz MA, Wojciechowski J, Wujtewicz M. Dexmedetomidine sedation for carotid endarterectomy. Anestezjol Intens Ter. 2009;41(2):78–83.

153. McCutcheon CA, Orme RM, Scott DA, Davies MJ, McGlade DP. A comparison of dexmedetomidine versus conventional therapy for sedation and hemodynamic control during carotid endarterectomy performed under regional anesthesia. Anesth Analg. 2006;102(3):668–75.

154. Rich JM. Dexmedetomidine as a sole sedating agent with local anesthesia in a high-risk patient for axillofemoral bypass graft: a case report. AANA J. 2005;73(5):357–60.

155. Hitt JM, Corcoran T, Michienzi K, Creighton P, Heard C. An evaluation of intranasal sufentanil and dexmedetomidine for pediatric dental sedation. Pharmaceutics. 2014;6(1):175–84.

156. Sheta SA, Al-Sarheed MA, Abdelhalim AA. Intranasal dexmedetomidine vs midazolam for premedication in children undergoing complete dental rehabilitation: a double-blinded randomized controlled trial. Paediatr Anaesth. 2014;24(2):181–9.

157. Surendar MN, Pandey RK, Saksena AK, Kumar R, Chandra G. A comparative evaluation of intranasal dexmedetomidine, midazolam and ketamine for their sedative and analgesic properties: a triple blind randomized study. J Clin Pediatr Dent. 2014;38(3):255–61.

158. Farah GJ, de Moraes M, Filho LI, Pavan AJ, Camarini ET, Previdelli IT, et al. Induced hypotension in orthognathic surgery: a comparative study of 2 pharmacological protocols. J Oral Maxillofac Surg. 2008;66(11):2261–9.

159. Ogawa S, Seino H, Ito H, Yamazaki S, Ganzberg S, Kawaai H. Intravenous sedation with low-dose dexmedetomidine: its potential for use in dentistry. Anesth Prog. 2008;55(3):82–8.

160. Hasan MS, Chan L. Dexmedetomidine and ketamine sedation for dental extraction in children with cyanotic heart disease. J Oral Maxillofac Surg. 2014;72(10):1920.e1–4.

161. Kim HS, Kim JW, Jang KT, Lee SH, Kim CC, Shin TJ. Initial experience with dexmedetomidine for dental sedation in children. J Clin Pediatr Dent. 2013;38(1):79–81.

162. Xu L, Bao H, Si Y, Wang X. Effects of dexmedetomidine on early and late cytokines during polymicrobial sepsis in mice. Inflamm Res. 2013;62(5):507–14.

163. Li S, Yang Y, Yu C, Yao Y, Wu Y, Qian L, et al. Dexmedetomidine analgesia effects in patients undergoing dental implant surgery and its impact on postoperative inflammatory and oxidative stress. Oxid Med Cell Longev. 2015;2015:186736.

164. Fan TW, Ti LK, Islam I. Comparison of dexmedetomidine and midazolam for conscious sedation in dental surgery monitored by bispectral index. Br J Oral Maxillofac Surg. 2013;51(5):428–33.

165. Taniyama K, Oda H, Okawa K, Himeno K, Shikanai K, Shibutani T. Psychosedation with dexmedetomidine hydrochloride during minor oral surgery. Anesth Prog. 2009;56(3):75–80.

166. Singh C, Pandey RK, Saksena AK, Chandra G. A comparative evaluation of analgo-sedative effects of oral dexmedetomidine and ketamine: a triple-blind, randomized study. Paediatr Anaesth. 2014;24:1252–9.

167. Eisenach JC, De Kock M, Klimscha W. alpha(2)-adrenergic agonists for regional anesthesia. A clinical review of clonidine (1984–1995). Anesthesiology. 1996;85(3):655–74.

168. Wu HH, Wang HT, Jin JJ, Cui GB, Zhou KC, Chen Y, et al. Does dexmedetomidine as a neuraxial adjuvant facilitate better anesthesia and analgesia? A systematic review and meta-analysis. PLoS One. 2014;9(3), e93114.

169. Saadawy I, Boker A, Elshahawy MA, Almazrooa A, Melibary S, Abdellatif AA, et al. Effect of dexmedetomidine on the characteristics of bupivacaine in a caudal block in pediatrics. Acta Anaesthesiol Scand. 2009;53(2):251–6.

170. El-Hennawy AM, Abd-Elwahab AM, Abd-Elmaksoud AM, El-Ozairy HS, Boulis SR. Addition of clonidine or dexmedetomidine to bupivacaine prolongs caudal analgesia in children. Br J Anaesth. 2009;103(2):268–74.

171. Tong Y, Ren H, Ding X, Jin S, Chen Z, Li Q. Analgesic effect and adverse events of dexmedetomidine as additive for pediatric caudal anesthesia: a meta-analysis. Paediatr Anaesth. 2014;24 (12):1224–30.

172. Huang Y, Lu Y, Zhang L, Yan J, Jiang J, Jiang H. Perineural dexmedetomidine attenuates inflammation in rat sciatic nerve via the NF-kappaB pathway. Int J Mol Sci. 2014;15(3):4049–59.

173. Konakci S, Adanir T, Yilmaz G, Rezanko T. The efficacy and neurotoxicity of dexmedetomidine administered via the epidural route. Eur J Anaesthesiol. 2008;25(5):403–9.

174. Lahdesmaki J, Sallinen J, MacDonald E, Sirvio J, Scheinin M. Alpha2-adrenergic drug effects on brain monoamines, locomotion, and body temperature are largely abolished in mice lacking the alpha2A-adrenoceptor subtype. Neuropharmacology. 2003;44 (7):882–92.

175. Quan N, Xin L, Ungar AL, Blatteis CM. Preoptic norepinephrine-induced hypothermia is mediated by alpha 2-adrenoceptors. Am J Physiol. 1992;262(3 Pt 2):R407–11.

176. Finkel JC, Quezado ZM. Hypothermia-induced bradycardia in a neonate receiving dexmedetomidine. J Clin Anesth. 2007;19 (4):290–2.

177. Pestieau SR, Quezado ZM, Johnson YJ, Anderson JL, Cheng YI, McCarter RJ, et al. The effect of dexmedetomidine during myringotomy and pressure-equalizing tube placement in children. Paediatr Anaesth. 2011;21(11):1128–35.

178. Hammer GB, Sam WJ, Chen MI, Golianu B, Drover DR. Determination of the pharmacodynamic interaction of propofol and dexmedetomidine during esophagogastroduodenoscopy in children. Paediatr Anaesth. 2009;19(2):138–44.

179. Makary L, Vornik V, Finn R, Lenkovsky F, McClelland AL, Thurmon J, et al. Prolonged recovery associated with dexmedetomidine when used as a sole sedative agent in office-based oral and maxillofacial surgery procedures. J Oral Maxillofac Surg. 2010;68(2):386–91.

180. Jalowiecki P, Rudner R, Gonciarz M, Kawecki P, Petelenz M, Dziurdzik P. Sole use of dexmedetomidine has limited utility for conscious sedation during outpatient colonoscopy. Anesthesiology. 2005;103(2):269–73.

181. Pestieau SR, Quezado ZM, Johnson YJ, Anderson JL, Cheng YI, McCarter RJ, et al. High-dose dexmedetomidine increases the opioid-free interval and decreases opioid requirement after tonsillectomy in children. Can J Anaesth. 2011;58(6):540–50.

182. Olutoye OA, Glover CD, Diefenderfer JW, McGilberry M, Wyatt MM, Larrier DR, et al. The effect of intraoperative dexmedetomidine on postoperative analgesia and sedation in pediatric patients undergoing tonsillectomy and adenoidectomy. Anesth Analg. 2010;111(2):490–5.

183. Mason KP. Sedation trends in the 21st century: the transition to dexmedetomidine for radiological imaging studies. Paediatr Anaesth. 2010;20(3):265–72.

184. Koroglu A, Teksan H, Sagir O, Yucel A, Toprak HI, Ersoy OM. A comparison of the sedative, hemodynamic, and respiratory effects of dexmedetomidine and propofol in children undergoing magnetic resonance imaging. Anesth Analg. 2006;103(1):63–7, table of contents.

185. Mason KP, Zgleszewski SE, Dearden JL, Dumont RS, Pirich MA, Stark CD, et al. Dexmedetomidine for pediatric sedation for computed tomography imaging studies. Anesth Analg. 2006;103 (1):57–62.

186. Heard CM, Joshi P, Johnson K. Dexmedetomidine for pediatric MRI sedation: a review of a series of cases. Paediatr Anaesth. 2007;17(9):888–92.

187. Alhashemi JA. Dexmedetomidine vs midazolam for monitored anaesthesia care during cataract surgery. Br J Anaesth. 2006;96 (6):722–6.

188. Munro HM, Tirotta CF, Felix DE, Lagueruela RG, Madril DR, Zahn EM, et al. Initial experience with dexmedetomidine for diagnostic and interventional cardiac catheterization in children. Paediatr Anaesth. 2007;17(2):109–12.

189. Char D, Drover DR, Motonaga KS, Gupta S, Miyake CY, Dubin AM, et al. The effects of ketamine on dexmedetomidine-induced electrophysiologic changes in children. Paediatr Anaesth. 2013;23 (10):898–905.

190. Tobias JD. Dexmedetomidine and ketamine: an effective alternative for procedural sedation? Pediatr Crit Care Med. 2012;13 (4):423–7.

191. Koruk S, Mizrak A, Gul R, Kilic E, Yendi F, Oner U. -Dexmedetomidine-ketamine and midazolam-ketamine combinations for sedation in pediatric patients undergoing extracorporeal shock wave lithotripsy: a randomized prospective study. J Anesth. 2010;24(6):858–63.

192. McVey JD, Tobias JD. Dexmedetomidine and ketamine for sedation during spinal anesthesia in children. J Clin Anesth. 2010;22 (7):538–45.

193. Zor F, Ozturk S, Bilgin F, Isik S, Cosar A. Pain relief during dressing changes of major adult burns: ideal analgesic combination with ketamine. Burns. 2010;36(4):501–5.

194. Shank ES, Sheridan RL, Ryan CM, Keaney TJ, Martyn JA. Hemodynamic responses to dexmedetomidine in critically injured intubated pediatric burned patients: a preliminary study. J Burn Care Res. 2013;34(3):311–7.

195. Barton KP, Munoz R, Morell VO, Chrysostomou C. Dexmedetomidine as the primary sedative during invasive procedures in infants and toddlers with congenital heart disease. Pediatr Crit Care Med. 2008;9(6):612–5.

196. Engelhard K, Werner C, Kaspar S, Mollenberg O, Blobner M, Bachl M, et al. Effect of the alpha2-agonist dexmedetomidine on cerebral neurotransmitter concentrations during cerebral ischemia in rats. Anesthesiology. 2002;96(2):450–7.

197. Eckenhoff JE, Kneale DH, Dripps RD. The incidence and etiology of postanesthetic excitment. A clinical survey. Anesthesiology. 1961;22:667–73.

198. Voepel-Lewis T, Malviya S, Tait AR. A prospective cohort study of emergence agitation in the pediatric postanesthesia care unit. Anesth Analg. 2003;96(6):1625–30.

199. Sikich N, Lerman J. Development and psychometric evaluation of the pediatric anesthesia emergence delirium scale. Anesthesiology. 2004;100(5):1138–45.

200. Kain ZN, Mayes LC, Caldwell-Andrews AA, Karas DE, McClain BC. Preoperative anxiety, postoperative pain, and behavioral recovery in young children undergoing surgery. Pediatrics. 2006;118(2):651–8.

201. Kain ZN, Caldwell-Andrews AA, Maranets I, McClain B, Gaal D, Mayes LC, et al. Preoperative anxiety and emergence delirium and postoperative maladaptive behaviors. Anesth Analg. 2004;99 (6):1648–54.

202. Vlajkovic GP, Sindjelic RP. Emergence delirium in children: many questions, few answers. Anesth Analg. 2007;104(1):84–91.

203. Ibacache ME, Munoz HR, Brandes V, Morales AL. Single-dose dexmedetomidine reduces agitation after sevoflurane anesthesia in children. Anesth Analg. 2004;98(1):60–3.

204. Isik B, Arslan M, Tunga AD, Kurtipek O. Dexmedetomidine decreases emergence agitation in pediatric patients after sevoflurane anesthesia without surgery. Paediatr Anaesth. 2006;16(7):748–53.

205. Guler G, Akin A, Tosun Z, Ors S, Esmaoglu A, Boyaci A. Single-dose dexmedetomidine reduces agitation and provides smooth extubation after pediatric adenotonsillectomy. Paediatr Anaesth. 2005;15(9):762–6.

206. Shukry M, Clyde MC, Kalarickal PL, Ramadhyani U. Does dexmedetomidine prevent emergence delirium in children after sevoflurane-based general anesthesia? Paediatr Anaesth. 2005;15 (12):1098–104.

207. Patel A, Davidson M, Tran MC, Quraishi H, Schoenberg C, Sant M, et al. Dexmedetomidine infusion for analgesia and prevention of emergence agitation in children with obstructive sleep apnea syndrome undergoing tonsillectomy and adenoidectomy. Anesth Analg. 2010;111(4):1004–10.

208. Doufas AG, Lin CM, Suleman MI, Liem EB, Lenhardt R, Morioka N, et al. Dexmedetomidine and meperidine additively reduce the shivering threshold in humans. Stroke. 2003;34 (5):1218–23.

209. Talke P, Tayefeh F, Sessler DI, Jeffrey R, Noursalehi M, Richardson C. Dexmedetomidine does not alter the sweating threshold, but comparably and linearly decreases the vasoconstriction and shivering thresholds. Anesthesiology. 1997;87 (4):835–41.

210. Bicer C, Esmaoglu A, Akin A, Boyaci A. Dexmedetomidine and meperidine prevent postanaesthetic shivering. Eur J Anaesthesiol. 2006;23(2):149–53.

211. Elvan EG, Oc B, Uzun S, Karabulut E, Coskun F, Aypar U. Dexmedetomidine and postoperative shivering in patients undergoing elective abdominal hysterectomy. Eur J Anaesthesiol. 2008;25(5):357–64.

212. Blaine Easley R, Brady KM, Tobias JD. Dexmedetomidine for the treatment of postanesthesia shivering in children. Paediatr Anaesth. 2007;17(4):341–6.

213. Frolich MA, Zhang K, Ness TJ. Effect of sedation on pain perception. Anesthesiology. 2013;118(3):611–21.

214. Schnabel A, Meyer-Friessem CH, Reichl SU, Zahn PK, Pogatzki-Zahn EM. Is intraoperative dexmedetomidine a new option for postoperative pain treatment? A meta-analysis of randomized controlled trials. Pain. 2013;154(7):1140–9.

215. Schnabel A, Reichl SU, Poepping DM, Kranke P, Pogatzki-Zahn EM, Zahn PK. Efficacy and safety of intraoperative dexmedetomidine for acute postoperative pain in children: a meta-analysis of randomized controlled trials. Paediatr Anaesth. 2013;23(2):170–9.

216. Riker RR, Shehabi Y, Bokesch PM, Ceraso D, Wisemandle W, Koura F, et al. Dexmedetomidine vs midazolam for sedation of critically ill patients: a randomized trial. JAMA. 2009;301 (5):489–99.

217. Pandharipande PP, Pun BT, Herr DL, Maze M, Girard TD, Miller RR, et al. Effect of sedation with dexmedetomidine vs lorazepam on acute brain dysfunction in mechanically ventilated patients: the MENDS randomized controlled trial. JAMA. 2007;298 (22):2644–53.

218. Tan JA, Ho KM. Use of dexmedetomidine as a sedative and analgesic agent in critically ill adult patients: a meta-analysis. Intensive Care Med. 2010;36(6):926–39.

219. Jakob SM, Ruokonen E, Grounds RM, Sarapohja T, Garratt C, Pocock SJ, et al. Dexmedetomidine vs midazolam or propofol for sedation during prolonged mechanical ventilation: two randomized controlled trials. JAMA. 2012;307(11):1151–60.

220. Ruokonen E, Parviainen I, Jakob SM, Nunes S, Kaukonen M, Shepherd ST, et al. Dexmedetomidine versus propofol/midazolam for long-term sedation during mechanical ventilation. Intensive Care Med. 2009;35(2):282–90.

221. Xia ZQ, Chen SQ, Yao X, Xie CB, Wen SH, Liu KX. Clinical benefits of dexmedetomidine versus propofol in adult intensive care unit patients: a meta-analysis of randomized clinical trials. J Surg Res. 2013;185(2):833–43.

222. Turunen H, Jakob SM, Ruokonen E, Kaukonen KM, Sarapohja T, Apajasalo M, et al. Dexmedetomidine versus standard care sedation with propofol or midazolam in intensive care: an economic evaluation. Crit Care. 2015;19:67.

223. Guinter JR, Kristeller JL. Prolonged infusions of dexmedetomidine in critically ill patients. Am J Health Syst Pharm. 2010;67(15):1246–53.

224. Shehabi Y, Ruettimann U, Adamson H, Innes R, Ickeringill M. Dexmedetomidine infusion for more than 24 hours in critically ill patients: sedative and cardiovascular effects. Intensive Care Med. 2004;30(12):2188–96.

225. Gerlach AT, Murphy CV, Dasta JF. An updated focused review of dexmedetomidine in adults. Ann Pharmacother. 2009;43 (12):2064–74.

226. Dasta JF, Kane-Gill SL, Durtschi AJ. Comparing dexmedetomidine prescribing patterns and safety in the naturalistic setting versus published data. Ann Pharmacother. 2004;38 (7–8):1130–5.

227. Czaja AS, Zimmerman JJ. The use of dexmedetomidine in critically ill children. Pediatr Crit Care Med. 2009;10(3):381–6.

228. Bejian S, Valasek C, Nigro JJ, Cleveland DC, Willis BC. Prolonged use of dexmedetomidine in the paediatric cardiothoracic intensive care unit. Cardiol Young. 2009;19(1):98–104.

229. Hammer GB, Philip BM, Schroeder AR, Rosen FS, Koltai PJ. Prolonged infusion of dexmedetomidine for sedation following tracheal resection. Paediatr Anaesth. 2005;15(7):616–20.

Mark G. Roback

Introduction

Ketamine was originally developed as a potent but safe intravenous anesthetic drug which has subsequently been used for premedication, sedation, induction, and maintenance of general anesthesia [1]. It is currently widely administered to children for dissociative sedation for painful procedures performed outside the operating room [2, 3]. Due to its unique and diverse properties, a large number of additional indications for ketamine have developed since it was derived from phencyclidine in 1963. There are two optical isomers of ketamine: S(+) ketamine and R(−) ketamine [1, 4, 5]. The S-ketamine isomer is two to four times more potent than the more commonly available, racemic ketamine [1, 6]. Doses listed in this chapter are for racemic ketamine. If S-ketamine is used, doses must be decreased by at least 50 % [4]. The chemical structures of phencyclidine and (S)-ketamine, the more potent of the two ketamine enantiomers, may be found in Fig. 14.1.

Ketamine is increasingly administered as a pure analgesic [7, 8], for induction of rapid sequence intubation performed outside the operating room [9], for bronchodilation in patients with asthma [10], as a pharmacologic restraint for agitated and combative patients in the emergency department as well as in the field [11], and more recently, for treatment of selected mental health disorders [12]. This chapter will review the history, pharmacology, clinical effects, and applications of ketamine. With each clinical effect of ketamine described, we will progress to the logical clinical applications and cautions for ketamine use that have resulted. We will examine the evidence for and against

traditional and expanding indications for ketamine administration. Due to ketamine's significant potential as a drug of abuse, we will explore the nonmedical use of ketamine as well [4, 13].

History

Over 50 years ago, ketamine was initially administered to humans under the original investigation number, CI-581 [4]. It was developed as a short-acting intravenous anesthetic due to the shortcomings of phencyclidine and cyclohexamine which resulted in long-lasting psychotomimetic activity (i.e., emergence delirium or recovery agitation) during the postanesthetic period [1, 4, 5]. Initial human studies of ketamine noted its ability to induce a trance-like, cataleptic state which inspired these investigators to coin the term "dissociative anesthetic" [4, 14, 15]. When compared to phencyclidine, ketamine was found to provide similar anesthetic effect but with a shorter half-life and with less problematic emergence delirium [6]. In addition, ketamine was found to preserve protective airway reflexes with minimal clinical respiratory or circulatory depression [16, 17]. Ketamine was approved by the Food and Drug Administration as an anesthetic and introduced into clinical practice in 1970 [5, 14] and due to its effectiveness and large margin of safety, was administered to injured American soldiers requiring anesthesia during the Vietnam War [1, 4].

In addition to its dissociative effects, ketamine also produces potent analgesia, at sub-anesthetic concentrations, and short-term amnesia [6]. The combination of these three properties (i.e., dissociative sedation/anesthesia, analgesia, and amnesia) makes ketamine a unique drug in clinical practice and, when coupled with its favorable safety profile, explains why ketamine use and indications have expanded so dramatically [1]. Ketamine is currently the single most commonly administered drug to children to facilitate the performance of painful procedures in the emergency

M.G. Roback, M.D.(✉)
Department of Pediatrics & Emergency Medicine, University of Minnesota Medical School and University of Minnesota Masonic Children's Hospital, M653 East Building, Minneapolis, MN 55454, USA
e-mail: mgroback@umn.edu

© Springer International Publishing AG 2017
A.R. Absalom, K.P. Mason (eds.), *Total Intravenous Anesthesia and Target Controlled Infusions*,
DOI 10.1007/978-3-319-47609-4_14

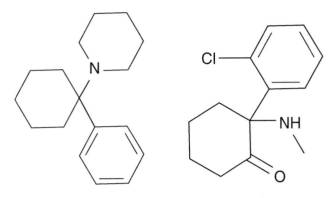

Fig. 14.1 Chemical structures of phencyclidine and (S)-ketamine

department [17, 18]. In addition to prominent clinical use, due to its unique dissociative and psychedelic properties, the potential for abuse of ketamine, like its parent drug phencyclidine, must also be considered [13, 19]. Ketamine was made a Schedule III controlled substance in the USA in 1999 [4, 6], and reports of ketamine abuse in the USA, Europe, and Southeast and East Asia are growing [6, 13].

Pharmacology

The dissociative state produced by ketamine is the result of a functional and electrophysiological dissociation between the thalamo-neocortical and limbic centers of the brain, preventing higher centers from perceiving visual, auditory, or painful stimuli [6, 16, 19]. Limbic system functions such as processing sensory information, regulating emotions, and facilitating the development of long- and short-term memory are affected by ketamine administration resulting in the dissociative state, analgesia, suppression of anxiety and fear, and amnesia [20]. The varied clinical effects of ketamine are believed to be mediated through its binding to multiple sites, primarily N-methyl-D-aspartate (NMDA) but also non-NMDA glutamate, nicotinic and muscarinic cholinergic, and opioid receptors in the central nervous system (CNS) [1, 5, 16, 20, 21]. Blockage of the excitatory neurotransmitter, glutamate, from binding NMDA receptors is the most likely etiology of ketamine dissociation [21]. The unique and diverse mechanisms of action of ketamine in the CNS result in a range of clinical effects and applications that we will discuss in this chapter.

Intravenous (IV) ketamine, 1.5–2 mg/kg, produces peak serum and CNS concentrations within 1 min of administration which reliably induces clinical dissociation [16, 17]. Due to the subsequent rapid, high CNS levels, recommendations for IV ketamine support administration over a 30–60 s time interval to prevent associated respiratory depression or apnea [17]. The duration of action of

traditionally administered IV dissociative-dose ketamine is about 10 min with full recovery observed between 1 and 2 h [22]. However, in a recent study of lower dose (0.7–0.8 mg/kg), rapid administration (less than 5 s) of IV ketamine, a shorter period of sedation was produced, and no respiratory depression was noted in this small sample of children who received ketamine for forearm fracture reduction [23]. Using this rapid administration, lower-dose method, the total time of sedation was reduced to about 25 min. While this method of ketamine administration is promising, especially in busy clinical settings where more rapid patient recovery from sedation will allow for quicker patient turn-around times, further study comparing rapid administration, lower-dose ketamine to traditional administration, dissociative-dose ketamine is required to fully elucidate the risks and benefits.

Intramuscular (IM) ketamine is dosed 4–5 mg/kg to induce dissociative sedation [17] and has an onset of action of 3–5 min [24]. The duration of action of IM ketamine is significantly longer than ketamine administered IV with time to full recovery exceeding 2 h [25]. Despite the increased length of sedation, one comparison of IM vs. IV ketamine found similar overall length of stay in the emergency department which suggests that the ease of IM administration, as compared to the time required for IV placement, proves to be a significant time saver [24]. IM ketamine has the distinct advantage of not requiring IV placement which results in more rapid administration of the drug and is important for patients in whom IV access is particularly problematic. A randomized, controlled trial of IV vs. IM ketamine in 225 children found those who received IM ketamine vomited significantly more frequently (26.3 % vs. 11.9 %) and had a longer length of sedation (129 vs. 80 min) than those who received IV ketamine. This study was terminated early because of nursing resistance to IM-administered ketamine based on increased vomiting and the longer recovery times observed in these patients, which resulted in a strong nursing preference for IV ketamine. Importantly, respiratory adverse events experienced by these patients were similar between the two routes of administration (4.0 % IM vs. 8.3 % IV), and IV access was not required to manage any adverse event [25]. In a recent review of the IV vs. IM ketamine literature, the authors conclude that IV ketamine "appears to have a better adverse events profile than IM ketamine…(and) has a shorter recovery." The authors recommend IV ketamine when intravenous access is readily available, but note that IM ketamine is acceptable for sedation and may be preferable when "it may be difficult to reliably establish IV access with minimal distress to the child." [26].

Although the bioavailability of intranasal (IN) ketamine has been reported to be poor, about 45 %, the onset of action is rapid and duration of action of 2–3 h makes IN ketamine administration popular among recreational users [6]. Studies describing the use of IN ketamine for pain and sedation have been published in a number of settings including prehospital, emergency department, postoperatively, and in dental practice [27]. IN ketamine has been successfully administered to adults and children for analgesia [28, 29]. Ketamine, 1 mg/kg IN, provided similar pain relief to children with moderate to severe pain from limb injuries as IN fentanyl, 1.5 mcg/kg, in a recent randomized controlled trial. Children in the IN ketamine group were more likely to experience drowsiness and dizziness and more frequently reported a bad taste in the mouth than those who received IN fentanyl [28]. While IN ketamine has been shown to be effective as a premedication or anxiolytic drug, [30, 31] IN ketamine for procedural sedation has not been found to be particularly effective [32]. In a randomized, controlled trial comparing three doses of IN ketamine (3 mg/kg vs. 6 mg/kg vs. 9 mg/kg) for sedation of children receiving laceration repair, only the 9 mg/kg group produced adequate sedation, and the study was suspended due to ineffectiveness of sedation, as per predetermined criteria. It is not clear whether such a high dose of IN ketamine will allow for reliable sedation given the high volume of drug required and degree of subsequent unabsorbed nasopharyngeal runoff which may be expected even with more concentrated ketamine formulations [32].

Orally ingested ketamine is poorly absorbed with bioavailability reported to be as low as 16 % [6]. The onset of action of oral ketamine is much slower than IV, IM, or IN routes with plasma concentrations detected about 30 min after administration. Peak plasma concentrations of oral ketamine are about 20 % of that obtained when a similar dose of ketamine is administered IM [6]. Oral ketamine, 5–10 mg/kg, has been used to augment laceration repair analgesia and sedation with positive results; however, this route is not commonly used for procedural sedation outside the operating room [33, 34]. Table 14.1 provides a summary of ketamine dosing by indication and route of administration.

Table 14.1 Ketamine dosing by indication and route of administration

Indication	Route	Dose
Dissociative sedation	IV	1.5–2 mg/kg
	IM	4–5 mg/kg
Brief sedation—rapid administration <5 s	IV	0.5–0.8 mg/kg
Analgesia	IV	0.2–0.75 mg/kg
	IM	1–3 mg/kg
	IN	0.5–1 mg/kg
Induction of rapid sequence intubation	IV	2 mg/kg
Moderate to severe asthma	IV	2 mg/kg
Pharmacologic restraint	IM	4–5 mg/kg

Clinical Effects and Applications

Protective Airway Reflexes and Laryngospasm

As mentioned previously, ketamine has become the most common agent used in the emergency department for children in need of painful procedures due to its desirable effects of sedation, analgesia, and amnesia but also because of its favorable safety profile [16–18]. Foremost, ketamine does not suppress normal upper airway protective reflexes such as coughing, sneezing, and swallowing, reducing the risk for pulmonary aspiration [16, 20]. For unfasted children who require emergent procedural sedation, ketamine may be the safest drug choice available due to the retention of airway protective reflexes [21]. Additionally, respiratory depression with ketamine is rare. In an individual patient data meta-analysis of 8282 children, apnea occurred in 63 (0.8 %) and laryngospasm in 22 (0.3 %), and the overall incidence of airway and respiratory adverse events defined as upper airway obstruction, oxygen desaturation less than or equal to 90 %, apnea, or laryngospasm was 3.9 % [2]. In this study, risk factors for ketamine-associated airway and respiratory adverse events were determined to be high intravenous doses (initial dose ≥2.5 mg/kg or total dose ≥5.0 mg/kg), administration to children younger than 2 years or aged 13 years or older, and the use of coadministered anticholinergics or benzodiazepines [2] (Table 14.2).

Ketamine is a sialagogue; it stimulates salivary and tracheobronchial mucous gland secretions and acts to exaggerate laryngeal reflexes [5, 17]. Anticholinergics such as atropine or glycopyrrolate have been coadministered with ketamine to reduce excessive salivation associated with ketamine which, it has been postulated, may precipitate laryngospasm [16, 21]. Recent study of the effects of anticholinergics on ketamine administered in the emergency department to children has shown that while hypersalivation decreases, anticholinergics have not been proven to provide a clinical benefit, that is, no difference in airway adverse events [35–37]. Coadministration of anticholinergics with ketamine is no longer routinely recommended and has been identified as a risk factor for ketamine-associated airway and respiratory adverse events, in one study, although the causative mechanism of this finding is not known [2, 17].

In one case-controlled study, the risk of laryngospasm in children undergoing general anesthesia was increased with active upper respiratory tract infection and in patients with an airway anomaly [38]. The incidence of ketamine-associated laryngospasm is unknown, although as mentioned previously, laryngospasm occurred in only 0.3 % of children in a meta-analysis of 8282 children [2]. A case-controlled analysis of this large ketamine data set found no evidence of association with laryngospasm based on age, dose,

Table 14.2 Risk factors for ketamine-associated adverse events

Adverse event	Risk factors	Comments
Airway and respiratory adverse events[a]	Independent predictors • Age less than 2 years • High IV dosing (initial dose $\geq$2.5 mg/kg or total dose $\geq$5 mg/kg) • Coadministered benzodiazepine • Coadministered anticholinergic	NOT independent predictors • Minor oropharyngeal procedures • Underlying physical illness (ASA class $\geq$III) • Route of administration IV vs. IM
Laryngospasm	• No association of age, dose, oropharyngeal procedure, underlying physical illness, route, or coadministered anticholinergics	• Laryngospasm appears to be idiosyncratic • Clinicians must be prepared for its rapid identification and management
Vomiting	• More common in children 5 years and older • Peak age is early adolescence • Increased when administered IM • Increased with high doses IV	• Incidence may be decreased with coadministered ondansetron
Unpleasant recovery reactions	• Not age related to a clinically important degree in children • Presence of significant presedation agitation may contribute	• Not decreased with coadministered midazolam in children • Decreased with coadministered midazolam in adults

[a]Airway and respiratory adverse events: upper airway obstruction (stridor, hypoventilation, or oxygen desaturation that resolved with repositioning of the airway), apnea (cessation of spontaneous respirations considered to be significant by observers and recorded as such), abnormal oxygen saturation (decrease in oxygen saturation to $\leq$90 % at any point), or laryngospasm (stridor or other evidence of airway obstruction that did not improve with airway alignment maneuvers) [2]

procedure performed (including minor intraoral procedures), the American Society of Anesthesiologists (ASA) risk classification status, route of administration (IV or IM), or the administration of anticholinergics [39]. The impact of an upper respiratory infection on ketamine-associated airway and respiratory adverse events was not studied. The authors conclude that laryngospasm occurrence is idiosyncratic and recommend that clinicians be prepared for laryngospasm anytime they administer ketamine.

Ketamine-associated laryngospasm may occur at any time from induction to emergence from sedation, and it may be brief or recurrent [39]. Cases of laryngospasm have been reported to have occurred with IV and IM ketamine. Laryngospasm in these cases was successfully managed with positive pressure ventilation delivered with simple bag-mask equipment and did not recur [39–42]. However, one report of two cases of recurrent, severe laryngospasm which were resistant to management with bag-mask ventilation has been reported [43]. In this case report, one patient required muscle relaxation with succinylcholine and endotracheal intubation. Although generally very safe, with low rates of airway and respiratory complications, clinicians administering ketamine must be prepared to provide advanced airway management on rare occasions.

Cardiovascular Effects

Unlike most sedative, anesthetic, and analgesic agents, ketamine is effectively a cardiovascular stimulant, producing increases in heart rate, cardiac output, and blood pressure in healthy patients [19, 20, 44, 45]. Although ketamine has a direct myocardial depressive effect, it indirectly stimulates the circulatory system by increasing circulating catecholamine levels [46]. The sympathomimetic effects of ketamine are believed to be primarily due to direct stimulation of CNS structures [5]. Ketamine blocks the reuptake of the catecholaminergic hormones norepinephrine, epinephrine, dopamine, and serotonin resulting in a 10–30 % increase in blood pressure and heart rate [21]. However, in critically ill patients, with severely depleted catecholamine stores, ketamine does not provide sympathomimetic effects [1]. In patients with limited myocardial reserve and increased demand as seen in shock, sepsis, and significant hypovolemia, ketamine may decrease cardiac output and may exacerbate or induce hypotension and bradycardia [21, 45]. In a recent, multicenter, prospective, randomized, controlled trial of critically ill adults, ketamine was compared to etomidate for induction of rapid sequence intubation. Both drugs performed similarly in facilitating rapid sequence intubation which resulted in patients having similar sequential organ failure assessment (SOFA) scores. The authors concluded that ketamine is a safe and valuable alternative to etomidate for endotracheal intubation in critically ill patients and should be considered in those with sepsis [47]. Based on these seemingly conflicting conclusions, it is not absolutely clear how the cardiovascular effects of ketamine will affect critically ill patients, and outcomes may be related to the degree of illness and severity of depletion of catecholamine stores. While ketamine appears to be a good option for induction of rapid sequence intubation for most critically ill patients, these conflicting findings must be taken into consideration when administering ketamine to critically ill patients with depleted catecholamine stores.

Due to its sympathomimetic effects, ketamine use has historically been discouraged for children or adults with known or possible coronary artery disease, congestive heart failure, or hypertension [5, 17, 19]. A recent clinical practice guideline for ketamine use in the emergency setting points out that the evidence suggesting that ketamine sympathomimetic effects may be problematic to patients with these conditions is inconclusive and that ketamine administration is not contraindicated in these patients [17]. However, the cardiovascular effects of ketamine are best tolerated in healthy individuals, and the risks and benefits to patients with coronary artery disease, congestive heart failure, or hypertension must be considered prior to ketamine administration.

Despite concerns for ketamine effects in critically ill patients with depleted catecholamine stores and underlying cardiac conditions, ketamine may prove to be the best option for these patients by providing less cardiovascular suppressive effects as compared to other commonly administered agents such as propofol, benzodiazepines, etomidate, and barbiturates.

Pulmonary Effects

In a study of ketamine, 2 mg/kg IV, administered to healthy (ASA I) children as a bolus, ketamine did not affect resting respiratory rate, tidal volume, end-tidal carbon dioxide (CO_2) tension, or minute ventilation [48]. At doses typically administered to patients for brief procedural sedation, ketamine does not produce significant respiratory depression and is a bronchodilator which has been shown to decrease bronchospasm [5, 17, 19]. The mechanism of diminished bronchospasm with ketamine administration is thought to be due to subsequent increase in circulating catecholamines, direct smooth muscle dilatation, and inhibition of vagal outflow [17]. Respiratory adverse events including oxygen desaturation <90 %, apnea, or laryngospasm, associated with ketamine sedation in children, have been shown to occur infrequently in one observational study (121 adverse events with 1791 ketamine administrations, 6.8 %) and a large, individual patient data meta-analysis (319 adverse events with 8282 ketamine administrations, 3.9 %) [2, 41]. In two studies of children, the addition of midazolam to emergency department ketamine sedation was associated with greater respiratory depression and increased respiratory adverse events as compared to ketamine alone [40, 41]. Respiratory adverse events in these two studies were predominantly managed with non-invasive maneuvers such as airway repositioning, verbal cues, tactile stimulation or oxygen administration. Positive pressure ventilation was applied using brief bag-mask ventilation in a few patients (less than 1 %), and no patients received endotracheal intubation [40, 41].

Although ketamine only rarely causes respiratory suppression or compromise, patients who receive dissociative doses of ketamine must be closely monitored and clinicians must be prepared to provide patients with airway repositioning, verbal cues, tactile stimulation, oxygen, and at least brief positive pressure ventilation with bag mask on infrequent occasions (slightly less than 1 % of the time).

Early work by Corssen et al. reported ketamine to be specifically beneficial in anesthesia for the asthmatic patient by diminishing existing bronchospasm and wheezing at time of induction [49]. In a case series of five adults with status asthmaticus in the emergency setting, four patients displayed immediate improvement of respiratory acidosis after receiving ketamine 1–2 mg/kg IV for intubation with succinylcholine. A fifth patient, intubated with diazepam and succinylcholine, experienced a dramatic rise in pCO_2 with intubation which was successfully treated with IV ketamine [46]. In a case report of two children with status asthmaticus, ketamine at dissociative doses, 2 mg/kg IV, followed by continuous infusion of 2 mg/kg/h was associated with improvement in bronchospasm which the authors report prevented intubation and mechanical ventilation [50]. Similar results were reported in an adult who received a dissociating dose of ketamine as a temporizing measure to avoid mechanical ventilation due to a severe asthma exacerbation [51]. While dissociative doses of ketamine provide bronchodilatory effects in patients with status asthmaticus and may be effective in assisting with intubation and even prevent mechanical ventilation, sub-dissociative doses of ketamine administered to adults and children have not been shown to be effective in significantly diminishing bronchospasm in asthma exacerbations [52, 53]. Although its bronchodilatory properties appear to make ketamine a promising addition to the treatment of patients with moderate to severe asthma, further study of the effects of dissociative and sub-dissociative doses of ketamine is needed to clarify the role of ketamine in the treatment of patients with asthma.

Effects on Intracranial and Intraocular Pressure

Ketamine increases cerebral blood flow and intracranial pressure in spontaneously breathing patients [1]. However, for ventilated patients, even those with head trauma, ketamine has not been shown to increase, and may actually decrease, intracranial pressure [21]. A large review of the effect of ketamine on intracranial and cerebral perfusion pressure and health outcomes concluded that the use of ketamine in critically ill patients did not appear to adversely affect patient outcomes [54]. Patients with head trauma may receive ketamine for induction of rapid sequence intubation which has the added benefit of providing blood pressure support to patients who may experience cardiovascular instability due to blood loss from associated injuries [17, 55, 56]. Given the recent evidence, patients with intracranial hypertension due to structural barriers to normal cerebrospinal fluid flow (i.e., hydrocephalus) would appear to be the only patients for whom ketamine administration is contraindicated due to concerns arising from intracranial pressure [17, 57].

A range of levels of increased intraocular pressure have been reported in association with ketamine [16]. However, two recent case series of healthy children, without eye injuries, found no significant change in intraocular pressure with ketamine administered for procedural sedation [58, 59]. While ketamine appears to have no effect on intraocular pressure in healthy children, further study of the effects of ketamine on intraocular pressure in patients with eye injuries or glaucoma is warranted before current guidelines which identify increased intraocular pressure as a relative contraindication to ketamine administration for emergency department procedural sedation may be revised [17].

Dissociative Effects

As mentioned previously, the dissociative sedation or anesthesia provided by ketamine is primarily the result of the excitatory effects which result with ketamine inhibition of glutamate binding to NMDA receptors in the CNS [1, 5, 16, 20, 21]. In the resulting state, patients do not respond purposely to external stimuli. Commonly, the patient's eyes remain open and nystagmus occurs [5]. Patients may make involuntary movements and sounds. It is important to inform patients and their families or care providers of these effects, which are generally harmless, but may be quite alarming to the uninitiated. The dissociative state lends itself very well to facilitating the completion of a wide range of procedures. However, due to ketamine-associated involuntary, non-purposeful movements, sedation for procedures which require the patient to be motionless for any meaningful length of time, such as magnetic resonance imaging (MRI), is better accomplished using other agents.

To reliably achieve the dissociative state, a range of dosing for ketamine has been proposed [5, 16, 17]. A recent emergency department clinical practice guideline recommends 1.5–2.0 mg/kg IV and 4–5 mg/kg IM for children and 1.0 mg/kg IV for adults for dissociative sedation [17]. To achieve analgesia, sub-dissociative, low-dose ketamine is recommended, 0.2–0.75 mg/kg IV, [5, 16, 60–62], 1–3 mg/kg IM [5, 62], and 0.5–1 mg/kg IN [28, 29] in children and adults.

The combination of dissociative sedation and analgesia with a favorable safety profile made ketamine ideal to provide care required for children and adults who experienced severe pain due to treatment of burns. Burn units used ketamine extensively for dressing changes, wound debridement, and skin grafting procedures [5, 63]. In 1971, Corssen et al. reported that ketamine was their drug of choice for the care of burn patients as ketamine ". . .does not depress respiratory function, while it stimulates the cardiovascular system. . .the protective laryngeal and pharyngeal reflexes (are maintained). . .thereby ensuring an unobstructed airway without the need for endotracheal intubation, regardless of the patient's position." [63].

The use of ketamine rapidly progressed from these beginnings. Starting in the 1970s, ketamine administered IM was used by "surgeon-anesthetists" for a variety of minor to major surgical procedures in developing countries [64, 65]. Phillips and Walker each describe their experience in the South Pacific of administering IM ketamine and performing surgery without the need for endotracheal intubation and without significant complication in most cases. Due to the ease of administration and its favorable cardiorespiratory effects, ketamine administration for painful procedures and surgeries spread to the battlefield and in disaster situations where supportive resources were severely limited [19, 66]. Ketamine use continued to expand from painful procedures in burn patients to obstetric procedures and "outpatient anesthesia" administered as an IV bolus or as a continuous IV infusion [5, 19, 67].

Ketamine has now been used successfully outside of the operating room for the sedation of children receiving a wide range of emergent and elective procedures including, but not restricted to, orthopedic reduction and arthrocentesis, incision and drainage of skin abscesses, laceration repair and wound care, lumbar puncture, bone marrow biopsy/aspiration, oropharyngeal procedures, foreign body removal, dental procedures, and diagnostic imaging [2, 3, 41, 68]. The sedative, analgesic, and amnestic properties of ketamine coupled with minimal respiratory depression and maintenance of intact airway protective reflexes make it an ideal agent for facilitating the performance of painful procedures in the emergency department [2, 3, 17].

A number of clinical trials which compare ketamine with other agents and combinations provide further insights into the strengths and weaknesses of sedation with ketamine. In a randomized, controlled trial of ketamine and midazolam vs. fentanyl and midazolam for emergent orthopedic reduction in children aged 5–15 years, Kennedy et al. found ketamine/midazolam to be more effective for pain and anxiety relief and to result in fewer respiratory complications than fentanyl/midazolam [69]. The authors further report that both regimens facilitated orthopedic reduction, produced amnesia, and rarely caused emergence delirium. The ketamine/midazolam group experienced more vomiting (3 % vs. 0 %) but less hypoxia (6 % vs. 25 %), less need for breathing cues (1 % vs. 12 %), and less need for supplemental oxygen (10 % vs. 20 %) than the fentanyl/midazolam group. Two patients (1.5 %) in the ketamine/midazolam group required brief positive pressure ventilation provided by bag mask. Orthopedic surgeons favored the ketamine/midazolam regimen despite the fact that recovery was 14 min shorter in the fentanyl/midazolam group [69].

Adverse events associated with IV ketamine alone, ketamine/midazolam, midazolam/fentanyl, and midazolam alone were compared in an observational case series of 2500 children who received sedation for emergency procedures [41]. Respiratory adverse events occurred less frequently in ketamine alone (6.1 %) and in the ketamine/midazolam (10 %) groups than in the midazolam/fentanyl group (19.3 %). As a single agent, midazolam use is limited as it provides no analgesia; however, patients who received midazolam alone experienced respiratory adverse events only slightly less commonly (5.8 %) than patients who received ketamine alone. As opposed to respiratory adverse events, vomiting was more common in children who received ketamine alone (10.1 %) than those who received ketamine/midazolam (5.4 %), midazolam/fentanyl (1.8 %), or midazolam alone (0.8 %). From the results of this study, it would appear that the addition of midazolam to ketamine increases respiratory adverse events and decreases the incidence of vomiting. These findings are consistent with the known respiratory suppressive and antiemetic properties of midazolam. Based on the results of this study and Kennedy's, we can conclude that ketamine, with or without midazolam, will provide more consistent sedation and analgesia and result in fewer respiratory adverse events but more vomiting than the commonly administered combination of midazolam/fentanyl when used for procedural sedation of children in the emergency department [41, 69].

Comparison of the longer-term effects of ketamine with or without midazolam vs. fentanyl/midazolam was performed through a prospective observational study of 554 children whose families were contacted to investigate the occurrence of adverse events after discharge [70]. The authors found post-discharge vomiting to be common (18 %) across all groups, and there was a low prevalence of adverse behavioral events in children once they returned to their homes. The fentanyl/midazolam group was associated with higher adverse behavioral scores than children who received ketamine alone or ketamine/midazolam [70].

The ultrashort-acting sedative agent propofol is commonly administered to children and adults for elective and emergent procedural sedation outside the operating room [71–74]. Godambe et al. compared propofol/fentanyl to ketamine/midazolam for sedation of children 3–18 years of age for emergent orthopedic procedures [75]. To assess efficacy of sedation, observers blinded to the agents administered scored patient distress during the procedure using a standardized scale. Distress scores were low in both groups, although recovery time was significantly shorter in the propofol/fentanyl group. Oxygen desaturations were more common in the propofol/fentanyl group as compared to the ketamine/midazolam group (30.5 % vs. 7.4 %). One patient in the propofol/fentanyl group experienced laryngospasm, and no patients had apnea in either group. Emesis occurred in 3.7 % of the ketamine/midazolam group and 0 % in the propofol/fentanyl group. The authors concluded that despite a greater potential of respiratory depression and airway obstruction as compared with ketamine, propofol offers unique advantages of quicker offset and smoother recovery [75].

In a randomized controlled trial of adults who received either propofol or midazolam/ketamine for painful orthopedic manipulation, the effectiveness of sedation outcomes was similar between groups [76]. Patients who received propofol experience a more rapid recovery (7.8 vs. 30.7 min) and shorter duration of sedation (16.2 min vs. 41.6 min) than the midazolam/ketamine group. The overall rate of respiratory and hemodynamic adverse events was 20 % for the propofol group and 10 % for the midazolam/ketamine group [76].

In a prospective, non-randomized study of sedation for oncology procedures (e.g. bone marrow biopsy or aspiration, lumbar puncture) in children, the first 25 patients received midazolam/ketamine and the second 25 propofol with or without morphine [77]. Both regimens were found to be efficacious for procedural sedation, and propofol, with or without morphine, was reported to have a quicker onset of action and a smoother recovery. Despite these advantages, propofol/fentanyl was also found to have significantly more side effects including oxygen desaturations in 36 % vs. 12 % in the midazolam/ketamine group.

From the comparison studies of ketamine, with or without midazolam, vs. propofol with or without an opioid in adults and children for elective and emergent procedures, we can conclude that both regimens have been shown to provide efficacious sedation and analgesia. In addition, patients who receive ketamine, with or without midazolam, may be expected to experience less respiratory adverse events, longer duration of sedation, and more vomiting than those who receive propofol without or without an opioid.

Based on a large body of literature investigating the administration of ketamine and propofol for procedural sedation outside the operating room, both have been shown to be efficacious and safe, with expected, associated adverse events which are readily managed by appropriately trained and experienced providers of sedation [2, 3, 17, 68, 71–74]. Since both have desirable and undesirable clinical effects, it has been proposed that the combination of ketamine and propofol will serve to decrease the total dose

Table 14.3 Coadministered adjuncts to ketamine administration

Adjunct drug	Rationale	Evidence of effects
Anticholinergics • Atropine • Glycopyrrolate	Believed to decrease hypersalivation associated with ketamine and therefore prevent laryngospasm	• Secretions are decreased with anticholinergics but no clinical benefits have been identified • Increases airway and respiratory adverse events
Midazolam	Postulated to decrease incidence of ketamine-associated unpleasant recovery reactions	• Decreases unpleasant recovery reactions in adults but **not** in children • Increases airway and respiratory adverse events • Decreases vomiting
Ondansetron	Vomiting is common with ketamine and administering an antiemetic will decrease the incidence of vomiting	• Ondansetron decreases vomiting • Most effective in children 5 years of age and older • Also decreases the incidence of post-discharge vomiting
Propofol	"Synergistic" relationship with ketamine will potentially make sedation more effective and decrease adverse effects	• No difference in objective measures of effectiveness or length of sedation • No difference in airway or respiratory adverse events • Decreases vomiting

required for each drug, potentiate both drugs' desirable properties, and ameliorate their shortcomings and undesirable qualities [78]. Propofol is an excellent sedative but lacks analgesic properties, while ketamine is a powerful analgesic. The sympathomimetic effects of ketamine will potentially counteract the respiratory depression and hypotension that may occur with propofol. The antiemetic effects of propofol may reduce vomiting commonly seen with ketamine, and emergence phenomena seen with ketamine may be diminished by the hypnotic properties of propofol which has been shown to produce quicker and smoother recovery from sedation. It is also been postulated that the addition of propofol to ketamine will decrease the dose of ketamine required which will result in shorter sedation time and ultimately, shorter lengths of stay [78] (Table 14.3).

Four observational case series of adults and children who received the propofol/ketamine combination referred to as "ketofol" support its efficacy and low rate of manageable adverse events when administered in the emergency department for painful procedures [79–82]. Three of these studies used a propofol to ketamine ratio of 1:1, while one administered propofol/ketamine at a 2:1 concentration.

The question remains whether ketofol provides clinical benefits over ketamine (with or without midazolam) or propofol (with or without an opioid). David and Shipp performed a randomized controlled trial of ketamine/propofol vs. propofol alone for emergency department procedural sedation of healthy children and adults [83]. Propofol/ketamine ratio in this study was 2:1, and the combination of ketamine and propofol did not reduce the incidence of respiratory depression but resulted in greater provider satisfaction, less propofol administered, and subjectively better sedation quality. Shah et al. performed a blinded, randomized controlled trial of ketamine/propofol vs. ketamine alone for procedural sedation in children [84]. Ketamine/propofol patients received an initial IV bolus dose of ketamine 0.5 mg/kg and propofol 0.5 mg/kg,

followed by propofol 0.5 mg/kg and saline solution placebo every 2 min, titrated to deep sedation. Ketamine patients received an initial IV bolus dose of ketamine 1.0 mg/kg and intralipid placebo (to ensure blinding), followed by ketamine 0.25 mg/kg and intralipid placebo every 2 min, as required. Sedation efficacy and airway complications were similar between groups, while the ketamine/propofol combination produced slightly faster recoveries with less vomiting (2 % vs. 12 %) and higher provider satisfaction scores than those in the ketamine alone group [84] (Table 14.3).

Two additional randomized, controlled trials comparing ketofol to propofol for procedural sedation are worth noting. Andolfatto et al. enrolled patients 14 years of age and older comparing a 1:1 mixture of ketofol to propofol alone for emergency department procedural sedation and analgesia [85]. In this study, ketofol was not found to reduce the incidence of adverse respiratory events as compared to propofol alone, and induction time, efficacy, and sedation time were similar in each group. Subjectively, sedation depth appeared to be more consistent with ketofol [85]. Miner et al. administered ketofol at 1:1 and 4:1 propofol/ketamine concentration ratios which were compared to propofol alone for emergency department deep procedural sedation in adults [86]. The authors found a similar frequency of airway and respiratory adverse events leading to intervention between propofol alone and either 1:1 or 4:1 ketofol. The authors conclude that ketofol, at either concentration, and propofol appear to be similarly safe and effective [86].

When compared to ketamine, patients who receive ketofol experience less vomiting and slightly shorter time of sedation with subjectively better sedation. As compared to propofol, ketofol performed very similarly at 1:1, 2:1, and 4:1 propofol to ketamine concentrations with regard to efficacy and complications of sedation. Importantly, ketofol was not found to improve the efficacy of sedation or decrease the incidence or severity of respiratory adverse events when compared to either propofol or ketamine. It is not clear whether ketofol provides any objective benefit over propofol. The objective benefits of ketofol over ketamine alone would appear to be limited to decreased vomiting and length of sedation which must be balanced with the increased risk of respiratory suppression. Additional studies are needed to clarify the advantages and disadvantages of ketofol procedural sedation as compared to ketamine or propofol [87].

As demonstrated in extensive investigations, the dissociative properties of ketamine make it an excellent choice for sedation outside the operating room for a wide variety of painful, elective, and emergent procedures. Patients who receive ketamine at recommended doses and routes of administration will have a predictable length of dissociation with typically manageable associated adverse effects. The serious airway and respiratory adverse events apnea and laryngospasm will occur in less than 1 % of children who receive IV ketamine and are usually managed effectively with brief bag-mask positive pressure ventilation [2].

Psychotomimetic Effects

Domino and Corssen reported the first pharmacologic and clinical experience with the phencyclidine derivative CI-581 (ketamine) in humans [14, 15]. In the pharmacologic study, they report the effects of CI-581 on 20 male volunteers from a prison population. The results of this study were consistent with the ketamine-associated sympathomimetic effects and transient respiratory depression with minimal clinical significance discussed previously. Most of the subjects showed changes in mood, body image and affect, and some reported vivid dreams and/or hallucinations. However, these effects were found to be short lasting and that some of the subjects experienced no undesirable psychotomimetic effects at all [14]. In their clinical study, 130 patients, ranging in age from 6 weeks to 86 years, received CI-581 for a variety of surgical procedures. Again, adverse cardiorespiratory events were minimal, and some of the adult patients had vivid dreams or frank hallucinations during recovery. The dreams lasted 5–15 min and were described by patients as ranging from amusing and pleasant to frightening. Their dreams frequently involved outer space and some patients experience frank hallucinations. Two middle-aged patients were reported to have displayed signs of schizoid behavior, and both experienced "traveling in outer space and thought that they had died and were flying to hell." In one of these patients, the experience lasted only a few minutes, but the other was affected for 40 min [15].

Adults emerging from the ketamine-induced dissociative state may experience psychotomimetic effects which have been described as schizophrenia-like symptoms and behaviors [5, 21]. Patients describe out-of-body experiences, floating sensations, vivid dreams, hallucinations, delusions, illogical thinking, agitation, disturbances of emotion and affect, decreases in memory, and occasionally, frank delirium [1, 4–6, 14–16, 19–21]. As ketamine acts to inhibit NMDA receptor binding of glutamate and functionally dissociate or disconnect the thalamo-neocortical and limbic centers of the brain, higher centers are prevented from normally perceiving visual, auditory, or painful stimuli [6, 16, 19]. This leads to a misperception or misinterpretation of auditory and visual stimuli which serves to explain many of the dreaming, floating, and out-of-body or flying sensations described by patients [5]. In preverbal and young or developmentally delayed children, who are unable to articulate the feelings they experience due to the psychotomimetic effects of ketamine, agitation may be the primary behavior seen [40].

The transient schizophrenia-like psychotic state that results from NMDA antagonist drugs like phencyclidine and ketamine has inspired Olney and others to investigate the potential role of the NMDA glutamate receptor system in schizophrenia [88]. They postulate that NMDA receptor blockade and subsequent hypofunction result in excessive release of excitatory transmitters (glutamate) and, consequentially, overstimulation of postsynaptic neurons. The result of this work is that pharmacologic models of schizophrenia now rely on glutamatergic rather than dopaminergic dysfunction to explain the symptoms of schizophrenia [89]. The glutamatergic dysfunction mechanism provides an explanation for the associated cognitive and behavioral disturbances seen with NMDA antagonists and in schizophrenia. Due to the similarity of the mechanism of action of ketamine and the pathologic process of schizophrenia, it is recommended to avoid using ketamine in patients with schizophrenia, and caution is advised in patients with other forms of psychosis [17, 21]. Ketamine may be administered to children with attention deficit and hyperactivity disorders (ADHD) as these conditions do not appear to increase the incidence or susceptibility to psychotomimetic effects [21].

Ketamine-induced psychotomimetic effects have been referred to by many names including emergence phenomena [16, 20, 21, 40, 90], emergence reactions [5, 91], emergence delirium [92], and recovery agitation [3, 93–95]. Lack of consistency in terms and definitions has led to a wide range in reporting the incidence of ketamine-induced psychotomimetic effects as some terms and definitions include pleasant dreams and euphoria, while others report only unpleasant reactions. To address the problem of inconsistent definitions and reporting of adverse events associated with procedural sedation, Bhatt led a panel of sedation researchers and experts in developing consensus-based recommendations for standardizing terminology and reporting of adverse events associated with procedural sedation and analgesia for children in the emergency department [96]. Since clinicians and families are most concerned about dysphoria, agitation, and adverse psychotomimetic effects of drugs, the consensus panel proposed the term "unpleasant recovery reactions" which they defined as "abnormal patient affect or behaviors during the recovery phase that requires additional treatment and a change or delay in patient discharge." The behaviors include one or more of the following:

(a) Crying—Inconsolable
(b) Agitation—Restless, continuous activity
(c) Delirium—State of severe confusion
(d) Dysphoria—Inappropriate mood of sadness
(e) Nightmares—Unpleasant dreams
(f) Hallucinations—Responds to sensory phenomena (i.e., seeing, hearing, or feeling) that are not physically present [96]

Although these guidelines were written to pertain to pediatric sedation research in the emergency department, as one editorial noted, ". . .despite the pediatric intent, each element applies readily to adults. The approach and the principles put forth also extrapolate to any setting. . ." [97].

The incidence of psychotomimetic effects associated with ketamine sedation in adults has been reported to have a wide range (partially due to inconsistent definitions and reporting) from less than 5 % to greater than 50 % [5, 16, 91]. In children, the incidence is believed to be significantly lower. One large, individual patient data meta-analysis of 8282 children found the incidence of recovery agitation to be 7.6 % with only 1.4 % of children experiencing a reaction that was felt to be clinically important (i.e., occurrences of abnormal behavioral responses that either led to specific treatment or were specially described by investigators as demonstrating substantial severity) [3].

Original reports found emergence reactions to be more common in patients over 16 year of age, in females than males, in subjects who normally dream, in those who received large doses of ketamine (>2 mg/kg IV) and rapid IV administration (>40 mg/min), and in patients with a history of personality problems [5, 19]. More recent studies have found unpleasant recovery reactions to not be related to age in children [3, 98] and to be infrequent and mild in patients aged 16–21 years [94]. Preprocedural agitation has been shown to increase the incidence of concerning recovery behaviors in children who receive procedural sedation in the emergency department as well as those who receive general anesthesia [93, 99] (Table 14.2). When ketamine was compared to fentanyl/midazolam for emergent procedural sedation, no difference in the incidence of associated unpleasant recovery reactions and post-discharge behavior problems was detected [21, 70, 90].

Many studies have reported decreased incidence of unpleasant recovery reactions in adults when benzodiazepines are coadministered with ketamine [5, 16, 19, 20]. A randomized controlled trial of ketamine with and without midazolam for emergency department sedation in adults found coadministered midazolam significantly reduced the incidence of recovery agitation (25 % in ketamine alone vs. 8 % in ketamine with midazolam) [95]. However, in children, midazolam has not been found to significantly affect the incidence of unpleasant recovery reactions. Two randomized controlled trials found no decrease in psychotomimetic effects of ketamine with administration of midazolam in children [40, 93] (Table 14.3). In both of these studies, midazolam and ketamine were administered simultaneously. It has been postulated that administering midazolam prior to ketamine, with the goal of decreasing preprocedural agitation, may prove beneficial in decreasing the incidence of unpleasant recovery reactions in children. However logical and promising the proposal to administer anxiolytic drugs prior to sedation to decrease agitation may be, further study is needed to explore this theory [100, 101]. For children who experience prolonged or particularly distressing unpleasant recovery reactions, midazolam, administered during recovery, has been shown to successfully diminish these symptoms [93].

Ketamine was developed as a short-acting intravenous anesthetic due to the shortcomings of phencyclidine and cyclohexamine which resulted in long-lasting psychotomimetic activity (i.e., emergence delirium, recovery agitation, or unpleasant recovery reactions) during the postanesthetic period [1, 4, 5]. Unpleasant recovery reactions associated with ketamine are more common in adults (10–25 %) than children (~7 %) and also appear to be uncommon in young adults (16–21 years of age) [3, 94, 102]. The incidence of clinically important (particularly distressing to the patient and resulting in additional treatment or length of stay) unpleasant recovery reactions in children is less than 2 % [3]. Unpleasant recovery reactions may be decreased in occurrence and severity in adults with the coadministration of midazolam [3, 95, 102]. In children, the incidence of unpleasant recovery reactions was not affected by the coadministration of midazolam in two randomized, controlled trials [40, 93]. Decreasing preprocedural agitation, educating patients of the expected psychotomimetic effects of ketamine such as a dream-like state of floating or flying, encouraging patients to prepare for their sedation by thinking pleasant thoughts, and inviting them to "dream well" appear to decrease the incidence of unpleasant recovery reactions [101]. For young children, providing them with a nonthreatening environment by allowing them to remain in a position of comfort, usually with their parents, will diminish presedation agitation and improve the sedation experience and outcomes. For all patients, informing them and their families of the effects and potential adverse effects of ketamine prior to administration will allow them to be informed, less surprised, and more prepared to handle ketamine-associated adverse events including unpleasant recovery reactions, if they occur.

Adverse Clinical Effects: Vomiting

The incidence of vomiting associated with ketamine in adults has been reported to be between 5 and 15 % [102], whereas the reported range of emesis in children is much wider, between 3 % and greater than 28 % [3, 25, 40, 41, 69, 103–108]. Ketamine-associated vomiting typically occurs during the late phase of recovery from sedation at which time patients are most able to respond in a manner which allows them to protect their airways and prevent pulmonary aspiration [17, 42, 69, 109]. As mentioned previously, ketamine does not suppress normal upper airway protective reflexes, further reducing the risk for pulmonary aspiration [16, 20]. In a case series of children who received ketamine for emergency department procedural sedation, prolonged preprocedural fasting time did not reduce the incidence of vomiting [107]. These findings are consistent with two larger case series of 2085 and 1014 children who received emergency department sedation, predominantly with ketamine (72 % and 47 %, respectively), and no association between preprocedural fasting and adverse events including vomiting was found in either study [110, 111]. The combination of intact airway protective reflexes and emesis occurring predominantly during the final stages of recovery makes aspiration unlikely with ketamine sedation regardless of preprocedural fasting status as is supported by these three studies as well as the large individual patient data meta-analysis which found no cases of pulmonary aspiration in 8282 ketamine administrations in children [3, 107, 110, 111].

The incidence of emesis with ketamine increases with age until early adolescence and then decreases [3, 17, 107]. In an individual patient data meta-analysis of 8282 children who received predominantly IV ketamine for emergency department procedural sedation, the incidence of vomiting was found to be 8.4 %. The most important independent predictors of vomiting in this study were unusually high IV dose (initial dose of $\geq$2.5 mg/kg or a total dose of $\geq$5.0 mg/kg), IM route, and increasing age (peak at 12 years) [3] (Table 14.2). In a separate meta-analysis of children who received IV ketamine, Thorp et al. found that vomiting was not related to either the initial loading dose or the total dose until the total dose exceeded 7 mg/kg [106]. In a randomized, controlled trial of IV vs. IM ketamine, vomiting occurred in 11.9 % of children who received ketamine

1 mg/kg IV and in 26.3 % of those who received ketamine 4 mg/kg IM [25]. It has been argued that the incidence of vomiting associated with parenteral ketamine is more dependent on the total dose of ketamine administered than actual route of administration. Kinder et al. found that children with high body mass indices (25 kg/m^2 or higher) who received larger total doses of ketamine were at greater risk of nausea and vomiting [105].

Coadministration of parenteral opioids has been reported to increase the incidence of emesis with ketamine; however, oral analgesics of any type were not associated with increased incidence of vomiting in one retrospective case series [21, 108]. Several studies have documented vomiting in children who received ketamine sedation after time of discharge [25, 40, 69, 103]. Vomiting after discharge was observed in between 3 and 12 % of these children, some of whom had not vomited during their stay in the emergency department.

Ketamine-associated vomiting at the time of sedation recovery and after discharge home may be decreased by the coadministration of ondansetron [103]. In a randomized, controlled trial of ketamine/ondansetron vs. ketamine/placebo, the addition of ondansetron decreased vomiting at the time of sedation recovery from 12.6 to 4.7 % in children who received IV ketamine for emergent procedures. Despite this decrease in emesis, 13 patients would need to be treated to prevent one episode of vomiting (number needed to treat equaled 13). Additionally, this study found increased rates of vomiting in children aged 5 years or older. When vomiting at home, as well as vomiting in the emergency department, was considered in children 5 years of age or older, the ondansetron group experienced a decrease in vomiting from 23.5 to 9.5 %. The number needed to treat to prevent one episode of vomiting in this highest-risk group was then decreased to seven [103] (Table 14.3).

Ketamine-associated vomiting occurs most commonly during the late phase of sedation recovery and after time of discharge. Vomiting is more common in older children, in those who received significantly higher doses IV and in those for whom ketamine was administered IM. Ondansetron coadministration will most effectively decrease the incidence of emesis with ketamine in children 5 years of age or older, especially when rates of vomiting during sedation recovery, as well as at home, are considered.

Adverse Clinical Effects: Hypertonicity and Random Movements

Ketamine has been shown to induce involuntary, rhythmic muscle contractions involving the arms and legs which have, in some instances, incorrectly been identified as seizures. These non-purposeful movements are extrapyramidal in nature and are not associated with EEG changes found in myoclonic seizures [112]. Ketamine is reported to have anticonvulsant properties [5, 16, 17] and has been used in adults to terminate malignant status epilepticus resistant to treatment with benzodiazepines, phenytoin, thiopental, and propofol [113]. Ketamine is not contraindicated in patients with seizure disorders. In a study of adults, Corssen et al. found no evidence that ketamine is likely to precipitate generalized convulsions, even in patients with both a history of epilepsy and an abnormal EEG [112]. Random, non-purposeful movements and increased muscle tone associated with ketamine administration are not related to painful stimuli and, although responsive to treatment with benzodiazepines, do not represent seizures.

Adverse Clinical Effects: Minor

Patients receiving ketamine have been reported to experience an erythematous rash on the face, neck, and chest. The rash does not appear to be allergic in nature, is transient, and resolves spontaneously requiring no specific treatment [16, 17]. Although hiccupping associated with ketamine has been reported, several studies support the successful use of ketamine to treat refractory hiccupping during anesthesia and in the postoperative period [114, 115]. As mentioned previously, hypersalivation occurs with ketamine, and although treatment with anticholinergic agents atropine or glycopyrrolate will decrease salivation, addition of these drugs has not been shown to decrease the incidence of laryngospasm or provide other significant clinical benefit [35–37].

Analgesic Effects

Early studies reported the acute analgesic effects of ketamine in adult human volunteers [14, 15]. The mechanism of ketamine's analgesic properties is believed to be through ketamine binding to the NMDA glutamate receptor complex on the neuronal membrane which effectively blocks the electrical propagation of pain. By blocking the binding of the neurotransmitter glutamate, ketamine induces inhibition of transmembrane calcium channels which interfere with calcium influx and prevents or decreases neurotransmission of pain [21].

NMDA receptor activation has been shown to be associated with pain perception due to peripheral tissue or nerve injury [116]. Central NMDA receptors such as those located in the spinal cord, but also NMDA receptors in peripheral somatic tissues and visceral pain pathways, play an important role in nociception, or the ability to perceive pain. It has been postulated that NMDA receptor antagonists, such as ketamine, will alleviate pain through inhibition of these mechanisms [4, 21, 116].

After trauma, changes at the site of the injury lead to peripheral sensitization and primary hyperalgesia. This hyperalgesia also has a central component. Central sensitization is propagated through the dorsal horn of the spinal cord with the result being that low-intensity stimuli produce a pain response that is augmented in amplitude and duration. In other words, after an injury, the state of central sensitization leaves the site of the injury susceptible to significant painful sensations (hyperalgesia) with only minimal stimulation [21].

The windup phenomenon is the progressive increase of the responses induced by repetitive nociceptive stimuli. It is believed that windup, this temporal summation of nociceptive inputs, may play a significant role in the development of central sensitization [117]. By binding to NMDA receptors and blocking windup and central sensitization, ketamine is believed to provide acute and prolonged analgesic effects [4, 21, 116, 117]. In addition, ketamine may provide effective analgesia in chronic pain syndromes that involve a windup mechanism such as postherpetic neuralgia, migraine, burns, neuropathies, and fibromyalgia [4].

There are several reasons clinicians may wish to use non-opioid analgesics such as ketamine, to treat pain in their patients. Opioid use for pain has been associated with side effects (particularly respiratory suppression), physical dependence, and addiction. Somewhat paradoxically, opioid therapy aimed at alleviating pain may render patients more sensitive to pain and potentially may aggravate their preexisting pain. Opioid-induced hyperalgesia has been described with opioid use for pain, especially with the administration of high or escalating doses [118]. Opioid-induced hyperalgesia is mediated by excitatory neurotransmission, making sustained NMDA receptor blocking, as occurs with ketamine, a potentially effective method of reducing this type of pain [21, 119].

In adult orthopedic surgical patients, intraoperative ketamine has been shown to result in less postoperative pain and to decrease opioid requirements [120, 121]. In another study, adults undergoing abdominal surgery received preemptive ketamine which decreased postoperative opioid requirements. This decreased opioid need was observed long after the normal expected duration of action of ketamine (day 2 post-op), demonstrating a prolonged analgesic effect [122]. However, in a study of children who received major urological surgery, intraoperative ketamine had no effect on morphine consumption during the first 72 h after surgery [123]. A qualitative review of randomized, controlled trials of adding ketamine to morphine for IV patient-controlled analgesia for acute postoperative pain found no clear benefit for patients after orthopedic or abdominal surgery [124].

The use of ketamine for acute pain has increased over the past decade in the emergency and prehospital settings. Three retrospective case series of sub-dissociative-dose ketamine (0.1–0.6 mg/kg IV) for adults with acute pain found ketamine to provide effective analgesia in the emergency setting with minimal adverse effects [62, 125, 126]. A recent randomized, controlled trial of sub-dissociative-dose ketamine vs. morphine for analgesia of acute abdominal, flank, or musculoskeletal pain in adults found ketamine 0.3 mg/kg IV provided analgesic effectiveness comparable to that of IV morphine [60]. In another randomized, controlled trial of ketamine 0.2 mg/kg added to morphine 0.1 mg/kg IV vs. a similar dose of morphine and placebo for acute pain in adult trauma patients, the addition of ketamine was found to decrease total morphine consumption [127]. Low-dose ketamine by subcutaneous infusion (0.1 mg/kg/h) was comparable to intermittent morphine (0.1 mg/kg IV) for adults with acute pain due to musculoskeletal trauma in a randomized, controlled trial [128]. In another randomized, controlled trial of sub-dissociative-dose ketamine vs. fentanyl in patients aged 14–65 years who received propofol for orthopedic reduction or abscess drainage, ketamine was found to induce less cardiorespiratory events and interventions than fentanyl [129]. Despite these studies which support the use of low-dose ketamine for pain, a systematic review of randomized controlled trials on the use of sub-dissociative-dose ketamine for acute pain in the emergency department determined that the four studies meeting their review criteria [69, 127–129] failed to provide convincing evidence to either support or refute the use of sub-dissociative-dose ketamine for acute pain control.

In a prospective observational study of mostly adult (three children) emergency patients with pain (75 % musculoskeletal, 10 % abdominal, 5 % dental, 10 % other), IN ketamine, 0.5–0.75 mg/kg, decreased pain in 88 % of patients [29]. In a randomized, controlled trial of children with moderate to severe isolated limb injury and pain, IN ketamine was shown to be as effective as IN fentanyl for pain reduction [28] (Table 14.1).

Ketamine has also been used for analgesia in the prehospital setting particularly for patients with hypotension and in those whose pain is unresponsive to opioid medications [130]. Prehospital case reports and case series provide preliminary data that supports the efficacy and safety of ketamine administered IV, IM, and IN for pain [130, 131]. Three prospective, randomized, controlled trials of IV ketamine for analgesia of adult trauma patients in the prehospital setting provide conflicting results [8, 132, 133]. Jennings et al. found IV ketamine, 10 or 20 mg bolus, added to morphine superior to morphine alone for pain [133]. However, Wiel et al. found that for patients who received bolus IV ketamine, 0.2 mg/kg, plus morphine, 0.1 mg/kg, and were randomized to either ketamine 0.2 mg/

kg/h or placebo, followed by morphine boluses as needed, no difference in total morphine administration was detected [8]. The third prehospital randomized controlled trial of adult trauma patients compared ketamine to morphine for pain and found ketamine to have an analgesic effect similar to morphine and carried a low risk of airway problems [132]. Two recent prospective, prehospital observational combat studies of pain medication use by US forces in Afghanistan found ketamine to be the most commonly administered analgesic drug for patients with blast, penetrating, and blunt trauma [134] and that ketamine was as safe as fentanyl or morphine in the prehospital setting [135].

There would appear to be great potential for the use of ketamine to ameliorate acute and long-term pain for patients postoperatively, in the hospital or the emergency department and in prehospital settings including combat. While many clinical studies support the effectiveness of ketamine as an effective analgesic, others have found less dramatic results. When administered at dissociative doses, ketamine is a powerful analgesic. The role of sub-dissociative-dose ketamine for the treatment of acute and prolonged pain in adults and children is promising and deserves further study.

Pharmacologic Restraint in Excited Delirium

According to the American College of Emergency Physicians Task Force, excited delirium syndrome is characterized by delirium, agitation, acidosis, and hyperadrenergic autonomic dysfunction, typically in the setting of acute-on-chronic drug abuse or serious mental illness or a combination of both [136, 137]. These patients present particularly challenging problems in the hospital, emergency department, or prehospital setting as they are commonly combative, violent, and dangerous to themselves as well as others. Additionally, patients with excited delirium or agitation are hypermetabolic and acidotic which may lead to metabolic derangements and potentially, lethal cardiac arrhythmias [138, 139]. Aggressive physical restraint is discouraged as increased muscle activity can lead to worsening acidosis and rhabdomyolysis. Pharmacologic restraint is commonly required to protect the patient and care providers. Historically administered benzodiazepines and antipsychotic drugs, such as haloperidol, have important limitations including an unpredictably long time to onset, especially when given IM, and important associated complications such as respiratory depression, hypotension, arrhythmias, and lowering of the seizure threshold [138, 139].

The literature contains several case reports and case series, mostly of adults, who received ketamine in the emergency department or prehospital setting emergently for out-of-control behavior associated with excited or agitated delirium of various etiologies [11, 140–145]. Ketamine was chosen in these patients due to its rapid, predictable onset of action IM (2–3 min) sympathomimetic effects and airway protective reflex sparing properties. Ketamine proved effective in calming patients; however, complications did occur. In a case series of 35 adults who received prehospital ketamine for control of severe agitation, eight (23 %) received endotracheal intubation, and six (17 %) required additional sedation post-ketamine administration [11]. After careful review of these cases, the authors concluded that secondary etiologies such as hemorrhagic cerebrovascular accident, ethanol intoxication, and aspiration pneumonia rather than side effects of ketamine were primarily responsible for endotracheal intubation in these patients [11]. A second case series of prehospital ketamine, dosed at 4 mg/kg IM, administered to violent and agitated adults found ketamine to effectively sedate 50 of 52 (96 %) patients [144]. Two of these patients subsequently received endotracheal intubation, and one required brief bag-mask ventilation. Ketamine use for adults and children with out-of-control behavior in the emergency department is also increasing. Isbister et al. report a case series of 1296 agitated adults in the emergency department, 49 of whom received ketamine as third-line therapy in treatment failure cases [145]. Ketamine 4–6 mg/kg IM was administered only after patients had already received two or three doses of droperidol 10 mg IM, as well as benzodiazepines in three cases. Adequate sedation was achieved in 44 (90 %) of these agitated adults, and inadequate dosing (200 mg or less) was believed to be the cause of sedation failure in four out of the five patients who required additional dosing. Two patients vomited and one experienced brief oxygen desaturation, but nightmares or recovery agitation was not observed in these 49 adult patients. In another recent case series of five children, ketamine was administered for management of agitation and delirium successfully in the emergency department without significant adverse events [139].

Adults and children with out-of-control behavior and excited or agitated delirium may benefit from acute treatment with parenteral (usually IM) ketamine with the goal of achieving the dissociative state to ensure the safety of patients and health care providers and so that patients may receive the medical and mental health care they require. The unique properties of ketamine support its use for this indication. However, these patients have significant comorbidities including polypharmacy substance abuse and mental illness which increase the risk of significant adverse events after ketamine administration. When ketamine is administered to treat excited delirium and out-of-control behavior, clinicians must be prepared to manage complications as well as the need for additional pharmaceutical restraint beyond an initial dose of ketamine. To reliably receive the desired effect, administration of a full 4 mg/kg of IM ketamine is recommended (Table 14.1).

Psychiatric Effects

In the 1990s, studies of sub-dissociative-dose ketamine in adults found that ketamine provided significant improvement in depressive symptoms in patients suffering from depression [146, 147]. Subsequently, a case report of two adults with major depressive disorder who benefitted from sub-anesthetic-dose ketamine infusions was reported [148]. A randomized, placebo-controlled trial of ketamine in treatment-resistant major depression in adults found rapid and robust antidepressant effects resulting within 2 h of a single IV infusion of 0.5 mg/kg which remained significant for 1 week [149].

Since this early work, several studies and reviews have supported a positive effect of ketamine for treatment-resistant major depression in adults [150–155] as well as posttraumatic stress disorder (PTSD) [12] and bipolar disorder [156]. Treatment with serial doses of IV and IN ketamine have been reported in adults with some success; however, the long-term effects of ketamine treatment are not well studied [151, 152] In children, only two case reports of ketamine for mental health indications exist; one reporting the use of IN ketamine for pediatric bipolar disorder and another in a child with behavioral dysregulation and PTSD [156, 157].

The neurobiological mechanisms of the antidepressant effects of ketamine are felt to be more complex than simple inhibition of glutamate binding to NMDA receptors. Further study is required to more definitively determine the mechanism of action of ketamine and to clarify indications and optimal treatment strategies for ketamine in the treatment of mental health disorders in adults and children [153, 154]. Additionally, chronic use of ketamine has been associated with short- and long-term memory impairment in recreational ketamine users, who self-administer significantly higher doses, more frequently, than has been used for mental health patients in the past [155]. The effects of ketamine administration over a longer period of time, under controlled, clinical situations, require further investigation.

Neurotoxicity

Clinical extremes as experienced by patients with hypoxic-ischemic head injuries, hypoglycemia, seizure activity, and surgery-related pain all induce excitatory neurotoxicity due to excessive NMDA receptor stimulation and ultimately, neuronal damage. Based on animal studies and preclinical trials, it has been proposed that under these noxious stimuli, ketamine, through blocking glutamate binding to NMDA receptors, has neuroprotective effects [1, 158–161]. The neuroprotective properties of NMDA receptor inhibition have led to speculation that drugs like ketamine may be used for therapeutic or prophylactic purposes in various neurodegenerative conditions [158].

Apoptosis, or programmed cell death, of neurons in the developing and aging adult brains of animals has been associated with inhaled anesthetics (isoflurane, halothane), nitrous oxide, ethanol, propofol, benzodiazepines, barbiturates, anticonvulsants, and ketamine [162–167]. To address growing concerns about the effects of anesthetic drugs on the developing brain, Strategies for Mitigating Anesthesia-Related Neurotoxicity in Tots (SmartTots) was established by the US Food and Drug Administration (FDA) in partnership with the International Anesthesia Research Society (IARS) in 2009 [168]. SmartTots, FDA, and the American Academy of Pediatrics developed a consensus statement which summarized current knowledge and recognized the limitations in data that preclude definitive statements on general anesthesia in young children; however, this group recommended that elective surgical procedures performed under anesthesia be avoided in children less than 3 years of age. Updates in 2014 and 2015 strengthened their previous statement; essentially, surgical procedures performed under general anesthesia should be avoided in children under 3 years of age unless urgently required or potentially harmful if not performed [164, 168]. The 2015 consensus statement emphasized that many questions regarding the effects of anesthetic drugs on developing brains, including which specific drugs and combinations of drugs, timing and duration of exposure represent the greatest risk, and how best to test for these effects, remain to be answered [168].

The neurotoxic and neuroprotective effects of ketamine in rats were first reported by Olney in 1989 [158]. Inadequate stimulation of NMDA receptors, as seen with ketamine blockade, is believed to accelerate neuroapoptosis in young, developing brains. Subsequent rodent and primate studies have implicated ketamine as a causative agent of neuronal degeneration and nerve cell death [159–162, 165, 167, 169–172]. These studies administered ketamine to animals at much higher doses (25–50 mg/kg), sequentially, and over lengthy periods of time as opposed to the one or two doses of ketamine, 1–2 mg/kg, which is typically administration to children outside the operating room for brief procedural sedation. Implications of the results of animal studies and the extrapolation of these results to humans are essentially unknown and have been rigorously debated [162].

The potential neurotoxic effects of ketamine on the developing brain have been demonstrated in a series of animal studies [158, 159, 167, 172]. In other animal studies, ketamine has been shown to have a CNS-protective effect by inhibiting inflammation [158, 160]. A recent review by Yan et al. concluded that the effects of ketamine on the brain varies not only on the basis of the dose and frequency of exposure but also the intensity of the noxious stimuli occurring at time of administration [160]. Repeated ketamine doses may be neurotoxic to immature brains in the absence of noxious stimuli, whereas it may be neuroprotective in the same brains in the presence of strong painful stimulation [160].

While it is clear that the effects of ketamine and other general anesthetic, sedative, and anticonvulsant drugs on the developing human brain represent a complex process, to determine the greatest risks and definitive answers to the many questions raised about neurotoxicity, prospective investigation of children with long-term neuropsychological follow-up will be required [17, 162]. In the meantime, recommendations by SmartTots and others [163, 164, 168] that general anesthesia and sedation be limited whenever possible seem appropriate. However, despite the potential risk of neurotoxicity, ketamine remains one of the best options available to facilitate the performance of relatively brief, painful procedures. The absence or restriction of ketamine availability for procedural sedation of emergent conditions would have major implications on care currently provided to children in the emergency department as well as the operating room [162]. Alternative agents, which may be less efficacious and safe than ketamine, would have to be found to facilitate the performance of painful procedures, and many children, who currently receive sedation in the emergency department for painful procedures, would subsequently require general anesthesia in the operating room were ketamine to become unavailable or its use restricted.

Nonmedical Use

As early as the first half of the 1970s, ketamine was being used recreationally in California, initially by Vietnam veterans who had experienced ketamine on the battlefield [6, 173]. Like other "club drugs" or "rave party" drugs such as MDMA (ecstasy), gamma-hydroxybutyric acid (GHB), and flunitrazepam, recreational ketamine abuse has been associated with dependence and adverse effects. Important adverse effects associated with recreational ketamine use include impairments of memory, hepatobiliary, and urinary pathology (K-cramps and cystitis), as well as sudden death [173–177]. Although death has been attributed to ketamine overdose alone, ketamine fatalities are generally related to polypharmacy ingestion or traumatic injuries from falls or traffic collisions associated with ketamine effects of disorientation and impairment of coordination and function [6, 173, 177].

The number of street names associated with ketamine provides insights into its growing popularity: K, Ket, Vitamin K, Super K, Special K, Lady K, KitKat, Kizzo, Keller, Cat Valium, Jet, Super Acid, Bump, Monkey Mix, Monkey Business, Special LA Coke, Barry Keddle, HOSS, The Hoos, Hossalar, kurdamin, and tranq have all been attributed to ketamine abuse [1, 4, 13]. Ketamine is available as a powder which is administered by snorting or inhaling lines [175]. Tablets may be ingested orally and ampoules of liquid ketamine injected intramuscularly or, less commonly, intravenously [6, 175, 178]. Recreational ketamine users report the most appealing aspects of ketamine to be a sense of dreaming or floating, a euphoric rush, tactile and visual distortion or hallucinations, sudden insights into the meaning of one's existence, and with larger doses, out-of-body experiences (dissociation) which are referred to as journeying into the "K-hole" [6, 13, 175, 179]. Unappealing effects of ketamine are memory loss, inability to speak, blurred vision (likely due to nystagmus), lack of coordination, and increased body temperature [175, 179]. The "K-hole" sensation can be frightening to some recreational users of ketamine who described it as a "near-death" experience [6]. Repeated doses of ketamine have been shown to produce chronic impairments to episodic memory after as few as three administrations [176].

Ketamine is commonly self-administered with other substances of abuse, primarily alcohol but also marijuana, benzodiazepines, ecstasy, GHB, cocaine, amyl nitrate, and LSD [6, 179]. Although ketamine is most commonly used for nonmedical purposes in recreationally settings, it has also been implicated as a "date rape" drug and may be used in combination with the other drugs listed above in this capacity [4, 6].

Summary

Ketamine is considered a core medicine (a minimum medical need for a basic health care system) both for adults and children according to the World Health Organization [180]. This statement is supported by ketamine's effectiveness in consistently achieving the dissociated state with powerful analgesia for patients in need of painful procedures coupled with a highly favorable safety profile that includes cardiorespiratory stability and maintenance of intact airway protective reflexes. Initially introduced as an IV anesthetic, ketamine may be administered IV, IM, IN, or orally to achieve dissociation, analgesia, and amnesia of painful procedures. Coadministration of anticholinergics and benzodiazepines does not appear to provide significant clinical benefit as opposed to ondansetron which does decrease ketamine-associated vomiting, especially in older children.

Ketamine use has expanded to effectively and safely provide analgesia at sub-dissociative doses for short- and long-term pain. Pharmacologic restraint with ketamine for patients with excited delirium and out-of-control behavior has proven effective; however, these patients' underlying conditions and ingestions/intoxications place them at significant risk for complications of this therapy. The sympathomimetic effects of ketamine make it an ideal induction agent for rapid sequence intubation in patients with septic shock and hypovolemic shock especially when due to trauma. Caution must be taken in patients who have completely depleted their catecholamine stores as ketamine administration may result in cardiovascular compromise in these patients.

The increased intracranial pressure effect of ketamine appears to only be significant in patients with obstructive lesions and hydrocephalus making ketamine an acceptable option for patients with head injuries. The bronchopulmonary dilatation effects of ketamine show promise in treating bronchospasm and perhaps preventing the need for intubation in patients with severe asthma. Early successes and enthusiasm for ketamine in treating patients with treatment-resistant depression, PTSD, and bipolar disease require further long-term study to clarify the role of ketamine, as well as potential for adverse effects, in the treatment of these mental health conditions.

Like a number of anesthetic, sedative, and anticonvulsant drugs, ketamine causes neurotoxicity in animals when administered in large doses with repeated exposures. The effects of ketamine on the developing and aging human brain when administered in the manner described in this chapter remain to be determined. Until future studies are able to more clearly define and describe the risks of ketamine and other anesthetic/sedative drugs, limiting their use whenever possible in the extremes of age has been recommended. Ketamine has become a drug of abuse with appealing and unappealing qualities as well as important side effects associated with its chronic, unmonitored use. As clinical use of ketamine increases, we can expect a similar increase in its nonmedical use.

The unique and diverse properties of ketamine make it an ideal agent for a wide variety of indications. Despite over 50 years of extensive clinical use and rigorous investigation, many questions remain regarding this commonly administered, indispensable, yet enigmatic drug.

Acknowledgments I wish to acknowledge Dr. Keira Mason for her unwavering support of the multidisciplinary approach to sedation for children outside the operating room and Drs. Bo Kennedy and Steve Green for being my ketamine mentors and colleagues.

References

1. Sinner B, Graf BM. Ketamine. Handb Exp Pharmacol. 2008;182:313–33.
2. Green SM, Roback MG, Krauss B, et al. Predictors of airway and respiratory adverse events with ketamine sedation in the

emergency department: an individual patient data meta-analysis of 8,282 children. Ann Emerg Med. 2009;54:158–68.

3. Green SM, Roback MG, Krauss B, et al. Predictors of emesis and recovery agitation with emergency department ketamine sedation: an individual-patient data meta-analysis of 8,282 children. Ann Emerg Med. 2009;54(2):171–80.e1–4.

4. Domino EF. Taming the ketamine tiger. 1965. Anesthesiology. 2010;113(3):678–84.

5. White PF, Way WL, Trevor AJ. Ketamine-its pharmacology and therapeutic uses. Anesthesiology. 1982;56:119–36.

6. Wolff K, Winstock AR. Ketamine. From medicine to misuse. CNS Drugs. 2006;20(3):199–218

7. Sin B, Ternas T, Motov SM. The use of subdissociative-dose ketamine for acute pain in the emergency department. Acad Emerg Med. 2015;22(3):251–7.

8. Wiel E, Zitouni D, Assez N. Continuous infusion of ketamine for out-of-hospital isolated orthopedic injuries secondary to trauma: a randomized controlled trial. Prehosp Emerg Care. 2015;19:10–6.

9. Patanwala AE, McKinney CB, Erstad BL, Sakles JC. Retrospective analysis of etomidate versus ketamine for first-pass intubation success in an academic emergency department. Acad Emerg Med. 2014;21:88–91

10. Kiureghian E, Kowalski JM. Intravenous ketamine to facilitate noninvasive ventilation in a patient with a severe asthma exacerbation. Am J Emerg Med. 2015;33:1720.e1–1720.e2.

11. Keseg D, Cortez E, Rund D, et al. The use of prehospital ketamine for control of agitation in a metropolitan firefighter-based EMS system. Prehosp Emerg Care. 2015;19:110–5.

12. Feder A, Parides MK, Murrough JW, et al. Efficacy of intravenous ketamine for treatment of chronic posttraumatic stress disorder: a randomized clinical trial. JAMA Psychiatry. 2014;1(6):681–8.

13. Li JH, Vicknasingam B, Cheung Y, et al. To use or not to use: an update on licit and illicit ketamine use. Subst Abuse Rehabil. 2011;2:11–20.

14. Domino EF, Chodoff P, Corssen G. Pharmacologic effects of CI-581, a new dissociative anesthetic, in man. Clin Pharmacol Ther. 1965;6(3):279–86.

15. Corssen G, Domino EF. Dissociative anesthesia: further pharmacologic studies and first clinical experience with the phencyclidine derivative CI-581. Anesth Analg. 1966;45(1):29–40.

16. Green SM, Johnson NE. Ketamine sedation for pediatric procedures: part 2, review and implications. Ann Emerg Med. 1990;19:1033–46.

17. Green SM, Roback MG, Kennedy RM, et al. Clinical practice guideline for emergency department ketamine dissociative sedation in children: 2011 update. Ann Emerg Med. 2011;57:449–61.

18. Bhargava R, Young KD. Procedural pain management patterns in academic pediatric emergency departments. Acad Emerg Med. 2007;14(5):479–82.

19. Reich DL, Silvay G. Ketamine: an update on the first twenty-five years of clinical experience. Can J Anaesth. 1989;36(2):186–97.

20. Bergman SA. Ketamine: a review of its pharmacology and its use in pediatric anesthesia. Anesth Prog. 1999;46:10–20.

21. Kennedy RM. Sedation in the emergency department: a complex and multifactorial challenge. In: Mason KP, editor. Pediatric sedation outside the operating room: a multispecialty international collaboration. New York: Springer; 2015.

22. Ramaswamy P, Babl FE, Deasy C, et al. Pediatric procedural sedation with ketamine: time to discharge after intramuscular versus intravenous administration. Acad Emerg Med. 2009;16:101–7.

23. Chinta SS, Schrock CR, McAllister JD, et al. Rapid administration technique of ketamine for pediatric forearm fracture reduction: a dose-finding study. Ann Emerg Med. 2015;65(6):640–8. e2.

24. Sahyoun C, Krauss B. Clinical implications of pharmacokinetics and pharmacodynamics of procedural sedation agents in children. Curr Opin Pediatr. 2012;24:225–32.

25. Roback MG, Wathen JE, Mackenzie T, Bajaj L. A randomized, controlled trial of iv vs. im ketamine for sedation of pediatric patients receiving emergency department orthopedic procedures. Ann Emerg Med. 2006;48:605–12.

26. Deasy C, Babl FE. Intravenous vs intramuscular ketamine for pediatric procedural sedation by emergency medicine specialists: a review. Pediatr Anesth. 2010;20:787–96.

27. Wolfe T. Sedation: intranasal sedatives. Available at: http://www.intranasal.net/. Accessed Jan 2016.

28. Graudins A, Meek R, Egerton-Warburton D. The PICHFORK (pain in children fentanyl or ketamine) trial: a randomized controlled trial comparing intranasal ketamine and fentanyl for the relief of moderate to server pain in children with limb injuries. Ann Emerg Med. 2015;65(3):248–54.

29. Andolfatto G, Willman E, Joo D, et al. Intranasal ketamine for analgesia in the emergency department: a prospective observational series. Acad Emerg Med. 2013;20:1050–4.

30. Diaz JH. Intranasal ketamine preinduction of paediatric outpatients. Paediatr Anaesth. 1997;7:273–8.

31. Weber F, Wulf H, el Saeidi G. Premedication with nasal s-ketamine and midazolam provides good conditions for induction of anesthesia in preschool children. Can J Anaesth. 2003;50:470–5.

32. Tsze DS, Steele DW, Machan JT, et al. Intranasal ketamine for procedural sedation in pediatric laceration repair. Pediatr Emerg Care. 2012;28:767–70.

33. Barkan S, Breitbart R, Brenner-Zada G, et al. A double-blind, randomized, placebo-controlled trial of oral midazolam plus oral ketamine for sedation of children during laceration repair. Emerg Med J. 2014;31(8):649–53.

34. Younge PA, Kendall JM. Sedation for children requiring wound repair: a randomized controlled double blind comparison of oral midazolam and oral ketamine. Emerg Med J. 2001;18:30–3.

35. Brown L, Christian-Kopp S, Sherwin TS, et al. Adjunctive atropine is unnecessary during ketamine sedation in children. Acad Emerg Med. 2008;15(4):314–8.

36. Kye YC, Rhee JE, Kim K, et al. Clinical effects of adjunctive atropine during ketamine sedation in pediatric emergency patients. Am J Emerg Med. 2012;30:1981–5.

37. Green SM, Roback MG, Krauss B. Anticholinergics and ketamine sedation in children: an observational analysis of atropine versus glycopyrrolate. Acad Emerg Med. 2010;17:157–62.

38. Flick RP, Wilder RT, Pieper SF, et al. Risk factors for laryngospasm in children during general anesthesia. Pediatr Anesth. 2008;18:289–96.

39. Green SM, Roback MG, Krauss B. Emergency department ketamine meta-analysis study group. Laryngospasm during emergency department ketamine sedation: a case control study. Pediatr Emerg Care. 2010;26(11):798–802.

40. Wathen J, Roback MG, Mackenzie T, Bothner JP. Does midazolam alter the clinical effects of intravenous ketamine sedation in children- a double blind, prospective, emergency department report. Ann Emerg Med. 2000;36:579–88.

41. Roback MG, Wathen JE, Bajaj L, Bothner JP. Adverse events with procedural sedation and analgesia in a pediatric emergency department: a comparison of common parenteral drugs. Acad Emerg Med. 2005;12:508–13.

42. Green SM, Rothrock SG, Lynch EL, et al. Intramuscular ketamine for pediatric sedation in the emergency department: safety profile with 1,022 cases. Ann Emerg Med. 1998;31:688–97.

43. Cohen VG, Krauss B. Recurrent episodes of intractable laryngospasm during dissociative sedation with intramuscular ketamine. Pediatr Emerg Care. 2006;22(4):247–9.

44. Lippmann M, Karnwal A, Julka IS. Cardiovascular effects of ketamine in sick patients: should physicians be concerned? J Clin Pharmacol. 2010;50:482.

45. Lippmann M, Appel PL, Mok MS, Shoemaker WC. Sequential cardiorespiratory patterns of anesthetic induction with ketamine in critically ill patients. Crit Care Med. 1983;11:730–4.

46. L'Hommedieu CS, Arens JJ. The use of ketamine for the emergency intubation of patients with status asthmaticus. Ann Emerg Med. 1987;16(5):568–71.

47. Jabre P, Combes X, Lapostolle F, et al. Etomidate versus ketamine for rapid sequence intubation in acutely ill patients; a multicentre randomised controlled trial. Lancet. 2009;374:293–300.

48. Hamza J, Ecoffey C, Gross JB. Ventilatory response to CO2 following intravenous ketamine in children. Anesthesiology. 1989;70(3):422–5.

49. Corssen G, Butierrez J, Feves JG, Huber FC. Ketamine in the anesthetic management of asthmatic patients. Anesth Anal. 1972;51(4):588–94.

50. Denmark TK, Crane HA, Brown L. Ketamine to avoid mechanical ventilation in severe pediatric asthma. J Emerg Med. 2006;30 (2):163–6.

51. Shlamovitz GZ, Hawthorne T. Intravenous ketamine in a dissociating dose as a temporizing measure to avoid mechanical ventilation in adult patient with severe asthma exacerbation. J Emerg Med. 2011;41(5):492–4.

52. Allen JY, Macias CG. The efficacy of ketamine in pediatric emergency department patients who present with acute severe asthma. Ann Emerg Med. 2005;46:43–50.

53. Howton JC, Rose J, Duffy S, et al. Randomized, double-blind, placebo-controlled trial of intravenous ketamine in acute asthma. Ann Emerg Med. 1996;27:170–5.

54. Cohen L, Athaide V, Wickham ME. The effect of ketamine on intracranial and cerebral perfusion pressure and health outcomes: a systematic review. Ann Emerg Med. 2015;65:43–51.

55. Bar-Joseph G, Guilburd Y, Tamir A, Guilburd JN. Effectiveness of ketamine in decreasing intracranial pressure in children with intracranial hypertension. J Neurosurg Pediatr. 2009;4:40–6.

56. Sehdev RS, Symmons DAD, Kindl K. Ketamine for rapid sequence induction in patients with head injury in the emergency department. Emerg Med Australas. 2006;18:37–44.

57. Green SM, Andolfatto G, Krauss BS. Ketamine and intracranial pressure: no contraindication except hydrocephalus. Ann Emerg Med. 2015;65:52–4.

58. Drayna PC, Estrada C, Wang W, et al. Ketamine sedation is not associated with clinically meaningful elevation of intraocular pressure. Am J Emerg Med. 2012;30:1215–8.

59. Halstead SM, Deakyne SJ, Bajaj L, et al. The effect of ketamine on intraocular pressure in pediatric patients during procedural sedation. Acad Emerg Med. 2012;19:1145–50.

60. Motov S, Rockoff B, Cohen V, et al. Intravenous subdissociative-dose ketamine versus morphine for analgesia in the emergency department: a randomized controlled trial. Ann Emerg Med. 2015;66:222–9.

61. Miller JP, Schauer SG, Ganem VJ. Low-dose ketamine vs morphine for acute pain in the ED: a randomized controlled trial. Am J Emerg Med. 2015;33:402–8.

62. Ahern TL, Herring AA, Anderson ES, et al. The first 500: initial experience with widespread use of low-dose ketamine for acute pain management in the ED. Am J Emerg Med. 2015;33:197–201.

63. Corssen G, Dget S. Dissociative anesthesia for the severely burned child. Anesth Analg. 1971;50:95–102.

64. Phillips LA, Seruvatu SG, Rika PN. Anaesthesia for the surgeon-anaesthetist in difficult situations. Anaesthesia. 1970;25:36–45.

65. Walker AK. Intramuscular ketamine in a developing country. Anaesthesia. 1972;27:408–14.

66. Trouwborst A, Weber BK, Dufour D. Medical statistics of battlefield casualties. Injury. 1987;18:96–9.

67. White PF. Use of continuous infusion versus intermittent bolus administration of fentanyl or ketamine during outpatient anesthesia. Anesthesiology. 1983;59:294–300.

68. Cravero J, Blike GT, Beach ML, et al. Incidence and nature of adverse events during pediatric sedation/anesthesia for procedures outside the operating room: a report from the Pediatric Sedation Research Consortium. Pediatrics. 2006;118:1087–96.

69. Kennedy RM, Porter FL, Miller P, et al. Comparison of fentanyl/midazolam with ketamine/midazolam for pediatric orthopedic emergencies. Pediatrics. 1998;102(4):956–63.

70. McQueen A, Wright RO, Kido MM, et al. Procedural sedation and analgesia outcomes in children after discharge from the emergency department: ketamine versus fentanyl/midazolam. Ann Emerg Med. 2009;54:191–7.

71. Miner JR, Burton JH. Clinical practice advisory: emergency department procedural sedation with propofol. Ann Emerg Med. 2007;50:182–7.

72. Cravero J, Beach ML, Blike GT, et al. The incidence and nature of adverse events during pediatric sedation/anesthesia with propofol for procedures outside the operating room: a report from the Pediatric Sedation Research Consortium. Anesth Analg. 2009;108(3):795–804.

73. Vespasiano M, Finkelstein M, Kurachek S. Propofol sedation: intensivists' experience with 7304 cases in a children's hospital. Pediatrics. 2007;120:e1411–7.

74. Kamat PP, McCracken CE, Gillespie SE, et al. Pediatric critical care physician-administered procedural sedation using propofol: a report from the pediatric sedation research consortium database. Pediatr Crit Care Med. 2015;16(1):11–20.

75. Godambe SA, Elliot V, Matheny D, et al. Comparison of propofol/fentanyl vs. ketamine/midazolam for brief orthopedic procedural sedation in a pediatric emergency department. Pediatrics. 2003;112:116–23.

76. Uri O, Behrbalk E, Haim A, et al. Procedural sedation with propofol for painful orthopaedic manipulation in the emergency department expedites patient management compared with a midazolam/ketamine regimen. A randomized prospective study. J Bone Joint Surg Am. 2011;93:2255–62.

77. Gottschling S, Meyer S, Krenn T, et al. Propofol versus midazolam/ketamine for procedural sedation in pediatric oncology. J Pediatr Hematol Oncol. 2005;27:471–6.

78. Green SM, Andolfatto G, Krauss B. Ketofol for procedural sedation? Pro and con. Ann Emerg Med. 2011;57:444–8.

79. Willman EV, Andolfatto G. A prospective evaluation of "ketofol" (ketamine/propofol combination) for procedural sedation and analgesia in the emergency department. Ann Emerg Med. 2007;49(1):23–30. Epub 2006 Oct 23.

80. Sharieff GQ, Trocinski DR, Kanegaye JT, et al. Ketamine-propofol combination sedation for fracture reduction in the pediatric emergency department. Pediatr Emerg Care. 2007;23 (12):881–4.

81. Andolfatto G, Willman E. A prospective case series of pediatric procedural sedation and analgesia in the emergency department using single-syringe ketamine-propofol combination (ketofol). Acad Emerg Med. 2010;17:194–201.

82. Andolfatto G, Willman E. A prospective case series of single-syringe ketamine-propofol combination (ketofol) for emergency department procedural sedation and analgesia in adults. Acad Emerg Med. 2011;18:237–45.

83. David H, Shipp J. Combined ketamine/propofol for emergency department procedural sedation. Ann Emerg Med. 2011;57:435–41.

84. Shah A, Mosdossy G, McLeod S, et al. A blinded, randomized controlled trial to evaluate ketamine-propofol versus ketamine

alone for procedural sedation in children. Ann Emerg Med. 2011;57:425–33.

85. Andolfatto G, Abu-Laban RB, Zed PJ, et al. Ketamine-propofol combination (ketofol) versus propofol alone for emergency department procedural sedation and analgesia: a randomized double-blind trial. Ann Emerg Med. 2012;59:504–12.

86. Miner JR, Moore JC, Austad EJ, et al. Randomized, double-blinded clinical trial of propofol, 1:1 propofol/ketamine, and 4:1 propofol/ketamine for deep procedural sedation in the emergency department. Ann Emerg Med. 2015;65:479–88.

87. Green SM, Andolfatto G, Krauss BS. Ketofol for procedural sedation revisited: pro and con. Ann Emerg Med. 2015;65 (5):489–91.

88. Olney J, Newcomer JW, Farber NB. NMDA receptor hypofunction model of schizophrenia. J Psychiatr Res. 1999;33:523–33.

89. Frohlich J, Van Horn JD. Reviewing the ketamine model for schizophrenia. J Psychopharmacol. 2014;28(4):287–302.

90. Treston G, Bell A, Cardwell R, Fincher G, Chand D, Cashion G. What is the nature of the emergence phenomenon when using intravenous or intramuscular ketamine for paediatric procedural sedation? Emerg Med Australas. 2009;21(4):315–22.

91. Morgan M, Loh L, Singer L, Moore PH. Ketamine as the sole anaesthetic agent for minor surgical procedures. Anaesthesia. 1971;26(2):158–65.

92. Vlajkovic GP, Sindjelic RP. Emergence delirium in children: many questions, few answers. Anesth Analg. 2007;104:84–91.

93. Sherwin TS, Green SM, Khan A, et al. Does adjunctive midazolam reduce recovery agitation after ketamine sedation for pediatric procedures? A randomized, double-blind, placebo-controlled trial. Ann Emerg Med. 2000;35(3):229–38.

94. Green SM, Sherwin TS. Incidence and severity of recovery agitation after ketamine sedation in young adults. Am J Emerg Med. 2005;23:142–4.

95. Sener S, Eken C, Schultz CH, et al. Ketamine with and without midazolam for emergency department sedation in adults: a randomized controlled trial. Ann Emerg Med. 2011;57 (2):109–114.e2.

96. Bhatt M, Kennedy R, Osmond MH, Krauss B, et al., Consensus Panel on Sedation Research of Pediatric Emergency Research Canada (PERC) and the Pediatric Emergency Care Applied Research Network (PECARN). Consensus-based recommendations for standardizing terminology and reporting adverse events for emergency department procedural sedation and analgesia in children. Ann Emerg Med. 2009;53:426–35.e4.

97. Green SM, Yealy DM. Procedural sedation goes Utstein: the Quebec guidelines. Ann Emerg Med. 2009;53:436–8.

98. Hostetler MA, Davis CO. Prospective age-based comparison of behavioral reactions occurring after ketamine sedation in the ED. Am J Emerg Med. 2002;20(5):463–8.

99. Kain ZN, Caldwell-Andrews AA, Maranets I, et al. Preoperative anxiety and emergence delirium and postoperative maladaptive behaviors. Anesth Analg. 2004;99(6):1648–54.

100. Kennedy RM, McAllister JD. Midazolam with ketamine: who benefits? Ann Emerg Med. 2000;35(3):297–9.

101. Kain ZN, Mayes LC, Wang SM, Hofstadter MB. Postoperative behavioral outcomes in children: effects of sedative premedication. Anesthesiology. 1999;90(3):758–65.

102. Strayer RJ, Nelson LS. Adverse events associated with ketamine for procedural sedation in adults. Am J Emerg Med. 2008;26:985–1028.

103. Langston WT, Wathen JE, Roback MG, et al. Effect of ondansetron on the incidence of vomiting associated with ketamine sedation in children—a double-blind, randomized placebo controlled trial. Ann Emerg Med. 2008;52(1):30–4.

104. Lee JS, Jeon WC, Park EJ, et al. Adjunctive atropine vs. metoclopramide: can we reduce ketamine-associated vomiting in young children? A prospective, randomized, open, controlled study. Acad Emerg Med. 2012;19:1128–33.

105. Kinder KL, Lehman-Huskamp KL, Gerard JM. Do children with high body mass indices have a higher incidence of emesis when undergoing ketamine sedation? Pediatr Emerg Care. 2012;28:1203–5.

106. Thorp AW, Brown L, Green SM. Ketamine-associated vomiting. Is it dose-related? Pediatr Emerg Care. 2009;25(1):15–8.

107. Treston G. Prolonged pre-procedure fasting time is unnecessary when using titrated intravenous ketamine for paediatric procedural sedation. Emerg Med Australas. 2004;16:145–50.

108. McKee MR, Sharieff GQ, Kanegaye JT, et al. Oral analgesia before pediatric ketamine sedation is not associated with an increased risk of emesis and other adverse events. J Emerg Med. 2008;35(1):23–8.

109. Pena BMG, Krauss B. Adverse events of procedural sedation and analgesia in a pediatric emergency department. Ann Emerg Med. 1999;34:483–90.

110. Roback MG, Bajaj LB, Wathen J, et al. Preprocedural fasting and adverse events in procedural sedation and analgesia in a pediatric emergency department—are they related? Ann Emerg Med. 2004;44:454–9.

111. Agrawal D, Manzi SF, Gupta R, et al. Preprocedural fasting state and adverse events in children undergoing procedural sedation and analgesia in a pediatric emergency department. Ann Emerg Med. 2003;42:636–46.

112. Corssen G, Little SC, Tavakoli M. Ketamine and epilepsy. Anesth Analg. 1974;53(2):319–35.

113. Pruss H, Holtkamp M. Ketamine successfully terminates malignant status epilepticus. Epilepsy Res. 2008;82:219–22.

114. Teodorowicz J, Zimny M. The effect of ketamine in patients with refractory hiccup in the postoperative period. Preliminary report. Anaesth Resusc Intensive Ther. 1975;3(3):271–2.

115. Shantha TR. Ketamine for the treatment of hiccups during and following anesthesia: a preliminary report. Anesth Analg. 1973;52 (5):822–4.

116. Petrenko AB, Yamakura T, Baba H, Shimoji K. The role of N-Methyl-D-Aspartate (NMDA) receptors in pain: a review. Anesth Analg. 2003;97:1108–16.

117. Guirimand F, Dupont X, Brasseur L, et al. The effects of ketamine on the temporal summation (wind-up) of the R_{III} nociceptive flexion reflex and pain in humans. Anesth Analg. 2000;90:408–14.

118. Angst MS, Clark JD. Opioid-induced hyperalgesia. A qualitative systematic review. Anesthesiology. 2006;104:570–87.

119. Laulin JP, Maurette P, Corcuff JB, et al. The role of ketamine in preventing fentanyl-induced hyperalgesia and subsequent acute morphine tolerance. Anesth Analg. 2002;94:1263–9.

120. Menigaux C, Fletcher D, Dupont X. The benefits of intraoperative small-dose ketamine on postoperative pain after anterior cruciate ligament repair. Anesth Analg. 2000;90:129–35.

121. Menigaux C, Guignard B, Fletcher D, et al. Intraoperative small-dose ketamine enhances analgesia after outpatient knee arthroscopy. Anesth Analg. 2001;93:606–12.

122. Fu ES, Miguel R, Scharf JE. Preemptive ketamine decreases postoperative narcotic requirements in patients undergoing abdominal surgery. Anesth Anal. 1997;84:1086–90.

123. Becke K, Albrecht S, Schmitz B, et al. Intraoperative low dose S-ketamine has no preventive effects on postoperative pain and morphine consumption after major urological surgery in children. Pediatr Anesth. 2005;15:484–90.

124. Carstensen M, Moller AM. Adding ketamine to morphine for intravenous patient-controlled analgesia for acute postoperative

pain: a qualitative review of randomized trials. Br J Anaesth. 2010;104(4):401–6.

125. Goltser A, Soleyman-Zomalan E, Kresch F, Motov S. Short (low dose) ketamine infusion for managing acute pain in the ED: case-report series. Am J Emerg Med. 2015;33:601.e5–601.e7.

126. Lester L, Braude DA, Niles C, Crandall CS. Low-dose ketamine for analgesia in the ED: a retrospective case series. Am J Emerg Med. 2010;28:820–7.

127. Galinski M, Dolveck F, Combes X. Management of severe acute pain in emergency settings: ketamine reduces morphine consumption. Am J Emerg Med. 2007;25:385–90.

128. Gurnani A, Sharma PK, Rautela RS, Bhattacharya A. Analgesia for acute musculoskeletal trauma: low-dose subcutaneous infusion of ketamine. Anaesth Intensive Care. 1996;24(1):32–6.

129. Messenger DW, Murray HE, Dungey PE, et al. Subdissociative dose ketamine versus fentanyl for analgesia during propofol procedural sedation: a randomized clinical trial. Acad Emerg Med. 2008;15:877–86.

130. Svenson JE, Abernathy MK. Ketamine for prehospital use: new look at an old drug. Am J Emerg Med. 2007;25:977–80.

131. Johansson J, Sjoberg J, Nordgren M, et al. Prehospital analgesia using nasal administration of s-ketamine- a case series. Scand J Trauma Resusc Emerg Med. 2013;21:38.

132. Tran KP, Nguyen Q, Truong XN, et al. A comparison of ketamine and morphine analgesia in prehospital trauma care: a cluster randomized clinical trial in rural Quang Tri Province, Vietnam. Prehosp Emerg Care. 2014;18:257–64.

133. Jennings PA, Cameron P, Bernard S, et al. Morphine and ketamine is superior to morphine alone for out-of-hospital trauma analgesia: a randomized controlled trial. Ann Emerg Med. 2012;59:497–503.

134. Petz LN, Tyner S, Barnard E, et al. Prehospital and en route analgesic use in the combat setting: a prospectively designed, multicenter, observational study. Mil Med. 2015;180(3):14–8.

135. Shackelford SA, Fowler M, Schultz K, et al. Prehospital pain medication use by U.S. forces in Afghanistan. Mil Med. 2015;180(3):304–9.

136. ACEP Excited Delirium Task Force. White paper report on excited delirium syndrome. September 10, 2009. Available at: http://www.academia.edu/1131068/ACEP_Excited_Delirium_ White_Paper_-_Contribution_via_CA_Hall_MD_FRCPC. Accessed 22 Feb 2016.

137. Vilke GM, BeBard ML, Chan TC, et al. Excited delirium syndrome (EXDS): defining based on a review of the literature. J Emerg Med. 2012;43(5):897–905.

138. Green SM, Andolfatto G. Let's "take 'em down" with a ketamine blow dart. Ann Emerg Med. 2016;67:588–90.

139. Kowalski JM, Kopec KT, Lavelle J, Osterhoudt K. A novel agent for management of agitated delirium. A case series of ketamine utilization in the pediatric emergency department. Pediatr Emerg Care. 2015 (Epub ahead of print).

140. Roberts JR, Geeting GK. Intramuscular ketamine for the rapid tranquilization of the uncontrollable, violent, and dangerous adult patient. J Trauma. 2001;51(5):1008–10.

141. Hick JL, Ho JD. Ketamine chemical restraint to facilitate rescue of a combative "jumper". Prehosp Emerg Care. 2005;9(1):85–9.

142. Ho JD, Smith SW, Nystrom PC. Successful management of excited delirium syndrome with prehospital ketamine: two case examples. Prehosp Emerg Care. 2013;17:274–9.

143. Burnett AM, Salzman JG, Griffith KR, et al. The emergency department experience with prehospital ketamine: a case series of 13 patients. Prehosp Emerg Care. 2012;16:553–9.

144. Scheppke KA, Braghiroli J, Shalaby M, et al. Prehospital use of im ketamine for sedation of violent and agitated patients. West J Emerg Med. 2014;15(7):736–41.

145. Isbister GK, Calver LA, Downes MA, Page CB. Ketamine as rescue treatment for difficult-to-sedate severe acute behavioral disturbance in the emergency department. Ann Emerg Med. 2016;67:581–7.

146. Krystal JH, Karper LP, Seibyl JP, Freeman GK, Delaney R, Bremner JD, Heninger GR, Bowers Jr MB, Charney DS. Subanesthetic effects of the noncompetitive NMDA antagonist, ketamine, in humans. Psychotomimetic, perceptual, cognitive, and neuroendocrine responses. Arch Gen Psychiatry. 1994;51:199–214.

147. Berman RM, Cappiello A, Anand A, Oren DA, Heninger GR, Charney DS, Krystal JH. Antidepressant effects of ketamine in depressed patients. Biol Psychiatr. 2000;47:351–4.

148. Correll GE, Futter GE. Two case studies of patients with major depressive disorder given low dose (subanesthetic) ketamine infusions. Pain Med. 2006;7:92–5.

149. Zarate CA, Singh JB, Carlson PJ, Brutsche NE, Ameli R, Luckenbaugh DA, Charney DS, Manji HK. A randomized trial of an N-methyl-D-aspartate antagonist in treatment resistant depression. Arch Gen Psychiatry. 2006;63:856–64.

150. Rasmussen KG, LIneberry TW, Galardy CW, et al. Serial infusion of low-dose ketamine for major depression. J Psychopharm. 2013;27(5):444–50.

151. Shiroma PR, Johns B, Kuskowski M, et al. Augmentation of response and remission to serial intravenous subanesthetic ketamine in treatment resistant depression. J Affect Dis. 2014;155:123–9.

152. Lapidus KA, Levitch CF, Perez AM, et al. A randomized controlled trial of intranasal ketamine in major depressive disorder. Biol Psychiatry. 2014;76(12):970–6.

153. Kavalali ET, Monteggia LM. Synaptic mechanisms underlying rapid antidepressant action of ketamine. Am J Psychiatry. 2012;169:1150–6.

154. Naughton M, Clarke G, O'Leary OF, et al. A review of ketamine in affective disorders: current evidence of clinical efficacy, limitation of use and preclinical evidence on proposed mechanism of action. J Affect Disord. 2014;156:24–35.

155. Salvadore G, Singh JB. Ketamine as a fast acting antidepressant: current knowledge and open questions. CNS Neurosci Ther. 2013;19(6):428–36.

156. Papolos DF, Teicher MH, Faedda GL, et al. Clinical experience using intranasal ketamine in the treatment of pediatric bipolar disorder/fear of harm phenotype. J Affect Disord. 2013;147:431–6.

157. Donohgue AC, Roback MG, Cullen KR. Remission from behavioral dysregulation in a child with PTSD after receiving procedural ketamine. Pediatrics. 2015;136(3):e694–6.

158. Olney JW, Labruyere J, Price MT. Science. 1989;244 (4910):1360–2.

159. Himmelseher S, Pfenninger E, Georgieff M. The effects of ketamine-isomers on neuronal injury and regeneration in rat hippocampal neurons. Anesth Analg. 1996;83:505–12.

160. Yan J, Jiang H. Dual effects of ketamine: neurotoxicity versus neuroprotection in anesthesia for the developing brain. J Neurosurg Anesthesiol. 2014;26:155–60.

161. Himmelseher S, Duriewx ME. Revising a dogma: ketamine for patients with neurological injury? Anesth Analg. 2005;101:524–34.

162. Green SM, Coté CJ. Ketamine and neurotoxicity: clinical perspectives and implications for emergency medicine. Ann Emerg Med. 2009;54:181–90.

163. Jevtovic-Todorovic V, Absalom AR, Blomgren K, et al. Anaesthetic neurotoxicity and neuroplasticity: an expert group report and statement based on the BJA Salzburg Seminar. Br J Anaesth. 2013;111:143–51.

164. Rappaport BA, Suresh S, Hertz S, et al. Anesthetic neurotoxicity – clinical implication of animal models. N Engl J Med. 2015;372 (9):796–7.

165. Yan J, Li Y, Zhang Y, Lu Y, Jiang H. Repeated exposure to anesthetic ketamine can negatively impact neurodevelopment in infants: a prospective preliminary clinical study. J Child Neurol. 2014;29(10):1333–8.

166. Loepke AW, Soriano SG. An assessment of the effects of general anesthetics on developing brain structure and neurocognitive function. Anesth Analg. 2008;106:1681–707.

167. Hayashi H, et al. Repeated administration of ketamine may lead to neuronal degeneration in the developing rat brain. Paediatr Anaesth. 2002;12:770–4.

168. SmartTots. Consensus Statement Supplement 11/2015. Available at: http://smarttots.org/consensus-statement-supplement/. Accessed 19 Feb 2016.

169. Jevtovic-Todorovic V, Wazniak DF, Benshoff ND, et al. A comparative evaluation of neurotoxic properties of ketamine and nitrous oxide. Brain Res. 2001;895:264–7.

170. Mellon RD, Simone AF, Rappaport BA. Use of anesthetic agents in neonates and young children. Anesth Analg. 2007;104:509–20.

171. Newcomer JW, Farber NB, Jevtovic-Todorovic V, et al. Ketamine-induced NMDA receptor hypofunction as a model of memory impairment and psychosis. Neuropsychopharmacology. 1999;20(2):106–18.

172. Zou X, Patterson TA, Bivine RL, et al. Prolonged exposure to ketamine increases neurodegeneration in the developing monkey brain. Int J Dev Neuosci. 2009;27:727–31.

173. Schifano F, Corkery J, Oyefeso A, et al. Trapped in the "K-hole": overview of deaths associated with ketamine misuse in the UK (1993–2006). J Clin Psychopharmacol. 2008;28:114–6.

174. Wang JW, Kivovich V, Gordon L. Ketamine abuse syndrome. Hepatobiliary and urinary pathology among adolescents in Flushing, NY. Pediatr Emerg Care. 2015 (Epub ahead of print).

175. Muetzelfeldt L, Kamboj SK, Rees H, et al. Journey through the K-hole: phenomenological aspects of ketamine use. Drug Alcohol Depend. 2008;95(3):219–29.

176. Morgan CJ, Riccelli M, Maitland CH, Curran HV. Long-term effects of ketamine: evidence for a persisting impairment of source memory in recreational users. Drug Alcohol Depend. 2004;75(3):301–8.

177. Gill JR, Stajic M. Ketamine in non-hospital and hospital deaths in New York City. J Forensic Sci. 2000;45(3):655–8.

178. Lankenau SE, Clatts MC. Drug injection practices among high-risk youths: the first shot of ketamine. J Urban Health. 2004;81 (2):232–48.

179. Dillon P, Copeland J, Jansen K. Patterns of use and harms associated with on-medical ketamine use. Drug Alcohol Depend. 2003;69:23–8.

180. WHO. WHO model lists of essential medicines. 2015 [updated 2015; cited February 11, 2016]; Available from: http://www.who.int/medicines/publications/essentialmedicines/en/.

Neuromuscular Blocking Drugs: Physiology, Pharmacology and Clinical Aspects

Claude Meistelman

Neuromuscular blocking agents (NMBAs) were introduced into clinical anaesthetic practice in 1942, by Griffith and Johnson. They changed the practice of anaesthesia and made possible the development of balanced anaesthesia [1]. The first relaxant was Intoconstrin which was obtained from the plant *Chondrodendron tomentosum*. In the 50 years that have elapsed, numerous compounds have been synthetised and introduced in clinical practice. As earlier stated by Cecil Gray in 1946: "The road lies open before us, we venture to say we have passed yet another milestone, and the distance to our goal is considerably shortened" [2]. NMBAs are a key component for general anaesthesia. The clinical use of muscle relaxants in routine improves intubating conditions and facilitates perioperative surgical conditions and controlled ventilation. It must be remembered that they should be administered to provide muscular relaxation and that they lack analgesic or anaesthetic effects. Recent publications have highlighted that proper use can improve clinical outcome after surgery. The development of new neuromuscular blocking agents (NMBAs), reversal agents and monitoring techniques leads to improved patient safety and outcome. This chapter reviews the physiology, pharmacology and clinical use of NMBA and reversal agents in clinical practice.

Physiology of Neuromuscular Transmission

Each muscle fibre is served by one or at the most three neuromuscular junctions. The nerve cell together with the muscle fibre it innervates is called the "motor unit". The axons make intimate contact with a single muscle fibre, lose their myelin sheath and then branch again to form neuromuscular junction. In mammals, the synapse is 40–60 μm in length and 32 μm in width. It is in close opposition to the muscle fibre, being separated from it by a narrow gap, the synaptic cleft which is 0.02–0.05 μm in width. There are two types of muscle fibres, slow-twitch fibres which tend to have slow contraction times and resistance to fatigue and fast-twitch fibres, which have fast contraction times and are less resistant to fatigue. The nerve terminal contains vesicles of the transmitter acetylcholine, mitochondria and cisternae which are involved in the recycling of the vesicles. Acetylcholinesterase is present in the synaptic cleft and is concentrated in the folds. Neuromuscular transmission starts with the arrival of a nerve action potential at the nerve terminal and concludes with depolarisation of the postjunctional membrane; the whole process takes only a few milliseconds. Nerve cells and muscle fibres are excitable. They can carry electrical impulses in response to an electrical or chemical stimulus. At rest, the internal electrical potential is negative (-90 mV). When a depolarisation above a certain threshold or a less potential occurs, sodium channels open. The density of sodium channels in the perijunctional area is richer than in more distal parts of the muscle membrane. This opening allows sodium to enter the cell. This influx of positive ions opposes the resting membrane potential causing a further depolarisation and hence the opening of more sodium channels in a positive manner. Duration of the action potential is short, less than 1 ms. Termination of the action potential is hastened by activation of voltage-sensitive gated potassium channels; the potassium efflux rapidly terminates the action potential and temporarily hyperpolarises the membrane. After the action potential, there is an increase in the activity of the sodium–potassium pumps to restore the ionic distributions. A peripheral nerve is made up of a large number of axons. Each axon responds in an all-or-none fashion to a stimulus, but axons differ in size or threshold. At low stimulating currents, depolarisation is insufficient in all axons. When the current

C. Meistelman(✉)
Department of Anesthesiology and Intensive Care Medicine, Hôpital de Brabois, Faculté de Médecine de Nancy, rue du Morvan, 54511 Vandœuvre, France
e-mail: c.meistelman@chu-nancy.fr

© Springer International Publishing AG 2017
A.R. Absalom, K.P. Mason (eds.), *Total Intravenous Anesthesia and Target Controlled Infusions*,
DOI 10.1007/978-3-319-47609-4_15

reaches a certain level, all axons will be depolarised and will propagate an action potential.

Release of Acetylcholine

Acetylcholine is the neurotransmitter present at the neuromuscular junction. It is synthetised from choline and acetyl coenzyme A under the influence of the enzyme choline acetyltransferase. About half of the acetylcholine present in each nerve terminal is contained in vesicles which are concentrated near the cell membrane opposite the crests of the junctional folds of the end plate. The rest is dissolved in the axoplasm. Each vesicle contains about 12,000 molecules of acetylcholine when full. The vesicles containing transmitter are arranged in repeating clusters alongside small, thickened, electron-dense patches of membrane, referred to as active zones or release sites.

In the absence of nerve impulses, acetylcholine is continually released spontaneously by packets or quanta from the nerve endings. Each quantum contains about 5000–10,000 molecules. This release causes a small depolarisation (0.5–1.0 mV) of the postjunctional motor end-plate membrane which is called miniature end-plate potential (MEPP). The MEPP is too small to produce a muscular contraction. Except for amplitude, these potentials resemble the end-plate potential in the time course. When acetylcholine is released by a nerve action potential, more than 100 quanta are released simultaneously and produce the full-sized EPP. When the EPP is above threshold (-50 mV), it triggers a muscle action potential. Release of acetylcholine is strongly dependent on extracellular calcium which enters through voltage-gated calcium channels [3]. The soluble N-ethylmaleimide-sensitive factor attachment receptor (SNARE) plays a role in the release of acetylcholine [4]. Then synaptotagmin, a protein of the vesicular membrane, acts as a calcium sensor and localises the synaptic vesicles to synaptic zones rich in calcium channels. If calcium is not present, depolarisation of the nerve, even by electrical stimulation, will not produce release of transmitter. Synaptotagmin fuses with a docking protein (syntaxin), in vesicles in the immediately available store. Binding produces opening of a pore which rapidly expands and release of acetylcholine ensues [5]. Acetylcholine action is very short-lived and is destroyed in less than 1 ms after being released.

Postjunctional Events

Following release and diffusion across the synaptic cleft, acetylcholine interacts with the end plate at the cholinergic receptor. The nicotinic acetylcholine receptor (nAChR) is a complex protein made up of five glycoprotein subunits arranged in a form of rosette. It belongs to the superfamily of Cys-loop ligand-gated ion channels. They are synthetised in muscle cells and anchored to the end-plate membrane by a special 43-kDa protein called rapsyn [6]. Two noncontiguous subunits are identical and called α. The initial receptor called foetal or immature consists of 2 $\alpha 1$ and one each of $\beta 1$, δ and γ subunits ($\alpha 1 \beta 1 \delta \gamma$). Development of innervation in the first weeks of life will lead to the replacement of the γ subunit by ϵ which creates the adult or mature receptor ($\alpha 1 \beta 1 \delta \epsilon$). Each subunit is built upon four transmembrane domains with the second transmembrane segment lining the pore (Fig. 15.1) [7]. Each subunit is composed of approximately 400–500 amino acids.

The receptor channel complex is roughly cylindrical in shape with a length of 11 nm and a diameter of 8.5–9.0 nm. The receptors are clustered on the crests of the junctional folds, the receptor; density in this area is 10,000–30,000/μm^2. There are about 5 million of them in each junction. Two molecules of acetylcholine must bind to the α subunits to induce the conformational changes, which will allow ionic flows. The ion channels of the end-plate region are chemically sensitive and when open cannot discriminate between sodium and potassium which will flow inward and outward. At resting potential the inward movement of sodium will be favoured because sodium will move along its electrical gradient. Accumulation of intracellular sodium makes the inside of the cell less negative. If a large number of receptors open simultaneously, the inside of the cell is depolarised sufficiently to trigger the action potential. The propagation of the action potential to the whole muscle is then independent of acetylcholine receptors. It produces opening of voltage-sensitive calcium channels. Intracellular calcium increases rapidly and binds with troponin which usually inhibits actin and myosin. The immature receptor has a smaller single-channel conductance and a much longer channel open time than the mature receptor.

Prejunctional Events

During high-frequency stimulation, under physiologic conditions, the release of acetylcholine decreases, but it is more than enough to depolarise the end plate above threshold. Small concentrations of acetylcholine increase the evoked release of acetylcholine, whereas D-tubocurarine and other nicotinic antagonists reduced the release, suggesting that acetylcholine may facilitate its own further release. The decrease in acetylcholine release during high-frequency stimulation (train-of-four (TOF), tetanus) in the presence of non-depolarising muscle relaxant (NDMR) drugs explains the progressive decrease in muscle response, i.e. fade. It is likely that this effect is mediated through

Fig. 15.1 Diagram of the
postsynaptic nicotinic
acetylcholine receptor at the
neuromuscular junction with the
five subunits. Each subunit
contains four transmembrane
domains labelled M1 to M4.
Reproduced from Naguib et al.
[7] with permission from Wolters
Kluwer Health, Inc.

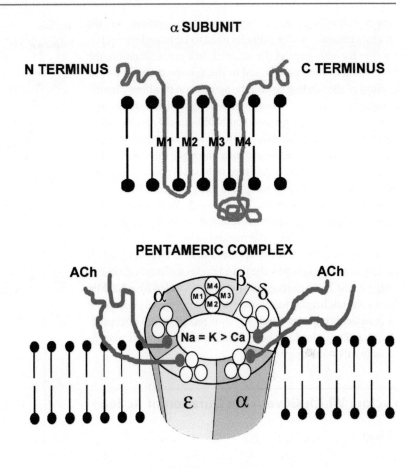

presynaptic receptors. These prejunctional receptors could mediate mobilisation of the reserve store into the readily releasable store in case of high-frequency stimulation [8]. Difference in potencies of nicotinic antagonists at pre- and postjunctional receptors suggests a difference between the two types [9].

Effects of Muscle Relaxants at the Neuromuscular Junction

Depolarising Muscle Relaxants: Succinylcholine

Succinylcholine produces a depolarisation of the end-plate region which is similar to, but more persistent than, that achieved by acetylcholine. This depolarisation induces desensitisation of the nAChR, inactivation of voltage-gated Na^+ channels at the neuromuscular junction and increase of the K^+ permeability in the surrounding membrane. Onset of neuromuscular blockade is characterised by an excitatory state with fasciculations of muscle fibres thought to represent random repetitive neuronal firing. It could be due to the depolarisation of prejunctional receptors; the abolition of fasciculations by D-tubocurarine may represent an action at the presynaptic receptor. The neuromuscular block is

characterised by a twitch response to indirect stimulation which is diminished but sustained with repetitive stimulation. It is associated with end-plate depolarisation and development of a surrounding zone of inexcitability through which a muscle action potential evoked by direct stimulation cannot propagate. During prolonged depolarisation, the muscle may gain sodium and chloride and lose significant amounts of potassium, sufficient to raise serum levels of this ion. Following continuous administration, a "phase II block" characterised by fade and post-tetanic facilitation occurs. One of the mechanisms could be an excessive activation of presynaptic nicotinic receptors, which could lead to reduced transmitter output. "Phase II block" could also be associated with a desensitisation of the end plate, which then becomes refractory to chemical stimulation. Succinylcholine depolarises immature receptors more easily, inducing a significant cation flux. Moreover, once depolarised, the immature receptor will stay open for a longer time.

Non-depolarising Muscle Relaxants (NDMRs)

NDMRs competitively bind at the same site as acetylcholine on the α subunit of the nicotinic postjunctional receptor. The binding of one nicotinic antagonist molecule to one of the two α subunits of the receptor prevents opening of the channel because both α subunits need to be bound by acetylcholine for activation of the channel. In a given situation, the proportion of receptors bound to the agonist depends on the affinity of the binding site for the agonist, on its affinity for the antagonist and on the concentration of agonist and antagonist. Some authors have suggested that NDMR could also block the open receptor because they can have access to the mouth of the open channel but cannot pass through, thus preventing further ionic movement. This type of block is non-competitive but its role is probably marginal. Only a small fraction of receptors need to bind to acetylcholine to produce depolarisation. This has been referred to as the "margin of safety" of the neuromuscular transmission. Non-depolarising neuromuscular block is not apparent until a large number of receptors are occupied by the muscle relaxant. Animal studies suggest that 75 % of receptors must be occupied by a NDMR before twitch height decreases. Blockade is usually complete in peripheral muscles when 92 % of receptors are occupied. Peripheral muscles have been found to have a smaller margin of safety than the diaphragm.

Factors Which Govern the Duration of Action

Onset

There is ample evidence that potent NDMRs have slower onset times than less potent drugs with similar physicochemical properties. These facts can be explained by the concept of the margin of safety. A critical number of receptors at the neuromuscular junction must be occupied before appearance of neuromuscular block, and at least 90 % of the receptors must be occupied before block is complete at the adductor pollicis. When the drug reaches the synaptic cleft, most molecules will bind to receptors which are present with a high density. As the concentration of free drug decreases, more molecules are driven in, and the process will continue until the concentrations of free drug within and outside the synaptic cleft are equal. This process is known as buffered diffusion [10]. When a potent drug is administered, fewer molecules are given than in a case of a less potent drug, and the onset will be slower compared to onset of weak potency NDMR [11]. This phenomenon is probably what contributes to the slower onset time for cisatracurium than atracurium. Based on theoretical calculations and experimental data, the ED95 to produce a short onset of action might be >0.3–0.5 mg/kg (Fig. 15.2) [9]. However, for very short-acting drugs, the ideal ED95 might be greater (0.5–1.0 mg/kg) because rapid metabolism destroys some of the muscle relaxant given before it reaches the neuromuscular junction [12]. This phenomenon can explain the relatively slow onset time for mivacurium.

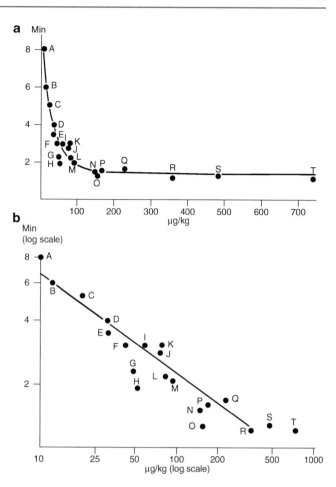

Fig. 15.2 The relationship between effective dose and onset time for 20 chemically related aminosteroidal neuromuscular blocking drugs. The effective dose (abscissa) is the mean dose to produce 50 % twitch depression of the tibialis anterior. Reproduced from Bowman et al. [9] with permission from Wolters Kluwer Health, Inc.

Plasma concentrations have only modest influence on onset time. Arterial plasma concentrations peak 25–35 s after administration thus before onset of neuromuscular block. This paradox can be explained by assuming that the site of action, the neuromuscular junction, is represented by the effect compartment in which the concentration of the NMBA is directly related to the magnitude of neuromuscular blockade [13]. As usual the model will include a rate constant for transfer into the effect compartment and another rate constant for transfer out of this compartment. The obtained k_{e0} or more appropriately the $T_{1/2ke0}$ is related to the time required to fill or empty the effect compartment for a constant plasma concentration. The k_{e0} is similar for most intermediate-duration action NMBAs and corresponds approximately to neuromuscular junction blood flow divided by neuromuscular junction/plasma partition coefficient. Whatever muscle relaxant, the limiting factor appears to be the time required for the drug to reach the neuromuscular junction which in turn depends on cardiac output, the distance of the muscle from the central circulation, and muscle blood flow. Therefore in most cases, the onset time will be dependent on blood flow to muscle. It has been demonstrated that in dogs time to maximum blockade was decreased when blood flow increased, whereas recovery was not affected by blood flow [14]. Under normal circumstances, muscle blood flow increases when cardiac output increases, with a direct relationship between speed of onset and cardiac output. This might explain why infants and children have a faster onset of action of NMB and elderly patients have a slower onset than younger individuals. It has been demonstrated that vecuronium-induced onset of NMB was shorter with etomidate than with either thiopental or propofol and onset time was longer if hypotension was present [15].

It is obvious that the intensity of maximum blockade is affected directly by the administered dose. However when the dose increases in the sub-paralysing range, that is, when maximum blockade is between 0 and 100 %, time to reach maximum effect is dose independent. This is because the time to peak concentration at the effect compartment is independent of the dose. When the administered dose is sufficient to obtain complete disappearance of the neuromuscular response, time to maximum blockade becomes dose dependent. For many years, it was believed that shorter-acting NMBA would have a faster onset time than long-acting NMBA. Many studies have shown that atracurium or vecuronium onset times were comparable to that of pancuronium. The lack of effect of elimination of these drugs on onset time is explained by the fact that these NMBAs are eliminated too slowly to see any difference.

Duration of Action

Although it is commonly believed that the rate of decline of NMBA plasma concentrations during recovery from neuromuscular blockade determines the duration of action and the rate of recovery, further explanations are needed. It has been suggested that muscle blood flow is, to a certain extent, a limiting factor for the termination of action. For long-acting NMBA, the dominant effect for the recovery from neuromuscular blockade is the rate of decrease of plasma concentration because there is a pseudoequilibrium between concentrations at the neuromuscular junction and the plasma. Therefore changing blood flow will not affect the duration of action. For intermediate-duration action NMBA, after a single bolus dose, plasma concentrations decrease at a rate that differs slightly from the equilibrium half-life with muscle. It can induce a significant

concentration gradient between neuromuscular junction and plasma during recovery, but provided that recovery rate is constant, the ratio of concentrations between the neuromuscular junction and plasma will remain relatively constant.

The most important issue is that the rate of decline of plasma concentration during recovery is not always related to the NMBA terminal half-life because after initial administration, plasma concentrations will decrease because of redistribution. It is only when redistribution will be complete that the decrease in plasma concentrations will be dependent of the terminal half-life and will decrease more slowly. For long-acting NMBA such as pancuronium, the recovery time will take place during the terminal half-life. In this situation, the duration of action will be dependent on the rate of decrease of plasma concentrations. It is different for intermediate-duration action NMBA. The terminal half-life of atracurium is around 20 min, whereas the elimination half-lives of both vecuronium and atracurium are between 60 and 120 min. Although such differences can be observed, the duration of action and recovery from neuromuscular block of these three drugs is very similar. These apparent discrepancies can be explained by the fact that the distribution phase is the most important factor and extends for a much longer period than for long-acting NMBA (Fig. 15.3) [16]. If their duration of action and recovery rates are almost identical, it is because plasma concentrations decrease to levels compatible with recovery during the redistribution phase.

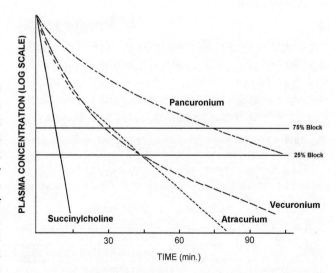

Fig. 15.3 Plasma concentrations after equipotent doses of pancuronium, vecuronium, atracurium and succinylcholine as a function of time. Reproduced from Donati F [16] with permission from Elsevier

Individual Drugs

Succinylcholine (Fig. 15.4)

Pharmacology

Succinylcholine is the only available NMBA with a rapid onset of effect and ultrashort duration of action. Succinylcholine is rapidly hydrolysed by plasma cholinesterase (Table 15.1) to choline and succinylmonocholine. Its estimated plasma half-life is about 2 min and a return of neuromuscular activity occurs quickly. The mean doses producing 50 % blockade (ED50) and 95 % blockade (ED95) at the adductor pollicis are close to 0.3 and 0.5–0.6 mg/kg, respectively, during oxygen–opioid anaesthesia. Following 0.5 mg/kg succinylcholine, onset time is within 60–90 s at the adductor pollicis and within 60 s at more central muscles such as the laryngeal adductor muscles [17] and the diaphragm. A dose of 1.0 mg/kg succinylcholine produces complete neuromuscular block in about 60 s. Time to 90 % recovery at the adductor pollicis, following 1 mg/kg succinylcholine, is within 6–12 min. When a small dose of NDMR is given before succinylcholine, the onset time is increased by about 30 %, and with the exception of pancuronium, which inhibits cholinesterase, the duration of action is decreased by 30–50 %. The dose of succinylcholine must be increased by 50–100 % to achieve comparable

acetylcholine

suxamethonium

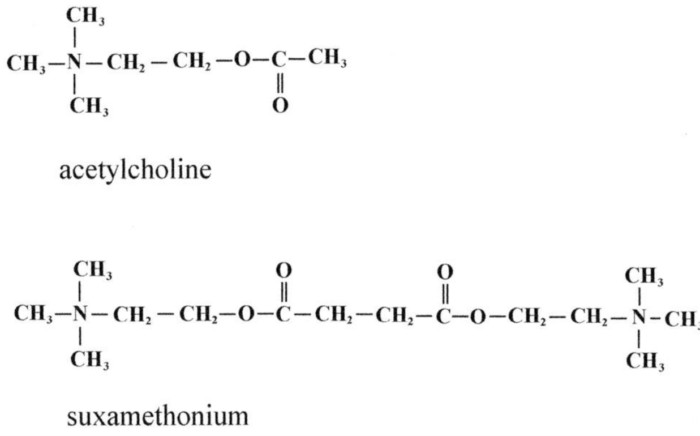

Fig. 15.4 Chemical structures of acetylcholine and succinylcholine

paralysis. Because little or no butyrylcholinesterase is present at the neuromuscular junction, the neuromuscular blockade is terminated by its diffusion away from the neuromuscular junction.

Butyrylcholinesterase is produced by the liver and is present in the plasma. Butyrylcholinesterase activity may be decreased during pregnancy, hepatic disease, burns, sepsis, malnutrition and treatment by cyclophosphamide, cytotoxic drugs or ecothiopate eye drops. The duration of action of succinylcholine may be increased by no more than 25–30 %. In clinical practice, esmolol can induce a slight and transient prolongation of succinylcholine-induced neuromuscular block.

A small proportion of patients have a genetically determined inability to metabolise succinylcholine. In white populations, 95–97 % of the population will have the normal cholinesterase genotype. The duration of action is slightly increased (10–20 min) in heterozygous patients. Neuromuscular block may be very prolonged (45–360 min) in patients homozygous for either the atypical or the silent gene [18]. Dibucaine is more active in inhibiting normal butyrylcholinesterase (80 %) than the abnormal variant (20 %). In clinical practice, the dibucaine number is recommended to confirm the deficit and the genetic profile [19].

Prolonged administration of succinylcholine leads to a change in the nature of the block from that of a depolarising drug to one resembling that of NDMR and called "phase II block". Appearance of fade after continuous administration of succinylcholine could be dependent on the affinity for the presynaptic $\alpha_3\beta_2$ neuronal subtype nAChR when the concentrations exceed the normal clinical concentration observed after a single bolus dose [20]. Its occurrence is dependent of the dose, the duration of administration and the patient; the specific contribution of each factor remains discussed.

Neostigmine and pyridostigmine inhibit acetylcholinesterase but may also inhibit butyrylcholinesterase. When succinylcholine is given, after neostigmine administration, the neuromuscular block will be more profound and prolonged.

Table 15.1 Metabolism and elimination of neuromuscular blocking agents

Muscle relaxant	Metabolism	Excretion	
		Kidney (%)	Liver (%)
Succinylcholine	Plasma cholinesterases (90 %)	1–2	–
Atracurium	Hofmann elimination + Ester hydrolysis (60–90 %)	10–40	
Cisatracurium	Hofmann elimination (80 %)	10–15	–
Pancuronium	Liver (10–20 %)	70	30
Pipecuronium	Liver (10 %)	70	20
Rocuronium	Liver (10 %)	30	70
Vecuronium	Liver (40 %)	20–30	70–80

Table 15.2 Clinical autonomic effects of neuromuscular blocking agents

Muscle relaxant	Autonomic ganglion	Cardiac muscarinic receptors	Histamine release
Succinylcholine	Stimulation	Modest stimulation	Slight
Atracurium	0	0	Moderate
Cisatracurium	0	0	None to slight
Mivacurium	0	0	Moderate
Pancuronium	0	Weak block	0
Pipecuronium	0	0	0
Rocuronium	0	Weak block	0
Vecuronium	0	0	0

Side Effects

Succinylcholine can produce a number of side effects, although these are usually of minor clinical importance. The life-threatening complications, malignant hyperthermia (MH), anaphylaxis and extreme hyperkalaemia, are rare but may arise without warning.

The frequency of fasciculations is high, especially in adults. It can be prevented by giving a small dose of NDMR before succinylcholine but care must be taken to avoid partial paralysis in awake patients. The reported incidence of muscle pain varies from 1.5 to 89 %. The importance of early postoperative mobility has been reported to be a factor in determining the severity of muscle pain. A relationship between fasciculations and muscle pain has not been established although it is considered that the unsynchronised contractions of muscle fibres before onset of neuromuscular block could play a significant role. It could also explain the rise of serum creatine kinase following succinylcholine administration [21].

The administration of succinylcholine is followed by a transient increase in serum potassium concentration which is usually less than 0.5 mmol/L. The increase in K^+ results from the depolarising action of the drug. It seems to be dependent of the anaesthetic technique used at induction. In children, halothane induction followed by succinylcholine produces an increase of serum potassium of 0.2–0.5 mmol/l, while the thiopental–succinylcholine sequence is associated with a small decrease of about 0.1–0.35 mmol/l. The rise usually occurs within 3–5 min after injection. Severe hyperkalaemia, producing arrhythmias or cardiac arrest, may occur in patients with burns, traumas, sepsis, severe metabolic acidosis and neurological and muscular disorders. The mechanism could be due to the extrajunctional spread of acetylcholine receptors. In burn patients, it has been suggested to avoid succinylcholine at least until several weeks to months after complete healing when the patient reverts to a normal metabolic state. In trauma patients the risk of hyperkalaemia occurs 2–7 days after the injury and can last at least 2 months after trauma. Therefore, the use of succinylcholine is contraindicated until complete healing of the muscular lesions and recovery of the patient [21].

Because of its structure similarity to acetylcholine, succinylcholine can stimulate cholinergic autonomic receptors on both sympathetic and parasympathetic ganglia and muscarinic receptors in the sinus node of the heat (Table 15.2). Therefore, succinylcholine can produce sinus bradycardia with nodal or ventricular escape beats, especially in children and infants when vagal tone is predominant. These changes in cardiac rhythm can be prevented by prior administration of atropine or glycopyrrolate. In adults bradycardia is more common after a second dose of succinylcholine. The mechanism of the bradycardia, in adults, following a second dose, is poorly understood. Succinylcholine increases catecholamine release, giving rise to tachycardia in adults. Ventricular escape beats may occur as a consequence of severe sinus bradycardia and atrioventricular nodal slowing. However a single bolus is not usually associated with any pronounced tachycardia in adults. Ventricular dysrhythmias can also be the consequence of hyperkalaemia.

Following succinylcholine, there is a mean increase in intraocular pressure of about 8 mmHg which peaks 2–4 min after administration and lasts for up to 10 min. This effect may be due to a sustained contraction of the extraocular muscles and is not reliably prevented by pretreatment with NDMR. Succinylcholine traditionally has been avoided in patients with a penetrating eye injury and the opening of the eye anterior chamber. However, there is a greater increase in intraocular pressure during laryngoscopy and intubation in lightly anaesthetised, poorly paralysed patients. When succinylcholine is contraindicated and in case of a patient with a full stomach and a penetrating eye injury, rocuronium can be used to perform a rapid sequence induction of anaesthesia.

Succinylcholine causes an increase in intragastric pressure which may be as high as 30-cm H_2O and is apparently related to the severity of the fasciculations of the abdominal wall muscles. It has been observed that the pressure in the lower oesophageal sphincter increases during fasciculations by more than the intragastric pressure, and this increase in pressure may lessen the risk of regurgitation and aspiration. However in case of pregnancy, hiatus hernia or bowel obstruction incompetence of the gastro-oesophageal junction can occur during an increase in intragastric pressure of less than 15-cm H_2O. The smaller increase in intragastric pressure in infants and children could be related to the less intense fasciculations in the first years of life [22].

The increase in intracranial pressure is poorly understood although it may be due to an increase in $PaCO_2$ during fasciculations. It can be prevented by pretreatment with NDMR. Masseter muscle rigidity (MMR) is a contracture of the masseter to a degree which interferes with tracheal intubation and despite the presence of adequate concentrations of succinylcholine. Several studies have demonstrated that an increase in masseter muscle tone of up to 500 g lasting 1–2 min is a normal finding [23]. Most cases of the so-called MMR may represent simply the extreme of a spectrum of tension changes in response to succinylcholine. The incidence of MMR is within 0.5–1 %, whereas the incidence of malignant hyperthermia is about 1:12,000 in children and 1:30,000 in adults. Traditionally, MMR has been taken to herald the development of malignant hyperthermia. Occasionally, MMR may precede malignant hyperthermia. Increasingly, an expected approach to the management of MMR is being advocated with monitoring for signs of hypermetabolism (hypercapnia, metabolic acidosis, hyperthermia, tachycardia, increased oxygen consumption, hyperthermia). Some authors have concluded that anaesthesia can be continued safely in isolated cases of MMR when careful monitoring is employed. Anaesthetic vapours will be avoided if the case is continued.

There is some controversy concerning the incidence of anaphylaxis following succinylcholine. Almost all the cases of anaphylaxis have been reported in Europe or Australia. The incidence of anaphylactic reactions may be close to 0.06 %. It has been shown that, of all muscle relaxants, succinylcholine was associated with the greatest number of serious reactions. The anaphylactic mechanism is the most frequent. When the muscle relaxant cross-links with IgE, degranulation and release of histamine, neutrophil chemotactic factor and platelet-activating factor occur. The release of these mediators can induce cardiovascular collapse, bronchospasm and skin reaction. Patients with a history of anaphylactic reaction to succinylcholine may exhibit a cross-reaction, at least in vitro, with other NMBAs in approximately 60–70 %. The cross-reactivity is related to the common structural features of these drugs, all of which contain quaternary ammonium ions [24]. In case of anaphylactic reaction to succinylcholine, it is mandatory to complete investigation for cross-reactivity with the other commercially available NMBAs to identify safe alternative regimens.

Steroidal Compounds (Fig. 15.5)

Vecuronium

Vecuronium is a synthetic steroid-based molecule which came from the demethylation of pancuronium. It is a monoquaternary compound. Vecuronium undergoes spontaneous deacetylation to 3- and 17-hydroxy metabolites. This process takes place principally in the liver, 40–80 % of the dose being taken up and excreted by the bile (Table 15.1). The most potent metabolite is the 3-OH derivative which is 50 % as potent as vecuronium. Vecuronium and the 3-OH derivative are eliminated through the kidneys [25]. The 17-OH and 3–17-dihydroxy metabolites retain almost no neuromuscular blocking activity.

In contrast to pancuronium, vecuronium has a relatively short duration of action which can be explained by a plasma clearance (3–5 ml/kg/min) double that of pancuronium (Table 15.3). Although the elimination half-life of vecuronium (50–80 min) [26] is larger than atracurium, the

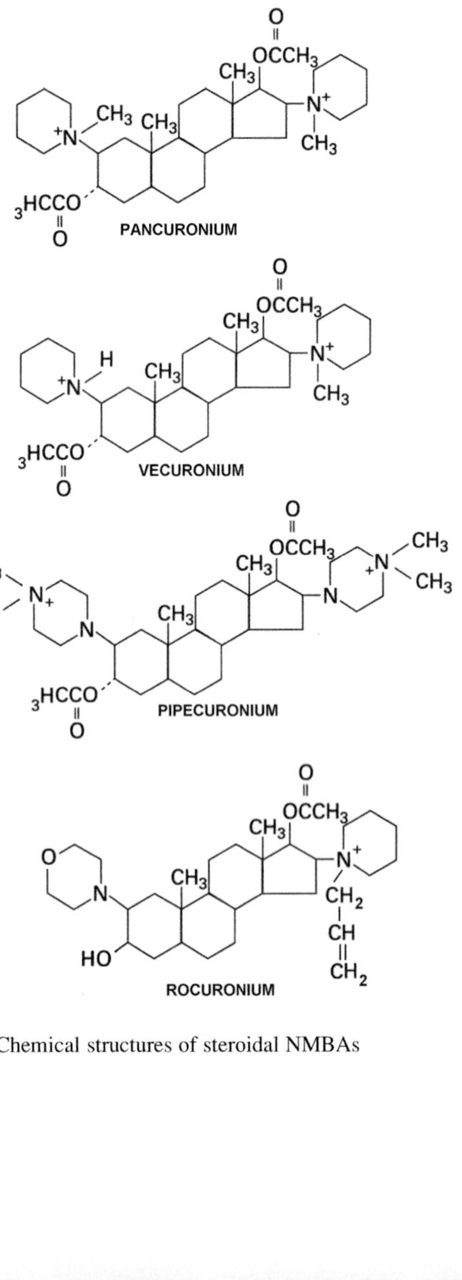

Fig. 15.5 Chemical structures of steroidal NMBAs

Table 15.3 Pharmacokinetic parameters of muscle relaxants

Drug	Vdss (ml/kg)	Clearance (ml/min/kg)	Elimination half-life (min)	Protein bound (%)
Succinylcholine	6–16	200–500	2–8	30
Pancuronium	260–280	1.9	110–135	30
Pipecuronium	340–425	1.6–3.4	100	–
Vecuronium	180–250	3.6–5.3	50–53	30–57
Rocuronium	170–210	3.4	70–80	25
Atracurium	180–280	5.5–10.8	17–20	51
Cisatracurium	110–200	4–7	18–27	–
Mivacurium				
cis–trans	146–588	26–147	1–5	–
trans–trans	123–338	18–79	2–8	–
cis–cis	191–346	2–5	41–200	–

Table 15.4 ED_{95} and clinical effects of NDMR at clinical doses (2 × ED95 at the adductor pollicis)

	ED_{95} (mg/kg)	Intubating dose (mg/kg)	Onset time (min)	Total duration of action (min)	Recovery index (min)
Atracurium	0.230	0.5	3–4	50–60	11–12
Cisatracurium	0.048	0.150	4–5	70–80	12–15
Mivacurium	0.080	0.200	3	30	6–7
Pancuronium	0.050	0.070–0.100	3.5–4	120	30–40
Pipecuronium	0.045	0.080	3.5–4	120	30–40
Rocuronium	0.300	0.600	1.5	60–70	14
Vecuronium	0.040	0.08–0.1	3	50–60	12

Onset time: Time from injection until maximum block at the adductor pollicis
Total duration of action: Time from injection to 90 % recovery of twitch height at the adductor pollicis
Recovery index: Time from 25 to 75 % spontaneous recovery of twitch height at the adductor pollicis

duration of action and the rate of recovery are similar. This discrepancy is explained by the fact that vecuronium has a more rapid initial distribution than atracurium. Plasma concentrations decrease rapidly, so that duration of action and recovery for vecuronium depend more on distribution than elimination. This also explains why larger doses are associated with a longer recovery index. In case of repeated dosing, accumulation may occur, especially in the presence of renal failure. The elimination half-life of vecuronium is increased from 55 to 73 min in cirrhotic patients as the result of a decrease in clearance, the volume of distribution being unchanged [27]. Similar findings were observed in patients with cholestasis [26].

The ED_{50} of vecuronium is 0.025–0.030 mg/kg and the ED_{95} about 0.04–0.05 mg/kg. The onset of action at one ED_{95} dose is within 5 and 6 min. It can be reduced considerably by increasing the intubating dose or by priming. A dose of 0.08–0.10 mg/kg will produce maximum block within 2–3 min (Table 15.4). As for other NDMRs, the onset of action is more rapid at the diaphragm and the laryngeal adductor muscles than at the adductor pollicis [28, 29]. Following twice the ED_{95}, the clinical duration of action is about 25–40 min at the adductor pollicis and minutes at the laryngeal muscles. The spontaneous recovery index is close to 12 min. Little accumulation is observed with vecuronium. Recovery from neuromuscular block can be accelerated by

neostigmine or edrophonium once the fourth response at the TOF is present. The dose–response of vecuronium is similar in elderly and young adults. Following a bolus of 0.07 mg/kg, the clinical duration of action is shorter in children than in adults and infants.

Even at high doses (8 times the ED_{95}), vecuronium does not have significant cardiovascular effects. It does not exhibit action at the autonomic ganglia or sympathetic nervous system exists and does not induce histamine release (Table 15.2). The intermediate duration of action following vecuronium administration makes it useful for most surgical procedures including day-care surgery. An initial dose of 0.07–0.10 mg/kg provides good intubating conditions within 2–3 min. During continuous infusion a dose of 1–2 μg/kg/min is necessary to maintain a 90 % block at the adductor pollicis. Large doses (0.2–0.4 mg/kg) have been used to provide rapid intubating conditions in place of succinylcholine. However the duration of action will be 90–120 min.

Rocuronium

Rocuronium's main characteristic is a short onset of action when compared with vecuronium, atracurium or cisatracurium.

In humans 33 % of the dose is eliminated unchanged by the kidneys. Metabolites are below the detection limit. There are no human data on biliary excretion; however in cats 50 % of the administered dose of rocuronium is recovered from the bile and only 9 % from the urine within 6 h after administration, indicating that elimination is mainly determined by hepatobiliary excretion [30] (Table 15.1). The pharmacokinetic parameters of rocuronium and vecuronium are of the same order of magnitude; the volume of the central compartment and the volume of distribution at steady state (Vdss) appear to be smaller than those for vecuronium in normal patients (Table 15.3). Pharmacokinetics of rocuronium have been reported in patients with or without renal failure after a single dose of 0.6 mg/kg. There were no significant differences between the two groups with respect to the neuromuscular parameters. The main difference in kinetic parameters was a decreased plasma clearance and an increased mean residence time in patients with renal failure. The duration of action is increased in patients with hepatic dysfunction (114 vs 47 min); this could be due to the larger volume of distribution when compared with healthy patients [31].

The potency of rocuronium is about one-seventh the potency of vecuronium. The ED_{95} is 0.300 mg/kg at the adductor pollicis. The low potency may explain its rapid onset of action when compared with other NDMRs [19, 20]. After a dose of 0.6 mg/kg, the onset of action is close to 90 s at the adductor pollicis [21] (Table 15.4). A relationship between potency and onset of action has been demonstrated by Bowman. When a less potent NDMR is administered, more molecules are administered than in the case of a more potent NDMR, and the receptors at the neuromuscular junction will be occupied more rapidly. Following equipotent doses, the duration of action of rocuronium is similar to that of atracurium and vecuronium. Minimal cumulative effects have been observed with up to three repeated doses under halogenated anaesthesia. Rocuronium has minimal vagolytic properties; its administration is associated with only small changes in haemodynamic variables (7 % increase in heart rate and 11 % increase in the cardiac index). Like other steroidal NDMRs, it does not cause histamine release (Table 15.2). The main advantage of rocuronium is its short onset of action which provides good intubating conditions 60–90 s after a bolus of 0.6 mg/kg [32]. Rocuronium can be used when rapid tracheal intubation is indicated and succinylcholine is contraindicated . However, it must be remembered that it is an intermediate-duration action NDMR with an onset of action less than 90 s at the laryngeal adductor muscles [33].

Long-Acting Steroidal Compounds

Long-acting NDMRs commercially available include, depending on the country, pancuronium and pipecuronium. Because of their clinical duration of action (time from injection until 25 % recovery of twitch height), the incidence of

residual block at the end of the procedure can be important (30–40 %). These compounds are specially designed for long surgical procedures or when mechanical ventilation is necessary in the postoperative period.

Pancuronium

Pancuronium is a synthetic bisquaternary aminosteroid compound. Pancuronium is metabolised mainly by acetylation in the liver to 3- and 17-OH derivatives which are excreted in the urine. The 3-OH metabolite which is 40–50 % as potent as pancuronium is the only one detected in humans. The 17-OH metabolite has about one-fiftieth the potency of pancuronium. Pancuronium is mainly eliminated through the kidney (40–70 % of the initial dose) (Table 15.1).

In normal patients volume of distribution is about 0.3 L/kg, corresponding to the extracellular fluid volume. Total plasma clearance is close to 2.0 ml/kg/min [34] (Table 15.3). In renal failure a decrease in clearance is observed leading to a prolonged duration of action, because biliary excretion cannot compensate for the decrease in glomerular filtration. Plasma clearance is reduced in patients with hepatic disease. However resistance to the initial dose is frequently observed in patients with liver cirrhosis. The resistance is explained by a larger distribution volume. No differences in pharmacokinetics have been observed between adults and children. In the elderly, the plasma clearance is lower than in young adults because glomerular filtration decreases with age.

The ED_{50} and ED_{95} at the adductor pollicis are 0.03 mg/kg and 0.05 mg/kg, respectively. The ED_{50} at the diaphragm is twice the ED_{50} at the adductor pollicis. Thus complete paralysis of the diaphragm is not expected with a dose that barely blocks the adductor pollicis [35]. Onset time of maximum neuromuscular block is about 3.5 min after administration of 0.10 mg/kg (Table 15.4). The use of a priming dose shortens the onset time. However, priming must be avoided, because of the risk of pulmonary aspiration and paralysis of upper airway muscles, which are more sensitive than the adductor pollicis to small doses of NDMR [36]. Following administration of twice the ED_{95}, the clinical duration of action and total duration of action are close to 70–80 and 120 min, respectively. Recovery at the diaphragm is faster than at the adductor pollicis because it is more resistant to NDMR than the adductor pollicis. Accumulation has been demonstrated with pancuronium inducing a progressive increase in the duration of action after repeated doses. Recovery is accelerated by neostigmine or edrophonium. In clinical practice, when the fourth response at the TOF is detected, neostigmine can be injected safely. Although edrophonium has a shorter duration of action than neostigmine, its use to antagonise residual neuromuscular block induced by pancuronium must be cautious because of its shorter duration of action. The halogenated agents induce a shift to the right of the dose–action curve. This interaction is concentration and duration of administration dependent. The potentiating effects of sevoflurane and desflurane are greater than that induced by other halogenated agents.

Pancuronium increases heart rate, arterial pressure and cardiac output. These cardiovascular effects are related to vagolytic and sympathomimetic effects (Table 15.2). The use of pancuronium in cardiovascular high-risk patients is discussed. Some authors recommend its use to counteract the bradycardia induced by high doses of opioids. Clinical use of pancuronium is now limited since the introduction of new compounds of intermediate duration of action. Due to its long duration of action, residual curarisation in the recovery room is more frequent with pancuronium when compared with vecuronium or atracurium. Its use is limited to long surgical procedures or when mechanical ventilation is needed in the postoperative period.

Pipecuronium

Pipecuronium bromide is a long-acting steroidal NDMR which resembles pancuronium in potency and duration of action. Pipecuronium is metabolised in the liver (Table 15.1) to a 3-OH derivative which has 40–50 % the potency of the parent drug. Renal elimination of this compound affects 37–41 % of the administered dose; biliary excretion is negligible (2 %). Pharmacokinetics of pipecuronium differs from pancuronium by a greater plasma clearance and a larger volume of distribution [37] (Table 15.3). Plasma clearance is decreased from 2.4 to 1.6 mL/min/kg in patients with renal failure, leading to a prolongation of the elimination half-life from 137 to 263 min. In humans, in the presence of cholestasis, neither the pharmacokinetics nor the time course of action was significantly different from those of normal patients.

The ED_{95} is approximately 0.045 mg/kg. Administration of a 0.070–0.08 mg/kg dose results in a complete block in 3.0–3.5 min, with a clinical duration of action of 70–110 min at the adductor pollicis (Table 15.3). Like other NDMRs, a bolus of pipecuronium exerts a greater effect in adults and infants than in children. In elderly patients (>70 years of age), the onset of action is longer than in younger patients, but the duration of action is not significantly prolonged if renal function is normal. Pipecuronium is comparable to other long-acting relaxants in terms of potentiation of neuromuscular block by halogenated agents and reversal by anticholinesterase drugs. Edrophonium is relatively ineffective against pipecuronium-induced neuromuscular block even when recovery has taken place.

Pipecuronium is devoid of cardiovascular side effects. It lacks the autonomic effects of pancuronium and does not cause histamine release (Table 15.2). Doses up to three times

the ED_{95} do not induce significant changes in heart rate or blood pressure in patients undergoing coronary artery bypass. Because of its long duration of action and interindividual variability in response, the use of pipecuronium is limited to long surgical procedures.

Benzylisoquinoline Compounds (Fig. 15.6)

Atracurium

Atracurium is a bulky diester with two positively charged nitrogen atoms. Atracurium presents four asymmetrical centres so that there are 16 possible isomers. It is metabolised by ester hydrolysis and Hofmann elimination (Table 15.1) which involves the conversion of an amide to an amine under alkaline conditions. Hofmann elimination for atracurium takes place at a pH of 7.4 and a temperature of 37 °C. Breakdown products of atracurium include laudanosine, acrylates and quaternary organic acids [38] (Fig. 15.7). High laudanosine plasma concentrations (17 mg/L) can be associated with convulsions in dogs but have never been implicated in humans. The acrylates are highly reactive substances which may be hepatotoxic although once again no problems have been reported in humans [39]. The ratio of ester hydrolysis to Hofmann elimination differs from species to species, but in humans up to about 60 % probably undergoes ester hydrolysis in the liver, although there is not a uniform agreement. The breakdown of atracurium is independent of plasma cholinesterase. The volume of distribution in normal patients is approximately 0.18 L/kg and clearance 5.5 ml/kg/min. The elimination half-life is 20 min and remains remarkably constant throughout studies (Table 15.3). In patients with renal failure, several pharmacokinetic and pharmacodynamic studies have shown no significant changes [40]. However recovery has been found to be prolonged following repeated doses in patients with renal failure. Laudanosine may accumulate in patients with renal failure, but the concentration attained after a continuous administration is ten times less than the toxic plasma level. In patients with fulminant hepatic failure, the volume of distribution is significantly increased but the elimination half-life (23 min) remains unchanged.

The ED_{50} of atracurium is 0.13 mg/kg, and the ED_{95} is 0.23 mg/kg (Table 15.3). The onset of action at the adductor pollicis of one ED_{95} is about 3–5 min. It can be reduced by increasing the dose, but doses above 3 times the ED_{95} can induce histamine release. The duration of action depends upon the dose administered; an intubating dose (0.50 mg/kg) provides muscular relaxation for 25–40 min in adults. Neuromuscular block is easily antagonised by neostigmine or edrophonium. Atracurium pharmacodynamics are very little affected in the elderly, probably because atracurium elimination is organ independent. The onset time is more

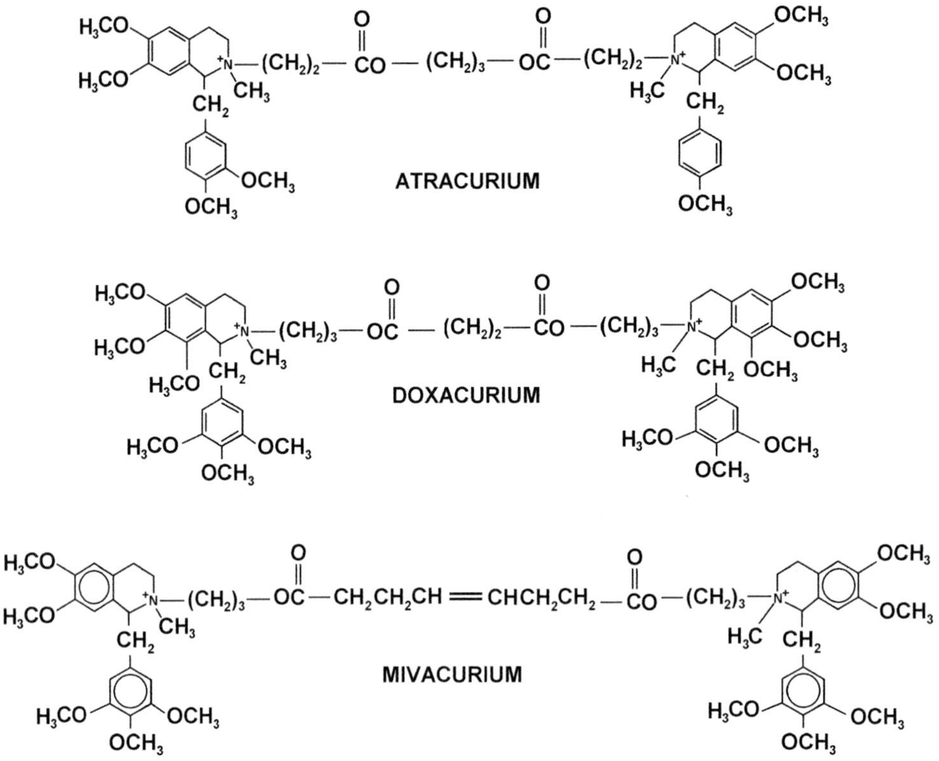

Fig. 15.6 Chemical structures of benzylisoquinoline NMBAs

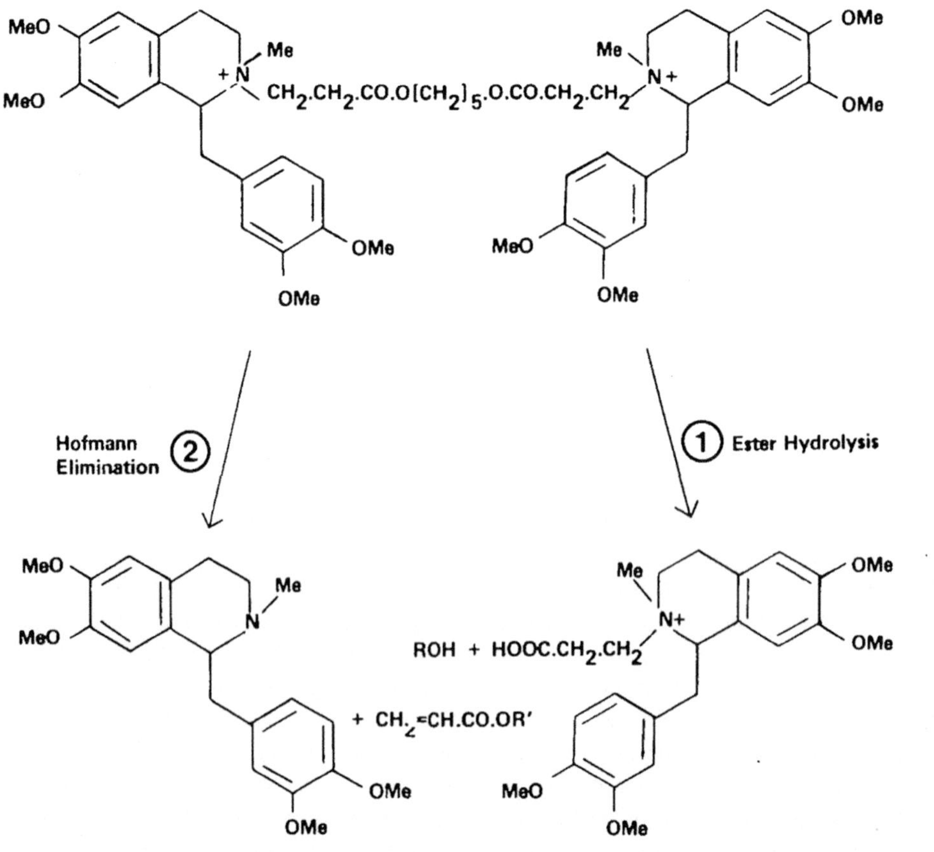

ATRACURIUM

DOXACURIUM

MIVACURIUM

Fig. 15.7 Metabolic pathways for atracurium degradation in humans. Reproduced from Hughes and Chapple [38] with permission from Oxford University Press

Hofmann Elimination ②

① Ester Hydrolysis

ROH + HOOC.CH₂.CH₂

+ CH₂=CH.CO.OR′

rapid and the duration of action slightly shorter in children than in adults. The breakdown of atracurium is decreased by hypothermia, causing a reduction in dose requirements during hypothermic cardiopulmonary bypass. Atracurium can induce histamine release (Table 15.2) and a drop in blood pressure at a dose of 3 times the ED_{95}. Histamine release can be reduced by slow IV injection.

Atracurium is indicated for intermediate to long duration of action procedures and for day case procedures. Due to its lack of accumulation, maintenance can be obtained by a continuous infusion at a rate of 5–10 µg/kg/min.

Cisatracurium

Cisatracurium is one of ten isomers of atracurium. Hofmann elimination is the predominant elimination pathway. Ester hydrolysis plays a limited role in humans (Table 15.1). The two metabolites are laudanosine and a monoquaternary alcohol. Urinary excretion is a minor elimination pathway but a major pathway for the elimination of laudanosine. Because of a greater potency than atracurium, the dose administered is lower, and the production of laudanosine is lower [41]. The mean clearance ranges from 4.5 to 5.7 mL/min/kg and the elimination half-life is 22–30 min [42] (Table 15.4).

The ED_{95} is 0.048 mg/kg. At twice the ED_{95}, the pharmacodynamic profile of cisatracurium is similar to that of an equipotent dose of atracurium apart from a slower onset of action (Table 15.4). A more rapid onset is produced when increasing the dose (2.7 min at 0.2 mg/kg). The clinical duration of action ranges from 45 min after twice the ED_{95} to approximately 90 min at eight times the ED_{95}. The recovery index is constant after repeated bolus doses or continuous infusions suggesting a lack of cumulation [43]. When neostigmine is given at 10 % of T1, a complete recovery from neuromuscular block is obtained in 7 min. The intensity of block and the clinical duration of action are not modified by renal failure. The same results are observed in patients with hepatic failure except for the onset of action which is significantly shorter in case of hepatic dysfunction. Contrary to atracurium, cisatracurium does not produce histamine release (Table 15.2) at doses up to 8 times the ED_{95}.

Mivacurium

Mivacurium is a benzylquinolinium diester with three isomers. It is hydrolysed by plasma cholinesterase. Clearance of the cis–trans and trans–trans isomers correlates with plasma pseudocholinesterase activity. The cis–cis isomer is more slowly hydrolysed (Table 15.3), but its potency is only one-tenth that of the two other isomers. Mivacurium is hydrolysed at 70–88 % of the rate of succinylcholine. The ED_{95} is 0.07–0.08 mg/kg at the adductor pollicis. Onset time is 3 min and the clinical duration of action is 20 min

following 0.2 mg/kg (Table 15.4). Mivacurium shows few cumulative effects; the recovery index is 6–7 min and does not change over a wide dose range nor after prolonged infusion up to 5 h. Administration of neostigmine or edrophonium, after the start of spontaneous recovery, reduces the recovery index by approximately 50 %. Prolonged block has been reported following its use in patients with low or abnormal plasma cholinesterase [44]. In patients heterozygous for the atypical and usual gene, the duration of action is about 50 % prolonged [45]. Mivacurium is four to five times more potent in homozygous abnormal patients than in patients with normal phenotype. In these patients the duration of action following 0.2 mg/kg may be very prolonged (6–8 h). Anticholinesterases should not be administered. Patients must be ventilated and sedated until spontaneous recovery occurs. Renal failure may reduce cholinesterase activity by 30–50 %; the duration of action may be prolonged in these patients. There is an inverse correlation between plasma cholinesterase activity and the duration of action of mivacurium in cirrhotic patients. Mivacurium may induce histamine release which is dose and rate of administration dependent (Table 15.2). A dose of 0.2 mg/kg can induce a drop in blood pressure which can be attenuated by slower injection (30 s).

The main advantage of mivacurium is a short duration of action which makes it suitable for short surgical procedures requiring tracheal intubation. A dose of 0.2 mg/kg is necessary to obtain good intubating conditions. Maintenance of neuromuscular block can be obtained by a continuous infusion at a rate of 5–10 µg/kg/min. Monitoring is mandatory during continuous administration to detect recovery or prolonged duration of action in patients with abnormal pseudocholinesterases.

Fumarate Compounds (Fig. 15.8)

These compounds share some structural properties with mivacurium. Gantacurium underwent clinical testing in humans a few years ago. It was shown that following 2–3 times the ED95 at the adductor pollicis, onset time at both the laryngeal muscles and the adductor pollicis was comparable to onset of block following succinylcholine administration. Gantacurium does not exhibit ganglionic blockade or vagolytic properties. However histamine release at 4 times the ED95 and a 17 % reduction in blood pressure in humans has hampered its clinical development [46]. Interestingly, gantacurium is metabolised by a slow pH-sensitive hydrolysis and also by adduction of the naturally occurring amino acid cysteine transforming gantacurium into an inactive compound. Administration of L-cysteine (10 mg/kg), 1 min after administration of gantacurium, results in return of complete neuromuscular function within 1–2 min [47].

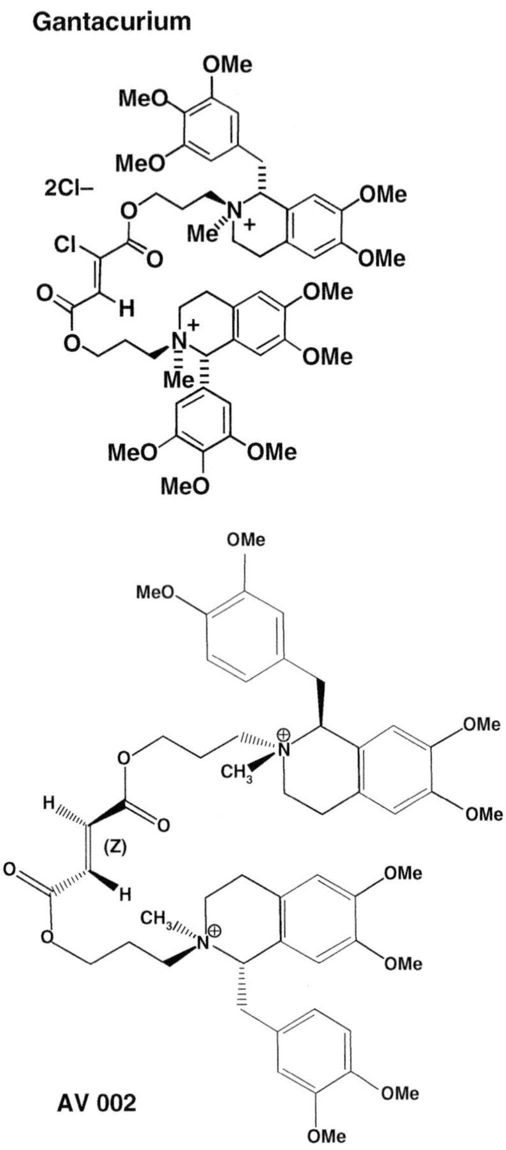

Gantacurium

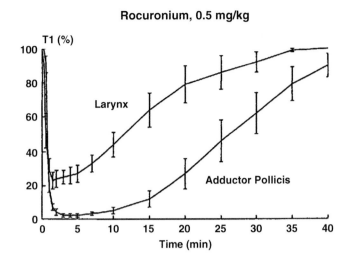

AV 002

Fig. 15.8 Chemical formulae of gantacurium and CW002 also named AV002. Reproduced from Lien et al. [46] with permission from Elsevier

CW002 is a gantacurium derivative of intermediate duration of action. Initial dose-finding studies in volunteers did not show any evidence of histamine release or bronchoconstriction. The resulting adduction of cysteine product retains some very low affinity for neuromuscular nAChR with potency for neuromuscular blockade decreased 70–100-fold [47]. CW002 is currently under clinical investigation.

Action of Relaxants on Different Muscle Groups

In man, several studies have reported some discrepancies between the level of peripheral paralysis and respiratory

Fig. 15.9 Onset and recovery of rocuronium-induced neuromuscular block at the laryngeal adductor muscles and the adductor pollicis. Reproduced from Meistelman et al. [33] with permission from Springer

depression or intubating conditions. Paton and Zaimis demonstrated in 1951 that some of the muscles of respiration, such as the diaphragm, were more resistant to curare than others. The dose of NDMR needed to block the diaphragm is 1.5–2 times that of the adductor pollicis. Thus, complete paralysis of the diaphragm is not expected with doses of neuromuscular blocking agents used to block neuromuscular transmission at the adductor pollicis [28]. Similarly, the laryngeal adductor muscles are more resistant to NDMR than the more peripheral muscles such as the adductor pollicis, for which all dosing recommendations for neuromuscular blocking agents and their antagonists have been made [29]. The sparing effect on the laryngeal adductor muscles has been documented with vecuronium, rocuronium (Fig. 15.9) [33], cisatracurium and mivacurium. Plaud et al. studied the pharmacokinetic–pharmacodynamic relationship of blocking agents at the adductor pollicis and the laryngeal adductors. They found that the concentration in the effect compartment producing 50 % of the maximum block was significantly greater at the laryngeal adductor muscles (1.5 µg/mL) than that at the adductor pollicis (0.8 µg/ml) (Fig. 15.10) [48]. There is convincing evidence that the EC_{50} for almost all drugs is 50–100 % higher at the diaphragm or larynx than it is at the adductor pollicis. These differences may be due to any of several factors. Waud and Waud found that following curare administration, neuromuscular transmission occurs when approximately 18 % of the receptors are free at the diaphragm, while it does not occur at the peripheral muscles unless 29 % of receptors are free [49]. This may be due to higher receptor density, greater release of acetylcholine or less acetylcholinesterase activity [50]. The lower density of acetylcholine receptors in slow muscle fibres, such as found in the peripheral muscles,

Fig. 15.10 Rocuronium plasma concentration and calculated concentration in the effect compartment at the laryngeal adductor muscles and the adductor pollicis versus time. Reproduced from Plaud et al. [48] with permission from John Wiley and Sons

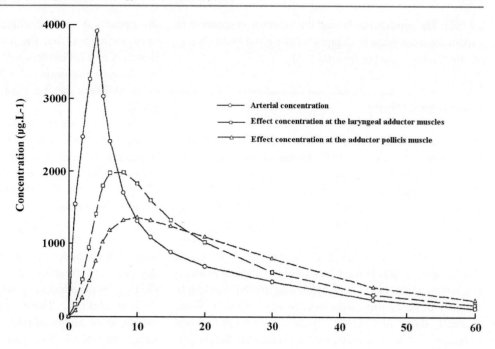

explains, at least in part, the lower margin of safety for neuromuscular transmission when compared to that in the faster muscle fibres in the laryngeal adductors. Interestingly, muscle sensitivity to succinylcholine is different than with other neuromuscular blocking agents [17]. It is the only muscle relaxant that, at equipotent doses, causes greater neuromuscular block at the vocal cords than at the adductor pollicis. Some data suggest that in contrast to NDMR, succinylcholine is more effective in blocking the muscles composed of primarily fast-contracting fibres [51].

In spite of their relative resistance to neuromuscular blockers, the onset of neuromuscular block is significantly faster at the diaphragm and the laryngeal adductors than at the adductor pollicis. Fisher et al. [52] postulated that a more rapid equilibration (shorter $t_{1/2}k_{e0}$) of the neuromuscular blocking agent between plasma and the effect compartment at these more centrally located muscles was the explanation for this observation. The accelerated rate of equilibrium probably represents little more than differences in regional blood flow. Therefore, muscle blood flow rather than a drug's intrinsic potency may be more important in determining the onset and offset time of NDMR. Greater blood flow per gram of muscle at the diaphragm or larynx results in them receiving a higher peak plasma concentration of drug in the brief period of time before rapid redistribution occurs. Plaud et al. have confirmed this hypothesis by demonstrating a faster transfer rate constant ($t_{1/2}k_{e0}$) at the laryngeal adductors (2.7 min) than at the adductor pollicis (4.4 min). Greater resistance to neuromuscular blockade accounts for the more rapid recovery of the respiratory muscles and the muscles of the abdominal wall than at the adductor pollicis. Recovery occurs more rapidly because blood concentration

of NMBA has to decrease more in the muscles of respiration than in the adductor pollicis for recovery of neuromuscular function to begin.

In contrast, the muscles of the upper airway are particularly sensitive to the effects of muscle relaxants. The masseter is 15 % more sensitive to NDMR agents than the adductor pollicis. Significant weakness of the muscles of the upper airway may exist even when strength at the adductor pollicis has recovered almost to baseline values. A train-of-four (TOF) ratio less than 0.9 at the adductor pollicis is associated with impaired pharyngeal function, reduced resting tone in the upper oesophageal sphincter muscle and decreased coordination of the muscles involved in swallowing which cause an increased incidence of misdirected swallows, or aspiration [53]. Because of the resistance of the muscles of respiration to neuromuscular block, patients may be weak but able to breathe as long as an endotracheal tube is in place. Once extubated, however, they may not be able to maintain a patent airway or protect their airway [54]. This is likely the reason that patients with a TOF <0.9 in the PACU are more likely to develop respiratory events than those whose TOF ratio is ≥0.9 [55].

The increase in ventilation during hypoxia is mainly governed by afferent neuronal input from peripheral chemoreceptors of the carotid body. Acetylcholine is involved in the transmission of afferent neuronal activity from the carotid bodies to the central nervous system. Eriksson et al. have shown that partial neuromuscular block (TOF ratio of 0.7) reduces specifically the ventilatory responses to isocapnic hypoxia without altering the response to hypercapnia. The ventilatory response to hypoxia returns to control values after recovery to a TOF ratio above

0.9 [56]. The mechanism behind this interaction seems to be a spontaneous reversible depression of carotid body chemoreceptor activity during hypoxia [57].

Drug Interactions

Simultaneous administration of two NDMR has either additive or synergistic effects [58]. The mechanism for synergy remains discussed, but it could include multiple binding sites at the neuromuscular junction or differences in binding activities of the α subunits. Some authors have suggested using simultaneously a combination of mivacurium and rocuronium to get both a rapid onset and a short duration of action. However this kind of interaction has almost no clinical interest and is used very rarely in clinical practice. The interaction between succinylcholine and NDMR can be antagonistic depending on the order of administration. When a small dose of NDMR, usually one-tenth of the recommended dose, is given before succinylcholine to prevent fasciculations and muscle pain, the duration of action and the effect of succinylcholine are decreased. On the other hand, the duration of action and the effects of NDMR are increased by prior administration of succinylcholine [59].

Sevoflurane, desflurane and isoflurane potentiate the neuromuscular effects of NDMR. It reflects a pharmacodynamic interaction. They induce a prolongation of the duration of action of neuromuscular block and of the recovery index. The effect is more important with the most recent halogenated agents (desflurane and sevoflurane) because they are less soluble [60]. Because equilibrium between the end-tidal concentration and the muscles is low (30–90 min), this potentiation is concentration but also time dependent.

Many other drugs may potentiate the effects of NMBA but most of these interactions have no significant clinical effects. Potentiation of neuromuscular block by aminoglycoside antibiotics is mainly observed in case of overdosage such as in patients with renal failure. Antiepileptic drugs, such as phenytoin, can induce a decrease in the release of acetylcholine at the neuromuscular junction and an upregulation of the cholinergic receptors inducing resistance to most of the NDMR [61].

Specific Populations

Paediatric Patients

In humans, maturation of neuromuscular transmission occurs after the first 2 months of age although immature junctions have been found up to 2 years of age. The main change during the first months of life is that the foetal receptors located outside the neuromuscular junction will disappear and will be replaced by mature receptors. These changes suggest that the neonate's neuromuscular junction may exhibit evidence of its immaturity by changes in response to neuromuscular blockers although neuromuscular blockers can be used safely in term and preterm infants.

The routine administration of succinylcholine to healthy children should be discontinued because there is a risk of intractable cardiac arrest with hyperkalaemia, rhabdomyolysis and acidosis after succinylcholine administration, particularly in patients with unsuspected muscular dystrophy of the Duchenne type.

There are significant age-related differences in the potency of NDMR in infants and children when compared with adults. Children require greater doses of NDMR than any other age group of patients. In infants less than 1 year, the ED_{95} at the adductor pollicis is approximately 30 % less than in children. These apparent discrepancies can be explained by studies of pharmacokinetics and pharmacodynamics of NMBA. Neonates and infants are more sensitive than adults to the neuromuscular blocking effects of NMBA. Plasma concentrations, required to achieve a desired level of neuromuscular blockade, are lower in neonates and infants when compared with children [62]. However, the dosage should not be decreased as much because neonates and infants have a larger volume of distribution at steady state [63]. This increased volume of distribution is due to the increase in extracellular fluid volume during the first months of life. This increase, in association with a lower elimination clearance, contributes to the longer elimination half-life, in the first months of life. The much greater range of response in neonates in association with a longer elimination half-life suggests that in neonates NDMR should be given in small additive doses until the required level of neuromuscular block is attained.

Atracurium, vecuronium, cisatracurium and rocuronium are commonly administered to children because many surgical procedures are of short duration in children and are compatible with the duration of action of a single intubating dose [64]. It must be highlighted that onset time of neuromuscular block is faster in infants (30 %) and children (40 %) when compared with adults [65]. This age-related effect is probably caused by circulatory factors such as the relative decrease of cardiac output and increase of circulation time with age. An age-dependent prolongation of action during vecuronium-induced neuromuscular block has been demonstrated in infants. A dose of 0.1 mg/kg produces a neuromuscular block >90 % of control value of almost 60-min duration in infants [66] but of only 20 min in children and adults. Vecuronium therefore acts as a long-acting muscle neuromuscular blocker in the neonate. In contrast, the duration of action of atracurium is not significantly different in the paediatric patient from that in the adult.

Therefore, the same dose (0.5–0.6 mg/kg) can be used in infants, children and adults for tracheal intubation without any major difference between the three groups in its duration of action. Recovery form atracurium-induced neuromuscular block is little affected by age in paediatric patients >1-month old. In children, a dose of 0.1 mg/kg of cisatracurium has an onset of just over 2 min and a clinical duration of approximately 30 min during balanced or halothane anaesthesia [67]. The calculated ED_{95} doses of cisatracurium in infants and children are 43 mg/kg and 47 mg/kg, respectively. It has been demonstrated that cisatracurium (0.1 mg/kg) when compared with atracurium (0.5 mg/kg) provides less good intubating conditions in children (69 %) than atracurium (98 %). The mean infusion rate necessary to maintain 90–99 % neuromuscular block is also similar in infants and children.

Rocuronium in adults is an intermediate-acting neuromuscular blocker with a faster onset of action than other NDMRs, and this is also true in infants and children. In children, 0.6 mg/kg of rocuronium produces better conditions for rapid tracheal intubation (60 s) [68] than does 0.1 mg/kg of vecuronium (100 s) or 0.5 mg/kg of atracurium (180 s). As with adults, for rapid sequence intubation (60 s) in the presence of a full stomach, a 1.2 mg/kg dose of rocuronium is suggested to provide excellent intubating condition in all the patients.

It has been frequently stated that dose requirements of neostigmine for reversal were greater in paediatric patients than in adults until it was demonstrated that neostigmine dose requirements were lower in infants and children than in adults [69]. Children can be reversed faster and by much smaller doses than adults. A dose of 30 μg/kg in children is quite comparable to the usual dose of 40 μg/kg in adults and provides satisfactory reversal of neuromuscular block. Neostigmine-assisted recovery of neuromuscular transmission is dependent of age and is slightly more rapid in children than either infants or adults [70]. Recovery is faster when neostigmine is administered after the beginning of spontaneous recovery. When neostigmine is administered at deeper levels of block in children, the total time from neostigmine administration to a 0.7 TOF recovery is longer than when neostigmine is given at 2–4 responses at the TOF. In all cases, tests of clinical recovery, such as head lift, leg lift and cry, can be misleading as in adults. Several studies have demonstrated that when children were extubated using clinical criteria of recovery, the TOF ratio did not exceed 0.5–0.6, whereas a 0.9 TOF ratio is required to guarantee full recovery from neuromuscular block. These results highlight the need for objective assessment of neuromuscular block, even in infants and children, at least at the time of extubation because of their increased sensitivity and variability in their responsiveness to NDMR.

Geriatric Patients

The pharmacodynamics of neuromuscular blockers may be altered in elderly patients. A number of physiological changes that accompany the ageing process will occur including decreases in total body water and lean body mass and increases in total body fat. Moreover, hepatic blood flow and hepatic enzyme activity decrease. Similarly, as a consequence of reduced renal blood flow, glomerular filtration rate decreases by about 20 % per year in adults. These changes may account for the altered responses of the elderly to neuromuscular blockers. Decreased muscular activity may lead to downregulation of nicotinic receptors at the neuromuscular junction.

Several studies found no differences in the initial dose requirement for NDMR in the elderly. The dose–response curves of atracurium, pancuronium and vecuronium were slightly to the right of the curves for the adult subjects; however, there were no significant differences. Several studies have confirmed that NDMRs are as potent in elderly as in young adult patients. The onset of neuromuscular block can be delayed and can be correlated with age. This age-related effect is probably caused by circulatory factors such as decrease in cardiac output and increase in circulation time in the elderly [65]. The onset of rocuronium neuromuscular block was prolonged to 3.7 from 3.1 min in the elderly. Similarly, the onset of cisatracurium is approximately 1 min longer in the elderly.

A prolongation of the duration of action of NDMR and a decrease in dose requirements for the maintenance of neuromuscular block have been observed with several currently available muscle relaxants in the elderly. These results are explained by pharmacokinetic changes in the elderly. The distribution and elimination may be altered by any of the multitude of physiological changes that accompany the ageing process. The effect of ageing alone, versus disease states often associated with the ageing process, may be difficult to distinguish in identifying mechanisms of altered neuromuscular blocker action in the elderly.

The steroidal NDMRs depend on the kidney and/or the liver for their metabolism and elimination. Therefore, they can show altered pharmacodynamics and pharmacokinetics in elderly patients [71, 72]. Vecuronium dose requirements to maintain a constant neuromuscular block are decreased by 36 % approximately in patients over 60 years and spontaneous recovery is significantly longer in the older patients. Lien et al. have shown that plasma clearance was reduced by more than 50 % and elimination half-life prolonged by 60 % in the elderly [72]. The prolongation of vecuronium action appears to be secondary to decreased drug elimination consistent with age-associated decrease in hepatic and renal blood flows. The duration of action of rocuronium and the recovery index are also increased in the elderly. The prolongation of action can be explained by a 27 % decrease in plasma clearance.

In the case of drugs whose elimination is independent of hepatic or renal blood flow, pharmacokinetics and pharmacodynamics should not be significantly altered by age. Atracurium has multiple routes of elimination. Degradation by Hofmann elimination and ester hydrolysis is independent of the liver and the kidney and is not affected with age. The only pharmacokinetic change is a slight increase of the volume of distribution at steady state leading to a modestly increased elimination half-life. Consequently, the duration of action, the recovery index and the dose requirement during a continuous infusion are independent of age [40]. Cisatracurium is mainly eliminated by Hofmann elimination. Unlike atracurium, cisatracurium does not undergo hydrolysis by nonspecific esterases. It exhibits a slightly delayed onset of effect in elderly patients because of slower biophase equilibration. The slight prolongation of the elimination half-life of the drug in the elderly is due to an increased volume of distribution at steady state (+10 %) [73]. These minor pharmacokinetic changes are not associated with changes in recovery profile in the elderly.

It has been demonstrated that the duration of action of neostigmine was prolonged in the elderly. The duration of maximal response to neostigmine increased from 11 to 32 min in the elderly. A shift to the right of the dose–response relationship has been shown for neostigmine antagonism of vecuronium-induced neuromuscular block in the elderly, the reason for the difference being uncertain.

Monitoring of neuromuscular block is of importance in the elderly because recovery of neuromuscular function can be delayed. It has been demonstrated that inadequate or incomplete recovery of muscle strength can be associated with an increased incidence of perioperative pulmonary complications in this patient population. The clear relation between incomplete recovery from neuromuscular block and occurrence of critical respiratory events in the PACU highlights the need for objective recovery of neuromuscular block in the elderly [74].

Patients with Severe Renal Disease

Muscle relaxants contain quaternary ammonium groups which make them very hydrophilic. They are therefore usually completely ionised at a 7.4 pH and poorly bound to plasma proteins. The predominant pathway of elimination of steroidal muscle relaxants is ultrafiltration by the glomeruli before urinary excretion. Only atracurium, cisatracurium and to some extent vecuronium are independent of renal function.

Succinylcholine is metabolised by pseudocholinesterases, the concentration of which may be slightly decreased in patients with severe renal failure. The decrease in plasma cholinesterase activity is always moderate (30 %) and does not result in prolongation of succinylcholine-induced neuromuscular block. Succinylcholine induces a transient increase in plasma potassium concentration (<0.5 mmol/L). Therefore, succinylcholine is not contraindicated in severe renal failure when K+ levels are within the normal range.

Sensitivity to the effects of NDMR remains unchanged in patients with renal failure [75, 76]. A longer onset of action in patients can be observed in patients with end-stage renal failure, because of the increase of the volume of distribution of any NDMR and a reduced cardiac output. Because of the potential for prolonged blockade and the availability of intermediate- and short-acting neuromuscular blockers, there is no longer any reason to recommend the use of the long-acting neuromuscular blockers in patients with renal failure.

The pharmacokinetics and duration of action of atracurium are unaffected by renal failure because Hofmann elimination and ester hydrolysis account for 50 % of its total clearance [77]. Laudanosine, the principal metabolite of atracurium, is eliminated unchanged by the kidney. However, during continuous administration of atracurium, laudanosine plasma concentrations are 10 times less than concentrations associated with convulsions in the dog. The same findings are observed when using cisatracurium, the duration of action remaining unchanged because Hofmann elimination accounts for 77 % of the total clearance and renal excretion accounts for 16 % of its elimination. The peak plasma laudanosine concentrations are 10 times lower than after equipotent doses of atracurium.

Vecuronium relies principally on hepatic, not renal, mechanisms for its elimination. However, its clearance is reduced, and its elimination half-life can be slightly increased in patients with renal failure [78]. However, in clinical use, in patients with renal failure, the duration of action and rate of recovery from vecuronium- or atracurium-induced neuromuscular blockade during surgery are similar. There is only one study where the duration of action of 0.1 mg/kg of vecuronium was both longer and more variable in patients with renal failure than in those with normal renal function. A small dose undergoes hepatic metabolism to, 3-desacetylvecuronium, which has 80 % of the neuromuscular blocking activity of vecuronium; it may cause prolonged paralysis in patients with renal failure in the intensive care unit.

Rocuronium is taken up by the liver and metabolised and excreted in bile and faeces in high concentrations although up to 33 % is eliminated through urinary excretion. After 0.6 mg/kg rocuronium, up to a fifth of the dose is recovered unchanged from the urine, and no active metabolites can be found in humans. The more recent pharmacokinetic studies have shown that the clearance of rocuronium is reduced by 33–39 % in patients with renal failure. Its distribution volume remains unchanged or slightly increased [79]. The elimination half-life was 70 vs 57 min in patients with and without renal failure, respectively. The duration of action of single and repeated doses is not significantly affected but the duration of action is less predictable.

In renal failure, there are no significant changes of the volume of distribution of neostigmine. The clearance of neostigmine is decreased by two-thirds and the elimination half-life is prolonged from 80 to 183 min in patients with renal failure. The clearance of edrophonium is also decreased and significantly reduced, and its elimination half-life is significantly prolonged in patients with end-stage renal failure.

Patients with Hepatobiliary Disease

Liver function is in most clinical situations a modest determinant of the pharmacology of NDMR. Therefore, prolonged neuromuscular block for drugs dependent on hepatic elimination will become apparent only with repeated doses or the use of continuous infusion. Cirrhosis is associated with an increased extracellular water compartment, oedema and often kidney dysfunction. Cholestasis decreases biliary excretion but is not associated with significant liver failure contrary to acute hepatic failure.

There is a delayed onset of action and an apparent resistance to NDMR in patients with cirrhosis although studies have demonstrated that the sensitivity of the neuromuscular junction was unaltered. This is the consequence of the increased volume of distribution inducing an increased dilution of muscle relaxants in cirrhotic patients. The increase of terminal half-life can be either due to the increased volume of distribution or to a decreased biliary excretion for muscle relaxants dependent on hepatic function for elimination [27]. Following a single dose of NDMR, in most cases, there is no prolongation of the duration of action because it is dependent on distribution.

Vecuronium elimination is mainly via the bile. The elimination half-life is increased in mildly decompensated cirrhotic patients as the result of a decreased clearance, while the volume of distribution at steady state can be increased [27]. In cirrhotic patients the duration of action of vecuronium is related to the dose. Cholestasis can increase plasma concentration of bile salts which will reduce the hepatic uptake of vecuronium [26]. This may be an explanation for the decreased clearance observed by some investigators. The duration of action of vecuronium is increased by 50 % in patients with biliary obstruction.

Rocuronium is mainly excreted into the bile. The volume of both the central compartments (33 %) and the volume of distribution at steady state (Vdss) (43 %) are increased in cirrhotic patients, whereas the clearance may be decreased. The duration of action is prolonged in patients with hepatic disease, and there is a correlation between the increased volume of distribution and the slower onset of action when compared to controls [80].

Due to their mode of elimination, the pharmacokinetics of atracurium and cisatracurium are little affected by hepatic disease. In fact, and in contrast to all other neuromuscular blockers, the plasma clearances of atracurium and cisatracurium are slightly increased in patients with liver disease [81]. Because elimination of atracurium and cisatracurium occurs outside of, as well as from within, the central compartment, it has been suggested that a larger distribution volume is associated with greater clearance. The increased clearance of the relaxant in patients with liver disease is not reflected in a decrease in the drugs' durations of action.

One concern raised about administering atracurium to patients with hepatic disease was the possible accumulation of laudanosine. Although laudanosine relies principally on hepatic mechanisms for its elimination, the concentrations encountered during liver transplantation are unlikely to be associated with clinical sequelae.

Because of the wide interindividual variations seen in response to NDMR in patients with hepatic disease, monitoring of neuromuscular block is required with titration of doses.

In patients with severe liver disease, butyrylcholinesterase activity is decreased because of decreased synthesis of the hepatic enzymes. Consequently, the plasma clearance of the isomers of mivacurium is decreased by approximately 50 %, and its duration of action is prolonged and may be almost tripled [82].

Obese Patients

The level of plasma pseudocholinesterase activity and the volume of extracellular fluid which are the main determinants of the duration of action of succinylcholine are increased in the obese patient. Therefore a 1 mg/kg dose based on total body weight (TBW) was recommended to get complete paralysis and predictable intubating condition [83].

Vecuronium doses based on TBW induce a prolonged duration of action in obese patients although vecuronium pharmacokinetics are unaltered by obesity. The prolonged recovery in the obese can be explained by the larger total dose administered in these patients. With larger doses, when administration is based on TBW, recovery will occur during the elimination phase when plasma concentrations decrease more slowly than during the distribution phase [84]. The pharmacokinetics of rocuronium are not altered by obesity. In the same way, the duration of action of rocuronium is significantly prolonged when the dose is calculated according to TBW. In contrast, when rocuronium is dosed according to ideal body weight (IBW), the clinical duration is less than half [85].

There is a correlation between the duration of action of atracurium and TBW when the dose is given as mg/kg of TBW. The clinical duration of action is doubled when the drug is given based on TBW vs IBW. Varin et al. reported the lack of difference between obese and normal patients in atracurium elimination half-life (19.8 vs 19.7 min), volume of distribution at steady state (8.6 vs 8.5 L) and total clearance (444 vs 404 ml/min) [86]. The finding that IBW avoids prolonged recovery of atracurium-induced block can be explained by an unchanged muscle mass and an unchanged volume of distribution in morbidly obese patients compared with normal weight patients. The duration of cisatracurium is also prolonged in obese patients when given on the basis of TBW vs IBW.

Reports on the effects of NDMR neuromuscular blockers in the obese recommend that they should be given on the basis of IBW rather than on actual body weight to ensure that these patients are not receiving relative overdoses with associated avoid prolonged recovery. Some authors did not find any influence of TBW or IBW, whereas some observed a delayed recovery after neostigmine when vecuronium was dosed on TBW. When using maintenance doses, objective monitoring is strongly recommended to avoid accumulation.

Clinical Use of NMBA

NMBAs are used routinely during induction of anaesthesia to provide optimal intubating conditions and paralysis of the diaphragm to facilitate controlled ventilation. During maintenance of anaesthesia, they must provide optimal surgical working conditions. It must be remembered that the intensity of maximum blockade is dependent of the dose. The recommended dose for any NDMR is twice the ED95 at the adductor pollicis because the laryngeal adductor muscles for which relaxation is needed to provide optimal intubating conditions, and the diaphragm, are the most resistant muscle of the body to NDMR. Such a dose will provide good intubating conditions in almost all patients and decrease the rate of vocal cord lesions following intubation [87]. Combes et al. have highlighted that the use of a muscle relaxant for tracheal intubation diminished the incidence of adverse postoperative upper airway symptoms and produces better tracheal intubation conditions and reduction of the

rate of adverse haemodynamic events [88]. Similar findings were even observed in paediatric patients where intubation conditions are usually favourable [68].

During surgery some authors have suggested that NDMRs do not need to be used routinely, for example, during retroperitoneal or retropubic surgery. A prospective controlled study has clearly demonstrated that NDMRs (vecuronium) very significantly decrease the rate of unacceptable conditions in patients undergoing retropubic surgery even if halogenated agents are used for maintenance of anaesthesia. Moreover, the surgeons found that abdominal muscle relaxation as estimated by clinical judgement increases with increasing doses of vecuronium [89]. In most cases, good perioperative conditions are obtained with shallow levels of neuromuscular block, i.e. one or two responses at the TOF at the adductor pollicis. In some cases, because the diaphragm and the abdominal wall muscles are the most resistant muscles of the body to NMBA, the surgeon may complain about the intensity of the block because the diaphragm has already started its recovery or the patient is coughing, whereas the peripheral muscles such as the adductor pollicis are still fully paralysed with no response to the TOF at the adductor pollicis [90]. During laparoscopic surgery it was demonstrated that deep neuromuscular block could reduce intra-abdominal pressure by almost 25 % [91]. In these situations a deep level (no more than three responses at the PTC) of neuromuscular block with abolition of the four responses at the TOF at the adductor pollicis can be indicated. In this case monitoring of the depth of block can be accomplished using the PTC (post-tetanic count) at the adductor pollicis or the TOF at the corrugator supercilii [92]. Up to now, anaesthesiologists have been rather reluctant to use these deep levels of neuromuscular block up to the very end of the surgical procedure because until now it was impossible to reverse deep neuromuscular block [93]. This kind of situation should not be a problem anymore because it is now possible to fully paralyse the diaphragm and the abdominal wall muscles with greater doses of steroidal NDMR [94, 95] and to maintain this deep block until the closure or the removal of the last device during laparoscopic surgery before reversal with new agents such as sugammadex [96].

Most anaesthesiologists prefer to maintain neuromuscular blockade by giving repeated doses and if possible by taking into account the information provided by monitoring such as the TOF at the adductor pollicis [97]. However, it can be tempting to maintain neuromuscular block by continuous infusion of intermediate-duration action NDMR. During continuous administration, there are risks of under- or overdosing when monitoring is not used. In most cases, it is recommended to avoid this risk by maintaining one or two responses at the TOF at the adductor pollicis. Due to the improvement and now simplicity of the new neuromuscular blockade monitors using acceleromyography, it is tempting to use closed-loop systems to maintain stable neuromuscular block and decrease the clinical workload. Another benefit would be to take into account a wide range of patient sensitivities. Different techniques using either PID controllers [98] or the fuzzy logic approach have been used [99]. Most of them are efficient, but these techniques have some drawbacks such as instability of the neuromuscular block in the first hour of administration or during a syringe change. Losses of the signal or interference with diathermy have also been described.

Monitoring Neuromuscular Blockade

Monitoring of neuromuscular blockade during anaesthesia is of great interest because subjective evaluation is often misleading leading to under- or overdosing. The large inter-individual variability in response to neuromuscular relaxants [100], whatever the drug used, makes the degree and the duration of action of a predetermined dose unpredictable. Moreover, the margin of safety is narrow and neuromuscular blockade will occur within a narrow range of receptor occupancy. The presence of residual neuromuscular block is a well-identified factor of postoperative respiratory depression and increases morbidity during general anaesthesia.

Stimulus Pattern

Train-of-Four (TOF)

TOF consists of four stimulations at a frequency of 2 Hz; it can be repeated at 10–12-s intervals. No control value is needed for TOF measurement, and there is a close relationship between single-twitch depression and the number of responses following TOF stimulation [101]. Sufficient neuromuscular blockade for common surgical procedures can be assumed until the reappearance of one or two responses at the TOF. When a deeper level of block is required, for example, during major laparoscopic surgery, a dose sufficient to cause disappearance of the TOF at the adductor pollicis is required. The TOF ratio is the ratio of the height of the first and the fourth response. However, visual or tactile evaluation of the TOF ratio can be misleading, because it is not always possible to detect fade until the TOF ratio is as low as 0.4–0.5, even for experienced observers. A TOF ratio of at least 0.9 is necessary to guarantee in all patients an adequate recovery of pharyngeal muscle function and respiratory function after neuromuscular blockade.

Tetanus, Post-tetanic Count (PTC)

For many years, tetanus has been used to detect fade during recovery, but it has recently been demonstrated that a 50-Hz tetanic stimulation for 5 s did not improve the detection of fade when compared with the TOF. The only remaining indication for tetanic stimulation is in performing a PTC when a deep neuromuscular blockade exists and no responses to TOF are detectable [102, 103]. It consists of a 50-Hz tetanic stimulation applied for 5 s, followed by single-twitch stimulations at 1 Hz after a 3-s pause. The reappearance of a twitch response when no TOF is observed accords with the principle of post-tetanic facilitation. For a given drug, the number of detectable responses correlates inversely with the time for spontaneous recovery of TOF [104, 105]. When five to seven responses are detectable, spontaneous return of the TOF response is imminent. It is usually recommended that PTC should not be performed more than once every 5 min.

Double-Burst Stimulation (DBS)

DBS has been introduced into clinical practice to improve the detection of fade during visual or tactile evaluation. DBS consists of two short bursts of 50-Hz tetanic stimulation separated by 750 ms. The duration of each burst is 0.2 ms. DBS3,3 consists of two bursts of three impulses. The two contractions induced by a DBS are of greater amplitude than the contractions after a TOF, and visual or tactile assessment of fade is easier than after a TOF [106]. A fading of the second impulse compared to the first correlates with an incomplete neuromuscular recovery with a comparable TOF ratio <60 % [107].

Assessment of the Muscular Response

Visual or tactile evaluation of muscular responses following nerve stimulation is the easiest way to assess neuromuscular blockade during anaesthesia. However, fade can be difficult to detect manually or visually and can lead to underestimation of neuromuscular block. Measurement of muscular strength using a force transducer is a more accurate method. Unfortunately, the force transducers available limit this technique to monitoring of the adductor pollicis. Tetanus or DBS is no longer helpful since a precise value of the TOF ratio is obtained. The use of electromyography has been proposed because it does not require bulky equipment and can be used in children. Monitoring is dependent of the muscle monitored. Monitoring the EMG of the hypothenar muscles overestimates the degree of recovery from neuromuscular blockade. Acceleromyography assumes that acceleration recorded by a piezoelectric transducer is proportional to force if mass remains unchanged [108]. The advantages of acceleromyography are an easy set-up of the transducer and the opportunity to monitor other muscles than the adductor pollicis. The acceleromyographic T4/T1 ratio can be greater than 1.0 in the absence of neuromuscular blockade although the new transducers are more accurate. Acceleromyography correlates well with techniques such as mechanomyography [109]. It is recommended to ensure correct fixation of the forearm and the fingers to avoid artefacts due to patient movements. The new generation of transducers usually provides improved set-up and the reduced variability of measurements.

Clinical Applications

Monitoring Onset

The adductor pollicis has been widely used to determine the onset of paralysis. However discrepancies have been described between tracheal intubating conditions and the intensity of peripheral paralysis. Although intubating conditions are affected by the depth of anaesthesia, the use of the adductor pollicis for monitoring, during onset to determine the time for good intubating conditions, could be misleading because paralysis of the adductor pollicis lags behind onset at the laryngeal adductor muscles and the diaphragm. Furthermore, the adductor pollicis may be blocked with a dose insufficient to block the laryngeal adductor muscles because the latter are more resistant to NDMR [29, 48, 110]. Since the sensitivity of the corrugator supercilii oculi is close to that of the respiratory and laryngeal muscles, monitoring the corrugator supercilii oculi may reliably detect when respiratory and vocal cords are paralysed [92].

Surgical Relaxation

When profound neuromuscular blockade is required, absence of the TOF response at the adductor pollicis does not eliminate the possibility that hiccups, cough or extrusion of the abdominal contents can occur because of the discrepancies between resistant muscles such as the diaphragm [90] or the abdominal wall muscles [111] and more sensitive muscles such as the adductor pollicis. Two techniques may allow the evaluation of intense neuromuscular blockade during the phase of the "period of no response" at the adductor pollicis and predict the time to the reappearance of the TOF at the adductor pollicis. The PTC at the adductor pollicis was the first technique described. For a given muscle relaxant, time until the return of the first response at the TOF is related to the PTC at a given time. The major drawback of this technique is that it cannot be repeated more often than every 5 min. Monitoring of the TOF at the corrugator supercilii also has a role because the response of the orbicularis oculi is a good reflector of diaphragmatic paralysis [92]. When profound blockade is not essential, monitoring of the adductor pollicis, with TOF, is sufficient.

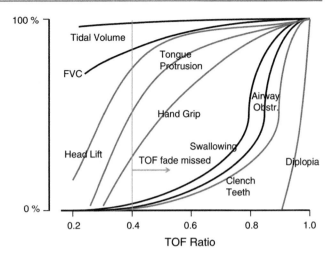

Fig. 15.11 Approximate behaviour of respiratory function, airway integrity and various tests as a function of train-of-four ratio. Reproduced from Donati [113] with permission from Springer

Monitoring Recovery

The adductor pollicis is preferable for the management of recovery because it is a sensitive muscle. When the adductor pollicis has almost completely recovered, it can be assumed that there is no residual paralysis of the more resistant muscles of the body such as the diaphragm, the abdominal wall muscles and the laryngeal muscles. However, recent studies have demonstrated that symptoms of residual paralysis may persist until the TOF ratio has returned to a value of 0.9 [53, 54, 112]. Therefore a TOF ratio above 0.9 is needed in the recovery room to avoid any respiratory problem secondary to residual neuromuscular blockade because the muscles of the upper airway are particularly sensitive to the effects of muscle relaxants (Fig. 15.11) [113]. Using DBS at the adductor pollicis, fade can only be detected at degrees of neuromuscular blockade corresponding to a TOF ratio of no more than 0.6 [114]. Recent studies have determined that TOF ratios <0.9 were observed in 30–60 % of postoperative patients who do not receive neuromuscular monitoring [115, 116]. These facts suggest that detection of residual paralysis can be improved by the use of objective monitoring such as acceleromyography [117] which can also decrease the rate of critical respiratory events due to residual paralysis in the PACU [74].

Anticholinesterase Drugs

In 1954, Beecher and Todd suggested that the use of NMBA could significantly increase the mortality rate during general anaesthesia [118]. These findings were due to the nonroutine use of controlled ventilation in these patients but also to residual paralysis and likely critical respiratory events (CRE) after surgery. Therefore, in the early 1950s, Cecil Gray suggested the routine administration of 5-mg neostigmine at the end of surgery to prevent residual paralysis, when long-acting NMBAs were used [2]. For over 40 years, anticholinesterases have been widely used to reverse neuromuscular block at the end of the case, the most commonly employed being neostigmine.

Anticholinesterase Drugs

The action of NMDR is reversed by anticholinesterase drugs, which temporarily inactivate acetylcholinesterase and increase the amount of acetylcholine at the postsynaptic membrane [119]. This causes an increase in the size and the duration of the end-plate potential. Anticholinesterases also have presynaptic effects, and in the absence of NMBA, they may potentiate the normal twitch response. Because anticholinesterase acts not only at the motor end plate but at all muscarinic receptors, they cause excessive salivation, increased bowel activity and bradycardia due to profound vagal stimulation. They are therefore combined with an anticholinergic agent such as atropine or glycopyrrolate which blocks the muscarinic but not the nicotinic effects of acetylcholine [120]. The concomitant use of atropine induces its own side effects such as tachycardia, dry mouth and blurred vision. Therefore neostigmine may be contraindicated in patients with cardiovascular disease or severe asthma. There are conflicting reports on the risk of bowel anastomotic leakage after reversal of neuromuscular blockade.

Neostigmine and pyridostigmine, but not edrophonium, bind to the anionic and esteratic sites and are hydrolysed by acetylcholinesterase. Edrophonium binds with the esterase site on acetylcholinesterase, forming a loose electrostatic bond, and there is a competition between it and acetylcholine for the site. The action of edrophonium is terminated as it simply diffuses away from the synaptic cleft. Neostigmine binds more strongly to both the anionic and esteratic sites on acetylcholinesterase. Neostigmine is approximately 12 times as potent as edrophonium. The durations of action of neostigmine, pyridostigmine and edrophonium are similar, but the onset times differ considerably: the peak effect of edrophonium occurs at 1–2 min [121], neostigmine at 7–11 min and pyridostigmine at greater than 16 min. The onset of pyridostigmine is too slow for clinical purposes. These differences in onset of action could be due to the different rates of binding to acetylcholinesterase. The anticholinesterase agents all have a ceiling effect, and there is

little benefit in administering more than 0.07 mg/kg neostigmine because of the limited amount of acetylcholine at the neuromuscular junction. Large doses, greater than those used in clinical practice, may produce neuromuscular blockade [122, 123].

The time to recovery from neuromuscular block depends on the rate of spontaneous recovery but essentially from the intensity of the block when the reversal agent is given [113]. It is recommended that at least two or even four visible twitches of a TOF be visible before reversing. When neostigmine is given without the use of neuromuscular monitoring, there is an increased incidence of postoperative respiratory complications [124]. Reversal with edrophonium is superior to neostigmine only if significant spontaneous recovery has occurred. Increasing neostigmine doses to shorten its onset is not a valuable option because neostigmine exhibits a ceiling effect. Moreover, recovery of shallow levels of neuromuscular block (at least two responses of the TOF at the adductor pollicis) following neostigmine is not as fast as usually thought. Kopman had demonstrated that when neostigmine was given during shallow rocuronium- or cisatracurium-induced neuromuscular block at two responses at the TOF, the TOF ratio was 0.76 and 0.72, respectively, 10 min after administration [125]. Blobner et al. have demonstrated that the median time to reach a 0.9 TOF ratio following neostigmine administered after reappearance of two twitches was 18.5 min. One major issue was the large interindividual variability; even 60 min after neostigmine administration, less than 90 % of the patients had reached a 0.9 TOF ratio [126]. When neostigmine or edrophonium has been administered at deep level of block, there is a chance of return of neuromuscular block particularly with the long-lasting NMBA such as pancuronium or pipecuronium. Elimination of anticholinesterases is delayed in patients with end-stage renal failure because they are eliminated by the kidney [127, 128]. Therefore they can be used safely in patients with renal failure and recurarisation cannot occur.

Reversal of Neuromuscular Blockade

Some authors have questioned the routine use of anticholinesterases drugs because it is considered that following the recommended intubating dose, i.e. twice the ED_{95} at the adductor pollicis, complete spontaneous recovery from intermediate-duration action NMBAs, will occur in less than 60–90 min after drug administration. Recent studies on a large number of young and healthy ASA I and II patients have clearly demonstrated that even 2 h after drug administration, around 30 % of patients receiving intermediate-duration action NMBAs still have a TOF ratio less than 0.9 [116]. Many studies have confirmed the efficiency of anticholinesterase agents. Baillard et al. have clearly demonstrated that the rate of residual paralysis in the recovery room has been decreased very significantly over 10 years by routine use of monitoring of neuromuscular block in association with administration of neostigmine when residual paralysis was detected [115]. The rate of residual blockade as defined as a TOF ratio <0.9 decreased from 62 to 3 %, confirming the benefit of reversal in routine anaesthetic practice.

Although some clinicians consider that muscle weakness is a rare event with few consequences, several studies have clearly demonstrated that a TOF ratio <0.9 is associated with critical respiratory events in the PACU such as airway obstruction, hypoxemia or even postoperative pulmonary complications [55]. Berg demonstrated that during pancuronium-induced neuromuscular blockade, patients with a TOF ratio less than 0.7 had mild or even severe episodes of desaturation in the PACU and were more likely to develop postoperative pulmonary complications [129]. More recent studies have clearly demonstrated that even after the use of intermediate-acting NMBA, the risk of postoperative pulmonary complications in the PACU when the TOF ratio was less than 0.9 was increased. Murphy studied 7459 patients arriving in the PACU. The patients who developed critical respiratory events such as severe hypoxemia and/or upper airway obstruction had a mean TOF ratio of 0.62. In contrast to the control group, the mean TOF ratio was 0.98, and no control patients had a TOF ratio less than 0.7 [55, 112]. When objective monitoring using acceleromyography is used instead of a conventional peripheral nerve stimulator, there is a significant reduction in the incidence of residual blockade [117] and associated unpleasant symptoms of muscle weakness in the PACU such as blurred vision or facial weakness or subjective difficulty speaking. In the same time, Arbous et al., by studying the morbidity and mortality rate in more than 850,000 patients in Holland, were able to demonstrate that the use of reversal agents at the end of the case could induce a very significant decrease in morbidity and mortality (odds ratio, 0.10; 95 % confidence interval, 0.032–0.314) [130].

After giving neostigmine, anaesthetists may be overconfident and extubate the patient, whereas a 0.9 TOF ration has not been yet reached. Therefore routine monitoring is strongly recommended to assess complete recovery from neuromuscular blockade. On the other hand, it has been demonstrated that 20 mcg/kg is as effective as 40 mcg/kg when TOF fade is no longer detectable, justifying the practice of giving a half dose if complete recovery cannot be ascertained [131, 132].

Sugammadex

Until recently, the action of NDMR could only be reversed by anticholinesterase drugs. However, as previously discussed, their use has several pitfalls due to their muscarinic effects, their relatively slow onset and their inability to reverse deep levels of neuromuscular block [113]. The release of sugammadex since 2009 provides a new approach in the management of neuromuscular blockade during surgery and the prevention of residual paralysis at the end of the case.

Pharmacology (Fig. 15.12)

Sugammadex is a modified γ cyclodextrin specifically designed to encapsulate rocuronium [133] and chemically similar aminosteroid muscle relaxants such as vecuronium. The underlying mechanism of action is new and differs

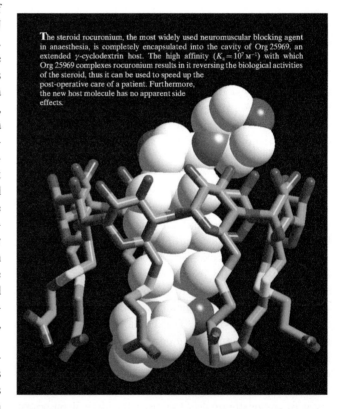

Fig. 15.12 Interaction of sugammadex (Org 25969) with rocuronium with rocuronium hydrophobic part with the cyclodextrin cavity. Reproduced from Bom et al. [133] with permission from John Wiley and Sons

completely from that of acetylcholine esterase inhibitors. When sugammadex is injected intravenously, the free molecules of rocuronium in plasma which are in equilibrium with the tissues are almost immediately captured by the sugammadex molecules, and the plasma-free rocuronium concentration decreases very rapidly [134–136]. This creates a gradient of rocuronium between tissue and plasma, with rocuronium molecules moving out of the tissue and into plasma where they are encapsulated by free sugammadex molecules. Following administration of sugammadex, the concentration of free rocuronium decreases rapidly in the plasma, but the total rocuronium plasma concentration (free and bound to sugammadex) increases rapidly [136]. The complex is then rapidly filtered by the glomerulus and eliminated through the kidney. Sugammadex has no direct effect on cholinergic transmission. It is considered as a selective relaxant binding agent (SRBA), and it does not exhibit intrinsic biological activity.

It does not have any affinity for more than 40 drugs that may be used during anaesthesia (hypnotics, analgesics, antibiotics, cardiovascular drugs). Affinity for cortisone, hydrocortisone and aldosterone has been extensively studied because sugammadex binds strongly to steroidal NMBA; affinity is 120-fold less than for rocuronium. Affinity for atropine, verapamil and ketamine is 400–700-fold lower than for rocuronium. Among many molecules studied, toremifene and flucloxacillin are the only molecules known to displace rocuronium or vecuronium from sugammadex. Sugammadex is ineffective when blockade is produced by mivacurium, atracurium or cisatracurium.

When compared with neostigmine for reversal of neuromuscular block at reappearance of four TOF responses, it has been shown that a 0.90 TOF ratio was obtained in approximately 2 min with sugammadex compared to a time of 17 min using neostigmine [137]. It was also shown that there are no differences in time taken to reach a 0.9 TOF ratio after anaesthesia maintained with halogenated agents when compared with propofol [138]. Although sugammadex was developed to antagonise rocuronium-induced block, it is also effective in reversing 0.1 mg/kg vecuronium-induced block [139] and even the long-acting steroidal NDMRs such as pipecuronium [140]. Jones et al. compared the efficacy of sugammadex versus neostigmine for reversal of deep level of rocuronium-induced paralysis. Sugammadex or neostigmine was given at reappearance of 1–2 responses at the PTC when no responses at the TOF at the adductor pollicis could be detected. A 0.9 TOF ratio was attained in 2.9 min with sugammadex versus 50.4 min in patients receiving neostigmine—glycopyrrolate. The most important finding was the reproducibility and the small range when sugammadex is given; 97 % of patients receiving

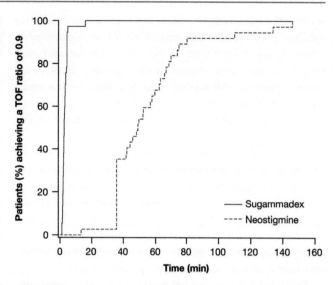

Fig. 15.13 Time to recovery of the TOF ratio to 0.9 from deep rocuronium-induced neuromuscular blockade after administration of sugammadex (4 mg/kg) or neostigmine (0.07 mg/kg). Reproduced from Jones et al. [141] with permission from Wolters Kluwer Health, Inc.

sugammadex had a TOF ratio above 0.9 within 5 min of administration, whereas a large number of patients receiving neostigmine did not recover until 30–60 min and 23 % did not recover to a 0.9 TOF ratio until more than 60 min (Fig. 15.13) [141].

It would be tempting to use lower doses of sugammadex to decrease costs, particularly when there are already four responses at the TOF with a measurable TOF ratio; however, due to the mechanism of action of sugammadex, using low doses could lead to reappearance of neuromuscular block after an initial and successful recovery. Such a risk was confirmed by Eleveld et al. who described reappearance of neuromuscular block following initial recovery, when using inadequate doses [142]. It is likely that when sugammadex is not administered at a sufficient dose, it can initially form complexes with rocuronium in blood and initiate initial recovery. However the dose will be insufficient to sustain redistribution of rocuronium from the neuromuscular junction to blood causing a reappearance of residual paralysis.

There are situations in which deep block must be reversed very rapidly, for example, when tracheal intubation has failed. When given, 3 min after 1.2 mg/kg rocuronium, 16 mg/kg sugammadex can completely reverse the block in less than 3 min. In this setting, recovery with sugammadex is significantly faster than spontaneous recovery from succinylcholine [143].

In elderly patients, the time needed to a 0.9 TOF ratio does not differ very much (2.9 min) when compared with younger patients [144]. As for any NMBA, this very mild slower onset of action in the elderly could be due to circulatory factors such as altered muscle perfusion or decreased cardiac output. There are few data in paediatric patients. Plaud et al. have demonstrated that sugammadex could be used safely at a dose of 2 mg/kg and that recovery times were similar in children and adolescents when compared with adults. Although there were a small number of infants studied, recovery time to obtain a 0.9 TOF ratio, after sugammadex, was rapid ranging from 0.6 to 3.7 min.

Because sugammadex does not act in the same way as neostigmine or edrophonium, by inhibition of acetylcholinesterase and an indirect action on receptors, but by encapsulation in the plasma, it is not expected to have the side effects associated with anticholinesterase agents. Dahl et al. have confirmed the lack of cardiovascular effects of both 2 and 4 mg/kg sugammadex in patients with cardiovascular disease undergoing noncardiac surgery [145].

The imprint of sugammadex has been recently supplemented with the notification of a longer clotting time in the first minutes following its administration without any documented clinical consequences. In an observational study, Raft et al. investigated before, 1 h after sugammadex administration and on the next day, clinical bleeding, haemoglobin concentration, haematocrit, activated partial thromboplastin time (aPTT) and prothrombin time (PT) in 142 patients scheduled for major abdominal cancer surgery and at risk of surgical bleeding. They did not find any significant differences between the control group (no sugammadex) and the groups receiving either 2 or 4 mg/kg sugammadex in terms of clinical bleeding [146]. Its administration was not associated with a longer clotting time nor decreased haemoglobin concentration. Rahe-Meyer confirmed that sugammadex produced limited transient (<1 h) increases in activated partial thromboplastin time and prothrombin time but was not associated with increased risk of bleeding versus usual care [147].

Any NMBA can cause anaphylactic reactions because quaternary ammonium ions are suggested to be the allergenic determinants in NMBAs. In most cases cross-reactivity can be observed even between steroidal and benzylisoquinoline NMBA. The use of sugammadex to capture rocuronium and to be an adjunct in the management of rocuronium-induced anaphylactic complications has been suggested. There are a few clinical cases where sustained haemodynamic improvement (increase in blood pressure and normalisation of heart rate) was observed during a rocuronium anaphylactic event, after administration of sugammadex. Baldo has suggested that sugammadex could eventually interact with mast cells [148]. However there is not yet enough scientific evidence to recommend sugammadex as the treatment of choice during anaphylactic reaction due to steroidal NMBAs [149].

Clinical Use

There has always been an unsatisfied need for a reversal agent that can rapidly reverse neuromuscular block regardless of its depth. This ability to reverse intense neuromuscular block very rapidly and reliably provides the opportunity to maintain it until the complete end of the procedure. There are clinical situations where the surgeon needs complete muscle relaxation until the end of the case (major abdominal or thoracic surgery, laparoscopic surgery) and where the anaesthetist is reluctant to provide full paralysis because it will delay significantly recovery and turnover of the patients in the operating room. Now it is possible to maintain paralysis of the diaphragm and the abdominal wall muscles until the very end of the procedure. The need for monitoring remains important since it is the only objective manner to follow the evolution of deep neuromuscular block and decide of the dose of sugammadex that need to be administered (2 or 4 mg/kg) at the end of the case (Fig. 15.14). There is a risk of a TOF ratio <0.9 in the PACU that can be as high as 10 % when sugammadex administration is not guided by neuromuscular monitoring [150].

Now that anaesthesiologists have available many drugs with a short offset (desflurane, sevoflurane, propofol, remifentanil), it will also be possible to have a very precise control of neuromuscular block when steroidal NMBAs are used to maintain relaxation and to obtain, for the first time, a rapid and reliable recovery from deep neuromuscular block.

Compared with neostigmine/atropine or edrophonium/glycopyrrolate, the costs for sugammadex are significantly higher. On the other hand, muscle weakness, significant delays in meeting PACU discharge criteria and achieving PACU discharge can be observed in patients with TOF ratios less than 0.9 after surgery. Taking into account the NHS Economic Evaluation Database assuming that time saved in the OR has a value of £4.44 per minute, Paton et al. were able to demonstrate that 2 or 4 mg/kg sugammadex was cost-effective for routine reversal of shallow and even deep neuromuscular blockade if reductions in recovery times were obtained in the operating room and associated with improvement in productivity and more efficient use of staff members [151]. In a teaching Australian hospital, following its introduction, the use of neostigmine nearly halved compared to that of the previous year. The cost of reversal increased significantly but a reduction in the median duration of stay was observed. From the author's point of view, the reduction in hospital stay could fully offset the observed increased costs [152]. However, it must be pointed out that neostigmine should not be withdrawn from clinical use, because it is the only reversal agent acting against residual paralysis induced by

Therapeutic Range of Neostigmine and Sugammadex

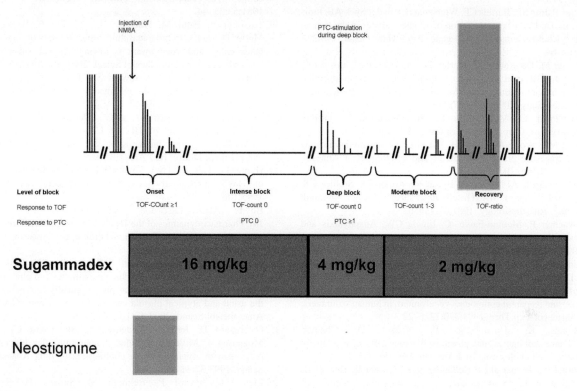

Fig. 15.14 Compared therapeutic window for neostigmine and sugammadex during rocuronium-induced neuromuscular block. Reproduced from Meistelman et al. [153] with permission from Springer

benzylisoquinoline NDMRs. Moreover, it use can still be discussed for the low levels of residual paralysis such as with a TOF >0.4 [131].

References

1. Griffith HR, Johnson GE. The use of curare in general anesthesia. Anesthesiology. 1942;3:418–20.
2. Gray TC, Halton J. Technique for the use of d-tubocurarine chloride with balanced anaesthesia. Br Med J. 1946;2:293–5.
3. Wang X, Engisch KL, Li Y, Pinter MJ, Cope TC, Rich MM. Decreased synaptic activity shifts the calcium dependence of release at the mammalian neuromuscular junction in vivo. J Neurosci. 2004;24(47):10687–92.
4. Lang T, Jahn R. Core proteins of the secretory machinery. Handb Exp Pharmacol. 2008;184:107–27.
5. Littleton JT, Bellen HJ. Synaptotagmin controls and modulates synaptic-vesicle fusion in a Ca(2+)-dependent manner. Trends Neurosci. 1995;18(4):177–83.
6. Cohen-Cory S. The developing synapse: construction and modulation of synaptic structures and circuits. Science. 2002;298 (5594):770–6.
7. Naguib M, Flood P, McArdle JJ, Brenner HR. Advances in neurobiology of the neuromuscular junction: implications for the anesthesiologist. Anesthesiology. 2002;96(1):202–31.
8. Bowman WC, Prior C, Marshall IG. Presynaptic receptors in the neuromuscular junction. Ann NY Acad Sci. 1990; 604:69–81.
9. Bowman WC, Rodger W, Houston J, Marshall RJ, McIndewar I. Structure:action relationships among some desacetoxy analogues of pancuronium and vecuronium in the anesthetized cat. Anesthesiology. 1988;69:57–62.
10. Glavinovic MI, Law Min JC, Kapural L, Donati F, Bevan DR. Speed of action of various muscle relaxants at the neuromuscular junction binding vs buffering hypothesis. J Pharmacol Exp Ther. 1993;265:1181–6.
11. Donati F, Meistelman C. A kinetic-dynamic model to explain the relationship between high potency and slow onset time for neuromuscular blocking drugs. J Pharmacokinet Biopharm. 1991;19:537–52.
12. Kopman AF. Pancuronium, gallamine, and d-tubocurarine compared: is speed of onset inversely related to drug potency. Anesthesiology. 1989;70:915–20.
13. Ducharme J, Varin F, Bevan DR, Donati F. Importance of early blood sampling on vecuronium pharmacokinetic and pharmacodynamic parameters. Clin Pharmacokinet. 1993;24:507–18.
14. Goat VA, Yeung ML, Blakeney C, Feldman SA. The effect of blood flow upon the activity of gallamine triethiodide. Br J Anaesth. 1976;48:69–73.
15. Szmuk P, Ezri T, Chelly JE, Katz J. The onset time of rocuronium is slowed by esmolol and accelerated by ephedrine. Anesth Analg. 2000;90(5):1217–9.
16. Donati F. Pharmacokinetic and pharmacodynamic factors in the clinical use of muscle relaxants. Semin Anesth. 1994;13:310–20.
17. Meistelman C, Plaud B, Donati F. Neuromuscular effects of succinylcholine on the vocal cords and adductor pollicis muscles. Anesth Analg. 1991;73:278–82.
18. Jensen FS, Viby-Mogensen J. Plasma cholinesterase and abnormal reaction to succinylcholine: twenty years' experience with the

Danish Cholinesterase Research Unit. Acta Anaesthesiol Scand. 1995;39:150–6.

19. Primo-Parmo SL, Bartels CF, Wiersema B, van der Spek AF, Innis JW, La Du BN. Characterization of 12 silent alleles of the human butyrylcholinesterase (BCHE) gene. Am J Hum Genet. 1996;58 (1):52–64.

20. Jonsson M, Dabrowski M, Gurley DA, Larsson O, Johnson EC, Fredholm BB, et al. Activation and inhibition of human muscular and neuronal nicotinic acetylcholine receptors by succinylcholine. Anesthesiology. 2006;104(4):724–33.

21. Meistelman C, McLoughlin C. Suxamethonium - current controversies. Curr Anaesth Crit Care. 1993;4:53–8.

22. Salem MR, Wong AY, Lin YH. The effect of suxamethonium on the intragastric pressure in infants and children. Br J Anaesth. 1972;44(2):166–70.

23. Van Der Spek AFL, Fang WB, Ashton-Miller JA, Stohler CS, Carlson DS, Schork MA. The effects of succinylcholine on mouth opening. Anesthesiology. 1987;67:459–63.

24. Dewachter P, Mouton-Faivre C, Emala CW. Anaphylaxis and anesthesia: controversies and new insights. Anesthesiology. 2009;111(5):1141–50.

25. Caldwell JE, Szenohradszky J, Segredo V, Wright PM, McLoughlin C, Sharma ML, et al. The pharmacodynamics and pharmacokinetics of the metabolite 3- desacetylvecuronium (ORG 7268) and its parent compound, vecuronium, in human volunteers. J Pharmacol Exp Ther. 1994;270:1216–22.

26. Lebrault C, Duvaldestin P, Henzel D, Chauvin M. Pharmacokinetics and pharmacodynamics of vecuronium in patients with cholestasis. Br J Anaesth. 1986;58:983–7.

27. Lebrault C, Berger JL, d'Hollander AA, Gomeni R, Henzel D, Duvaldestin P. Pharmacokinetics and pharmacodynamics of vecuronium (ORG NC 45) in patients with cirrhosis. Anesthesiology. 1985;62:601–5.

28. Donati F, Meistelman C, Plaud B. Vecuronium neuromuscular blockade at the diaphragm, the orbicularis oculi, and adductor pollicis muscles. Anesthesiology. 1990;73:870–5.

29. Donati F, Meistelman C, Plaud B. Vecuronium neuromuscular blockade at the adductor muscles of the larynx and adductor pollicis. Anesthesiology. 1991;74:833–7.

30. Khuenl-Brady KS, Castagnoli KP, Canfell PC, Caldwell JE, Agoston S, Miller RD. The neuromuscular blocking effects and pharmacokinetics of ORG 9426 and ORG 9616 in the cat. Anesthesiology. 1990;72:669–74.

31. Magorian T, Wood P, Caldwell J, Fisher D, Segredo V, Szenohradszky J, et al. The pharmacokinetics and neuromuscular effects of rocuronium bromide in patients with liver disease. Anesth Analg. 1995;80:754–9.

32. Magorian T, Flannery KB, Miller RD. Comparison of rocuronium, succinylcholine, and vecuronium for rapid- sequence induction of anesthesia in adult patients. Anesthesiology. 1993;79:913–8.

33. Meistelman C, Plaud B, Donati F. Rocuronium (ORG 9426) neuromuscular blockade at the adductor muscles of the larynx and adductor pollicis in humans. Can J Anaesth. 1992;39:665–9.

34. Agoston S, Vermeer GA, Kersten UW, Meijer DKF. The fate of pancuronium bromide in man. Acta Anaesthesiol Scand. 1973;17:267–75.

35. Donati F, Antzaka C, Bevan DR. Potency of pancuronium at the diaphragm and the adductor pollicis muscle in humans. Anesthesiology. 1986;65:1–5.

36. Smith CE, Donati F, Bevan DR. Differential effects of pancuronium on masseter and adductor pollicis muscles in humans. Anesthesiology. 1989;71:57–61.

37. Ornstein E, Matteo RS, Schwartz AE, Jamdar SC, Diaz J. Pharmacokinetics and pharmacodynamics of pipecuronium bromide (Arduan) in elderly surgical patients. Anesth Analg. 1992;74 (6):841–4.

38. Hughes R, Chapple DJ. The pharmacology of atracurium: a new competitive neuromuscular blocking agent. Br J Anaesth. 1981;53:31–44.

39. Tassonyi E, Fathi M, Hughes GJ, Chiodini F, Bertrand D, Muller D, et al. Cerebrospinal fluid concentrations of atracurium, laudanosine and vecuronium following clinical subarachnoid hemorrhage. Acta Anaesthesiol Scand. 2002;46(10):1236–41.

40. Parker CJ, Hunter JM, Snowdon SL. Effect of age, sex and anaesthetic technique on the pharmacokinetics of atracurium. Br J Anaesth. 1992;69(5):439–43.

41. Eastwood NB, Boyd AH, Parker CJR, Hunter JM. Pharmacokinetics of 1R- cis 1'R- cis atracurium besylate (51W89) and plasma laudanosine concentrations in health and chronic renal failure. Br J Anaesth. 1995;75:431–5.

42. Hunter JM, Eastwood NB, Boyd AH, Parker CJ. Pharmacokinetics of 51W89: preliminary data. Acta Anaesthesiol Scand Suppl. 1995;106:94.

43. Boyd AH, Eastwood NB, Parker CJ, Hunter JM. Pharmacodynamics of the 1R cis-1'R cis isomer of atracurium (51W89) in health and chronic renal failure. Br J Anaesth. 1995;74 (4):400–4.

44. Ostergaard D, Viby-Mogensen J, Rasmussen SN, Gatke MR, Pedersen NA, Skovgaard LT. Pharmacokinetics and pharmacodynamics of mivacurium in patients phenotypically heterozygous for the usual and atypical plasma cholinesterase variants (UA). Acta Anaesthesiol Scand. 2003;47(10):1219–25.

45. Ostergaard D, Jensen FS, Jensen E, Skovgaard LT, Viby-Mogensen J. Mivacurium-induced neuromuscular blockade in patients with atypical plasma cholinesterase. Acta Anaesthesiol Scand. 1993;37:314–8.

46. Lien CA, Savard P, Belmont M, Sunaga H, Savarese JJ. Fumarates: unique nondepolarizing neuromuscular blocking agents that are antagonized by cysteine. J Crit Care. 2009;24 (1):50–7.

47. Savarese JJ, McGilvra JD, Sunaga H, Belmont MR, Van Ornum SG, Savard PM, et al. Rapid chemical antagonism of neuromuscular blockade by L-cysteine adduction to and inactivation of the olefinic (double-bonded) isoquinolinium diester compounds gantacurium (AV430A), CW 002, and CW 011. Anesthesiology. 2010;113(1):58–73.

48. Plaud B, Proost JH, Wierda JM, Barre J, Debaene B, Meistelman C. Pharmacokinetics and pharmacodynamics of rocuronium at the vocal cords and the adductor pollicis in humans. Clin Pharmacol Ther. 1995;58(2):185–91.

49. Waud BE, Waud DR. The margin of safety of neuromuscular transmission in the muscle of the diaphragm. Anesthesiology. 1972;37:417–22.

50. Nguyen-Huu T, Molgo J, Servent D, Duvaldestin P. Resistance to D-tubocurarine of the rat diaphragm as compared to a limb muscle: influence of quantal transmitter release and nicotinic acetylcholine receptors. Anesthesiology. 2009;110(5):1011–5.

51. Ibebunjo C, Srikant CB, Donati F. Morphological correlates of the differential responses of muscles to vecuronium. Br J Anaesth. 1999;83(2):284–91.

52. Fisher DM, Szenohradszky J, Wright PM, Lau M, Brown R, Sharma M. Pharmacodynamic modeling of vecuronium-induced twitch depression. Rapid plasma-effect site equilibration explains faster onset at resistant laryngeal muscles than at the adductor pollicis. Anesthesiology. 1997;86(3):558–66.

53. Sundman E, Witt H, Olsson R, Ekberg O, Kuylenstierna R, Eriksson LI. The incidence and mechanisms of pharyngeal and upper esophageal dysfunction in partially paralyzed humans: pharyngeal videoradiography and simultaneous manometry after atracurium. Anesthesiology. 2000;92(4):977–84.

54. Eikermann M, Vogt FM, Herbstreit F, Vahid-Dastgerdi M, Zenge MO, Ochterbeck C, et al. The predisposition to inspiratory upper

airway collapse during partial neuromuscular blockade. Am J Respir Crit Care Med. 2007;175(1):9–15.

55. Murphy GS, Szokol JW, Marymont JH, Greenberg SB, Avram MJ, Vender JS. Residual neuromuscular blockade and critical respiratory events in the postanesthesia care unit. Anesth Analg. 2008;107(1):130–7.

56. Eriksson LI, Sato M, Severinghaus JW. Effect of a vecuronium-induced partial neuromuscular block on hypoxic ventilatory response. Anesthesiology. 1993;78(4):693–9.

57. Wyon N, Eriksson LI, Yamamoto Y, Lindahl SG. Vecuronium-induced depression of phrenic nerve activity during hypoxia in the rabbit. Anesth Analg. 1996;82(6):1252–6.

58. Naguib M, Samarkandi AH, Bakhamees HS, Magboul MA, Magboul MA, el-Bakry AK. Comparative potency of steroidal neuromuscular blocking drugs and isobolographic analysis of the interaction between rocuronium and other aminosteroids. Br J Anaesth. 1995;75:37–42.

59. Naguib M, Abdulatif M, Selim M, al-Ghamdi A. Dose–response studies of the interaction between mivacurium and suxamethonium. Br J Anaesth. 1995;74:26–30.

60. Wulf H, Kahl M, Ledowski T. Augmentation of the neuromuscular blocking effects of cisatracurium during desflurane, sevoflurane, isoflurane or total i.v. anaesthesia. Br J Anaesth. 1998;80(3):308–12.

61. Ornstein E, Matteo RS, Schwartz AE, Silverberg PA, Young WL, Diaz J. The effects of phenytoin on the magnitude and duration of neuromuscular block following atracurium or vecuronium. Anesthesiology. 1987;67:191–6.

62. Fisher DM, Castagnoli K, Miller RD. Vecuronium kinetics and dynamics in anesthetized infants and children. Clin Pharmacol Ther. 1985;37:402–6.

63. Fisher DM, Canfell PC. Pharmacokinetics and pharmacodynamics of atracurium in infants and children. Anesthesiology. 1990;73:33–7.

64. Meretoja OA, Wirtavuori K, Neuvonen PJ. Age-dependence of the dose–response curve of vecuronium in pediatric patients during balanced anesthesia. Anesth Analg. 1988;67:21–6.

65. Koscielniak-Nielsen ZJ, Bevan JC, Popovic V, Baxter MR, Donati F, Bevan DR. Onset of maximum neuromuscular block following succinylcholine or vecuronium in four age groups. Anesthesiology. 1993;79:229–34.

66. Meretoja OA. Is vecuronium a long-acting neuromuscular blocking agent in neonates and infants? Br J Anaesth. 1989;62:184–7.

67. Erkola O, Rautoma P, Meretoja OA. Mivacurium when preceded by pancuronium becomes a long-acting muscle relaxant. Anesthesiology. 1996;84:562–5.

68. Devys JM, Mourissoux G, Donnette FX, Plat R, Schauvliege F, Le Bigot P, et al. Intubating conditions and adverse events during sevoflurane induction in infants. Br J Anaesth. 2011;106(2):225–9.

69. Meistelman C, Debaene B, d'Hollander A, Donati F, Saint-Maurice C. Importance of the level of paralysis recovery for a rapid antagonism of vecuronium with neostigmine in children during halothane anesthesia. Anesthesiology. 1988;69(1):97–9.

70. Debaene B, Meistelman C, d'Hollander A. Recovery from vecuronium neuromuscular blockade following neostigmine administration in infants, children, and adults during halothane anesthesia. Anesthesiology. 1989;71(6):840–4.

71. Duvaldestin P, Saada J, Berger JL, d'Hollander A, Desmonts JM. Pharmacokinetics, pharmacodynamics and dose–response relationships of pancuronium in control and elderly subjects. Anesthesiology. 1982;56:36–40.

72. Lien CA, Matteo RS, Ornstein E, Schwartz AE, Diaz J. Distribution, elimination, and action of vecuronium in the elderly. Anesth Analg. 1991;73:39–42.

73. Sorooshian SS, Stafford MA, Eastwood NB, Boyd AH, Hull CJ, Wright PM. Pharmacokinetics and pharmacodynamics of cisatracurium in young and elderly adult patients. Anesthesiology. 1996;84:1083–91.

74. Murphy GS, Szokol JW, Avram MJ, Greenberg SB, Shear TD, Vender JS, et al. Residual neuromuscular block in the elderly incidence and clinical implications. Anesthesiology. 2015;123(6):1322–36.

75. Bevan DR, Donati F, Gyasi H, Williams A. Vecuronium in renal failure. Can Anaesth Soc J. 1984;31:491–6.

76. Ward S, Boheimer N, Weatherley BC, Simmonds RJ, Dopson TA. Pharmacokinetics of atracurium and its metabolites in patients with normal renal function, and in patients in renal failure. Br J Anaesth. 1987;59:697–706.

77. Hunter JM, Jones RS, Utting JE. Comparison of vecuronium, atracurium and tubocurarine in normal patients and in patients with no renal function. Br J Anaesth. 1984;56:941–51.

78. Bencini AF, Scaf AH, Sohn YJ, Meistelman C, Lienhart A, Kersten UW, et al. Disposition and urinary excretion of vecuronium bromide in anesthetized patients with normal renal function or renal failure. Anesth Analg. 1986;65:245–51.

79. Szenohradszky J, Fisher DM, Segredo V, Caldwell JE, Bragg P, Sharma ML, et al. Pharmacokinetics of rocuronium bromide (ORG 9426) in patients with normal renal function or patients undergoing cadaver renal transplantation. Anesthesiology. 1992;77:899–904.

80. Khalil M, D'Honneur G, Duvaldestin P, Slavov V, De Hys C, Gomeni R. Pharmacokinetics and pharmacodynamics of rocuronium in patients with cirrhosis. Anesthesiology. 1994;80:1241–7.

81. Parker CJ, Hunter JM. Pharmacokinetics of atracurium and laudanosine in patients with hepatic cirrhosis. Br J Anaesth. 1989;62(2):177–83.

82. Devlin JC, Head-Rapson AG, Parker CJ, Hunter JM. Pharmacodynamics of mivacurium chloride in patients with hepatic cirrhosis. Br J Anaesth. 1993;71:227–31.

83. Lemmens HJ, Brodsky JB. The dose of succinylcholine in morbid obesity. Anesth Analg. 2006;102(2):438–42.

84. Schwartz AE, Matteo RS, Ornstein E, Halevy JD, Diaz J. Pharmacokinetics and pharmacodynamics of vecuronium in the obese surgical patient. Anesth Analg. 1992;74:515–8.

85. Leykin Y, Pellis T, Lucca M, Lomangino G, Marzano B, Gullo A. The pharmacodynamic effects of rocuronium when dosed according to real body weight or ideal body weight in morbidly obese patients. Anesth Analg. 2004;99(4):1086–9. table of contents.

86. Varin F, Ducharme J, Theoret Y, Besner JG, Bevan DR, Donati F. Influence of extreme obesity on the body disposition and neuromuscular blocking effect of atracurium. Clin Pharmacol Ther. 1990;48:18–25.

87. Mencke T, Echternach M, Kleinschmidt S, Lux P, Barth V, Plinkert P, et al. Laryngeal morbidity and quality of tracheal intubation: a randomized controlled trial. Anesthesiology. 2003;98(5):1049–56.

88. Combes X, Andriamifidy L, Dufresne E, Suen P, Sauvat S, Scherrer E, et al. Comparison of two induction regimens using or not using muscle relaxant: impact on postoperative upper airway discomfort. Br J Anaesth. 2007;99(2):276–81.

89. King M, Sujirattanawimol N, Danielson DR, Hall BA, Schroeder DR, Warner DO. Requirements for muscle relaxants during radical retropubic prostatectomy. Anesthesiology. 2000;93(6):1392–7.

90. Cantineau JP, Porte F, D'Honneur G, Duvaldestin P. Neuromuscular effects of rocuronium on the diaphragm and adductor pollicis in anesthetized patients. Anesthesiology. 1994;81:585–90.

91. Van Wijk RM, Watts RW, Ledowski T, Trochsler M, Moran JL, Arenas GW. Deep neuromuscular block reduces intra-abdominal pressure requirements during laparoscopic cholecystectomy: a prospective observational study. Acta Anaesthesiol Scand. 2015;59(4):434–40.

92. Plaud B, Debaene B, Donati F. The corrugator supercilii, not the orbicularis oculi, reflects rocuronium neuromuscular blockade at the laryngeal adductor muscles. Anesthesiology. 2001;95 (1):96–101.

93. Kopman AF, Naguib M. Laparoscopic surgery and muscle relaxants: is deep block helpful? Anesth Analg. 2015;120(1):51–8.

94. Martini CH, Boon M, Bevers RF, Aarts LP, Dahan A. Evaluation of surgical conditions during laparoscopic surgery in patients with moderate vs deep neuromuscular block. Br J Anaesth. 2014;112 (3):498–505.

95. Dubois PE, Putz L, Jamart J, Marotta ML, Gourdin M, Donnez O. Deep neuromuscular block improves surgical conditions during laparoscopic hysterectomy: a randomised controlled trial. Eur J Anaesthesiol. 2014;31(8):430–6.

96. Puhringer FK, Rex C, Sielenkamper AW, Claudius C, Larsen PB, Prins ME, et al. Reversal of profound, high-dose rocuronium-induced neuromuscular blockade by sugammadex at two different time points: an international, multicenter, randomized, dose-finding, safety assessor-blinded, phase II trial. Anesthesiology. 2008;109(2):188–97.

97. Shorten GD, Merk H, Sieber T. Perioperative train-of-four monitoring and residual curarization. Can J Anaesth. 1995;42 (8):711–5.

98. Mason DG, Linkens DA, Edwards ND, Reilly CS. Development of a portable closed-loop atracurium infusion system: systems methodology and safety issues. Int J Clin Monit Comput. 1996;13(4):243–52.

99. Mason DG, Ross JJ, Edwards ND, Linkens DA, Reilly CS. Self-learning fuzzy control of atracurium-induced neuromuscular block during surgery. Med Biol Eng Comput. 1997;35 (5):498–503.

100. Katz RL. Neuromuscular effects of d-tubocurarine, edrophonium and neostigmine in man. Anesthesiology. 1967;28:327–36.

101. Viby-Mogensen J, Jensen NH, Engbaek J, Ording H, Skovgaard LT, Chraemmer-Jorgensen B. Tactile and visual evaluation of the response to train-of-four nerve stimulation. Anesthesiology. 1985;63:440–3.

102. Eriksson LI, Lennmarken C, Staun P, Viby-Mogensen J. Use of post-tetanic count in assessment of a repetitive vecuronium-induced neuromuscular block. Br J Anaesth. 1990;65:487–93.

103. ØStergaard D, Viby-Mogensen J, Pedersen NA, Holm H, Skovgaard LT. Pharmacokinetics and pharmacodynamics of mivacurium in young adult and elderly patients. Acta Anaesthesiol Scand. 2002;46(6):684–91.

104. Viby-Mogensen J, Howardy-Hensen P, Chraemmer-Jorgensen B, Ording H, Engbaek J, Nielsen A. Posttetanic count (PTC): a new method of evaluating an intense non depolarizing neuromuscular blockade. Anesthesiology. 1981;55:458–61.

105. Bonsu AK, Viby-Mogensen J, Fernando PUE, Muchhal K, Tamilarasan A, Lambourne A. Relationship of post-tetanic-count and train-of-four response during intense neuromuscular blockade caused by atracurium. Br J Anaesth. 1987;59:1089–92.

106. Drenck NE, Ueda N, Olsen NV, Engbaek J, Jensen E, Skovgaard LT, et al. Manual evaluation of residual curarization using double burst stimulation: a comparison with train-of-four. Anesthesiology. 1989;70:578–81.

107. Samet A, Capron F, Alla F, Meistelman C, Fuchs-Buder T. Single acceleromyographic train-of-four, 100-Hertz tetanus or double-burst stimulation: which test performs better to detect residual paralysis? Anesthesiology. 2005;102(1):51–6.

108. Viby-Mogensen J, Jensen E, Werner M, Kirkegaard-Nielsen H. Measurement of acceleration: a new method of monitoring neuromuscular function. Acta Anaesthesiol Scand. 1988;32:45–8.

109. Capron F, Alla F, Hottier C, Meistelman C, Fuchs-Buder T. Can acceleromyography detect low levels of residual paralysis? A probability approach to detect a mechanomyographic train-of-four ratio of 0.9. Anesthesiology. 2004;100(5):1119–24.

110. Meistelman C. Effects on laryngeal muscles and intubating conditions with new generation muscle relaxants. Acta Anaesthesiol Belg. 1997;48(1):11–4.

111. Kirov K, Motamed C, Dhonneur G. Differential sensitivity of abdominal muscles and the diaphragm to mivacurium: an electro-myographic study. Anesthesiology. 2001;95(6):1323–8.

112. Murphy GS, Szokol JW, Avram MJ, Greenberg SB, Shear T, Vender JS, et al. Postoperative residual neuromuscular blockade is associated with impaired clinical recovery. Anesth Analg. 2013;117(1):133–41.

113. Donati F. Residual paralysis: a real problem or did we invent a new disease? Can J Anaesth. 2013;60(7):714–29.

114. Fruergaard K, Viby-Mogensen J, Berg H, el Mahdy AM. Tactile evaluation of the response to double burst stimulation decreases, but does not eliminate, the problem of postoperative residual paralysis. Acta Anaesthesiol Scand. 1998;42 (10):1168–74.

115. Baillard C, Clec'h C, Catineau J, Salhi F, Gehan G, Cupa M, et al. Postoperative residual neuromuscular block: a survey of management. Br J Anaesth. 2005;95(5):622–6.

116. Debaene B, Plaud B, Dilly MP, Donati F. Residual paralysis in the PACU after a single intubating dose of nondepolarizing muscle relaxant with an intermediate duration of action. Anesthesiology. 2003;98(5):1042–8.

117. Murphy GS, Szokol JW, Avram MJ, Greenberg SB, Marymont JH, Vender JS, et al. Intraoperative acceleromyography monitoring reduces symptoms of muscle weakness and improves quality of recovery in the early postoperative period. Anesthesiology. 2011;115(5):946–54.

118. Beecher HK, Todd DP. A study of the deaths associated with anesthesia and surgery: based on a study of 599, 548 anesthesias in ten institutions 1948–1952, inclusive. Ann Surg. 1954;140 (1):2–35.

119. Bevan DR, Donati F, Kopman AF. Reversal of neuromuscular blockade. Anesthesiology. 1992;77(4):785–805.

120. Plaud B, Debaene B, Donati F, Marty J. Residual paralysis after emergence from anesthesia. Anesthesiology. 2010;112 (4):1013–22.

121. Mirakhur RK, Gibson FM, Lavery GG. Antagonism of vecuronium-induced neuromuscular blockade with edrophonium or neostigmine. Br J Anaesth. 1987;59:473–7.

122. Payne JP, Hughes R, Al Azawi S. Neuromuscular blockade by neostigmine in anaesthetized man. Br J Anaesth. 1980;52 (1):69–76.

123. Herbstreit F, Zigrahn D, Ochterbeck C, Peters J, Eikermann M. Neostigmine/glycopyrrolate administered after recovery from neuromuscular block increases upper airway collapsibility by decreasing genioglossus muscle activity in response to negative pharyngeal pressure. Anesthesiology. 2010;113(6):1280–8.

124. Sasaki N, Meyer MJ, Malviya SA, Stanislaus AB, MacDonald T, Doran ME, et al. Effects of neostigmine reversal of nondepolarizing neuromuscular blocking agents on postoperative respiratory outcomes: a prospective study. Anesthesiology. 2014;121(5):959–68.

125. Kopman AF, Zank LM, Ng J, Neuman GG. Antagonism of cisatracurium and rocuronium block at a tactile train-of-four count of 2: should quantitative assessment of neuromuscular function be mandatory? Anesth Analg. 2004;98:102–6.

126. Blobner M, Eriksson LI, Scholz J, Motsch J, Della Rocca G, Prins ME. Reversal of rocuronium-induced neuromuscular blockade with sugammadex compared with neostigmine during sevoflurane anaesthesia: results of a randomised, controlled trial. Eur J Anaesthesiol. 2010;27(10):874–81.

127. Cronnelly R, Stanski DR, Miller RD, Sheiner LB, Sohn YJ. Renal function and the pharmacokinetics of neostigmine in anesthetized man. Anesthesiology. 1979;51(3):222–6.

128. Morris RB, Cronnelly R, Miller RD, Stanski DR, Fahey MR. Pharmacokinetics of edrophonium in anephric and renal transplant patients. Br J Anaesth. 1981;53(12):1311–4.

129. Berg H, Viby-Mogensen J, Roed J, Mortensen CR, Engbaek J, Skovgaard LT, et al. Residual neuromuscular block is a risk factor for postoperative pulmonary complications. A prospective, randomised, and blinded study of postoperative pulmonary complications after atracurium, vecuronium and pancuronium. Acta Anaesthesiol Scand. 1997;41(9):1095–103.

130. Arbous MS, Meursing AE, van Kleef JW, de Lange JJ, Spoormans HH, Touw P, et al. Impact of anesthesia management characteristics on severe morbidity and mortality. Anesthesiology. 2005;102(2):257–68.

131. Fuchs-Buder T, Meistelman C, Alla F, Grandjean A, Wuthrich Y, Donati F. Antagonism of low degrees of atracurium-induced neuromuscular blockade: dose-effect relationship for neostigmine. Anesthesiology. 2010;112(1):34–40.

132. Fuchs-Buder T, Baumann C, De Guis J, Guerci P, Meistelman C. Low-dose neostigmine to antagonise shallow atracurium neuromuscular block during inhalational anaesthesia: a randomised controlled trial. Eur J Anaesthesiol. 2013;30(10):594–8.

133. Bom A, Bradley M, Cameron K, Clark JK, Van Egmond J, Feilden H, et al. A novel concept of reversing neuromuscular block: chemical encapsulation of rocuronium bromide by a cyclodextrin-based synthetic host. Angew Chem. 2002;114(2):275–80.

134. Adam JM, Bennett DJ, Bom A, Clark JK, Feilden H, Hutchinson EJ, et al. Cyclodextrin-derived host molecules as reversal agents for the neuromuscular blocker rocuronium bromide: synthesis and structure-activity relationships. J Med Chem. 2002;45(9):1806–16.

135. de Boer HD, Van Egmond J, van de Pol A, Booij LH. Sugammadex, a new reversal agent for neuromuscular block induced by rocuronium in the anaesthetized Rhesus monkey. Br J Anaesth. 2006;96(4):473–9.

136. Epemolu O, Bom A, Hope F, Mason R. Reversal of neuromuscular blockade and simultaneous increase in plasma rocuronium concentration after the intravenous infusion of the novel reversal agent Org 25969. Anesthesiology. 2003;99(3):632–7.

137. Sacan O, White PF, Tufanogullari B, Klein K. Sugammadex reversal of rocuronium-induced neuromuscular blockade: a comparison with neostigmine-glycopyrrolate and edrophonium-atropine. Anesth Analg. 2007;104(3):569–74.

138. Vanacker BF, Vermeyen KM, Struys MM, Rietbergen H, Vandermeersch E, Saldien V, et al. Reversal of rocuronium-induced neuromuscular block with the novel drug sugammadex is equally effective under maintenance anesthesia with propofol or sevoflurane. Anesth Analg. 2007;104(3):563–8.

139. Duvaldestin P, Kuizenga K, Saldien V, Claudius C, Servin F, Klein J, et al. A randomized, dose–response study of sugammadex given for the reversal of deep rocuronium- or vecuronium-induced neuromuscular blockade under sevoflurane anesthesia. Anesth Analg. 2010;110(1):74–82.

140. Tassonyi E, Pongracz A, Nemes R, Asztalos L, Lengyel S, Fulesdi B. Reversal of pipecuronium-induced moderate neuromuscular block with sugammadex in the presence of a sevoflurane anesthetic: a randomized trial. Anesth Analg. 2015;121(2):373–80.

141. Jones RK, Caldwell JE, Brull SJ, Soto RG. Reversal of profound rocuronium-induced blockade with sugammadex: a randomized comparison with neostigmine. Anesthesiology. 2008;109(5):816–24.

142. Eleveld DJ, Kuizenga K, Proost JH, Wierda JM. A temporary decrease in twitch response during reversal of rocuronium-induced muscle relaxation with a small dose of sugammadex. Anesth Analg. 2007;104(3):582–4.

143. Lee C, Jahr JS, Candiotti KA, Warriner B, Zornow MH, Naguib M. Reversal of profound neuromuscular block by sugammadex administered three minutes after rocuronium: a comparison with spontaneous recovery from succinylcholine. Anesthesiology. 2009;110(5):1020–5.

144. McDonagh DL, Benedict PE, Kovac AL, Drover DR, Brister NW, Morte JB, et al. Efficacy, safety, and pharmacokinetics of sugammadex for the reversal of rocuronium-induced neuromuscular blockade in elderly patients. Anesthesiology. 2011;114(2):318–29.

145. Dahl V, Pendeville PE, Hollmann MW, Heier T, Abels EA, Blobner M. Safety and efficacy of sugammadex for the reversal of rocuronium-induced neuromuscular blockade in cardiac patients undergoing noncardiac surgery. Eur J Anaesthesiol. 2009;26(10):874–84.

146. Raft J, Guerci P, Harter V, Fuchs-Buder T, Meistelman C. Biological evaluation of the effect of sugammadex on hemostasis and bleeding. Korean J Anesthesiol. 2015;68(1):17–21.

147. Rahe-Meyer N, Fennema H, Schulman S, Klimscha W, Przemeck M, Blobner M, et al. Effect of reversal of neuromuscular blockade with sugammadex versus usual care on bleeding risk in a randomized study of surgical patients. Anesthesiology. 2014;121(5):969–77.

148. Baldo BA. Sugammadex and hypersensitivity. Anaesth Intensive Care. 2014;42(4):525–7.

149. Raft J, Belhadj-Tahar N, Meistelman C. Slow recovery after sugammadex bolus after rocuronium-induced anaphylaxis. Br J Anaesth. 2014;112(6):1115–6.

150. Kotake Y, Ochiai R, Suzuki T, Ogawa S, Takagi S, Ozaki M, et al. Reversal with sugammadex in the absence of monitoring did not preclude residual neuromuscular block. Anesth Analg. 2013;117(2):345–51.

151. Paton F, Paulden M, Chambers D, Heirs M, Duffy S, Hunter JM, et al. Sugammadex compared with neostigmine/glycopyrrolate for routine reversal of neuromuscular block: a systematic review and economic evaluation. Br J Anaesth. 2010;105(5):558–67.

152. Ledowski T, Hillyard S, Kozman A, Johnston F, Gillies E, Greenaway M, et al. Unrestricted access to sugammadex: impact on neuromuscular blocking agent choice, reversal practice and associated healthcare costs. Anaesth Intensive Care. 2012;40(2):340–3.

153. Meistelman C, Fuchs-Buder T, Raft J. Sugammadex development and use in clinical practice. Curr Anesthesiol Rep. 2013;3(2):122–9.

New and Upcoming Drugs: Intravenous Anesthetic Agents

16

John William Sear

The first of the modern generation of intravenous agents for the induction (and maintenance) of anesthesia dates back to the introduction and evaluation of thiopental in 1934 (Lundy and others). Since then, there have been a large number of intravenous agents introduced and in parallel a number which have undergone clinical usage and then withdrawn when found wanting.

The concept of the ideal properties of an intravenous hypnotic agent for induction of anesthesia has been defined by many different researchers, but the first list of desirable characteristics was probably that defined by the late John Dundee in 1979 [1] (Table 16.1).

The present use of modern intravenous agents to provide an alternate to the volatile agents for the maintenance of anesthesia has stemmed from the development of four intravenous agents which fulfilled most of these properties (ketamine, Althesin (alfaxalone-alfadolone acetate), etomidate, and propofol), as well as showing the important pharmacokinetic-pharmacodynamic features needed. The latter features ideally include being water soluble and hence no likelihood of solvent toxicity; rapid blood-brain equilibration, high potency, and a steep dose-response curve to enhance titratability; rapid plasma clearance and small volume of distribution to minimize the potential for tissue accumulation; and the absence of active metabolites. Other desirable features are minimal cardiovascular and respiratory depression and low potential for histamine release.

Of those drugs listed above, propofol is considered by many present-day observers to be near to the ideal. However, time and experience have shown its use to be associated with a number of important issues and side effects. Because of its water insolubility, the drug must be formulated in a lipid solution, with the added issue of the risk of bacterial contamination if vials are left open to the air. Early on in the evaluation of the agent, there was noted to be significant pain on intravenous injection, especially when administered into small veins on the back of the hand. Although all intravenous agents have cardiovascular effects, the dose-related cardiovascular and respiratory depression seen with propofol, especially when the drug is given in conjunction with opioid drugs, was greater than with the other agents. Propofol also has a liability to development of the propofol infusion syndrome (PRIS), with hyperlipidemia and metabolic acidosis, when given for prolonged sedation especially in the intensive care unit [2]. Other issues that have been researched include the stability of the solvent and the need for antimicrobials to prevent bacterial contamination.

Because of the drawbacks associated with the use of the original 10 % soy bean oil emulsion for the formulation of propofol, there have been a number of different solutions investigated—these include solutions with a lower quantity of soy bean oil, the use of solutions containing both short-chain and long-chain fatty acids, the use of albumen emulsions, the use of cyclodextrins, and the development of aqueous formulations by presentation of the drug as a phosphate or other salt.

The observation of these side and untoward effects associated with the use of propofol has led to considerable effort over the last decade or so by both the pharmaceutical industry and other researchers to develop either new formulations of existing agents or new chemical entities able to provide both induction and maintenance of anesthesia.

These researches have been addressed in this chapter by considering the researches to improve the profile of the archetypal IV agent propofol and then to consider other new chemical entities for the induction and maintenance of anesthesia. Discussion of these has been divided into those that have undergone or are undergoing clinical evaluation and other drugs presently at the preclinical phase.

J.W. Sear, MA, BSc, MBBS, PhD, FFARCS(✉)
Nuffield Department of Anaesthetics, University of Oxford, Headington, Oxford, Oxfordshire OX3 9DU, UK
e-mail: john.sear@gtc.ox.ac.uk

© Springer International Publishing AG 2017

A.R. Absalom, K.P. Mason (eds.), *Total Intravenous Anesthesia and Target Controlled Infusions*,
DOI 10.1007/978-3-319-47609-4_16

Table 16.1 Ideal properties of an intravenous hypnotic agent

Water soluble
Stable in solution
Long shelf life
No pain on intravenous injection
Nonirritant if given subcutaneously
Painful on arterial injection
No sequelae after intra-arterial injection
Low incidence of venous sequelae (thrombophlebitis)
Small injection volume
Lack of hypersensitivity reactions
Lack of intravascular hemolysis
Does not necessarily need to have analgesic properties
No induction complications such as excitatory effects, tremor, spontaneous movements, or hypertonus
No muscular reaction as maintenance of jaw tone may facilitate airway maintenance
No effect on uterine tone
Does not induce episode of malignant hyperpyrexia nor induce acute porphyria
Ideally free of fetal teratogenicity

New Propofol Formulations

The aim for any new propofol formulation must be to show an improved pharmacologic profile compared with the original "Diprivan" formulation. To do this, there must be a reduced incidence of pain on injection and an improved profile of the other minor untoward side effects. But reformulation must not cause any significant change in the drug's PK-PD profile. If the incidence of PRIS is to be reduced, a non-lipid formulation should ideally be developed. It will also be desirable that any new formulation achieved a faster onset of effect. The one other key adverse effect is the risk of bacterial contamination; however, support of bacterial growth can be obtunded by addition of benzyl alcohol, sulfite, or EDTA.

The problem of pain on injection is more debatable as the lipid solvent is not associated with pain when given alone or when used to solubilize other agents [3], suggesting that the pain may be due to the propofol itself. New formulations have focused either on the choice of lipid or other solvent used to solubilize propofol or on the formulation of water-soluble preparations of the drug. The Lipuro formulation of propofol is solubilized in medium-chain triglycerides rather than long-chain triglycerides. It has an identical pharmacokinetic-pharmacodynamic profile to the "Diprivan" formulation but is associated with less pain on injection. However, this formulation is not available in the USA because of the lack of EDTA in the solvent. Propofol emulsions contain oil droplet average sizes of 0.15–0.5 μm (**fine macroemulsions**) [4]. If the droplet size is less than 0.1

um, the emulsion is known as **a microemulsion;** these are more highly stable in solution because of a larger droplet size, but they require the addition of surfactants to retain the drug in solution [5]. Examples of these microemulsions include *Aquafol* (Daewon Pharmaceutical Co., Ltd, Seoul, Korea) which contains 1 % propofol, 8 % polyethylene glycol 600 hydroxystearate (solutol HS 15; BASP Co. Ltd., Seoul, Korea) as a nonionic surfactant, and 5 % Glycofurol (Roche, Basel, Switzerland) as a cosurfactant. Its use has been compared with Diprivan 1 % in volunteers with similar pharmacokinetic and pharmacodynamic properties and safety profiles [5]. However the doses of surfactant and cosurfactant used in this formulation limited its administration to a maximum of 100 ml Aquafol per day.

This has led to the microemulsion being reformulated with another, better tolerated cosurfactant (Purified poloxamer 188; PP188). When investigated in the rat, the kinetics of this formulation were found to be nonlinear [6]. There are no studies to date in man which report on the incidence or not of pain on injection to this formulation. It has been suggested that this might increase with microemulsion formulations due to a greater amount of free propofol in the aqueous phase [7].

Three aqueous formulations of propofol solubilized using cyclodextrins have been studied in various animal species [8]. These use hydroxypropyl-gamma-cyclodextrin, hydroxypropyl-β-cyclodextrin (HP-βCD), or sulfobutyl-β-cyclodextrin as the solvent. The hydroxypropyl-β-cyclodextrin formulation showed favorable physicochemical and biological properties as a water-based formulation. Early porcine studies show an equivalent PK-PD profile to "Diprivan." Again, there are no reported studies in patients. However, when formulations were used containing large amounts of a cyclodextrin complexing agent (20 % w/v), IV dosing of propofol-hydroxypropyl-β-cyclodextrin in rats caused immediate bradycardia of variable duration, while the solvent alone had no effect [9]. Hence, safety issues were highlighted which might be improved by minimizing the amount of the cyclodextrin. The sulfobutyl-β-cyclodextrin is more soluble and safer than hydroxypropyl-β-cyclodextrin, and, while many of these formulations showed improved pharmacodynamic profiles, there was often an increased duration of effect and stability problems.

Other propofol formulations use cosolvent mixtures with propofol solubilized in propylene glycol-water (1:1 v/v) or the prolinate ester of propofol and its water-soluble derivative dissolved in water at equimolar concentrations. However, studies with the prolinate ester in rats showed the formulation to have a longer induction time and longer duration of action [10].

A more recent water-based formulation of propofol is in a poly(N-vinyl-2-pyrrolidone) block polymer (Labopharm

Inc., Quebec, Canada) in which propofol is dissolved inside micelles which are 30–60 nm in diameter [11, 12]. This solution is then lyophilized to form Propofol-PM (propofol polymeric micelle) that instantaneously reconstitutes to a clear solution upon addition of an aqueous medium. This formulation does not support the growth of microorganisms [11]. Micellar propofol has been examined in rats and shown to produce anesthesia. There were no differences in propofol kinetics compared with the "Diprivan" formulation [12]. There are no reported data on its use in higher species.

Propofol Analogs and Prodrugs

Other approaches have also been used to overcome some of the major disadvantages of propofol, specifically its hydrophobicity, cardiovascular and respiratory depression especially when given in association with opioids, and pain on injection. The physicochemical features of several propofol prodrugs have been described by Banaszczyk and colleagues [13]. The first attempt was a propofol sodium hemisuccinate prodrug, but this was unsuitable for commercialization as a stable aqueous solution. A phosphate ester formulation has been studied in mice, rats, rabbits, and pigs

[13]. Metabolism by phosphatases yielded inorganic phosphate and propofol with a similar kinetic profile to the parent compound. Propofol concentrations greater than 1 ug.ml^{-1} were associated with sedation in rats and pigs. The median hypnotic dose of the propofol phosphate in mice was about ten times than seen when using propofol alone; and there was a similar increase in median lethal dose. Other highly water-soluble derivatives of propofol, formulated as cyclic amino acid esters, have been described [10]. The anesthetic properties of the most promising of these, the prolinate, have been described following intraperitoneal injection in rats and showed a faster loss of righting reflex than after "Diprivan."

Fospropofol

Fospropofol (previously known as GPI-15715, Aquavan, Lusedra®) is the only clinically approved propofol analogue. It is a water-soluble phosphate ester of propofol (phosphono-O-methyl-2,6-diisopropylphenol). It is moderately rapidly and completely broken down in vivo to propofol, inorganic phosphate, and formaldehyde by alkaline phosphatases which are widely distributed in the body (Fig. 16.1). Based on the molecular weights of propofol and fospropofol, 1 mg

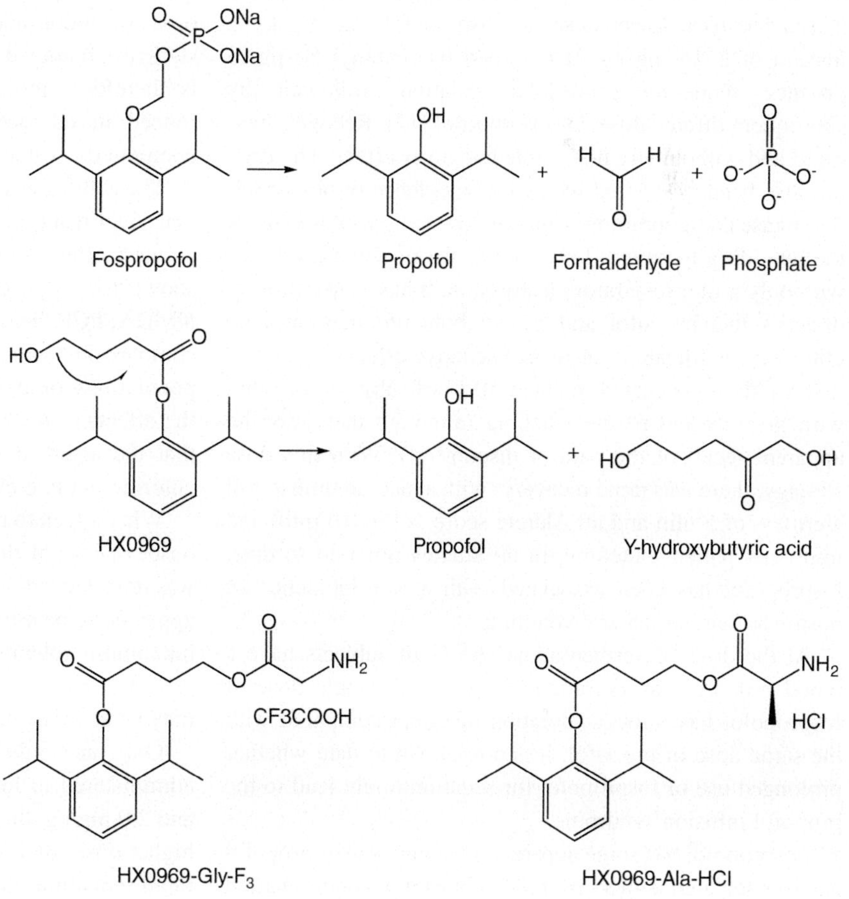

Fig. 16.1 Structures of fospropofol and HX0969w; together with their metabolic breakdown pathways. Also shown are the structures of HX0969-Gly-F$_3$ and HX0969-Ala-HCl

of the latter should liberate 0.54 mg propofol. The formaldehyde is further broken down to formate which has not been shown to date to be associated with systemic toxicity.

Administration of fospropofol is associated with a slow onset of effect (over 4–13 min depending on the dose used and much slower than the parent compound propofol—about 40 s). In man, the in vitro hydrolysis of fospropofol has a half-life of about 8 min. One of the issues to date is the absence of reliable pharmacokinetics (due to assay methodological problems). However preliminary data have suggested a short half-life (as might be expected from a drug undergoing plasma hydrolysis) and small apparent volume of distribution. The ED_{50} effective dose is about 6.5 mg kg^{-1}, while the maximum recommended dose (12.5 mg kg^{-1}) produces loss of consciousness in about 4 min.

The side effect profile of the drug is interesting—it has a lower incidence of hypotension, respiratory depression and apnea, and loss of airway patency than is seen with propofol at similar levels of sedation or anesthesia. This probably relates to the slower onset of effect of the drug. Although there have been no reports of pain on injection, a major side adverse effect is the onset of transient paresthesia and pruritus in the perineal region at the start of the infusion! Not surprisingly, these burning sensations were accompanied by a transient increase in heart rate [14]. A multicenter phase 3 trial has used lower doses of fospropofol (6.5 mg kg^{-1} instead of 5–14 mg kg^{-1}) preceded by fentanyl 50 μg to produce moderate procedural sedation, followed by subsequent titrated doses of fospropofol [15]. Recovery was rapid and without any noticeable hangover effect. The drug has also been associated with a low incidence of postoperative nausea and vomiting. Comparison with propofol shows the new drug to have a lower incidence of adverse effects, with only minor respiratory depression. It has a slower onset of action than propofol, and the metabolic products cause no clinically significant drug-related sedative effects.

Paresthesia occurred in about 50 % of subjects, together with pruritus and perineal itching (although there was no apparent recall of the pain or discomfort). With this dose strategy, there was rapid recovery (with a median time to full alertness of 5 min and an Aldrete score >9 by 10 min) and improved patient outcome. In all studies reported to date, fospropofol has been associated with a low incidence of postoperative nausea and vomiting.

At the doses described above, 95 % of subjects have a blood propofol concentration <2 μg/ml. A single dose of fospropofol has a longer duration of effect compared with the same dose of propofol. It is not known to date whether prolonged use of fospropofol for sedation might lead to the propofol infusion syndrome.

Fospropofol has some apparent advantages over propofol and is associated with a lower risk of bacterial contamination as well as the absence of the infused lipid load that has been associated with organ toxicity during long-term infusions of Diprivan. Fospropofol was approved by the US FDA in December 2008 for use in monitored anesthesia care sedation in adult patients undergoing diagnostic or therapeutic procedures. But fospropofol can only be given by persons trained in the administration of general anesthesia and not involved in the conduct of procedure. Because of the slow-onset kinetics, the main utility of fospropofol will probably be for sedation in the intensive care unit, for procedural sedation outside of the operating room, and for sedation during monitored anesthesia care or regional anesthesia per se where its slow onset is less critical [16–18]. Present comparative studies have evaluated fospropofol against propofol and midazolam; further studies are needed for the drug's true profile needs to be better established.

Other New Chemical Entities Studied (To Date—2016) in Man

PF0713

PF0713 is a water-insoluble 2'6'dialkylphenol formulated as a 1 % lipid emulsion. It is a potent $GABA_A$ receptor agonist which, in the animal species so far tested, shows a hypnotic potency comparable to that of propofol, but with a slower onset of action and duration of effect. Structurally, it is a sterically hindered phenol (R,R 2'6' di-sec-butylphenol) and is therefore similar in structure to propofol (Fig. 16.2). Indeed in its racemic form, it was one of the original compounds evaluated during the development of propofol.

The actions of PF0713 have been examined at the molecular level using rat cerebral cortex binding assays, with the greatest effect found on the chloride channel (as has been shown for propofol) and a lack of interaction with alpha$_2$, NMDA, PCP, benzodiazepine, or opioid receptors [19]. In a comparison with the effects of propofol on the CA1 populations of pyramidal neurons, both drugs potentiated the effects of muscimol at the $GABA_A$ receptor, suggesting that the agent acts via the picrotoxin-binding site on the chloride binding channel.

When given to rats by the intravenous route, there is rapid onset of loss of the righting response, with a duration that was dose related over the range of 1.9–15.2 mg/kg. The drug appeared to be more potent than propofol in the rat, with the maximum tolerated dose being greater than that for propofol. However, after high doses (>7.0 mg/kg), PF0713 may be accompanied by prolonged recovery times [20].

Only one study has described the profile of PF0713 when administered to human subjects. At doses between 0.0156 and 2.0 mg/kg, there were no notable adverse events. At the higher doses of 1.0 mg/kg and 2.0 mg/kg, PF0713 produced rapid induction of general anesthesia without injection pain

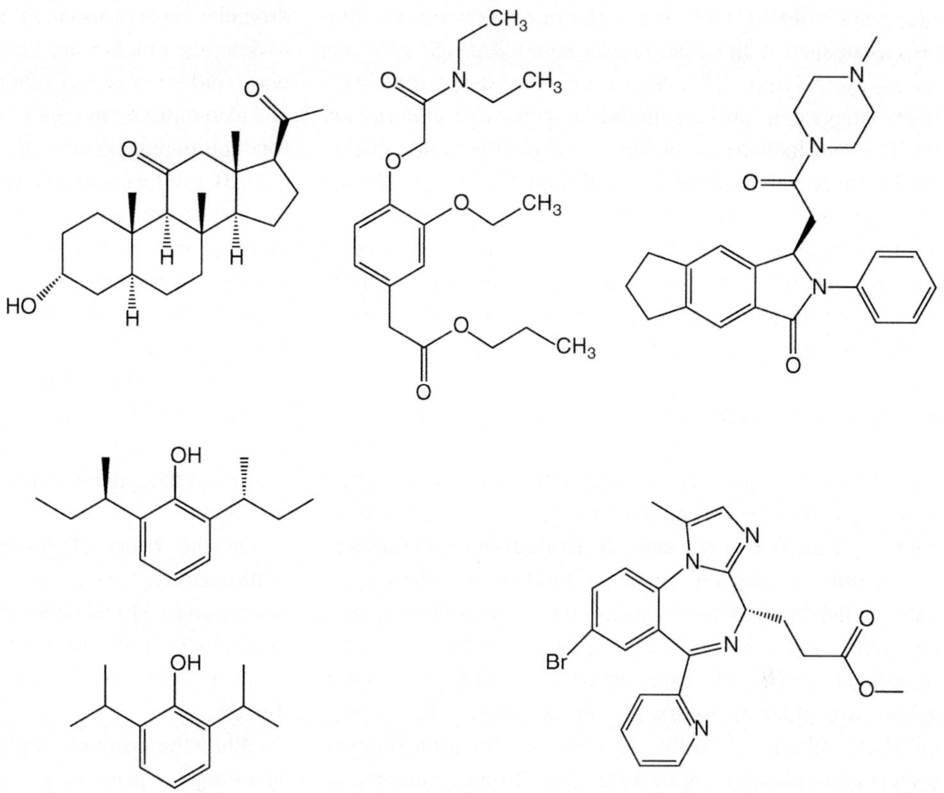

Fig. 16.2 Chemical structures of hypnotic drugs that have undergone evaluation in man. *Top row*—alfaxalone (Phaxan-CD), AZD 3043, and JM-1232 (also known as MR04A3). *Second row*—PF0713 (and structure of propofol for comparison) and remimazolam (CNS-7056X)

or agitation. When the depth and duration of anesthetic effect were assessed by the bispectral index and the Richmond Agitation and Sedation Score, the drug showed dose-related effects, with maintenance of blood pressure and heart rate. Preliminary kinetic data suggest that the drug has a high plasma clearance [21]. When given as a bolus dose, recovery was predictable. There are no data describing the drug's profile when given by infusion; and further assessments of the agent have not been forthcoming.

JM-1232(−)

JM-1232(−) is one of a series of water-soluble sedative-hypnotics being evaluated by the Maruishi Pharmaceutical Company (Osaka, Japan) [22]. The lead compound [JM-1232(−)] is an isoindolin-1-one derivative which was shown to be active in mice (Fig. 16.2). It has a wide margin of safety—with a hypnotic ED_{50} of 3.1 mg/kg and LD_{50} of >120 mg/kg (giving a therapeutic index >35). In vitro binding data suggest the compound has a high affinity for the benzodiazepine receptor, but at a different binding site to midazolam. In vitro studies examining the effects of JM-1232(−) in a brain stem-spinal cord preparation of neonatal rats showed no effect on the C4 burst rate and amplitude at concentrations between 10 and 500 μM. However, at higher concentrations, there was depression of central respiratory activity which could be reversed by the addition of 100 μM flumazenil [23].

Recent studies have also examined the drug when given intrathecally to the rat, where it produces antinociception by an action thought to be on synaptic transmission at spinal nerves in the substantia gelatinosa. In vitro experiments suggest that JM-1232 enhances inhibitory transmission by prolonging the decay phase of the GABAergic sIPSCs. This effect might either be through benzodiazepine receptor activation or by increasing the spontaneous release of GABA and glycine from nerve terminals. This enhancement of the GABAergic effect could contribute to the antinociception seen in these animals [24].

JM-1232 has undergone limited clinical evaluation. When given as a 10 min infusion to male volunteers, it had a rapid onset and short duration of action [25]. Doses between 0.05 and 0.8 mg/kg caused sedation, with the higher doses producing a deeper and longer reduction in the bispectral index. There was no significant excitation associated with the onset of hypnosis (which is a common feature seen with neurosteroids and some other sedative-hypnotic agents). When given as a 1 or 10 min infusion at doses between 0.025 and 0.8 mg/kg, there were minimal effects on heart rate and blood pressure.

The drug produces dose-dependent sedation with rapid onset and recovery, although some volunteers showed upper airway obstruction at deeper levels of sedation. The population PK model indicates plasma clearance (for a 70 kg male) of 654 ml/min and apparent volume of distribution at steady state of 91.6 l per 70 kg. The plasma drug concentration associated with sedation was about 200 ng/mL^{-1} and the $t_{1/2}k_{e0}$ 5.1 min [25]. Simulated context-sensitive half-times suggest a profile similar to propofol. Preliminary PK-PD data indicate an estimated EC$_{50}$ effect-site concentration for anesthesia of 162 ng/mL and a $t_{1/2}k_{e0}$ of 4.2 min. The value for $t_{1/2}k_{e0}$ compares with 0.9 to 5.6 min for midazolam and 1.2–3.3 min for propofol. One unanswered question is whether the main metabolite of JM-1232 (so-called metabolite 3) has any hypnotic properties—especially at higher doses or during prolonged infusion.

Remimazolam (CNS 7056)

In animal studies, remimazolam is a benzodiazepine (Fig. 16.2) with a very predictable onset and offset of effect with a low risk of oversedation. The effects of the agonist are readily reversed by the benzodiazepine antagonist flumazenil. In vitro, remimazolam binds to benzodiazepine sites in the brain with a high affinity. Its carboxylic acid metabolite has a 300 times lower binding affinity. Neither the parent drug nor the main metabolite shows any binding affinity for other receptors, nor any selectivity for specific GABA$_A$ subtypes. In this respect, the pharmacological effects of remimazolam are similar to those of midazolam. Remimazolam causes dose-dependent inhibition of neuronal firing of the substantia nigra pars reticulata.

Remimazolam undergoes biotransformation by hydrolysis in human, rat, mouse, and minipig liver tissue, yielding CNS 7054 as the major metabolite. Metabolism also occurs in organs other than the liver (kidney, lung, brain), but there is no evidence of metabolism by plasma in human, minipig, or dog. The metabolite profile is therefore in keeping with remimazolam being a substrate for carboxylesterases rather than butyrylcholinesterase [26].

When given IV, 25 mg/kg midazolam and remimazolam both produced immediate loss of righting reflex in rats, but recovery of the righting reflex was faster with remimazolam [25 vs. 10 min, respectively]. The effect of remimazolam is inhibited by pretreatment with flumazenil [27]. In a kinetic and dynamic comparison with midazolam in the pigs [28], both drugs rapidly induced sedation, but recovery was faster after remimazolam. This slower recovery after midazolam can be related to the drug being eliminated more slowly (33 vs. 18 min half-life) and was more widely distributed with a larger apparent volume of distribution at steady state (1038 vs. 440 ml/kg), although the clearance rates of the two sedatives were similar (35.4 and 32.2 ml/kg/min, respectively).

Early human studies with remimazolam showed it to be well tolerated in doses between 0.05 and 0.35 mg/kg; at higher doses, episodes of hypoxia may be observed. However unlike other benzodiazepines, sedative doses are not accompanied by significant hypo- or hypertension. Plasma

drug clearance is about 3× that of midazolam, and in studies to date, the kinetics are linear over a wide dose range. There was rapid onset of sedation (after 1 min with a peak at 4 min) and also rapid recovery (10 min compared with about 40 min for equipotent doses of midazolam). At higher doses (>0.20 mg/kg), studies have reported episodes of blood oxygen desaturation [29]. A recent PK-PD assessment of remimazolam in doses from 0.01 to 0.3 mg/kg given by infusion over 1 min shows a population kinetic model with clearance of 66.7 l/h and apparent volume of distribution at steady state of 37.3 l, terminal half-life of 0.92 h, and mean residence time of 0.57 h [30]. The $t_{1/2}k_{e0}$ was 0.25 min−1 for remimazolam (compared with 0.05 min^{-1} for midazolam). The IC50 for BIS was 0.26 µg/mL. Over the wide dose range studied to date, there is a linearity between dose and AUC to infinity.

On the basis of present knowledge, the CSHT for remimazolam appears to be short (15–16 min) for infusions lasting up to 3 h; this compares with values of 45–50 min for midazolam. However there are no presently published kinetics or dynamics of the agent in patients with liver and renal disease.

While this benzodiazepine was initially developed for use as a drug for procedural sedation, more recent studies have focused on use of the drug for both induction and maintenance of general anesthesia—especially within the fields of cardiovascular and cardiac anesthesia. When used in conjunction with analgesic agents (usually remifentanil), the drug has been compared with propofol. Remimazolam was infused at a dose of 1 mg/kg/h for maintenance after induction of anesthesia with an infusion rate of either 6 or 12 mg/kg/h. At these doses, all patients achieved satisfactory anesthesia for operative surgery. There were no major adverse effects, but the decrease in blood pressure following induction of anesthesia was about 50 % of that seen with the comparator propofol group. Recovery data are not presently available.

AZD3043

AZD3043 (previously known as THRX-918661 and TD4756) is a water-insoluble drug which is a congener of the hypnotic agent propanidid, but with about twice the potency of the latter. Its structure is that of an acetic acid propyl ester which is broken down through the action of plasma and tissue (mainly hepatic) esterases (Fig. 16.2). In vitro AZD 3043 undergoes rapid hydrolysis in whole blood of rat and guinea pig with half-lives of 0.4 and 0.1 min, respectively. There are no reported data on the activity of the main metabolites.

When given intravenously to rats, doses of 5–30 mg/kg caused dose-dependent loss of righting reflex and short-lived EEG suppression. After infusions ranging from 20 min to 5 h, the time to recovery of the righting reflex was about 3 min. In contrast, the recovery from propofol anesthesia ranged between 30 and 60 min. Faster recovery was also seen when AZD 3043 was compared with propofol in a pig model [31]. In the rat, an infusion of 2.5 mg/kg/min (in conjunction with remifentanil) was needed to maintain a surgical plane of anesthesia. After a 3 h continuous infusion in rats, kinetic studies showed a rapid loss of the parent compound within about 5 min. Comparable studies in the pig revealed that after a 3 h continuous infusion, clearance was about 3.4 l/kg/h and the elimination half-life was 0.4 h. Again, recovery was faster than after propofol when given at equipotent doses [31]. However one major concern about this agent is the low potency with doses for maintenance of anesthesia in the pig of the order of 1.5 mg/kg/min.

Clinical studies of the PK-PD relationships of remimazolam in man have been conducted in a single center series during which the pharmacology of the drug has been assessed based on bolus dosing (1–6 mg/kg) and 30 min infusions of the drug at doses ranging from 1 to 81 mg/kg/h [32–34]. The depth of sedation-hypnosis was measured using the BIS monitor. The aim of the studies was also to examine the sedation profile and safety of bolus doses and the combination of bolus and infusion to provide sedation (and anesthesia). The 30 min infusions of 1–81 mg/kg/h were associated with rapid onset of sedation or anesthesia at doses >12 mg/kg/h. All doses were accompanied by rapid and complete recovery although after the higher doses, recovery was associated with some involuntary movements and limb hypertonus.

Based on the blood concentration data from all 125 subjects, a kinetic model has been developed. This shows that in man AZD 3043 has a high clearance rate (with a mean value of 2.2 L/min) and a low apparent volume of drug distribution (which appears from the studies to date to be dose dependent ranging from about 15 L at low doses to 37 L at the highest doses). The main metabolites of AZD are the carboxylic acid metabolite (THRXZ-108893) and 1-propanol. Only a small fraction of the parent drug (0.02 %) is excreted unchanged. Breakdown occurs due to the action of both plasma and tissue (mainly hepatic) esterases with the metabolites being either inactive or showing only weak hypnotic properties. There is no evidence to date of any analgesic properties of the drug.

During the infusions of AZD 3043, drug effects on the processed EEG (BIS) were studied and the 50 % effective plasma concentration for hypnosis determined to be about 15 µg/mL (again, supporting the concept of the drug being of low potency). The blood-brain equilibration time was rapid ($t_{1/2}k_{eO}$ about 1.1 min) but the slope of the concentration-effect relationship (gamma) was steep (1.7).

However from these series of studies, the drug appears to have a number of properties that may render it less than the ideal. It has a low potency and is formulated as a lipid emulsion similar to that used for propofol, so there is the risk of contamination by bacteria. In the three studies described, one or more adverse effects of the drug were observed in 29 % of the volunteers. Of greatest concern is that there were the signs or symptoms suggesting an adverse allergic-type reaction in three subjects (erythema, chest discomfort, and dyspnea after drug dosing). But, there were no accompanying ECG changes and no pulmonary rhonchi on auscultation. Furthermore, serial blood samples for plasma tryptase activity were negative in the one subject where samples were taken. Of advantage to its profile was the finding that even at the highest doses administered, the majority of subjects recovered orientation within 5 min of the end of the bolus-infusion regimens, with all subjects oriented to a MOAA/S score of 4 or greater within 25 min and able to walk unaided by 30 min. At time of writing, there appear to be no plans for the further evaluation of this drug.

Pregnane Steroid Anesthetics

The hypnotic properties of steroid molecules have been long known being first recognized by Cashin and Moravek [35] following the infusion of colloidal suspensions of cholesterol into cats. It was clear that there exists no relationship between the anesthetic and hormonal properties of the steroids; indeed the most potent anesthetic steroid being pregnan-3,20-dione [pregnanedione] is virtually devoid of endocrine activity. Although a number of steroid agents have been assessed in vitro and in man, one of the main problems of these agents has been their lack of water solubility [36]. Most steroids have high therapeutic indices in animals but a variable effect in man on the speed or onset of hypnosis and the rapidity and completeness of recovery.

Althesin (introduced to clinical practice in 1972 as a mixture of alfaxalone and alfadolone acetate formulated in a 20 % solution of polyoxyethylated castor oil surfactant (Cremophor EL); the alfadolone acetate being present to increase alfaxalone solubility) has been the only steroid anesthetic to have achieved clinical use outside of trials programs and then only in some countries of the world. Althesin had a number of positive features (minimal cardiovascular and respiratory depression and a low incidence of postoperative nausea and vomiting). Its use was associated with few venous sequelae; but induction of anesthesia with Althesin was often accompanied by a dose-related incidence of hiccoughs, coughing, involuntary muscle movements, and some laryngospasm.

Following the finding that repeat doses of the drug in laboratory animals were not associated with prolongation of recovery (in contrast to the main comparator at the time—thiopental), there were early reports of the drug's use when administered by continuous infusion [37, 38]. Formal studies showing the marked hemodynamic sparing effects of infusions of Althesin in combination with nitrous oxide and fentanyl as analgesia were then reported in both spontaneously breathing and ventilated patients by Sear and Prys-Roberts [39, 40]. Only minimal cardiovascular depression was found when the drug was given at infusion rates of up to four times the ED50 infusion rate (MIR: minimum infusion rate) in the spontaneously breathing patients and to 8× the MIR in the ventilated subjects. Furthermore, there was little effect of the drug on baroreflex activity [41]—in contrast to the later findings with propofol infusions [42]. Respiratory depression in the spontaneously breathing subjects was only minimal with the paCO2 in patients receiving an infusion rate of 4× MIR rising to 52.5 mmHg.

The pharmacokinetics of both steroid components of the drug have been reported for man [43–45]. Following bolus dosing, alfaxalone has an elimination half-life of about 30 min, systemic clearance of approximately 20 ml/kg/min, and an apparent volume of distribution at steady state of 0.79 l/kg. The kinetics of alfadolone acetate were also studied and showed no significant difference to those of alfaxalone [45]. Alfaxalone and alfadolone are mainly bound to albumin although alfaxalone also binds to β-lipoproteins, with total protein binding in animals and man being 96–97 % [46]. When given as Althesin by continuous infusion, the kinetics of alfaxalone showed differences to data from bolus dose studies, with evidence of a dose-related effect on drug kinetics (with plasma clearance of 10.9 ml/kg/min (757 mL/min), apparent volume of distribution at steady state of 92.1 L, and elimination half-life of 90.5 min) [44]—longer when compared with data for bolus dosing [43, 45].

As observed in patients receiving Althesin for induction of anesthesia, continuous infusions were accompanied by some minor side effects—including excitatory movements and limb hypertonus. However a major adverse effect of Althesin was the development of perioperative allergic reactions, with an incidence of between 1/1000 and 1/18000. These were of three main types of reaction—histaminoid, bronchospasm, and cardiovascular collapse. Evidence suggests that the solvent Cremophor EL may have been at least partly responsible for these adverse effects. Because of these side effects, Althesin was withdrawn from clinical practice in 1984; other solvents have been assessed for the continued use of the drug in various animal species.

More recently, the efficacy of alfaxalone alone in other solvents has been assessed in some animal species and in man (Fig. 16.2) Using 2-hydroxypropyl-beta-cyclodextrin as the solubilizing agent (Alfaxan), studies in the dog show the alfaxalone-cyclodextrin formulation to have a high plasma clearance (48–64 ml/kg/min) and an apparent volume of distribution at steady state of 2.5–3.0 l/kg. No adverse effects have been associated with injection of the steroid, although some excitation was seen at the time of awakening [47]. Repeat dosing shows no apparent accumulation in the dog. Studies in the cat by Whittem et al. and Goodwin et al. in the horse confirm similar kinetics for alfaxalone but a slower recovery profile for the cat [48–50]. Evidence of dose-related kinetics for this formulation of alfaxalone has been seen with Alfaxan in the cat [48].

Because 2-hydroxypropyl-beta-cyclodextrin has been shown to be toxic in humans [51], a different formulation, currently being assessed in man, has been solvented in the 7-sulfo-butyl-ether-beta-cyclodextrin (Phaxan-CD; Drawbridge Pharmaceuticals, Melbourne, Australia). This solvent has a low toxicity and hypersensitivity profile in man and has been used to solubilize a number of other drugs being used in clinical practice (including propofol) [52]. Neither of these new formulations of alfaxalone appear to be associated with causing histamine release and anaphylaxis or anaphylactoid reactions.

In a comparative study using Phaxan-CD, propofol, and the Cremophor EL formulation of Althesin in the rat, there was rapid onset of effect and rapid recovery with all agents. Limited hemodynamic studies showed similar changes in heart rate and blood pressure to those seen after equipotent doses of propofol, although there was some evidence to suggest that Phaxan-CD was associated with less cardiovascular depression. Another important difference was the higher therapeutic index of Phaxan when compared with both propofol and Althesin [53].

In a first-in-man randomized double-blind study (again comparing Phaxan-CD with propofol), the primary aim was to determine the dose equivalence of the two hypnotic agents for their effects on the bispectral index (BIS) [54]. In groups of 12 male volunteers, anesthesia was induced with alfaxalone (Phaxan) or propofol. The aim was achievement of BIS value of <50. Physiological parameters (blood pressure, heart rate) were assessed for 80 min after drug injection and in addition evidence of pain on injection, involuntary movement, and need for airway support. Recovery from sedation was evaluated using the Richmond Agitation and Sedation Scale and the Digit Symbol Substitution Test.

No subject complained of pain on injection with Phaxan-CD, whereas 8 of the 12 subjects given propofol did. Nine of the Phaxan and eight of the propofol subjects achieved a target BIS value of ≤50, with the median doses being 0.5 mg/kg for Phaxan-CD and 2.9 mg/kg for propofol. There was no difference between treatment groups in the lowest median BIS and also no significant differences on the timing of the onset and recovery of the BIS. The accompanying median changes in systolic and diastolic blood pressures were −11 % vs. −19 % for systolic and −25 % vs. −37 % for diastolic in Phaxan-CD- and propofol-treated subjects, respectively. Nine of the 12 propofol-treated subjects, but none of Phaxan-CD-treated subjects, required airway support.

In subjects where a BIS value of ≤ 50 was attained, the Richmond Agitation and Sedation Scale score of 0 was reached at a median of 5 and 15 min after Phaxan-CD and propofol, respectively. The BIS value returned to >90 at a mean of 21 min in the two treatment arms, while the Digit Symbol Substitution Test scores returned to predrug injection values at median times of 50 and 42.5 min after Phaxan and propofol. There were no changes in biochemical or hematological indices with either treatment and no evidence of complement activation after either drug.

From these data, the authors conclude that Phaxan-CD causes fast-onset, short-duration anesthesia with rapid cognitive recovery similar to propofol. However, there was less cardiovascular depression following induction of anesthesia with Phaxan-CD, with no episodes of airway obstruction and no pain on injection. Further studies in man are awaited.

Etomidate Congeners

Etomidate is a useful intravenous anesthetic agent but has the adverse effects of adrenocortical suppression, myoclonus, and postoperative nausea and vomiting. In an attempt to overcome these problems, a series of novel etomidate derivatives were developed and studied in the laboratory by researchers at the Massachusetts General Hospital. These compounds which combine etomidate with a covalent group are subject to rapid ester hydrolysis (and are thus termed "soft") so limiting their duration of effect. The initial "first-generation" compounds were MOC-etomidate [MOC = methoxycarbonyl], carboetomidate, and MOC-carboetomidate (Fig. 16.3) [55, 56]. Studies showed

Etomidate

MOC-etomidate

Carboetomidate

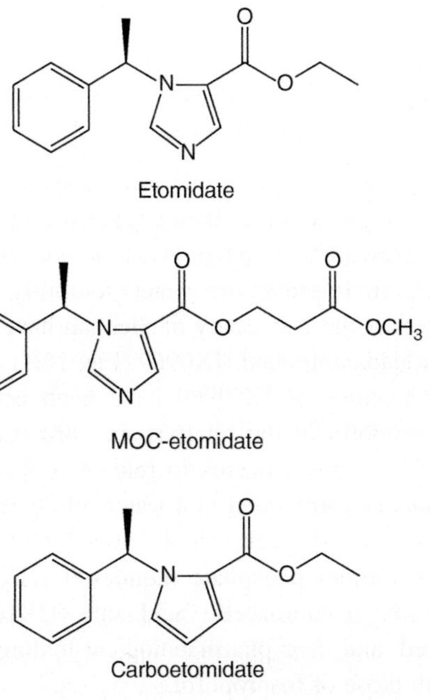

Fig. 16.3 Etomidate and its congeners: MOC-etomidate; carboetomidate

that the occurrence of adrenocortical suppression could be minimized by two different approaches: either by the synthesis of analogs that are rapidly breakdown by ester hydrolysis or by structural change within the etomidate molecule.

The aim of the researches was to avoid the prolonged adrenocortical depression following bolus doses and infusions of etomidate. MOC-etomidate (MOC-E) was the first analog to be evaluated [55]. It was designed to maintain the critical properties of the parent compound, but with the advantage of being rapidly metabolized by esterases in different tissues. The ester moiety attached to etomidate was both sterically unhindered and electronically isolated from the pi electron systems in the imidazole ring. In Xenopus oocytes, MOC-E enhanced submaximal GABA-evoked currents in α_1, β_2, gamma$_{2L}$ GABAA receptors but was less potent than etomidate. MOC-E had an in vitro metabolic half-life of 4.2 min in rat liver homogenate. This compared with little breakdown of etomidate even after 40 min of incubation. In tadpoles, the EC50 for loss of the righting reflex (LORR) for MOC-E was 8 μM (compared with 2 μM for etomidate), while in the rat, the ED50s for LORR were 5.2 mg/kg for MOC-E, 1.00 mg/kg for etomidate, and 4.1 mg/kg for propofol. The hemodynamic effects of MOC-E were similar for etomidate and MOC-E at $2\times$ the ED50 dose; however the duration of effect was less (about 30 s) with MOC-E.

In the rat, MOC-E caused no suppression of ACTH-stimulated corticosterone production at 30 min after dosing, when compared with a 58 % suppression following an equipotent dose of etomidate. After dosing either as an intravenous bolus or a continuous infusion, adrenocortical function after MOC-E recovered more rapidly than after etomidate. For comparison, studies showed that those doses of etomidate in man needed to produce hypnosis could lead to adrenocortical suppression persisting for more than 4 days after discontinuing a prolonged infusion and for 24 h or more after a single induction dose [57–60].

However, recovery in the rat was delayed after prolonged MOC-E infusions. The exact mechanism involved here is not clearly understood but may be due to an increased flux of a metabolite into the central nervous system [61]. No further development of this congener has been undertaken.

A second analog, carboetomidate, where removal of one nitrogen atom from the imidazole ring reduced drug binding and hence adrenocortical suppression by about three orders of magnitude compared with etomidate has also been evaluated [56]. Although Carbo-E did not bind to the enzyme and hence inhibit 11β-hydroxylase activity (and so did not depress cortisol formation), it was shown in Xenopus oocytes to inhibit neural AcH receptors at concentrations close to the EC$_{50}$ for LORR in animals. In addition, it was far more hydrophobic than the parent compound (with the olive oil-buffer partition coefficients being 7700 for Carbo-E

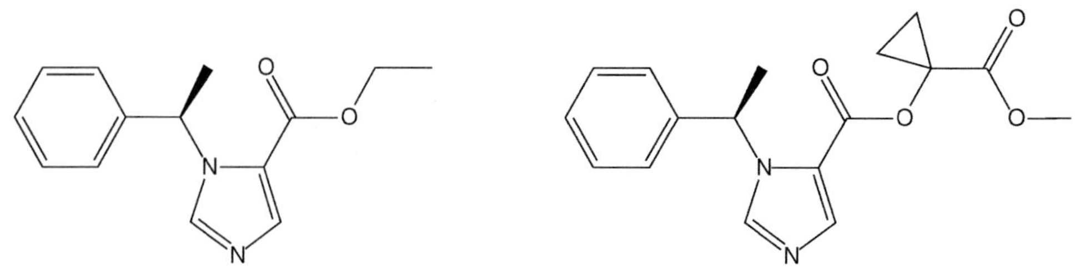

Fig. 16.4 Etomidate and the second-generation congener, cyclopropyl-methoxycarbonyl metomidate (CPMM—ABP-700)

compared with 2100 for etomidate). Hence, this formulation did not provide the water-soluble compound that was the aim of the researches and it too has not undergone further evaluation. In comparison with MOC-E, which is a kinetic solution to the adrenocortical suppressive effects of etomidate, carboetomidate was seen as a dynamic solution.

In order to increase water solubility and low potency of other congeners (especially of MOC-E), a series of "second-generation" etomidate congeners were developed: dimethyl-methoxycarbonyl metomidate (DMMM) and cyclopropyl-methoxycarbonyl metomidate (CPMM) (Fig. 16.4) [62]. In the rat, both compounds were associated with faster EEG and hypnotic recovery following a 2 h infusion when compared with both MOC-E and etomidate itself. In the case of CPMM, the recovery time was about 4 min and appeared to be context insensitive [63]. Although CPMM when infused in the rat caused a depression of adrenocortical function, the agent was associated with rapid recovery [64]. In the dog, again after a 120 min infusion of 0.5 mg/kg/min, there was a parallel recovery of the adrenal depression and hypnosis, with a normal response to IV ACTH seen at 180 min post-infusion compared with an obtunded response to ACTH at more than 300 min after etomidate. The half-times for recovery were 215 min for CPMM compared with 1623 min for etomidate. Another feature of CPMM was myoclonus—seen in 8/8 dogs receiving CPMM compared with 2/8 following infusions of etomidate [65]. There was an obtunding of this adverse effect by midazolam (but without the benzodiazepine having any apparent significant influence on the recovery profile from CPMM).

Pharmacokinetic studies in the dog have been conducted following both bolus dosing and a 120 min infusion [65]. After the single dose, the elimination half-life of CPMM was 16.1 min (compared with 60.1 min for etomidate), with a significantly greater clearance 211 vs. 14.7 ml/kg/min. This rate of clearance is greater than liver blood flow, indicating that hydrolysis to the carboxylic acid metabolite must be primarily extrahepatic. After a 2 h infusion, there was a longer half-life for CPMM of 96.8 min.

More recently, the drug (known as ABP-700) has been evaluated in human subjects. In 60 patients receiving either ABP-700 or the solventing vehicle, there was no evidence of adrenal suppression. Clinical studies have shown that with doses of 0.03–1.00 mg/kg, the drug is well tolerated with minimal cardiovascular and respiratory effects and no adverse effect on adrenal function. Sedation was seen with drug doses $\geq$0.175 mg/kg. The safety of the drug has also been assessed in two more cohorts of patients receiving ABP-700 0.25 or 0.35 mg/kg preceded by 1 µg/kg fentanyl.

At doses of 1 mg/kg, ABP-700 caused an increase in blood pressure following induction of anesthesia. There was also an increased heart rate at lower doses but not in those patients receiving anesthetic doses (0.75 or 1.0 mg/kg). Preliminary kinetics show linearity over the dose range studied, with an elimination half-life of 10.5–18.7 min and dose-related proportionality for AUC. Further studies are being undertaken to examine more fully the PK-PD characteristics of this drug.

Preclinical Studies of Other Potential New Intravenous Anesthetics

These compounds are mainly water-soluble versions of propofol.

HX0969w

Because of the significant side effects associated with the use of fospropofol for sedation (paresthesia and perineal tingling), researchers have used a number of other approaches to improve the water solubility of propofol. Researchers at the University of Sichuan have produced an important lead compound HX0969 (Fig. 16.1). The pharmacological features of HX0969 have been compared with those of propofol in the rat [64]. In vitro studies showed that rapid breakdown occurs to release propofol when the compound was formulated in a water-oil emulsion. To render the compound ester soluble, two further compounds HX0969 disodium phosphate monoester (HX0969W) and glycine ester trifluoroacetic acid salt (HX101230) were synthesized, and their pharmacological features were compared with those of fospropofol.

Results show that HX0969 can produce an anesthetic effect within a few seconds (mean: 3.6 s) in the rat, and its

Fig. 16.5 Rates of conversion to propofol from propofol prodrugs—fospropofol, HX0969, HX0969w, HX0969-Gly-F₃, and HX0969-Ala-HCl

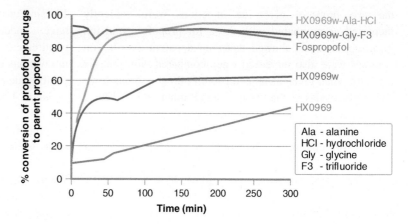

therapeutic index was 4.66. The pharmacodynamic characteristics of HX0969W were similar to those of fospropofol. A second compound, HX101230, also produced anesthesia within 60s in the rat, but the therapeutic index was not so high (TI = 2.96). Unlike fospropofol, HX0969w is a prodrug designed to release propofol and gamma-hydroxybutyrate (GHB), without the formation of formaldehyde.

When in vitro hydrolysis studies were carried out in the plasma from mice and rats, there was a prompt release of propofol (Fig. 16.5). In vivo studies determined the half-maximal effective doses (ED50) and half-maximal lethal doses (LD50) of fospropofol and HX0969w [65]. For HX0969w, the ED50 values in mice and rats were 133.03 and 53.79 mg kg⁻¹, respectively, with LD50 values of 607.11 and 283.79 mg kg⁻¹, respectively. The therapeutic indices were calculated as 4.56 and 5.28 for mice and rats. A pharmacodynamic comparison showed that HX0969w had a longer onset time and shorter duration than fospropofol [66].

The prodrugs of fospropofol and HX0969w both contain phosphate ester groups. It has been suggested that accumulation of a phosphate ester component might be the cause of the paresthesia and pruritus. To exclude this potential risk, the same group of researchers has designed 2 amino acid propofol prodrugs (HX0969-Gly-F3, HX0969-Ala-HCl) (Fig. 16.1). Again the bioconversion of the esters to give propofol was examined in vitro, and then the drugs were tested in vivo to determine the 50 % effective dose (ED50) of the four propofol prodrugs. Their action onset time and duration time were also measured after their equipotent doses were given.

The water solubilities of fospropofol, HX0969W, HX0969-Gly-F3, and HX0969-Ala-HCl are 461.2 mg/mL, 189.5 mg/mL, 49.9 mg/mL, and 246 mg/mL, respectively. Hydrolysis experiments using the plasma of both rat and rhesus monkey showed that the two amino acid prodrugs released propofol to a greater extent and at a more rapid rate than the two phosphate prodrugs during the testing period of 5 h (Fig. 16.5). Overall all 4 prodrugs released propofol

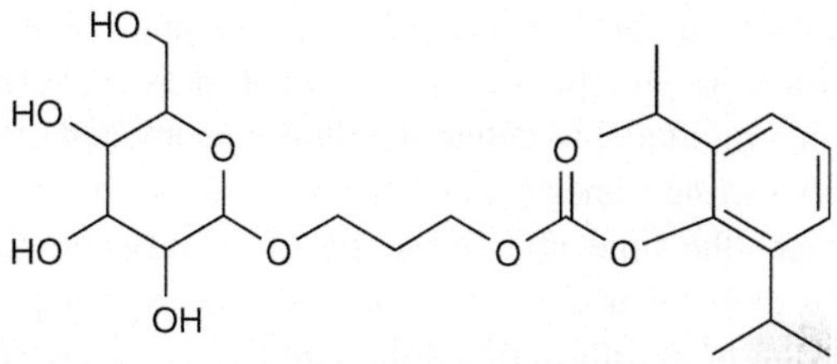

Fig. 16.6 Chemical structure of propofol glycoside

rapidly in the presence of rat hepatic enzymes. However, when the two amino acid ester compounds were compared with fospropofol, and HX0969W, the two novel compounds (HX0969-Gly-F3, HX0969-Ala-HCl) had a much shorter onset time and were more potent.

Further studies have shown that HX0969w, fospropofol disodium, and propofol emulsion can also produce sedative-hypnotic effects and are safe when administered by oral route. The ED50 of oral HX0969w, fospropofol disodium, and propofol emulsion was 96.5 mg/kg, 130.0 mg/kg, and 113.8 mg/kg, respectively. The two propofol prodrugs HX0969w and fospropofol disodium have a shorter time to loss of the righting reflex than was seen with propofol emulsion (10.0 min, 7.5 min, and 16.0 min, respectively). HX0969w, fospropofol disodium, and propofol emulsion caused the loss of righting reflex for mean times of 66.9 min, 131.9 min, and 198.9 min, respectively [66], with HX0969w having a shorter time to restoration of the righting reflex than either fospropofol disodium or propofol emulsion. This suggests that HX0969w may have a role as an oral sedative drug.

Propofol Glycoside

Another approach to the recent formulation of propofol is to make the agent water soluble in the form of a propofol glycoside (Fig. 16.6). Following intravenous dosing in rats, the pharmacokinetics of the two propofol glycosides exhibited the same pharmacokinetic behavior. However, the clearance and area under curve values of propofol for the two propofol glycoside injections were evidently increased as compared with those for propofol emulsion injection. Analysis showed that their apparent distribution volumes were also increased when compared with that for propofol when given as an emulsion. Following breakdown of the glycosides in the plasma, the elimination half-life of the derived propofol (t1/2) was the same as that of commercial propofol emulsion injection (approximately 1.5 h) [67].

This formulation will hopefully be examined in higher species.

Ketamine Esters

Researchers at the University of Auckland have been evaluating the structure-activity relationships of ketamine esters in a rat model to determine their potency and efficacy as short-acting anesthetics. Two indices have been measured—the time after cessation of an infusion for the animals to recover from both loss of the righting reflex (a measure of anesthesia) and the duration of response to a noxious stimulus (pedal withdrawal—the analgesic effect).

The esters were formed by conjugation of ketamine with a methyl, ethyl, or propyl group. The potency of the esters as sedatives was not significantly related to chain length, but methyl, ethyl, and iso-propyl esters were the more potent (although up to twofold less than ketamine), whereas n-propyl esters were less potent (from two- to sixfold less than ketamine). All five ester compounds produced a rapid loss of the righting reflex and diminished pedal withdrawal with an ultrarapid offset (the mean offset for the lead compound being 87 s compared with 996 s for the parent drug ketamine). The LD50s for the esters were similar to that found for ketamine. All the esters underwent rapid in vivo biodegradation by hydrolysis to carboxylic acid derivatives.

For recovery from anesthesia, the methyl, ethyl, and iso-propyl esters were considerably faster than the recovery seen from ketamine itself. The n-propyl esters were 20–25-fold faster than from ketamine. Another new dimethylamino ketamine derivative (homoketamine) had ketamine-like sedative effects but was slightly less potent. The ester analogues of homoketamine had very weak sedative effects [68].

Limited kinetic studies in the rabbit show that the lead compound (N-alkylated norketamine methyl ester) has a large clearance (0.72 l/kg/min) and a small volume of distribution (0.65 l/kg). There are no studies to date in larger mammals.

Concluding Remarks

The development of intravenous anesthesia and the associated target controlled infusion devices has arisen largely on the back of the introduction of propofol into clinical practice in 1986 in Europe and soon after in many other countries. As we have understood more about the pharmacological requirements of a drug for maintenance of anesthesia by the intravenous route, we have found areas where present drugs exhibit side effects or undesirable features.

Since 1986, several other drugs have been evaluated clinically as possible contenders to the "throne" occupied by propofol. To date, none has stood the test of time or surpassed it. Despite the increasing costs of drug development, several new chemical entities are being evaluated. Whether any will join propofol as the hypnotic component of intravenous anesthesia remains to be evaluated.

Speaking from the position of a researcher who has been privileged to study the potential of five such compounds over the last 40 years, I look on with expectation—but not without trepidation—at the road ahead.

References

1. Dundee JW. In 'Intravenous Anaesthetic Agents'. Current Topics in Anaesthesia Series, No 1. London: Edward Arnold; 1979.
2. Wysowski DK, Pollock ML. Reports of death with use of propofol (Diprivan) for nonprocedural (long-term) sedation and literature review. Anesthesiology. 2006;105:1047–51.
3. Doenicke AW, Roizen MF, Hoernecke R, Lorenz W, Ostwald P. Solvent for etomidate may cause pain and adverse effects. Br J Anaesth. 1999;83:464–6.
4. Baker MT, Naguib M. Propofol: the challenges of formulation. Anesthesiology. 2005;103:860–76.
5. Kim KM, Choi BM, Park SW, Lee SH, Christensen LV, Zhou J, Yoo BH, Shin HW, Bae KS, Kern SE, Kang SH, Noh GJ. Pharmacokinetics and pharmacodynamics of propofol microemulsion and lipid emulsion after an intravenous bolus and variable rate infusions. Anesthesiology. 2007;106:924–34.
6. Lee EH, Lee SH, Park DY, Ki KH, Lee EK, Lee DH, Noh GJ. Physicochemical properties, pharmacokinetics, and pharmacodynamics of a reformulated microemulsion propofol in rats. Anesthesiology. 2008;109:436–47.
7. Dubey PK, Kumar A. Pain on injection of lipid-free propofol and propofol emulsion containing medium-chain triglyceride: a comparative study. Anesth Analg. 2005;101:1060–2.
8. Trapani A, Laquintana V, Lopedota A, Franco M, Latrofa A, Talani G, Sanna E. Evaluation of new propofol aqueous solutions for intravenous anesthesia. Int J Pharm. 2004;278:91–8.
9. Bielen SJ, Lysko GS, Gough WB. The effect of a cyclodextrin vehicle on the cardiovascular profile of propofol in rats. Anesth Analg. 1996;82:920–4.
10. Altomare C, Trapani G, Latrofa A, Serra M, Sanna E, Biggio G, Liso G. Highly water-soluble derivatives of the anaesthetic agent propofol: in vitro and in vivo evaluation of cyclic amino acid esters. Eur J Pharm Sci. 2003;20:17–26.
11. Ravenelle F, Gori S, Le Garrec D, Lessard D, Luo L, Palusova D, Sneyd JR, Smith D. Novel lipid and preservative-free propofol formulation: properties and pharmacodynamics. Pharm Res. 2008;25:313–9.
12. Ravenelle F, Vachon P, Rigby-Jones AE, Sneyd JR, Le Garrec D, Gori S, Lessard D, Smith DC. Anaesthetic properties of propofol polymeric micelle: a novel water soluble propofol formulation. Br J Anaesth. 2008;101:186–93.
13. Banaszczyk MG, Carlo AT, Millan V, Lindsey A, Moss R, Carlo DJ, Hendler SS. Propofol phosphate. A water-soluble propofol prodrug: in vivo evaluation. Anesth Analg. 2002;95:1285–92.

14. Struys MM, Vanluchene AL, Gibiansky E, Gibiansky L, Vornov J, Mortier EP, Van Bortel L. AQUAVAN injection, a water-soluble prodrug of propofol, as a bolus injection: a phase I dose-escalation comparison with DIPRIVAN (part 2): pharmacodynamics and safety. Anesthesiology. 2005;103:730–43.

15. Campion ME, Gan TJ. Fospropofol disodium for sedation. Drugs Today (Barcelona, 1998). 2009;45:567–76.

16. Liu R, Luo C, Liu J, Zhang W, Li Y, Xu J. Efficacy and safety of fospropofol _{FD} compared to propofol when given during the induction of general anaesthesia: a phase II, multicenter, randomized, parallel-group, active-controlled, double-blind, double-dummy study. Basic Clin Pharmacol Toxicol. 2016;119:93–100.

17. Yen P, Prior S, Riley C, Johnston W, Smiley M, Thikkurissy S. A comparison of fospropofol to midazolam for moderate sedation during outpatient dental procedures. Anesth Prog. 2013;60:162–77.

18. Cohen LB, Cattau E, Goetsch A, Shah A, Weber JR, Rex DK, Kline JM. A randomized, double-blind, phase 3 study of fospropofol disodium for sedation during colonoscopy. J Clin Gastroenterol. 2010;44:345–53.

19. Siegel LC, Wray J. Initial studies on the mechanism of action of PF0713, an investigational anesthetic agent. Anesthesiology. 2008; ASA abstracts: A642.

20. Siegel LC, Pelc LR, Shaff K. Dose response of PF0713, a novel investigational intravenous anesthetic agent. Anesthesiology. 2008; ASA abstracts: A869.

21. Siegel LC, Konstantatos A. PF0713 produced rapid infusion of general anesthesia without injection pain in a phase 1 study. Anesthesiology. 2009; ASA abstracts: A463.

22. Kanamitsu N, Osaki T, Itsuji Y, Yoshimura M, Tsujimoto H, Soga M. Novel water-soluble sedative-hypnotic agents: isoindolin-1-one derivatives. Chem Pharm Bull (Tokyo). 2007;55:1682–8.

23. Kuribayashi J, Kuwana S, Hosokawa Y, Hatori E, Takeda J. Effect of JM-1232(−), a new sedative on central respiratory activity in newborn rats. Adv Exp Med Biol. 2010;669:115–8.

24. Uemura E, Fujita T, Sakaguchi Y, Kumamoto E. Actions of a novel water-soluble benzodiazepine-receptor agonist JM-1232(−) on synaptic transmission in adult rat spinal substantia gelatinosa neurons. Biochem Biophys Res Commun. 2012;418:695–700.

25. Sneyd JR, Rigby-Jones AE, Cross M, Tominaga H, Shimizu S, Ohkura T, Grimsehl K. First human administration of MR04A3: a novel water-soluble nonbenzodiazepine sedative. Anesthesiology. 2012;116:385–95.

26. Tilbrook GS, Kilpatrick CJ. CNS 7056X, an ultra-short acting benzodiazepine: In vitro metabolism. Anesthesiology 2006; ASA abstracts A 1611.

27. Kilpatrick GJ, McIntyre MS, Cox RF, Kilpatrick GJ, McIntyre MS, Cox RF, Stafford JA, Pacofsky GJ, Lovell GG, Wiard RP, Feldman PL, Collins H, Waszczak BL, Tilbrook GS. CNS 7056: a novel ultra-short acting benzodiazepine. Anesthesiology. 2007;107:60–6.

28. Mutter C, Rudolf G, Diemunsch PA, Tilbrook GS, Borgeat A. CNS 7056X an ultra-short-acting benzodiazepine: pharmacokinetic and pharmacodynamic study in pig. Anesthesiology 2006;105:A1610 (abstract).

29. Worthington MT, Antonik LJ, Goldwater DR, Lees JP, Wilhelm-Ogunbiyi K, Borkett KM, Mitchell MC. A phase Ib, dose-finding study of multiple doses of remimazolam (CNS 7056) in volunteers undergoing colonoscopy. Anesth Analg. 2013;117:1093–100.

30. Wiltshire HR, Kilpatrick GJ, Tilbrook GS, Borkett KM. A placebo- and midazolam-controlled phase I single ascending-dose study evaluating the safety, pharmacokinetics, and pharmacodynamics of remimazolam (CNS 7056): Part II. Population pharmacokinetic and pharmacodynamic modeling and simulation. Anesth Analg. 2012;115:284–96.

31. Egan TD, Obara S, Jenkins TE, Jaw-Tsai SS, Amagasu S, Cook DR, Steffensen SC, Beattie DT. AZD-3043: a novel, metabolically labile sedative-hypnotic agent with rapid and predictable emergence from hypnosis. Anesthesiology. 2012;116:1267–77.

32. Kalman S, Koch P, Ahlén K, Kanes SJ, Barassin S, Björnsson MA, Norberg Å. First human study of the investigational sedative and anesthetic drug AZD3043: a dose-escalation trial to assess the safety, pharmacokinetics, and efficacy of a 30-minute infusion in healthy male volunteers. Anesth Analg. 2015;121:885–93.

33. Norberg Å, Koch P, Kanes SJ, Björnsson MA, Barassin S, Ahlén K, Kalman S. A bolus and bolus followed by infusion study of AZD3043, an investigational intravenous drug for sedation and anesthesia: safety and pharmacodynamics in healthy male and female volunteers. Anesth Analg. 2015;121(4):894–903.

34. Björnsson MA, Norberg Å, Kalman S, Simonsson US. A recirculatory model for pharmacokinetics and the effects on bispectral index after intravenous infusion of the sedative and anesthetic AZD3043 in healthy volunteers. Anesth Analg. 2015;121:904–13.

35. Cashin MF, Moravek V. The physiological action of cholesterol. Am J Physiol. 1927;82:294–8.

36. Sear JW. ORG 21465, a new water-soluble steroid hypnotic: more of the same or something different? Br J Anaesth. 1997;79:417–9.

37. Du Cailar J. The effects in man of infusions of Althesin with particular regard to the cardiovascular system. Postgrad Med J. 1972;48 Suppl 2:72–9.

38. Savege TM, Ramsay MA, Curran JP, Cotter J, Walling PT, Simpson BR. Intravenous anaesthesia by infusion. A technique using alphaxolone/alphadolone (althesin). Anaesthesia. 1975;30:757–64.

39. Sear JW, Prys-Roberts C. Dose-related haemodynamic effects of continuous infusions of Althesin in man. Br J Anaesth. 1979;51:867–73.

40. Sear JW, Prys-Roberts C. Plasma concentrations of alphaxalone during continuous infusion of Althesin. Br J Anaesth. 1979;51:861–5.

41. Jones DF, Prys-Roberts C. Baroreflex effects of althesin infusions to supplement nitrous oxide anaesthesia in man. Br J Anaesth. 1983;55:849–53.

42. Cullen PM, Turtle M, Prys-Roberts C, Way WL, Dye J. Effect of propofol anesthesia on baroreflex activity in humans. Anesth Analg. 1987;66:1115–20.

43. Simpson ME. Pharmacokinetics of althesin--comparison with lignocaine. Br J Anaesth. 1978;50:1231–5.

44. Sear JW, Prys-Roberts C, Gray AJ, Walsh EM, Curnow JS, Dye J. Infusions of minaxolone to supplement nitrous oxide-oxygen anaesthesia. A comparison with althesin. Br J Anaesth. 1981;53:339–50.

45. Sear JW, Sanders RS. Intra-patient comparison of the kinetics of alphaxalone and alphadolone in man. Eur J Anaesthesiol. 1984;1:113–22.

46. Visser SA, Smulders CJ, Reijers BP, Van der Graaf PH, Peletier LA, Danhof M. Mechanism-based pharmacokinetic-pharmacodynamic modeling of concentration-dependent hysteresis and biphasic electroencephalogram effects of alphaxalone in rats. J Pharmacol Exp Ther. 2002;302:1158–67.

47. Ferré PJ, Pasloske K, Whittem T, Ranasinghe MG, Li Q, Lefebvre HP. Plasma pharmacokinetics of alfaxalone in dogs after an intravenous bolus of Alfaxan-CD RTU. Vet Anaesth Analg. 2006;33:229–36.

48. Whittem T, Pasloske KS, Heit MC, Ranasinghe MG. The pharmacokinetics and pharmacodynamics of alfaxalone in cats after single and multiple intravenous administration of Alfaxan at clinical and supraclinical doses. J Vet Pharmacol Ther. 2008;31:571–9.

49. Pasloske K, Sauer B, Perkins N, Whittem T. Plasma pharmacokinetics of alfaxalone in both premedicated and unpremedicated Greyhound dogs after single, intravenous administration of Alfaxan at a clinical dose. J Vet Pharmacol Ther. 2009;32:510–3.

50. Goodwin WA, Keates HL, Pasloske K, Pearson M, Sauer B, Ranasinghe MG. The pharmacokinetics and pharmacodynamics of the injectable anaesthetic alfaxalone in the horse. Vet Anaesth Analg. 2011;38:431–8.

51. Brewster ME, Estes KS, Bodor N. An intravenous toxicity study of 2-hydroxypropyl-β-cyclodextrin, a useful drug solubilizer, in rats and monkeys. Int J Pharmaceut. 1990;59:231–43.

52. Egan TD, Kern SE, Johnson KB, Pace NL. The pharmacokinetics and pharmacodynamics of propofol in a modified cyclodextrin formulation (Captisol) versus propofol in a lipid formulation (Diprivan): an electroencephalographic and hemodynamic study in a porcine model. Anesth Analg. 2003;97:72–9.

53. Goodchild CS, Serrao JM, Kolosov A, Boyd BJ. Alphaxalone reformulated: a water-soluble intravenous anesthetic preparation in sulfobutyl-ether-β-cyclodextrin. Anesth Analg. 2015;120:1025–31.

54. Monagle J, Siu L, Worrell J, Goodchild CS, Serrao JM. A phase 1c trial comparing the efficacy and safety of a new aqueous formulation of alphaxalone with propofol. Anesth Analg. 2015;121:914–24.

55. Cotton JF, Husain SS, Forman SA, Miller KW, Kelly EW, Nguyen HH, Raines DE. Methoxycarbonyl-etomidate: a novel rapidly metabolized and ultra-short-acting etomidate analogue that does not produce prolonged adrenocortical suppression. Anesthesiology. 200;111(2):240–9.

56. Cotten JF, Forman SA, Laha JK, Cuny GD, Husain SS, Miller KW, Nguyen HH, Kelly EW, Stewart D, Liu A, Raines DE. Carboetomidate: a pyrrole analog of etomidate designed not to suppress adrenocortical function. Anesthesiology. 2010;112:637–44.

57. Wagner RL, White PF, Kan PB, Rosenthal MH, Feldman D. Inhibition of adrenal steroidogenesis by the anesthetic etomidate. N Engl J Med. 1984;310:1415–21.

58. Wagner RL, White PF. Etomidate inhibits adrenocortical function in surgical patients. Anesthesiology. 1984;61:647–51.

59. Moore RA, Allen MC, Wood PJ, Rees LH, Sear JW. Peri-operative endocrine effects of etomidate. Anaesthesia. 1985;40:124–30.

60. Absalom A, Pledger D, Kong A. Adrenocortical function in critically ill patients 24 h after a single dose of etomidate. Anaesthesia. 1999;54:861–7.

61. Ge R, Pejo E, Husain SS, Cotton JF, Raines DE. Electroencephalographic and hypnotic recoveries after brief and prolonged infusions of etomidate and optimized soft etomidate analogs. Anesthesiology. 2012;117:1037–43.

62. Campagna JA, Pojasek K, Grayzel D, Randle J, Raines DE. Advancing novel anesthetics: pharmacodynamic and pharmacokinetic studies of cyclopropyl-methoxycarbonyl metomidate in dogs. Anesthesiology. 2014;121:1203–16.

63. Ge R, Pejo E, Cotton JF, Raines DE. Adrenocortical suppression and recovery after continuous hypnotic infusion: etomidate versus its soft analogue cyclopropylmethoxycarbonyl metomidate. Crit Care. 2012;17:R20.

64. Yang J, Yin W, Liu J, Wang Y, Zhou C, Kang Y, Zhang WS. Synthesis and characterization of novel quick-release propofol prodrug via lactonization. Bioorg Med Chem Lett. 2013;23:1813–6.

65. Zhou Y, Yang J, Liu J, Wang Y, Zhang WS. Efficacy comparison of the novel water-soluble propofol prodrug HX0969w and fospropofol in mice and rats. Br J Anaesth. 2013;111:825–32.

66. Wang HY, Yang J, Yin W, Yang LH, Zhang WS. The sedative-hypnotic effects and safety of oral administrated propofol prodrugs hx0969w and fospropofol disodium in comparison with propofol emulsion in rats. Xue Xue Bao Yi Xue Ban. 2015;46:214–7 [in Chinese].

67. Zhang Z, Ju RJ, Li XT, Zhang DX, Wu RR, Chen XJ, Lu WL. Pharmacokinetics for the solutable type injections of propofol glycoside in rats. Sichuan Da Beijing Da Xue Xue Bao. 2015;47:846–52 [in Chinese].

68. Harvey M, Sleigh J, Voss L, Jose J, Gamage S, Pruijn F, Liyanage S, Denny W. Development of rapidly metabolized and ultra-short-acting ketamine analogs. Anesth Analg. 2015;121:925–33.

Drug Interactions in Anesthesia

Jaap Vuyk

Introduction

Context-sensitive halftime, time to peak effect, and effect site equilibration half-life are parameters that were introduced over the past three decades to improve the understanding of the clinical pharmacology of anesthetic agents when given as single agents. In addition, anesthesiologists have become increasingly aware of the pharmacokinetic and pharmacodynamic drug interactions that play an important role in the clinical dose–effect relationship of drugs used in anesthesia.

Drug interactions may be beneficial or detrimental to the patient involved. A drug interaction may be used to the benefit of a patient when the interaction is used to reduce the dose or drug concentration of the individual agents to diminish the magnitude of side effects of the combination. In contrast, patients may take drugs that interact in a harmful way, leading to a change in the efficacy and/or toxicity of one of the agents. Epidemiological data suggest that the incidence of possible drug interactions is increasing in the population with estimates of the order of 5–63 % [1, 2]. Especially, with regard to the use of opioids for chronic and oncological pain, concern is mounting with respect to the growing use of opioids itself and with respect to the thus increasing possibility of interactions between opioids and concurrent medication such as antidepressants, sedatives, or other opioids that may lead to detrimental effects on the patient. Over the past two decades, the prescription of opioids for noncancer pain has doubled with a prevalence in some populations of up to 10 % [3].

With regard to intraoperative anesthesia, drug interactions may be viewed differently. Anesthesia today is seldom accomplished through the action of a single agent.

This is because mono-agent anesthesia is often associated with significant side effects such as hemodynamic and respiratory depression. Total intravenous anesthesia (TIVA), therefore, is provided using combinations of hypnotic and analgesic agents, often combined with muscle relaxants, sometimes in the presence of central neuraxial blockade or locoregional anesthesia. The combination of agents is often chosen such that the desired effects are optimal in the presence of minimal side effects.

This chapter aims to shed light on the magnitude and the mechanisms of action of the pharmacokinetic and pharmacodynamic interactions between intravenous hypnotic and analgesic agents and between perioperative-administered agents and the anesthetics given intraoperatively. With this knowledge, the anesthesiologist may be better equipped to choose the optimal combination of agents to assure the most stable anesthetic, optimal operating conditions with the shortest possible induction and recovery, and the lowest incidence of adverse effects [4]. In 2004 Lichtenbelt and colleagues [5] described three tools that may help the anesthesiologist to do so. These tools include optimal pharmacological knowledge of the agents used, state-of-the-art administration techniques like target-controlled infusion (TCI), and lastly the most recent pharmacodynamic monitoring techniques such as bispectral index monitoring (BIS). The use of these three tools will play a role in this chapter as well.

Pharmaceutical Interactions

A pharmaceutical interaction is defined as a direct chemical reaction between two drugs. An example of such an interaction is the interaction between thiopental, being highly alkaline, and an acidic solution such as succinylcholine. Similarly, combining thiopental and vecuronium in a single infusion line results in the precipitation of a white thiopental dust that may obstruct the intravenous tubing and result in a

J. Vuyk, MD, PhD(✉)
Department of Anesthesiology, Leiden University Medical Center (LUMC), 2333 RZ, Leiden, The Netherlands
e-mail: j.vuyk@lumc.nl

© Springer International Publishing AG 2017
A.R. Absalom, K.P. Mason (eds.), *Total Intravenous Anesthesia and Target Controlled Infusions*,
DOI 10.1007/978-3-319-47609-4_17

less than expected dose and effect of thiopental [6]. Pulmonary emboli have even been described as a result of this interaction, in animal studies [7].

Pharmacokinetic Interactions Between Anesthetics

Whereas pharmaceutical drug interactions occur rarely and may be prevented easily, pharmacokinetic drug interactions occur during almost every anesthetic, often cannot be prevented, and may cause significant changes in the effect of the anesthetics used. A pharmacokinetic interaction may be defined as the process in which a drug alters the distribution, redistribution, clearance, or excretion of another agent [8, 9]. Pharmacokinetic interactions between anesthetic agents may occur as a result of hemodynamic changes, changes in protein binding, or shifts in metabolism resulting from enzyme induction or inhibition [10]. Pharmacokinetic interactions between anesthetics often are the result of changes in clearance and distribution. Pharmacokinetic interactions between anesthetic agents and concomitant home medication often are the result of changes in anesthetic drug metabolism resulting from cytochrome P450 enzyme induction or inhibition. Interactions between anesthetics result in relatively small changes in the drug concentration (of the order of 25 %), whereas enzyme inhibition or induction caused by drugs such as some antibiotics or anticonvulsants may cause much larger anesthetic agent concentration shifts.

The analysis of pharmacokinetic drug interactions may be performed by a paired analysis of the dose–concentration relationship of the pharmacokinetic parameter set of the agent when given in the absence and in the presence of the second agent. A more refined method, offering greater insight in the actual mechanism of the interaction, is through a population pharmacokinetic analysis in which the influence of the second agent is modeled as covariate on the various parameters of the pharmacokinetic model. Computer simulation may then reveal the interaction throughout the full concentration range of both agents.

Opioid–Hypnotic Pharmacokinetic Interaction

During TIVA for general surgery, propofol or midazolam is almost always combined with an opioid to assure adequate analgesia as well as surgical hypnosis. The interaction between the opioids and intravenous hypnotic agents is therefore of great clinical importance and the subject of many studies.

Propofol reduces peripheral vascular resistance and is associated with a decrease in blood pressure and blood

flow during induction and maintenance of anesthesia. Similarly, most opioids, albeit to a smaller degree, also affect hemodynamics via their vagotonic effects, resulting in small changes in cardiac output and blood pressure. The hemodynamic changes inflicted by propofol and the opioids make these agents susceptible to pharmacokinetic interactions because changes in cardiac output and peripheral vascular resistance may result in changes in distribution and clearance [11].

Due to its hemodynamic effects, propofol, at clinical relevant concentrations, increases the plasma remifentanil concentration. Propofol does so through a reduction in the central volume of distribution and distributional clearance of remifentanil of over 40 % and a reduction of the elimination clearance by 15 %, in a non-concentration dependent manner [12]. As a consequence, the combined administration of propofol and remifentanil reduces the required remifentanil induction dose but does not affect the remifentanil maintenance infusion rate required to achieve and maintain a given analgesic level. In a similar manner, propofol affects the pharmacokinetics of alfentanil [13]. Alfentanil is extensively metabolized through CYP3A4 and CYP3A5 via 2 pathways, forming noralfentanil and N-phenylpropionamide. Propofol coadministration, by causing a decrease in mean arterial blood pressure, systemic vascular resistance, and stroke volume, significantly reduces the fast and slow distribution clearances and metabolic clearances of alfentanil in volunteers. In the end, at blood concentrations sufficient for general anesthesia, this propofol hemodynamic-induced pharmacokinetic interaction leads to an elevation of the plasma alfentanil concentration by about 25 %. Propofol probably influences the metabolic clearance of alfentanil through a reduction of liver blood flow. The hepatic extraction ratio of alfentanil is 0.3–0.5, making its clearance only moderately sensitive to changes in hepatic blood flow. Secondly, propofol is known as an inhibitor of the cytochrome P450 3A4 subenzyme and may thus affect the clearance of alfentanil as well in this manner [14]. Clinically this means that in the presence of propofol at concentrations assuring surgical hypnosis, alfentanil requirements are diminished by 25 % due to elevation of the plasma alfentanil concentration. This is in line with earlier observations of Gepts and Pavlin who also report on the elevated plasma alfentanil concentrations in the presence of propofol [15, 16]. Propofol not only affects Cyp 450 3A4 but also inhibits other cytochrome subenzymes like CYP 1A2, 2C9, and 2D6, thus allowing for other pharmacokinetic interactions as well, such as that with sufentanil [17, 18].

In addition to the fact that propofol affects the pharmacokinetics of opioids, various studies comment on the influence of the opioids on the pharmacokinetics of propofol. Remifentanil is often combined with propofol and is known to have a negative influence on heart rate, arterial blood pressure, and cardiac output. Changes in cardiac output and the concomitant change in liver blood flow have been shown to affect the distribution and clearance of propofol [19]. This is because the hepatic extraction ration exceeds 0.7, making propofol's metabolic clearance highly sensitive to hepatic flow changes. Consequently, remifentanil may well have an effect on the pharmacokinetics of propofol. Yufune et al. recently studied the influence of remifentanil on propofol TCI pharmacology during gynecological surgery. These authors describe how remifentanil reduces cardiac index and is associated with a decrease in indocyanine green clearance and an elevation of the blood propofol concentration [20]. This was despite the fact that remifentanil appeared to have no effect on the BIS. Remifentanil infusion at a constant rate of $1~\mu g~kg^{-1}~min^{-1}$ reduced the clearance of propofol by about 25 % and elevated plasma propofol concentrations accordingly. The changes in indocyanine clearance strongly suggest that remifentanil affects hepatic blood flow and thus the hepatic clearance of propofol. Interestingly, Boullion and colleagues found no effect of remifentanil on the pharmacokinetics of propofol in a non-steady-state situation [12].

Mertens et al. studied the influence of alfentanil on propofol pharmacokinetics in volunteers. In line with previous studies, the authors describe how alfentanil coadministration results in a 20–25 % increase in the blood propofol concentration [21]. This elevation in the blood propofol concentration resulted from an alfentanil-induced decrease in cardiac output and heart rate. Both cardiac output and heart rate proved to be significant parameters in the propofol pharmacokinetic parameter set affecting metabolic clearance and the slow distribution volume.

Hypnotic–Hypnotic Pharmacokinetic Interactions

In addition to the opioids, other sedative agents may affect the pharmacokinetics of propofol. Because midazolam is used in many hospitals as a sedative premedication before TIVA, the interaction between propofol and midazolam is highly clinically relevant. Already many studies have described the fact that midazolam as a preoperative sedative reduces propofol requirements. However, the nature of this interaction—pharmacokinetic, pharmacodynamic, or both—remained unclear for a long time [22, 23].

In a study by Lichtenbelt et al., propofol significantly increased plasma midazolam concentrations [24]. This was effectuated predominantly through a decrease in the central compartment volume and the metabolic and rapid distribution clearances of midazolam. With an increase in the propofol concentration, this effect became more prominent. The clinical consequence of this interaction is that the midazolam induction dose and maintenance requirements

may be reduced by 25 % when combined with propofol, for purely pharmacokinetic reasons. The influence of propofol on midazolam pharmacokinetics possibly is the result from both cytochrome P450 inhibition by propofol and hemodynamic alterations that may cause a reduction in midazolam metabolic clearance, in line with the intermediate hepatic extraction ratio of midazolam. The inhibitory effects of propofol on the cytochrome P450 enzyme system was explored in closer detail by Hamaoka et al. [25]. These authors showed in vitro and in vivo evidence that propofol inhibits CYP 3A4 which leads, after combined propofol–midazolam administration, to 50 % higher plasma midazolam concentrations with an increase of the elimination half-life of midazolam from 132 to 212 min.

Propofol's own metabolic oxidation involves predominantly CYP 2B6, whereas part of the propofol hydroxylase activity is mediated by CYP2C9 in the human liver, especially at low substrate concentration [5]. Propofol is metabolized by additional isoforms such as CYP2A6, 2C8, 2C18, 2C19, and 1A2, especially when substrate concentrations are high. This low specificity among cytochrome P450 isoforms may contribute to the low pharmacokinetic interindividual variability (70 %). Propofol produces inhibition of CYP1A2 (phenacetin O-deethylation), CYP2C9 (tolbutamide 4′-hydroxylation), CYP2D6 (dextromethorphan O-demethylation), and CYP3A4 (testosterone 6beta-hydroxylation) activities at an IC50 of 40, 49, 213, and 32 µM, respectively [17, 26].

In addition to the influence of propofol on the pharmacokinetics of midazolam, midazolam affects the pharmacokinetics of propofol [27]. In the presence of midazolam at sedative concentrations, the blood propofol concentration becomes elevated by about 25 %. This probably is not the result of an interaction at the cytochrome P450 enzyme family but purely the result of the moderate hemodynamic effects of midazolam. One may conclude that midazolam as a preoperative sedative not only supports the anesthetic through the sedative effect itself but also by elevating the intraoperative propofol concentration.

Lastly, pharmacokinetic interactions with ketamine also occur. Ketamine is known as an inducer of various CYP450 subenzymes such as CYP450 1A, 2B, 2E, and 3A. Cytochrome P450 2B is particularly important in the metabolism of propofol. It is therefore not surprising that in rats the repetitive administration of ketamine is associated with an increase in the metabolic clearance of propofol, and a reduction in blood propofol concentrations and a reduction in sleeping time [28].

In the clinical setting, combinations of propofol and midazolam may favor hemodynamic stability compared to propofol alone [29]. Also Carrasco et al. describe a greater hemodynamic stability in ICU patients with propofol–midazolam compared to propofol alone [30]. Midazolam

316 J. Vuyk

may, however, increase ventilation weaning time, when compared to pure propofol sedation [31, 32]. From the midazolam point of view, adding propofol to reduce the required midazolam dose improves the induction and recovery profile for sedation for ERCP. The overall clinical conclusion thus may be that adding propofol to midazolam improves the clinical profile of the combined drug effect, especially regarding induction and recovery times, whereas when adding midazolam to propofol, the combination may be favorable from a hemodynamic point of view, but recovery times may be delayed compared to when propofol is used alone.

Central Neuraxial Blockade Affects the Pharmacokinetics of Anesthetic Agents

Central neuraxial blockade is often administered to patients receiving general anesthesia or undergoing sedation [33]. Local anesthetics have been shown to enhance sedation and reduce the hypnotic dose requirements for these purposes in animal studies [34, 35]. Doherty et al. found that intravenous lidocaine decreased the MAC of halothane in a dose-dependent fashion in animals. In man, intravenous lidocaine is increasingly advocated for its perioperative opioid sparing effect. A recent Cochrane review [36], though, concludes that only limited evidence exists that lidocaine has any effect on postoperative pain, postoperative opioid consumption, and postoperative nausea. Poor evidence exists as well that lidocaine may affect gastrointestinal recovery, length of hospital stay, or opioid requirements. Possible mechanisms for the lidocaine effects are unrelated to the direct sodium channel blocking effects of lidocaine. Possible mechanisms of action may be inhibition of the NMDA receptor, inhibition of NF-kB, or protein kinase C [37].

In addition to intravenously administered local anesthetics, epidurally administered local anesthetics do reduce the hypnotic dose requirements [33]. Studies by Hodgson et al. support the hypothesis that epidural anesthesia reduces volatile anesthetic requirements [38, 39]. In addition, the level of sensory blockade in spinal anesthesia is associated with an increase in the degree of sedation [40, 41]. In the presence of epidural blockade, the dose of midazolam and propofol to induce loss of consciousness was found to be reduced by up to 25 % [39–41].

Until recently, the mechanism and the magnitude of the sedative sparing effect of central neuraxial blockade remained poorly understood. Central neuraxial blockade may affect both the pharmacokinetics and the pharmacodynamics of sedative agents. The proposed mechanisms of the sedative sparing effect of central neuraxial blockade include systemic effects of local anesthetic agents, rostral spread of the spinal local anesthetic concentration, reduced afferent input deactivating the central nervous system, and lastly, the hemodynamic side effects of central neuraxial blockade that

may change the pharmacokinetics of intravenous hypnotics such that elevated hypnotic concentrations clarify the interaction [33].

The pharmacokinetics of intravenous sedatives may be affected by a change in distribution or clearance induced by epidural anesthesia, whereas the pharmacodynamics of intravenous agents may be affected through the deafferentation that occurs when central neuraxial blockade is installed. Most studies published so far show a considerable reduction in sedative requirements but, due to the study set up, cannot differentiate whether the described effect is a result of pharmacokinetic or pharmacodynamic interactions. Despite this, most authors suggest that the interaction may be predominantly of pharmacodynamic origin.

Recently, though, a study could differentiate between the effect of epidural ropivacaine on the pharmacokinetics and pharmacodynamics of propofol. Sitsen et al. [42] studied the pharmacokinetics and pharmacodynamics of propofol in 28 patients scheduled for general surgery in the presence of an epidural blockade with 0, 50, 100, or 150 mg of ropivacaine. These authors found that with increasing ropivacaine dose and with a corresponding increasing number of blocked epidural segments, the blood propofol concentration increased by up to 32 %, compared to when no epidural blockade was present. Population pharmacokinetic modeling showed that epidural blockade with 150 mg of ropivacaine significantly reduced the metabolic clearance of propofol (Fig. 17.1) by up to 30 % with an epidural blockade of 20 segments up to the fourth thoracic dermatome. The authors hypothesize that the hemodynamic changes induced by the epidural blockade are responsible for this pharmacokinetic interaction. High epidural blockade is associated with venous pooling, a reduction in cardiac output, and a reduction in hepatic blood flow [43]. A reduction in hepatic blood flow is associated with a reduction in clearance for an agent like propofol which has a high hepatic extraction ratio (>0.7). The authors conclude that in the presence of high epidural blockade, propofol requirements for surgical hypnosis may be reduced by 30 %, compared to when no epidural blockade is present, purely due to this pharmacokinetic interaction. Now that epidural blockade has been clearly shown to affect the pharmacokinetics of propofol, it remains yet unclear if a pharmacodynamic interaction also remains present between central neuraxial blockade and intravenous sedatives. Further studies are needed to unravel this question.

Pharmacokinetic Interactions Between Anesthetics and Concomitant Home Medication

Apart from the pharmacokinetic interactions between the agents given perioperatively, anesthetic agent pharmacology may be influenced by agents that patients use preoperatively

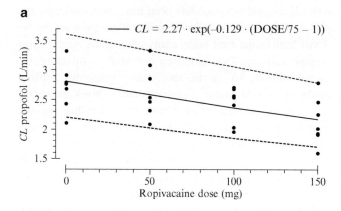

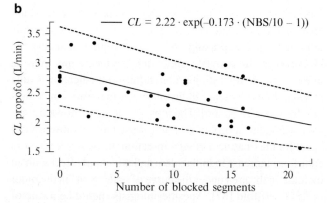

Fig. 17.1 The influence of epidural ropivacaine dose (**a**) and the number of blocked epidural segments (**b**) on the elimination clearance (CL) of propofol. An epidural dose of 150 mg ropivacaine decreases the propofol clearance from 2.58 to 2.0 L/min; 20 blocked epidural segments reduce the clearance of propofol from 2.64 to 1.87 L/min. The discontinuous line shows the 95 % confidence intervals. The dots are the empirical Bayesian estimates of clearance for each patient (Adapted from Sitsen et al. [42] With permission from Wolters Kluwer Health, Inc.)

at home. Phase I drug elimination includes oxidation, hydrolysis, and reduction of the parent drug. Oxidation is generally catalyzed by one or more of the nearly 60 cytochrome P450 members of this isoenzyme family. For the metabolic clearance of drugs, cytochrome P450 3A4 is probably the most important cytochrome isoenzyme. This subenzyme is, for example, important for the oxidation of midazolam and alfentanil. Other important subenzymes for anesthetic agent breakdown are CYP 2B6, 3A3, 3A5, and 2E1. The 60 isoenzymes are subject to induction and inhibition, causing a possible increase or decrease of their catalyzing capacity, thus affecting the clearance of agents and thereby drug effect. Many agents are known to be potent cytochrome P450 inducers and cytochrome P450 inhibitors and may greatly alter the dose–concentration time relationship of sedatives and opioid analgesics. The clinical impact of enzyme induction and inhibition may be huge. Whereas anesthetic–anesthetic drug interactions generally cause plasma concentration changes in the order of 25 %, certain

antibiotics, antifungal agents, or anticonvulsants may increase or decrease anesthetic opioid or sedative concentrations by two- to tenfold through enzyme induction or inhibition.

The clinical consequences of cytochrome P450 inhibition and induction thus may be significant. Numerous case reports describe the unpleasant effects of enzyme inhibitors and/or inducers on opioid effect. Discontinuation of carbamazepine and thus termination of the cytochrome enzyme-inducing effect caused a woman taking methadone, 210 mg PO daily for lung cancer pain relief, to lose consciousness and experience severe respiratory depression 11 days later [44]. Similarly, a male and female patient taking methadone per os on a daily basis went into coma and respiratory depression several days after the start of the intravenous administration of fluconazole and cimetidine, respectively, both being cytochrome P450 3A4 inhibitors [45, 46].

Cytochrome P450 Enzyme Inhibition

Inhibition of cytochrome P450 by one agent may lead to a reduced clearance and thereby to an increase in desired effects and adverse effects of a second agent. The increase in adverse effects may lead to potentially hazardous consequences. Enzyme inhibition occurs when a cytochrome enzyme is unable to metabolize its substrate due to the interference of another substrate [47]. Often this is the case when the cytochrome simply reaches its maximal metabolizing potential, is competitively blocked, or results from a negative feedback induced by a substrate [47]. Enzyme inhibition develops fast, sometimes within 24 h, and may last for weeks after the discontinuation, for example, as in the case of cimetidine [48, 49]. Well-known cytochrome P450 enzyme inhibitors include macrolide antibiotics like erythromycin and troleandomycin, antifungal agents like ketoconazole, Ca-channel blockers like verapamil and diltiazem, anticancer agents like tamoxifen, and omeprazole, cimetidine, grapefruit juice, and propofol [50]. Except for remifentanil, the clearance of opioids is, besides redistribution, predominantly dependent on hepatic metabolism. Drug interactions with opioids involving cytochrome inhibition may cause significant drug concentration changes and may therefore be of great clinical relevance.

Erythromycin and troleandomycin cause significant inhibition of CYP 3A4 through the formation of an inactive complex. The result is that with increasing erythromycin intake over days, the clearance of alfentanil gradually decreases, causing the plasma alfentanil concentration, after a similar dose, to increase. The clearance of alfentanil may decrease by 25 % with an increase in the elimination half-life of over 50 % [51]. Alfentanil thus shows prolonged activity in the presence of erythromycin, causing prolonged analgesia but also prolonged respiratory depression [51, 52]. Similarly, the available drug concentration of midazolam over time after oral midazolam intake increases by a factor of 3.8 after pretreatment with oral erythromycin, 500 mg for 5 days [53, 54]. Olkkola and colleagues reported the potential harmful interaction between erythromycin and midazolam, observing prolonged sedation and amnesia after the intake of erythromycin 3 times daily 500 mg for a week [55]. Similarly, an 8-year-old boy lost consciousness during an erythromycin infusion after premedication with midazolam as a result of unexpectedly high plasma midazolam concentrations due to cytochrome P450 inhibition [56].

Antifungal agents are frequently used in the intensive care for the treatment and prevention of fungal infections. Antimycotics like fluconazole, ketoconazole, and itraconazole all strongly inhibit cytochrome P450 3A [57]. Ketoconazole is the most potent inhibitor, predominantly on CYP 3A. CYP 3A is the most important cytochrome for catalyzation of drug metabolism and accounts for 40–50 % of cytochrome activity in the liver but is also present in the small intestine. Antifungal agent use in ICU patients may strongly prolong the effect of midazolam with plasma peak midazolam concentrations increasing by three- to fourfold [58]. Sedation with midazolam in the presence of azole agents in ICU patients thus may cause hazardous consequences. Also ketamine that is metabolized through CYP 2B6, 3A4, and 2C9 may be subject to a clearance reduction by the concomitant use of antifungal agents. The same is true for alfentanil, fentanyl, and oxycodone. No data suggest that propofol, which is subject to metabolism through CYP 2B6 and 2C, interacts with antifungal agents. The calcium-channel blockers verapamil and diltiazem show similar interaction to the antifungal agents and also affect the pharmacokinetics of benzodiazepines [59].

Lastly, grapefruit juice is also known as a potent cytochrome P450 inhibitor. Several studies report on the inhibition of benzodiazepine clearance through grapefruit juice [60–62]. Grapefruit juice has been reported to increase the plasma concentration of oral midazolam by over 50 %. Apart from grape fruit juice, many other fruits inhibit cytochrome activity. The inhibitory potential of human cytochrome P450 3A is in the order: grapefruit > black mulberry > wild grape > pomegranate > black raspberry [63]. All the abovementioned fruit juices are thus capable of inhibiting midazolam 1-hydroxylation. These fruit juices may thus potentiate the effect of oral benzodiazepines when used for sleep medication in the home situation or as premedication for surgery. Grapefruit juice also increases the area under the curve of S-ketamine by threefold [64].

Other inhibitors of cytochrome enzymes include the proton pump inhibitors like omeprazole and pantoprazole. Diazepam and midazolam are substrates for CYP 2C19, which is inhibited by omeprazole [65]. In a similar manner, the H_2-receptor antagonist cimetidine affects the plasma midazolam concentrations. Cimetidine co-medication results in a significant increase in the plasma midazolam concentration by about 30 % [66]. The most potent now known inhibitor is ritonavir, a protease inhibitor used as an antiretroviral agent for the treatment of HIV infection. Ritonavir leads to an enormous increase in midazolam and alfentanil effect with an increase in the area under the curve of both agents in the order of 25- to 30-fold [67]. Anesthesiologists should be aware of this interaction when opioids or benzodiazepines are used in the presence of ritonavir.

Cytochrome P450 Enzyme Induction

Enzyme induction is defined as the process of an increase in metabolizing enzyme quantity or activity as the result of the administration of another agent. Induction of a cytochrome P450 subenzyme by one agent may lead to an increased clearance and thereby to a reduced effect of a second agent (Fig. 17.2), or it may lead to an unexpected inactivation or

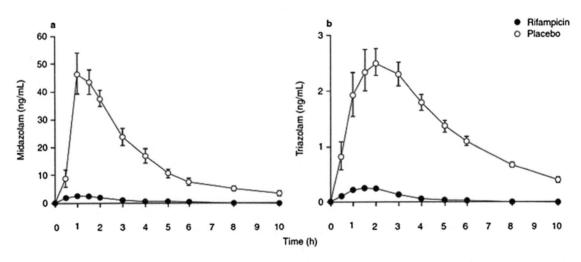

Fig. 17.2 Mean plasma midazolam (**a**) and triazolam concentration (**b**) after a 15 mg oral midazolam dose or an 0.5 mg oral triazolam dose, after treatment with placebo or rifampicin 600 mg daily, for 5 days (Adapted from Niemi et al. [69] with permission from Springer; Backman et al. [91] with permission from John Wiley and Sons; and Villikka et al. [92] with permission from John Wiley and Sons)

detoxification. The sometimes unexpected decrease in effect may lead to potentially hazardous consequences when the agent is not titrated to effect. Enzyme induction is dose and agent dependent, often occurring at the higher ranges of clinical drug administration. Enzyme induction involves receptor binding, gene encoding, mRNA transcription, and synthesis of the new protein and may be effective within hours after administration [47, 68]. Well-known cytochrome P450 enzyme inducers include (Table 17.1) barbiturates, tobacco smoke, antiepileptics like phenytoin and carbamazepine, rifampicin, and ethanol [50]. Enzyme induction may also be caused by ingestion of char-grilled meat, dexamethasone, St John's wort, alcohol, or by obesity and fasting [47]. The influence of enzyme induction may be significant. The enhanced clearance may lead to a tenfold reduction in the plasma concentration of a drug leading to close to no effect at a normal drug dose and an area under the curve of only 0.3–0.4 of the control. In Fig. 17.2 illustrates the influence of the cytochrome P450 inducer rifampicin on the concentration–time relationships of midazolam and triazolam after oral intake of clinically significant doses of 15 mg and 0.5 mg, respectively. In the absence of rifampicin, these benzodiazepine dosages assure hypnosis or deep sedation, while with rifampicin, the plasma concentration of these agents drop dramatically, leaving the patients awake [69].

Hepatic enzyme induction is furthermore important for the metabolism of inhalational agents. Cytochrome P450 2E1 catalyzes the oxidation of halothane to trifluoroacetyl. This compound is excreted through the urine, but some binds to hapten and may result in halothane-induced hepatitis. Hepatic enzyme inducers may induce P450 2E1 and enhance the formation of this hepatotoxic compound during halothane anesthesia, whereas cimetidine, through enzyme inhibition, may protect against halothane-associated hepatotoxicity [70].

Pharmacodynamic Interactions Between Anesthetics

Because of the small therapeutic window, a detailed characterization of the concentration–effect relationships of anesthetic agents and their interactions is required to allow a proper selection of the various intravenous agents and their combinations, to obtain an optimal therapeutic pharmacological effect while avoiding significant side effects [5].

Bovill reviewed the methodology of the analysis of drug interaction and described four ways of interaction analysis: fractional analysis, isobolographic analysis, method of Plummer and Short, and the parallel line assay [71]. From these, isobolographic analysis and, in parallel, response surface modeling have become the most important methods of

Table 17.1 Enzymes, substrates, inhibitors, and inducers of cytochrome P450 enzymes relevant to anesthetic practice

CYP subenzyme	Substrate	Inhibitors	Inducers
CYP 1A2	Caffeine	Cimetidine	Smoking
	Haloperidol	Erythromycin	Phenytoin
	Theophylline	Grapefruit juice	Phenobarbitone
	Paracetamol	Amiodarone	Omeprazole
	Lignocaine		Insulin
	Ondansetron		Char-grilled meat
	Ropivacaine		Ketamine
	Naproxen		
	Amitriptyline		
CYP 2C9	Phenytoin	Ketoconazole	Rifampicin
	Irbesartan	Fluconazole	Phenobarbitone
	Losartan	Metronidazole	
	Amitriptyline	Amiodarone	
	Ibuprofen	Lovastatin	
	Diclofenac		
CYP 2C19	Diazepam	Cimetidine	Rifampicin
	Phenytoin	Omeprazole	Phenobarbitone
	Omeprazole	Indomethacin	
	Pantoprazole	Ketoconazole	
	Propranolol		
	Indomethacin		
	Progesterone		
CYP 2D6	Haloperidol	Cimetidine	Dexamethasone
	Amitriptyline	Ranitidine	Rifampicin
	Flecainide	Chlorpromazine	Tramadol
	Codeine	Amiodarone	
	Lignocaine	Celecoxib	
	Metoclopramide	Methadone	
	Ondansetron		
	Tramadol		
CYP 2E1	Alcohol	Disulfiram	Acetone
	Enflurane		Alcohol
	Halothane		Isoniazid
	Isoflurane		Obesity
	Sevoflurane		Fasting
	Paracetamol		Ketamine
	Ropivacaine		
	Theophylline		
CYP 3A4	Nifedipine	Grapefruit juice	Rifampicin
	Diltiazem	Erythromycin	Carbamazepine
	Amiodarone	Clarithromycin	Phenytoin
	Fentanyl	Ciprofloxacin	Phenobarbitone
	Alfentanil	Fluconazole	St John's wort
	Sufentanil	Ketoconazole	Ketamine
	Codeine	Cimetidine	
	Lignocaine	Propofol	
	Bupivacaine	Verapamil	
	Ropivacaine		
	Midazolam		
	Triazolam		
	Diazepam		

Adapted from Sweeney et al. [47] with permission from John Wiley and Sons analysis of pharmacodynamics interactions. More recently, Shafer and colleagues wrote two landmark papers [72, 73] on the analysis of pharmacodynamic drug interactions in anesthesia. These authors explored the analysis of the interaction of drugs that compete for a single receptor and postulated that agents that act at a similar receptor must be additive in their combined effects. This is why inhalational anesthetic agents interact in an additive manner. In contrast, the authors state that synergy implies multiple sites of action by definition and that additivity among drugs acting on different receptors is only likely if the concentrations responsible for the drug effect of interest are well below the concentration associated with 50 % receptor occupancy.

Four types of pharmacodynamic interaction may be distinguished. Zero interaction, or additivity, is said to occur when a combination exerts an effect that is exactly the sum of the action of the individual agents. Combinations of inhalational anesthetics generally exert an additive interaction. The combination of 0.5 MAC halothane and 0.5 MAC sevoflurane exerts an effect of 1 MAC. Supra-additivity, synergism, or potentiation is said to occur when a combination of drugs exerts an effect that is stronger than the sum of the action of the individual agents. One then needs relatively less of the combination compared to the use of the individual agents. The interaction between inhalational agents and opioids, and between intravenous hypnotic agents and opioids, is generally synergistic in nature. Infra-additivity is said to occur when a combination exerts less effect than the sum of the action of the individual agents. Lastly, antagonism takes place when the effect of the combination is less than that of the action of one of its constituents [74].

Pharmacodynamic Interaction Between Intravenous Hypnotics and Opioids

Pharmacodynamic interactions between agents given intraoperatively may affect the pharmacodynamic profile of the combination considerably. Opioids exhibit strong analgesic effects, but also cause sedation at high drug concentration. Intravenous hypnotic agents, like propofol, induce and maintain surgical hypnosis but at a high concentration also suppress nociception. It is therefore no surprise that intravenous hypnotics and opioids support each other's action in safeguarding general anesthesia. Propofol diminishes the opioid requirements needed for suppression of nociception, whereas opioids diminish the propofol concentration that is needed for induction and maintenance of surgical hypnosis. The interaction between intravenous hypnotics and intravenous opioids generally is found to be synergistic [5]. Alfentanil and fentanyl affect the blood propofol concentration needed to induce loss of

consciousness in a synergistic manner [75, 76]. The EC_{50} for loss of consciousness with propofol is reduced by 50 % from 3.6 µg/ml to 1.8 µg/ml in the presence of a plasma alfentanil concentration of 300 ng/ml. The hemodynamic depression of the combination of propofol and alfentanil is more or less similar compared to when propofol is administered alone to induce loss of consciousness. The blood propofol concentration needed for loss of consciousness could not be reduced below 1.2 µg/ml, no matter how high the alfentanil concentration, exhibiting a ceiling in the hypnotic sparing effect by alfentanil.

This is different for the maintenance of anesthesia. With a fivefold increase in the blood propofol concentration from 2 to 10 µg/ml, the alfentanil requirements are reduced by over tenfold. Alfentanil at high concentrations postpones recovery. In the presence of a significant plasma alfentanil concentration of 150 ng/ml, the blood propofol concentration has to decrease to as low as 0.5–1 µg/ml before patients regain consciousness [4, 5, 8, 9, 77–81]. In contrast, in the presence of a plasma alfentanil concentration below 50 ng/ml, patients are already awake postoperatively at blood propofol concentrations of 2–3 µg/ml. For remifentanil [82] and propofol, the interaction for intraoperative end points and awakening run parallel to those between alfentanil and propofol (Fig. 17.3) [83–85]. Fentanyl and propofol also interact in this synergistic manner [76, 86, 87]. One may conclude that propofol concentrations at which patients regain consciousness are affected by the degree of painful stimulation at awakening postoperatively and by concurrent opioid concentration. The propofol EC_{50} reduction for intraoperative anesthetic stability by alfentanil and remifentanil is similar with a potency ratio of alfentanil/remifentanil of 35:1 [5].

By means of computer simulations, based both on pharmacokinetic and pharmacodynamic interaction data, the optimal propofol–opioid concentration combination has been defined that assures both adequate anesthesia and the most rapid possible recovery in 50 % of patients [4]. This optimal propofol–alfentanil concentration combination has been determined to be a blood propofol concentration of 3.5 µg/ml in the presence of 85 ng/ml of alfentanil. The optimal propofol concentration is much lower when combined with remifentanil compared to when combined with fentanyl, sufentanil, or alfentanil [4]. Whereas the optimal propofol concentration (EC_{95}) when combined with fentanyl is of the order of 5 µg/ml, the optimal propofol concentration is 2.5 µg/ml in the presence of remifentanil (Fig. 17.4). From the optimal propofol–opioid concentrations, optimal propofol and opioid infusion schemes have been derived that assure adequate anesthesia and the most rapid return of consciousness after termination of the infusion when propofol is combined with one of the opioids fentanyl, alfentanil, sufentanil, or remifentanil (Table 17.2). These

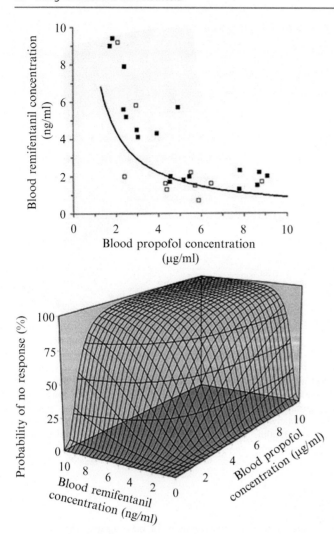

Fig. 17.3 Concentration–effect relation of the combination of propofol and remifentanil for suppression of responses to intubation. The iso-effect *curve* (=isobole) in the upper graph was obtained by response surface modeling of the response (*open squares*)–no response (*closed squares*) data on intubation versus the corresponding measured blood propofol concentrations and blood remifentanil concentrations. The displayed iso-effect *curve* represents remifentanil and propofol concentrations associated with a 50 % probability of no response to intubation, describing the synergistic interaction model. In the concentration–response surface (*bottom*) for the combination of propofol and remifentanil, the isoboles for 25, 50, and 75 % probability of no response are shown (Adapted from Mertens et al. [83] with permission from Wolters Kluwer Health, Inc.)

infusion schemes should be used as guidelines, and adjustments should be made to the individual needs of the patient in anticipation of factors such as age, gender, and stimulus intensity related to the type of surgery. The overall message, though, remains clear; the propofol–opioid interaction is synergistic and the optimal propofol infusion regimen is different for the various opioids.

Lastly, in spontaneously breathing patients, propofol and remifentanil also exhibit a synergistic interaction on resting ventilation (Fig. 17.5), resting end-tidal PCO_2, ventilation at a fixed PCO_2 of 55 Torr, and the ventilation–PCO_2 response slope [88]. Nieuwenhuijs et al. concluded that while remifentanil shifts the ventilation–CO_2 response curve in a parallel fashion to higher $P_{ET}CO_2$ levels, propofol reduces the slope of the response rather than shifting its position. When propofol and remifentanil are combined, the depressant effect involves a shift to the right and includes a flatting of the ventilation–CO_2 response curve.

The depressant effect of remifentanil and propofol on blood pressure and heart rate is modest, when given separately; when combined, their depressant effect is additive [89]. Clinically, respiratory depression already occurs at rather low concentrations when propofol and remifentanil are combined, especially in the absence of nociception. Propofol at a sedative concentration of 1–2 µg/ml only reduces resting minute ventilation from 9 to 8 L/min, a respiratory depressant effect similarly induced by a plasma remifentanil concentration of 1 ng/ml. When propofol and remifentanil are combined at these low concentrations, resting ventilation drops by 80 % to 1–2 L/min (Fig. 17.5). This, while the respiratory drive remains rather strong with propofol alone up until deep levels of sedation [90]. When combining propofol and remifentanil in spontaneously breathing patients, the doses should thus be carefully titrated to the individual needs of the patients and in close relation to the level of nociception under proper respiratory monitoring.

Conclusion

The extensive variability in the dose–response relationship of intravenous anesthetics and opioids remains a challenge for the clinical anesthesiologist. Some patients need ten times the dose of others to experience the same hypnotic or analgesic effect. Pharmacokinetic and pharmacodynamic interactions explain part of this wide pharmacokinetic–dynamic variability.

Two groups of interactions deserve special attention from the anesthesiologist. The first are the pharmacokinetic interactions caused by cytochrome P450 inhibition and induction and the second the pharmacodynamic interactions between intravenous hypnotic agents and opioids. The anesthesiologist should be aware of the inhibitory and inductive influence of some agents on cytochrome P450 activity as displayed in Table 17.1. The impact of a modification in cytochrome P450 activity on the clinical action of benzodiazepines and opioids may be huge, causing either no effect or a vastly exaggerated effect of a normal clinical dose.

In addition, the anesthesiologist should be aware of the optimal propofol–opioid concentration combinations and

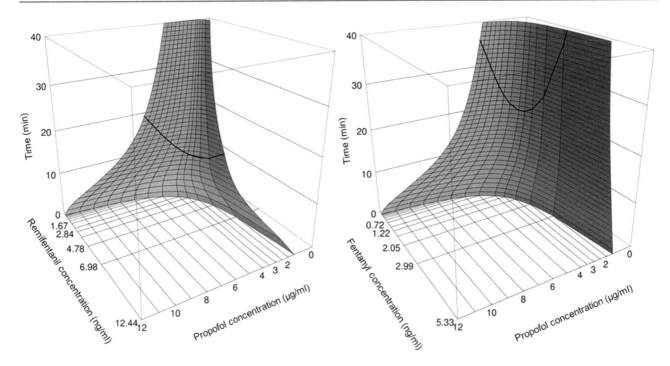

Fig. 17.4 The decrease in the propofol–remifentanil and propofol–fentanyl concentrations (from *bottom* to *top*) after termination of a 300 min simulated infusion of these agents at concentrations needed to assure adequate anesthesia in 50 % of patients (EC$_{50}$). The *bold line* within the response surface exhibits the simulated propofol–remifentanil and propofol–fentanyl plasma concentrations at which 50 % of patients regain consciousness after termination of these 300 min infusions. The optimal propofol concentration that assures adequate anesthesia and the most rapid return to consciousness is 2 µg/ml when combined with remifentanil and 4 µg/ml in combination with fentanyl (Adapted from Vuyk [4] with permission from Wolters Kluwer Health, Inc. and Lichtenbelt [5] with permission from Springer)

Table 17.2 Infusion schemes of propofol and the opioids required to maintain effect site concentrations of these agents, when given in combination, within +/− 15 % of the effect site concentrations that are associated with a 50 and 95 % probability of no response to surgical stimuli and the most rapid possible return of consciousness after termination of the infusions [4, 5]

Opioid	Alfentanil EC$_{50}$–EC$_{95}$	Fentanyl EC$_{50}$–EC$_{95}$	Sufentanil EC$_{50}$–EC$_{95}$	Remifentanil EC$_{50}$–EC$_{95}$
Bolus	25–35 µg/kg in 30 s	3 µg/kg in 30 s	0.15–0.25 µg/kg in 30 s	1.5–2 µg/kg in 30 s
	50–75 µg/kg/h for 30 min	1.5–2.5 µg/kg/h for 30 min	0.15–0.22 µg/kg thereafter	13–22 µg/kg/h for 20 min
Infusion 2	30–42.5 µg/kg/h thereafter	1.3–2 µg/kg/h up to 150 min		11.5–19 µg/kg/h thereafter
Infusion 3		0.7–1.4 µg/kg/h thereafter		
Propofol	Propofol EC$_{50}$–EC$_{95}$	Propofol EC$_{50}$–EC$_{95}$	Propofol EC$_{50}$–EC$_{95}$	Propofol EC$_{50}$–EC$_{95}$
Bolus	2.0–2.8 mg/kg in 30 s	2.0–3.0 mg/kg in 30 s	2.0–2.8 mg/kg in 30 s	1.5 mg/kg in 30 s
Infusion 1	9–12 mg/kg/h for 40 min	9–15 mg/kg/h for 40 min	9–12 mg/kg/h for 40 min	7–8 mg/kg/h for 40 min
Infusion 2	7–10 mg/kg/h for 150 min	7–12 mg/kg/h for 150 min	7–10 mg/kg/h for 150 min	6–6.5 mg/kg/h for 150 min
Infusion 3	6.5–8 mg/kg/h thereafter	6.5–11 mg/kg/h thereafter	6.5–8 mg/kg/h thereafter	5–6 mg/kg/h thereafter

Adapted from Vuyk et al. [4] With permission from Wolters Kluwer Health, Inc
These optimal infusion schemes have been derived from data in female patients undergoing lower abdominal surgery
These should be used as guidelines and be adjusted to the individual needs of the patient

optimal propofol–opioid infusion regimen as displayed in Table 17.2. The propofol infusion regimen during general anesthesia or sedation should be adjusted to the opioid used. Patients will benefit from this alertness, for it allows them to receive an anesthetic with optimal intraoperative nociceptive control as well as experience the most rapid possible return to consciousness thereafter.

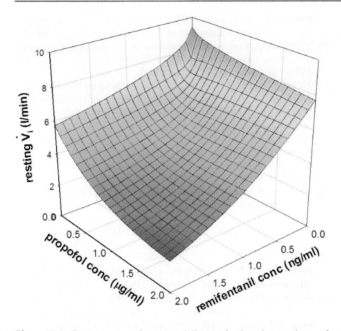

Fig. 17.5 Response surface modeling of the interaction of remifentanil and propofol on resting ventilation. Population response surface showing that the propofol–remifentanil interaction is synergistic. Also, the dose–response relationship between drugs and effect was not linear (Adapted from Nieuwenhuijs et al. [89] with permission from Wolters Kluwer Health, Inc.)

References

1. Pergolizzi JV. Quantifying the impact of drug-drug interactions associated with opioids. Am J Manag Care 2011;17 Suppl 11: S288–92.
2. Pergolizzi Jr JV, Labhsetwar SA, Puenpatom RA, Joo S, Ben-Joseph RH, Summers KH. Prevalence of exposure to potential CYP450 pharmacokinetic drug-drug interactions among patients with chronic low back pain taking opioids. Pain Pract. 2011;11:230–9.
3. Ackerman SJ, Mordin M, Reblando J, Xu X, Schein J, Vallow S, Brennan M. Patient-reported utilization patterns of fentanyl transdermal system and oxycodone hydrochloride controlled-release among patients with chronic nonmalignant pain. J Manag Care Pharm. 2003;9:223–31.
4. Vuyk J, Mertens MJ, Olofsen E, Burm AG, Bovill JG. Propofol anesthesia and rational opioid selection: determination of optimal EC50-EC95 propofol-opioid concentrations that assure adequate anesthesia and a rapid return of consciousness. Anesthesiology. 1997;87:1549–62.
5. Lichtenbelt BJ, Mertens M, Vuyk J. Strategies to optimise propofol-opioid anaesthesia. Clin Pharmacokinet. 2004;43:577–93.
6. Taniguchi T, Yamamoto K, Kobayashi T. The precipitate formed by thiopentone and vecuronium. Can J Anaesth. 1996;43:511–3.
7. Taniguchi T, Yamamoto K, Kobayashi T. Precipitate formed by thiopentone and vecuronium causes pulmonary embolism. Can J Anaesth. 1998;45:347–51.
8. Vuyk J. Drug interactions in anaesthesia. Minerva Anestesiol. 1999;65:215–8.
9. Vuyk J. TCI: supplementation and drug interactions. Anaesthesia. 1998;53 Suppl 1:35–41.
10. Lotsch J, Skarke C, Tegeder I, Geisslinger G. Drug interactions with patient-controlled analgesia. Clin Pharmacokinet. 2002;41:31–57.

11. Kurita T, Uraoka M, Jiang Q, Suzuki M, Morishima Y, Morita K, Sato S. Influence of cardiac output on the pseudo-steady state remifentanil and propofol concentrations in swine. Acta Anaesthesiol Scand. 2013;57:754–60.
12. Bouillon T, Bruhn J, Radu-Radulescu L, Bertaccini E, Park S, Shafer S. Non-steady state analysis of the pharmacokinetic interaction between propofol and remifentanil. Anesthesiology. 2002;97:1350–62.
13. Mertens MJ, Vuyk J, Olofsen E, Bovill JG, Burm AG. Propofol alters the pharmacokinetics of alfentanil in healthy male volunteers. Anesthesiology. 2001;94:949–57.
14. Baker MT, Chadam MV, Ronnenberg Jr WC. Inhibitory effects of propofol on cytochrome P450 activities in rat hepatic microsomes. Anesth Analg. 1993;76:817–21.
15. Pavlin DJ, Coda B, Shen DD, Tschanz J, Nguyen Q, Schaffer R, Donaldson G, Jacobson RC, Chapman CR. Effects of combining propofol and alfentanil on ventilation, analgesia, sedation, and emesis in human volunteers. Anesthesiology. 1996;84:23–37.
16. Gepts E, Jonckheer K, Maes V, Sonck W, Camu F. Disposition kinetics of propofol during alfentanil anaesthesia. Anaesthesia. 1988;43(Suppl):8–13.
17. McKillop D, Wild MJ, Butters CJ, Simcock C. Effects of propofol on human hepatic microsomal cytochrome P450 activities. Xenobiotica. 1998;28:845–53.
18. Janicki PK, James MF, Erskine WA. Propofol inhibits enzymatic degradation of alfentanil and sufentanil by isolated liver microsomes in vitro. Br J Anaesth. 1992;68:311–2.
19. Kurita T, Morita K, Kazama T, Sato S. Influence of cardiac output on plasma propofol concentrations during constant infusion in swine. Anesthesiology. 2002;96:1498–503.
20. Yufune S, Takamatsu I, Masui K, Kazama T. Effect of remifentanil on plasma propofol concentration and bispectral index during propofol anaesthesia. Br J Anaesth. 2011;106:208–14.
21. Mertens MJ, Olofsen E, Burm AGL, Bovill JG, Vuyk J. Mixed-effects modeling of the influence of alfentanil on propofol pharmacokinetics. Anesthesiology. 2004;100:795–805.
22. Short TG, Chui PT. Propofol and midazolam act synergistically in combination. Br J Anaesth. 1991;67:539–45.
23. Short TG, Plummer JL, Chui PT. Hypnotic and anaesthetic interactions between midazolam, propofol and alfentanil. Br J Anaesth. 1992;69:162–7.
24. Lichtenbelt BJ, Olofsen E, Dahan A, van Kleef JW, Struys MM, Vuyk J. Propofol reduces the distribution and clearance of midazolam. Anesth Analg. 2010;110:1597–606.
25. Hamaoka N, Oda Y, Hase I, Mizutani K, Nakamoto T, Ishizaki T, Asada A. Propofol decreases the clearance of midazolam by inhibiting CYP3A4: an in vivo and in vitro study. Clin Pharmacol Ther. 1999;66:110–7.
26. Guitton J, Buronfosse T, Desage M, Flinois JP, Perdrix JP, Brazier JL, Beaune P. Possible involvement of multiple human cytochrome P450 isoforms in the liver metabolism of propofol. Br J Anaesth. 1998;80:788–95.
27. Vuyk J, Lichtenbelt BJ, Olofsen E, van Kleef JW, Dahan A. Mixed-effects modeling of the influence of midazolam on propofol pharmacokinetics. Anesth Analg. 2009;108:1522–30.
28. Chan WH, Chen TL, Chen RM, Sun WZ, Ueng TH. Propofol metabolism is enhanced after repetitive ketamine administration in rats: the role of cytochrome P-450 2B induction. Br J Anaesth. 2006;97:351–8.
29. Lim YS, Kang DH, Kim SH, Jang TH, Kim KH, Ryu SJ, Yu SB, Kim DS. The cardiovascular effects of midazolam co-induction to propofol for induction in aged patients. Korean J Anesthesiol. 2012;62:536–42.
30. Carrasco G, Cabre L, Sobrepere G, Costa J, Molina R, Cruspinera A, Lacasa C. Synergistic sedation with propofol and midazolam in intensive care patients after coronary artery bypass grafting. Crit Care Med. 1998;26:844–51.

31. Walder B, Borgeat A, Suter PM, Romand JA. Propofol and midazolam versus propofol alone for sedation following coronary artery bypass grafting: a randomized, placebo-controlled trial. Anaesth Intensive Care. 2002;30:171–8.

32. Walder B, Elia N, Henzi I, Romand JR, Tramer MR. A lack of evidence of superiority of propofol versus midazolam for sedation in mechanically ventilated critically ill patients: a qualitative and quantitative systematic review. Anesth Analg. 2001;92:975–83.

33. Ingelmo PM, Ferri F, Fumagalli R. Interactions between general and regional anesthesia. Minerva Anestesiol. 2006;72:437–45.

34. Doherty TJ, Frazier DL. Effect of intravenous lidocaine on halothane minimum alveolar concentration in ponies. Equine Vet J. 1998;30:300–3.

35. Valverde A, Gunkelt C, Doherty TJ, Giguere S, Pollak AS. Effect of a constant rate infusion of lidocaine on the quality of recovery from sevoflurane or isoflurane general anaesthesia in horses. Equine Vet J. 2005;37:559–64.

36. Kranke P, Jokinen J, Pace NL, Schnabel A, Hollmann MW, Hahnenkamp K, Eberhart LH, Poepping DM, Weibel S. Continuous intravenous perioperative lidocaine infusion for postoperative pain and recovery. Cochrane Database Syst Rev. 2015;7:CD009642.

37. Brinkrolf P, Hahnenkamp K. Systemic lidocaine in surgical procedures: effects beyond sodium channel blockade. Curr Opin Anaesthesiol. 2014;27:420–5.

38. Hodgson PS, Liu SS. Epidural lidocaine decreases sevoflurane requirement for adequate depth of anesthesia as measured by the Bispectral Index monitor. Anesthesiology. 2001;94:799–803.

39. Hodgson PS, Liu SS, Gras TW. Does epidural anesthesia have general anesthetic effects? A prospective, randomized, double-blind, placebo-controlled trial. Anesthesiology. 1999;91:1687–92.

40. Gentili M, Huu PC, Enel D, Hollande J, Bonnet F. Sedation depends on the level of sensory block induced by spinal anaesthesia. Br J Anaesth. 1998;81:970–1.

41. Gentili ME, Enel D, Bonnet FJ. Spinal anesthesia-induced sedation may obviously facilitate general anesthesia. J Clin Anesth. 2011;23:79.

42. Sitsen E, Olofsen E, Lesman A, Dahan A, Vuyk J. Epidural blockade affects the pharmacokinetics of propofol in surgical patients. Anesth Analg. 2015; published ahead of print.

43. Simon MJ, Reekers M, Veering BT, Boer F, Burm AG, van Kleef JW, Vuyk J. Cardiovascular parameters and liver blood flow after infusion of a colloid solution and epidural administration of ropivacaine 0.75%: the influence of age and level of analgesia. Eur J Anaesthesiol. 2009;26:166–74.

44. Benitez-Rosario MA, Salinas MA, Gomez-Ontanon E, Feria M. - Methadone-induced respiratory depression after discontinuing carbamazepine administration. J Pain Symptom Manage. 2006;32:99–100.

45. Tarumi Y, Pereira J, Watanabe S. Methadone and fluconazole: respiratory depression by drug interaction. J Pain Symptom Manage. 2002;23:148–53.

46. Sorkin EM, Ogawa GS. Cimetidine potentiation of narcotic action. Drug Intell Clin Pharm. 1983;17:60–1.

47. Sweeney BP, Bromilow J. Liver enzyme induction and inhibition: implications for anaesthesia. Anaesthesia. 2006;61:159–77.

48. Somogyi A, Muirhead M. Pharmacokinetic interactions of cimetidine 1987. Clin Pharmacokinet. 1987;12:321–66.

49. Somogyi A, Gugler R. Drug interactions with cimetidine. Clin Pharmacokinet. 1982;7:23–41.

50. Bovill JG. Adverse drug interactions in anesthesia. J Clin Anesth. 1997;9:3S–13.

51. Bartkowski RR, Goldberg ME, Larijani GE, Boerner T. Inhibition of alfentanil metabolism by erythromycin. Clin Pharmacol Ther. 1989;46:99–102.

52. Bartkowski RR, McDonnell TE. Prolonged alfentanil effect following erythromycin administration. Anesthesiology. 1990;73:566–8.

53. Yeates RA, Laufen H, Zimmermann T. Interaction between midazolam and clarithromycin: comparison with azithromycin. Int J Clin Pharmacol Ther. 1996;34:400–5.

54. Zimmermann T, Yeates RA, Laufen H, Scharpf F, Leitold M, Wildfeuer A. Influence of the antibiotics erythromycin and azithromycin on the pharmacokinetics and pharmacodynamics of midazolam. Arzneimittelforschung. 1996;46:213–7.

55. Olkkola KT, Aranko K, Luurila H, Hiller A, Saarnivaara L, Himberg JJ, Neuvonen PJ. A potentially hazardous interaction between erythromycin and midazolam. Clin Pharmacol Ther. 1993;53:298–305.

56. Hiller A, Olkkola KT, Isohanni P, Saarnivaara L. Unconsciousness associated with midazolam and erythromycin. Br J Anaesth. 1990;65:826–8.

57. Saari TI, Olkkola KT. Azole antimycotics and drug interactions in the perioperative period. Curr Opin Anaesthesiol. 2010;23:441–8.

58. Olkkola KT, Backman JT, Neuvonen PJ. Midazolam should be avoided in patients receiving the systemic antimycotics ketoconazole or itraconazole. Clin Pharmacol Ther. 1994;55:481–5.

59. Backman JT, Olkkola KT, Aranko K, Himberg JJ, Neuvonen PJ. Dose of midazolam should be reduced during diltiazem and verapamil treatments. Br J Clin Pharmacol. 1994;37:221–5.

60. Bailey DG, Malcolm J, Arnold O, Spence JD. Grapefruit juice-drug interactions. Br J Clin Pharmacol. 1998;46:101–10.

61. Bailey DG, Arnold JMO, Spence JD. Grapefruit juice and drugs - how significant is the interaction. Clin Pharmacokinet. 1994;26:91–8.

62. Bailey DG, Edgar B, Spence JD, Munoz C, Arnold JMO. Felodipine and nifedipine interactions with grapefruit juice. Clin Pharmacol Ther. 1990;47:180.

63. Kim H, Yoon YJ, Shon JH, Cha IJ, Shin JG, Liu KH. Inhibitory effects of fruit juices on CYP3A activity. Drug Metab Dispos. 2006;34:521–3.

64. Peltoniemi MA, Saari TI, Hagelberg NM, Laine K, Neuvonen PJ, Olkkola KT. S-ketamine concentrations are greatly increased by grapefruit juice. Eur J Clin Pharmacol. 2012;68:979–86.

65. Li G, Klotz U. Inhibitory effect of omeprazole on the metabolism of midazolam in vitro. Arzneimittelforschung. 1990;40:1105–7.

66. Klotz U, Arvela P, Rosenkranz B. Effect of single doses of cimetidine and ranitidine on the steady-state plasma levels of midazolam. Clin Pharmacol Ther. 1985;38:652–5.

67. Hohmann N, Haefeli WE, Mikus G. CYP3A activity: towards dose adaptation to the individual. Exp Opin Drug Metab Toxicol. 2016

68. Sweeney BP, Grayling M. Smoking and anaesthesia: the pharmacological implications. Anaesthesia. 2009;64:179–86.

69. Niemi M, Backman JT, Fromm MF, Neuvonen PJ, Kivisto KT. Pharmacokinetic interactions with rifampicin - clinical relevance. Clin Pharmacokinet. 2003;42:819–50.

70. Wood M, Uetrecht J, Phythyon JM, Shay S, Sweetman BJ, Shaheen O, Wood AJ. The effect of cimetidine on anesthetic metabolism and toxicity. Anesth Analg. 1986;65:481–8.

71. Bovill JG. Analysis of drug interactions, drug interactions. In: Bovill JG, editor. Baillierre Tindall; 1998. pp. 153–68.

72. Shafer SL, Hendrickx JF, Flood P, Sonner J, Eger EI. Additivity versus synergy: a theoretical analysis of implications for anesthetic mechanisms. Anesth Analg. 2008;107:507–24.

73. Hendrickx JF, Eger EI, Sonner JM, Shafer SL. Is synergy the rule? A review of anesthetic interactions producing hypnosis and immobility. Anesth Analg. 2008;107:494–506.

74. Minto C, Vuyk J. Response surface modelling of drug interactions. Adv Exp Med Biol. 2003;523:35–43.

75. Vuyk J, Engbers FH, Burm AGL, Vletter AA, Griever GE, Olofsen E, Bovill JG. Pharmacodynamic interaction between

propofol and alfentanil when given for induction of anesthesia. Anesthesiology. 1996;84:288–99.

76. Smith C, McEwan AI, Jhaveri R, Wilkinson M, Goodman D, Smith LR, Canada AT, Glass PS. The interaction of fentanyl on the Cp50 of propofol for loss of consciousness and skin incision. Anesthesiology. 1994;81:820–8.

77. Vuyk J, Hennis PJ, Burm AG, de Voogt JW, Spierdijk J. Comparison of midazolam and propofol in combination with alfentanil for total intravenous anesthesia. Anesth Analg. 1990;71:645–50.

78. Vuyk J, Engbers FH, Lemmens HJ, Burm AG, Vletter AA, Gladines MP, Bovill JG. Pharmacodynamics of propofol in female patients. Anesthesiology. 1992;77:3–9.

79. Vuyk J, Lim T, Engbers FH, Burm AG, Vletter AA, Bovill JG. Pharmacodynamics of alfentanil as a supplement to propofol or nitrous oxide for lower abdominal surgery in female patients. Anesthesiology. 1993;78:1036–45.

80. Vuyk J, Lim T, Engbers FH, Burm AG, Vletter AA, Bovill JG. The pharmacodynamic interaction of propofol and alfentanil during lower abdominal surgery in women. Anesthesiology. 1995;83:8–22.

81. Vuyk J. Pharmacokinetic and pharmacodynamic interactions between opioids and propofol. J Clin Anesth. 1997;9:23S–6.

82. Bouillon TW, Bruhn J, Radulescu L, Andresen C, Shafer TJ, Cohane C, Shafer SL. Pharmacodynamic interaction between propofol and remifentanil regarding hypnosis, tolerance of laryngoscopy, bispectral index, and electroencephalographic approximate entropy. Anesthesiology. 2004;100:1353–72.

83. Mertens MJ, Olofsen E, Engbers FHM, Burm AGL, Bovill JG, Vuyk J. Propofol reduces perioperative remifentanil requirements in a synergistic manner - response surface modeling of perioperative remifentanil-propofol interactions. Anesthesiology. 2003;99:347–59.

84. Johnson KB, Syroid ND, Gupta DK, Manyam SC, Egan TD, Huntington J, White JL, Tyler D, Westenskow DR. An evaluation of remifentanil propofol response surfaces for loss of responsiveness, loss of response to surrogates of painful stimuli and laryngoscopy in patients undergoing elective surgery. Anesth Analg 2008;106:471–9, table.

85. Lapierre CD, Johnson KB, Randall BR, White JL, Egan TD. An exploration of remifentanil-propofol combinations that lead to a loss of response to esophageal instrumentation, a loss of responsiveness, and/or onset of intolerable ventilatory depression. Anesth Analg. 2011

86. Kazama T, Ikeda K, Morita K, Katoh T, Kikura M. Propofol concentration required for endotracheal intubation with a laryngoscope or fiberscope and its interaction with fentanyl. Anesth Analg. 1998;86:872–9.

87. Kazama T, Ikeda K, Morita K. Reduction by fentanyl of the Cp50 values of propofol and hemodynamic responses to various noxious stimuli. Anesthesiology. 1997;87:213–27.

88. Olofsen E, Boom M, Nieuwenhuijs D, Sarton E, Teppema L, Aarts L, Dahan A. Modeling the non-steady state respiratory effects of remifentanil in awake and propofol-sedated healthy volunteers. Anesthesiology. 2010;112:1382–95.

89. Nieuwenhuijs DJ, Olofsen E, Romberg RR, Sarton E, Ward D, Engbers F, Vuyk J, Mooren R, Teppema LJ, Dahan A. Response surface modeling of remifentanil-propofol interaction on cardiorespiratory control and bispectral index. Anesthesiology. 2003;98:312–22.

90. Dahan A, Nieuwenhuijs DJF, Olofsen E. Influence of propofol on the control of breathing. Adv Exp Med Biol. 2003;523:81–92.

91. Backman JT, Olkkola KT, Neuvonen PJ. Rifampin drastically reduces plasma concentrations and effects of oral midazolam. Clin Pharmacol Ther. 1996;59:7–13.

92. Villikka K, Kivisto KT, Backman JT, Olkkola KT, Neuvonen PJ. Triazolam is ineffective in patients taking rifampin. Clin Pharmacol Ther. 1997;61:8–14.

Pump Pitfalls and Practicalities

18

Frank Engbers

Introduction

Planning to give the right drug with the right dose to the right patient is mandatory for a successful application of intravenous anaesthesia. Making sure that this dose will be delivered to the patient at all times in the course of an anaesthetic procedure is of equal importance. This requires knowledge of the infusion device and how to control it. It requires thoughtful setup of infusion systems including the lines to avoid disturbances in the flow of the drug to the patient. As no system can be guaranteed to be fail-safe, back up plans need to be available to cope with situations not expected when starting the anaesthesia. In addition, inexperienced clinicians with to use intravenous techniques need to be properly trained and educated. In this chapter, syringe driving infusion pumps will be discussed in general but particularly in relation to target (TCI) and effect target-controlled infusion (ETCI). Issues to be discussed include the effect of occlusions and alarm settings and how to connect the syringe to the patient. Possible pitfalls caused by, for example, dead space in the infusion line and how to deal with situations like a failing TCI system or an inadvertently reset or not reset TCI device will be addressed.

The Infusion Device

There are a variety of different mechanical principles used for devices that aim to deliver a fluid in a controllable way, but in the end, they all come down to the same principle: creating a pressure in the outflow of the device that is high enough to establish a user selectable flow rate out of that device [1]. For intravenous anaesthesia, the system most frequently used is a syringe driving pump. Another available infusion device in the operating theatre and specially the intensive care is the volumetric infusion pump. In contrast to a syringe pump where a definite amount of drug solution is loaded inside the pump, the volumetric infusion device is connected to a reservoir that is not part of the driving mechanism of the pump. The obvious advantage of the volumetric pump is that the size of the reservoir and so the available amount of drug or fluid can be adjusted to requirements. The driving mechanism in a volumetric pump usually involves controlled compression of the infusion tubing with an external chamber where drops are counted. Even if this tubing is specially developed for the device, the accuracy and reliability at low flow rates is less than syringe infusion pumps in particular when rapid adjustments to the flow rate are required as is the case with TCI. Volumetric pumps can oscillate around the set value even more than syringe driving pumps. If used as a carrier infusion in a multi-infusion setup, they may influence the delivery of highly concentrated drugs delivered by syringe driving pump [Fig. 18.1]. The example given here demonstrates that the complexity of multidrug infusions should not be underestimated.

For the delivery of intravenous anaesthetic drugs, predominantly syringe pumps are used as over a large range of infusion rates the accuracy is considered to be adequate. But syringe-driven infusion pumps also have their disadvantages. Several conditions can cause an infusion device not to deliver the expected infusion rate and volume.

The source of these deviations can be the pump, the syringe and infusion setup or the user and his interaction with the infusion device.

The Syringe Pump

Basic components of an infusion pumps are the electrical motor, one or more displacement sensors and a pressure sensor. A sensor will measure the movement of the plunger

F. Engbers, MD, FRCA(✉)
Department of Anesthesiology, Leiden University Medical Centre,
Albinusdreef 2 Leiden, Leiden, ZH 2333 ZA, The Netherlands
e-mail: fengbers@me.com

© Springer International Publishing AG 2017
A.R. Absalom, K.P. Mason (eds.), *Total Intravenous Anesthesia and Target Controlled Infusions*,
DOI 10.1007/978-3-319-47609-4_18

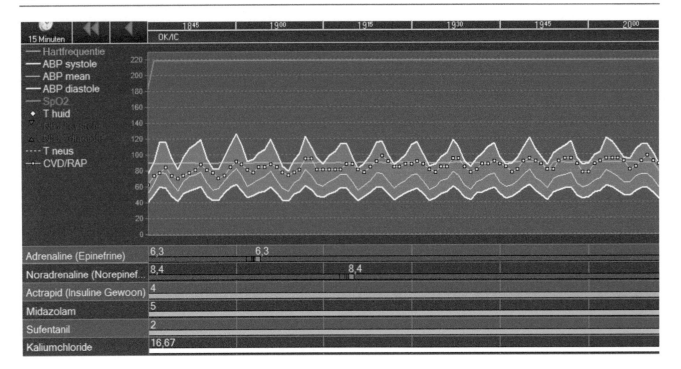

Fig. 18.1 Oscillating blood pressure in a real patient with a frequency of about 1 cycle every 6 min. Highly concentrated norepinephrine and epinephrine solutions (200 μg/ml) were being infused by syringe driving pumps, while a volumetric pump provided a carrier infusion. Oscillations in the carrier fluid flow rate caused oscillations in vasopressor administration

of the installed syringe. Speed of the motor is controlled by electronic circuitry that uses this sensor output for feedback. In the past, analogue circuits were used. Today most controlling circuits will contain microprocessors which highly increase the accuracy. Feedback mechanisms need time to optimise the control and hence will create fluctuations around the set point. The lower the infusion rate and the shorter the time of measurement or observation, the higher the deviation of set infusion rate will be. In order to assess the final error in the infusion rate, trumpet curves are constructed [Fig. 18.2] that show the percentage error related to the time of observation of measurement. When the observation window enlarges, the effect of the fluctuation is damped out and the bias relative to the set rate of the pump becomes apparent. The trumpet curve is in essence a statistical analysis of the error of the pump over time and belongs to one particular flow rate. To get a good impression of the infusion pump, trumpet curves at different flow rates should be judged, dependent on the clinical use of the infusion pump. Modern infusion pumps with microprocessor control can be so accurate that the trumpet curves almost become irrelevant. Trumpet curves do *not* reflect the startup behaviour of the device and possible under or overshoot.

For intravenous anaesthesia, flow rates from 1 to 1000 ml/h are necessary, but requirements on a neonatology department will differ from an adult department and may require accurate flow rates less than 1 ml/h. Not only mechanical parts like gear boxes but also electronic

components like capacitors will wear out over time. This may influence the accuracy of the infusion pump, and it is a good practice to check infusion pumps on a scheduled time base.

Pumps used in Europe must comply with CE (Conformitée Européene) marking. For CE-marked pumps, the measurements of flow rate accuracy conform to standards developed by the International Electrotechnical Commission and are described in standard IEC 60601-2-24. There are more standards issued by the IEC that concern the electrical safety and reliability of infusion pumps that are both adopted by the CE marking and the federal agency for Food and Drug Administration (FDA).

For target-controlled infusion, no specific standards exist yet. The aforementioned trumpet curves are not sufficient to determine the accuracy of the target-controlled infusion pumps as the impact of rate deviations on the calculated concentrations is difficult to predict and are dependent on the characteristics of the applied pharmacokinetic model. Furthermore, adequate startup performance is important for target-controlled infusion and effect-controlled infusion as this influences the loading of the central volume of the pharmacokinetic model. Trumpet curves do not describe the startup performance.

During the first commercialisation of target-controlled infusion pumps, Astra Zeneca sold a separate microprocessor module (Diprifusor®) that could be implemented in existing infusion pumps for the target-controlled infusion

Fig. 18.2 Typical results from testing conventional rate-controllable syringe driver pumps. Fluctuations around the mean infusion rate are caused by positive and negative feedback of the control mechanism, giving the typical funnel shape curve after several repeated tests. Usually the observation window starts when the output is stable and therefore does not give information on the startup performance

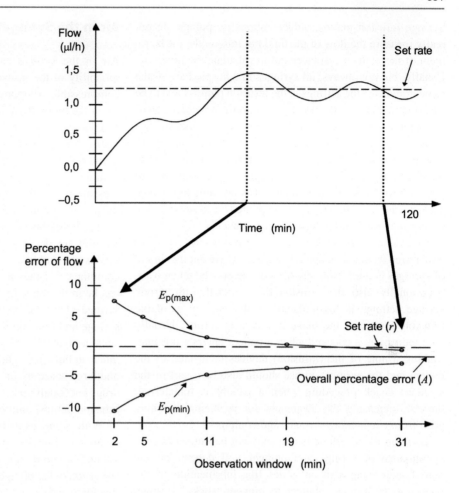

of propofol [2]. Accuracy and precision of the combination of module and pump was guarded by standards and testing requirements, issued internally by the manufacturer of the module (personal communication). The performance of the module-pump combination was confirmed in laboratory settings [3].

The coming of the so-called open TCI devices has opened the possibility of implementing more drugs and models but also opened the door for other errors.

The pharmacokinetic calculations may be erroneous or based on inappropriate parameters, but also the interplay between the computational software layer that handles the pharmacokinetic calculations and the layer that handles the flow rate control can influence the performance of the TCI system [4, 5].

There are a multitude of pharmacokinetic models in use these days. For some drugs, the users of target-controlled infusion pumps even have more than one model to choose from. Even pharmacokinetic data coming from the same publication can have a different implementation of the pharmacokinetic model due to different interpretation of the data by the pump manufacturer (see target-controlled infusion).

Compartmental models have an inherent problem of being unable to correctly predict the early phase in fast changing concentrations because the model assumes immediate mixing of the drug in the compartments [6]. The discussion of the most appropriate model for propofol still continues. It is however important to emphasise that from a clinical point of view, only the predictability of the drug effect, which is the result of the correctly chosen dose and not the drug's theoretical blood concentration, is important [7].

The electronic circuitry in modern infusion pumps mostly consist of an embedded microprocessor. Together with the improved sensor technology, this allows for a much better accuracy of the mechanical performance of the syringe-based infusion pump. Unless not appropriately programmed, the biggest deviation from the set infusion rate, when controlled manually, is not to be expected from the mechanical and electronic controlling part of the device but from external equipment like the syringe and infusion lines.

The Syringe

The syringe can be an important source of deviation from the intended amount of fluid or drug delivery.

First of all, syringes are not standardised in sizes, even if the volume indication of different brands is the same.

Syringe infusion pumps, unlike volumetric pumps, do not really measure the flow of the fluid but rely on the measurement of the plunger displacement to calculate the flow rate. Usually, but not always, all syringes in a hospital are of the same brand, and the settings in the infusion pumps have to be adjusted to this specific brand. The automatic recognition of different syringe sizes by the infusion pump is not always reliable especially when differences in diameter are small like in the case of 20 and 30 ml syringes. When the procurement department of a hospital changes syringe supplier, all pumps have to be reprogrammed. It is not unlikely that in such a case not all pumps are updated because infusion pumps may travel a lot between departments.

An even more frequent source of error is when a patient is transferred from one hospital to another where another brand of syringes is used. Not only the syringe may be taken over, occasionally also the infusion device itself with wrong syringe settings is 'assimilated' in the bulk of available infusion devices if the make and type is similar. Usually the medication is checked when a patient enters a hospital. Making a note of the (infusion) devices connected to the patient and the syringes in use should also be a part of the standard check procedure when a patient is transferred, thereby increasing the awareness for problems that may arise from exchanging syringes and equipment.

Differences in syringe brands may not be limited to size. Compliance of syringe and plunger will depend on the manufacturer and also on issues like lubrification of the inside of the syringe plunger to prevent 'sticky' syringe, which will play a role in the performance of syringe-pump combination [8].

Fitting of the Syringe

Because infusion pumps will have to accommodate different syringes with different sizes, the fitting of the flange of the syringe and the plunger is often somewhat loose. This is especially true for pumps that have no automatic syringe loading. An easy way of assessing the amount of fluid involved in the play in the syringe flange fitting is to put the infusion pump in pressure display mode and press some fluid retrogradely into the syringe via a stopcock at the end of the syringe. The amount measured is also dependent on the compliance of the syringe. Deformation of the rubber plunger is for a large part responsible for the initial low stiffness of the syringe, allowing for about 1–2 ml of extra fluid to enter a syringe of 50 ml without substantial increase in pressure. With higher pressures, the syringe may move a little bit if the part where the flange of the syringe is fitted is flexible. Using this simple test, the consequence of air in the syringe can also be demonstrated.

Air in the Syringe

Air in the syringe can have great consequences for the reliability of the infusion and alarm functioning [9]. Air is compressible, as opposed to fluids. This will have an impact when the pressure in the syringe changes due to obstruction or change of height of pump position. Usually occlusion alarms are set around 100 kPa (1 Bar). This is about twice the atmospheric pressure, so according to Boyle's law the volume of the air bubble will be halved at the time the pressure inside the syringe will be at the level that triggers the alarm. For an air bubble of 1 ml, and an infusion rate of 1 ml/h, it will take 30 min before an occlusion is noticed. At 10 ml/h, the delay is still 3 min [Fig. 18.3]. To be added to this is the volume extension that occurs because of the compliance of the whole infusion system and pump which can be in the range of 1–2 ml. It is important always deair a syringe. This has to be done just before connecting the syringe and infusion line to the patient. If there are multiple small air bubbles, the initial visual inspection may not reveal much air but after light tapping these bubbles will merge into one large space of air. Not only for intravenous anaesthetic drugs but for all highly concentrated drugs in syringe-driven infusion pumps, uninterrupted flow is essential.

With some exceptions where the pressure inside the syringe is directly measured in the infusion line, most syringe-driven pumps derive the pressure from the force on the piston or the plunger of the syringe. The relation between this force and the actual pressure inside the syringe is dependent on the size of the surface of the plunger. A 50 ml syringe has a radius of about 30 mm, whereas a 20 ml syringe has a radius of about 20 mm. The surfaces of these plungers are 28.3 cm^2 and 12.5 cm^2 (πr^2), respectively. To obtain the same pressure in the syringes, the force has to be reduced for the 20 ml syringe to 0.44 of the force of the 50 ml syringe. Or in other words, if not adjusted, the level of the pressure alarm would be more than doubled in the 20 ml syringe.

Syringe pumps reduce the force that will activate the high pressure alarm, usually according to this relationship of the plunger areas. The problem is that the force is not only used for building the pressure inside the syringe but also to overcome the resistance of the friction of the plunger inside the syringe. This friction is related the circumference of the plunger which is 9.4 cm and 6.3 cm, respectively ($2\pi r$), and hence the part of the force responsible for overcoming the friction should be only reduced to 0.67 of the value for a 50 ml syringe. As the friction is unknown and cannot be taken into the adjustment, smaller syringes tend to alarm on overpressure much earlier than bigger syringes when the pressure alarm limits are set sensitive and may even tend to give false alarms on line occlusion. This should however

Fig. 18.3 Effect of air in the syringe on delay in activation of occlusion alarm set at 1 bar. Usually at least 1 ml must be added for the compliance in plunger and play of the syringe fitting in the case of a 50 ml syringe

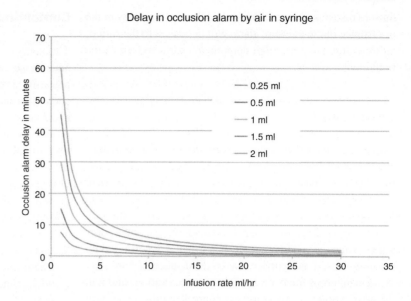

not influence the decision to select the appropriate syringe for clinical circumstances such as paediatric intravenous anaesthesia, as compliance of the smaller syringes is better and amount of undissolved air in the syringe is less.

Positioning of the Pump

It is clear that pressure changes inside the syringe will cause fluctuations in the flow of fluid towards the patient. As explained above, the easy compressibility of the rubber part of the plunger together with residual air is mainly responsible. Pressure changes can result from obstruction of the flow but also may be caused by a change in the height of the infusion pump in respect to the level of the patient [10]. Accurate measurements show that lowering and lifting of the pump even over relative small distances will influence the constant flow rate of the infusion. When the position of the syringe pump is 80 cm below the patient, a pressure of 80 cm H_2O will exist inside the syringe. When the position is changed to 80 cm above the patient, the pressure will change to negative: −80 cm water. It is inevitable that some fluid will spontaneously flow into the patient with an amount that is dependent on all the above-mentioned factors: play in the mechanics of the pump, fitting of the syringe, compliance of syringe and plunger and the existence of air. If the plunger is not retained by the pump, the negative pressure will force the syringe to empty itself. If that happens, then once the initial resistance of the plunger has been overcome, a 50 ml syringe will empty itself in a view minutes. This process is called syphoning or free flow and can be prevented by putting an *anti-syphoning valve* in the infusion line [11]. This valve will only open at a certain overpressure, thereby preventing this free flow. Syphoning is a dangerous situation that can

easily occur in the hectic environment of a surgical procedure or in the emergency room. This can happen if, for example, someone takes the syringe out of an infusion pump and puts it on top of a monitor or if the syringe is not properly placed in the pump because the contents of the syringe are temporarily not required and pump and syringe are put in an elevated position relative to the patient.

When there is a possibility of air entering the syringe, for example, by cracks or a not appropriately closed stopcock, the level of the pump only needs to be a few centimetres above the venous pressure to allow drug to free flow into the patient as no friction of the plunger will play a role in such a situation. Although these possible deleterious situations must have occurred numerous times in emergency rooms, intensive care units, operation theatres and other places in the hospital where patients are transported while being connected to a syringe infusion pumps, very little is known on the real incidence, and reports are incidental [12]. Closing the stopcock when an infusion is temporarily not required should be a habit of all care providers.

The opposite of syphoning is back flow into the syringe. This can happen when the pump is positioned lower than the patient or when more pumps are connected to a manifold. When an infusion line is occluded downstream from connected infusion pumps, then contents from the infusion system with the lowest compliance will flow into the infusion system with the highest compliance until the pressure rise is large enough to trigger the occlusion alarm in one of the connected devices. This can be prevented by one-way valves in the infusion line [13]. One-way valves should definitely be used when a gravity infusion is part of a multi-infusion setup. Not doing so will effectively remove the occlusion alarm from the infusion pumps. If no one-way valves are used in the individual infusion lines, then one must realise that in case of a distal occlusion, the delay in the occurrence of the pressure alarm will be related to the sum of all the volumes of the high compliance parts and air in the individual syringes.

Dead Space

Dead space in infusion systems is by far the most unpredictable cause of flow change when infusion pumps and infusion lines are connected to one single entry point into the patient [14]. Dependent on the bore and length of an infusion line, dead spaces of 5 ml or more can easily be created if extension lines are placed between the point where infusion lines come together and the venous cannula. In particular, when a gravity infusion is used as a carrier, such a dead space of 5 ml may create dangerous fluctuations in drug concentrations and will disturb the objective of a targeted-controlled infusion system when used. Especially in the early phase of an anaesthetic procedure, for most drugs unintentional interruption of drug administration will cause a much faster decrement in blood concentration than when the drug has been administered for hours (context-sensitive decrement time).

Another complicating factor at the start of an anaesthetic procedure is the fact that individual pharmacokinetic and pharmacodynamic properties of the patient are initially unknown while there is a great change required in the patients' conscious and anaesthetic state to cope with another unknown factor: the surgical stimulation of the patient. Based on monitored patient data, the anaesthesiologist will try to get an idea of the sensitivity of the patient for the administered drugs in relation to the applied stimulus. Unnoticed changes in the drug flow caused by dead space and the other above-mentioned phenomena will disturb this feedback process and may lead to over or under drug dosing not only immediately but also later on.

Drug infusion is not only about the physics of flow, compliance and dead space [15]. Pharmacodynamic interactions may exaggerate the influence of the above-mentioned phenomena especially when high drug concentrations are used. Therefore, even intentional changes in drug administration like the change of a target in TCI may lead to unintended changes in the anaesthetic state when these high drug concentrations are used in the presence of dead space [Fig. 18.4].

> **Practical Advice**
> *For intravenous anaesthesia, use dedicated infusion systems with low dead space and one-way valves in each individual line to avoid possible problems with dead space and occlusion alarm delays.*
> *Use the lowest concentrations of IV drugs that are clinically acceptable.*

Contamination

The success and increasing use over time of intravenous anaesthesia and TCI is for a large part attributable to propofol. Propofol has an advantageous pharmacokinetic and pharmacodynamic profile, but it also has its disadvantages. With respect to the equipment and handling, probably the biggest disadvantage is the ease of contamination. For this reason, some manufacturers offer propofol in pre-filled syringes, and/or preservatives have been added. Originally, ethylenediaminetetraacetic acid (EDTA) was used, but other manufacturers used sulphite for marketing reasons. The latter has been withdrawn because of predictable bronchospasm problems that sulphite caused in patients that had a history of heavy smoking [16].

There are a couple of reports on sepsis in patients that could be traced back to handling open vials and reusing syringes of propofol [17]. Even the presence of preservatives will not prevent contamination of the propofol and the growth of bacteria after 6 h. Despite these risks, in many hospitals, the use of pre-filled syringes has been abandoned because of the higher costs involved. Selection of the infusion systems and composition of the connections may seem trivial but can have a major impact on the safety and the post-operative morbidity of the patient. Especially for propofol, unnecessary access points like stopcocks should be avoided as accumulations of propofol in the dead spaces of the infusion line are dangerous sources of contamination and infection [18]. With modern infusion pumps and target-controlled infusion, there is no need to prepare separate syringes for bolus administration when a continuous infusion of propofol for anaesthesia or sedation is planned. When the infusion of propofol is stopped and is not necessary anymore, it is advisable to remove the infusion line completely as small amounts of propofol may stay behind, even in the threads of the Luer-Lock connections between the lines. Another reason to remove the infusion line that is used for propofol is the fact that propofol may cause or aggravate cracks in some plastics used in Luer-Lock connections [19].

> **Practical Advice**
> *Prepare syringes with drugs for intravenous anaesthesia close to the time of administration.*
> *Prepare the syringes under sterile circumstances.*
> *Consider the use of pre-filled syringes when available.*

Target-Controlled Infusion

As explained above, target-controlled infusion and effect target-controlled infusion are dependent on a computational layer on top of the rate-controlling software of the infusion

Fig. 18.4 Effect of dead space and high drug concentration [33]. Propofol (P) TCI 10 mg/ml target 4 µg/ml after 3 h changed to 2 µg/ml. Remifentanil (R) 100 µg/ml fixed rate at 0.25 µg/kg/min. Dead space (DP) volume: 1 ml. No mixing inside DP assumed [14]. A. Mixture of propofol remifentanil runs into the patient—at 180 min P target is changed from 4 µg/ ml to 2 µg/ml: TCI pump stops. B. Flow in DP equals flow R. Existing mixture is pushed out slowly; R and P concentrations drop. Probability of wakening up rises. A small amount of propofol is still delivered. C. Mixture does not contain P anymore. Concentration R rises. D. P reaches new target of 2 µg/ml. TCI pump starts again. No propofol delivered because of DP. R is flushed by P, causing concentration to overshoot. E. DP filled by mixture again. R concentration stabilises to initial concentration

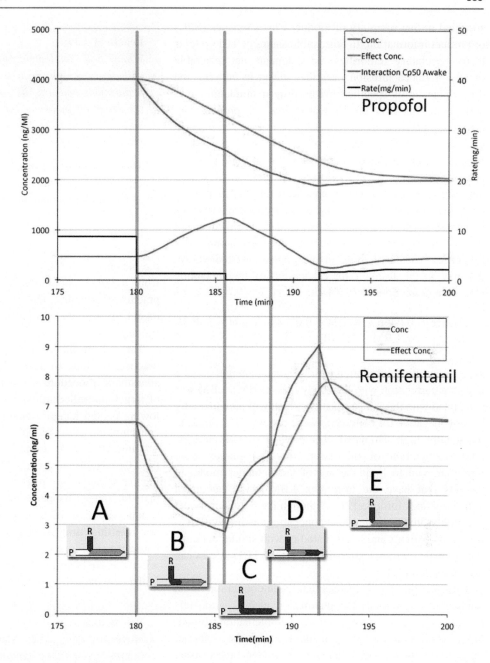

pump. Unintended disturbances in the drug flow to the patient for reasons described above are not incorporated in the pharmacokinetic model as the controlling computer has no knowledge of these disturbances. This will affect the accuracy of the predicted concentrations in blood or at the effect site in a way that is dependent on the pharmacokinetic and pharmacodynamic properties of the drug involved. For example, a delayed occlusion alarm because of air in the syringe may affect the difference between predicted and real drug concentration and clinical effect of a drug like remifentanil more than sufentanil because remifentanil has a larger clearance and a shorter blood-brain equilibration half-life.

There is as yet no standard that specifies clinically acceptable deviations from the ideal infusion profile for the different drugs. To make the issue even more complicated, interactions, often non-linear, between anaesthetic drugs are common. This makes it very difficult to predict what the final effect of these flow influencing factors will be. The worked out example in Fig. 18.4 is context sensitive: the influence of the target change is dependent on the concentration in the different pharmacokinetic compartments and hence the history of the selected targets.

It is usually the responsibility of the drug manufacturer to give dosing guidance in the prescription advice. For some drug-model-device combinations, specific targets have been specified in the Summary of Product Characteristics (SPC) or Product Information. In other submissions of TCI systems to the regulatory authorities, the statement that selectable targets produced infusion rates that stayed in between the dose range limits specified by the drug manufacturer was sufficient. This may be the reason that for propofol six different pharmacokinetic models are implemented in commercially available target-controlled infusion systems: four for adults and two for children. Very few of these pharmacokinetic datasets were developed and tested for use in a target-controlled infusion system. Most published pharmacokinetic data are optimally parameterised to describe the behaviour of the drug in the study population. This does not mean that they are suited for a broader population with properties outside of those of the population studied. An example is the formula for calculation of the metabolic clearance in the Schnider [20] set:

$$\text{Clearance} = 0.0456 \times \text{weight} + 0.0264 \times \text{height} - 0.0681 \times \text{LBM} - 2.2761$$

Note the positive correlation with weight and height and the negative correlation with lean body mass (LBM). LBM was calculated with the James equation which will paradoxly become negative for extremely obese patients. This leads to irrationally high estimated clearances in obese patients. After recognition of this error, the TCI pumps were reprogrammed to limit the use of the Schnider model to patients that have the maximum LBM when calculated with the James formula [21]. Although the Schnider model accurately predicted the blood concentrations in the derivation study patients and in other studies with similar patients, the rationale for its selection in commercial TCI systems can be questioned [22].

A further problem is the fact that the interpretation of the publication containing the pharmacodynamic parameters has lead to two different methods of implementing blood-brain equilibration rate constants, K_{eo}, for the Schnider model. One interpretation is based on a fixed time to peak effect (TTPE) method. As the clearance is highly dependent on the patient's height and weight, it follows that in order to keep the TTPE fixed, the K_{eo} differs between patients. In the other interpretation, the K_{eo} is constant and patient independent. Because of the relatively small central volume and the corresponding small induction dose when used in blood control mode, it has been advised to only use the Schnider model in effect site mode. In effect site mode, the blood-brain equilibration constant becomes a determinant of the induction dose. Therefore, the induction dose will differ between the different brands of pumps even when selecting a pharmacokinetic model with a similar name.

Practical Advice

When first implementing TCI, agree with your colleagues which drug and model to use in your department and ask the pump manufacturer to limit the selection in the TCI system to that specific drug and model.

These examples illustrate the fact that when a drug and a specific model are available in a commercial TCI pump, this does not implicitly mean that the model is suitable for every patient.

Use of computers for controlling infusions offers the potential of automatic selection of the optimal model for the patient. With the development of new models derived from a larger population and appropriately evaluated in practice, this undesirable necessity of selecting the correct model for drug and patient will hopefully disappear in the future.

Target-controlled infusion has its own pitfalls in clinical practice. Failure to reset the pump at the end of an anaesthetic procedure sometimes happens if the principle of target-controlled infusion is not understood and the following patient has the same proportions and the displayed concentration in the blood is close to zero.

Quite often in departments where TCI is frequently used, the TCI systems are prepared by anaesthetic nurses. Assuming that someone else reset the TCI system without verifying that this indeed happened is a mistake easily made in the frantic situation of a patient change. Because of this non-resetting, drug is assumed to be still in the peripheral compartments. Infusion rates calculated to obtain set targets will therefore be lower than required leading to underdosing in the new patient.

Practical Advice

Make sure that a TCI system has been switched off in between patients by making this part of the standard device check.

The opposite will be the case when a TCI system shuts down or when anaesthesia has to be restarted after the TCI system has been switched off during a case. Generally the best advice is to continue the anaesthetic with a manually controlled infusion (in ml/h or mg/kg/h) at roughly the same rate as that present when the pump shut down. If you do want to continue to use TCI a couple of minutes after it has been switched of, and all the previous infusion administration history has been erased, then one solution is to restart the pump and infusion at the same target, but with an empty syringe, not connected to the patient. Once the pump display estimates that the set target has been reached, replace that syringe with a drug containing one and connect it to the patient. This will avoid the administration of an extra loading bolus dose. It should be remembered that dependent on the drug pharmacokinetics and infusion history, the infusion rates will be somewhat higher than necessary; therefore, the attained blood concentrations will initially be higher than calculated too but will slowly converge to the concentration present before shutdown of the pump.

TCI and the Heart Lung Machine

When initiating the cardiopulmonary bypass, there is a dilution of the circulating volume with the priming volume of the heart lung machine. Techniques like pre-donation may alter this volume. One would expect that this dilution would lower the concentration of anaesthetic drugs and hence influence the level of anaesthesia and analgesia. Although this is indeed the case when measuring total blood concentration, in practice, an adaptation of the target concentration is seldom required when the decision to change targets is based on depth of anaesthesia monitoring and other clinical parameters. For propofol the explanation for this discrepancy between theory and practice is found in the fact that although the total concentration may be reduced, the unbound free fraction of the drug is unaffected [23]. It is the free fraction that is capable of acting on the receptors. After the initial loss of drug by the dilution, drug will be redistributed from peripheral compartments back to the central compartment. Remember that the compartments in the pharmacokinetic model are purely mathematical and not physiological compartments, but a lipophilic drug will have a large third compartment, and in the case of propofol, this is more than 200 l. It is clinical experience that, once the appropriate individual target has been determined and maintained, very few changes are required even in extreme haemodynamically challenging procedures like left-left perfusion as used in thoraco-abdominal aneurysm surgery.

> **Practical Advice**
> *Expected hemodynamic and circulatory disturbances are not a contraindication for the use of intravenous anaesthesia and target-controlled infusion.*

While the above-mentioned circulatory disturbances usually do not require large changes in the targets in TCI or infusion rates in TIVA applications, the temperature of the patient may be of greater influence. The temperature usually affects pharmacokinetics of the drug by lowering the

clearance which in time will cause an increase in the concentration. The protein binding will also be affected, causing an increase of the free fraction. The influence on pharmacodynamic properties of the drug is even more complex: the receptor affinity may be lowered, but temperature also has its own physiologic effect on pain perception and consciousness. The net effect in a real clinical situation is therefore difficult to predict, and titration of drug dosing should be based on the usual clinical observations and guided by publications that have studied this effect in a clinical setting [24].

Paediatric IV Anaesthesia

Traditionally paediatric anaesthesia was performed using inhalational agents. There are no calculations required to operate a vaporiser, and this made this type of anaesthesia the easiest to perform for the anaesthesiologist. Properties and advantages of intravenous agents and the possibility to deliver sedation and anaesthesia anywhere in the hospital have caused a shift towards intravenous anaesthesia. The availability of new pharmacokinetic models and increasing knowledge on how to 'size' paediatric patients [25] has supported this shift. What is true for adult intravenous anaesthesia in terms of flow accuracy influencing factors is *a fortiori* applicable to paediatric anaesthesia. Smaller syringes have a larger plunger displacement at equal flow rates and therefore have shorter startup delays than larger syringes, especially at low infusion rates. Also the time before an alarm may indicate an occlusion is much shorter [26]. For patients weighing less than 10 kg, it is therefore advisable to use smaller syringes (e.g. 20 ml) with Luer Locks to allow the highest precision in pump performance. Even a normal stopcock can cause unacceptable delays in required drug effect. Diluting the drug to increase the flow rate is often not possible for the very young patients because of the possibility of fluid overload. Special multi-lumen infusion sets with small bores and low dead space are highly recommended for use in paediatric anaesthesia.

For intravenous anaesthesia with propofol for paediatric patients, two models are available in commercial TCI pumps—the Peadfusor [27] model and the Kataria [28] model. As with the Schnider model, the Kataria model will produce erroneous values when used outside the properties of the original patient population: the volume of the second (redistribution) compartment becomes negative for a child of 2 years below 12.75 kg. The Paedfusor model is the only model that has been prospectively tested with TCI in a paediatric patient population.

The possibility of entering the patient demographic data on pump start up does not guarantee that the model is suitable for the patient. For example, using adult pharmacokinetic models, the smallest and youngest patient that can be entered in the Arcomed pump is 50 cm tall, 12 years old and weighs 10 kg. Selecting these parameters for remifentanil with the Minto model will produce a pharmacokinetic model with a clearance that is in absolute values similar to the clearance from an adult patient with a weight of 60 kg, height 160 cm and an age of 60 years. Because of the large clearance and the limited influence of the distribution in the pharmacokinetic model for remifentanil, after a short while, about 15 min, both patients will get the same amount of drug for a specific target concentration. For example, for a target of 4 ng/ml, the adult patient will receive 0.145 µg/kg/min. For the same target, the patient for which the above-mentioned limits of the pump settings are used will receive 0.86 µg/kg/min which is about six times more when dose is scaled to weight and about four times more than when allometric scaling [29] is used.

The availability of dedicated paediatric models for propofol and lack of knowledge on the parameters of the remifentanil pharmacokinetic model may beguile the anaesthesiologist to accept the above irrational values when he is trying to use the TCI system for a child. Limits on patient data are different between the different brands of pumps. Different limits on the patient population between pumps may confuse the user. Some pumps limit the patient demographics universally for all models with the exception of the models where the lean body mass calculation with the James equation becomes erroneous. Others adjust limits to specific models, but without scientific support for some populations. For example, with the Alaris PK, it is possible to use the Gepts sufentanil model that does not incorporate patient parameters, not even the weight, down to a patient weight of 1 kg. Although the lower age limit is 12 years, the anaesthesiologist may know that just like in some other models, the age is not a parameter in the model, and if he assumes that the model is scaled to weight, he may be tempted to use the TCI system with sufentanil for a neonate. By doing so, he will overdose his patient massively because this neonate of 1 kg will get a dose that is suited for an adult! Even when the Gepts model is scaled to weight so that the neonate of 1 kg would continuously receive 1/70th of the dose of a patient of 70 kg, there would be overdosing because of the much lower clearance of sufentanil in a neonate [30]. This is the result of immaturity of the metabolisation capacity of the liver which will be the case up to 3 or 4 months of age.

But even if the anaesthesiologists limit the use of TCI sufentanil to patients above 12 years, then it is still unlikely that a patient of 12 years with a normal weight of 40 kg will have similar blood concentrations as a patient of 40 years with a weight of 100 kg when given the same non-weight-adjusted dose. None of the current target-controlled infusion pumps have algorithms that prevent obvious erroneous data entries like a height of 200 cm with a weight of 10 kg.

> **Practical Advice**
> *Do not assume that when the pump accepts the patient data, the selected model is appropriate for your patient. Knowledge on the parameters that are incorporated in the model is indispensable.*

Time to Awakening

All commercial TCI systems display a 'decrement time', which is the time it will take for the blood concentration to a prespecified lower concentration, if the infusion is switched off. Often this time is called the 'time to awakening'. This feature of the TCI systems should be looked at with caution. Obviously the moment a patient will wake up is not only dependent on the concentration of the hypnotic but also on the stimulus and the presence of stimulus-suppressing agents like opioids and other analgesics. Displaying a time to awakening in case of an opioid, like some TCI systems do, makes no sense.

One of the problems with calculating the time to reach a lower concentration is that the error in this estimation is highly non-linear. When there is a small difference between the estimated pharmacokinetic model and the 'real' patient model, then the error will be small in the fast decay phase of the drug. When the decay curve starts deflecting and approaches the x-axis, asymptotically the prediction error of the wakening time will increase dramatically [Fig. 18.5].

Although the wakening concentration may vary widely in a patient population, there is some evidence that there is a correlation between the concentration at loss of consciousness and regaining consciousness even in the individual patient. But this is highly dependent on the technique of induction: with or without analgesics and premedication and depending on which model was used. The best correlation has been found in the Marsh model when used in blood control mode [31].

> **Practical Advice**
> *The clinical value of 'time to awakening' or 'time to concentration' is dependent on many factors and should be judged in the context of these factors.*

Training and Education

Emphasis on patient safety has increasingly caused hospitals and departments to focus attention on training in handling complex devices such as ventilators, ultrasound machines, etc. In some hospitals, the confirmation of the existence of this knowledge is part of the check procedure before each case in theatre. Infusion devices and the operation of infusion systems however are not often considered as 'new' and

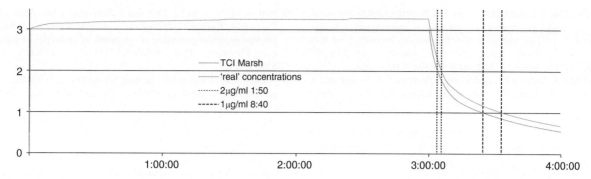

Fig. 18.5 Non-linear increase in error of 'time to concentration'. Pharmacokinetics used for 'real' concentration differ from the Marsh kinetics by a decrease of 10 % in the central clearance. This will increase the concentration after 3 h on a target from 3 to 3.25 µg/ml. When the infusion is switched off, the concentration is decreased to 2 µg/ml in 3:40 and 5:30, respectively, a difference of 1:50. For a decrease to 1 µg/ml, these times are 24:40 and 33:20, a difference of 8:40

therefore are quite often not well explained and trained. Consequences of irregularities in the administration of highly potent and fast-acting drugs caused by flushes and dead space can be seen every day in high- and low-tech departments in the hospital but often stay unnoticed. It is, for example, quite common to disconnect the gravity infusion for transport or delay replacement of an empty infusion bag, while this infusion may function as a carrier for a patient-controlled analgesia (PCA) system.

Several parts in the training of intravenous anaesthesia can be identified and separated. The handling and training of the control of the infusion devices and information on the device can, for example, be done by instructors of the company that produces the device. Training on local implementation of protocols for handling drugs and infusion systems could be done by trainers from the department or from the pharmacology department. Finally training on the use of intravenous anaesthesia, which involves target-controlled infusion, should be performed by specialist trainers. This should involve a course on basic pharmacology and how the concepts are implemented in the smart infusion pumps. Unfortunately a survey in the UK revealed that even in departments where target-controlled infusion was used on a regular base, the knowledge of the users of these systems was limited [32]. This is not only caused by a lack in education: the understanding and use of target-controlled infusion systems have been made unnecessarily complex by implementing different models and different implementations of these models. In the ideal system, only drug and patient parameters should be the required entries so that for employing TCI, mainly knowledge on the appropriate target is needed.

References

1. Peterfreund RA, Philip JH (2013) Critical parameters in drug delivery by intravenous infusion. Exp Opin Drug Deliv. 10 (8):1095–108. doi:10.1517/17425247.2013.785519.

2. Struys MMRF, De-Smet T, Glen JIB, Vereecke HEM, Absalom AR, Schnider TW. The history of target-controlled infusion. Anesth Analg. 2016;122(1):56–69. doi:10.1213/ANE.0000000000001008.

3. Schraag S, Flaschar J. Delivery performance of commercial target-controlled infusion devices with diprifusor module. Eur J Anaesthesiol. 2002;19(5):357–60. doi:10.1017/S0265021502000571.

4. Sarraf E, Mandel JE. Time-delay when updating infusion rates in the Graseby 3400 pump results in reduced drug delivery. Anesth Analg. 2014;118(1):145–50. doi:10.1213/01.ane.0000438349.21617.2f.

5. Engbers FHM. Total intravenous anaesthesia: the equipment. In: Vuyk J, Mulder S, Engbers F, editors. On the study and practice of intravenous anaesthesia. Dordrecht: Kluwer Academic Publishers; 2000. p. 71–81.

6. Chiou WL. Potential pitfalls in the conventional pharmacokinetic studies: effects of the initial mixing of drug in blood and the pulmonary first-pass elimination. J Pharmacokinet Biopharm. 1979;7:527–36.

7. Glen JIB, Engbers FHM. The influence of target concentration, equilibration rate constant (ke0) and pharmacokinetic model on the initial propofol dose delivered in effect-site target-controlled infusion. Anaesthesia. 2016;71(3):306–14. doi:10.1111/anae.13345.

8. Chan E, Hubbard A, Sane S, Maa Y-F. Syringe siliconization process investigation and optimization. J Pharm Sci Technol. 2012;66(2):136–50. doi:10.5731/pdajpst.2012.00856.

9. Schulz G, Fischer J, Neff T, Bänziger O, Weiss M. The effect of air within the infusion syringe on drug delivery of syringe pump infusion systems. Anaesthesist. 2000;49(12):1018–23.

10. Kern H, Kuring A, Redlich U, Döpfmer UR, Sims NM, Spies CD, Kox WJ. Downward movement of syringe pumps reduces syringe output. Br J Anaesth. 2001;86(6):828–31.

11. McCarroll C, McAtamney D, Taylor R. Alteration in flow delivery with antisyphon devices. Anaesthesia. 2000;55(4):355–7.

12. Sundaram R, Dell AE. Interaction between infusion equipment resulting in drug overdose in a critically ill patient. Anaesthesia. 2005;60(1):88–91. doi:10.1111/j.1365-2044.2004.04012.x.

13. Lannoy D, Décaudin B, Dewulf S, Simon N, Secq A, Barthélémy C, et al. Infusion set characteristics such as antireflux valve and dead-space volume affect drug delivery: an experimental study designed to enhance infusion sets. Anesth Analg. 2010;111(6):1427–31. doi:10.1213/ANE.0b013e3181f66ee3.

14. Lovich MA, Doles J, Peterfreund RA. The impact of carrier flow rate and infusion set dead-volume on the dynamics of intravenous drug delivery. Anesth Analg. 2005;100(4):1048–55. doi:10.1213/01.ANE.0000146942.51020.88.

15. Lovich MA, Kinnealley ME, Sims NM, Peterfreund RA. The delivery of drugs to patients by continuous intravenous infusion: modeling predicts potential dose fluctuations depending on flow rates and infusion system dead volume. Anesth Analg. 2006;102 (4):1147–53. doi:10.1213/01.ane.0000198670.02481.6b.

16. Rieschke P, LaFleur BJ, Janicki PK. Effects of EDTA- and sulfite-containing formulations of propofol on respiratory system resistance after tracheal intubation in smokers. Anesthesiology. 2003;98 (2):323–8.

17. Muller AE, Huisman I, Roos PJ, Rietveld AP, Klein J, Harbers JBM, Dorresteijn JJ, van Steenbergen JE, Vos MC. Outbreak of severe sepsis due to contaminated propofol: lessons to learn. J Hosp Infect. 2010;76(3):225–30.

18. Cole DC, Baslanti TO, Gravenstein NL, Gravenstein N. Leaving more than your fingerprint on the intravenous line: a prospective study on propofol anesthesia and implications of stopcock contamination. Anesth Analg. 2015;120(4):861–7. doi:10.1213/ANE. 0b013e318292ed45.

19. Nakao M, Yamanaka S, Iwata M, Nakashima M, Onji I. [The cracks of polycarbonate three-way stopcocks are enhanced by the lubricating action of fat emulsion of propofol]. Masui. 2003;52 (11):1243–7.

20. Schnider TW, Minto CF, Shafer SL, Gambus PL, Andresen C, Goodale DB, Youngs EJ. The influence of age on propofol pharmacodynamics. Anesthesiology. 1999;90(6):1502–16.

21. Absalom AR, Mani V, De Smet T, Struys MMRF. Pharmacokinetic models for propofol--defining and illuminating the devil in the detail. Br J Anaesth. 2009;103(1):26–37. doi:10.1093/bja/aep143.

22. Engbers FH, Sutcliffe N, Kenny G, Schraag S. Pharmacokinetic models for propofol: defining and illuminating the devil in the detail. Br J Anaesth. 2010;104(2):261–2, author reply 262–4. doi:10.1093/bja/aep385.

23. Dawson PJ, Bjorksten AR, Blake DW, Goldblatt JC. The effects of cardiopulmonary bypass on total and unbound plasma concentrations of propofol and midazolam. Yjcan. 1997;11 (5):556–61. doi:10.1016/S1053-0770(97)90003-3.

24. Peeters MYM, Bras LJ, DeJongh J, Wesselink RMJ, Aarts LPHJ, Danhof M, Knibbe CAJ. Disease severity is a major determinant for the pharmacodynamics of propofol in critically ill patients. Clin Pharmacol Ther. 2008;83(3):443–51. doi:10.1038/sj.clpt. 6100309.

25. Anderson BJ, Meakin GH. Scaling for size: some implications for paediatric anaesthesia dosing. Paediatr Anaesth. 2002;12 (3):205–19.

26. Donmez A, Araz C, Kayhan Z. Syringe pumps take too long to give occlusion alarm. Pediatr Anesth. 2005;15(4):293–6. doi:10.1111/ pan.2005.15.issue-4.

27. Absalom A. Accuracy of the "Paedfusor" in children undergoing cardiac surgery or catheterization. Br J Anaesth. 2003;91 (4):507–13. doi:10.1093/bja/aeg220.

28. Kataria BK, Ved SA, Nicodemus HF, Hoy GR, Lea D, Dubois MY, et al. The pharmacokinetics of propofol in children using three different data analysis approaches. Anesthesiology. 1994;80 (1):104–22.

29. Knibbe CAJ, Zuideveld KP, Aarts LPHJ, Kuks PFM, Danhof M. Allometric relationships between the pharmacokinetics of propofol in rats, children and adults. Br J Clin Pharmacol. 2005;59(6):705–11. doi:10.1111/j.1365-2125.2005.02239.x.

30. Greeley WJ, de Bruijn NP, Davis DP. Sufentanil pharmacokinetics in pediatric cardiovascular patients. Anesth Analg. 1987;66 (11):1067–72.

31. Iwakiri H, Nishihara N, Nagata O, Matsukawa T, Ozaki M, Sessler DI. Individual effect-site concentrations of propofol are similar at loss of consciousness and at awakening. Anesth Analg. 2005;100(1):107–10. doi:10.1213/01.ANE.0000139358. 15909.EA.

32. McGlone and Peck. Bulletin RCoA 91, 2015. p. 47–9. https://www. rcoa.ac.uk/system/files/CSQ-Bulletin91_1.pdf. Accessed 11 Mar 2016.

33. Barvais L, Lobo FA, Engbers FHM, Irwin MG, Schnider TW, Schraag S. Tips and tricks to optimize total intravenous anesthesia. Acta Anaesthesiol Belg. 2013;64(4):137–46.

EEG Monitoring of Depth of Anesthesia

19

Michael R.J. Sury

Learning Points

- During anaesthesia the spinal cord is more important than the cortex in the control of movement.
- Depth monitoring is not necessary or practical in patients who are sedated and able to move.
- EEG depth monitoring is not useful for rapid changes in consciousness: propofol sedation is likely to be in this category.
- In the sedated patient observation alone is likely to be better than relying on an EEG.
- If anaesthesia depth changes slowly, perhaps the EEG could be useful.
- Neuromuscular blocking drugs make the patient vulnerable to accidental awareness during general anaesthesia (AAGA).
- Depth monitoring is indicated for patients given NMBs.
- EEG effects of anaesthesia are broadly similar and are not difficult to understand.
- Changes in processed EEG are related to depth and dose.
- Raw EEG has utility because of its speed of response.
- EEG depth monitoring, alone, is unreliable, but may have utility in the prevention of AAGA if conventional propofol doses are used and analgesia is used to counter autonomic signs of pain.

Overview This chapter explores the potential of how EEG monitoring can assess depth of anaesthesia (DoA) in patients receiving TIVA. It has four sections:

- Theoretical constructs
  - Discussing the problem of uncertainty about the relationship between dose and depth of anaesthesia
  - Examining concepts that help to explain when monitors are, and are not, of value
- Essential EEG knowledge
  - Summarising the theory and in practice of EEG monitoring describes the problems of research
- Evidence for and against using EEG DoA monitoring
  - A selective review of the evidence for and against EEG monitoring during propofol sedation and anaesthesia
- Potential for clinical utility
  - Discussing how EEG monitoring could be useful to prevent AAGA and excessive depth

Introduction

The anaesthetist has two priorities: controlling consciousness and ensuring survival. The first demonstration of ether anaesthesia[1] made history in 1846, because ether kept the patient both insensible and alive. Likewise, modern anaesthesia is accepted because patients are highly likely to both remain unconscious and survive. These favourable outcomes are related to anaesthetic dose, and there is confidence about the effective and safe dose range largely through the experience from large numbers of patients. We are also reassured by the knowledge that the effective dose can be exceeded, up to a point, without harming the patient. Obviously, vital physiological functions may need to be supported, and for the sake of simplicity in this discussion, it is assumed that anaesthesia does not have delayed or long-lasting toxic effects. In essence therefore we can, within wide yet reasonable limits, expose patients to excessive doses and expect the vast majority to be unharmed.

[1] Anaesthesia, general anaesthesia or GA.

M.R.J. Sury, FRCA, PhD (✉)
Department of Anaesthesia, Great Ormond Street Hospital for Children NHS Foundation Trust, London, UK

Portex Department of Anaesthesia, Great Ormond Street Hospital Insitute of Child Health, University College London, Great Ormond Street, London WC1N 3JH, UK
e-mail: mike.sury@gosh.nhs.uk

© Springer International Publishing AG 2017
A.R. Absalom, K.P. Mason (eds.), *Total Intravenous Anesthesia and Target Controlled Infusions*,
DOI 10.1007/978-3-319-47609-4_19

341

Table 19.1 Summary of findings of NAP5

Reports	Reports of AAGA had to be of procedures in which the patient expected to be unconscious	First reports (irrespective of when the AAGA occurred) collected over 12 months	Reports gathered by local coordinators across the whole of the UK (NHS only) and Republic of Ireland (all hospitals)
Type of report	300 reports	• 141 certain/probable • 17 awake paralysis due to drug error • 7 ICU • 32 after sedation	*The 141 certain/probable and possible reports were the basis of in-depth analysis (the following summary applies to these)*
Incidence	Estimated incidence of reports of AAGA was ~1:19,000	Incidence varied considerably in different settings	• 1:8000 with NMB • 1:136,000 without
Psychological experiences	Wide range, most reports lasting <5 min	Distress particularly likely when patients experienced paralysis	Longer-term psychological effects identified in approximately 50 %
Risk factors: four categories were identified	1/ Drug factors: neuromuscular blockade, thiopental, TIVA	2/ Patient factors: female gender, age (younger adults but not children); obesity; previous AAGA and possibly difficult airway management	3/ Subspecialties: obstetric, cardiac, thoracic, neurosurgical 4/ Organisational factors: emergencies, out of hours operating, junior anaesthetists
TIVA	AAGA approximately twice as likely during TIVA as during volatile anaesthesia	However, many AAGA cases during TIVA involved use of non-TCI techniques: inadequate dosing using non-TCI regimens was common	High-risk situations were conversion of a volatile anaesthetic to TIVA and transfer of paralysed patients outside theatres
NMB	*93 % of reports to NAP5 concerned patients who had received an NMB*		
Depth of anaesthesia monitoring	Specific monitors are rarely used during general anaesthesia in UK practice—processed EEG in 2.8 % of general anaesthetics	*The overall findings are supportive of the use of depth monitors during TIVA with NMB*	End-tidal anaesthetic gas monitoring is an alternative to depth monitoring, but in ~75 % of reports to NAP5, it would likely have been impractical or ineffective at preventing AAGA

Summary of main findings of the Fifth National Audit Project of The Royal College of Anaesthetists and the Association of Anaesthetists of Great Britain and Ireland: Accidental Awareness during General Anaesthesia (AAGA) in the UK and Ireland [2, 3]

If we accept that this is the common situation, the precise dose is much less important than supporting vital functions, and therefore the anaesthetist will give most of their attention to monitoring and managing the airway, breathing and circulation. Capnography and pulse oximetry are the most useful and reliable monitors, and blood pressure, ECG and gas analysis monitors are also crucial. If the patient is stable, there may be time to consider other monitors, but there is a limit to the number of monitors that can be assessed simultaneously. If there is blood loss for example, the anaesthetist may not be able to take account of more than three or four monitors at a time. The anaesthetist has to prioritise his or her tasks, and this includes the observation and interpretation of the information presented by the monitoring. How should, therefore, depth of anaesthesia (DoA) monitors relying on electroencephalography (EEG) be prioritised. How useful are they?

The Problem

Current Opinion and Practice

Accidental awareness during general anaesthesia (AAGA) can be a very distressing experience. A large survey of spontaneous reporting of AAGA was undertaken in the UK by the NAP5 project [1, 2], and its main findings are summarised in Table 19.1. It showed that the incidence of AAGA depends on the procedure and that overall the incidence of spontaneous reports of AAGA was 1:19,000 [2]. Such a low incidence is surprising but was related to the method of enquiry. If patients are asked direct questions after they have recovered, the incidence is much higher, and if the dose of anaesthetic has to be restricted, the incidence may be as high as 1 in 100 cases [4].

A survey of anaesthesia activity in the UK in 2013 estimated that there were approximately 2.8 million GAs that year and that only 2.8 % had depth of anaesthesia (depth) monitoring [5]. There are several likely reasons to explain this low percentage. First, there are practical difficulties. During surgery, the scalp is often inaccessible and the sensors readily detect electrical interference especially from diathermy. The EEG itself is a random waveform which changes rapidly. Its interpretation is complicated and depends on the circumstances of the patient. In an attempt to simplify the situation, monitors have been developed that process the EEG (pEEG) and present to the anaesthetist a score related to central nervous system (CNS) suppression (usually a score from 100 to 0). The score however is derived from a complex algorithm, and the ordinary anaesthetist will not understand the process within the monitor and may treat the score with suspicion. The process calculating the score requires a length of EEG and therefore takes time. A delay, perhaps of 15 or 30 s, may be considered to be unacceptable in some circumstances. Finally there is an easier alternative to pEEG monitoring. In contrast to pEEG, the inspired anaesthetic vapour concentration monitoring is reliable and practical in all patients having an inhalational anaesthetic via a tracheal tube or supraglottic airway device.

Immobility

There has also been a misunderstanding of what the EEG monitor can achieve. It was a common assumption that a patient who moved was awake, and therefore a monitor was wanted that would warn of movement. We now appreciate that all pEEG monitors will fail to reliably predict movement because movement during anaesthesia is controlled primarily through the spinal cord. In rodents the dose required to immobilise decorticate animals is same as that for intact animals [6]. In goats, the cerebral and spinal cord circulations can be isolated, and by adjusting anaesthesia levels separately in the brain and spinal cord, it has been demonstrated that almost always immobility is related to spinal cord effect [7]. In humans halothane suppresses movement at lower BIS values than sevoflurane which could mean that the EEG effects of the agents are different or that halothane suppresses the spinal cord more than sevoflurane [8]. These studies support the idea that in respect of the relationship of dose of anaesthetic to movement, the spinal cord is more important than the cortex (which is where consciousness is assumed to lie). EEG monitors, therefore, cannot measure the effect of anaesthesia in respect of the likelihood of movement. The anaesthetist, on the other hand, may wish to deliver anaesthesia to the endpoint of immobility, and for this task, EEG monitors are not useful.

The dose that causes immobility however may be so high that it is close to the dose that could cause cardiovascular depression in vulnerable patients. Consequently, neuromuscular blocking drugs (NMBs) may be indicated but such a step makes the patient vulnerable to AAGA. Inhalational anaesthesia can be monitored by gas analysis, but total intravenous anaesthesia (TIVA) cannot as yet be monitored continuously. It is the scenario of TIVA therefore, in the presence of NMBs, that a depth monitor may be most useful. In the UK in 2013, 23 % of patients managed with TIVA and NMBs had depth monitoring [5].

AAGA: Unmet Need

EEG depth monitors have been available widely for two decades. Electrode placement and cabling have been simplified and are less impractical than before. In a survey of opinions Myles et al. [9] found that anaesthetists were prepared to use depth monitoring if there was evidence that it prevented AAGA. To date the evidence is not clear enough to be certain, but as the technology improves, the potential for utility may increase.

In the UK NAP5 study [2], the likely causes of AAGA were examined in a large group of patients reporting AAGA in 2013 (see Table 19.1). Of the 300 patients with reliable reports, 28 were managed with TIVA (and NMB). This was a surprisingly large group, but the main problem with TIVA was that the propofol doses were clearly too low. Four groups could be identified:

- Sick patients in whom the dose has been reduced to prevent cardiovascular depression
- Transfer of patients to from resuscitation or surgery to intensive care
- Poor dosing—failure of technique
- Infusion errors (disconnection, extravasation, syringe driver failure)

In 7 % of reports (all techniques including TIVA and inhalational techniques), the reason for AAGA was not determined inferring that the doses used were within accepted practice and yet were inadequate.

The clinician needs a monitor to warn of both inadequate and excessive depths of anaesthesia. The following discusses the uncertainty of propofol anaesthesia and prepares the way for understanding the need for more routine use of depth monitoring.

Uncertainty About Propofol Dose and Effect

Pharmacodynamics

It is generally accepted that anaesthetic effect is related, at least in part, to the concentration of drug at ligand-gated receptors at the target site. The main target receptors are GABA-A which are rapidly acting membrane ion channels that inhibit action potentials. However, other receptor types may also be involved, and there are intracellular mechanisms that regulate and modify the number and effect of the activated receptors. The true relationship between receptor site drug concentration and drug effect therefore is variable both between and within individuals.

The target receptors are in the CNS not the blood. The relationship between blood and target propofol concentration is unknown but is inferred by the EEG. The assumption is that the EEG effect is related to blood level because it is assumed that target concentration will match the blood level, albeit after a short delay. This is the principle of effect-site concentration.

Pharmacokinetics

Blood levels of propofol cannot be measured continuously. Rapid near patient blood testing is possible but not widely available yet [10, 11]. Expired gas monitoring can detect propofol but is not yet accurate enough for clinical use [12, 13]. Tracking blood levels frequently over time, therefore, has been achieved only from a limited number of patients. The majority of pharmacokinetic data have been derived from much larger samples of patients in whom only a few blood levels have been obtained [14], and in these studies the relationship of dose to blood level, even with target controlled infusions, varies widely [15].

Cardiovascular Depression

Propofol reduces both cardiac contractility and peripheral vascular resistance [16]. Consequently, the dose has to be reduced in patients with cardiovascular disease or instability, but by how much it should be reduced is uncertain. Neuromuscular blocker drugs (NMBs) and potent opioids remove the possibility of movement and modify the autonomic reaction to pain so that patients who cannot move may not change their heart rate and blood pressure appreciably to alert the anaesthetist of AAGA [2].

Mortality

Sick and elderly patients are vulnerable to cause cardiovascular depression. One hopes that serious problems are rare. In the common situation however, the certainty of propofol dose and effect can also be challenged. A worrying association has been found between mortality and three coincident features of anaesthesia: EEG suppression, low blood pressure and low doses of anaesthesia (so-called triple low) [17, 18]. In sedated patients in intensive care, burst suppression is associated with high mortality. Such concepts are concerning and make EEG monitoring desirable.

In summary, the dose of propofol that achieves anaesthesia in sick patients managed with NMBs is uncertain. Measuring blood levels would help but there would still be a degree of uncertainty. Depth monitors may help these patients, and their use is increasing.

The remainder of this chapter explores the potential of how EEG monitoring can assess depth in TIVA patients. It has four sections:

- Concepts
- Essential EEG knowledge for the clinician
- Evidence for and against EEG DoA monitoring
- Future directions and the potential for clinical utility

Concepts

What Is Depth of Anaesthesia?

The concept of depth has not always been accepted. It can be said that a patient is either anaesthetised or not and that depth is therefore a false construct [19]. Whereas this statement is reasonable from the patient's perspective in terms of their consciousness, there are additional neurological effects that take place beyond the point of loss of consciousness, and these effects constitute a progressive suppression of the CNS. The stages of ether anaesthesia originally described by Guedel in 1937 show that increasing the dose of anaesthesia progressively suppresses important neurological reflexes and functions [20]. For example, the dose causing suppression of the response to pain is less than that which causes apnoea. A more recent example is the demonstration that after consciousness has been lost, increasing the blood propofol concentration, tracked by processed electroencephalography (pEEG), can prevent a response to defined painful stimuli of increasing severity [21] (Table 19.2). In a recent editorial Pandit [23] described anaesthesia as being "a spectrum of brain states" because not all parts of the brain, and its associated functions, are suppressed similarly and this will lead to variation in the characteristics of CNS suppression at various doses.

Table 19.2 Clinical markers of depth of anaesthesia

Score	Description	Level of sedation or anaesthesia
5	Responds readily to name spoken	Minimal
4	Lethargic response to name spoken	Moderate
3	Responds after name called loudly/repeatedly	Moderate
2	Purposeful response to mild-to-moderate shaking	Moderate
1	Responds to trapezius squeeze	Deep
0_T	No response to trapezius squeeze[a]	Light general anaesthesia
0_E	No response to electrical stimulation[b]	Deeper general anaesthesia

The Extended Observer's Assessment of Alertness and Sedation (EOAA/S) score, which is a modification of the OAAS (originally described by Chernik et al. [22]) and modified by Kim et al. [21]
[a]10 pounds per square inch ($\sim$0.7 kg cm^{-2}) for 5 s
[b]50 mA tetanus for 5 s

In principle, increasing the dose of an anaesthetic beyond that needed to cause unconsciousness has two related effects.

1. It increases brain suppression. There are, however, a few minor exceptions: ether anaesthetics have an excitement phase (notorious with diethyl ether, but only at induction and at low doses), benzodiazepines can cause clinical paradoxical excitement during sedation, and nitrous oxide and ketamine cause paradoxical EEG excitement.
2. It reduces the likelihood of AAGA. There are no known analeptic effects of anaesthesia, and it may be assumed that increasing the dose will reduce the chance of any reaction to an arousing stimulus.

If these two statements are accepted, anaesthesia depth is related to dose. Yet how certain is this principle?

Is Depth Related to Anaesthesia Blood Level?

Before an operation begins, the patient is given an effective blood level and appears adequately anaesthetised. When the operation begins, the patient often reacts by moving or having a tachycardia (or other autonomic responses). The blood level of anaesthetic has to be increased to stop the patient reacting. The certainty of effect is therefore only temporary, and anaesthesia depth varies even when the blood level of anaesthetic remains constant. Blood levels will need to be increased, or decreased, appropriately to match the stimuli. Whereas it is true that increasing the blood level increases the depth, we cannot be certain about the depth at a specified blood level. It is helpful to know the blood level, but information about the effect on the target organ may be useful.

How Can Consciousness and Depth Be Described?

Consciousness and anaesthesia, two commonly used terms, are both difficult to describe, and their measurement is elusive. However descriptions or definitions of various levels of consciousness are generally accepted [24]. The levels of sedation (minimal, moderate and deep) leading to anaesthesia have been defined within a so-called continuum of level of consciousness [24]. The continuum infers that the boundaries between the levels are blurred. In principle the levels are useful but in practice the patient can move from one level to the next quickly and subtle changes are difficult to chart accurately. The levels of sedation have been used to create a widely used scale of sedation known as the Observer's Assessment of Alertness and Sedation (OAA/S) scale: a scale ranging from 5 (full consciousness) down to 0 (unconscious, or anaesthesia, as defined by no response to painful stimulus) [22].

There are few descriptors of depth of unconsciousness. The Extended Observer's Assessment of Alertness and Sedation (EOAA/S) score has recently been proposed (see Table 19.2) by Kim et al. [21]. It uses two painful stimuli, one more intense than the other and depth of unconsciousness is described by the lack of response to these.

Diagrammatic Representation of Consciousness and Depth

Increasing CNS suppression can be represented on a line (Fig. 19.1). The line represents the *consciousness-anaesthesia depth* continuum: the state of full wakefulness is on the extreme left and total cortical suppression on the extreme right. In this model a drug such as propofol is given to

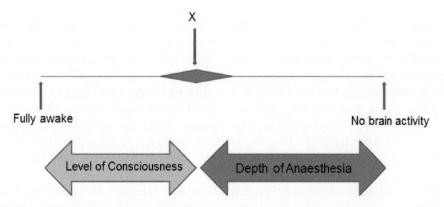

Fig. 19.1 Consciousness and depth. A *horizontal line* representing the continuum of cortical depression related to the blood level of propofol. The midpoint (X) marks the point of loss of consciousness and separates consciousness from of anaesthesia. The terms "level of consciousness" and "depth of anaesthesia" are therefore distinct. The line length is proportional to the dose of an anaesthetic drug such as propofol. The *blue horizontal diamond* illustrates that X has variability: X may represent the median dose of propofol causing unconsciousness in a population, or it could represent the variability within an individual over time.

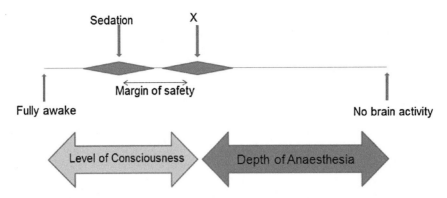

Fig. 19.2 Sedation and margin of safety. A *horizontal line* representing the continuum of cortical depression related to the blood level of propofol. The line length is proportional to the dose of an anaesthetic drug such as propofol. The midpoint (X) marks the point of loss of consciousness and separates consciousness from of anaesthesia.

The distance between the points marked by sedation and X is proportional to the difference between the doses required to cause sedation and unconsciousness. This describes margin of safety of a moderate sedation technique. The *blue horizontal diamonds* illustrate potential variation of the points marked by "sedation" and X.

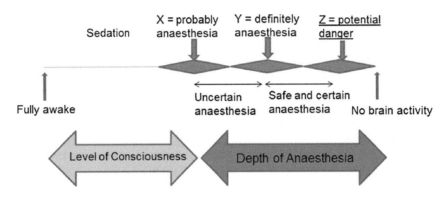

Fig. 19.3 Depth of anaesthesia and margin of safety. A *horizontal line* representing the continuum of cortical depression related to the blood level of propofol. The line length is proportional to the dose of an anaesthetic drug such as propofol. X (loss of consciousness) could be considered to be "probably anaesthesia". Higher doses are needed to ensure the patient is definitely anaesthetised (Y). Excess doses beyond

this point could expose the patient to harm (Z). The distance between X and Y could be termed a margin of uncertainty (within anaesthesia). The distance between Y and Z could represent the margin of safety of anaesthesia. The *blue horizontal diamonds* indicate potential variation of X, Y and Z.

achieve increasing blood levels. The distance between the far left point and any other point on the line is proportional to the blood level of propofol. The points on the line represent the blood level of propofol but these are arbitrary and have no units or scale. The patient begins at the extreme left, and the brain will be progressively suppressed so that consciousness is lost at some point X on the line. X separates consciousness from anaesthesia. Further travel along the line to the right beyond X represents increasing depth.

On the *consciousness* part of the line lie the levels of sedation. The line (see Fig. 19.2) shows the distance between moderate sedation (known as or conscious sedation in the UK) and loss of consciousness, and this represents the difference between the blood levels required to cause sedation and loss of consciousness; it represents the width of the margin of safety of sedation.

What happens to the right of X is less clear. As CNS suppression progresses, I propose that there are three zones (Fig. 19.3). In the zone centred on X, the patient appears anaesthetised, yet they can, in theory, react to stimuli and move back into sedation and consciousness. In this zone therefore the patient is only probably anaesthetised; their unconsciousness is uncertain. Y marks the point of definite anaesthesia in which the patient can be stimulated but does not react and therefore is safe from a return to unwanted consciousness. In the zone centred on Y is a state that could be termed *definitely* anaesthesia. The final zone has danger. Z is the point at which the patient is unnecessarily deep and they are in danger of cardiovascular depression or other unspecified damaging effects. The distances between these points or zones are unknown and could be investigated. The distance between Y and Z could represent the margin of safety for depth of anaesthesia. The distances between X and Y could be termed a margin of uncertainty of anaesthesia.

Is EEG Related to Consciousness?

The EEG changes according to the position on this line. The rapidity of change of consciousness is a major problem because usually an EEG monitor reacts too slowly to be of use. Often the EEG can do no more than confirm the observation that a patient has changed their conscious level. For example, if target controlled infusion (TCI) of propofol is set at a low target blood level (e.g. 1 mcg/ml), a patient may become deeply sedated before the EEG can detect it. Likewise, if a procedure is undertaken on deeply sedated patient, they could awaken before the EEG changes. The EEG is not useful in either situation. In practical terms, therefore, the EEG is not useful for rapid changes in consciousness: propofol sedation is likely to be in this category. Some studies have shown a relationship between EEG and conscious level [25], but there is considerable variation and the association is loose and unreliable.

In the sedated patient observation alone is likely to be better than relying on an EEG. If an EEG could warn of impending loss of consciousness or unanticipated awakening, then it would have utility. The evidence (below) shows that the EEG is poor at this task for sedation. Other monitors, such as capnography, have a higher priority in this situation, and the observer would need to intervene to maintain a patent airway rather than wait for the EEG to change.

Is EEG Related to Depth?

The anaesthesia zone concept is theoretical and, as yet, has no accepted descriptors or markers. Can the EEG help? The EEG is a measure of cortical suppression, and this is a strong reason to consider the EEG as a useful surrogate marker of both consciousness and depth. The validity of this statement is difficult to prove beyond doubt but it has a degree of truth. Conscious level too often changes too quickly during propofol sedation, but if depth changes less quickly, perhaps the EEG could be useful.

Is EEG Related to Dose?

This depends on several factors, the most important being the type of EEG, the drug or combination of drugs and the presence of painful stimulation. Testing the relationship of EEG to dose would require steady-state conditions and these are often impractical. Possibly, there is a strict relationship

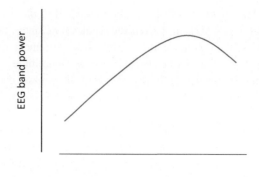

Fig. 19.4 Common relationship of EEG band power to concentration of anaesthetic

between propofol blood level and EEG effect, but this might only apply to unstimulated patients. Once the patient is stimulated, there could be a rapid change in EEG. Possibly, the relationship between propofol blood level and EEG effect is non-linear (see Fig. 19.4) so that within a certain range of blood level, the EEG remains relatively unchanged with stimulation, but if the blood level is lower than this range, stimulation could cause awakening. Nevertheless, the effective blood level range would depend upon pain, analgesia and other sedative drugs.

Essential EEG Knowledge for the Clinician

General EEG Knowledge

The EEG detects electrical activity of the outer layer of cerebral cortex from scalp electrodes. The signals are considered to be postsynaptic potentials originating from groups of axons. The waveform is random, complex and of variable and low amplitude (usually less than 100 µV). Signals from muscle are much larger (up to 500 µV) and easily hide the EEG in a moving patient. Visual inspection of an EEG shows oscillations between 1 and 20 Hz. The EEG is unequal over the scalp: parietal, central and frontal positions are most accessible and give highest amplitude signals. An EEG specialist can describe these and interpret them. There are three features: a continuous waveform, transients and periods of electrical silence. Transients are seen in natural sleep. The continuous waveform changes with consciousness and depth [26]. Electrical silence occurs with deep anaesthesia (and coma).

Unprocessed EEG in Natural Sleep

The EEG in awake and natural sleep is irregular. Conventional classification of EEG frequency bands are *gamma*

($>$30 Hz), *beta* (14–30 Hz), *alpha* (8–13 Hz), *theta* (4–7) and *delta* ($<$4 Hz). In the relaxed awake state, intermittent *alpha* oscillations are common, but these disappear in the alert state—the EEG becomes low amplitude with frequencies between 30 and 50 Hz. Sleepiness usually begins with large slow waves, and as sleep progresses five EEG stages can be seen. In stage 1 alpha oscillations become less regular and eventually disappear; background amplitude decreases. Sleep spindles characterise stage 2 (these are prominent transients of 12–14 Hz lasting more than 0.5 s, beta and theta activity become obvious and other transients appear (vertex sharp waves and K-complexes)). Stages 3 and 4 are marked by increasing prominent theta waves. Stages 1–4 are termed slow wave sleep (SWS). Stage 4 SWS progresses to a fifth stage known as rapid eye movement (REM) sleep in which eye movements cause large voltage shifts in frontal channels. REM has background low amplitude gamma activity and looks similar to that seen in the alert state.

Unprocessed EEG in Anaesthesia

The EEG under anaesthesia is relatively regular. There are methodological problems when comparing different drugs (and doses) because efficacy is usually assessed by suppression of movement to a painful stimulus, which is known to be mainly influenced by the spinal cord. High doses of propofol are needed to suppress movement unless an opioid is used, and the different inhalational agents have different spinal cord suppression effects. Therefore it is difficult to be sure that the EEG effects of various drugs have been compared under equal depth doses. Nevertheless the differences between the vapour anaesthetics and propofol are probably not important. EEG changes during progressively increasing doses of propofol [27], sevoflurane [28] and isoflurane [29] anaesthesia are broadly similar.

At induction the waveform becomes low amplitude and prominent oscillations disappear. Oscillations of 8–20 Hz appear and these become slower and more regular and increase in amplitude as doses increase. At deeper levels there are periods of EEG suppression alternating with bursts of high amplitude slow waves: this is *burst suppression* [30]. Further increasing the dose causes electrical silence. All these changes are reversed as anaesthesia dose reduces, and pain also causes some reversal [31].

The dose of propofol that causes EEG suppression will vary between patients and also within individuals according to the state of stimulation and the combination of other drugs: it is context dependent. The dose causing onset of burst suppression has recently been described. Pilge et al. [32] studied anaesthetised healthy patients immediately before surgery and found that the median effective blood level to cause the onset of burst suppression was 4.9 μg ml (-1) (compared with 2.9 vol.% for sevoflurane and 1.5 vol.% for isoflurane). The use of median infers that there was a non-parametric distribution of blood level.

Processed EEG: Power Spectrum

The EEG can be considered to be composed of many sinusoidal waves varying in frequency, amplitude and phase. The early EEG monitors (1970–1985) excluded unwanted low and high frequencies by filters, and then the amplitude of the remaining signal was calculated. The cerebral function monitor (CFM) [33] measured the minimum and maximum amplitude of a wide frequency band and the cerebral functioning analysing monitor (CFAM) [34] added the power of conventional frequency bands. As soon as personal computers became available, the EEG could be analysed using digital signal processing to calculate band power. Band power was found to change in proportion to anaesthesia blood level, but the relationship deteriorated with burst suppression. Usually, therefore, any specified band power had a biphasic change with deepening anaesthesia [27]. For example, low-frequency band power increases and then decreases as anaesthesia deepens (Fig. 19.5). Power in the highest frequencies (gamma) tend to discriminate awakening from anaesthesia best, but these are the hardest signals to measure because of their small amplitude [36, 37].

Other potentially useful descriptors of the power spectrum were total power and the spectral edge frequency (SEF). SEF90 is the frequency below which 90 % of the total power lies; the median frequency is equivalent to SEF50, i.e. the frequency below which 50 % of the power lies. Single variables were not considered reliable indicators of depth, and gradually, it became clear that combining more than one EEG descriptor could improve reliability.

Another method of EEG analysis uses short signals in "wavelet" analysis which has the potential for fast response [38]. Recent advances in characterising the EEG changes that could distinguish consciousness and anaesthesia have been made by Ní Mhuircheartaigh and colleagues [39] and Purdon and colleagues [40].

Processed EEG: Spontaneous Cortical Activity

Since the 1990s processed EEG (pEEG) monitors have been developed such as "BIS", "Entropy" and the "Narcotrend". In these, several EEG variables have been combined, for example, the band power, burst suppression, muscle activity and frequency synchronisation. All use forehead electrodes and process the signals to achieve a score. In respect of BIS the score is from 100 (fully alert) down to 0 (electrical silence—

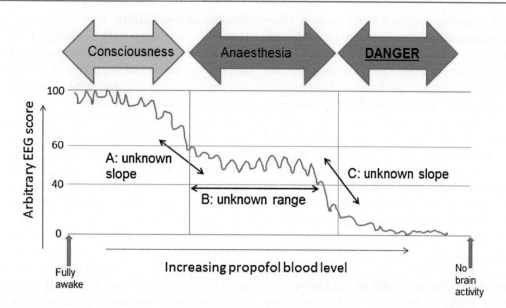

Fig. 19.5 Non-linear relationship between propofol blood level and EEG score. A probable relationship between increasing blood level of propofol and an arbitrary EEG score. For this construction it is proposed that the anaesthesia range of EEG score is between 60 and 40, and a score less than 25 may be dangerous. If these are accepted, the range of propofol blood level (B) capable of keeping an EEG score in the anaesthesia range is unknown: it may be narrow or very wide. The slopes at A and C represent the changes in EEG score leading into and out of the anaesthesia range, and these are also unknown. Similar ideas about variability of the dose response have been discussed by Escallier et al. [35]

deepest coma possible). Notwithstanding the complexity of the algorithms of these monitors, the scores decrease with both decreasing conscious level (as defined by a validated scale of behaviour) [25]; and also with increasing blood levels of propofol [41, 42]. Modification of the algorithms may improve the performance of monitors, and a recent example of such a study is by Shoushtarian and colleagues [43].

Processed EEG: Auditory Evoked Potential

An EEG signal provoked by a "click" noise is known as an auditory evoked potential (AEP). Background EEG is removed by averaging the EEG after many clicks. A typical diagnostic AEP waveform takes 2–3 min to achieve and has characteristic peaks and troughs that are related to transmission of the auditory signal through the brainstem and the cortex [44]. The brainstem is resistant to anaesthesia. The cortex has early and late components. The late cortical component is very sensitive and disappears at low blood levels of anaesthetic. The early cortical waveform however is suppressed by anaesthesia in a dose-dependent manner [45] and may be useful. Commercial monitors use headphones and frontal EEG electrodes and can obtain a waveform, suitable for anaesthesia depth assessment, within 2–6 s; from this a score is calculated (ranging from 100 to 0 as for pEEG). Unfortunately, this promising technique is spoiled by muscle activity in the posterior auricular muscle,

which is itself triggered by noise. AEP therefore is of value only in patients having NMBs [44].

In a study comparing AEP with BIS, Kreuer and colleagues [46] found that both behaved similarly during propofol TIVA (with NMB and remifentanil) but that the variation in scores was wide particularly during consciousness which reduced the ability of the monitors to differentiate between consciousness and unconsciousness.

The Evidence

Methodological Issues

There are two important considerations in testing utility: 1/ what the monitor is trying to detect and 2/ how it is assessed.

Assessment of Detection

The statistics of detection should be appreciated before a study is designed. The following methods have been used in the investing EEG detection of depth.

Positive and Negative Prediction

A diagnostic test can be described in terms of sensitivity and specificity. These are the proportion of positive and negative situations that are correctly predicted by the monitor. These terms can be confusing. To be clear, sensitivity considers the number of true positive predictions first and compares these to the total number of positives (specificity considers the negatives). Positive and negative predictions, in contrast, are the proportion of predictions by the monitor that are correct, and these are more relevant to the practical question of whether a depth monitor has utility—i.e. this means that we look at the monitor first, assess the prediction and then find out from the patient whether the prediction is correct or not. The problem is that the prediction value is affected by prevalence. For example, the low prevalence of AAGA will mean that the positive prediction test proportions are unlikely to be high and that negative predictions are more likely to be true.

Receiver Operating Characteristic (ROC) Curve

A ROC curve is a graphical representation of how sensitivity (number of positive findings correctly predicted) and 1-specificity (number of positive findings incorrectly predicted) change as the value of the "cut-off" varies (Fig. 19.6). The ROC was developed as a useful method to illustrate the viability of radar to detect aircraft in the 1950s. Radar operators were tasked with trying to tell the difference between incoming aircraft and, for example, a flock of geese. Sensitivity is plotted against 1-specificity and if the ROC gradient is close to 45 % the "test" is not useful. The problem with this method is that the number of "aircraft" and "flocks of geese" should be similar. Finding similar numbers of awake and anaesthetised patients in similar situations is a practical problem.

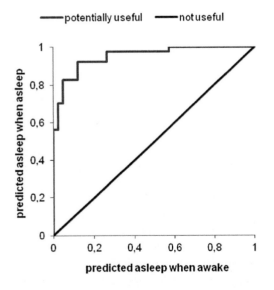

Fig. 19.6 Receiver operating characteristic curve

Prediction Probability

Prediction probability (Pk), described by Smith and colleagues [47], has become a standard tool to estimate the ability of an anaesthetic depth indicator to detect or predict the *depth*. The test outcome is the probability that the predictor variable correctly predicts the rank order of any pair of observed *depths*. Commonly, in the literature, the model to be tested has both the predictor variable and the depth ideally monotonically (=always) increasing during emergence (e.g. BIS increases as the patient awakens). Under this assumption, if, in any data pair, both the predictor variable and the observed depth change in the same direction, the pairs are considered concordant. The Pk is a statistic that is based on the ratio of the probability of concordance to the combined probabilities of concordance, dis-concordance and tied predictor variables. Pk varies between one (all pairs concordant) and zero (all pairs dis-concordant). The problem with this method is that it always tests a depth monitor around the point of return of consciousness and cannot test utility at deeper levels of anaesthesia. Also, the test is applied in patients who awaken (or the converse—become unconscious) and does not include a similar number who do not.

What Is the Monitor Trying to Detect?

The question "Is the patient awake, or not?" is not as simple as it might seem. The following scenarios are different:

- Wakefulness during anaesthesia
- Timing of awakening during emergence
- Anaesthesia during sedation
- Prediction of the above

All are related, but a monitor may be useful for only one of these tasks rather than all of them. They all, to some extent, suffer from the problem that consciousness can occur (or be lost) too quickly for the monitor to detect it, let alone predict it. If depth, also, changes quickly monitors may be too slow and have limited utility. Nevertheless if they can detect consciousness (or anaesthesia), then the distress (or harm) may at least be minimised.

All of the above involve taking the patient to a state of near wakefulness (or near anaesthesia) termed the "X" zone (a dose of propofol that probably, but not certainly, causes anaesthesia). The anaesthetist might wish the patient to be in the "Y" zone. That is that they are certainly anaesthetised, unlikely to react to stimuli and not at risk of wakefulness. Such an idea has been explored by Pilge and colleagues [32] who have measured the propofol blood level required to reach EEG suppression at the onset of burst suppression (the blood level causing onset of BS in 50 % of subjects before surgery was 4.9 µg/ml).

I propose that the monitor should be able to:

- Detect reacting during anaesthesia
- Prediction of (and therefore prevention of) reacting during anaesthesia

Obstacles

An ideal test of a monitor would involve testing its ability to follow a change in consciousness in patients who are made conscious and unconscious, repeatedly. Such a test may only be reasonably applied, ethically, in volunteers.

A clinical trial designed would need to involve enough patients who were at risk of the specified problem. The number of patients in the trial would depend on the desired reduction in risk. We know, already, that risk of AAGA is very small, and therefore the size of the trial would need to be very large.

If the specified problem was of wakefulness, then the patients would need to be tested in the "X" zone, and there may be ethical implications of this kind of research. Certainly, patients would have to receive conventional doses of anaesthetic to make the test useful. If the monitor detected wakefulness, it may be unethical to deprive the patient of higher doses of anaesthesia, but, if the patient is not awake, this may cause unwanted cardiovascular effects.

A target score of the monitor would have to be agreed. A target score thought to represent the anaesthesia has been suggested by the manufacturers, and some investigators have reported patients who were awake at these scores. This target score may therefore be only suitable for the detection of the "X" zone. A lower target score may be suitable for detection of the "Y" zone; for example, the presence of short periods of burst suppression may have utility [32]. Finally, it would also be useful for a monitor to warn that the patient was in the dangerous and potentially harmful "Z" zone.

Protocol Objectives

A protocol would have to be developed that could determine if the monitor could assist the anaesthetist in decisions about whether to increase or decrease the dose of anaesthetic. I propose that research needs to be directed to answer two main questions:

1. Can the monitor determine if (or when) a patient will awaken or remain anaesthetised?
   NB: These patients are close to the point of loss consciousness on the consciousness-anaesthesia continuum (i.e. uncertain anaesthesia ~ the "X" zone)

2. Can it be used to help decision making to prevent AAGA and, if so, how?
   NB: These patients should be to the right of the point of loss consciousness on the consciousness-anaesthesia continuum (i.e. safe and certain anaesthesia ~ the "Y" zone)

Evidence Against Utility

Sedation Studies

Earlier in this chapter, the utility of pEEG for monitoring consciousness has been discounted on a theoretical basis. The following three papers were in children, who may be a difficult group to study, but they show that BIS has either poor utility or is no better than clinical observation alone.

Mason et al. [48] showed that there was a very wide range of BIS scores in children (over 1 year old) sedated for painless imaging with barbiturate alone (BIS ranged from 31 to 90) and that there was no statistical difference between scores for moderate versus deep sedation. Powers et al. [49] showed that in children who underwent painful procedures, propofol was administered to achieve a BIS score of 50 but produced only 90 % success for adequate sedation (defined as being unrousable); there were no failures if the score was 45 or less (but there were only ten children with these low BIS scores). The important problem was that the patients were anaesthetised rather than sedated, and several children had oxygen desaturations. Gill et al. [50] used BIS in the emergency department to monitor sedation for painful procedures and found that even though children were only moderately sedated, the BIS score varied between 40 and 98.

Isolated Forearm Technique Studies

If muscle relaxants are not used, movement should warn the anaesthetists of the possibility of awareness. If muscle relaxants are used, communication is possible by using the isolated forearm technique (IFT) [51]. In this technique a tourniquet isolates the forearm so that its muscles are not affected by the relaxant drug. The patient therefore has the capacity of non-verbal communication by hand movement. At least 31 published trials have shown that anaesthetised patients can respond to verbal commands (IFT responders) but that very few remember anything afterwards [52, 53]. A surprising observation is that patients who do respond to commands do not respond to surgical stimuli. This had led to a suggestion that there is an unconscious state, within anaesthesia, called dysaesthesia [54]. Since IFT responses are abolished by increasing anaesthesia, dose dysaesthesia is considered a feature of light depth of anaesthesia (a feature of the "X" zone).

Russell has used the IFT to test the ability of BIS to identify IFT responders [55]. He studied 22 women undergoing major surgery and guaranteed full analgesia by a remifentanil infusion and extradural local anaesthesia. He then adjusted the blood level of propofol to achieve a BIS of 55–60. Under these conditions 16 patients responded, and in these, if the BIS was >60 for at least 60 s within the time period extending from 2 min before to 2 min after the patient responded, this was considered a potential marker of wakefulness: it matched an IFT response with a sensitivity of 59 % and specificity of 85 %. Therefore, a BIS of 55–60 was too often found in IFT responders and was not a reliable method of preventing IFT responses. Interestingly, even though the median effect-site propofol concentration during IFT responses and emergence was similar (2 mcg/ml compared with 2.1 mcg/ml), the median BIS value at emergence was significantly higher than that associated with IFT responses (75 vs. 61 ($p < 0.001$). Russell concluded that "The manual control of propofol intravenous anaesthesia to target a BIS index range of 55–60 may result in an unacceptable number of patients who are conscious during surgery (albeit without recall)" [55]. These important findings show that BIS alone is not reliable enough and is not wholly dependent on the blood level of propofol. BIS was dependent on both the propofol blood level and the situation: i.e. BIS is context dependent. There were similar findings in an earlier study of the Narcotrend [56].

The company who sells BIS monitoring advises that at a score of 60–80, the patient may respond to mild prodding or shaking, whereas at values of 45–60, the patient has a "low probability" of explicit recall (see www.covidien.com). These are helpful albeit imperfect markers of the boundaries of zones "X" and "Y".

Muscle Relaxants Affect pEGG

Messner and colleagues [57] have given muscle relaxants to three awake volunteers monitored with BIS. BIS reduced to less than 60 in two, but only briefly. Almost certainly this finding relates to the EMG component in the BIS algorithm and is another example of how the BIS is context dependent. More recently, Schuller and colleagues [58] tested suxamethonium and rocuronium in ten awake volunteers and showed that the BIS score reduced to the anaesthesia range. These studies demonstrate that the EMG can have a misleading effect in the presence of neuromuscular blockade. It is possible however that the volunteers were made to be comfortable during the experiments and that if they had been distressed the BIS score may have been higher.

Additional Anaesthetic Agents

In the presence of steady-state propofol anaesthesia, other drugs may affect BIS either directly or indirectly. Indirect suppression of EEG is likely to follow analgesia because the stimulation of surgery will be reduced. In these circumstances ketamine creates effective analgesia without reducing the BIS [59]. Nitrous oxide seems to have little effect or a paradoxical effect on BIS. In a study of a closed-loop propofol-remifentanil BIS system designed to keep the BIS steady, nitrous oxide had no effect on remifentanil infusion rate and a minor effect on propofol doses [60].

Rarity of AAG

Given that AAGA is variable and its severest form is usually related to the use of NMB, how many patients would need to be monitored to save one from being distressed? This number would also be related to the scenario—for example, the highest incidence of AAGA is in obstetric patients at induction where the priority would be airway management rather than EEG monitoring. Sandin and others determined the incidence of AAGA (by Brice interview) in almost 12,000 patients and calculated that 861 would need to be monitored to prevent one case of AAGA [61]. In this series only 3 % of patients were managed with TIVA.

Evidence for Utility of DoA

Target BIS Studies

Rigouzzo and colleagues [62] used propofol TCI (with fixed rate remifentanil infusion) to show that the target concentration of propofol was strongly correlated with the BIS score. When propofol was given to achieve a target BIS score of 50, the measured blood propofol concentration varied widely between 1.5 and 5.5 mcg/ml. West et al. [63] also showed that an EEG-based system can drive a propofol infusion to achieve a steady EEG target and provide safe and effective anaesthesia in 85 % of children ($n = 102$) having endoscopy procedures. There was wide variation in the propofol effect-site concentration showing that EEG-driven system may help to adjust the propofol administration to take account of pharmacodynamics and pharmacokinetic variability.

Both of these studies show that propofol blood levels (in the presence of adequate remifentanil to prevent reacting to stimuli) are correlated to pEEG effect but both show that it is difficult to predict an EEG effect from a certain dose. Targeting an EEG effect also needs a variable dose, and this confirms that constant alterations to the propofol dose are needed to maintain a steady pEEG during the stimulation of surgery. pEEG therefore may have utility, but is a success rate of 85 % useful in the clinical area? Certainly a monitor that controls propofol dosing better than the judgement of an anaesthetist has the potential for utility and could be applied to patients receiving NMBs. There is danger however that a monitor may reduce the blood propofol level to an unnecessarily low level.

Large Clinical Trials

BIS-directed anaesthesia can reduce the incidence of explicit recall. In a study of adults who were at risk of awareness, Myles and colleagues randomised patients to receive either anaesthesia directed by BIS or by clinical judgement alone. BIS reduced explicit recall from 11 in 1238 patients to 2 in 1225 [4]. In both groups approximately 40 % of patients received TIVA. In a study by Avidan and colleagues, patients were randomised to receive either BIS-directed anaesthesia or anaesthesia in which end-tidal anaesthesia vapour concentration was maintained greater than 0.7 MAC [64]. In each group of almost 1000 patients, 2 had explicit recall, and it is likely therefore that either BIS-directed or MAC-directed anaesthesia is equally effective [65]. A larger study by Avidan and colleagues [66] confirmed that BIS-directed inhalational anaesthesia was no better than end-tidal vapour monitoring.

Cases Reports

The NAP5 project identified 28 cases of AAGA during intravenous anaesthesia and at least 75 % of these were preventable [3]. A common feature was low dose. Blood levels compatible with anaesthesia are known to vary widely

and are believed to lie between 1.5 and 6.0 μg/ml [67]. Some of the NAP5 reports had doses that were unlikely to have achieved adequate blood propofol levels.

NAP5 Recommendation 18.3 states that "Depth of anaesthesia monitoring should be considered in circumstances where patients undergoing TIVA may be at higher risk of AAGA. These include use of neuromuscular blockade, at conversion of volatile anaesthesia to TIVA and during use of TIVA for transfer of patients" [3]. There were two cases caused by extravasation or "failure" of the IV cannula, and in at least one of these the cannula was not visible during surgery, and it is very likely that a BIS device could have provided warning of the accident to minimise the time spent being aware.

Conclusions and Future Directions

The NAP5 study [3] and other case series [68, 69] have shown how AAGA can occur with TIVA. To date, no reliable continuous non-invasive method exists for measuring blood levels of propofol. To measure the effect of propofol is therefore logical and potentially useful. Even if blood level monitoring was available, the variability in dose required to cause anaesthesia is so great that an EEG monitor should have utility.

The NAP5 study made four recommendations about depth monitors (see Table 19.3) and helped to define which patients (having TIVA) should benefit most from monitoring depth. The first two recommendations were that depth monitoring should be considered in patients:

- Having tracheal intubation and NMBs
- With uncertain propofol pharmacokinetics (obese, sick patients at risk of cardiovascular depression)

Table 19.3 NAP5 recommendations

20.1	Familiarity and training	Anaesthetists should be familiar with the principles, use and interpretation of: • Specific depth of anaesthesia monitoring techniques: – The available EEG-based monitors – The isolated forearm technique Relevant anaesthetic organisations should include this monitoring in their core training programmes
20.2	Pragmatic protocols	The relevant anaesthetic organisations should: • Develop pragmatic protocols or algorithms for the use of all available information about depth of anaesthesia (including information from DOA to guide anaesthetic dosing)
20.3	Use depth monitors with NMB	Anaesthetists should recognise that: • Neuromuscular blockade constitutes a particular risk for AAGA • Use of a specific form of depth of anaesthesia monitor (e.g. pEEG or IFT) is logical to reduce risk of AAGA in patients who are judged to have high risk of AAGA for other reasons • In whom neuromuscular blockade is then used
20.4	Apply depth monitors before induction	If specific depth of anaesthesia monitoring is to be used (e.g. pEEG or IFT), then it should logically commence, if feasible: • Before/at induction of anaesthesia • Continue until it is known that the effect of the neuromuscular blocking drug has been reversed sufficiently

Summary of NAP5 recommendations on depth of anaesthesia monitoring [2, 3]

The last two recommendations are related to:

- Training: the anaesthetist should know when and how to use the monitor.
- Pragmatic guidance on how to use the monitors to guide better decision making on drugs doses.

Pragmatic "How best to use the monitor to guide better decisions" will take time to achieve. We do not have sufficient information yet about safe ranges of depth monitor scores that are compatible with secure and safe anaesthesia. Until we do, anaesthetists should use depth monitors to confirm that patients are receiving standard doses of anaesthetics in the presence of controlled or minimal painful stimulation. I propose that the priorities of tasks to ensure effective delivery of TIVA are:

1. Ensure that propofol is being administered in a dose to achieve a blood level compatible with anaesthesia. The lower limit of effective dose range may vary between patient groups: awakening may be unlikely over 3 mcg/ml. Check that the infusion pump is working and that the infusion is being delivered via a cannula in a vein.
2. That sufficient analgesia is given to minimise signs of autonomic stimulation (such as high heart rate and blood pressure).
3. That a depth monitor is applied and used to check that the scores are compatible with deep sedation or anaesthesia. Depth monitoring is most likely to protect against AAGA if the patient has received a NMB.
4. If the EEG depth monitor indicates excessive cortical suppression, this suggests that propofol blood level is too high; however, if the patient's cardiovascular system is not depressed, a reduction of propofol blood may not be necessary and may reduce the protection against AAGA.

Research should continue until we have accepted reliable markers of anaesthesia depth.

References

1. Fifth National Audit Project of the Royal College of Anaesthetists and the Association of Anaesthetists of Great Britain and Ireland: Accidental Awareness during General Anaesthesia in the United Kingdom and Ireland. Report and findings September 2014 Editors Pandit J & Cook T. http://www.nationalauditprojects.org.uk/NAP5report#pt.
2. Pandit JJ, Andrade J, Bogod DG, Hitchman JM, Jonker WR, Lucas N, Mackay JH, Nimmo AF, O'Connor K, O'Sullivan EP, Paul RG, Palmer JH, Plaat F, Radcliffe JJ, Sury MR, Torevell HE, Wang M, Hainsworth J, Cook TM. Royal College of Anaesthetists and the Association of Anaesthetists of Great Britain and Ireland. Fifth National Audit Project (NAP5) on accidental awareness during general anaesthesia: summary of main findings and risk factors. Br J Anaesth. 2014;113(4):549–59.
3. NAP5 Fifth National Audit Project of the Royal College of Anaesthetists in collaboration with the Association of Anaesthetists of Great Britain and Ireland. 2014. http://www.nationalauditprojects.org.uk/NAP5report#pt. Accessed Mar 2016.
4. Myles PS, Leslie K, McNeil J, Forbes A, Chan MT. Bispectral index monitoring to prevent awareness during anaesthesia: the B-Aware randomised controlled trial. Lancet. 2004;363 (9423):1757–63.
5. Sury MR, Palmer JH, Cook TM, Pandit JJ. The state of UK anaesthesia: a survey of national health service activity in 2013. Br J Anaesth. 2014;113(4):575–84.
6. Rampil IJ, Mason P, Singh H. Anesthetic potency (MAC) is independent of forebrain structures in the rat. Anesthesiology. 1993;78 (4):707–12.
7. Antognini JF, Carstens E. In vivo characterization of clinical anaesthesia and its components. Br J Anaesth. 2002;89(1):156–66.
8. Schwab HS, Seeberger MD, Eger EI, Kindler CH, Filipovic M. Sevoflurane decreases bispectral index values more than does halothane at equal MAC multiples. Anesth Analg. 2004;99:1723–7.
9. Myles PS, Symons JA, Leslie K. Anaesthetists' attitudes towards awareness and depth-of-anaesthesia monitoring. Anaesthesia. 2003;58(1):11–6.
10. Cowley NJ, Laitenberger P, Liu B, Jarvis J, Clutton-Brock TH. Evaluation of a new analyser for rapid measurement of blood propofol concentration during cardiac surgery. Anaesthesia. 2012;67(8):870–4.
11. Liu B, Pettigrew DM, Bates S, Laitenberger PG, Troughton G. Performance evaluation of a whole blood propofol analyser. J Clin Monit Comput. 2012;26(1):29–36.
12. Harrison GR, Critchley AD, Mayhew CA, Thompson JM. Real-time breath monitoring of propofol and its volatile metabolites during surgery using a novel mass spectrometric technique: a feasibility study. Br J Anaesth. 2003;91(6):797–9.
13. Perl T, Carstens E, Hirn A, Quintel M, Vautz W, Nolte J, et al. Determination of serum propofol concentrations by breath analysis using ion mobility spectrometry. Br J Anaesth. 2009;103(6):822–7.
14. Schuttler J, Ihmsen H. Population pharmacokinetics of propofol: a multicenter study. Anesthesiology. 2000;92(3):727–38.
15. Eleveld DJ, Proost JH, Cortínez LI, Absalom AR, Struys MM. A general purpose pharmacokinetic model for propofol. Anesth Analg. 2014;118(6):1221–37.
16. Kakazu C, Lippmann M. Bispectral index monitors, non-invasive cardiac output monitors, and haemodynamics of induction agents. Br J Anaesth. 2014;112(1):169.
17. Kertai MD, Pal N, Palanca BJ, Lin N, Searleman SA, Zhang L, Burnside BA, Finkel KJ, Avidan MS, B-Unaware Study Group. Association of perioperative risk factors and cumulative duration of low bispectral index with intermediate-term mortality after cardiac surgery in the B-Unaware trial. Anesthesiology. 2010;112:1116–27.
18. Sessler DI, Sigl JC, Kelley SD, Chamoun NG, Manberg PJ, Saager L, Kurz A, Greenwald S. Hospital stay and mortality are increased in patients having a "triple low" of low blood pressure, low bispectral index, and low minimum alveolar concentration of volatile anesthesia. Anesthesiology. 2012;116:1195–203.
19. Prys-Roberts C. Anaesthesia: a practical or impractical construct? Br J Anaesth. 1987;59:1341–5.
20. Galla SJ, Rocco AG, Vandam LD. Evaluation of the traditional signs and stages of anesthesia: an electroencephalographic and clinical study. Anesthesiology. 1958;19:328–38.
21. Kim TK, Niklewski PJ, Martin JF, Obara S, Egan TD. Enhancing a sedation score to include truly noxious stimulation: the extended

observer's assessment of alertness and sedation (EOAA/S). Br J Anaesth. 2015;115:569–77.

22. Chernik DA, Gillings D, Laine H, et al. Validity and reliability of the observer's assessment of alertness/sedation scale: study with intravenous midazolam. J Clin Psychopharmacol. 1990;10:244–51.

23. Pandit JJ. Monitoring (un)consciousness: the implications of a new definition of 'anaesthesia'. Anaesthesia. 2014;69:801–15.

24. American Society of Anesthesiologists Task Force on Sedation and Analgesia by Non-Anesthesiologists. Practice Guidelines for Sedation and Analgesia by Non-Anesthesiologists. Anesthesiology. 2002;96:1004–17.

25. Kato T, Suzuki A, Ikeda K. Electroencephalographic derivatives as a tool for predicting the depth of sedation and anesthesia induced by sevoflurane. Anesthesiology. 1998;88(3):642–50.

26. Jones JG. Awareness during general anaesthesia-what are we monitoring? In: Jordan C, Vaughan DJA, Newton DEF, editors. Memory and awareness in anaesthesia IV. London: Imperial College Press; 2000. p. 3–40.

27. Koskinen M, Mustola S, Nen T. Relation of EEG spectrum progression to loss of responsiveness during induction of anesthesia with propofol. Clin Neurophysiol. 2005;116(9):2069–76.

28. Gugino LD, Chabot RJ, Prichep LS, John ER, Formanek V, Aglio LS. Quantitative EEG changes associated with loss and return of consciousness in healthy adult volunteers anaesthetized with propofol or sevoflurane. Br J Anaesth. 2001;87(3):421–8.

29. Schwender D, Daunderer M, Klasing S, Finsterer U, Peter K. Power spectral analysis of the electroencephalogram during increasing end-expiratory concentrations of isoflurane, desflurane and sevoflurane. Anaesthesia. 1998;53(4):335–42.

30. Doyle PW, Matta BF. Burst suppression or isoelectric encephalogram for cerebral protection: evidence from metabolic suppression studies. Br J Anaesth. 1999;83(4):580–4.

31. Bennett C, Voss LJ, Barnard JP, Sleigh JW. Practical use of the raw electroencephalogram waveform during general anesthesia: the art and science. Anesth Analg. 2009;109:539–50.

32. Pilge S, Jordan D, Kreuzer M, Kochs EF, Schneider G. Burst suppression-MAC and burst suppression-CP$_{50}$ as measures of cerebral effects of anaesthetics. Br J Anaesth. 2014;112:1067–74.

33. Schwartz MS, Colvin MP, Prior PF, Strunin L, Simpson BR, Weaver EJ, et al. The cerebral function monitor. Its value in predicting the neurological outcome in patients undergoing cardiopulmonary by-pass. Anaesthesia. 1973;28(6):611–8.

34. Maynard DE, Jenkinson JL. The cerebral function analysing monitor. Initial clinical experience, application and further development. Anaesthesia. 1984;39(7):678–90.

35. Escallier KE, Nadelson MR, Zhou D, Avidan MS. Monitoring the brain: processed electroencephalogram and peri-operative outcomes. Anaesthesia. 2014;69:899–910

36. Dressler O, Schneider G, Stockmanns G, Kochs EF. Awareness and the EEG power spectrum: analysis of frequencies. Br J Anaesth. 2004;93(6):806–9.

37. Dubois M, Savege TM, O'Carroll TM, Frank M. General anaesthesia and changes on the cerebral function monitor. Anaesthesia. 1978;33(2):157–164.

38. Zikov T, Bibian S, Dumont GA, Huzmezan M, Ries CR. Quantifying cortical activity during general anesthesia using wavelet analysis. IEEE Trans Biomed Eng. 2006;53:617–32.

39. Ní Mhuircheartaigh R, Warnaby C, Rogers R, Jbabdi S, Tracey I. Slow-wave activity saturation and thalamocortical isolation during propofol anesthesia in humans. Sci Transl Med. 2013;55 (208):208ra148.

40. Purdon PL, Pierce ET, Mukamel EA, Prerau MJ, Walsh JL, Wong KF, Salazar-Gomez AF, Harrell PG, Sampson AL, Cimenser A, Ching S, Kopell NJ, Tavares-Stoeckel C, Habeeb K, Merhar R, Brown EN. Electroencephalogram signatures of loss and recovery of consciousness from propofol. Proc Natl Acad Sci U S A. 2013;110:E1142–51.

41. Struys M, Versichelen L, Mortier E, Ryckaert D, De Mey JC, De DC, et al. Comparison of spontaneous frontal EMG, EEG power spectrum and bispectral index to monitor propofol drug effect and emergence. Acta Anaesthesiol Scand. 1998;42(6):628–36.

42. Vanluchene AL, Vereecke H, Thas O, Mortier EP, Shafer SL, Struys MM. Spectral entropy as an electroencephalographic measure of anesthetic drug effect: a comparison with bispectral index and processed midlatency auditory evoked response. Anesthesiology. 2004;101(1):34–42.

43. Shoushtarian M, Sahinovic MM, Absalom AR, Kalmar AF, Vereecke HE, Liley DT, Struys MM. Comparisons of electroencephalographically derived measures of hypnosis and antinociception in response to standardized stimuli during target-controlled propofol-remifentanil anesthesia. Anesth Analg. 2016;122:382–92.

44. Thornton C, Sharpe RM. Evoked responses in anaesthesia. Br J Anaesth. 1998;81(5):771–81.

45. Gajraj RJ, Doi M, Mantzaridis H, Kenny GN. Comparison of bispectral EEG analysis and auditory evoked potentials for monitoring depth of anaesthesia during propofol anaesthesia. Br J Anaesth. 1999;82(5):672–8.

46. Kreuer S, Bruhn J, Larsen R, Hoepstein M, Wilhelm W. Comparison of alaris AEP index and bispectral index during propofol-remifentanil anaesthesia. Br J Anaesth. 2003;91:336–40.

47. Smith WD, Dutton RC, Smith NT. Measuring the performance of anesthetic depth indicators. Anesthesiology. 1996;84(1):38–51.

48. Mason KP, Michna E, Zurakowski D, Burrows PE, Pirich MA, Carrier M, Fontaine PJ, Sethna NF. Value of bispectral index monitor in differentiating between moderate and deep Ramsay sedation scores in children. Paediatr Anaesth. 2006;16 (12):1226–31.

49. Powers KS, Nazarian EB, Tapyrik SA, Kohli SM, Yin H, van der Jagt EW, Sullivan JS, Rubenstein JS. Bispectral index as a guide for titration of propofol during procedural sedation among children. Pediatrics. 2005;115(6):1666–74.

50. Gill M, Green SM, Krauss B. A study of the Bispectral Index Monitor during procedural sedation and analgesia in the emergency department. Ann Emerg Med. 2003;41(2):234–41.

51. Tunstall ME. Detecting wakefulness during general anaesthesia for caesarean section. Br Med J. 1977;1:1321.

52. Pandit JJ, Russell IF, Wang M. Interpretations of responses using the isolated forearm technique in general anaesthesia: a debate. Br J Anaesth. 2015;115 suppl 1:i32–45.

53. Russell IF, Wang M. Absence of memory for intra-operative information during surgery with total intravenous anaesthesia. Br J Anaesth. 2001;86:196–202.

54. Pandit JJ. Isolated forearm – or isolated brain? Interpreting responses during anaesthesia – or 'dysanaesthesia'. Anaesthesia. 2013;68:995–1009.

55. Russell IF. The ability of bispectral index to detect intra-operative wakefulness during total intravenous anaesthesia compared with the isolated forearm technique. Anaesthesia. 2013;68:502–11.

56. Russell IF. The Narcotrend 'depth of anaesthesia' monitor cannot reliably detect consciousness during general anaesthesia: an investigation using the isolated forearm technique. Br J Anaesth. 2006;96(3):346–52.

57. Messner M, Beese U, Romstock J, Dinkel M, Tschaikowsky K. The bispectral index declines during neuromuscular block in fully awake persons. Anesth Analg. 2003;97(2):488–91, table.

58. Schuller PJ, Newell S, Strickland PA, Barry JJ. Response of bispectral index to neuromuscular block in awake volunteers. Br J Anaesth. 2015;115 Suppl 1:i95–103.

59. Sakai T, Singh H, Mi WD, Kudo T, Matsuki A. The effect of ketamine on clinical endpoints of hypnosis and EEG variables during propofol infusion. Acta Anaesthesiol Scand. 1999;43:212–6.

60. Liu N, Le Guen M, Boichut N, Genty A, Hérail T, Schmartz D, Khefif G, Landais A, Bussac J, Charmeau A, Baars J, Rehberg B, Tricoche S, Chazot T, Sessler DI, Fischler M. Nitrous oxide does not produce a clinically important sparing effect during closed-loop delivered propofol–remifentanil anaesthesia guided by the bispectral index: a randomized multicentre study. Br J Anaesth. 2014;112(5):842–51.

61. Sandin RH, Enlund G, Samuelsson P, Lennmarken C. Awareness during anaesthesia: a prospective case study. Lancet. 2000;355:707–11.

62. Rigouzzo A, Girault L, Louvet N, Servin F, De-Smet T, Piat V, Seeman R, Murat I, Constant I. The relationship between bispectral index and propofol during target-controlled infusion anesthesia: a comparative study between children and young adults. Anesth Analg. 2008;106(4):1109–16.

63. West N, Dumont GA, van Heusden K, Petersen CL, Khosravi S, Soltesz K, Umedaly A, Reimer E, Ansermino JM. Robust closed-loop control of induction and maintenance of propofol anesthesia in children. Paediatr Anaesth. 2013;23(8):712–9.

64. Avidan MS, Zhang L, Burnside BA, Finkel KJ, Searleman AC, Selvidge JA, et al. Anesthesia awareness and the bispectral index. N Engl J Med. 2008;358(11):1097–108.

65. Sneyd JR, Mathews DM. Memory and awareness during anaesthesia. Br J Anaesth. 2008;100(6):742–4.

66. Avidan MS, Jacobsohn E, Glick D, et al. Prevention of intraoperative awareness in a high-risk surgical population. N Engl J Med. 2011;365:591–600.

67. Reves JG, Glass PSA, Lubarsky DA, MvEvoy MD, Martinez-Ruiz R. Intravenous anesthetics. In: Miller RD, editor. Miller's Anesthesia. Philadelphia: Churchill Livingston; 2007. p. 719–68.

68. Nordström O, Engström AM, Persson S, Sandin R. Incidence of awareness in total i.v. anaesthesia based on propofol, alfentanil and neuromuscular blockade. Acta Anaesthesiol Scand. 1997;41:978–84.

69. Sandin R, Norström O. Awareness during total i.v. anaesthesia. Br J Anaesth. 1993;71:782–7.

Monitoring the Analgesic Component of Anesthesia

20

Isabelle Constant

Anesthesia Results from Anesthetic Effects on Cortical and Subcortical Brain Areas

Despite different mechanisms and sites of action, most of the anesthetics act on the central nervous system as a whole, including the cortical and subcortical brain areas and the spinal cord. Basically the conscious processes are integrated at the level of the cortical network, while the nonconscious processes such as nociception or implicit memory, which are of particular interest under anesthesia, are integrated in the subcortical areas. Among the subcortical structures, we can mention the limbic system involved in emotional modulation; the thalamus which receives sensory information and relays them to the cortex; the medulla where the controls of blood pressure, heart rate, and respiration are located; and the midbrain where ocular reflexes are controlled. The spinal cord is also a major target for the anesthetic agents, mainly responsible for the motor response to nociception [1] (Fig. 20.1).

Schematically, anesthetic agents induce in a dose-dependent manner a loss of consciousness (cortical inhibition), followed by a loss of motor response to nociceptive stimulation (spinal inhibition), and lastly a loss of autonomic response to nociception (subcortical inhibition) [2] (Fig. 20.2).

Nociceptive information is transmitted through the spinal cord to the thalamus and then to the cortex. In an awake subject, a number of responses are triggered: firstly, the motor response; then, the cardiovascular autonomic response with a possible emotional component; and, finally, a cognitive response. Anesthetics induce inhibition of these different processes, and this inhibition depends on both the agent and the dose. If the stimulus is greater than expected or

the analgesia insufficient, a partial activation of the brain networks may occur with firstly the reappearance of autonomic responses (pupillary or cardiovascular reactivity), then a motor response is possible, and finally a cortical activation may be observed. The assessment of nociception is based on monitoring of these possible responses, especially the autonomic responses which are, up to now, the most investigated.

The EEG Gives Mainly Information About Cortical Inhibition and Loss of Consciousness

Up to now the concept of monitoring the depth of anesthesia is mainly based on EEG analysis, using devices providing automatically calculated indices which are supposed to vary with the hypnotic concentrations [3].

High doses of analgesic agents may cause a slowing of EEG with large amplitude waveforms and without burst suppression. These effects are only seen with high concentrations, well above those used for routine balanced anesthesia. In routinely used doses, these agents do not influence the EEG to a noticeable degree. The weakness of this effect is also dependent on the intensity of the painful stimulus (and on the balance between pain-related activation and analgesic related inhibition).

The value of the EEG or an EEG-derived parameter in predicting movement attributed to a painful stimulus under hypnotic anesthesia depends on the profile of the relationship between the anesthetic agent and the EEG parameter; thus, if the concentration being examined lies in the horizontal portion of the dose–response curve, the relationship will be weak, but if it lies in the steep part, the predictive value will be better. This explains why the BIS is more predictive during propofol infusion than under sevoflurane anesthesia. The motor response to each hypnotic agent, which is mediated by cortical and spinal mechanisms, is in proportion to the agent's specific cortical, subcortical, and spinal

I. Constant, MD, PhD(✉)
Armand Trousseau Hospital, Anesthesiology and Intensive Care, 26 rue du Docteur Arnold Netter, Paris 75012, France
e-mail: isabelle.constant@aphp.fr

© Springer International Publishing AG 2017
A.R. Absalom, K.P. Mason (eds.), *Total Intravenous Anesthesia and Target Controlled Infusions*,
DOI 10.1007/978-3-319-47609-4_20

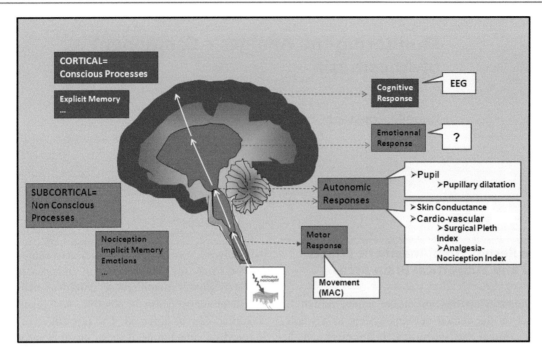

Fig. 20.1 A schematic representation of the brain. The cortical area or cortex (shown in deep *blue*) is where conscious processes are integrated, and the subcortical areas (shown in *red*) are where a number of nonconscious processes such as implicit memory or nociception are integrated. The subcortical structures include the limbic system involved in emotional modulation, the thalamus which receives sensory information and relays them to the cortex, and also the medulla where the controls of blood pressure, heart rate, and respiration are located Nociceptive information is transmitted through the spinal cord to the thalamus and then to the cortex. In awake subject, a number of responses are triggered: firstly the motor response, then the

cardiovascular autonomic response with a possible emotional component, and finally a cognitive response. Anesthetics induce inhibition of these different processes, and this inhibition depends on both the agent and the dose
If the stimulus is greater than expected or the analgesia insufficient, a partial activation of the brain networks, may occur with firstly the reappearance of autonomic responses (pupils or cardiovascular reactivity), then a motor response is possible and finally a cortical awakening may be observed. The assessment of nociception is based on monitoring of these possible responses, especially the autonomic responses which are, up to now, the most investigated

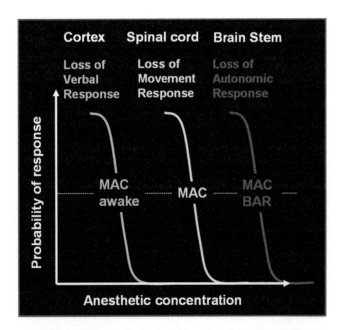

Fig. 20.2 Anesthetic agents induce in a dose-dependent manner a loss of consciousness (cortical inhibition), followed by a loss of motor response to nociceptive stimulation (spinal inhibition), and lastly a loss of autonomic response to nociception (subcortical inhibition)

actions (spinal effects of sevoflurane are more marked than for propofol) [4].

In a schematic sense, pain causes EEG activation in the deeply asleep patient, similar to a startle reaction, with a decrease in slow delta and augmentation of fast alpha and beta activity. This depends on the type of stimulus and on the degree of pain (articular > muscular > cutaneous) [5]. In the anesthetized patient, the same response is observed, similar to a startle reaction, and is diminished by increasing the depth of anesthesia or by increasing the dose of analgesic agent. This activation of rapid frequencies in response to pain (cortical awakening) is the basis of the decision algorithms that generate a higher BIS score and indicate a lack of analgesia.

In the same way, increase of EEG and EMG variability seems to be associated with the occurrence of intraoperative somatic events in anesthetized adults [6]. Some authors have proposed a composite variability index (CVI) derived from the standard deviations of the bispectral index and the electromyogram, to assess the level of analgesia/nociception during general anesthesia [7]. However, if the CVI appears to correlate with somatic responses to noxious stimuli, the unstimulated CVI depends more on the hypnotic drug effect than on opioid concentration [8].

The noxious stimulation response index (NSRI) is a newer index under development. It is a novel index, ranging between 100 and 0, computed from estimated hypnotic and opioid effect-site concentrations using a hierarchical interaction model [9]. The NSRI provides a prediction of the probability of a response to a standardized noxious stimulus (laryngoscopy). However given the unreliability of currently available PKPD modeling data in children, this index will require specific validation in pediatric populations.

Based on cortical and subcortical recordings of EEG in patients undergoing neurosurgery, the study by Velly went further and deeper, providing important findings regarding the monitoring of depth of anesthesia. The authors have demonstrated that quantitative parameters derived from the cortical EEG but not from the subcortical EEG were able to predict consciousness versus unconsciousness. Conversely, quantitative parameters derived from the subcortical EEG but not from the cortical EEG were able to predict movement in response to laryngoscopy [10]. They conclude that in humans, unconsciousness mainly involves the cortical brain, but that suppression of movement in response to noxious stimuli is mediated through the effect of anesthetic agents on subcortical structures. These data support Kissin's view that "the search for a reliable index of anesthetic depth" should be transformed into a search for separate indices of different components of anesthesia [11]. These conclusions suggest that besides monitoring of the hypnotic component of general anesthesia, the analgesic component should also be assessed, for instance, by using investigating and analyzing the subcortical effects of anesthesia.

Monitoring Nociception Requires Assessment of Subcortical Activity

The EEG-derived parameters can improve our ability to detect consciousness or unconsciousness. However the probability of movement in response to a noxious stimulus seems to be much more difficult to assess because it is under the control of brain structures not monitored by the EEG. Thus we need an index allowing the assessment of subcortical activity, and this activity may be approached at multiple levels, for instance, diencephalic, mesencephalic, and brain stem (Fig. 20.1). The best way might be to use subcortical electrodes, as in Velly's study; however this invasive method obviously cannot be considered in routine clinical practice. Conversely, a simple (and old) way to assess the nociceptive response is to look at the motor response to a painful stimulus; however we know that the motor response may have disappeared while the autonomic response, including cardiovascular response, persists (Fig. 20.2). This

persistence of autonomous responsiveness suggests that subcortical brain regions may not be completely inhibited, and this lack of inhibition might be responsible for a deleterious stress response or a nonconscious mnesic trace. On the other hand, the possibility of opioid-induced postoperative hyperalgesia should lead us to refine opioid administration by targeting a relevant clinical end point [12, 13].

Consequently monitoring of the nociception–antinociception balance in routine practice appears to be an important challenge for anesthesiologists [14].

During the last decade, a variety of monitoring systems were developed in order to assess the nociceptive balance. Up to now, all these devices are based on the assessment of the autonomic response to nociceptive stimulation. The emerging clinical devices include those which assess peripheral sympathetic response (skin conductance), cardiac and vascular sympathetic response (surgical pleth index), parasympathetic cardiac response (analgesia/nociception index), and finally pupillometry which is based on the assessment of the pupillary reflex dilatation (PRD) induced by nociceptive stimuli.

Assessment of Peripheral Sympathetic Responses to Nociceptive Stimuli

Skin Conductance Measurement

The sudoral glands in the palms of the hands and the soles of the feet are exclusively innervated by sympathetic nervous fibers. Sympathetic stimulation generates an efflux of sweat at the surface of the skin. Sweat is mainly composed of salt and water; thus after a sympathetic stimulation, an electric current can be transmitted faster from one point to another at the surface of the skin, that reflects an increase of skin conductance. The interval between a sympathetic stimulation and an elevation of skin conductance is very short (approximately 2 s).

A noninvasive device based on these changes of skin conductance has been developed by the team of Hanne Storm, in Norway [15, 16]. Skin conductance fluctuations are recorded by three cutaneous electrodes attached to the palm or sole of the patient, and connected to a monitor.

This device intends to evaluate the intensity of nociception by measuring the intensity of the peripheral sympathetic activation through the changes of skin conductance.

This noninvasive device has been initially designed and tested in infants including neonates. The evolution of the values of skin conductance parameters during the first year of life was assessed by Hernes [17]: in full-term healthy children, skin conductance parameters increase during the first 10 weeks, then reach values close to those observed in adults. In neonatology units, the skin conductance monitor showed very interesting results: the value of skin conductance parameters increased during heel stick procedures in awake premature infants [15], but on the contrary, it did not increase during non-painful stimuli (such as changing and feeding) [18]. In infants, skin conductance is probably not influenced by hemodynamic variations, muscle relaxants, ventilation, or temperature (except in extreme conditions) [19]. Inter- and intraindividual variability was described as low in infants [20].

Used in 1–16-year-old children to assess postoperative pain, skin conductance fluctuations were correlated to standard clinical pain assessment tools with a good sensitivity and a moderate specificity [21]. Another study, performed in school-aged children after surgery, found that the number of fluctuations of skin conductance per second (NFSC) correlated weakly with numeric rating scale pain scores; the authors concluded that NFSC measurement was feasible in a perioperative setting but was not specific for postoperative pain intensity and was unable to identify analgesia requirements when compared with self-report measures [22]. In a prospective observational study, skin conductance was not found to be more sensitive or faster than a clinical scale for the assessment of pain or stress in critically ill children undergoing painful procedures [23].

Fewer data are available about skin conductance variations in anesthetized children. In sedated children under mechanical ventilation in intensive care units, skin conductance was the parameter that correlated best to COMFORT scale scores, compared to heart rate or blood pressure during endotracheal suctioning [24]. During the maintenance of inhaled desflurane anesthesia in children, at BIS 50, tetanic stimulations of 60 milliamps performed at different levels of remifentanil analgesia induced low-amplitude variations of skin conductance [25]. These mild variations were only observed at the lower infusion rates of remifentanil. Indeed, at this deep and constant level of hypnosis, with halogenated agents, the sympathetic nervous system activity is likely to be virtually abolished. And as sympathetic activity is the source of skin conductance variations, deep halogenated anesthesia might prevent the occurrence of significant skin conductance fluctuations for moderate nociceptive stimulations.

In adult patients, changes in skin conductance partially reflected changes in plasma noradrenaline levels and were not affected by a bolus of opioids [26]. Several studies from the team of Ledowski investigated the usefulness of the NFSC to assess post-operative pain. The authors found that NFSC were weakly correlated with postoperative VAS ratings [27–29]. Taken together, these results led to some questioning about the sensitivity and above all the specificity of this device used in the particular context of awake cooperating adults for whom self-evaluation of pain by means of a VAS remains the gold standard.

Regarding assessment of skin conductance in anesthetized adults, skin conductance parameters were correlated to the variations of catecholamine serum concentrations during intubation [19] and to a clinical score of stress [30]. At emergence [31] or during peroperative stimulations inducing a rise in the bispectral index above 50 [32], skin conductance parameters increased. The ability of skin conductance to predict clinical reactions or response to extubation, however, is still debated [31, 33, 34]. In critically ill adults, NFSC might be more useful at evaluating emotional distress than pain assessment alone [35].

Taken together, these findings suggest that skin conductance may provide a noninvasive and quick assessment of sympathetic activation induced by emotional stress or nociception, in children, and even in neonates, as well as in adults. Skin conductance measured in healthy subjects may provide a useful parametric prediction of pain for many experimental settings [36]. One of the major interests of this monitor is to propose an evaluation of nociception which does not imply an involvement of the patient: it might improve pain assessment in patients whose communication abilities are poor. However the relevance of this monitor might be weaker when the sympathetic activity is strongly inhibited, for instance, under general anesthesia.

Pulse Wave Amplitude Measurement Using Photoplethysmography

The activation of the peripheral sympathetic nervous system induces a distal vasoconstriction. The degree of vasoconstriction is determined by the intensity of the sympathetic stimulation. By measuring the absorption of light at the tip of the finger, the photoplethysmographic monitor intends to quantify this distal vasoconstriction and thus to evaluate the peripheral sympathetic nervous activity. Basically, the photoplethysmographic pulse wave amplitude (PPGA) is inversely correlated to the intensity of sympathetic activation [37].

This noninvasive monitor is routinely used in anesthesia, because the digital absorption of light also provides vital information about the patient's arterial blood oxygenation (SpO2). In the operating room, the variability of the beat-to-beat amplitude of the plethysmographic signal is often masked by the auto-scaling processes of the monitor.

In the context of monitoring of analgesia, to increase the specificity of the index, photoplethysmography was associated to the measure of RR interval. Indeed, the changes in pulse wave amplitude provide information about the peripheral sympathetic vasomotor tone, while heart rate changes result from autonomic influences on the sinus node. These two parameters are normalized and processed in a unique algorithm that creates an index, scaled between 0 and 100: the surgical stress index (SSI), later renamed surgical pleth index (SPI), presented in 2007 by Huiku [38].

Although the performance of the SPI to evaluate postoperative pain in awake adults seems to be poor [39], many studies are in favor of its usefulness in the assessment of the peroperative balance between nociception and analgesia. In anesthetized adults, it has been demonstrated that the SSI increases after nociceptive stimulation [40, 41] and that it decreases in a dose-dependent manner after the administration of opioids [38, 42, 43]. During balanced anesthesia, the SSI correlated with the target concentration of remifentanil, but not with the concentration of hypnotics [42, 44]. Regarding regional anesthesia, the SSI does not increase if a nociceptive stimulation is applied in a site covered by a peripheral nerve block [45].

The SSI is the first monitor to have been tested as a pharmacodynamic assessment of the analgesia/nociception balance and used to guide the administration of remifentanil infusions: in adults under BIS-guided propofol TCI, compared to a "standard practice" group, SSI guidance for remifentanil (with SSI target 20–50) was associated with significantly decreased total remifentanil consumption of 30 % [46]. SSI also decreased the incidence of movement, and of peroperative major hemodynamic variations. This unexpected association between "less analgesic" and "less hypertension, less tachycardia, less movement" could be explained by a greater overall stability of the analgesia/nociception balance during the surgical procedure, thus providing a more stable level of hypnosis. Recovery and postoperative pain were similar in both groups. These important findings were later confirmed by a second study comparing SPI-guided remifentanil infusion to standard practice in adults anesthetized with entropy-guided propofol infusion for day-case surgery [47]. Again, SPI monitoring resulted in a reduced total consumption of remifentanil, but also of propofol. Postoperative pain and complications were similar in both groups. Finally, this last study showed a faster recovery and hence a better cost-effectiveness associated to the SPI guidance of remifentanil administration.

Interestingly, SSI has been shown to increase after noxious stimulations even in patients receiving β-blocking agents, when compared with those receiving an appropriate dose of fentanyl [48]. However, other factors known to influence autonomic reactions independently of a noxious stimulus might interfere with the accuracy of the SSI in evaluating the nociception–antinociception balance. Factors that may be relevant include intravascular volume status, diabetes, or chronic high arterial pressure and antihypertensive medications. Local vasoconstriction (hypothermia, severe hypovolemia) or vasodilation (regional anesthesia) might also influence the value of the SSI. Lastly, in fully awake patients under spinal anesthesia, the SSI does not reflect the nociception–antinociception balance [49].

In children, however, very few studies have focused on the interest of the SSI in the assessment of peroperative nociception. As in adults, the SSI increased significantly during nociceptive stimulation in 22 patients aged 4–17 undergoing strabismus surgery under sevoflurane [50]. Recently the potential interest of the SPI was investigated in children from 3 to 10 years, scheduled for adenotonsillectomy. The authors found that SPI-guided analgesia reduced opioid consumption during surgery compared with conventional analgesia practices, whereas it also led to more frequent postoperative hypertension and higher emergence agitation and pain scores in the recovery room; they concluded that SPI was inadequate to guide preoperative analgesia in children [51].

Up to now, no study on the SSI included a patient younger than 3 years. In neonates or infants, because of the very high physiological levels of heart rate at rest, the reliability of the SSI still requires investigations.

Assessment of Cardiac Parasympathetic Responses to Nociceptive Stimuli

The autonomic response to noxious stimulation can be investigated at the cardiac level, by studying heart rate variability. Basically heart rate variability results from sympathetic and parasympathetic modulation of the sinus node. When the sympathetic influence increases, the parasympathetic influence decreases and vice versa. This autonomic equilibrium is classically called the sympathovagal balance. Noxious stimulations induce changes in this balance with a shift toward the sympathetic activity associated with a decrease of the parasympathetic influence.

When HR is continuously recorded beat-to-beat, regular oscillations are found. Among these constitutive rhythms, it can be interesting to focus on the respiratory oscillations of HR. Indeed the latter result from changes in the parasympathetic drive exerted on the sinus node in response to respiratory movements (Fig. 20.3). Consequently quantification of these respiratory oscillations of HR allows an indirect assessment of cardiac parasympathetic modulation [52].

Using continuous recordings of HR in anesthetized adults, it has been observed that the respiratory sinus arrhythmia pattern changed when a surgical stimulation was associated with clinical signs of insufficient analgesia, even though the patient was not conscious [53, 54]. A nociception/analgesia algorithm based on the magnitude of the respiratory fluctuations in the RR series was developed and tested in adults anesthetized with propofol [55]. The parameters computed from this algorithm were recorded, and the calculated index was found to be related to pain/analgesia and relatively independent from other anesthesia-related events like hypnosis and hemodynamic conditions.

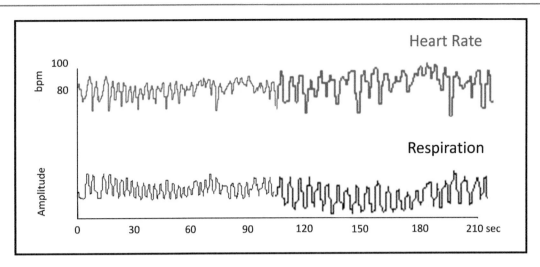

Fig. 20.3 Beat-to-beat continuous recording of heart rate (in *red*) and respiratory movements (in *black*). Respiratory oscillations of HR are generated by the reflex modulation of cardiac parasympathetic activity, due to the distension of pulmonary stretch receptors. Indeed, at the end of inspiration, there is an increase of HR due to PS inhibition, followed by a slowing down during expiration due to the comeback of the vagal control on the sinus node. This phenomenon is called respiratory sinus arrhythmia (RSA). The quantification of RSA allows parasympathetic assessment

Therefore the analgesia/nociception index (ANI) was designed to give an online index calculated from the ECG signal, providing a quantification of the respiratory variability of heart rate. This index is supposed to reflect the cardiac parasympathetic activity and thus to decrease in response to a nociceptive stimulation under general anesthesia [56]. Its accuracy for predicting analgesia/nociception balance is still under investigation. Previous studies, carried out to validate the device, have suggested that in anesthetized adults, the ANI seems more sensitive than HR and SBP to moderate nociceptive stimuli in propofol anesthetized patients [57, 58]. The ANI could be also used to assess the parasympathetic tone in various clinical conditions, for instance, it might be a useful indicator of parasympathetic tone changes in emotional situations [59, 60].

In a recent study, the ability of the ANI was compared with that of the SPI to detect standardized noxious stimulation during propofol–remifentanil anesthesia. The authors demonstrated that ANI and SPI may improve detection but not prediction of a possible inadequate nociception–antinociception balance [61]. The same conclusions were found in adults anesthetized with sevoflurane [41, 62]. Regarding prediction of movement during laryngoscopy, the performance of the ANI might be interesting [63]. Interestingly, low doses of ketamine administered during standardized sevoflurane anesthesia did not influence the ANI reactivity to nociceptive stimulation [64]. Regarding postoperative pain assessment, the value of the ANI is still being debated: Boselli et al. demonstrated in adults that a measurement of ANI during the immediate postoperative period after general anesthesia was significantly correlated with pain intensity on arrival in the postanesthesia care unit [65, 66]. However on the other hand, Ledowski concluded that ANI did not reflect different states of acute postoperative pain measured on a NRS scale after adult sevoflurane-based general anesthesia [67]. Therefore further studies are required to conclude on the value of the ANI in awake subjects.

Recently, a prospective randomized study performed in adults failed to show any advantages of ANI-guided morphine administration in elective laparoscopic cholecystectomy, compared to the current standard of care [68]. This nevertheless highlights the difficulties in designing such studies; indeed the results depend on both the targeted threshold of the ANI number and the administrated opioid.

This noninvasive monitor might be useful in anesthetized children. For example, it could be used under general anesthesia to assess the sensory blockade induced by regional anesthesia [69]. In anesthetized children receiving different remifentanil infusion rates, the ANI provided a more sensitive assessment of nociception than hemodynamic parameters or skin conductance [25]. The current ANI was not designed for analyzing high respiratory frequencies and high heart rate level and so was not adapted to pain assessment in infants. However a further approach was developed to assess high-frequency variability of heart rate. The algorithm was adapted to the typical physiological parameters of the neonate. Indeed in full-term newborn infants, postoperative pain seems to be associated with a decrease in high-frequency heart rate variability. These findings suggest that assessment of HRV could provide a useful indicator to assess prolonged pain in newborn infants [70, 71]. Another new version of the ANI monitor dedicated specifically to assess well-being in neonates is in progress [70, 72].

The main advantage of this monitor is its usability. If the concept is physiologically attractive, its reliability under different anesthetic agents and conditions interacting with the autonomic nervous system activity should be investigated. Indeed parasympathetic activity could be decreased by stress (including nociceptive stress), anxiety, and all the factors or drugs which are known to increase the sympathetic activity. Consequently ANI may not be considered as a specific and robust measure for assessment of pain intensity [73].

Assessment of Pupillary Response to Nociceptive Stimulation

Besides the cardiovascular response, the autonomic response to nociception may be investigated at the level of the pupil.

The pupil is an orifice limited by the iris, which is a motor anatomic entity composed of two antagonistic muscles (constrictor/dilator). Pupillary size therefore results from a balance between the sympathetic dilator tone and the constrictor parasympathetic tone.

Among the pupillary reflexes, the pupillary reflex dilation (PRD) in response to nociceptive stimulation (the ciliospinal reflex) is of a particular interest for anesthesiologists. In awake healthy subjects, standardized nociceptive stimulation induces an increase in pupillary diameter correlated with both the intensity of the stimulus and the pain rating by the investigated subjects [74]. In many experimental and clinical settings, the pupil diameter response is considered as an objective indicator of pain in human subjects [36].

Regarding the physiological mechanisms, stimulus-induced dilatation is primarily sympathetically mediated in the awake subject. However, because this reflex is not present in organ donors, the neural pathway requires a supraspinal component for completion [75]. This reflex persists in subjects anesthetized with isoflurane, desflurane, sevoflurane, or propofol. However, Larson and colleagues have shown that pupillary dilatation in response to noxious electrical stimulation results from a different neurological pathway during anesthesia when compared to the awake state [76]. Indeed this PRD persists after local alpha1 adrenergic blockade during desflurane anesthesia, suggesting that the sympathetic contribution to pupil size is negligible during the anesthetized state. Thus the mechanism of the PRD in response to nociception under anesthesia remains unclear, as some experimental animal findings suggest that an inhibition of the constrictor parasympathetic nucleus might be involved.

In awake subjects, opioid administration induces a decrease in pupillary diameter. These pupillary diameter changes can be used for investigating the pharmacodynamics of opioids [77, 78].

The interesting point is that under hypnotic anesthesia, the pupillary diameter decreases, but the PRD in response to noxious stimuli persists. In subjects anesthetized by TCI of propofol, the amplitude of pupillary dilation in response to a tetanic stimulus was attenuated by intravenous opioids in a dose-dependent manner [79]. Therefore, the amplitude of pupillary dilatation has been proposed as a tool to guide opioid administration during general anesthesia. Used in subjects having a peripheral nerve block under propofol–remifentanil anesthesia, the measurement of pupillary dilation allows assessment of the sensory blockade caused by locoregional anesthesia [80]. When continuously monitored during maintenance of anesthesia for cardiac surgery, the pupillary diameter may reveal acute tolerance to remifentanil [81].

Recently some authors have investigated the possible ability of the PRD measurement to predict postoperative analgesia in adults. They found that pupillary dilatation correlates with the verbal pain rating scale and concluded that pupillometry could be a relevant tool to guide morphine administration in the immediate postoperative period [82]. In pregnant women in labor, pupillary diameter changes have been demonstrated to correlate with the intensity of pain due to uterine contraction [83]. In contrast to assessment of PRD, the simple measurement of pupillary diameter failed to predict acute postoperative pain [84].

The monitoring of pupillary diameter might also be relevant in the intensive care unit. Indeed in deeply sedated mechanically ventilated patients, a pupil diameter variation $\geq 5\%$ during a 20 mA tetanic stimulation was highly predictable of insufficient analgesia during endotracheal suction [85].

Some studies have investigated the influence of some currently used anesthetic drugs. The muscle relaxants do not modify the PRD, as they have no effect on smooth muscles [86]. The antiemetics with dopaminergic antagonist properties, such as metoclopramide and droperidol, inhibit the PRD. At the contrary ondansetron, a selective antagonist of 5HT3 receptors does not influence the PRD [87]. Dexmedetomidine, an alpha2-adrenoceptor agonist, significantly reduces the amplitude of PRD to noxious stimulus, in healthy subjects anesthetized with propofol and remifentanil [88].

In children, it has been demonstrated that the assessment of the PRD, enabled testing of the sensory blockade induced by epidural anesthesia and regional anesthesia [69, 89].

In children anesthetized with 1.5 MAC sevoflurane, a standardized skin incision was associated with a rapid and large increase of pupillary diameter, without any other clinical changes [90]. The IV administration of alfentanil rapidly inhibited the pupillary dilatation. The amplitude of pupillary dilatation was not influenced by the age of children

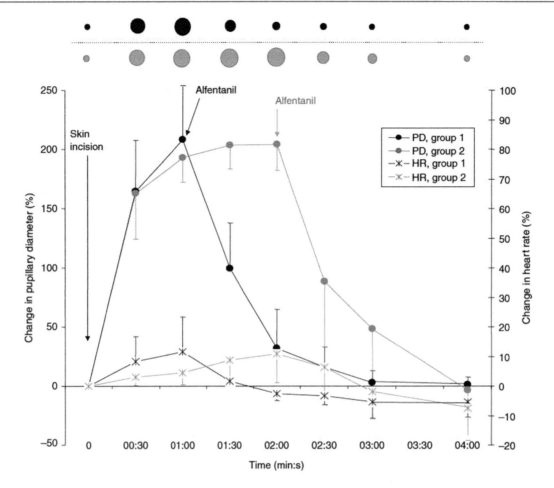

Fig. 20.4 Changes in pupillary diameter (PD) and heart rate (HR) measured after skin incision and alfentanil injection at 1 min (group 1, *black circles*) and 2 min (group 2, *gray circles*), expressed in percentage of pre-stimulation values [mean (SD)]. The pupillary size corresponding to each studied point in the two groups is illustrated on the top portion of the figure

(from 2 to 18 years) (Fig. 20.4). The authors concluded that pupillary dilatation is a more sensitive measure of noxious stimulation than the commonly used variables of heart rate, arterial blood pressure, and BIS in children anesthetized with sevoflurane [90].

Recently it has been demonstrated in children, that the minimal alveolar concentration of sevoflurane inhibiting the PRD in 50 % of subjects in response to skin incision (MACpup) was higher than the surgical MAC and close to the MACBAR. Inhibition of PRD in prepubertal children required higher sevoflurane concentrations compared to young adults. In prepubertal children receiving high concentrations of sevoflurane, significant PRD in response to noxious stimulation was frequently associated with lack of HR response and subtotal cortical inhibition. These findings might suggest that for a given level of cortical inhibition, young children require higher anesthetic doses to inhibit the subcortical structures compared to teenagers [91] (Fig. 20.5).

Using incremental intensity tetanic stimulations, it has been demonstrated that the pupillary dilatation increased with the intensity of stimulation in anesthetized children. An increase of 20–30 % of the pupillary diameter may be considered as clinically relevant in children as well as in adults [82, 92].

Recently a strong association between baseline pupillary diameter and daily dose of morphine was shown in children after surgical correction of pectus excavatum [93].

Measurement of the pupillary diameter changes in response to noxious stimulus seems to be a reliable parameter to assess specifically the analgesia/nociception balance in children as well as in adults. This measurement can be performed in routine practice by using a pupillometer which allows intermittent monitoring of the pupil size. Compared to the previously described devices, the pupillometer probably provides more accurate and specific information; however its ergonomics may be considered as less simple, especially in infants.

Fig. 20.5 Consecutive target sevoflurane concentrations in prepubertal children (*top*) and postpubertal subjects (*bottom*). When a patient showed a significant pupillary dilatation (increase in pupillary diameter of more than 100 %) at skin incision (PRD+), the sevoflurane concentration for the next patient was increased by 0.2 %. Conversely, when a patient showed a lack of significant pupillary dilatation (PRD), the sevoflurane concentration for the next patient was decreased by the same amount. The *horizontal lines* represent the MACpup values

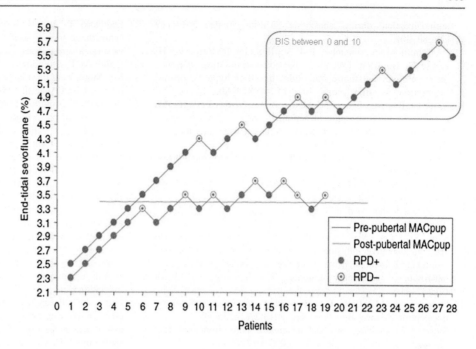

Conclusions

Anesthesia results from several inhibitory processes, which interact to lead to loss of consciousness, amnesia, immobility, and analgesia. The anesthetic agents act on the whole brain and the cortical and subcortical areas according to their receptor targets. The conscious processes are rather integrated at the level of the cortical neuronal network, while the nonconscious processes such as nociception or implicit memory require subcortical processing. A reliable and meaningful monitor of depth of anesthesia should provide assessment of these different processes. Besides EEG monitoring which gives mainly information on cortical anesthetic effects, it would be relevant to also have feedback on subcortical activity allowing an assessment of nociception. Several devices have been proposed in this last decade, to give us an idea of the analgesia/nociception balance. Up to now, most of these devices are based on the assessment of the autonomic response to noxious stimulation.

Basically skin conductance seems to best be able to assess stress in the awake or sedated neonate, while the performance of this method appears disappointing under anesthesia. The surgical pleth index is still poorly investigated especially in young children. The analgesia/nociception index showed promising results in adults to assess emotional or nociceptive stress, but these findings have to be confirmed, especially in children and in infants. And lastly pupillometry can be considered to be as reliable and reactive to noxious stimuli in children as well as in adults but is still sometimes slightly complicated to use.

Further studies are required to improve, if possible, the performances of these devices to predict the analgesia/nociception balance instead of measuring the nociceptive response.

References

1. Sonner JM, Antognini JF, Dutton RC, Flood P, Gray AT, Harris RA, et al. Inhaled anesthetics and immobility: mechanisms, mysteries, and minimum alveolar anesthetic concentration. Anesth Analg. 2003;97(3):718–40.
2. Aranake A, Mashour GA, Avidan MS. Minimum alveolar concentration: ongoing relevance and clinical utility. Anaesthesia. 2013;68 (5):512–22.
3. Constant I, Sabourdin N. The EEG signal: a window on the cortical brain activity. Paediatr Anaesth. 2012;22(6):539–52.
4. Mourisse J, Lerou J, Struys M, Zwarts M, Booij L. Multi-level approach to anaesthetic effects produced by sevoflurane or propofol in humans: 2. BIS and tetanic stimulus-induced withdrawal reflex. Br J Anaesth. 2007;98(6):746–55.
5. Drewes AM, Nielsen KD, Arendt-Nielsen L, Birket-Smith L, Hansen LM. The effect of cutaneous and deep pain on the electroencephalogram during sleep--an experimental study. Sleep. 1997;20(8):632–40.
6. Mathews DM, Clark L, Johansen J, Matute E, Seshagiri CV. Increases in electroencephalogram and electromyogram variability are associated with an increased incidence of intraoperative somatic response. Anesth Analg. 2012;114 (4):759–70.
7. Ellerkmann RK, Grass A, Hoeft A, Soehle M. The response of the composite variability index to a standardized noxious stimulus during propofol-remifentanil anesthesia. Anesth Analg. 2013;116 (3):580–8.
8. Sahinovic MM, Eleveld DJ, Kalmar AF, Heeremans EH, De Smet T, Seshagiri CV, et al. Accuracy of the composite variability index as a measure of the balance between nociception and

antinociception during anesthesia. Anesth Analg. 2014;119 (2):288–301.

9. Luginbuhl M, Schumacher PM, Vuilleumier P, Vereecke H, Heyse B, Bouillon TW, et al. Noxious stimulation response index: a novel anesthetic state index based on hypnotic-opioid interaction. Anesthesiology. 2010;112(4):872–80.

10. Velly LJ, Rey MF, Bruder NJ, Gouvitsos FA, Witjas T, Regis JM, et al. Differential dynamic of action on cortical and subcortical structures of anesthetic agents during induction of anesthesia. Anesthesiology. 2007;107(2):202–12.

11. Kissin I. Depth of anesthesia and bispectral index monitoring. Anesth Analg. 2000;90(5):1114–7.

12. Crawford MW, Hickey C, Zaarour C, Howard A, Naser B. Development of acute opioid tolerance during infusion of remifentanil for pediatric scoliosis surgery. Anesth Analg. 2006;102(6):1662–7.

13. Kim SH, Lee MH, Seo H, Lee IG, Hong JY, Hwang JH. Intraoperative infusion of 0.6–0.9 microg.kg(-1).min(-1) remifentanil induces acute tolerance in young children after laparoscopic ureteroneocystostomy. Anesthesiology. 2013;118 (2):337–43.

14. Gruenewald M, Ilies C. Monitoring the nociception-antinociception balance. Best Pract Res. 2013;27(2):235–47.

15. Storm H. Skin conductance and the stress response from heel stick in preterm infants. Arch Dis Child. 2000;83(2):F143–7.

16. Storm H. The development of a software program for analyzing skin conductance changes in preterm infants. Clin Neurophysiol. 2001;112(8):1562–8.

17. Hernes KG, Morkrid L, Fremming A, Odegarden S, Martinsen OG, Storm H. Skin conductance changes during the first year of life in full-term infants. Pediatr Res. 2002;52(6):837–43.

18. Harrison D, Boyce S, Loughnan P, Dargaville P, Storm H, Johnston L. Skin conductance as a measure of pain and stress in hospitalised infants. Early Hum Dev. 2006;82(9):603–8.

19. Storm H, Myre K, Rostrup M, Stokland O, Lien MD, Raeder JC. Skin conductance correlates with perioperative stress. Acta Anaesthesiol Scand. 2002;46(7):887–95.

20. Roeggen I, Storm H, Harrison D. Skin conductance variability between and within hospitalised infants at rest. Early Hum Dev. 2011;87(1):37–42.

21. Hullett B, Chambers N, Preuss J, Zamudio I, Lange J, Pascoe E, et al. Monitoring electrical skin conductance: a tool for the assessment of postoperative pain in children? Anesthesiology. 2009;111 (3):513–7.

22. Choo EK, Magruder W, Montgomery CJ, Lim J, Brant R, Ansermino JM. Skin conductance fluctuations correlate poorly with postoperative self-report pain measures in school-aged children. Anesthesiology. 2010;113(1):175–82.

23. Solana MJ, Lopez-Herce J, Fernandez S, Gonzalez R, Urbano J, Lopez J, et al. Assessment of pain in critically ill children. Is cutaneous conductance a reliable tool? J Crit Care. 2015;30 (3):481–5.

24. Gjerstad AC, Wagner K, Henrichsen T, Storm H. Skin conductance versus the modified COMFORT sedation score as a measure of discomfort in artificially ventilated children. Pediatrics. 2008;122 (4):e848–53.

25. Sabourdin N, Arnaout M, Louvet N, Guye ML, Piana F, Constant I. Pain monitoring in anesthetized children: first assessment of skin conductance and analgesia-nociception index at different infusion rates of remifentanil. Paediatr Anaesth. 2013;23(2):149–55.

26. Ledowski T, Pascoe E, Ang B, Schmarbeck T, Clarke MW, Fuller C, et al. Monitoring of intra-operative nociception: skin conductance and surgical stress index versus stress hormone plasma levels. Anaesthesia. 2010;65(10):1001–6.

27. Ledowski T, Ang B, Schmarbeck T, Rhodes J. Monitoring of sympathetic tone to assess postoperative pain: skin conductance vs surgical stress index. Anaesthesia. 2009;64(7):727–31.

28. Ledowski T, Bromilow J, Paech MJ, Storm H, Hacking R, Schug SA. Monitoring of skin conductance to assess postoperative pain intensity. Br J Anaesth. 2006;97(6):862–5.

29. Ledowski T, Bromilow J, Wu J, Paech MJ, Storm H, Schug SA. The assessment of postoperative pain by monitoring skin conductance: results of a prospective study. Anaesthesia. 2007;62(10):989–93.

30. Gjerstad AC, Storm H, Hagen R, Huiku M, Qvigstad E, Raeder J. Comparison of skin conductance with entropy during intubation, tetanic stimulation and emergence from general anaesthesia. Acta Anaesthesiol Scand. 2007;51(1):8–15.

31. Ledowski T, Bromilow J, Paech MJ, Storm H, Hacking R, Schug SA. Skin conductance monitoring compared with Bispectral Index to assess emergence from total i.v. anaesthesia using propofol and remifentanil. Br J Anaesth. 2006;97(6):817–21.

32. Storm H, Shafiei M, Myre K, Raeder J. Palmar skin conductance compared to a developed stress score and to noxious and awakening stimuli on patients in anaesthesia. Acta Anaesthesiol Scand. 2005;49(6):798–803.

33. Ledowski T, Paech MJ, Storm H, Jones R, Schug SA. Skin conductance monitoring compared with bispectral index monitoring to assess emergence from general anaesthesia using sevoflurane and remifentanil. Br J Anaesth. 2006;97(2):187–91.

34. Ledowski T, Preuss J, Ford A, Paech MJ, McTernan C, Kapila R, et al. New parameters of skin conductance compared with bispectral Index monitoring to assess emergence from total intravenous anaesthesia. Br J Anaesth. 2007;99(4):547–51.

35. Gunther AC, Bottai M, Schandl AR, Storm H, Rossi P, Sackey PV. Palmar skin conductance variability and the relation to stimulation, pain and the motor activity assessment scale in intensive care unit patients. Crit Care (Lond). 2013;17(2):R51.

36. Geuter S, Gamer M, Onat S, Buchel C. Parametric trial-by-trial prediction of pain by easily available physiological measures. Pain. 2014;155(5):994–1001.

37. Korhonen I, Yli-Hankala A. Photoplethysmography and nociception. Acta Anaesthesiol Scand. 2009;53(8):975–85.

38. Huiku M, Uutela K, van Gils M, Korhonen I, Kymalainen M, Merilainen P, et al. Assessment of surgical stress during general anaesthesia. Br J Anaesth. 2007;98(4):447–55.

39. Thee C, Ilies C, Gruenewald M, Kleinschmidt A, Steinfath M, Bein B. Reliability of the surgical pleth index for assessment of postoperative pain: a pilot study. Eur J Anaesthesiol. 2014;13.

40. Bonhomme V, Uutela K, Hans G, Maquoi I, Born JD, Brichant JF, et al. Comparison of the surgical pleth Index with haemodynamic variables to assess nociception-anti-nociception balance during general anaesthesia. Br J Anaesth. 2011;106(1):101–11.

41. Gruenewald M, Herz J, Schoenherr T, Thee C, Steinfath M, Bein B. Measurement of the nociceptive balance by analgesia nociception index (ANI) and surgical pleth index (SPI) during sevoflurane - remifentanil anaesthesia. Minerva Anestesiol. 2014;17.

42. Gruenewald M, Meybohm P, Ilies C, Hocker J, Hanss R, Scholz J, et al. Influence of different remifentanil concentrations on the performance of the surgical stress index to detect a standardized painful stimulus during sevoflurane anaesthesia. Br J Anaesth. 2009;103(4):586–93.

43. Mustola S, Parkkari T, Uutela K, Huiku M, Kymalainen M, Toivonen J. Performance of surgical stress index during sevoflurane-fentanyl and isoflurane-fentanyl anesthesia. Anesthesiol Res Pract. 2010;2010.

44. Struys MM, Vanpeteghem C, Huiku M, Uutela K, Blyaert NB, Mortier EP. Changes in a surgical stress index in response to standardized pain stimuli during propofol-remifentanil infusion. Br J Anaesth. 2007;99(3):359–67.

45. Wennervirta J, Hynynen M, Koivusalo AM, Uutela K, Huiku M, Vakkuri A. Surgical stress index as a measure of nociception/ antinociception balance during general anesthesia. Acta Anaesthesiol Scand. 2008;52(8):1038–45.

46. Chen X, Thee C, Gruenewald M, Wnent J, Illies C, Hoecker J, et al. Comparison of surgical stress index-guided analgesia with standard clinical practice during routine general anesthesia: a pilot study. Anesthesiology. 2010;112(5):1175–83.

47. Bergmann I, Gohner A, Crozier TA, Hesjedal B, Wiese CH, Popov AF, et al. Surgical pleth index-guided remifentanil administration reduces remifentanil and propofol consumption and shortens recovery times in outpatient anaesthesia. Br J Anaesth. 2013;110 (4):622–8.

48. Ahonen J, Jokela R, Uutela K, Huiku M. Surgical stress index reflects surgical stress in gynaecological laparoscopic day-case surgery. Br J Anaesth. 2007;98(4):456–61.

49. Ilies C, Gruenewald M, Ludwigs J, Thee C, Hocker J, Hanss R, et al. Evaluation of the surgical stress index during spinal and general anaesthesia. Br J Anaesth. 2010;105(4):533–7.

50. Kallio H, Lindberg LI, Majander AS, Uutela KH, Niskanen ML, Paloheimo MP. Measurement of surgical stress in anaesthetized children. Br J Anaesth. 2008;101(3):383–9.

51. Park JH, Lim BG, Kim H, Lee IO, Kong MH, Kim NS. Comparison of surgical pleth index-guided analgesia with conventional analgesia practices in children: a randomized controlled trial. Anesthesiology. 2015;122(6):1280–7.

52. Pomeranz B, Macaulay RJ, Caudill MA, Kutz I, Adam D, Gordon D, et al. Assessment of autonomic function in humans by heart rate spectral analysis. Am J Physiol. 1985;248(1 Pt 2): H151–3.

53. Jeanne M, Logier R, De Jonckheere J, Tavernier B. Validation of a graphic measurement of heart rate variability to assess analgesia/ nociception balance during general anesthesia. Conf Proc IEEE Eng Med Biol Soc. 2009;2009:1840–3.

54. Logier R, Jeanne M, Tavernier B, De Jonckheere J. Pain/analgesia evaluation using heart rate variability analysis. Conf Proc IEEE Eng Med Biol Soc. 2006;1:4303–6.

55. Jeanne M, Logier R, De Jonckheere J, Tavernier B. Heart rate variability during total intravenous anesthesia: effects of nociception and analgesia. Auton Neurosci. 2009;147(1–2):91–6.

56. Logier R, Jeanne M, De Jonckheere J, Dassonneville A, Delecroix M, Tavernier B. PhysioDoloris: a monitoring device for analgesia/nociception balance evaluation using heart rate variability analysis. Conf Proc IEEE Eng Med Biol Soc. 2010;2010:1194–7.

57. Jeanne M, Clement C, De Jonckheere J, Logier R, Tavernier B. Variations of the analgesia nociception index during general anaesthesia for laparoscopic abdominal surgery. J Clin Monit Comput. 2012;26(4):289–94.

58. Jeanne M, Delecroix M, De Jonckheere J, Keribedj A, Logier R, Tavernier B. Variations of the analgesia nociception index during propofol anesthesia for total knee replacement. Clin J Pain. 2014;30 (12):1084–8.

59. De Jonckheere J, Logier R, Jounwaz R, Vidal R, Jeanne M. From pain to stress evaluation using heart rate variability analysis: development of an evaluation platform. Conf Proc IEEE Eng Med Biol Soc. 2010;2010:3852–5.

60. De Jonckheere J, Rommel D, Nandrino JL, Jeanne M, Logier R. Heart rate variability analysis as an index of emotion regulation processes: interest of the analgesia nociception index (ANI). Conf Proc IEEE Eng Med Biol Soc. 2012;2012:3432–5.

61. Gruenewald M, Ilies C, Herz J, Schoenherr T, Fudickar A, Hocker J, et al. Influence of nociceptive stimulation on analgesia nociception index (ANI) during propofol-remifentanil anaesthesia. Br J Anaesth. 2013;110(6):1024–30.

62. Ledowski T, Averhoff L, Tiong WS, Lee C. Analgesia Nociception Index (ANI) to predict intraoperative haemodynamic changes: results of a pilot investigation. Acta Anaesthesiol Scand. 2014;58(1):74–9.

63. Boselli E, Bouvet L, Begou G, Torkmani S, Allaouchiche B. Prediction of haemodynamic reactivity during total intravenous anaesthesia for suspension laryngoscopy using Analgesia/ Nociception Index (ANI): a prospective observational study. Minerva Anestesiol. 2014.

64. Bollag L, Ortner CM, Jelacic S, Rivat C, Landau R, Richebe P. The effects of low-dose ketamine on the analgesia nociception index (ANI) measured with the novel PhysioDoloris analgesia monitor: a pilot study. J Clin Monit Comput. 2014;26.

65. Boselli E, Bouvet L, Begou G, Dabouz R, Davidson J, Deloste JY, et al. Prediction of immediate postoperative pain using the analgesia/nociception index: a prospective observational study. Br J Anaesth. 2014;112(4):715–21.

66. Boselli E, Daniela-Ionescu M, Begou G, Bouvet L, Dabouz R, Magnin C, et al. Prospective observational study of the non-invasive assessment of immediate postoperative pain using the analgesia/nociception index (ANI). Br J Anaesth. 2013;111 (3):453–9.

67. Ledowski T, Tiong WS, Lee C, Wong B, Fiori T, Parker N. Analgesia nociception index: evaluation as a new parameter for acute postoperative pain. Br J Anaesth. 2014;111(4):627–9.

68. Szental JA, Webb A, Weeraratne C, Campbell A, Sivakumar H, Leong S. Postoperative pain after laparoscopic cholecystectomy is not reduced by intraoperative analgesia guided by analgesia nociception index (ANI(R)) monitoring: a randomized clinical trial. Br J Anaesth. 2015;114(4):640–5.

69. Migeon A, Desgranges FP, Chassard D, Blaise BJ, De Queiroz M, Stewart A, et al. Pupillary reflex dilatation and analgesia nociception index monitoring to assess the effectiveness of regional anesthesia in children anesthetised with sevoflurane. Paediatr Anaesth. 2013;23(12):1160–5.

70. De Jonckheere J, Rakza T, Logier R, Jeanne M, Jounwaz R, Storme L. Heart rate variability analysis for newborn infants prolonged pain assessment. Conf Proc IEEE Eng Med Biol Soc. 2011;2011:7747–50.

71. Faye PM, De Jonckheere J, Logier R, Kuissi E, Jeanne M, Rakza T, et al. Newborn infant pain assessment using heart rate variability analysis. Clin J Pain. 2010;26(9):777–82.

72. Alexandre C, De Jonckheere J, Rakza T, Mur S, Carette D, Logier R, et al. Impact of cocooning and maternal voice on the autonomic nervous system activity in the premature newborn infant. Arch Pediatr. 2013;20(9):963–8.

73. Jess G, Pogatzki-Zahn EM, Zahn PK, Meyer-Friessem CH. Monitoring heart rate variability to assess experimentally induced pain using the analgesia nociception index: a randomised volunteer study. Eur J Anaesthesiol. 2015;11.

74. Ellermeier W, Westphal W. Gender differences in pain ratings and pupil reactions to painful pressure stimuli. Pain. 1995;61(3):435–9.

75. Yang LL, Niemann CU, Larson MD. Mechanism of pupillary reflex dilation in awake volunteers and in organ donors. Anesthesiology. 2003;99(6):1281–6.

76. Larson MD, Tayefeh F, Sessler DI, Daniel M, Noorani M. Sympathetic nervous system does not mediate reflex pupillary dilation during desflurane anesthesia. Anesthesiology. 1996;85 (4):748–54.

77. Lotsch J. Pharmacokinetic-pharmacodynamic modeling of opioids. J Pain Symptom Manage. 2005;29(5 Suppl):S90–103.

78. Brokjaer A, Olesen AE, Kreilgaard M, Graversen C, Gram M, Christrup LL, et al. Objective markers of the analgesic response to morphine in experimental pain research. J Pharmacol Toxicol Methods. 2015;73:7–14.

79. Barvais L, Engelman E, Eba JM, Coussaert E, Cantraine F, Kenny GN. Effect site concentrations of remifentanil and pupil response to noxious stimulation. Br J Anaesth. 2003;91(3):347–52.

80. Isnardon S, Vinclair M, Genty C, Hebrard A, Albaladejo P, Payen JF. Pupillometry to detect pain response during general anaesthesia following unilateral popliteal sciatic nerve block: a prospective, observational study. Eur J Anaesthesiol. 2013;30(7):429–34.

81. Coquin J, Tafer N, Mazerolles M, Pouquet O, Pfeiff R, Richebe P, et al. Pupillary dilatation monitoring to evaluate acute remifentanil tolerance in cardiac surgery. Ann Fr Anesth Reanim. 2009;28(11):930–5.

82. Aissou M, Snauwaert A, Dupuis C, Atchabahian A, Aubrun F, Beaussier M. Objective assessment of the immediate postoperative analgesia using pupillary reflex measurement: a prospective and observational study. Anesthesiology. 2012;116(5):1006–12.

83. Guglielminotti J, Mentre F, Gaillard J, Ghalayini M, Montravers P, Longrois D. Assessment of pain during labor with pupillometry: a prospective observational study. Anesth Analg. 2013;116(5):1057–62.

84. Kantor E, Montravers P, Longrois D, Guglielminotti J. Pain assessment in the postanaesthesia care unit using pupillometry: a cross-sectional study after standard anaesthetic care. Eur J Anaesthesiol. 2014;31(2):91–7.

85. Paulus J, Roquilly A, Beloeil H, Theraud J, Asehnoune K, Lejus C. Pupillary reflex measurement predicts insufficient analgesia before endotracheal suctioning in critically ill patients. Crit Care (Lond). 2013;17(4):R161.

86. Gray AT, Krejci ST, Larson MD. Neuromuscular blocking drugs do not alter the pupillary light reflex of anesthetized humans. Arch Neurol. 1997;54(5):579–84.

87. Larson MD. The effect of antiemetics on pupillary reflex dilation during epidural/general anesthesia. Anesth Analg. 2003;97(6):1652–6.

88. Larson MD, Talke PO. Effect of dexmedetomidine, an alpha2-adrenoceptor agonist, on human pupillary reflexes during general anaesthesia. Br J Clin Pharmacol. 2001;51(1):27–33.

89. Emery J, Ho D, MacKeen L, Heon E, Bissonnette B. Pupillary reflex dilation and skin temperature to assess sensory level during combined general and caudal anesthesia in children. Paediatr Anaesth. 2004;14(9):768–73.

90. Constant I, Nghe MC, Boudet L, Berniere J, Schrayer S, Seeman R, et al. Reflex pupillary dilatation in response to skin incision and alfentanil in children anaesthetized with sevoflurane: a more sensitive measure of noxious stimulation than the commonly used variables. Br J Anaesth. 2006;96(5):614–9.

91. Bourgeois E, Sabourdin N, Louvet N, Donette FX, Guye ML, Constant I. Minimal alveolar concentration of sevoflurane inhibiting the reflex pupillary dilatation after noxious stimulation in children and young adults. Br J Anaesth. 2012;108(4):648–54.

92. Louvet N, Sabourdin N, Guye ML, Giral T, Constant I. Evolution of the pupillary reflex dilatation, of the analgesia nociception index and of heart rate variations during tetanic stimulations of increasing intensity, in anesthetized children. ASA Meeting. 2011;A829.

93. Connelly MA, Brown JT, Kearns GL, Anderson RA, St Peter SD, Neville KA. Pupillometry: a non-invasive technique for pain assessment in pediatric patients. Arch Dis Child. 2014;3.

Intravenous Drugs for Sedation: Target-Controlled, Patient-Controlled and Patient-Maintained Delivery

Keith J. Anderson and Gavin N.C. Kenny

Definition of Sedation

Sedation has become a very popular technique to help patients tolerate unpleasant medical procedures. Sedation has been termed as the act or process of calming. The desired components of this are anxiolysis, amnesia and/or altered conscious level [1]. Analgesia may also be required if the procedure is painful. Whereas some sedatives have intrinsic analgesia properties, such as ketamine or nitrous oxide; often sedatives are given with opioid analgesics to avoid or mitigate the pain of the procedure itself. This may be termed "analgo-sedation".

There are many definitions of sedation; however it is really a spectrum of consciousness from fully awake to general anaesthesia [1]. In the United Kingdom (UK), conscious sedation is defined as "a technique in which the use of a drug or drugs produces a state of depression of the central nervous system enabling treatment to be carried out, but during which verbal contact with the patient is maintained throughout the period of sedation. The drugs and techniques used should carry a margin of safety wide enough to render loss of consciousness unlikely" [1, 2]. The end point is clearly defined and wide margins of safety stipulated. The airway is normally unaffected and spontaneous ventilation adequate. The desired target for non-anaesthetists is always conscious sedation, which relies on the maintenance of verbal contact. This is intended to ensure patients are kept awake enough to avoid cardiorespiratory depression, particularly airway obstruction. The Safe Sedation Practice document produced in the UK is quite typical in mandating that loss of verbal contact means general anaesthesia and this should only be provided by individuals with training in anaesthesia and access to anaesthetic equipment [1, 2]. The American Society of Anesthesiologists (ASA) uses different terms (Table 21.1) [3]. Moderate sedation is roughly akin to conscious sedation: it describes a state where there is a purposeful response to verbal commands, either alone, or accompanied by light tactile stimulation. No airway intervention is required, spontaneous ventilation is adequate, and cardiovascular function is usually maintained. The ASA makes great emphasis that this is a continuum from minimal to deep sedation and eventually to general anaesthesia. As a patient passes along this continuum, depression of physiological systems occurs which require intervention to avoid adverse outcomes. The competency required increases, as does the depth of sedation. The unpredictability of individual patient response means a sedationist may inadvertently take a patient to a level of sedation greater than that intended. Therefore, if practicing moderate sedation, one should be able to support the patient in deep sedation and return them to the intended level of sedation safely. Similarly, if delivering deep sedation, one should be able to deal with an anaesthetised patient.

The Academy of Medical Royal Colleges (UK) is more simplistic: "If verbal responsiveness is lost the patient requires a level of care identical to that needed for general anaesthesia". Hence, if propofol is ever to be self-administered by patients without an anaesthetist present, the methods of delivery must have some way of limiting drug administration to avoid loss of verbal contact.

Indications and Demand for Sedation

Patients request sedation for many types of invasive procedures, e.g. gastrointestinal endoscopy, bronchoscopy, dental surgery, interventional radiology, emergency

K.J. Anderson, BSc (Hons), MB, ChB, FRCA (✉)
Department of Anesthesiology, Foothills Medical Centre, University of Calgary, C222, 1403 29th Street NW, Calgary, AB, Canada T2N 2T9,
e-mail: Keith.Anderson@albertahealthservices.ca;
keithanderson@doctors.net.uk

G.N.C. Kenny
Department of Anaesthesia, University of Glasgow, Scotland, UK
e-mail: gavinkenny@talktalk.net

© Springer International Publishing AG 2017
A.R. Absalom, K.P. Mason (eds.), *Total Intravenous Anesthesia and Target Controlled Infusions*,
DOI 10.1007/978-3-319-47609-4_21

Table 21.1 The ASA continuum of depth of sedation

	Minimal sedation	Moderate sedation	Deep sedation	General anaesthesia
Responsiveness	Normal response to verbal stimulation	Purposeful response to verbal or tactile stimulation	Purposeful response following repeated or painful stimulation	Unrousable even with painful stimulus
Airway	Unaffected	No intervention required	Intervention may be required	Intervention often required
Spontaneous ventilation	Unaffected	Adequate	May be inadequate	Usually inadequate
Cardiovascular function	Unaffected	Usually maintained	Usually maintained	May be impaired

Reproduced from Reference [3] with permission from the American Society of Anesthesiologists

Table 21.2 Hospital episode statistics Department of Health 2000–2001

Procedure	Three-digit OPCS4 code	Completed episodes	% As day case
Upper GI endoscopy	G01-25	561,572	72
ERCP	J38-45	33,504	21
Colonoscopy	H04-30	331,646	75
Bronchoscopy	E01-63	205,984	61

department procedures and oocyte retrieval for assisted fertility. Patients request sedation for a variety of reasons: anxiolysis, amnesia and reduced consciousness. Regardless of the reason, provision of sedation generally improves patient satisfaction [4, 5]. For example, the scale of sedation occurring in the UK is vast (Table 21.2).

Given the large numbers of patients receiving sedation, it is not practical that anaesthetists provide all sedation. Indeed, it seems that anaesthetists already do not provide the majority of sedation. For instance, the National Confidential Enquiry into Patient Outcome and Deaths (NCEPOD) 2004 studied deaths associated with invasive gastrointestinal endoscopy surgical procedures in the UK [6]. An estimated 128,000 procedures were performed in 2003, with a 3 % 30-day mortality. In approximately 85 % of cases, the operator or nurse administered sedation.

Dentistry

Historically general anaesthesia was used to treat the severely anxious patient in general dental practice; however, there were serious concerns about the safety of this and was highlighted in the Poswillo report [7]. The subsequent **reduction** in general anaesthetic numbers was not sustained [8]. Eventually in 1998 the General Dental Council banned general anaesthesia by all non-anaesthetists [9]. This led to a large increase in the sedation required in primary care [10].

A survey of primary care dentists revealed around 75 % felt a need for sedation in their practice, with around half providing sedation for their patients [11]. Only about 10 % of these had any training in sedation. The sedation techniques being used were mainly i.v. sedation with midazolam, oral sedation with temazepam and nitrous oxide. One dentist was using propofol routinely. Most patients were monitored using pulse oximetry, with few using blood pressure and electrocardiography (ECG) [11]. There has been development of general dental practitioners with special interests in anxiety and sedation, this is likely to develop further, and training is likely to become standard for undergraduates and encouraged for those already in practice [12]. There is also a parallel secondary care service [13], which provides both primary and secondary restorative dental care for patients under sedation [14]. There are also patients who are medically compromised who may require sedation but are not considered suitable for treatment in primary care. The majority of those using sedation in secondary care used i.v. midazolam, with a minority using propofol and diazepam. An overwhelming majority of 80 % of these had a separate operator and sedationist. Secondary care sedation in dentistry is more developed than in many other specialties with systems of training and accreditation [15]. Realising the likely increase in demand for sedation the British Dental Association was proactive in instituting guidelines for sedation practice and coordinated training for this via the Dental Sedation Teachers Group.

Gastrointestinal Endoscopy

Sedation is widely used in endoscopy. Older reports suggested that benzodiazepines were predominantly used, often in conjunction with opioids [16, 17].

Practice appears to have changed recently, and propofol has been used increasingly. Although primarily an anaesthetic drug, it has been given with a surprisingly good safety profile by non-anaesthetists, such as general practitioners [18]. It is popular with non-anaesthetists because of its many desirable qualities [19, 20]. There are numerous studies examining its efficacy in colonoscopy [21], and emerging data that in this environment morbidity is relatively rare [22]. Its use by non-anaesthetists is however controversial to say the least. For example, the European Society of Anaesthesiologists after trying to control its use has come out quite strongly against its use by non-anaesthetists [23]. The Academy of Medical Royal Colleges in the UK has been more pragmatic and tried to improve standards of care and training.

Emergency Medicine

Historically sedation in the emergency department was mainly based using a benzodiazepine, with limited monitoring, training and knowledge [24]. More recently it has been proposed strongly that propofol use in emergency medicine is safe, a better sedative than benzodiazepines, and that serious complications are acceptably rare [25]. The use for sedation in the UK by emergency departments has become popular; it seems mainly administered by physicians (most of whom) have at least some anaesthetic experience. Early reports were, however, worryingly naive in their proclamations of safety [26] and came in for strong criticism by our group [27].

In fact some patients were almost certainly receiving general anaesthesia, and with a far worse safety record than other published experience. In defence, the criticism has been taken on board and larger case series are being reported. In addition, there has been a serious attempt at clinical governance with regard to index incidents using the World Society for Intravenous Anaesthesia Sedation Index Events framework [28, 29]. The Academy of Medical Royal Colleges Sedation publications are almost certainly helping, but it has been pointed out again that even with a more conservative dose regimen, many patients are still receiving anaesthesia [30].

The Main Options for Sedative Agents

Benzodiazepines

Theoretically any benzodiazepine can be used to provide sedation. However midazolam is the most popularly used agent owing to its relatively rapid onset and offset compared to the alternatives diazepam and lorazepam [31]. It seems most logical to give midazolam intravenously. However, it is also possible to give it sublingually or intranasally. Though popular in children, the volume required in adults limits its usefulness.

Midazolam gives good amnesia and anxiolysis [32, 33] though it is also associated with delayed return of cognitive function and discharge. The most common regimens involve relatively frequent titration of small doses until the patient reaches the desired sedation level either by a physician [34] or even using patient-controlled sedation (PCS) [32] or target-controlled infusion (TCI) [35]. It is recognised that the elderly are more sensitive [36], and most titrate such patients much more cautiously. It seems that recovery from midazolam is the fastest of the benzodiazepines, but longer than propofol [32, 37]. The main unrecognised problem with midazolam is that its pharmacodynamics have a relatively slow onset and longer than appreciated offset [38]. The $t_{1/2ke0}$ (the half-life for midazolam in the plasma equilibrating with the brain) is relatively slow, one estimate being around 9 min [39]. This means that when the patient has reached the desired sedation level, and drug administration stops, the clinical effect of the drug (effect-site concentration (Ce)) is still rising for 10–20 min (Fig. 21.1) [38].

This perhaps explains the reports of prolonged hypoxia after the use of midazolam in conjunction with opioids in the elderly for upper GI endoscopy (Fig. 21.2) [40]. Common problems are respiratory depression, reduction in blood pressure and paradoxical excitement [41].

A major advantage of midazolam is the availability of the reversal agent flumazenil, which can reverse the sedative and respiratory depressant effects. However, sedationists should be wary that the half-life of flumazenil is relatively short, and its effects may wear off before the midazolam has been eliminated [42].

Many of the adverse events in previous studies of morbidity and mortality were attributed to inappropriate use of benzodiazepines and poor monitoring and recovery [16, 17]. The NCEPOD report in 2004 still identified about 14 % of deaths for endoscopy where sedation was a factor, predominantly excessive doses and combinations of drugs, particularly in the elderly. Although recently its safety profile has improved [43], there are still warnings of adverse events with midazolam from the National Patient Safety Agency [44].

Propofol

Propofol has been used in sub-anaesthetic doses for over 25 years [45]. Propofol is an excellent sedative due to its pharmacokinetics and dynamics [45]. Its onset is rapid [46] and recovery faster than midazolam [32, 34, 37, 47]. It has long been known to have anxiolytic and sedative properties with minimal amnesia at plasma concentrations less than 1.0 µg·ml^{-1} [48]. It seems to offer excellent anxiolysis and has even been used as a

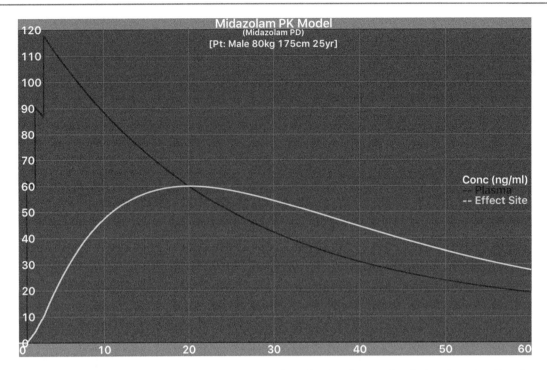

Fig. 21.1 Typical titration of midazolam i.v. with 2 mg followed by 1 mg, 1 mg at minute intervals. Note the effect-site concentration significantly lags behind plasma concentration. Hence if clinical sedation is judged to be adequate after the last dose, the effect-site concentration continues to rise for the next 17 min. This is calculated with a pharmacokinetic simulator using the Zomorodi model and a recent estimate of k_{e0}

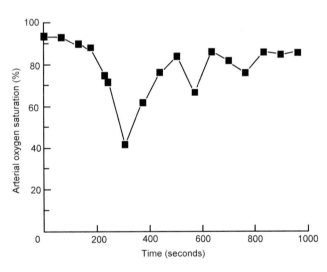

Fig. 21.2 Example of prolonged arterial oxygen desaturation after sedation with midazolam and pethidine (meperidine) [40]

premedication using target-controlled infusions (TCI) before surgery, significantly reducing state anxiety visual analogue scores [49]. A subset of these patients rated propofol superior to previous benzodiazepine premedication. Interestingly subsequent analysis of these data revealed that those with the highest visual analogue anxiety score before sedation had the largest drop in anxiety after propofol (Fig. 21.3).

The benefits of propofol delivered by patient-maintained sedation compared to standard sedation with midazolam were compared in a large randomised controlled trial by our group [50]. This study was powered to detect a difference in arterial oxygen saturation, and indeed there was a statistically higher SpO_2 in the propofol compared to midazolam patients, with the only patient reaching an unsafe level in the midazolam group. Perhaps the most striking result was that propofol was shown to be a superior anxiolytic to midazolam. The VAS recordings of anxiety taken after sedation immediately prior to surgery were compared with baseline anxiety measurements. The propofol patients had almost double the mean reduction in anxiety compared to the midazolam patients (Fig. 21.4). Despite this superior anxiolysis in the propofol group, there was significantly less depression of psychomotor function (as measured by digit-symbol substitution scores) when the patients felt adequately sedated and faster return to baseline after cessation of sedation. Furthermore, despite taking longer to reach readiness for the start of surgery, the faster recovery to meet discharge criteria more than offset this reducing overall sedation time.

Propofol has potential problems with respiratory depression, reduction in blood pressure and paradoxical excitement [51]. However, experience in over 4000 patients receiving true conscious sedation with TCI propofol and alfentanil analgesia for oocyte retrieval suggests that

Fig. 21.3 Individual patients ranked by baseline state anxiety measured by visual analogue scale (*dark grey* column), with subsequent anxiety measurement after propofol premedication. Of note is that the patients with the highest baseline state anxiety had the greatest reduction in anxiety with propofol [49]

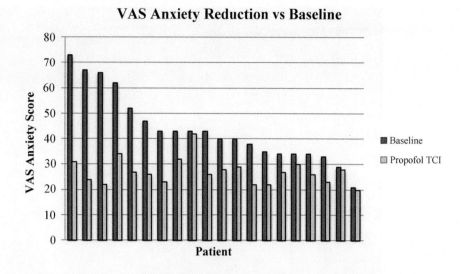

Fig. 21.4 Reduction in baseline anxiety score measured by VAS after receiving sedation with midazolam and propofol delivered by patient-maintained sedation (PMS) [50]

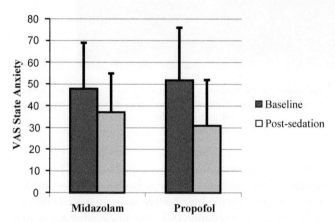

respiratory and airway events are extremely rare (0.5/1000), as is paradoxical excitement (1.4/1000) [52]. There is no reversal agent for propofol, so with oversedation the drug administration must be stopped, and supportive care provided until the plasma drug level reduces. This reinforces the need for reliable prevention of oversedation and loss of verbal contact.

Its main limitation is that it generally needs a quite sophisticated mechanism of delivery. Intermittent bolus provides fleeting sedation with possible over and undersedation. It has been delivered by patient-controlled sedation [46, 53, 54], by manual infusions [37, 45] and more recently with target-controlled infusions [55, 56]. The measured plasma concentration required to reach a standard sedation level (approximating the loss of verbal contact) varies hugely between individuals, 0.2–2.7 $\mu g \cdot ml^{-1}$ range [55]. Even after temazepam premedication, this wide range did not change much, but the elderly were more sensitive [56].

Pharmacokinetics: The Difficulty with Propofol Administration for Sedation [57]

Although propofol has many desirable properties, the main problem with its use for sedation is deciding the best mode of delivery. Its three-compartment pharmacokinetics make it obvious that for anything except a simple induction of anaesthesia (bolus dose), quite complicated dose regimens are required to achieve and then maintain a steady plasma concentration [58].

It is known that intermittent boluses provide oscillating plasma concentrations (Cp) and predicted brain concentrations or effect-site concentrations (Ce), and thus alternating overdose and underdose is quite possible (Fig. 21.5). A combination of bolus and continuous infusions is more useful as they provide steadier Cp, Ce and clinical effects. It is relatively easy to calculate a loading dose if we know the desired plasma concentration ($C_{desired}$) and the volume of distribution (Vd). Maintenance infusions require knowledge of clearance and the rate constant values between the compartments of the appropriate pharmacokinetic model. The concept of context-sensitive half-time (the principle that observed half-life is dependent on the duration of the infusion) and its relationship to published redistribution half-life ($t_{1/2}\alpha$) and elimination half-life ($t_{1/2}\beta$) are not straightforward and make matters more complex [59, 60]. In short, the pharmacokinetics involved are complicated and difficult in practice for the clinician [60].

Target-Controlled Infusions [61]

These use a pharmacokinetic model and a microprocessor to control delivery of the sedative or anaesthetic drug via a syringe pump. The anaesthetist enters some patient factors

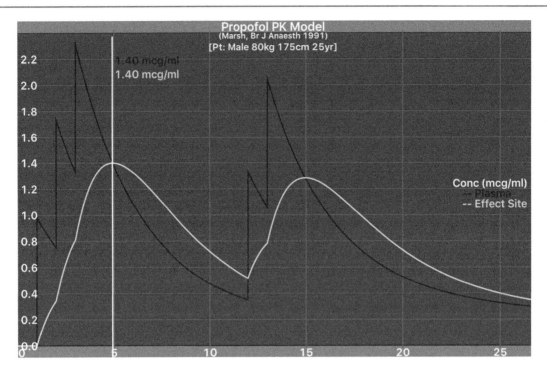

Fig. 21.5 Intermittent boluses of propofol for sedation showing oscillating predicted plasma concentrations and the effect-site concentration (*y*-axis) lagging behind. Note when the last bolus is given, there is a shorter lag in effect-site concentration than with

midazolam. However, after the last dose, both plasma and effect-site concentration fall rapidly. These are calculated using a pharmacokinetic simulator using the Marsh model

such as weight, age, sex and height, some drug factors such as drug concentration and the desired plasma (Cp) or effect-site (Ce) concentration—the "target concentration". The microprocessor calculates the amount of drug required to achieve that concentration, automatically administering a loading dose, and varying the infusion rate to keep the Cp_{target} steady. The anaesthetist observes the patient and alters the target up or down if required depending on the clinical response of that patient. The development of TCI techniques using microprocessors and pharmacokinetic models such as the Diprifusor™ revolutionised the delivery of propofol infusions in anaesthesia. This made simple delivery of propofol infusions possible for the average anaesthetist.

The actual plasma concentration may not be the same as the calculated concentration; however, it is generally more stable and predictable compared with a manual infusion regimen. Although, there is little evidence for anaesthesia that outcomes are better with TCI [62], anaesthetists have to make fewer adjustments and seem to prefer it [63, 64]. TCI pumps can also calculate predicted brain concentration or "effect-site concentration" [65]. For this it uses a rate constant k_{e0} that describes equilibration of plasma concentration and clinical effect (usually measured by a depth of anaesthesia monitor). It can also calculate time to reach a predetermined concentration, which can be set by the user.

It seems clear that delivery is simpler using TCI technology and practitioners prefer this to manual infusions. Indeed it did not take long for anaesthetists to apply this technology to the provision of sedation [56], and anaesthetist-controlled sedation using TCI propofol remains a popular technique. Similarly to data from studies providing general anaesthesia with TCI propofol, when it is used for conscious sedation during monitored anaesthetic care, anaesthetists have to make fewer pump adjustments than with manual infusions [66]. The main problem is that non-anaesthetists deliver the majority of sedation in our healthcare system, and they generally do not have access to TCI pumps or training in their use.

Patient-Activated Drug Delivery Systems: PCA, PCS and PMS

Patient-Controlled Analgesia

At a similar time to the development of TCI techniques, patient-controlled analgesia (PCA) was becoming popular in the control of postoperative pain with opioids. The premise being that the patient could self-administer small doses of an opioid when experiencing pain, giving them control over their own pain relief. The main safety feature is the "lock-out" which is the period of time when they can't self-administer any further drug, until the first dose had begun to achieve its effect. PCA opioid was a revolution. Despite patients using similar amounts of drugs to when administered by a nurse and consequently having very similar pain scores and adverse event rates [67], patient satisfaction with these techniques was much better [67, 68].

Patient-Controlled Sedation

The first application of the PCA principle to sedation, and the first report of patient self-administered sedation with propofol "patient-controlled sedation" (PCS), was in 1991 [53]. When compared with midazolam, propofol seemed a better choice of agent as patients had a feeling of well-being [32, 54], higher satisfaction [34, 54] and faster recovery [32, 34, 54], despite less amnesia and less suppression of psychometric testing [32, 54]. There have been some concerns about restlessness or disinhibition with the use of propofol by PCS [33]; however, others have rated patient cooperation higher [34].

Patient satisfaction seems higher with PCS than when propofol is administered by a physician or nurse either by infusion or bolus [55, 69–71]. Generally anaesthetists give more drug and titrate to deeper levels of sedation [69, 70, 72, 73] and higher plasma concentrations [55]. Accordingly there is less oversedation [55, 69, 70, 72] and less amnesia [70] with PCS. Patients generally prefer self-administration when they try both as a crossover trial [55, 69] or have higher levels of satisfaction when group comparisons are done [70]. This higher satisfaction occurs, even when exactly the same PCS pump with the same dose and lockout is self-administered, compared with when given by a nurse for them [71].

Various approaches have been made to vary the "bolus" dose administered with each button press and the "lockout" period between boluses to achieve optimum sedation, patient satisfaction without oversedation. The first report described a 0.7 mg·kg^{-1} bolus and a 1 min lockout [54]. There are two broad approaches: a small bolus dose generally less than 10 mg and short or no lockout [46, 74, 75], a larger dose 20–40 mg with a longer lockout of 3–5 min [4, 33, 76–78]. There is also an in-between approach of moderate dose 18–20 mg with a short 1 min lockout [32, 69, 79]. Even within the same group, settings have changed study to study, presumably searching for the perfect balance of access to drug and safety [32, 53, 54, 69]. In the end there are lots of opinions on what is best, but no direct comparisons.

The zero lockout patient-controlled sedation (ZLPCS) is interesting [80]. With this instead of using the lockout to limit the dose of sedative, the maximum infusion rate of the pump is used. The dose rate depends on the physical maximum rate of travel of the plunger on the pump, and to add complexity also depends on the cross-sectional area of the syringe used [81]. Surprisingly it seems that even with unlimited access to propofol, patients deliver less than if an anaesthetist was controlling a TCI pump [55]. Some have made the concept of PCS even more complicated by advocating the principle of fuzzy logic demonstrated in PCA [82] applied to PCS [81].

Many PCS settings use a fixed dose making no attempt to individualise drug administration to the patient. Even using rudimentary pharmacokinetic principles, one would expect patient factors, e.g. weight, to affect the relationship between dose and plasma concentration hence effect.

Patient-Maintained Sedation

Patient-maintained sedation (PMS) combines the steady plasma concentrations of TCI with the patient-controlled function of PCS [83]. Initially, the system is set to administer propofol to a predetermined target Cp (or more recently Ce). The first reported initial target 1.0 μg·ml^{-1} was based on experience of range of Cp that patients obtain adequate anxiolysis and sedation. It then allows the patient to increase the TCI target by pressing the button. The size of the stepwise increase is determined by the "increment" and was originally described as 0.2 mg·ml^{-1} up to a preset maximum 3.0 μg·ml^{-1}. There is a lockout period (originally 2 min) that prevents the patient increasing the target concentration until the clinical effect has had a chance to equilibrate after an increase in Cp. There is usually some programmed condition, e.g. a period of no button presses (6–12 min), that prompts the pump to reduce the target. There is an implied safety feature, similar to the premise used in PCS, that an oversedated patient would not be able to press the button and demand more drug. This was modified to make it more difficult for an uncoordinated sedated patient to increase the Cp. The original versions of PMS required a double click of the button within 1 s to activate an increased Cp. Despite this sedation scores in volunteers encouraged to take as much propofol as possible reflected some oversedation. Subsequent experience in a younger cohort of real patients having dental surgery revealed no loss of verbal contact, high patient satisfaction and cooperation with the surgeon [84]. However, there was one patient desaturated to less than 90 % and an epileptic patient who had three grand mal seizures. Attempts were then made to alter the settings to prevent possible oversedation as reported in the initial study. Despite these technical problems in the early studies, a crossover comparison was performed with PCS; patients seem to prefer PMS [85]. PMS patients reached adequate sedation faster, but this was at the cost of some oversedation. It seems that the theoretical benefits of steadier plasma concentration improved patient satisfaction with the quality of sedation.

Pharmacokinetics and Pharmacodynamics Relevant to Propofol Sedation

The main pharmacological issues when using any microprocessor-delivered drug system (such as TCI or PMS) are the choice of pharmacokinetic model, choice of k_{e0}, and deciding whether to deliver drug to target plasma or effect-site concentration. All versions of the PMS system used the same PK and PD models as the Diprifusor™. It is important to know the suitability of this model in contrast to alternatives.

Pharmacokinetic Models

Most anaesthetists globally became familiar with the use of TCI to deliver propofol with the Diprifusor™ system. The first description of the prototype Diprifusor™ [86] used the Marsh propofol PK model [87] as its basis for drug delivery. The Diprifusor's PK model was first explicitly described in a study looking at the performance of the adult model used in children [88].

This study reported that this adult PK model was unsuitable for use in children and detailed an alternative data set for use in children. This became known as the Marsh model.

Subsequently other models have been suggested, the main rival model being the Schnider model [89]. This was proposed considerably after the clinical introduction of the Diprifusor™ and about the same time that the first estimates of Cp_{50} were being reported [90]. Confusingly some of the first open TCI systems available in the UK allowed the Schnider model to be chosen to deliver TIVA even though the predictive performance was not clear at the time, and there were major errors in the implementation in that with a heavy patient, the calculated lean body mass could decrease to zero or less. The importance of knowing the features of the models available and the relative merits of each has been stressed [91]. The major difference between the Marsh/

Diprifusor™ model and the Schnider model is the small fixed volume of distribution of the Schnider model, which therefore gives a considerably smaller bolus at induction than the Marsh. Because of the small central volume, the Schnider must be used in so-called "effect" mode, but in reality this model still delivers less drug than the Marsh model in plasma mode. The result is that the calculated effect-site concentration for the Schnider model is incorrect for the first 15 min after changing a target concentration [115]. So an anaesthetist inadvertently using the Schnider model when used to using the Marsh will deliver **significantly less drug** than they intended. A further major factor is that the Marsh PK model is the only one which has been approved for clinical use by regulatory authorities throughout the world. All of our studies used the Marsh model.

Predictive Performance of Pharmacokinetic Models

It was acknowledged from an early stage that the target concentration (Cp_{target}) was an *estimate* of the individual patient's actual plasma concentration and that measured plasma concentration ($Cp_{measured}$) would be different [92]. The predictive performance of TCI systems should be described in terms of the magnitude and direction of this inaccuracy [93]. The terms used to describe performance error are defined in Table 21.3. The initial study to establish the magnitude of these errors with the Diprifusor™ was published in 1998 [92]. Measured and predicted concentrations from the Diprifusor™ were compared in 46 patients of both sexes between 18 and 80 years old, at different phases of propofol infusion (induction, maintenance and recovery). The performance of the Diprifusor™ system was established by comparing the predicted concentration Cp_{target} with a laboratory measured value $Cp_{measured}$, for each patient at each time point. The inaccuracy (MDAPE) was 24 %, bias (MDPE) +15 %, divergence

Table 21.3 Glossary of terms used in describing the performance of a TCI system [93]

Performance error		Plain language description
Bias Median performance error (MDPE)	$(Cp_{measured} - Cp_{target}) \times 100/Cp_{target}$ The median value as a % and direction	Systematic over or under prediction of a device
Precision Median absolute performance error (MDAPE)	Median $(Cp_{measured} - Cp_{target})$	Size of error/inaccuracy
Divergence	1. Slope of the linear regression of absolute performance error (APE) versus time 2. Regression of signed PE against time	Change in performance error over time
Wobble	The median absolute deviation of PE from MDPE	Failure to keep a steady plasma concentration over time
Accuracy		Size of the average difference between $Cp_{measured} + Cp_{target}$

-8 % h^{-1} and wobble at steady state 22 %. These were felt to be clinically acceptable and of similar magnitude to the difference between end-tidal and arterial anaesthetic gas monitoring [94]. The most interesting observation was pattern of errors: measured concentration was higher than predicted during induction and lower than predicted during emergence.

More recently other models have been proposed: the Schüttler model [95] which was defined after studying the largest number of recruited subjects, 270, and an adapted Diprifusor™ model proposed by White [96] which addresses the difference in clearance between men and women, especially related to aging. Comparisons have been made of these four main pharmacokinetic candidates: Diprifusor™ (Marsh), Schnider, Schüttler and White [97]. Overall median bias (MDPE) was lowest for Schnider at -0.1 % and then Diprifusor™ $+2.3$ % and worst for White at -12.6 % although the range of bias in patients was remarkably similar. The devil is as always in the detail, as the bias is negligible for the Schnider model because measured concentration is less than predicted in the early phase and greater than predicted at termination of infusion phase cancelling each other out. The Diprifusor™ is the opposite, measured concentration is greater than predicted in the early phase (by around half of the level of Schnider prediction error) and less than predicted at termination of infusion. The overall median inaccuracy (MDAPE) was very similar between all groups at 20–24 % as was the wobble at 14–19 %; however divergence was worst for the Schnider model at $+13$ %.h^{-1} compared to 1–2 % for the other models. More recently a similar comparison was performed between Diprifusor™, White and Schnider using the original data from the Swinhoe study [98]. Essentially, overall Diprifusor™ and Schnider have very similar levels of bias (MDPE) 16 and 15 %, respectively, and of inaccuracy (MDAPE) of 26 and 23 %, respectively. The pattern of over and under-reads was the same. The newer White model appears better with a bias of 5 % and inaccuracy of 19 % [98]. None of the models accounted fully for the extent of interindividual variation in propofol clearance, but the improved performance with the White model suggests it may have some advantages over the others. Eleveldt and colleagues have taken an innovative approach to defining the "best" PK model [99]. The models discussed generally describe the best PK parameters for the (often small) group of patients studied in the situation studied. They rightly point out that there is uncertainty of the accuracy of the models with different patients and clinical conditions, and caution should be applied when extrapolating a model to a population different to that from which it was developed. To this end they have created a large data set from 21 previously published studies using opentci.org data and collaborative data sharing between groups. This gave them over 10,000 data points from 660 individuals of with widely varying patient features such as age, BMI and clinical situations. A new PK model was generated using allometric scaling, which when retrospectively tested performed better than all other models for the complete data set. This may be a model that has wider applicability in clinical practice. This needs to be tested prospectively, but initial indicators are that it could be very useful in clinical practice [100].

Applying Population Pharmacokinetics to Individuals

The transformation of a drug dose profile to a plasma or effect-site concentration is done by each individual patient's body, and drug concentration achieved is a result of their variation from the summary values of the PK model used to guide drug administration. This is present whether using standard dose regimens or TCI technology. Shafer's group has published simulation studies of a population bearing the same variation as reference pharmacokinetic data and described the coefficient of variation (CV) after bolus dose, fixed rate infusion and TCI. They show that CV is highest for bolus dosing and identical for both types of infusion [101]. These simulation data are backed up with limited retrospective animal data. He addresses the criticism of the performance of TCI systems by pointing out that this is what we would expect by biological variation and less variation than we accept every day with intravenous induction of anaesthesia by bolus dose. Measuring the predictive performance of TCI devices shows the magnitude of biologic variability. However they do not cause the biological variability. It is completely understandable that investigators strive to compare and refine models and produce systems with minimal bias, inaccuracy, wobble and divergence. It is likely that TCI will in fact *reduce* the impact of biologic variability by accounting for patient factors that influence the concentration achieved from the same dose with increasingly complex models. For instance, a vast array of patient factors have been shown to influence the accuracy of PK and PD models for propofol: from the common known and accepted weight [88, 102]and age [89, 95, 96, 103] to the less known but interesting smoking status [104], alcoholism [105], cirrhosis [106], use of anticonvulsants [107], ethnicity [108] and even phase of the menstrual cycle [109], to the controversial obesity [110–113] and to the speculative cardiac output [114] and eventually perhaps even pharmacogenetics.

Pharmacodynamics: Using Measures of Drug Effects

No matter how sophisticated PK and PD models become, it is probable, however, that these will always be limited by biologic variability. It has been shown that using some form of assessment of the clinical effect of the drug to control administration reduces unwanted side effects [115]. It is likely that this adjusts for pharmacodynamic variability, by defining whether that individual patient requires less than average drug dose (nearer Ce_{05}), average drug dose (nearer Ce_{50}) or above average drug dose (nearer Ce_{95}) by allowing the patient to be titrated to defined clinical effect within the range of effect-site concentrations described by an investigated population. Sophisticated simulation studies confirm that using some defined clinical end point entered by the operator reduces the impact of biological variability [116]. This equally applies to measuring patient clinical effect directly.

A novel way to decide on choice of PK model is, rather than looking at how the predicted concentration compares to measured concentration, to look at the how different model estimation of Ce compares to a measured clinical effect of the drug. Sutcliffe's group compared the performance of the Marsh and Schnider models with patients who were administered with propofol to a Ce_{target} using the Schnider model (and simulated Ce with Marsh) and administered to a Cp_{target} using the Marsh model (and simulated Ce with Schnider) [117]. Correlation of Ce was made with measured sedation score (observer's assessment of alertness/sedation scale, OAAS) and Bispectral Index (BIS). Correlation was considerably better between the predicted Ce and the surrogate markers of effect for both groups with the Marsh model. Indeed, the Schnider model in so-called "effect" mode produced a Ce profile that matched those achieved by the Marsh model used in "plasma" mode. This could reflect a more suitable PK model, k_{e0} (rate constant describing

equilibration between plasma and brain or effect site), or both with the Marsh model (Fig. 21.6).

Defining k_{e0}

The use of effect-site-driven drug delivery is more than just choosing the "correct" or best estimate (for the population) of k_{e0}. It also changes the pattern of drug delivery, increasing Cp over the desired Ce to speed up drug movement to the site of action and achieving the effect-site target. It increases the complexity of the system, increasing choices for the end user and increasing the likelihood of significantly altering the amount of drug delivered, for good or bad [91]. Traditionally k_{e0} was determined by measuring time to peak effect with a surrogate of drug effect (BIS or auditory evoked potentials (AEP)) and assuming plasma and effect site had equilibrated at this point [118]. Mathematical modelling may be done with these data to determine the k_{e0} that causes the flattest concentration-effect hysteresis curve. It is still an average of a biological parameter that varies by a factor of up to four in the population [65] and is subject to variability with patient factors such as age [103]. There are a wide variety of values quoted; Schnider calculated 0.45 min^{-1} [103]. Whereas the original work used for the Diprifusor™ k_{e0} was 0.20 min^{-1} [65] and later found as 0.26 min^{-1} in the commercially available TCI pumps, an adjustment which gave the same Ce at induction and recovery [119, 120]. These different values could reflect the best fit for each particular PK model; however even using the Marsh model, it has been suggested the faster k_{e0} of 1.2 min^{-1} is a better fit for the time to peak effect observed with BIS, perhaps reflecting the use of a different

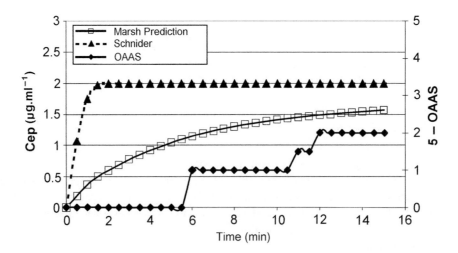

Fig. 21.6 Propofol effect-site concentration versus sedation score in Schnider-driven TCI group (20 patients). The *triangles* represent the propofol effect-site concentration predicted by the Schnider model. The *squares* represent the propofol effect-site concentration as predicted by the Marsh model as calculated by the Tivatrainer when the same bolus and infusion rates are used. Predicted propofol concentration (Cep) is plotted on the primary y-axis. The *diamonds* represent the median sedation score on an inverted scale as calculated by 5-OAAS plotted on a secondary y-axis. It can be seen that observed sedation score correlates better with the Marsh estimate of Ce propofol. The Schnider model predicts sedation should be maximal at 1–2 min (reproduced from Reference [117] with permission from John Wiley and Sons)

EEG monitor [121]. There is debate over how best to determine k_{e0}, acknowledging that the delay in data acquisition with depth of anaesthesia monitors could have a significant effect on the measured k_{e0}. The use of a direct clinical measure seems more logical than a surrogate. Loss of eyelash reflex [122] and more recently by defining which value delivers stable sedation level have been used [123]. When using stable sedation assessed by OAAS and choice reaction time, a faster k_{e0} than that we used on our model of 0.6 min^{-1} seemed the best fit. The observed clinical effect is probably a combination of PK and PD factors [124]. All in all, when using effect-site-driven sedation, it is perhaps difficult to see how variation in clinical effect would not be greater by adding another factor with biological variability to a system. Certainly our data from the safety study described below using Ce-driven propofol delivery suggested clinical effect was more unpredictable, with more oversedation than our earlier plasma-driven systems [125–127]. This may reflect the way in which propofol is delivered: increasing Cp over Ce$_{target}$ and then turning the pump rate to zero so that Cp and Ce meet (Cp falling, Ce rising) while no drug is actually being delivered. This is in contrast to others who have shown no excess haemodynamic effects in an effect-site-driven mode of propofol delivery for general anaesthesia [121]. The fact that haemodynamic effects take longer to equilibrate than hypnosis may confound this observation [128].

Safety Studies for Patient-Maintained Sedation

Asking volunteers to deliberately attempt to oversedate themselves was used as a "stress test" to assess the safety of the PMS system [126]. The premise being if volunteers could not accidentally oversedate themselves when deliberately trying to "defeat" the system, then patients could not do this when the systems were in clinical use. However, a small proportion of volunteers with this original system could oversedate, calling into question the safety of the button

press as the main method of limiting increase in Cp in oversedated patients.

Changes were made to the settings to slow the increase in sedation level. Despite reducing the initial concentration, increment dose and increasing the lockout, one volunteer from 20 still achieved an unsafe SpO$_2$ [127].

Methods to Attempt to Prevent Oversedation

Using Effect-Site-Driven PMS

Our initial studies confirmed the benefits of propofol sedation by PMS over midazolam [50] and showed the utility and high patient satisfaction in dental surgery [50, 84]. Our main focus was to achieve a method of preventing oversedation as we had reported in our safety studies where volunteers deliberately attempted to oversedate using plasma concentration-delivered PMS [126]. Our analysis of the reason for the oversedated volunteers was that they likely demanded more propofol when the clinical effect was lagging behind the plasma concentration. Hence when they stopped pressing the button, the effect site/clinical effect of propofol continued to rise after they could not manage to press the button leading to loss of verbal contact. Initial attempts to prevent this scenario were tried by reducing the initial Cp target (0.5 μg·ml^{-1}), increasing the lockout time (4 min) and reducing the increments with each button press (0.1 μg·ml^{-1}) [127]. Surprisingly a volunteer still reached an unsafe end point (desaturation) without losing verbal contact. Hence we hypothesised that if we delivered to predicted effect-site concentration, this would make the system safer. We tested this with a very similar study design except using an effect-site-controlled PMS system [125]. This system delivered propofol to an initial Ce target of 1.0 μg·ml^{-1} by increasing Cp up to 100 % higher than the target Ce (Fig. 21.7). This was to speed up drug delivery to the brain and then reducing the Cp as the predicted Ce approached the target.

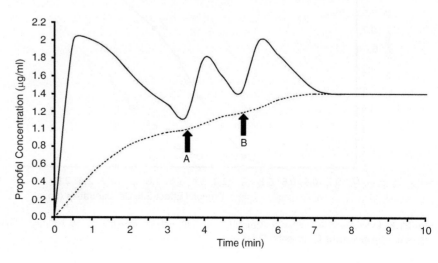

Fig. 21.7 Demonstration of how an effect-site-driven PMS system increased Cp (*solid line*) to a level 100 % higher than Ce target to speed up drug movement in to the brain (Ce). It reduces this Cp/Ce gradient as Ce (*dotted line*) approaches target and allows further drug demand when Ce and Cp are within 10 % at points A and B

However, we found that this made unsafe sedation *more likely* not less; 20 % of the volunteers desaturated and 20 % lost verbal contact. Although others have suggested that effect-site control delivery of propofol anaesthesia does not cause extra morbidity, our study design is somewhat artificial in that volunteers are deliberately trying to oversedate. Furthermore, it was clear that some volunteers could press the demand button even when sedated enough to forget to press the button. While we were initially surprised by these results, in retrospect, it was perhaps understandable.

With effect-site control, the system uses higher Cp values than plasma control. This probably exacerbates any variations of clinical effect in individuals who differ from the population mean PK and PD values. Oversedation is likely to occur if a patient's actual measured Cp is greater than target (positive bias), and their k_{e0} is faster (fast equilibrators). Hence they have a higher concentration gradient for blood-brain equilibration and a faster equilibration constant. The main danger here is early during sedation.

With plasma control, the Cp is titrated to the target the anaesthetist considers necessary to achieve the required clinical effect, and the effect-site concentration "catches up" based on that patients k_{e0}. The main danger here is in those with a slow k_{e0} such as the elderly. The anaesthetist (or patient controlling the system) may think they require more drug for the desired clinical effect and titrates the target upwards when in reality it is simply the slow k_{e0} which has not allowed the drug to achieve its full effect on the patient. When this happens there may be delayed oversedation when the effect site catches up with the plasma control. This is obviously a complex area and highlights why PK and PD models and using average sedation requirements are always likely to cause a few unexpected clinical effects. It is clear that either careful titration is required by an anaesthesiologist in attendance or a method of individual feedback that detects that the clinical effect is close to oversedation and reduces propofol dose is required to prevent oversedation and adverse outcomes.

Using Reaction Time as Patient Feedback

It became obvious to us that individual variability means that application of population pharmacokinetics and simply limiting increments in drug dose and/or the lockout time between these increments are unlikely to provide a system with which accidental oversedation can be prevented. Our group had previously studied the effects of alcohol and propofol on complex measures of reaction time [129, 130]. The involvement of a psychologist expert in psychometric measurement encouraged us to pursue reaction time as a means of providing individual patient feedback to the PMS system. And whereas our study of the effects of propofol on reaction time (RT) is perhaps not novel, our study of the reaction time right up to the point of onset of anaesthesia, and the way we interpreted these data, is unique. In summary there is a huge range of predicted Ce that causes each individual to become sedated to the point of losing verbal contact (Fig. 21.8) [131].

However, the pattern of slow deterioration of RT initially with an exponential slowing just before loss of verbal contact was the key in our understanding of how best to prevent oversedation. The observation that there is a threefold variation in Ce at this point (Fig. 21.9), whereas there was very little variation in the pattern of RT slowing (Fig. 21.10) suggested that this could be an effective warning of impending loss of verbal contact. Comparison of the EC_{50} from the dose–response curves of Ce increment immediately

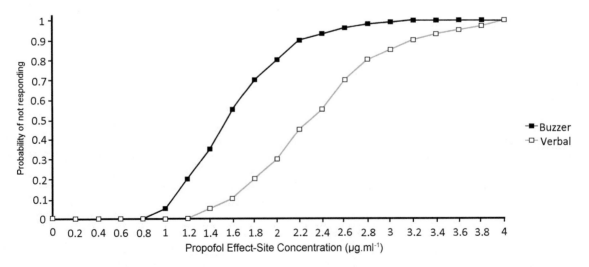

Fig. 21.8 Dose–response curves constructed by probit analysis showing the probability of not responding to vibrating handset and verbal response with increasing Ce propofol [131]

Fig. 21.9 The change in reaction time from baseline (100 %) with increasing Ce propofol. Note the interpatient variation in the dose required to stop the patient responding to the vibrating handset [131]

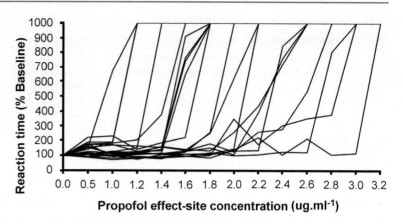

Fig. 21.10 Mean change in patient reaction time from baseline measurement (100 %) at the five changes of the calculated effect-site concentration of propofol before the concentration at which loss of response to the vibrating handset (CeLOR) occurred in that patient [131]. Error bars are SD

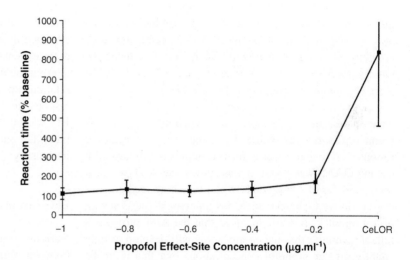

before the rapid increase in RT with the Ce at loss of verbal contact suggests there is a reasonable separation of 0.7 µg·ml^{-1} or 3 PMS increments. This shows that RT *could* be a suitable patient feedback mechanism. We tested this hypothesis by performing our standard "stress test" safety study using RT-controlled PMS. This study demonstrated that for the first time, volunteers could not use the PMS system to oversedate despite trying and confirmed the utility of this approach [132].

We are not the first to report the effect of sedative drugs in general and propofol in particular on reaction time. Members of our own group studied the effect of alcohol [129] and propofol [130] on psychomotor measures relevant to driving. This used a sophisticated computer system and monitor to measure changes in dual-task tracking, secondary reaction time and choice reaction time. Increasing Cp propofol from 0.2 to 0.8 µg·ml^{-1} caused a significant deterioration in all measures, with quite high individual variation (wide 95 % confidence intervals). Another group used complicated goggles with light-emitting diode lights and headphone system to measure visual and auditory reaction time [133]. They showed that both deteriorated with increasing Ce propofol with a rapid slowing RT before loss of responsiveness

(no response for 10 s). The mean propofol level at which patients stopped responding to visual stimulus was a mean of Ce 1.2 µg·ml^{-1} and for auditory stimulus a mean of Ce 1.4 µg·ml^{-1}. Again, there was considerable interpatient variability. More recently another group measured the choice RT using a mobile phone during propofol sedation [134]. This required the volunteer to use both hands. Again they found that RT slowed gradually initially then rapidly before loss of response between Ce 1.1 and 2.5 µg·ml^{-1}. The same pattern of large inter-volunteer variation in Ce propofol at loss of response was again noted. All of these methods of using RT as a measure of sedation are novel, interesting research approaches, but more cumbersome than our system which measures RT via the patient demand button which is integrated with the infusion pump.

Response to Verbal Stimulus as Patient Feedback

It has previously suggested that using a clinical measure in addition to PK/TCI improves the delivery of sedation [116]. Using response to a verbal stimulus has been proposed

Table 21.4 Observer's assessment of alertness/sedation scale

Subscore	Responsiveness	Speech	Facial expression	Eyes
5	Responds readily to name spoken in normal tone	Normal	Normal	Clear, no ptosis
4	Lethargic response to name spoken in normal tone	Mild slowing or thickening	Mild relaxation	Glazed or mild ptosis
3	Responds only after name is spoken loudly and repeatedly or both	Slurring or prominent slowing	Marked relaxation (slack jaw)	Glazed and marked ptosis
2	Responds only after mild prodding or shaking	Few recognised words		
1	Does not respond to mild prodding or shaking			

Reproduced from Reference [136] with permission from Wolters Kluwer Health, Inc.

as a method of patient feedback as the automated responsiveness test (ART) [135]. This system automatically prompts the patient to press a button up to five times with increasingly louder voice and stronger handset vibration; lack of response (in 10 s) is used to indicate too deep sedation. This was compared to a score out of 20 using the Observer's Assessment of Alertness/Sedation Scale (OAAS) [136] scoring all subcategories (Table 21.4), a score of 10/20 was defined as a loss of consciousness. Twenty volunteers were studied during TCI propofol sedation (controlled by Stanpump software) while breathing 30 % oxygen or Entonox. A linear inverse relationship between propofol Ce and OAAS was noted. It was shown that ART was lost at a mean Ce of 1.6 $\mu g \cdot ml^{-1}$ while breathing oxygen; this was at a lower Ce level than the loss of consciousness at a Ce of 1.9 $\mu g \cdot ml^{-1}$. It was concluded that the ART provides a reliable warning that unconsciousness will develop at only slightly greater propofol concentrations, but this is in the area of sedation where "red alert events" (physiological derangement, mostly apnoea) occur.

This occurred in 4/20 breathing oxygen and 5/20 breathing nitrous oxide. The most obvious criticism is that by definition, when a patient was failed to respond to ART, they have lost verbal contact and by the UK definition are unconscious or anaesthetised. The fact that physiological adverse events were occurring in 20 % of volunteers at this point strengthens the UK advice to maintain verbal contact. Also their definition of unconsciousness of 10/20 OAAS is significantly more sedated than our definition. They must score 3/5 eyes, glazed eyes with marked ptosis; 3/5 facial expression, marked relaxation and slack jaw; 2–3/5 speech, marked slurring or few recognisable words; and 1–2/5 responsiveness, responds after mild prodding or shaking or does not respond at all. Subsequently the same group changed their definition of unconsciousness to be more simply calculated using just the responsiveness score and has taken a score of 2/5 only responding to mild prodding or shaking as being unconscious [137]. Furthermore they added "ART delay" defining the number of prompts required to respond. They then tested this new system during propofol sedation again with patients breathing Entonox and after washout, oxygen alone. They correlated the new ART delay with sedation scale (OAAS) and BIS monitoring. ART and ART delay had a worse prediction probability than BIS for distinguishing OAAS 3 (acceptable/moderate sedation) from 2 (excessive/deep sedation). Although more sensitive than BIS of 70 at detecting oversedation, this was at the expense of poor specificity. A more recent study, again altering the ART delay (to 4 prompts in 10 s), confirmed the relationship of ART and OAASS [138]. The Ce_{50} for loss of response to ART was at Ce 1.7 $\mu g \cdot ml^{-1}$, OAASS 12–13 and BIS 75. Furthermore ART was lost and returned at essentially the same Ce, within acceptable limits of bias and inaccuracy.

EEG Monitors as Patient Feedback

Various groups have sought to define the relationship between sedation level and measures of EEG: BIS [137–143], spectral edge frequency [139, 144], auditory evoked potential [142, 143] and spectral entropy [144, 145]. Milne showed nicely the relationship between clinically important end points [143]: loss of verbal contact "unconsciousness" and anaesthesia "no response to pain", with propofol dose (predicted Cp and Ce) and the changes in BIS and AEP associated with these. Of note the Ce_{50} for loss of verbal contact was 2.8 (95 % CI 2.7–2.9) $\mu g \cdot ml^{-1}$. The Ce propofol at this clinical end point varied significantly between individuals from low end of the dose–response curve Ce_{05} 1.5 $\mu g \cdot ml^{-1}$ (95 % CI 1.3–1.7) and high end of the dose–response curve Ce_{95} 4.1 $\mu g \cdot ml^{-1}$ (95% CI 3.9–4.3), almost a threefold difference. The BIS and AEPindex (AEPex) at loss of verbal contact show similar dose–response patterns with similarly impressive p values for linear regression goodness of fit test. The values at Cp_{50} are quite different BIS of 71 (95% CI 69–72) and AEPex 54 (95% CI 53–56). Similarly there is a large population variation at loss of verbal contact in BIS between Ce_{05} 89 (95% CI 86–92) and Ce_{95} 53 (95% CI 47–57), effectively 47–92, i.e. twofold, and also for AEPex between Ce_{05} 69 (95% CI 67–71) and Ce_{95} 40 (95 % CI 35–43) effectively 35–71, i.e. twofold. Given that this study used the same PK and PD settings as we used in our studies, the results are particularly relevant. However, one interpretation of their data is of course that it suggests that these EEG monitors correlate with drug dose rather than a clinical end point. A premise re-enforced by the observations that the BIS value at which consciousness is lost is higher in the elderly than the young [146], and the dose required for loss of consciousness is lower in the elderly [103].

In addition to the inherent problem with large variation in the EEG monitor levels that the population lose verbal contact at, others have pointed to 7 % BIS probe failure rate [115] and slow acquisition time [116] as making them inherently unsuitable for controlling sedation. However, the more practical consideration of the cost of disposables and poor availability of machines will always make it a difficult technique to convince non-anaesthetists to use.

Commercially Available Sedation System (SEDASYS)

Recently the ART monitor has been incorporated into the commercially available sedation system SEDASYS [147]. This system is a computer-assisted propofol infusion and bolus delivery system controlled by an endoscopist, with integrated patient monitoring (Fig. 21.8). This was approved by the FDA in 2013 but with several restrictions: the use in ASA grade 1 and 2 patients older than 18 years only, use for minimal and moderate sedation only, use for colonoscopy and esophagogastroduodenoscopy procedures only and use only by physicians who have received training (propofol pharmacology, identifying high-risk patients, identification of levels of sedation, use of capnometry and assessment of adequacy of ventilation and management of airways obstruction and hypoventilation). Finally it is only approved in institutions where there is an anaesthesiologist immediately available to assist or consult. Sales have been disappointing, and the owners Johnson and Johnson indicated their intention to stop selling SEDASYS in March 2016 [148].

SEDASYS Sedation Protocol

After a loading dose of up to 0.5 mg·kg^{-1} given over 3 min, the propofol infusion rate can be commenced between 25 and 75 µg·kg min^{-1} as determined by the endoscopist. Extra bolus doses of 0.25 mg·kg^{-1} can be given by the physician to treat transient unpleasant procedures. The propofol infusion is allowed to increase and is reduced, or suspended in response to ART. All patients receive a minimum 2 l·min^{-1} of nasal oxygen, which is increased automatically in response to arterial oxygen saturation: 8 l·min^{-1} under 96 % and 12 l·min^{-1} under 88 %.

Depth of Sedation and Adverse Events with SEDASYS

The initial version of SEDASYS published pilot data with the same propofol dosage in 24 patients [149]. Patients were more sedated than would be considered acceptable in the UK, with around 10 % of all sedation measurements at OAAS 3 or less. Adverse event rates were high, with 38 % suffering transient apnoea (less than 30 s) and 6 % oxygen desaturation below 90 %, but no airway interventions. The later version of SEDASYS used the automated responsiveness test [138] to limit increases in infusion rate, and automatically turn the infusion off, then on at a lower rate if ART was lost [147]. This was a randomised controlled unblinded trial in 469 patients comparing sedation for gastrointestinal endoscopy administered with SEDASYS-delivered propofol (average infusion rate around 50 µg·kg.min^{-1}) and current standard of care sedation (CSC) using midazolam (average dose around 5 mg) with opioid used in both groups. There was a large reduction in area under the curve for oxygen desaturation (AUC$_{Desat}$) for SEDASYS compared with the CSC group, with 8 % of SEDASYS group desaturating (to SpO$_2$ less than 90 %) compared to 17 % for CSC. The average desaturation to less than SpO$_2$ of 90 % was 23.6 s (95 % CI 11–36). Secondary outcomes were faster recovery, higher patient and clinician satisfaction and less adverse events despite deeper sedation in the SEDASYS group. These were similar benefits of propofol over midazolam to our comparison (though we had less desaturation and didn't use supplementary oxygen) [50]. Although the majority of patients were sedated appropriately to an OAASS levels of 4 or 5. Closer inspection of sedation levels reveals 2.5 % with SEDASYS had response only to painful stimulus for an average of 5 min (OAASS 1–2), thus the ASA definition of deep sedation or anaesthesia in the UK. There were less adverse events in this group than one might expect; the predominant effect was apnoea without desaturation of 2–25 s (95% CI). It seems likely desaturation rates would have been significantly higher without supplementary oxygen. It is notable that the definitions of adverse events were somewhat unclear or lax: it is unclear what made an oxygen desaturation an adverse event, and apnoea was only considered significant if it lasted 30 s.

Is SEDASYS Patient Feedback Appropriate?

It is likely using *failure* of response to auditory stimulus or the vibrating handset as the trigger a reduction of dose is too deep a plane of sedation to avoid adverse physiological events. If we consider that 15 % reached OAASS 3 or less, a significant amount is in the transition zone between moderate sedation and deep sedation/anaesthesia. The fundamental problem is when aiming for a certain sedation level, biological variability means that the sedationist must be trained and prepared to deal with a deeper than intended level [3].

SEDASYS Post-market Approval Studies

The FDA required more safety data before lifting the current restrictions on the SEDASYS [150]. Accordingly, they have requested that Ethicon prospectively study the response of users to yellow and red alarms (SpO$_2$ less than 92 and 85 %, respectively) in 866 patients. Furthermore, a large post-market study of anaesthesiology intervention rates (bag-mask ventilation, artificial airway), and all adverse and serious adverse events in 7240 patients, is also required. Given they are aiming for a similar level of sedation (OAASS level 4 and 5), but using a deeper level of sedation to trigger reduction in dose than in our study of sedation delivery by non-anaesthetists using TCI propofol augmented by alfentanil, it seems likely that they will have a higher rate of patients requiring airway intervention than we reported of 0.25/1000 patients [52]. This would be unlikely to encourage the lifting of the restriction of the use in an environment with immediate access to anaesthesiology. A significant proportion of patients would fail the UK definition of conscious sedation, making the SEDASYS unsuitable for providing true conscious sedation.

Comparison of SEDASYS Safety Data

If one compares the safety data with SEDASYS with published large series of non-anaesthetist-delivered sedation, we had airway/respiratory events at a rate of 0.5/1000 patients [52], Australian general practitioners 4.1/1000 and 2.6/1000 for Australian anaesthetists [18]. The SEDASYS causes oxygen desaturation at a rate of 78/1000 even with significant amounts of supplementary oxygen and apnoea (less than 30 s) in 24/1000. In this context the safety data seems somewhat less than impressive and at similar levels to which we have been critical of studies by emergency medicine physicians [27]. We currently only have limited safety data for the reaction time monitored PMS where under extreme stressing of the system with deliberate attempts at oversedation none lost verbal contact [132]. These data while limited are encouraging enough to warrant a large-scale safety study.

Table 21.5 Published values Cp and Ce of self-administered propofol by patients to obtain adequate sedation

Situation	Propofol concentration (μg·ml^{-1})		Reference
	Mean	Range	
Plasma pre-med (General surgery)	1.3	0.6–1.6	[49]
Plasma pre-op (Dental surgery)	1.4	0.8–2.3	[50]
Plasma intra-op (Dental surgery)	1.9	1.0–3.0	[50]
Effect-site pre-op (Dental surgery)	1.5	1.0–2.5	[151]
Effect-site intra-op (Dental surgery)	1.6	1.0–2.6	[152]

Use of Patient-Maintained Sedation in Clinical Practice

Despite the difficulties in preventing oversedation in the very artificial situation of volunteers actively trying to defeat the system, all of our experience of its use clinically has been very positive. When patients use it for its intended use to deal with procedural anxiety, it has proved effective and safe, with high patient and operator satisfaction [49, 50, 79, 83, 151, 152]. Despite the alterations that have been made to attempt to prevent the highly undesirable situation of accidental oversedation, there has never been a problem with the quality of sedation propofol provides when the patient has limited control over a PMS system. Indeed these studies have allowed us to characterise what the mean and range of plasma concentrations and effect-site concentrations that the patient decides they need for procedural sedation. These data are extremely useful regardless of the mode of delivery and are summarised in Table 21.5.

Opioid Sedation

Remifentanil TCI

Remifentanil is an ultra-short-acting opioid analgesic with a context-sensitive half-time of around 3 min [153]. It offers good analgesia but less anxiolysis and amnesia than alternative sedatives such as propofol [154, 155]. Despite this remifentanil has become popular for sedation in specific scenarios in recent years. Many of the publications describe standard infusions at a specific μg·kg^{-1}·min^{-1} rate. The newer generation of TCI syringe pumps offers TCI with various drugs other than propofol, including remifentanil. TCI remifentanil seems particularly suited to awake fibreoptic intubation after local anaesthesia is applied to the airway; this may be because suppression of cough is more important than anxiolysis [156].

Remifentanil causes measurable effects on respiratory rate, end-tidal carbon dioxide and ventilatory variability at relatively low Ce levels 1.5 ng·ml^{-1} [157]. It causes more frequent respiratory events than propofol. However, it may be well suited for supplementing an incomplete regional block [155] or in a situation where complete regional anaesthesia is difficult and rapid recovery from sedation is necessary. A good example is the dissection phase of awake carotid endarterectomy under cervical plexus block. This is followed by carotid cross clamping which necessitates neurological and cognitive assessment unclouded by residual sedatives [158].

There is little argument about the best pharmacokinetic model to use for remifentanil, which is the Minto model [159]. The main covariates that are used in programming a TCI system are height, weight (calculating lean body mass), age and sex. There are recent comparisons of TCI versus manual infusion remifentanil published [160, 161]. It appears there is less variation in plasma concentration, easier titration and fewer respiratory events with TCI.

Reasonable Dose Regimens for Remifentanil

It seems that hypoventilation and apnoea are unlikely under a TCI remifentanil target of 2.0 ng·ml^{-1} and more likely above 3.0 ng·ml^{-1} [162]. Many awake fibreoptic intubation (AFOI) studies use it in the dose range 3–6 ng·ml^{-1}. High doses are required if it is used in isolation and lower doses if used in conjunction with a hypnotic such as midazolam or propofol, where it may be prudent to start at a lower level, e.g. 1 ng·ml^{-1}, then titrate up. Patient-maintained analgesia with remifentanil has also been described postoperatively when a patient can control the TCI target by pressing a patient demand button [163]. Generally they achieve adequate analgesia at around 2.0 ng·ml^{-1} but with the expected wide variability of several hundred percent for the optimum target concentration required by individual patients.

If using manual infusions, you must be aware the variation in Cp/Ce is greater [161], and titration should be cautious. However, a bolus dose of 0.25 µg·kg^{-1} followed by an infusion of 0.05 µg·kg^{-1}·min^{-1} will yield a final Cp and Ce of approximately 1–1.2 ng·ml^{-1} at steady state. Whereas higher rates such as 0.5 µg·kg^{-1} bolus followed by 0.1 µg·kg^{-1}·min^{-1} will yield Cp/Ce in the 2–2.5 ng·ml^{-1} range.

Many still consider that because its offset is so predictable regardless of the infusion rate, there is little to be gained from TCI remifentanil. This might well be true for its use in general anaesthesia, but inadvertent overdose during sedation without a secured airway is more of an issue. However, if one is to use a manual infusion regimen, there are a few tips to do this successfully.

1. Ideal body weight: we should really use the patient's ideal body weight not actual body weight. This can be done with a rough calculation (height in cm −100 for men or −105 in women), e.g. a 40-year-old 165 cm, 80 kg female at steady state after 0.1 µg·ml^{-1}·min^{-1} remifentanil will have a Cp of 3.2 ng·kg^{-1} if we use her actual body weight. But would only have a Cp of 2.5 ng·ml^{-1} if we used her ideal body weight (165 cm, 105 = 60 kg).

2. Age: be aware that elderly will have a much higher plasma concentration than a young person for the same infusion rate, e.g. if we compare a 20-year-old 178 cm 80 kg male and an 80-year-old 178 cm 80 kg male. At steady state after 0.1 µg·kg^{-1}·min^{-1} remifentanil, the 21 year old will have a Cp of 2.8 ng·ml^{-1} and the 80 year old a Cp of 4.0 ng·ml^{-1}. *In addition, older patients are more sensitive to any given plasma concentration.*

3. Also be aware that when changing infusion rates, it will take 5–6 half-lives, i.e. 15–30 min, to reach steady state. The use of boluses (0.25–0.5 µg·kg^{-1}) can speed this up but make inadvertent apnoea more likely.

Other TCI Opioids for Sedation

Alfentanil TCI has also been reported for postoperative analgesia showing large interindividual variation in the plasma concentration required for analgesia (<1–175 ng·ml^{-1}) [164] but mostly in the 26–52 range [165]. Minor improvements have been shown in pain scores [166] and time to adequate analgesia compared to PCA morphine. TCI alfentanil has also been used to facilitate burn dressings [167]. Other methods of alfentanil analgesia have been explored: a simple patient-controlled analgesia with a background infusion [168] and a hybrid PCA and TCI combination, essentially patient-maintained analgesia with alfentanil where the patient can increase the TCI target by pressing a patient demand button [169, 170].

Hypnotic Opioid or Both?

Propofol is an excellent choice for anxiolysis, but remifentanil may be a better choice for an imperfect regional block or in specific situations like AFOI. It seems reasonable to make individual choices based on the patient and procedure factors [171]. All the while bear in mind that when given together, remifentanil and propofol behave synergistically, not in an additive manner [172]. Careful incremental titration of one agent at a time, allowing some time to allow effect-site/clinical effect and plasma concentration to equilibrate, would be prudent. TCI may make this easier for the average clinician with no specific expertise in the pharmacodynamics or pharmacokinetics of these extremely useful agents.

References

1. Academy of Medical Royal Colleges. Safe Sedation Practice for Healthcare Procedures. 2013.
2. UK Academy of Medical Royal Colleges and their Faculties. Implementing and ensuring safe sedation practice for healthcare procedures in adults. Report of an Intercollegiate working party chaired by the Royal College of Anaesthetists. 2001.
3. American Society of Anesthesiologists. Continuum of Depth of Sedation: Definition of General Anesthesia and Levels of Sedation/Analgesia. 2009.
4. Ekin A, Donmez F, Taspinar V, Dikmen B. Patient-controlled sedation in orthopedic surgery under regional anesthesia: a new approach in procedural sedation. Rev Bras Anestesiol. 2013;63:410–4.
5. Wu CL, Naqibuddin M, Fleisher LA. Measurement of patient satisfaction as an outcome of regional anesthesia and analgesia: a systematic review. Reg Anesth Pain Med. 2001;26:196–208.
6. NCEPOD. Scoping Our Practice. NCEPOD. 2004.
7. Poswillo D. General anaesthesia, sedation and resuscitation in dentistry. Report of an Expert Working Party for the Standing Dental Advisory Committee. London: Department of Health; 1990.
8. Department of Health. Dental general anaesthesia. Report of a clinical standards advisory committee on general anaesthesia for dentistry. London: Department of Health; 1995.
9. General Dental Council. Maintaining standards. Guidance to dentists on professional and personal conduct. London: General Dental Council; 1998.
10. Whittle JG. The provision of primary care dental general anaesthesia and sedation in the north west region of England, 1996–1999. Br Dent J. 2000;189:500–2.
11. Foley J. The way forward for dental sedation and primary care? Br Dent J. 2002;193:161–4.
12. The Standing Committe for Sedation in Dentistry. Standards for Conscious Sedation in Dentistry: Alternative Techniques. 2007.
13. Morris AJ, Burke FJ. Primary and secondary dental care: the nature of the interface. Br Dent J. 2001;191:660–4.
14. Morgan CL, Skelly AM. Conscious sedation services provided in secondary care for restorative dentistry in the UK: a survey. Br Dent J. 2005;198:631–5. discussion 25.
15. The Dental Teachers Sedation Group. Conscious Sedation in Dentistry Standards for Postgraduate Education. 2008.
16. Daneshmend TK, Bell GD, Logan RF. Sedation for upper gastrointestinal endoscopy: results of a nationwide survey. Gut. 1991;32:12–5.
17. Quine MA, Bell GD, McCloy RF, Charlton JE, Devlin HB, Hopkins A. Prospective audit of upper gastrointestinal endoscopy in two regions of England: safety, staffing, and sedation methods. Gut. 1995;36:462–7.
18. Clarke AC, Chiragakis L, Hillman LC, Kaye GL. Sedation for endoscopy: the safe use of propofol by general practitioner sedationists. Med J Aust. 2002;176:158–61.
19. Dumonceau JM, Riphaus A, Aparicio JR, et al. European Society of Gastrointestinal Endoscopy, European Society of Gastroenterology and Endoscopy Nurses and Associates, and the European Society of Anaesthesiology Guideline: non-anaesthesiologist administration of propofol for GI endoscopy. Eur J Anaesthesiol. 2010;27:1016–30.
20. Cote GA. The debate for nonanesthesiologist-administered propofol sedation in endoscopy rages on: who will be the "King of Prop?". Gastrointest Endosc. 2011;73:773–6.
21. Singh H, Poluha W, Cheung M, Choptain N, Baron KI, Taback SP. Propofol for sedation during colonoscopy. Cochrane Datab Syst Rev 2008:CD006268.
22. Slagelse C, Vilmann P, Hornslet P, Hammering A, Mantoni T. Nurse-administered propofol sedation for gastrointestinal endoscopic procedures: first Nordic results from implementation of a structured training program. Scand J Gastroenterol. 2011;46:1503–9.
23. Perel A. Non-anaesthesiologists should not be allowed to administer propofol for procedural sedation: a consensus statement of 21 European National Societies of Anaesthesia. Eur J Anaesthesiol. 2011;28:580–4.
24. Hewitt SM, Hartley RH. Manipulation under sedation in the accident and emergency department. J Accid Emerg Med. 1994;11:186–8.
25. Green SM. Propofol in emergency medicine: further evidence of safety. Emerg Med Australas. 2007;19:389–93.
26. Mathieu N, Jones L, Harris A, et al. Is propofol a safe and effective sedative for relocating hip prostheses? Emerg Med J. 2009;26:37–8.
27. Anderson KJ, Sim M, Puxty A, Kinsella J. Propofol is not safe for sedation for hip relocation. Emerg Med J. 2010;27:885.
28. Newstead B, Bradburn S, Appelboam A, et al. Propofol for adult procedural sedation in a UK emergency department: safety profile in 1008 cases. Br J Anaesth. 2013;111:651–5.
29. Mason KP, Green SM, Piacevoli Q, International Sedation Task F. Adverse event reporting tool to standardize the reporting and tracking of adverse events during procedural sedation: a consensus document from the World SIVA International Sedation Task Force. Br J Anaesth. 2012;108:13–20.
30. Wade CN. Journal club response. Br J Anaesth. 2014;112:939.
31. Olkkola KT, Ahonen J. Midazolam and other benzodiazepines. Handb Exp Pharmacol. 2008;182:335–60.
32. Rudkin GE, Osborne GA, Finn BP, Jarvis DA, Vickers D. Intraoperative patient-controlled sedation. Comparison of patient-controlled propofol with patient-controlled midazolam. Anaesthesia. 1992;47:376–81.
33. Herrick IA, Gelb AW, Tseng PS, Kirkby J. Patient-controlled sedation using propofol during interventional neuroradiologic procedures. J Neurosurg Anesthesiol. 1997;9:237–41.
34. Ng JM, Kong CF, Nyam D. Patient-controlled sedation with propofol for colonoscopy. Gastrointest Endosc. 2001;54:8–13.
35. Zomorodi K, Donner A, Somma J, et al. Population pharmacokinetics of midazolam administered by target controlled infusion for sedation following coronary artery bypass grafting. Anesthesiology. 1998;89:1418–29.
36. Chauhan M, Carter E, Rood P. Intravenous midazolam dose ranges in older patients sedated for oral surgery--a preliminary retrospective cohort study. Br Dent J. 2014;216:E12.
37. Wilson E, David A, MacKenzie N, Grant IS. Sedation during spinal anaesthesia: comparison of propofol and midazolam. Br J Anaesth. 1990;64:48–52.
38. Sneyd JR, Rigby-Jones AE. New drugs and technologies, intravenous anaesthesia is on the move (again). Br J Anaesth. 2010;105:246–54.
39. Rigby-Jones A. Comparison of KeO Half-Life for MR04A3, midazolam and propofol: a study in healthy male volunteers. Anesthesiology. 2010;113 Suppl:A348.
40. Murray AW, Morran CG, Kenny GN, Macfarlane P, Anderson JR. Examination of cardiorespiratory changes during upper gastrointestinal endoscopy. Comparison of monitoring of arterial oxygen saturation, arterial pressure and the electrocardiogram. Anaesthesia. 1991;46:181–4.

41. Weinbroum AA, Szold O, Ogorek D, Flaishon R. The midazolam-induced paradox phenomenon is reversible by flumazenil. Epidemiology, patient characteristics and review of the literature. Eur J Anaesthesiol. 2001;18:789–97.

42. Weinbroum AA, Flaishon R, Sorkine P, Szold O, Rudick V. A risk-benefit assessment of flumazenil in the management of benzodiazepine overdose. Drug Saf. 1997;17:181–96.

43. Gavin DR, Valori RM, Anderson JT, Donnelly MT, Williams JG, Swarbrick ET. The national colonoscopy audit: a nationwide assessment of the quality and safety of colonoscopy in the UK. Gut. 2013;62:242–9.

44. The National Patient Safety Agency. Reducing risk of overdose with midazolam injection in adults. Rapid Response Report (and supporting information). NPSA. 2008.

45. Mackenzie N, Grant IS. Propofol for intravenous sedation. Anaesthesia. 1987;42:3–6.

46. Cook LB, Lockwood GG, Moore CM, Whitwam JG. True patient-controlled sedation. Anaesthesia. 1993;48:1039–44.

47. White PF, Negus JB. Sedative infusions during local and regional anaesthesia: a comparison of midazolam and propofol. J Clin Anesth. 1991;3:32–9.

48. Smith I, Monk TG, White PF, Ding Y. Propofol infusion during regional anesthesia: sedative, amnestic, and anxiolytic properties. Anesth Analg. 1994;79:313–9.

49. Murdoch JA, Kenny GN. Patient-maintained propofol sedation as premedication in day-case surgery: assessment of a target-controlled system. Br J Anaesth. 1999;82:429–31.

50. Leitch JA, Anderson K, Gambhir S, et al. A partially blinded randomised controlled trial of patient-maintained propofol sedation and operator controlled midazolam sedation in third molar extractions. Anaesthesia. 2004;59:853–60.

51. Hohener D, Blumenthal S, Borgeat A. Sedation and regional anaesthesia in the adult patient. Br J Anaesth. 2008;100:8–16.

52. Edwards JA, Kinsella J, Shaw A, Evans S, Anderson KJ. Sedation for oocyte retrieval using target controlled infusion of propofol and incremental alfentanil delivered by non-anaesthetists. Anaesthesia. 2010;65:453–61.

53. Rudkin GE, Osborne GA, Curtis NJ. Intra-operative patient-controlled sedation. Anaesthesia. 1991;46:90–2.

54. Osborne GA, Rudkin GE, Curtis NJ, Vickers D, Craker AJ. Intra-operative patient-controlled sedation. Comparison of patient-controlled propofol with anaesthetist-administered midazolam and fentanyl. Anaesthesia. 1991;46:553–6.

55. Oei-Lim VL, Kalkman CJ, Makkes PC, Ooms WG. Patient-controlled versus anesthesiologist-controlled conscious sedation with propofol for dental treatment in anxious patients. Anesth Analg. 1998;86:967–72.

56. Skipsey IG, Colvin JR, Mackenzie N, Kenny GN. Sedation with propofol during surgery under local blockade. Assessment of a target-controlled infusion system. Anaesthesia. 1993;48:210–3.

57. Gepts E. Pharmacokinetic concepts for TCI anaesthesia. Anaesthesia. 1998;53 Suppl 1:4–12.

58. Roberts FL, Dixon J, Lewis GT, Tackley RM, Prys-Roberts C. Induction and maintenance of propofol anaesthesia. A manual infusion scheme. Anaesthesia. 1988;43 Suppl:14–7.

59. Hughes MA, Glass PS, Jacobs JR. Context-sensitive half-time in multicompartment pharmacokinetic models for intravenous anesthetic drugs. Anesthesiology. 1992;76:334–41.

60. Keifer J, Glass P. Context-sensitive half-time and anesthesia: how does theory match reality? Curr Opin Anaesthesiol. 1999;12:443–8.

61. Glen JB. The development of 'Diprifusor': a TCI system for propofol. Anaesthesia. 1998;53 Suppl 1:13–21.

62. Leslie K, Clavisi O, Hargrove J. Target-controlled infusion versus manually-controlled infusion of propofol for general anaesthesia or sedation in adults. Cochrane Datab Syst Rev. 2008;CD006059.

63. Russell D. Intravenous anaesthesia: manual infusion schemes versus TCI systems. Anaesthesia. 1998;53 Suppl 1:42–5.

64. Servin FS. TCI compared with manually controlled infusion of propofol: a multicentre study. Anaesthesia. 1998;53 Suppl 1:82–6.

65. White M, Schenkels MJ, Engbers FH, et al. Effect-site modelling of propofol using auditory evoked potentials. Br J Anaesth. 1999;82:333–9.

66. Newson C, Joshi GP, Victory R, White PF. Comparison of propofol administration techniques for sedation during monitored anesthesia care. Anesth Analg. 1995;81:486–91.

67. Walder B, Schafer M, Henzi I, Tramer MR. Efficacy and safety of patient-controlled opioid analgesia for acute postoperative pain. A quantitative systematic review. Acta Anaesthesiol Scand. 2001;45:795–804.

68. Ballantyne JC, Carr DB, Chalmers TC, Dear KB, Angelillo IF, Mosteller F. Postoperative patient-controlled analgesia: meta-analyses of initial randomized control trials. J Clin Anesth. 1993;5:182–93.

69. Osborne GA, Rudkin GE, Jarvis DA, Young IG, Barlow J, Leppard PI. Intra-operative patient-controlled sedation and patient attitude to control. A crossover comparison of patient preference for patient-controlled propofol and propofol by continuous infusion. Anaesthesia. 1994;49:287–92.

70. Wahlen BM, Kilian M, Schuster F, Muellenbach R, Roewer N, Kranke P. Patient-controlled versus continuous anesthesiologist-controlled sedation using propofol during regional anesthesia in orthopedic procedures--a pilot study. Expert Opin Pharmacother. 2008;9:2733–9.

71. Yun MJ, Oh AY, Kim KO, Kim YH. Patient-controlled sedation vs. anaesthetic nurse-controlled sedation for cataract surgery in elderly patients. Int J Clin Pract. 2008;62:776–80.

72. Alhashemi JA, Kaki AM. Anesthesiologist-controlled versus patient-controlled propofol sedation for shockwave lithotripsy. Can J Anaesth. 2006;53:449–55.

73. Mazanikov M, Udd M, Kylanpaa L, et al. A randomized comparison of target-controlled propofol infusion and patient-controlled sedation during ERCP. Endoscopy. 2013;45:915–9.

74. Hamid SK, McCann N, McArdle L, Asbury AJ. Comparison of patient-controlled sedation with either methohexitone or propofol. Br J Anaesth. 1996;77:727–30.

75. Mandel JE, Tanner JW, Lichtenstein GR, et al. A randomized, controlled, double-blind trial of patient-controlled sedation with propofol/remifentanil versus midazolam/fentanyl for colonoscopy. Anesth Analg. 2008;106:434–9, table of contents.

76. Herrick IA, Gelb AW, Nichols B, Kirkby J. Patient-controlled propofol sedation for elderly patients: safety and patient attitude toward control. Can J Anaesth. 1996;43:1014–8.

77. Gan TJ, El-Molem H, Ray J, Glass PS. Patient-controlled antiemesis: a randomized, double-blind comparison of two doses of propofol versus placebo. Anesthesiology. 1999;90:1564–70.

78. Janzen PR, Christys A, Vucevic M. Patient-controlled sedation using propofol in elderly patients in day-case cataract surgery. Br J Anaesth. 1999;82:635–6.

79. Rodrigo C, Irwin MG, Yan BS, Wong MH. Patient-controlled sedation with propofol in minor oral surgery. J Oral Maxillofac Surg. 2004;62:52–6.

80. Mandel JE. A method for producing predictable transitions in response probability for mixed-effect models of propofol/remifentanil using single syringe infusion. Soc Technol Anesth. 2008;S29.

81. Atkins JH, Mandel JE. Recent advances in patient-controlled sedation. Curr Opin Anaesthesiol. 2008;21:759–65.

82. Shieh JS, Chang LW, Wang MS, Sun WZ, Wang YP, Yang YP. Pain model and fuzzy logic patient-controlled analgesia in shock-wave lithotripsy. Med Biol Eng Comput. 2002;40:128–36.

83. Irwin MG, Thompson N, Kenny GN. Patient-maintained propofol sedation. Assessment of a target-controlled infusion system. Anaesthesia. 1997;52:525–30.

84. Leitch JA, Sutcliffe N, Kenny GN. Patient-maintained sedation for oral surgery using a target-controlled infusion of propofol - a pilot study. Br Dent J. 2003;194:43–5.

85. Rodrigo MR, Irwin MG, Tong CK, Yan SY. A randomised crossover comparison of patient-controlled sedation and patient-maintained sedation using propofol. Anaesthesia. 2003;58:333–8.

86. White M, Kenny GN. Intravenous propofol anaesthesia using a computerised infusion system. Anaesthesia. 1990;45:204–9.

87. Gepts E, Jonckheer K, Maes V, Sonck W, Camu F. Disposition kinetics of propofol during alfentanil anaesthesia. Anaesthesia. 1988;43(Suppl):8–13.

88. Marsh B, White M, Morton N, Kenny GN. Pharmacokinetic model driven infusion of propofol in children. Br J Anaesth. 1991;67:41–8.

89. Schnider TW, Minto CF, Gambus PL, et al. The influence of method of administration and covariates on the pharmacokinetics of propofol in adult volunteers. Anesthesiology. 1998;88:1170–82.

90. Stuart PC, Stott SM, Millar A, Kenny GN, Russell D. Cp50 of propofol with and without nitrous oxide 67%. Br J Anaesth. 2000;84:638–9.

91. Absalom AR, Mani V, De Smet T, Struys MM. Pharmacokinetic models for propofol--defining and illuminating the devil in the detail. Br J Anaesth. 2009;103:26–37.

92. Swinhoe CF, Peacock JE, Glen JB, Reilly CS. Evaluation of the predictive performance of a 'Diprifusor' TCI system. Anaesthesia. 1998;53 Suppl 1:61–7.

93. Varvel JR, Donoho DL, Shafer SL. Measuring the predictive performance of computer-controlled infusion pumps. J Pharmacokinet Biopharm. 1992;20:63–94.

94. Landon MJ, Matson AM, Royston BD, Hewlett AM, White DC, Nunn JF. Components of the inspiratory-arterial isoflurane partial pressure difference. Br J Anaesth. 1993;70:605–11.

95. Schuttler J, Ihmsen H. Population pharmacokinetics of propofol: a multicenter study. Anesthesiology. 2000;92:727–38.

96. White M, Kenny GN, Schraag S. Use of target controlled infusion to derive age and gender covariates for propofol clearance. Clin Pharmacokinet. 2008;47:119–27.

97. Glen JB, Servin F. Evaluation of the predictive performance of four pharmacokinetic models for propofol. Br J Anaesth. 2009;102:626–32.

98. Glen JB, White M. A comparison of the predictive performance of three pharmacokinetic models for propofol using measured values obtained during target-controlled infusion. Anaesthesia. 2014;69:550–7.

99. Eleveld DJ, Proost JH, Cortinez LI, Absalom AR, Struys MM. A general purpose pharmacokinetic model for propofol. Anesth Analg. 2014;118:1221–37.

100. Vereecke HE, Eleveld DJ, Colin P, Struys MM. Performance of the eleveld pharmacokinetic model to titrate propofol in an obese Japanese patient population. Eur J Anaesthesiol. 2016;33:58–9.

101. Hu C, Horstman DJ, Shafer SL. Variability of target-controlled infusion is less than the variability after bolus injection. Anesthesiology. 2005;102:639–45.

102. Gepts E, Camu F, Cockshott ID, Douglas EJ. Disposition of propofol administered as constant rate intravenous infusions in humans. Anesth Analg. 1987;66:1256–63.

103. Schnider TW, Minto CF, Shafer SL, et al. The influence of age on propofol pharmacodynamics. Anesthesiology. 1999;90:1502–16.

104. Lysakowski C, Dumont L, Czarnetzki C, Bertrand D, Tassonyi E, Tramer MR. The effect of cigarette smoking on the hypnotic efficacy of propofol. Anaesthesia. 2006;61:826–31.

105. Liang C, Chen J, Gu W, Wang H, Xue Z. Chronic alcoholism increases the induction dose of propofol. Acta Anaesthesiol Scand. 2011;55:1113–7.

106. Servin F, Cockshott ID, Farinotti R, Haberer JP, Winckler C, Desmonts JM. Pharmacokinetics of propofol infusions in patients with cirrhosis. Br J Anaesth. 1990;65:177–83.

107. Choi EM, Choi SH, Lee MH, Ha SH, Min KT. Effect-site concentration of propofol target-controlled infusion at loss of consciousness in intractable epilepsy patients receiving long-term antiepileptic drug therapy. J Neurosurg Anesthesiol. 2011;23:188–92.

108. Dahaba AA, Zhong T, Lu HS, et al. Geographic differences in the target-controlled infusion estimated concentration of propofol: bispectral index response curves. Can J Anaesth 2011;58:364–70.

109. Fu F, Chen X, Feng Y, Shen Y, Feng Z, Bein B. Propofol EC50 for inducing loss of consciousness is lower in the luteal phase of the menstrual cycle. Br J Anaesth. 2014;112:506–13.

110. La Colla L, Albertin A, La Colla G, et al. No adjustment vs. adjustment formula as input weight for propofol target-controlled infusion in morbidly obese patients. Eur J Anaesthesiol. 2009;26:362–9.

111. Echevarria GC, Elgueta MF, Donoso MT, Bugedo DA, Cortinez LI, Munoz HR. The effective effect-site propofol concentration for induction and intubation with two pharmacokinetic models in morbidly obese patients using total body weight. Anesth Analg. 2012;115:823–9.

112. Albertin A, Poli D, La Colla L, et al. Predictive performance of 'Servin's formula' during BIS-guided propofol-remifentanil target-controlled infusion in morbidly obese patients. Br J Anaesth. 2007;98:66–75.

113. Coetzee JF. Total intravenous anaesthesia to obese patients: largely guesswork? Eur J Anaesthesiol. 2009;26:359–61.

114. Johnson KB, Egan TD, Kern SE, McJames SW, Cluff ML, Pace NL. Influence of hemorrhagic shock followed by crystalloid resuscitation on propofol: a pharmacokinetic and pharmacodynamic analysis. Anesthesiology. 2004;101:647–59.

115. Mandel JE, Lichtenstein GR, Metz DC, Ginsberg GG, Kochman ML. A prospective, randomized, comparative trial evaluating respiratory depression during patient-controlled versus anesthesiologist-administered propofol-remifentanil sedation for elective colonoscopy. Gastrointest Endosc. 2010;72:112–7.

116. Mandel JE, Sarraf E. The variability of response to propofol is reduced when a clinical observation is incorporated in the control: a simulation study. Anesth Analg. 2012;114:1221–9.

117. Barakat AR, Sutcliffe N, Schwab M. Effect site concentration during propofol TCI sedation: a comparison of sedation score with two pharmacokinetic models. Anaesthesia. 2007;62:661–6.

118. Cortinez LI. What is the ke0 and what does it tell me about propofol? Anaesthesia. 2014;69:399–402.

119. Milne SE, Kenny GN, Schraag S. Propofol sparing effect of remifentanil using closed-loop anaesthesia. Br J Anaesth. 2003;90:623–9.

120. Iwakiri H, Nishihara N, Nagata O, Matsukawa T, Ozaki M, Sessler DI. Individual effect-site concentrations of propofol are similar at loss of consciousness and at awakening. Anesth Analg. 2005;100:107–10.

121. Struys MM, De Smet T, Depoorter B, et al. Comparison of plasma compartment versus two methods for effect compartment--controlled target-controlled infusion for propofol. Anesthesiology. 2000;92:399–406.

122. Lim TA. A novel method of deriving the effect compartment equilibrium rate constant for propofol. Br J Anaesth. 2003;91:730–2.

123. Thomson AJ, Nimmo AF, Engbers FH, Glen JB. A novel technique to determine an 'apparent ke0' value for use with the Marsh pharmacokinetic model for propofol. Anaesthesia. 2014;69:420–8.

124. Thomson AJ, Morrison G, Thomson E, Beattie C, Nimmo AF, Glen JB. Induction of general anaesthesia by effect-site target-controlled infusion of propofol: influence of pharmacokinetic model and ke0 value. Anaesthesia. 2014;69:429–35.

125. Anderson KJ, Leitch JA, Green JS, Kenny GN. Effect-site controlled patient maintained propofol sedation: a volunteer safety study. Anaesthesia. 2005;60:235–8.

126. Murdoch JA, Grant SA, Kenny GN. Safety of patient-maintained propofol sedation using a target-controlled system in healthy volunteers. Br J Anaesth. 2000;85:299–301.

127. Henderson F, Absalom AR, Kenny GN. Patient-maintained propofol sedation: a follow up safety study using a modified system in volunteers. Anaesthesia. 2002;57:387–90.

128. Jack ES, Shaw M, Harten JM, Anderson K, Kinsella J. Cardiovascular changes after achieving constant effect site concentration of propofol. Anaesthesia. 2008;63:116–20.

129. Grant SA, Millar K, Kenny GN. Blood alcohol concentration and psychomotor effects. Br J Anaesth. 2000;85:401–6.

130. Grant SA, Murdoch J, Millar K, Kenny GN. Blood propofol concentration and psychomotor effects on driving skills. Br J Anaesth. 2000;85:396–400.

131. Anderson KJ, Allam S, Chapman R, Kenny GN. The effect of propofol on patient reaction time and its relationship with loss of verbal contact before induction of anaesthesia. Anaesthesia. 2013;68:148–53.

132. Allam S, Anderson KJ, O'Brien C, et al. Patient-maintained propofol sedation using reaction time monitoring: a volunteer safety study. Anaesthesia. 2013;68:154–8.

133. Kim KM, Jeon WJ, Lee DH, Kang WC, Kim JH, Noh GJ. Changes in visual and auditory response time during conscious sedation with propofol. Acta Anaesthesiol Scand. 2004;48:1033–7.

134. Thomson AJ, Nimmo AF, Tiplady B, Glen JB. Evaluation of a new method of assessing depth of sedation using two-choice visual reaction time testing on a mobile phone. Anaesthesia. 2009;64:32–8.

135. Doufas AG, Bakhshandeh M, Bjorksten AR, Greif R, Sessler DI. Automated responsiveness test (ART) predicts loss of consciousness and adverse physiologic responses during propofol conscious sedation. Anesthesiology. 2001;94:585–92.

136. Chernik DA, Gillings D, Laine H, et al. Validity and reliability of the observer's assessment of alertness/sedation scale: study with intravenous midazolam. J Clin Psychopharmacol. 1990;10:244–51.

137. Doufas AG, Bakhshandeh M, Haugh GS, Bjorksten AR, Greif R, Sessler DI. Automated responsiveness test and bispectral index monitoring during propofol and propofol/N2O sedation. Acta Anaesthesiol Scand. 2003;47:951–7.

138. Doufas AG, Morioka N, Mahgoub AN, Bjorksten AR, Shafer SL, Sessler DI. Automated responsiveness monitor to titrate propofol sedation. Anesth Analg. 2009;109:778–86.

139. Billard V, Gambus PL, Chamoun N, Stanski DR, Shafer SL. A comparison of spectral edge, delta power, and bispectral index as EEG measures of alfentanil, propofol, and midazolam drug effect. Clin Pharmacol Ther. 1997;61:45–58.

140. Struys M, Versichelen L, Byttebier G, Mortier E, Moerman A, Rolly G. Clinical usefulness of the bispectral index for titrating propofol target effect-site concentration. Anaesthesia. 1998;53:4–12.

141. Singh H. Bispectral index (BIS) monitoring during propofol-induced sedation and anaesthesia. Eur J Anaesthesiol. 1999;16:31–6.

142. Bonhomme V, Plourde G, Meuret P, Fiset P, Backman SB. Auditory steady-state response and bispectral index for assessing level of consciousness during propofol sedation and hypnosis. Anesth Analg. 2000;91:1398–403.

143. Milne SE, Troy A, Irwin MG, Kenny GN. Relationship between bispectral index, auditory evoked potential index and effect-site EC50 for propofol at two clinical end-points. Br J Anaesth. 2003;90:127–31.

144. Mahon P, Greene BR, Greene C, Boylan GB, Shorten GD. Behaviour of spectral entropy, spectral edge frequency 90%, and alpha and beta power parameters during low-dose propofol infusion. Br J Anaesth. 2008;101:213–21.

145. Mahon P, Kowalski RG, Fitzgerald AP, et al. Spectral entropy as a monitor of depth of propofol induced sedation. J Clin Monit Comput. 2008;22:87–93.

146. Lysakowski C, Elia N, Czarnetzki C, et al. Bispectral and spectral entropy indices at propofol-induced loss of consciousness in young and elderly patients. Br J Anaesth. 2009;103:387–93.

147. Pambianco DJ, Vargo JJ, Pruitt RE, Hardi R, Martin JF. Computer-assisted personalized sedation for upper endoscopy and colonoscopy: a comparative, multicenter randomized study. Gastrointest Endosc. 2011;73:765–72.

148. Rockoff JD. J&J to stop selling automated sedation system Sedasys. Wall Street J. 2016.

149. Pambianco DJ, Whitten CJ, Moerman A, Struys MM, Martin JF. An assessment of computer-assisted personalized sedation: a sedation delivery system to administer propofol for gastrointestinal endoscopy. Gastrointest Endosc. 2008;68:542–7.

150. US Food and Drug Administration USFaD. SEDASYS Computer-Assisted Personalized Sedation System – P0800092013.

151. Chapman RM, Anderson K, Green J, Leitch JA, Gambhir S, Kenny GN. Evaluation of a new effect-site controlled, patient-maintained sedation system in dental patients. Anaesthesia. 2006;61:345–9.

152. O'Brien C, Urquhart CS, Allam S, et al. Reaction time-monitored patient-maintained propofol sedation: a pilot study in oral surgery patients. Anaesthesia. 2013;68:760–4.

153. Glass PS, Hardman D, Kamiyama Y, et al. Preliminary pharmacokinetics and pharmacodynamics of an ultra-short-acting opioid: remifentanil (GI87084B). Anesth Analg. 1993;77:1031–40.

154. Mingus ML, Monk TG, Gold MI, Jenkins W, Roland C. Remifentanil versus propofol as adjuncts to regional anesthesia. Remifentanil 3010 Study Group. J Clin Anesth. 1998;10:46–53.

155. Servin FS, Raeder JC, Merle JC, et al. Remifentanil sedation compared with propofol during regional anaesthesia. Acta Anaesthesiol Scand. 2002;46:309–15.

156. Johnston KD, Rai MR. Conscious sedation for awake fibreoptic intubation: a review of the literature. Can J Anaesth. 2013;60:584–99.

157. Mitsis GD, Governo RJ, Rogers R, Pattinson KT. The effect of remifentanil on respiratory variability, evaluated with dynamic modeling. J Appl Physiol. (1985) 2009;106:1038–49.

158. Marrocco-Trischitta MM, Bandiera G, Camilli S, Stillo F, Cirielli C, Guerrini P. Remifentanil conscious sedation during regional anaesthesia for carotid endarterectomy: rationale and safety. Eur J Vasc Endovasc Surg. 2001;22:405–9.

159. Minto CF, Schnider TW, Egan TD, et al. Influence of age and gender on the pharmacokinetics and pharmacodynamics of remifentanil. I. Model development. Anesthesiology. 1997;86:10–23.

160. Yeganeh N, Roshani B, Azizi B, Almasi A. Target-controlled infusion of remifentanil to provide analgesia for awake nasotracheal fiberoptic intubations in cervical trauma patients. J Trauma. 2010;69:1185–90.

161. Moerman AT, Herregods LL, De Vos MM, Mortier EP, Struys MM. Manual versus target-controlled infusion remifentanil administration in spontaneously breathing patients. Anesth Analg. 2009;108:828–34.

162. Byun SH, Hwang DY, Hong SW, Kim SO. Target-controlled infusion of remifentanil for conscious sedation during spinal anesthesia. Korean J Anesthesiol. 2011;61:195–200.

163. Schraag S, Kenny GN, Mohl U, Georgieff M. Patient-maintained remifentanil target-controlled infusion for the transition to early postoperative analgesia. Br J Anaesth. 1998;81:365–8.

164. van den Nieuwenhuyzen MC, Engbers FH, Burm AG, et al. Computer-controlled infusion of alfentanil for postoperative analgesia. A pharmacokinetic and pharmacodynamic evaluation. Anesthesiology. 1993;79:481–92; discussion 27A.

165. Van den Nieuwenhuyzen MC, Engbers FH, Burm AG, Vletter AA, Van Kleef JW, Bovill JG. Target-controlled infusion of alfentanil for postoperative analgesia: a feasibility study and pharmacodynamic evaluation in the early postoperative period. Br J Anaesth. 1997;78:17–23.

166. van den Nieuwenhuyzen MC, Engbers FH, Burm AG, Vletter AA, van Kleef JW, Bovill JG. Computer-controlled infusion of alfentanil versus patient-controlled administration of morphine for postoperative analgesia: a double-blind randomized trial. Anesth Analg. 1995;81:671–9.

167. Gallagher G, Rae CP, Kenny GN, Kinsella J. The use of a target-controlled infusion of alfentanil to provide analgesia for burn dressing changes A dose finding study. Anaesthesia. 2000;55:1159–63.

168. Sim KM, Hwang NC, Chan YW, Seah CS. Use of patient-controlled analgesia with alfentanil for burns dressing procedures: a preliminary report of five patients. Burns. 1996;22:238–41.

169. Irwin MG, Jones RD, Visram AR, Kenny GN. Patient-controlled alfentanil. Target-controlled infusion for postoperative analgesia. Anaesthesia. 1996;51:427–30.

170. Checketts MR, Gilhooly CJ, Kenny GN. Patient-maintained analgesia with target-controlled alfentanil infusion after cardiac surgery: a comparison with morphine PCA. Br J Anaesth. 1998;80:748–51.

171. Raeder J. Opioid or propofol: what kind of drug for what kind of sedation? Manual dosing or target-controlled infusion? Anesth Analg. 2009;108:704–6.

172. Mertens MJ, Olofsen E, Engbers FH, Burm AG, Bovill JG, Vuyk J. Propofol reduces perioperative remifentanil requirements in a synergistic manner: response surface modeling of perioperative remifentanil-propofol interactions. Anesthesiology. 2003;99:347–59.

Pediatric TIVA/TCI: Case Presentations and Discussion

Vivian Man-ying Yuen

Case Presentation and Discussion on Children with Total Intravenous Anesthesia

Despite the advantages of total intravenous anesthesia (TIVA) in children, TIVA is not yet a popular anesthetic technique in children [1]. This may be related to the availability of target control infusion (TCI) systems and unfamiliarity with this technique. Practical tips of using TIVA in children are provided with the following case presentation.

TIVA by Manual Infusion

TIVA in children is most commonly administered by manual infusion. Previous studies have revealed that the loading dose and maintenance infusion rate are higher in children than in adults secondary to the larger volume of distribution in children [2]. By using a pharmacokinetic simulation program to predict propofol concentrations during infusion to achieve plasma concentration of propofol of 3 μg/ml in young children, the initial loading dose required is 2.5 mg/kg with subsequent infusion rate at 15-13-11-10-9 mg/kg/h in children aged between 3 and 11 years [3]. The loading dose and dose rate may still be higher in children younger than 3 years of age [4]. Moreover, there is evidence that children may have different pharmacodynamics responses to propofol comparing to adult; therefore, plasma concentration of propofol required to achieve adequate anesthesia may tend to be higher in children [5]. Since the interindividual variability of propofol requirement is high in adults as well as in children [5, 6], one may find the above regimen is inadequate in some patients. The following cases illustrate

how propofol-maintained anesthesia by manual infusion may be used in minor surgeries in children.

Case 1

A 4-year-old 16 kg boy with acute leukemia was scheduled for lumbar puncture and intrathecal drug injection. He was anxious and his mother held him in her lap sitting next to the operating table. The child had a permanent central catheter (Boviac), which could be used for anesthesia induction.

Intravenous propofol bolus of 2 mg/kg and fentanyl 0.5 μg/kg was administered before the child was separated from her mother and transferred to operating table. Standard monitor and end-tidal CO_2 (ETCO2) were applied (Figs. 22.1 and 22.2). Repeated bolus of propofol 1 mg/kg was administered before the child was put to left lateral position. Oxygen supplementation was given via a face mask placed in front of the patient. Infusion of propofol was commenced at 18 mg/kg/h, while surgeon cleaned and draped her surgical site. After another bolus of fentanyl 1 μg/kg, local anesthetic was infiltrated. The child moved when the pediatrician injected local anesthetic; hence, injection was stopped until another bolus of 1 mg/kg propofol was given. Propofol infusion was stopped when the successful placement of needle into intrathecal space was confirmed. Patient was recovered in lateral position with ETCO2 until awake.

Case 2

A 6-year-old 25 kg healthy boy was scheduled for circumcision. Gas induction with sevoflurane 4–6 % in oxygen was administered followed by intravenous cannulation on his right dorsum. IV propofol 2.5 mg/kg and IV fentanyl 1 μg/kg were given. Sevoflurane was stopped and propofol infusion commenced at 15 mg/kg/h. Another IV bolus of

V.M.-y. Yuen, MD, MBBS, FANZCA, FHKCA, FHKAM(✉)
Department of Anaesthesiology, University of Hong Kong Shenzhen Hospital, No. 1 Haiyuan 1st Road, Futian District, Shenzhen, Guangdong 518053, China
e-mail: vtang131@hku.hk

© Springer International Publishing AG 2017
A.R. Absalom, K.P. Mason (eds.), *Total Intravenous Anesthesia and Target Controlled Infusions*,
DOI 10.1007/978-3-319-47609-4_22

propofol at 2 mg/kg was given before the attempt for dorsal penile nerve block. The nerve block is performed with 4 ml of 0.5 % ropivacaine. Another 25 µg IV fentanyl was given before surgical procedure. During the procedure, the patient breathed spontaneously. ETCO2 was monitored, and oxygen supplementation was given via face mask placed loosely over his face (Fig. 22.3). The procedure took 10 min and propofol infusion was stopped before the last few stitches were done.

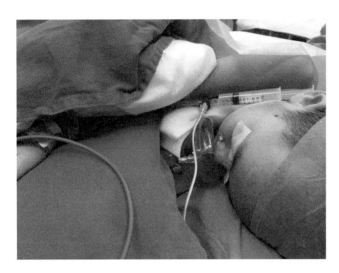

Fig. 22.1 A child in right lateral position for lumbar puncture. The airway was ensured patent and the child was breathing spontaneously. A face mask and breathing circuit were prepared and ready in case he needed support for his ventilation. A small extension was connected to the gas sampling line, and it was placed at the nostril to serve as capnography monitoring

Fig. 22.2 ETCO2 and capnograph were continuously monitored during the procedure, and it serves as a sensitive monitor of patient's ventilation

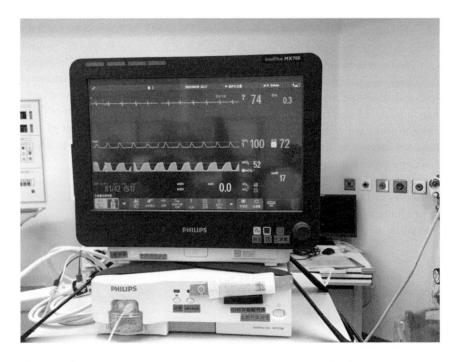

Discussion

Traditionally, it is common that anesthesia for simple procedures be maintained with inhalation agents via face mask or supraglottic airway devices. When face mask is used, airway support is often required, and face mask should be tightly fitted over patient's face to avoid leakage of inhalation agent; otherwise, supraglottic airway device would be used to achieve tight seal around the airway and to ensure effective delivery of inhalation agent.

It is shown in the above examples that TIVA techniques may be used in children undergoing minor diagnostic and surgical procedures. The child may maintain spontaneous breathing with minimal need of airway support. This obviates the need of a tight-fitting face mask and supraglottic airway device. Not only would this be more cost-effective, the risk associated with insertion and removal of supraglottic airway device can be avoided. Moreover, this would improve the turnaround time, and anesthetist is freed to manage anesthetic record or to prepare drug for the subsequent patients.

Although tight face mask or laryngeal mask airway is not used, ETCO2 monitoring is still applied and highly recommended as it is the best monitor for ventilation. ETCO2 gives information on ventilation and respiratory rate. Slow respiratory rate indicates hypoventilation, and propofol infusion rate may be decreased and vice versa. ETCO2 can be easily monitored by placing a small extension tube connected to the sampling line of a sidestream anesthetic gas monitor at the nostril (Fig. 22.1). Good signal may be obtained with the sampling line placed just at the outside of

Fig. 22.3 A child undergoing circumcision under propofol-maintained anesthesia. A face mask and breathing circuit were ready in case the child required ventilatory support. Gas sampling line is placed at his nostril for capnography monitoring during the procedure

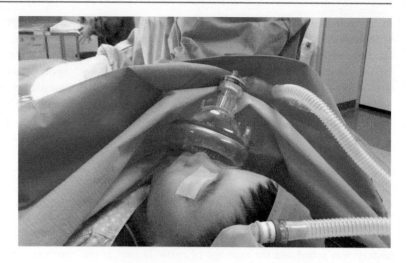

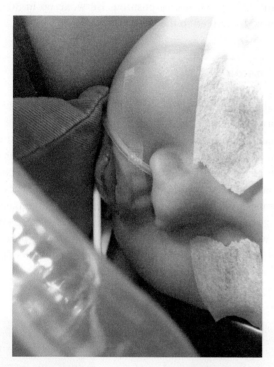

Fig. 22.4 Sampling line of capnography is placed just outside of the child's nostril for good signal. Signal can be lost easily if the sampling line is inserted into the nostril as the line would be blocked by touching the nasal mucosal wall

the nostril without entering into the nasal cavity, as this would prevent the interference of capnograph signal from the extension tube touching against the nasal mucosa (Fig. 22.4).

Although oxygen supplementation is not necessary in most children, it is good practice to have it readily available as it is not possible for children to become bradypneic or apneic with propofol or opioid boluses. It is recommended that face mask and breathing circuit are easily accessible so that you are ready to support ventilation whenever it is necessary. Airway support may be necessary in children with large tonsils, in children with obstruction sleep apnea, or in obese children.

When anesthesiologists start to use TIVA propofol technique to maintain anesthesia, movement secondary to surgical stimulation may be commonly encountered and problematic. This can be overcome by adequate dosing of propofol and good analgesia and regional block. When movement occurs, stimulation should be withheld, and propofol bolus is administered before surgery should be proceeded again. Since there is great interindividual variability in propofol requirement, one has to titrate to individual need. Vital signs including respiratory frequency and pulse rate are good indicators of adequate depth of anesthesia.

TIVA by TCI for Minor Surgeries

Since the initial dose rate of propofol is usually higher in young children, it is important to remember to titrate down the dose rate with time when manual infusion is used for TIVA in children. Manual titration may be avoided by TCI propofol. Currently two models of TCI of propofol are available and used commonly. The Kataria model is a model derived from a study of 53 healthy patients aged between 3 and 11 years, with body weight of 15–61 kg. It has been validated for used in children aged between 3 and 16 years with body weight of 15–61 kg [7]. The other commonly used model is the Paedfusor model which developed from the Marsh model for adults [8]. This model was subsequently validated in children undergoing cardiac surgery [9], and it is a model for children aged 1–16 years with lowest body weight of 5 kg. Both of these models are validated for plasma TCI and to date there is no effect-site TCI for children. Although there is a published pharmacokinetic and pharmacodynamics model by Choi et al. [10] for children aged 2–12 years which may allow effect-site TCI in children, this model is not yet made available in commercial TCI pumps. As discussed previously, due to the pharmacokinetic and pharmacodynamics differences in children, the target plasma concentration (Cp) required to induce and maintain anesthesia is usually higher in children.

In an open pilot study of 30 healthy children, a target Cp of 8 µg/ml was used to induce anesthesia, and the mean calculated effect-site concentration was 4.29 µg/ml for insertion of laryngeal mask airway [11]. A recent study has shown that the ED50 and ED95 of Cp propofol are 4–6 and 6–7 µg/ml, respectively, in young children and they are inversely related to age of child [12]. The following cases illustrate how TCI may be used in children undergoing minor surgical procedures.

Case 3

A 1-year-old 8 kg boy with unremarkable past medical history was scheduled for drainage of cystic lesions at the posterior neck under ultrasound guidance by intervention radiologist at radiology suite. Inhalational induction with 4–6 % sevoflurane in oxygen was conducted. Intravenous access was placed after anesthesia. TCI with Paedfusor model was commenced at Cp of 6 µg/ml when sevoflurane was stopped. Patient was turned to lateral position. IV fentanyl 1 µg/kg was given. ETCO2 monitor was placed. Local anesthetic was infiltrated before the start of the procedure. The procedure took 15 min and Cp propofol was maintained at 5.5 µg/ml during the procedure.

Case 4

A 3-year-old 12 kg boy was planned for change of portacath at radiology suite (Fig. 22.5). Intravenous cannula was placed uneventfully while the child was held in his mother's lap. TCI propofol with Paedfusor model was administered with Cp of 6 µg/ml. IV fentanyl at 1 µg/kg was given before supraglottic airway device was placed. Patient maintained spontaneous breathing throughout the procedure. Local anesthetic was infiltrated by radiologist before painful intervention. The old portacath was removed and a new one was replaced under ultrasound and fluoroscopic guidance. Propofol Cp was kept at 4–5 µg/ml 10 min after the procedure has started. Another bolus of IV fentanyl at 1 µg/kg was given before the procedure commenced. IV dexmedetomidine was given as small intermittent 2 µg boluses, and a total of 8 µg was given before the procedure ended 40 min after start of the procedure. 5 min before the procedure was completed, TCI was stopped. Supraglottic airway device was removed when the dressing was applied. Patient was put on lateral position. He woke up in 30 min and was discharged to the ward.

Discussion

The above cases illustrate how TCI propofol may be used in children for minor procedures. Supraglottic airway device maybe placed if procedure is relatively prolonged. The more common choice of anesthesia maintenance would be inhalational anesthetic. Patients may act as their own control for the depth of anesthesia with inhalational agents when spontaneous respiration is preserved. Nevertheless, laryngospasm and respiratory adverse event is more common with inhalation anesthesia when compared to propofol [13–15]. Propofol is a safe and feasible alternative to inhalation anesthesia in spontaneous ventilation [11, 16].

Fig. 22.5 A child undergoing portacath replacement in radiological suite. The airway was secured with supraglottic airway device, and spontaneous ventilation was maintained throughout the procedure

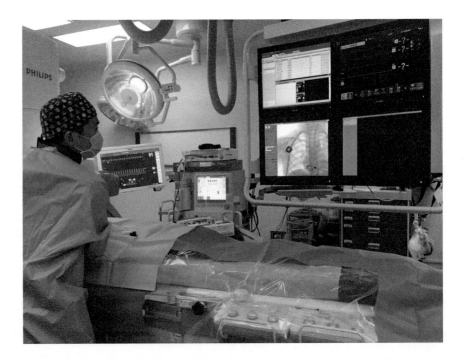

Timing of removal of supraglottic airway devices in children with inhalation anesthesia is controversial, and both deep and awake removal have been advocated. While awake removal ensures return of protective airway reflexes, problems of patient movement, retching, coughing, and biting on the devices are commonly encountered. It is generally agreed that supraglottic airway devices should not be removed in light planes of inhalation anesthesia as this is associated with high risk of coughing and laryngospasm [17, 18]. Deep removal avoids the problems of coughing and biting, but adequate depth of anesthesia level for safe removal could be difficult to judge [19, 20]. Since propofol-maintained anesthesia is associated with lower risk of laryngospasm and respiratory adverse events, the timing of removal of airway device is less critical. Propofol infusion may be stopped when it is close to the end of surgical procedure or when stimulation is low or minimal, and supraglottic airway device may be removed at the completion of the procedure before the patient is awake. Similar technique may be used in extubation of endotracheal tube except in patient at risk of gastric aspiration.

TIVA in Controlled Ventilation

The previous cases illustrate that spontaneous ventilation may be maintained in children undergoing minor procedures with TIVA using propofol and intermittent bolus fentanyl. Propofol is also commonly used with remifentanil in TIVA. Remifentanil is a potent opioid and it can cause significant respiratory depression. Although it is not impossible, maintaining spontaneous respiration with propofol and remifentanil is technically more challenging. In situation of controlled ventilation when respiratory depression is not a concern, combining remifentanil with propofol is less demanding TIVA technique. Since remifentanil is ultrashort acting with context-sensitive half-time remaining stable and predictable despite dose and duration of infusion, its use in TIVA would reduce the dose requirement of propofol [21, 22] and hasten recovery time [21–24] secondary to the synergistic effect of propofol and remifentanil.

Case 5

A 23-month-old 14 kg boy with suprasellar arachnoid cyst and obstructive hydrocephalus was scheduled for endoscopic truncation of suprasellar arachnoid cyst and ventriculostomy. The child was anxious as he has had many procedures before this. Inhalational induction was achieved with 4–5 % sevoflurane in oxygen followed by intravenous cannulation. The Cp of TCI propofol with Paedfusor model was set at 5 μg/ml, with IV remifentanil

administer at 0.2 μg/kg/min. Sevoflurane was stopped. The child was intubated at 2 min after IV cisatracurium and fentanyl; minimal hemodynamic changes were observed during intubation. The patient was then positioned and put on headrest. During patient positioning, the Cp of propofol was kept at 4 μg/ml. After positioning, surgeons spent time on checking the endoscopic equipment, so Cp of propofol was decreased to 3 μg/ml and remifentanil decreased to 0.1 μg/kg/min until surgery began. Local infiltration of scalp was performed by surgeon with 1.5 ml of 1 % lignocaine in 1:400,000 adrenaline. Cp of propofol and remifentanil was increased to 5 μg/ml and 0.25 μg/kg/min at 5 min before skin incision. Another IV bolus of fentanyl was given to prepare for surgical stimulation. Thirty minutes into surgery Cp of propofol was decreased to 4 μg/ml. When it was decreased to 3.5 μg/ml at 40 min, patient was noted to have increase heart rate from 90 to 110/min, so it was kept at 4 μg/ml until 10 min before the end of surgery. During the procedure, intermittent boluses of IV dexmedetomidine at 2 μg were given, and 10 μg of dexmedetomidine in total was administered before the end of surgery. IV nonsteroidal anti-inflammatory drug (NSAID) and rectal paracetamol were used before the patient was awake. The child was extubated 5 min after cessation of TCI propofol and remifentanil. He was initially restless after extubation; therefore, IV fentanyl 1 μg/kg was given. He could clearly communicate and expressed that he wanted his mother's company after he was calm.

Case 6

A 3-year-old 14 kg girl was scheduled for laparoscopic hernia repair. With topical anesthetic cream and distraction with video game, intravenous cannula was inserted with no distress. IV fentanyl 1 μg/kg was given. TCI propofol with Paedfusor model was started at Cp of 6 μg/ml; remifentanil was also infused at 0.15 μg/kg/min. IV atracurium 5 mg was given. IV bolus of remifentanil 15 μg was administered prior to intubation. Repeated dose of IV fentanyl 15 μg was given at skin incision. IV NSAID and rectal paracetamol were also used for pain relief. IV dexmedetomidine 0.7 μg/kg was administered as intermittent 2 μg boluses. The procedure lasted for 30 min. During the procedure, propofol was titrated down to 4.5 μg/ml. Propofol was stopped 5 min before completion of surgery. Local anesthetic was infiltrated by surgeon during skin closure. Remifentanil was stopped when surgery was completed. Secretion of the oropharynx was cleared, and the child was extubated at 5 min after cessation of remifentanil infusion, when spontaneous and adequate ventilation resumed. The child was still drowsy after extubation; therefore, he was turned to lateral position and transferred to PACU. He was discharged from the ward at 30 min in PACU. No additional analgesia was required. Postanesthesia emergency delirium (PAED) score was less than 2, and Aldrete score was 9 upon discharge.

Case 7

A 9-year-old 24 kg boy with chronic diarrhea and hepatosplenomegaly was planned for liver biopsy and diagnostic gastroscopy and colonoscopy. He was underweight and malnourished. Endotracheal intubation was elected for this patient as he has distended abdomen and the surgeon anticipated difficult colonoscopy. Anesthesia was induced with sevoflurane 4 % in oxygen as he has difficult intravenous access. 22G intravenous cannula was inserted after gas induction. TCI propofol with Paedfusor model at Cp of 4 µg/ml and remifentanil at 0.15 µg/kg/min was commenced when sevoflurane was ceased. Bispectral index (BIS) monitor was applied and the first BIS value was 45. TCI propofol was decreased to 3.5 µg/ml for the rest of the examination, and BIS was kept at 55–60 throughout the procedure. Propofol and remifentanil were stopped 5 min before the end of the procedure. Patient woke up 5 min after procedure was stopped. He was awake and cooperative during recovery, and Aldrete score was 10 at 5 min after extubation.

Case 8

A 36-day-old 4.4 kg boy with right lung mass for video-assisted thoracoscopic lung biopsy. Since the infant has a 24G intravenous cannula, anesthesia was induced with IV fentanyl 1 µg/kg and propofol 3.5 mg/kg, in three divided doses. After patient was anesthetized, IV atracurium 1 mg was given. Propofol and remifentanil infusion was commenced at 18 mg/kg/h and 0.2 µg/kg/min, respectively. After endotracheal tube was secured, another 22G intravenous cannula was inserted. Propofol infusion was decreased to 10 mg/kg/h since systolic blood pressure decreased from 75 to 55 mmHg after induction. Patient was turned to left lateral position. Before procedure was commenced, IV fentanyl 1 µg/kg and atracurium 0.5 mg were given. Propofol infusion increased to 18 mg/kg/h transiently before skin incision. It was titrated down to 15 mg/kg/h and then 13 mg/kg/h at 10 and 20 min into surgical procedure. Propofol was stopped during wound closure. Local anesthetic was infiltrated by the surgeon before the patient woke up. Remifentanil was stopped when surgery was completed. Spontaneous ventilation was resumed at 5 min after the procedure was completed. When he was judged to have adequate ventilation and awake, he was extubated at 15 min after completion of surgery. He was transferred to PACU before he was escorted to pediatric intensive care unit.

Discussion

During the surgical procedures, Cp may be reduced and titrated according to patient's clinical sign and surgical stimulation. Generally the use of remifentanil as part of the TIVA regimen in controlled ventilation would allow lower dose of propofol [21]. Keidan et al. have shown that the propofol dose may be reduced by up to 25 % when 0.025 µg/kg/min of remifentanil is used in children undergoing esophagogastroduodenoscopy [22]. The use of BIS in children older than 2 years of age may allow more accurate titration and shorten recovery time. Its use may be especially beneficial in children with comorbidities as the propofol requirement in these patients may be unpredictable and excessive anesthesia can potentially lead to hemodynamic instability and delay recovery.

TIVA with Propofol and Remifentanil for Spontaneous Respiration

In endoscopic airway procedures in small children, maintaining spontaneous breathing without airway device is essential for surgeon to assess for the cause of respiratory symptoms, be able to evaluate dynamic airway function and the degree of airway obstruction, so as to decide on, and to carry out, the appropriate interventions. Since administration of anesthesia is independent of airway device, sharing airway with surgeons and pollution is not a concern when TIVA is used in this type of procedures. Surgical access is unobstructed, and titration of depth of anesthesia would not be affected by patient's ventilation. Deepening of anesthesia is easily achieved by increasing the infusion rate or giving a bolus dose of propofol. Propofol has shown to be associated with less laryngospasm and apneic episodes when compared with sevoflurane, and this would translate to less interruption of surgical procedures [13–15]. Although propofol was shown to be associated with more body movement and breath holding in one study on rigid bronchoscopy for foreign body retrieval in young children [25], this could be mitigated by adequate dosing of propofol.

Remifentanil has been shown to be an excellent adjunct to propofol anesthesia in young children undergoing endoscopic airway procedures requiring preservation of spontaneous respiration [26]. Although it is a potent opioid with significant respiratory depressant effect, its antitussive properties would provide an excellent condition for airway examination and intervention as it would obtund airway reflexes during surgical manipulation. With careful titration, remifentanil infusion may be used and spontaneous ventilation is maintained [16]. Usually the author starts at 0.05 µg/kg/min and may titrate up to 0.1 µg/kg/min during painful and stimulating intervention. It was shown in a prospective study that the median tolerated dose of remifentanil without causing apnea was 0.127 µg/kg/min [27] and it was shown to be inversely related to age [28].

Both respiratory rate and heart rate can be used as endpoints to titration of depth anesthesia. Patient may be induced with either intravenous propofol or sevoflurane, depending on the availability of intravenous access. Spontaneous respiration should be preserved as far as possible, and this may be achieved by slow induction. After intravenous access is achieved, anesthesia may be maintained with intravenous agent. While the infusion rate of remifentanil is kept relatively constant to avoid severe hypoventilation and apnea, there is great interindividual variability of propofol requirement [5]. Propofol may be titrated until there is 30–50 % reduction of respiratory rate in neonates and infants or in the range of 10–15 breaths/min in older children. Topical lidocaine should be applied to the pharynx and larynx by direct laryngoscopy, and it would be a good opportunity to assess the depth of anesthesia. If the child is adequately anesthetized, there should be minimal to no movement in response to direct laryngoscopy; moreover, the heart rate and respiratory rate should remain stable throughout the procedure. Propofol bolus may be given, and infusion rate should be raised if movement, coughing, or gagging is encountered during direct laryngoscopy.

Case 9

A 2-month-old 4 kg girl with stridor was scheduled for laryngotracheal bronchoscopic assessment and possibly supraglottoplasty. Her stridor was mild at rest and more severe when she was crying or feeding. She has no intravenous access, and inhalational induction with sevoflurane 4 % in oxygen was commenced after standard monitor was placed. Intravenous cannula was placed after induction. Sevoflurane was stopped when propofol and remifentanil infusion was started. Propofol was administered at 18 mg/kg/h and remifentanil at 0.05 µg/kg/min. Spontaneous breathing was maintained throughout the procedure. Xylometazoline nasal drops were administered to both nostrils. Since the maximum dose of lignocaine for this infant was 12 mg, 1.2 ml of 1 % lignocaine was prepared in a 2-ml syringe. Direct laryngoscopy by anesthesiologists was performed, and 1 % lignocaine was sprayed to the pharynx and vocal cords with mucosal atomization device. If mucosal atomization device was not available, an 18-gauge cannula could be used for topical application of the local anesthetic. During the first attempt of direct laryngoscopy the infant reacted, so the procedure was withheld

and anesthesia was deepen with 1 mg/kg propofol. Direct laryngoscopy was reattempted, and 0.5 ml of 1 % lignocaine was applied to the pharynx and vocal cords. The rest of the lignocaine was saved for later when the surgeon needed to topicalize the lower part of the airway. A 3.0 uncuffed endotracheal tube was inserted via one nostril to the pharynx and used as nasal airway for oxygen insufflation before the surgeon started endoscopic assessment. The infant's airway was examined with flexible and rigid laryngobronchoscopes. It was decided that supraglottoplasty by laser should be carried out under rigid suspension laryngoscope. During the suspension laryngoscopy, laryngospasm was encountered, and IV propofol at 1 mg/kg was given. Remifentanil was kept at 0.05 µg/kg/min throughout the procedure, whereas propofol infusion was decreased to 15, 13, and 10 mg/kg/h gradually. The fraction of inspired oxygen decreased to 25 %, and the flow rate decreased to 2 L/min during the laser procedure. The whole procedure lasted for 40 min. The patient was put onto a lateral position during recovery, and the nasal airway was removed when she was awake.

Troubleshooting with TIVA in Children

TIVA is a relatively new and uncommon technique to be used in young children. Apart from understanding the pharmacokinetic and pharmacodynamics differences of propofol in children, provision of flawless TIVA in young children could be demanding and tedious. In order to ensure proper delivery of intravenous anesthesia, there would be a number of tasks anesthesiologists need to go through. Anesthesiologist should ensure the equipment and pumps are functioning and prepared at the correct setting, the drugs are prepared with appropriate dilution, the syringes are connected to the patient's intravenous cannula with nonreturn valve, all the connections are secure and tight with no leakage, and the intravenous cannula is functioning. Moreover, the anesthesiologist should ensure the appropriate model for drug delivery is chosen and the correct patient parameters are used. Repeated checking of syringe pump and intravenous site during the procedure should be performed to ensure safe drug delivery during the surgical procedures. For this reason, it is recommended to keep the intravenous infusion sites visible so that they may be monitored regularly for leakage, disconnection, or extravasation. To guarantee the above task is accomplished, the use of TIVA checklist should be considered, and this may be especially useful for novice TIVA anesthesiologists. A template of TIVA checklist is provided in Table 22.1. The following cases illustrate how one may get into trouble with TIVA in young children.

Table 22.1 TIVA checklist template

Infusion pumps
☐ Pump functioning with battery or power cable
☐ Familiar with the pump
☐ Setting checked and correct
Syringes
☐ Syringes recognized by the pump
Drugs
☐ Propofol 1%
☐ Remifentanil (~BW in µg/ml)
Three-way stopcock and extension
☐ Three-way extension
☐ Extension of adequate length
☐ Three-way stopcock and extension connected and functioning with no leak
☐ Nonreturn valve if this is not dedicated IV line
IV access
☐ Well secured
☐ Visible during surgery otherwise use another extension so that patency can be checked intraoperatively

Case 10

A very anxious 5-year-old boy who weighed 16 kg was scheduled for circumcision for which anesthesia was induced with sevoflurane 4 % in oxygen. After an intravenous cannula was placed, TCI propofol with Paedfusor model was commenced at 5 µg/ml and fentanyl 1 µg/kg was given. Sevoflurane was stopped subsequently. The patient breathes spontaneously without the need of airway support. After ETCO2 was monitored, resident anesthesiologist attempted to do dorsal penile nerve block. Patient moved in response to painful stimulation; hence, TCI propofol Cp target was increased to 6 µg/ml. However, patient did not respond to increase propofol infusion, his movement increased, and he raised his arm. It was noted that the noninvasive blood pressure cuff was on the same side as the intravenous access site and the inflation of blood pressure cuff caused venous stasis. Blood pressure cuff was deflated immediately and patient movement ceased. Dorsal penile nerve block was performed when patient was adequately anesthetized again. TCI Cp target was adjusted to 5 µg/ml until the end of the procedure. Another bolus dose of fentanyl 0.5 µg/kg, IV NSAID, and rectal paracetamol was administered for analgesia. Dexmedetomidine 12 µg was administered as intermittent boluses before the end of the procedure. Patient was put in lateral position and was escorted to PACU.

Case 11

A 3-year-old 15 kg boy was planned for bone marrow biopsy. This child has an intravenous cannula placed in the ward. While he was still in his mother's lap, IV propofol

2.5 mg/kg and fentanyl 0.5 µg/kg were given. The patient was separated from his mother; standard monitor was applied while oxygen was administered with face mask by anesthetic resident. The child resisted face mask application and moved his limbs. IV was dislodged with movement; hence, sevoflurane via face mask was commenced. IV was reinserted once the child was adequately anesthetized. Propofol bolus at 1 mg/kg and infusion commenced at 20 mg/kg/h while sevoflurane was stopped. After ETCO2 monitor was placed, the patient was turned to lateral position for the procedure. The patient maintained spontaneous breathing throughout the procedure. Oxygen supplementation was given via a face mask put in front of the patient's face. Local anesthetic was infiltrated before painful stimulation. Propofol was decreased to 15 mg/kg/h 15 min after commencement of surgical procedure. The procedure was completed at 20 min and the patient recovered uneventfully.

Discussion

These cases illustrated that ensuring a well-secured and functioning vascular access is extremely important in TIVA. Moreover, anesthetists need to be especially careful when managing small children whose vascular accesses are covered by surgical drapes. Dislodgement, disconnection, kinking, extravasation, or syringe pump problems can lead to inadequate depth of anesthesia. When patient is light in anesthesia, apart from increasing the infusion rate of propofol or giving extra analgesic, it is also important to rule out problems arising from delivery of intravenous drugs.

It is important to ensure that intravenous cannula is well secured before and during induction (Fig. 22.5). Movement during induction, especially if dose of propofol is inadequate, is common. Ask an anesthetic assistant or nurse to help to gently stabilize the limb of intravenous site, and ensure IV drugs are administered (Fig. 22.6). Anesthesiologist should also be familiar with the syringe pumps in use and be ready to troubleshoot in case problems arise. Nowadays good pumps with sensitive malfunction alarms are available. Nevertheless, good pumps cannot replace the vigilance of anesthesiologists.

TIVA for Radiotherapy

Radiotherapy in young children requires moderate to deep level of sedation [29, 30]. It is crucial to keep the child motionless during the 5–20 min procedure to allow precise delivery of radiation, as any movement would decrease treatment efficacy and cause damage to normal tissues [31]. For this reason, the children needed to be kept under an immobilization device which could be uncomfortable and

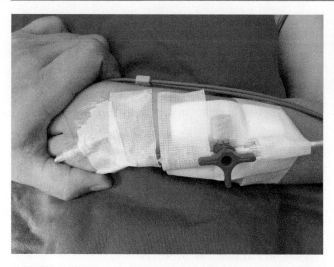

Fig. 22.6 Ensure intravenous access is well secured and functioning. Gentle restraint on patient's hand with intravenous access would prevent the IV from kinking or dislodgement during induction

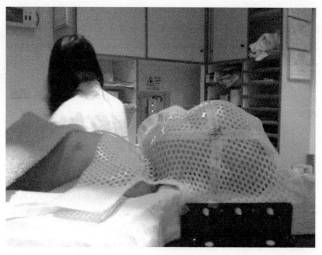

Fig. 22.7 Radiotherapy in supine position. Capnography monitoring is feasible during the procedure

frightening. In addition, radiotherapy in prone position for craniospinal irradiation may demand an even deeper level of sedation. Propofol could be an ideal agent as it is possible to titrate to the depth of sedation required while the child maintains spontaneous respiration [32]. However, there is concern of adverse respiratory events such as airway obstruction, apnea, and desaturation with propofol sedation [33]. During the radiotherapy treatment, anesthesiologist can only observe the patient in the control room; therefore, prompt reaction to adverse respiratory events may be delayed. After patient is in position and immobilization device is placed, the actual radiotherapy is non-painful and noninvasive. Since dexmedetomidine has minimal effect on respiration and ventilation [34, 35], it may be a good alternative to propofol in this setting. The following case illustrates how intravenous dexmedetomidine is used in sedation for children undergoing radiotherapy.

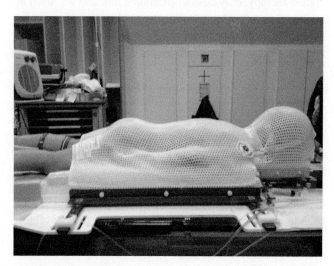

Fig. 22.8 Craniospinal irradiation in prone position

Case 12

A 5-year-old 15 kg child who had surgical excision of medulloblastoma required craniospinal irradiation in prone and supine position. A total of 30 sessions of irradiation was planned. She has a Boviac indwelling catheter which was used for induction and maintenance of sedation and anesthesia. For each session similar regimen was used. Intravenous dexmedetomidine at 12 µg/kg/min was commenced until the child appeared drowsy. Usually this took 5 min and about 1 µg/kg of dexmedetomidine was administered. Subsequently, intravenous dexmedetomidine would be reduced to 1 µg/kg/min; pulse oximetry and blood pressure cuff were applied, and child was transferred to the operating table. Subsequently, intravenous propofol was given in small aliquots at 0.5–1 mg/kg, titrated to allow patient positioning and placement of immobilization devices (Fig. 22.7). Usually the child needed 0.5–1.5 mg/kg of propofol in total to allow successful positioning. Supplemental oxygen was given via nasal cannula. After ensuring sufficient sedation and stable cardiorespiratory conditions in the child, dexmedetomidine infusion was decreased to 0.7 µg/kg/h, and all staff would leave the treatment room. The child would be continuously monitored through video system which enabled staff to visualize the child and the physiological monitor from control room. Blood pressure and heart rate often decreased by 10–15 % from the baseline after sedation. SpO2 was always maintained above 96 % with oxygen. ETCO2 and capnography was used in supine position, but it was not feasible in prone position (Figs. 22.7 and 22.8). The child usually woke up 30 min after the radiotherapy.

Discussion

In this case, propofol is used as an adjunct to dexmedetomidine sedation. Dexmedetomidine has been used and investigated extensively as sedative agent for radiological imaging studies in children [36]. When intravenous dexmedetomidine is used as sole agent for sedation in computer tomography imaging studies or magnetic resonance imaging studies, the loading dose required is about 2 μg/kg and 3 μg/kg, respectively [37, 38]. The maintenance infusion rate ranged from 1 to 2 μg/kg/h. Although the dose of dexmedetomidine required is high when it is used as sole agent for moderate to deep sedation, it is associated with excellent safety record because of its wide margin of safety. When intravenous dexmedetomidine was used in the above case, since small bolus dose of propofol was used in the most simulative part of the procedure, the dose of dexmedetomidine required is relatively lower. During irradiation therapy, only dexmedetomidine infusion was used as maintenance of sedation when the peak effect of propofol has already worn off; therefore, the chance of adverse respiratory events would be quite low.

Summary

TIVA is a feasible and good alternative technique to inhalation anesthesia. Secondary to the pharmacokinetic and pharmacodynamics difference of young children from adults, the dose required with manual infusion or the target Cp for TCI is higher. Although recovery from anesthesia tends to be prolonged, it is associated with a number of beneficial effects including decreased incidence of laryngospasm, emergence of delirium, postoperative nausea and vomiting, and possibly pain. Since TIVA is a relatively new technique of anesthesia in children, when anesthesiologists begin to practice TIVA in children, they are encouraged to prepare a checklist for TIVA to serve as an aid and reminder of important steps and issues in carrying out safe TIVA in children.

References

1. Hill M, Peat W, Courtman S. A national survey of propofol infusion use by paediatric anaesthetists in Great Britain and Ireland. Paediatr Anaesth. 2008;18:488–93.
2. Murat I, Billard V, Vernois J, Zaouter M, Marsol P, Souron R, Farinotti R. Pharmacokinetics of propofol after a single dose in children aged 1–3 years with minor burns. Comparison of three data analysis approaches. Anesthesiology. 1996;84:526–32.
3. McFarlan CS, Anderson BJ, Short TG. The use of propofol infusions in paediatric anaesthesia: a practical guide. Paediatr Anaesth. 1999;9:209–16.
4. Steur RJ, Perez RS, De Lange JJ. Dosage scheme for propofol in children under 3 years of age. Paediatr Anaesth. 2004;14:462–7.
5. Rigouzzo A, Girault L, Louvet N, Servin F, De-Smet T, Piat V, Seeman R, Murat I, Constant I. The relationship between bispectral index and propofol during target-controlled infusion anesthesia: a comparative study between children and young adults. Anesth Analg. 2008;106:1109–16, table of contents.
6. Iwakiri H, Nishihara N, Nagata O, Matsukawa T, Ozaki M, Sessler DI. Individual effect-site concentrations of propofol are similar at loss of consciousness and at awakening. Anesth Analg. 2005;100:107–10.
7. Kataria BK, Ved SA, Nicodemus HF, Hoy GR, Lea D, Dubois MY, Mandema JW, Shafer SL. The pharmacokinetics of propofol in children using three different data analysis approaches. Anesthesiology. 1994;80:104–22.
8. Marsh B, White M, Morton N, Kenny GN. Pharmacokinetic model driven infusion of propofol in children. Br J Anaesth. 1991;67:41–8.
9. Absalom A, Amutike D, Lal A, White M, Kenny GN. Accuracy of the 'Paedfusor' in children undergoing cardiac surgery or catheterization. Br J Anaesth. 2003;91:507–13.
10. Choi BM, Lee HG, Byon HJ, Lee SH, Lee EK, Kim HS, Noh GJ. Population pharmacokinetic and pharmacodynamic model of propofol externally validated in children. J Pharmacokinet Pharmacodyn. 2015;42:163–77.
11. Varveris DA, Morton NS. Target controlled infusion of propofol for induction and maintenance of anaesthesia using the paedfusor: an open pilot study. Paediatr Anaesth. 2002;12:589–93.
12. Fuentes R, Cortinez I, Ibacache M, Concha M, Munoz H. Propofol concentration to induce general anesthesia in children aged 3–11 years with the Kataria effect-site model. Paediatr Anaesth. 2015;25:554–9.
13. Heard C, Harutunians M, Houck J, Joshi P, Johnson K, Lerman J. Propofol anesthesia for children undergoing magnetic resonance imaging: a comparison with isoflurane, nitrous oxide, and a laryngeal mask airway. Anesth Analg. 2015;120:157–64.
14. von Ungern-Sternberg BS, Boda K, Chambers NA, Rebmann C, Johnson C, Sly PD, Habre W. Risk assessment for respiratory complications in paediatric anaesthesia: a prospective cohort study. Lancet. 2010;376:773–83.
15. Oberer C, von Ungern-Sternberg BS, Frei FJ, Erb TO. Respiratory reflex responses of the larynx differ between sevoflurane and propofol in pediatric patients. Anesthesiology. 2005;103:1142–8.
16. Ansermino JM, Magruder W, Dosani M. Spontaneous respiration during intravenous anesthesia in children. Curr Opin Anaesthesiol. 2009;22:383–7.
17. Al-alami AA, Zestos MM, Baraka AS. Pediatric laryngospasm: prevention and treatment. Curr Opin Anaesthesiol. 2009;22:388–95.
18. Hampson-Evans D, Morgan P, Farrar M. Pediatric laryngospasm. Paediatr Anaesth. 2008;18:303–7.
19. Lee JR, Kim SD, Kim CS, Yoon TG, Kim HS. Minimum alveolar concentration of sevoflurane for laryngeal mask airway removal in anesthetized children. Anesth Analg. 2007;104:528–31.
20. Pappas AL, Sukhani R, Lurie J, Pawlowski J, Sawicki K, Corsino A. Severity of airway hyperreactivity associated with laryngeal mask airway removal: correlation with volatile anesthetic choice and depth of anesthesia. J Clin Anesth. 2001;13:498–503.
21. Drover DR, Litalien C, Wellis V, Shafer SL, Hammer GB. Determination of the pharmacodynamic interaction of propofol and remifentanil during esophagogastroduodenoscopy in children. Anesthesiology. 2004;100:1382–6.
22. Keidan I, Berkenstadt H, Sidi A, Perel A. Propofol/remifentanil versus propofol alone for bone marrow aspiration in paediatric haemato-oncological patients. Paediatr Anaesth. 2001;11:297–301.
23. Hayes JA, Lopez AV, Pehora CM, Robertson JM, Abla O, Crawford MW. Coadministration of propofol and remifentanil for lumbar puncture in children: dose-response and an evaluation of two dose combinations. Anesthesiology. 2008;109:613–8.

24. Tsui BC, Wagner A, Usher AG, Cave DA, Tang C. Combined propofol and remifentanil intravenous anesthesia for pediatric patients undergoing magnetic resonance imaging. Paediatr Anaesth. 2005;15:397–401.

25. Chen LH, Zhang X, Li SQ, Liu YQ, Zhang TY, Wu JZ. The risk factors for hypoxemia in children younger than 5 years old undergoing rigid bronchoscopy for foreign body removal. Anesth Analg. 2009;109:1079–84.

26. Malherbe S, Ansermino JM. Total intravenous anesthesia and spontaneous ventilation for foreign body removal in children: how much drug? Anesth Analg. 2010;111:1566. author reply 1566.

27. Ansermino JM, Brooks P, Rosen D, Vandebeek CA, Reichert C. Spontaneous ventilation with remifentanil in children. Paediatr Anaesth. 2005;15:115–21.

28. Barker N, Lim J, Amari E, Malherbe S, Ansermino JM. Relationship between age and spontaneous ventilation during intravenous anesthesia in children. Paediatr Anaesth. 2007;17:948–55.

29. Seiler G, De Vol E, Khafaga Y, Gregory B, Al-Shabanah M, Valmores A, Versteeg D, Ellis B, Mustafa MM, Gray A. Evaluation of the safety and efficacy of repeated sedations for the radiotherapy of young children with cancer: a prospective study of 1033 consecutive sedations. Int J Radiat Oncol Biol Phys. 2001;49:771–83.

30. Scheiber G, Ribeiro FC, Karpienski H, Strehl K. Deep sedation with propofol in preschool children undergoing radiation therapy. Paediatr Anaesth. 1996;6:209–13.

31. Harris EA. Sedation and anesthesia options for pediatric patients in the radiation oncology suite. Int J Pediatr. 2010;2010:870921.

32. McFadyen JG, Pelly N, Orr RJ. Sedation and anesthesia for the pediatric patient undergoing radiation therapy. Curr Opin Anaesthesiol. 2011;24:433–8.

33. Cravero JP, Beach ML, Blike GT, Gallagher SM, Hertzog JH, Pediatric Sedation Research C. The incidence and nature of adverse events during pediatric sedation/anesthesia with propofol for procedures outside the operating room: a report from the Pediatric Sedation Research Consortium. Anesth Analg. 2009;108:795–804.

34. Yuen VM. Dexmedetomidine: perioperative applications in children. Paediatr Anaesth. 2010;20:256–64.

35. Ebert TJ, Hall JE, Barney JA, Uhrich TD, Colinco MD. The effects of increasing plasma concentrations of dexmedetomidine in humans. Anesthesiology. 2000;93:382–94.

36. Mahmoud M, Mason KP. Dexmedetomidine: review, update, and future considerations of paediatric perioperative and periprocedural applications and limitations. Br J Anaesth. 2015;115:171–82.

37. Mason KP, Zgleszewski SE, Dearden JL, Dumont RS, Pirich MA, Stark CD, D'Angelo P, Macpherson S, Fontaine PJ, Connor L, Zurakowski D. Dexmedetomidine for pediatric sedation for computed tomography imaging studies. Anesth Analg. 2006;103:57–62, table of contents.

38. Mason KP, Zurakowski D, Zgleszewski SE, Robson CD, Carrier M, Hickey PR, Dinardo JA. High dose dexmedetomidine as the sole sedative for pediatric MRI. Paediatr Anaesth. 2008;18:403–11.

TCI/TIVA Adult Case Studies

23

Nicholas Sutcliffe

Introduction

Total intravenous anesthesia (TIVA) has many potential benefits. Indeed some situations mandate the use of an intravenous technique. However, rates of TIVA use in many countries remain low, compared with the use of volatile anesthesia. The recent NAP5 study from the UK and Ireland suggested that some anaesthesiologists lack appropriate knowledge of dosing and that training needs to be improved [1]. Recommendation four from the NAP5 report states: "All anesthetists should be trained in the maintenance of anesthesia with intravenous infusions". The current situation in the UK and Ireland likely falls far short of this simple goal. Madhivathanan and colleagues published the results of a survey of UK anaesthesiologists in training. The responses revealed the following results: 78 % of trainees had no formal teaching or training in TIVA; 60 % of trainees occasionally, rarely or never use TIVA; and 48 % of trainees were not competent using TIVA unsupervised [2].

The benefits of TIVA are dealt with elsewhere in this publication, as are the detailed pharmacokinetics (PK) and pharmacodynamics (PD) of intravenous agents and their delivery. As many of the case studies involve TCI, this chapter will briefly consider the potential merits of target-controlled infusion (TCI) versus manual-controlled infusion (MCI). It will also deal briefly with the concept of the effect site and measure of potency of intravenous agents equivalent to the MAC for volatile agents. We will then move on to detailed case studies to highlight appropriate doses in real-life clinical scenarios and emphasise key learning points.

TCI vs. MCI for TIVA

There have been a number of studies comparing TCI with MCI. In general no major advantage has been demonstrated with regard to patient outcomes [3]. However, more recently the NAP5 study suggested a lower incidence of awareness when using TCI, compared to manual drug delivery [1]. Studies looking at ease of use and operator preference show that anaesthesiologists tend to subjectively score TCI highly, in this respect [4]. To look for differences between the two techniques in terms of patient benefits is to misunderstand the utility of TCI. The benefits to patients from the use of TIVA derive mainly from the drugs themselves rather than the delivery methodology. It is possible to deliver "bad" or "good" anesthesia with both TCI and MCI. What is important for the quality of anesthesia delivered by TIVA is the knowledge and experience of the anesthetist concerned. Appropriate dosing and ability to titrate the dose to individual patients and differing levels of surgical stimulus will determine the quality of surgical anesthesia and recovery in an individual patient. It is in the training of the anaesthesiologist that TCI has its major utility.

Let us consider an induction and initial maintenance strategy with the two methodologies. Figure 23.1 shows a TCI with a plasma target set at 3 µg/ml and a MCI designed to achieve a similar plasma concentration, in a patient weighing 70 kg. Now examine the anesthetist's task in each of these examples. The anaesthesiologist delivering the TCI infusion inputs the patient data into the TCI system, selects a target of 3 and presses start. The anesthetist delivering the MCI takes the patients weight, calculates the bolus and calculates the initial, second and third infusion rates.

Electronic supplementary material: The online version of this chapter (https://doi.org/10.1007/978-3-319-47609-4_23) contains supplementary material, which is available to authorized users.

N. Sutcliffe, BSc Phys, MBChB, MRCP, FRCA (✉)
Hamad Medical Corporation, Hamad Medical City,
P.O. Box 3050 Doha, Qatar
e-mail: nick.sut@doctors.org.uk

A.R. Absalom, K.P. Mason (eds.), *Total Intravenous Anesthesia and Target Controlled Infusions*,
DOI 10.1007/978-3-319-47609-4_23

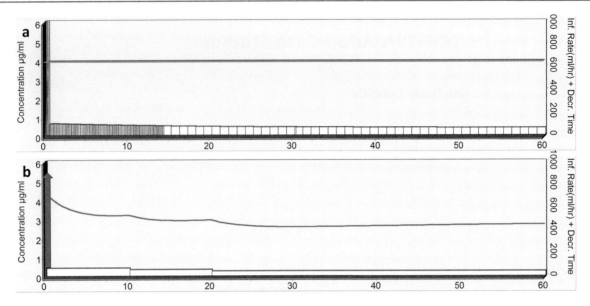

Fig. 23.1 **a** Propofol TCI set at 3 µg/ml, **b** MCI propofol infusion regimen, designed to give a plasma concentration of 3 µg/ml: 1 mg/kg bolus, 10 mg/kg/h, reduced to 8 mg/kg/h at 10 min, reduced to 6 mg/kg/h at 20 min. *Large arrow* bolus dose, *solid line* plasma concentration µg/ml, *white boxes* infusion rate ml/h

He then delivers the bolus, starts the initial infusion and sets a timer or relies on remembering to change the infusion after 10 min and again after 20 min. During this induction phase, he also has to preoxygenate, look after the airway and intubate the patient, as well as be vigilant for any cardiovascular compromise which may need prompt treatment.

Now, consider a further thought experiment in which we communicate these two methodologies to a first year resident and, even more challenging, a senior colleague not familiar with intravenous anesthesia practice.

For TCI the simple instructions are easy to follow: enter the patient details and propofol concentration into the pump, select a target of 3 and press start.

In comparison the instructions for the MCI involve the following steps:

1. Calculate the bolus dose as follows:

   70 kg × 1 mg/kg := 70 mg = 7 ml of 1% propofol or 3.5 ml 2% of propofol.

2. Calculate initial infusion rate as follows:

   70 kg × 10 mg/kg/h = 700 mg/h = 70 ml/h for 1% propofol or 35 ml/h for 2% propofol.

3. Enter these details and press start.
4. Calculate the second infusion rate as follows:

   70 kg × 8 mg/kg/h = 560 mg/h = 56 ml/h for 1% propofol or 28 ml/h for 2% propofol.

5. Calculate the third infusion rate as follows:

   70 kg × 6 mg/kg/h = 420 mg/h = 42 ml/h for 1% propofol or 21 ml/h for 2% propofol.

At this point our senior colleague is likely to decide that TIVA does not suit his clinical practice. Our resident, who is keen to learn a new technique, is likely to point out that the bolus and initial infusion rate, using 1 % propofol, are numerically the same as the patient's weight in kg. He notes that after 10 min the infusion rate is reduced by one fifth and then by one quarter after 20 min and is likely to conclude this as relatively straightforward.

Now we need to consider titration of our hypnotic infusion and infusion of an opiate. With TCI the anaesthesiologist simply selects a lower or higher target depending on the response of the patient and can likewise start a TCI of opiate. With MCI, if the infusion rate is doubled at 10 min, it will take approximately 10 min before the plasma concentration has doubled. Halving the infusion rate at this point will not result in a halving of the plasma concentration, no matter how long we wait. This is because of the drug that is already in the body and the fact that a fixed infusion rate of propofol will result in plasma concentrations that rise until steady state is reached. This will take more than 24 h in the case of propofol. In contrast doubling the set target concentration with a TCI at 10 min results in a doubling of the plasma concentration in less than 1 min. Halving the TCI target at 20 min results in a halving of the plasma concentration in less than 5 min. This is because the TCI system switches off the infusion, allowing the plasma concentration of propofol to fall as rapidly as possible, as dictated by the kinetics of the drug (see Fig. 23.2) and then restarts the infusion at an appropriate lower concentration. In order to achieve a similar rapidity of titration with MCI, for an increase in the desired plasma concentration, the anaesthesiologist would have to calculate a small supplementary bolus size and a new infusion rate. For a decrease in the desired plasma concentration, he will have to calculate an interval of zero infusion and a new infusion rate thereafter. All these calculations are complex for propofol (and all other anesthetic drugs) as they depend on the interplay between three exponential processes, how much

drug has been delivered and the duration of infusion (see Chaps. 6—Raeder and 25—Anderson on PK/PD).

At this point our keen resident should logically concede that the TCI methodology will be easier to learn and implement than MCI. With the MCI methodology the anaesthesiologist's focus is on drug calculations, infusion rates and timings, at a time when the he should be focusing on his patient. The TCI methodology allows rapid stepwise changes in the plasma propofol concentration, in a manner analogous to the use of a calibrated vaporiser. The anaesthesiologist needs to only decide if more, less or the same target is required, and titration is simply achieved by changing one number, the target concentration.

There is also brevity in the description of dosing with TCI. What response do I give if a colleague asks "what sedative dose of propofol do I need for conscious sedation"? When describing TCI dosing, I can say "around 1–2 µg/ml titrated to effect". This description includes the automatically calculated loading dose and rate adjustment over time, which will be identical for all patients with the same characteristics and for the same target concentrations. With MCI I would have to specify a loading dose range in mg/kg and a maintenance infusion regimen with a wide range in mg/kg/h, to account not only for interindividual differences in pharmacokinetics and pharmacodynamics but also for the changing relationship between infusion rate and plasma concentration (as the propofol concentration gradient between the central and other compartments gradually decreases). As we will see in the case studies that follow, TCI dosing facilitates easy communication and understanding of dosing strategies for TIVA, in a wide range of cases.

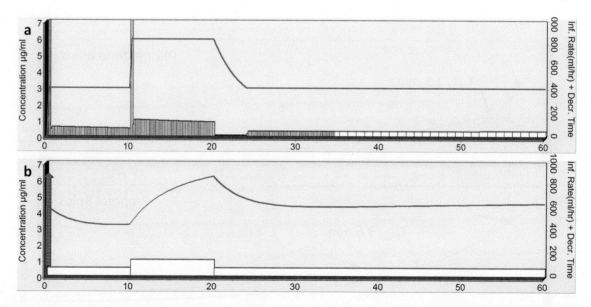

Fig. 23.2 Comparison of titration with TCI and MCI: **a** propofol TCI 3 µg/ml initial target increased to 6 µg/ml at 10 min, decreased back to 3 µg/ml at 20 min; **b** MCI propofol infusion regimen 1 mg/kg bolus, 10 mg/kg/h increased to 20 mg/kg/h at 10 min, reduced back to 10 mg/kg/h at 20 min. *Large arrow* bolus dose, *solid line* plasma concentration µg/ml, *white boxes* infusion rate ml/h

The illustrations we have looked at so far have only considered the blood (or plasma) concentration of propofol, whereas the blood compartment is not the site of action of propofol. While we know that the site of action of the hypnotics is somewhere in the brain, it is by no means certain where and how in the brain this action occurs. Therefore the site of action is commonly referred to rather vaguely as the effect site (see Fig. 23.2, Chap. 25 [Anderson]).

Before continuing to the case studies, we will therefore briefly consider the modelling and relevance of the effect-site concentration.

Effect-Site Concentration

I can clearly remember an incident during my first few weeks as an anesthesia senior house officer in the UK. A senior colleague was teaching me about induction of anesthesia, at the time using thiopentone (as propofol was a new drug that was then considered to be expensive and not regularly used). He informed me that if I injected an appropriate dose, anesthesia would be induced within one "arm-brain circulation time". The underlying assumption made was that equilibration across the blood-brain barrier is instantaneous. Now that we have a better understanding of drug PK/PD, we know this to be untrue. In fact thiopentone does equilibrate more rapidly with the brain than propofol (this is one of the reasons why some still recommend thiopentone for rapid sequence induction of anesthesia), but this equilibration is by no means instant.

Each drug appears to have a unique equilibration profile presumably related to its physiochemical properties and mechanism of receptor interaction. Hypnotic agents have to diffuse across the blood-brain barrier (BBB) and then to their site of action. At the site of action, a hypnotic/receptor interaction occurs which then induces changes within the brain, resulting in a change in conscious level. The time taken for this process can be modelled by objectively measuring the clinical effect—usually by means of a form of processed EEG. One of the parameters derived from this PD modelling is a rate constant (K_{e0}), which can be used to calculate a theoretical effect-site concentration. This assumes that the drug has maximal effect when blood and brain concentrations equilibrate. This assumption cannot be tested in practice, as we don't currently have the means to measure the hypnotic concentration at the site of its action (the brain). We rely instead on a derived surrogate measure of drug effect. As there is no standardised effect measure, or agreed methodology in the literature, and significant variation is seen between subjects within individual studies, various values for the K_{e0} of propofol have been published in the literature.

As mentioned, using PD modelling we can derive a K_{e0} and estimate an effect-site concentration of the hypnotic, which should better relate to conscious level and depth of anesthesia. Figure 23.3 shows a simulation of the time course of plasma and effect-site concentrations following a bolus dose of propofol and thiopentone. Both drugs rapidly achieve a peak plasma concentration. Thiopentone has a more rapid initial decay due to its rapid redistribution, but it also has a more rapid effect-site equilibration rate due to a "faster K_{e0}". The result of both these factors is a more rapid time to peak effect (T_{PEAK}). The T_{PEAK} for thiopentone is about 1.5 min compared to about 3.5 min for propofol using

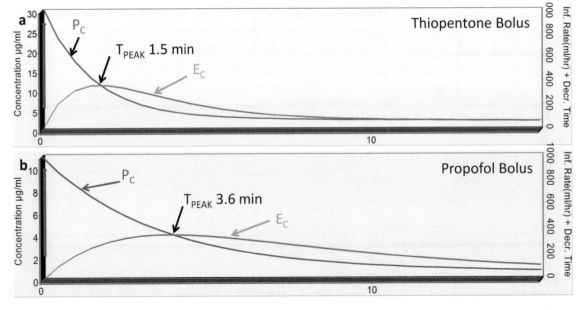

Fig. 23.3 Bolus dose of **a** thiopentone and **b** propofol. Effect-site concentration (C_e): plasma concentration (C_p), time to peak effect (T_{PEAK})

the Marsh PK/PD model[1] [5]. The clinical consequence is that in experienced hands thiopentone can achieve rapid and safe induction of anesthesia. The longer delay to peak effect seen with propofol means that an anaesthesiologist is more likely to overdose during bolus induction, particularly if he is thinking in terms of "one arm-brain" circulation time and is overhasty in administering subsequent doses. The rapid initial decrement in blood concentration seen with thiopentone, and this, coupled for the fast K_{e0} is the reason for the short duration of effect of a single bolus. While this has some benefits, it has been implicated in awareness during rapid sequence induction, when difficulties with the airway may result in delays in attaining adequate inhalational agent levels [1]. Anesthesiologists considering administering additional boluses of thiopentone should of course remember that it is slowly metabolised. This results in a long elimination half-life, so that significant accumulation occurs with multiple boluses or infusions and may result in delayed awakening.

Clearly, among other pharmacokinetic and pharmacodynamic issues, the anaesthesiologist also needs to consider the speed of equilibration between plasma and effect site during TIVA administration and in particular at induction, during titration and during emergence.

---

[1] *The K_{e0} used in the Diprifusor and implemented in Tivatrainer is 0.26 published in a poster at the WCA Australia 1996.

MAC Equivalence EC$_{50}$

No new volatile agents have been developed in recent decades. Nonetheless, if an anesthetist is faced with an unfamiliar or new volatile agent, he will soon want to know the MAC$_{50}$ or MAC of the agent. The MAC$_{50}$ is the minimum alveolar concentration associated with a 50 % probability of movement in response to skin incision. This will immediately allow an assessment of potency of the new agent and give a guide to dosing. An analogous measure for intravenous agents is the effective concentration resulting in a 50 % probability of movement in response to skin incision (EC$_{50}$). This can be determined for an intravenous agent for a single drug or a combination of agents, and we will discuss this in more detail later in this chapter. For now we will concentrate on a single agent used for induction of anesthesia. The EC$_{50}$ for loss of consciousness (EC$_{50}$ LOC) can be determined for both plasma and effect-site concentrations. These values may differ substantially depending on the method of induction. The faster the induction dose is given, the more the effect-site concentration (C_e) and plasma concentration (C_p) will differ at various clinical end points. Figure 23.4 illustrates induction of anesthesia with 3 different infusion rates 1200, 600 and 300 ml/h. The data are also presented in Table 23.1 [6]. The lowest infusion rate results in the longest induction time and the lowest induction dose. As can be seen from the data, the C_p at LOC varies from 4.3 µg/ml at the 300 ml/h induction rate up to 9.2 µg/ml at the 1200 ml/h induction rate. However, the calculated C_e for

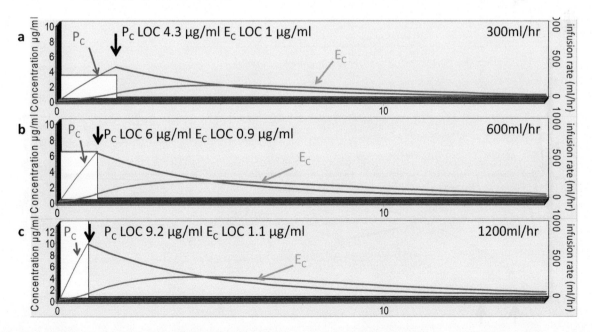

Fig. 23.4 Induction of anesthesia with different rates of infusion: **a** 300 ml/h, **b** 600 ml/h, **c** 1200 ml/h. Effect-site concentration (C_e), plasma concentration (C_p), plasma concentration at loss of concentration (C_p LOC), effect-site concentration at loss of consciousness (C_e LOC). *White boxes* infusion rate ml/h. Data re-simulated from the infusion rate and induction times from Peacock and co-workers [6] using Tivatrainer with Marsh PK/PD

LOC is similar for all three infusion rates at around 1 µg/ml and essentially rate independent. Thus it is more appropriate to consider the C_e LOC when comparing induction strategies in our case studies to follow.

Case Studies

All the cases detailed below are taken from real patients to whom I or my colleagues have administered TIVA. All propofol TCI infusions were delivered using the standard Marsh model in plasma control mode with 1 % propofol. Remifentanil TCI infusions were delivered using the Minto model in plasma control mode with a syringe concentration of 20 µg/ml (1 mg in 50 ml 0.9 % NaCl). The timeline displayed in the text is in the format hh:mm:ss, and time 00:00:00 is the start time of anesthesia. The C_p and C_e time course presented in the figures are simulated using Tivatrainer©[2]. For a video of the TIVAtrainer output, and a sound recorded during the case, see the online material.

---

[2] Tivatrainer© F. Engbers: http://www.eurosiva.org/Tivatrainer/tivatrainer_main.htm.

Table 23.1 Blood and effect-site concentration at loss of consciousness for 3 different infusion rates

	C_p LOC	C_e LOC (µ/ml)
1200 ml/h	9.2	1.1
600 ml/h	6.0	0.9
300 ml/h	4.3	1.0

Induction of Anesthesia

Case Study 1

First let us consider a simple single agent induction of anesthesia with propofol, in a 68-year-old male who weighs 82 kg and is 170 cm tall, attending for inguinal hernia repair surgery. He has a history of stable angina on beta-blocker therapy and as required nitroglycerine spray. He is otherwise fit and healthy. In this case we started a TCI of propofol at 4 µg/ml, using the Marsh model in plasma control. Figure 23.5 and Video 23.1 show the time course of the C_p and C_e. Below is the clinical course from induction (time zero).

00:00:00

Haemodynamics: blood pressure (BP) 122/77 mmHg, heart rate (HR) 69/min, pulse oximeter oxygen saturation (SpO$_2$) 98 %. Initial propofol TCI target set at 4 µg/ml.

00:00:28

The C_p is now calculated to have reached the target of 4 µg/ml, achieved with a loading dose of 8 ml (80 mg). I speak to the patient and he responds with no discernible change in conscious level; the temptation is to increase the target, but if we look at the calculated C_e, it is still only 0.2 µg/ml, so we wait without changing the target.

00:00:50

The patient yawns and is not as attentive to his surroundings. The C_p has not changed, but the C_e has risen to 0.6 µg/ml.

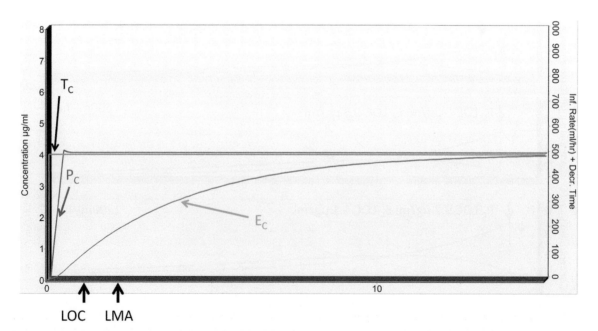

Fig. 23.5 Case study 1: propofol TCI induction of anesthesia 4 µg/ml. Target concentration (T_C), effect-site concentration (C_e), plasma concentration (C_p), loss of consciousness (LOC), loss of eyelash reflex (LER), laryngeal mask airway insertion (LMA)

The total dose given to the patient at this stage is 87 mg; BP is now 112/71, HR 62 and SpO$_2$ 99 %.

00:01:01
The patient looses response to verbal contact, but eyelash reflex remains, the C_e is now 0.8 μg/ml and 90 mg of drug has been delivered.

00:01:36
The eyelash reflex is lost and the patient's airway is supported by face mask with 100 % O$_2$; BP 97/58, HR 55 and SpO$_2$ 97 %, the C_e has now risen to 1.2 μg/ml and 102 mg of propofol has been delivered. At this point the anaesthesiologist checks the slackness of the jaw but feels the patient is not yet ready for insertion of the laryngeal mask airway (LMA).

00:02:26
The C_p is still 4 μg/ml as we have not changed the target; the C_e is now 1.7 μg/ml and 118 mg of propofol has been delivered. The jaw is now slack and a LMA is inserted successfully at first attempt; repeat haemodynamics reveal a BP of 105/65 and HR 72, following the mild stimulation of the LMA insertion.

In this example we have achieved a smooth induction of anesthesia and LMA insertion with minimal effect on haemodynamics in an elderly patient with a history of cardiovascular disease. The system delivered a total induction dose of almost 120 mg (1.46 mg/kg) of propofol over 2.5 min, in keeping with dosing recommendations in the elderly (1.5–1.75 mg/kg) [7]. Delivering this dose over a longer time frame is likely to result in less cardiovascular depression. The high peak blood concentration seen with bolus dosing has been avoided, at the expense of prolonging the induction time. The same dose given as a bolus would result in a peak blood concentration of 6.4 μg/ml. If we assume that the patient would lose consciousness at the same effect-site concentration of 0.8 μg/ml, then this would be achieved at 38 s. However, we would likely see a bigger decline in BP, as propofol has a direct vasodilatory effect on the vasculature, as well as a centrally mediated cardiovascular depressant action.

It is important to realise that there is variability between patients with respect to both PK and PD. Typically PK variability results in 30–35 % variation in blood concentrations given the same dosing regimen. However, PD differences mean that the effect a given blood concentration can vary as much as 100 % between individuals. Some of this variability is predictable from patient factors such as age and previous exposure to drugs. In practice it is always important to titrate to drug effect in an individual patient, rather than giving the same dose to all patients. Table 23.2 illustrates the difference in two patients of similar age with respect to their response to a TCI of propofol set at 4 μ/ml. Patient 1 is the patient we discussed in the example above. Patient 2 is a 69-year-old male of similar body habitus. The second patient loses consciousness at a higher effect-site concentration 1.5 μ/ml compared with the first patient 0.8 μ/ml, showing almost a 100 % difference. Some of this difference may be due to PK differences, but it is more likely to be related to PD variability.

Case Study 2
Now we will consider a younger male patient aged 28, with weight 75 Kg, height 179 cm and no comorbidity. In this case we would expect the patient to be less sensitive to propofol and to have more cardiovascular reserve. In order to have a shorter induction phase in this patient, we select a higher initial target of 8 μg/ml to drive the drug into the effect site. Once loss of consciousness is achieved, the target concentration of propofol is reduced to 4 μg/ml. Figure 23.6 and Video 23.2 show the time course of the blood and effect-site concentrations of propofol during this case, and the induction doses and times are presented in Table 23.2.

00:00:00
The initial propofol target concentration is set at 8 μg/ml. BP is 122/77, HR 69 and SpO$_2$ 97 %.

00:00:47
A loading dose of 152 mg has been delivered. The infusion rate is now 238 ml/h, the C_p is 8 μg/ml but the C_e is still only 0.8 μg/ml. The patient's eyes are open, he is looking around, the BP has dropped to 112/71 and HR is 62 and SpO$_2$ 99 %.

00:01:10
The patient's eyes are closed, but he responds to the question "are you feeling sleepy" in the affirmative. The C_p is

Table 23.2 Comparison of propofol induction dose requirements and induction time, for two patients of similar age and weight, together with a younger patient

	C_e LOC (μ/ml)	C_e LER (μ/ml)	T LOC (mm:ss)	T LER (mm:ss)	Propofol LOC (mg)	Propofol LER (mg)
Case study 1 age 68, weight 82 kg, height 176	0.8	1.2	01:01	01:36	90	102
Similar patient age 69, weight 82 kg, height 174	1.5	1.9	02:01	02:35	110	122
Young patient age 28, weight 75, height 179	1.8	2.2	01:02	01:36	172	182

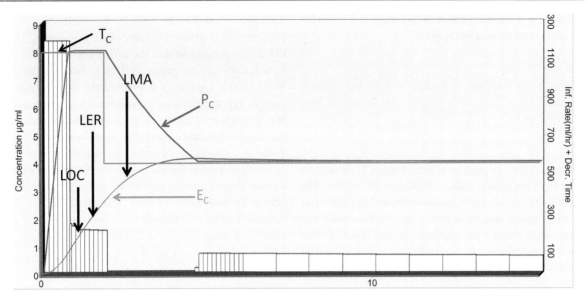

Fig. 23.6 Case study 2: induction with TCI propofol 8 µg/ml reduced to 4 µg/ml following induction of anesthesia. Target concentration (T_C), effect-site concentration (C_e), plasma concentration (C_p), *white boxes* infusion rate ml/h, loss of consciousness (LOC), loss of eyelash reflex (LER), laryngeal mask airway insertion (LMA)

maintained at 8 µg/ml (this calculated value will not change until a new target is set), the C_e has risen to 1.6 µg/ml and the infusion rate is now 219 ml/h.

00:01:20

The patient looses response to verbal communication at a C_e of 1.8 µg/ml, a total of 172 mg of propofol have been delivered and BP is 97/58, HR 56 and SpO$_2$ 98 %.

00:01:36

The eyelash reflex is lost, the C_e is 2.2 µg/ml and bag mask ventilation is commenced; infusion rate is 217 ml/h and 182 mg of propofol has been delivered.

00:01:50

The target concentration is reduced to 4 µg/ml, the C_e is currently 2.6 µg/ml and a total of 190 mg of propofol has been infused. The infusion rate is now 0 ml/h, as the system has switched off the infusion to allow the C_p to fall as quickly as possible to the new target. BP is 85/54, HR 48 and SpO$_2$ 98 %.

00:02:20

The infusion rate is still zero as the calculated C_p of 7 µg/ml is above the set target of 4 µg/ml. The C_e is now 3.3 µg/ml and continues to rise despite the infusion rate being zero, as there is still a concentration gradient between plasma and effect-site concentrations. The jaw is now relaxed and an LMA is inserted. Following this mild stimulus the BP is 107/67, HR 55 and SpO$_2$ 97 %.

00:04:50

The C_p and C_e have now equilibrated at 4 µg/ml, the system has restarted and the infusion is at 95.7 ml/h. A total of 194 mg of propofol has been delivered. Before surgery starts an opiate TCI will be started to blunt the response to surgical stimulation. The plan would be to have the C_e of hypnotic/opiate combination at around the EC$_{95}$ as a starting point for maintenance. However, the clinician always needs to adjust these values according to the patient's response, to the induction phase and proposed surgery and to its associated degree of stimulation. We will consider the concept of hypnotic/opiate EC$_{95}$ in more detail in the case studies to follow.

In this case we have started with a high initial target concentration, which results in a larger loading dose, achieving a high C_p to drive the drug into the brain. In this healthy young individual who has a reasonable cardiovascular reserve, this is well tolerated. However, this is not a technique to use in the elderly or cardiovascularly compromised patients, as such patients are likely to have a steep decline in their blood pressure. In these patients a more cautious approach is merited. We have seen such an approach in case one. In more fragile patients, it is often better to select an even lower target and titrate up slowly, allowing time for effect-site equilibration. This technique will result in a more stable haemodynamic response, but will also result in a slow induction phase. The patient will pass through progressively deeper levels of sedation before losing consciousness. An alternative approach for such patients is to use a lower dose of hypnotic combined with an opiate. We will consider these combinations for both induction and maintenance in the

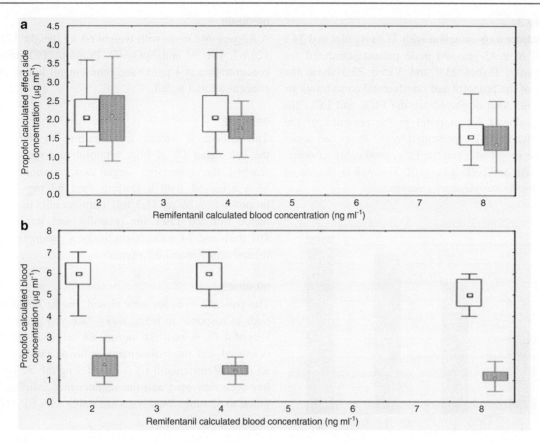

Fig. 23.7 **a** Propofol plasma concentration at loss of and recovery of consciousness, **b** propofol effect-site concentration at loss of and recovery of consciousness [8]

cases that follow. However, many colleagues prefer to use TCI propofol as a sole induction agent, in order to gauge the individual patient's response, as a guide to dosing and an indication of the wakening concentration of hypnotic. The C_e at loss of consciousness (C_e LOC) can indicate if the patient is sensitive or relatively resistant to propofol and guide initial maintenance dosing. There is also some evidence to support the fact that the C_e LOC but not the C_p LOC is a guide to the C_e at recovery of consciousness (C_e ROC). Milne and colleagues determined the values for calculated plasma and effect-site concentrations of propofol at LOC and ROC in three remifentanil groups, low, medium and high [8]. The data is presented in Fig. 23.7. The mean value for C_e LOC was 2.08 (1.85–2.32) μg ml^{-1} and that for C_e ROC 1.85 (1.68–2.00) $\mu g/ml$. These are calculated values using the Marsh model for propofol; however, this relationship does not hold up using the Schnider model for propofol, which predicts a much higher C_e LOC than C_e ROC. Of course there are many potentially compounding factors; the level of stimulus from the wound during recovery will have a profound effect on the C_e ROC. If a good-quality regional block is in place, the patient is likely to wake up at a lower C_e, than if there is significant pain from the wound. Also the nature of surgery, body surface vs. body cavity procedures. Finally the

concomitant concentration of opiate in the patient will also affect the recovery concentration. Interestingly this study showed little difference in propofol C_e ROC, between the three remifentanil groups; testament to the unique and rapid metabolism of this drug even after prolonged infusion.

Drug Interactions and Induction of Anesthesia

Milne and co-workers also studied the interaction between remifentanil and propofol during induction of anesthesia. They found a calculated C_e propofol of around 2 $\mu g/ml$ at LOC, in the presence of a calculated C_e remifentanil of 2 ng/ml, and this was reduced to around 1.5 $\mu g/ml$ with an associated C_e remifentanil of 8 ng/ml. However, there was a large range with almost 300 % interindividual variation, again emphasising the need to titrate the dose to the individual.

Similarly a concurrent dose of a second hypnotic such as midazolam reduces the propofol requirements for loss of consciousness. Tzabar and colleagues showed an increasing success rate of induction of anesthesia in response to a TCI of propofol set at 4 $\mu g/ml$, with increasing doses of midazolam, as represented in Fig. 23.8 [9].

Case Study 3

We will consider a co-induction with TCI propofol and TCI remifentanil in a 42-year-old male patient scheduled for septorhinoplasty. Figure 23.9 and Video 23.3 show the time course of the propofol and remifentanil concentrations in this patient. Also displayed are the EC_{50} and EC_{95} for adequate anesthesia for propofol in the presence of the current remifentanil C_e, represented by the lower and upper border of the grey band, and the EC_{50} awakening as determined by Vuyk and colleagues [10]. This will be discussed further during the maintenance case studies.

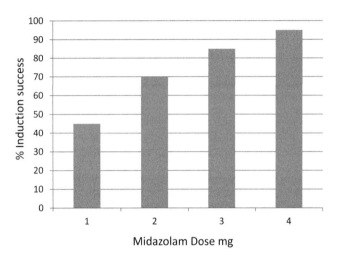

Fig. 23.8 Co-induction midazolam and TCI propofol: percentage success rate for induction of anesthesia with a TCI propofol set at 3 µg/ml, with different concomitant doses of midazolam

00:00:00

A 42-year-old male with weight 65 kg, height 175 cm, BP 123/67, HR 90 and SpO_2 99. Propofol TCI initial target concentration is 4 µg/ml and remifentanil initial TCI target concentration 4 ng/ml.

00:00:22

The patient is awake and chatting to the staff, and the calculated C_p of both propofol and remifentanil has reached the respective target concentrations. This has been achieved with a loading dose 62 mg (6.2 ml) of propofol and 26 µg (1.3 ml) remifentanil. Initial maintenance infusion rates for propofol and remifentanil are 161 ml/h and 54 ml/h, respectively; C_e propofol is 0.2 µg/ml and remifentanil 0.7 ng/ml.

00:00:45

The patient's eyes are now closed, but he opens them and nods in response to being asked "are you getting sleepy"? Propofol C_e is now 0.6 µg/ml, 68 mg (6.8 ml) has been delivered and the maintenance infusion rate has fallen to 95 ml/h. Remifentanil C_e is now 1.3 ng/ml, 32 µg (1.6 ml) has been delivered and the maintenance infusion rate has fallen to 52 ml/h. Vital signs are stable with BP 110/56, HR 76 and SpO_2 99.

00:01:00

The patient has now lost response to verbal stimulation at an C_e propofol of 0.8 µg/ml and remifentanil C_e 1.7 ng/ml.

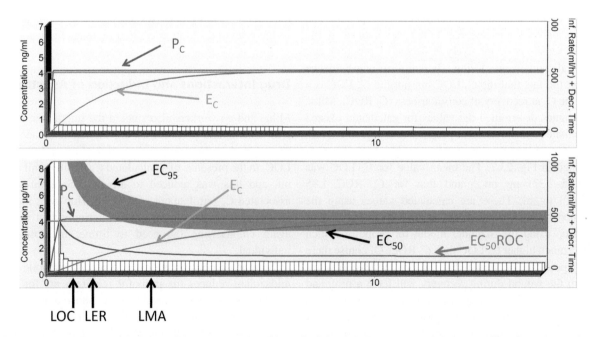

Fig. 23.9 Case study 3: co-induction with TCI propofol and remifentanil of 4 µg/ml. Target concentration (T_C), effect-site concentration (C_e), plasma concentration (C_p), loss of consciousness (LOC), loss of eyelash reflex (LER), laryngeal mask airway insertion (LMA)

0001:26

The patient has now lost his eyelash reflex at C_e of 1.2 μg/ml and 2.2 ng/ml for propofol and remifentanil, respectively. This has been achieved with a dose of 8 ml (80 mg) propofol and 2.2 ml (44 μg) remifentanil; infusion rates are 94 and 50 ml/h, respectively. The patient is apneic and gentle bag mask ventilation is commenced. The anaesthesiologist is waiting for jaw relaxation prior to LMA insertion.

00:02:20

LMA insertion is performed at a propofol C_e of 1.8 μg/ml and remifentanil C_e of 2.9 ng/ml, which has been achieved with a total dose 92 mg of propofol and 60 μg of remifentanil; BP has fallen to 90/48, HR is 62 and SpO_2 97 %.

00:02:48

Local anesthetic agent is injected by the surgeon to the site of operation; no response is seen in the patient despite the drug concentrations being below the EC_{50} interaction prediction depicted in Fig. 23.9. This illustrates the difference between body surface and body cavity surgery. In general, body surface surgery involves a less severe surgical stimulus, and thus the interaction model of Vuyk and co-workers derived from lower abdominal surgery is not directly applicable to body surface surgery. Following this stimulation repeat vital signs are BP 110/60, HR 70 and SpO_2 99 %.

In this relative young and fit patient, we have achieved LOC at a C_e propofol of 0.8 μg/ml similar to our first case study, which involved an elderly patient. This concentration is half that of our second case, but with a simultaneous remifentanil C_e of 1.7 ng/ml. LOC has been achieved with relatively small doses 74 mg propofol and 38 μg remifentanil. Also apparent is the low volume of remifentanil delivered even at a concentration of 20 μg/ml, which is less than half the standard recommended concentration for adults in the data sheet for this drug. So, had we used the recommended remifentanil (syringe) concentration, then LOC would have occurred after a dose 0.76 ml and LMA insertion with a dose of 1.2 ml. There are practical considerations relating to this. With such a co-induction method and indeed during maintenance, the depth of anesthesia of the patient is dependent upon delivery of both agents. The low volume of drug delivered during induction means that any compliance in the delivery system will compromise the accuracy of delivery. Air in the delivery syringe or the use of pumps with a slow "response motor" may result in only a proportion of the dose reaching the patient, particularly in the initial stages of the infusion. Fortunately all current TCI pumps have a rapid response motor, but some older devices used for MCI may cause problems. Also any redundant dead space in the delivery lines may lead to a delay in drug arriving to the patient. TIVA sets are now available with low dead space volume and anti-reflux and anti-siphon valves to reduce this problem. Even so, TIVA should be delivered into a free flowing IV line with a continuous infusion of a "carrier fluid" or into a separate dedicated line. Anaesthesiologists sometimes administer TIVA with "home-made" administration setups with multiple three-way taps and a large dead space volume. This is unwise. At best this will result in delayed induction, but it may increase the risk of light anesthesia and awareness particularly if combined with the use of muscle relaxants before LOC.

Maintenance of Anesthesia

Drug Interactions and Maintenance

The EC_{50} for propofol was determined by Davidson and colleagues [11]. They found the EC_{50} for propofol alone to be 6 μg/ml, with a 25 % reduction to 4.5 μg/ml for patients breathing 67 % nitrous oxide. These values were predicted blood concentrations using the Marsh model, and in common with MAC determination, there is significant interindividual variation.

Vuyk and co-workers took a more sophisticated approach to defining the EC_{50} for the combination of propofol with opiate, in a series of publications in female patients undergoing lower abdominal surgery [10, 12, 13]. These studies determined the EC_{50} of opiate in the presence of varying concentrations of propofol, using measured plasma concentrations. A supra-additive relationship was found between opiate and hypnotic in these studies. Figure 23.10 shows the EC_{50} for propofol/alfentanil and propofol/remifentanil; as one would expect the higher the blood propofol concentration, the lower the corresponding opiate requirement to achieve EC_{50}. Clearly administration of other analgesics and regional anesthesia and the degree of surgical stimulus will have an effect on this relationship. However, these studies provide a good starting point for dosing strategies using TIVA. The authors also determined the EC_{50} at return of consciousness (EC_{50} ROC) and the optimum anesthetic concentration for rapid awakening (by calculating the EC_{50} and EC_{95} concentrations for both associated drugs with the most rapid transition to EC_{50} ROC, following termination of infusion). This data is presented in Table 23.3. Naturally practicing anaesthesiologists do not want 50 % of their patients to move in response to surgery, and so the EC_{95} concentrations are a better guide to initial dosing during the maintenance of anesthesia. However, if we are to achieve a rapid transition from anesthesia to wakefulness, then the targets should be reduced towards the EC_{50} values towards the end of surgery, perhaps even lower, particularly if there is little stimulation at this time. The reader needs to appreciate that these numbers are only a

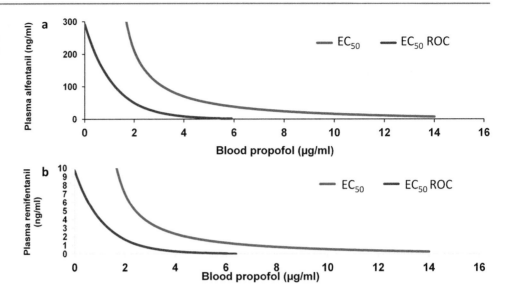

Fig. 23.10 Propofol/opioid interaction: **a** propofol/alfentanil; **b** propofol/remifentanil. Effective concentration for 50 % response to surgical stimulus (EC_{50}), effective concentration for 50 % recovery of consciousness (EC_{50} ROC) [10, 12]

Table 23.3 Propofol and remifentanil concentrations required for adequate anesthesia from [8, 10]

	EC_{50} propofol/ remifentanil (μ/ml/ng/ml)	EC_{95} propofol/ remifentanil (μ/ml/ng/ml)	EC_{50} ROC propofol/ remifentanil (μ/ml/ng/ml)
Vuyk et al. [10]	2.51/4.78	2.7/7.7	1.59/2.39
Milne et al. [8]	2.6/5	3/8	1.7/2

guide and that the PK/PD variability seen between patients means that dosing always needs to be titrated to the individual patient's response. However looking at Table 23.3 and rounding the numbers suggests that initial maintenance targets for the propofol/alfentanil combination would be 4.5 μg/ml and 120 ng/ml, respectively, reducing towards the end of surgery to 3.5 μg/ml and 90 ng/ml. For the propofol/remifentanil combination, the corresponding optimum concentrations are 3 μg/ml and 8 ng/ml, respectively, reducing to 2.5 μg/ml and 5 ng/ml towards the end of surgery. These numbers and recipes will be discussed further in the following case studies.

Milne and co-workers showed a similar synergistic relationship between calculated propofol and remifentanil concentrations, using a closed-loop system, in patients undergoing day-case surgery [8]. Three levels of remifentanil were used to represent low, medium and high doses given by TCI at 2, 4 and 8 ng/ml, respectively. An auditory evoked potential index (APEX) was used as an input signal for the closed-loop system, which then controlled a TCI of propofol to maintain an APEX value of 35. Figure 23.11 shows the relationship between propofol and remifentanil for EC_{50} and EC_{95} for loss of response to intraoperative stimulus (IOP) and EC_{50}, ROC described in this study. Interestingly looking at the data in this and the Vuyk studies, although the data are produced by totally different methods, the data are remarkably similar. We can estimate the C_p propofol concentrations associated with the optimal remifentanil concentrations taken from Vuyk's paper [10]. This gives an EC_{50} of 5 ng/ml and 2.6 μg/ml and EC_{95} of 8 ng/ml and 3 μg/ml for remifentanil and propofol, respectively (data also presented in Table 23.3).

Case Study 4

We will now consider a patient presenting for coronary artery bypass surgery; he is a 61-year-old male from Algeria with weight 65 Kg and height 172 cm. He is on a beta-blocker and an ACE inhibitor. The latter was stopped the day before surgery. A thoracic epidural catheter was placed at T3/T4 prior to induction through which 10 ml of 0.5 % bupivacaine was administered in divided doses to establish a block between T2 and T8. Standard monitoring for cardiac surgery including an arterial line, 5 lead ECG and pulse oximetry was established prior to activation of the epidural. TCI propofol and remifentanil were used for induction and maintenance of anesthesia. An initial TCI of propofol was commenced at 1 μg/ml to relax the patient while IV fluids were attached, and the patient received preoxygenation. Figure 23.12 details the time course of the TCI infusions and the patient's clinical response.

00:00:00

TCI propofol 1 μg/ml commenced with preoxygenation. Baseline BP is 110/65, HR 65 and SpO_2 97 %. Patient is alert with his eyes open.

00:00:20

C_p propofol is now at 1 μg/ml; 1.6 ml propofol has been delivered, the C_e is only 0.1 μg/ml and there is no discernible clinical effect.

Fig. 23.11 Drug interaction
between propofol and
remifentanil: *curves* describe the
effective concentration for 50 %
(EC$_{50}$ IOP) and 95 % (EC$_{95}$ IOP)
for lack of response to
intraoperative stimulation and
effective concentration for 50 %
recovery of consciousness (EC$_{50}$
ROC) [8]

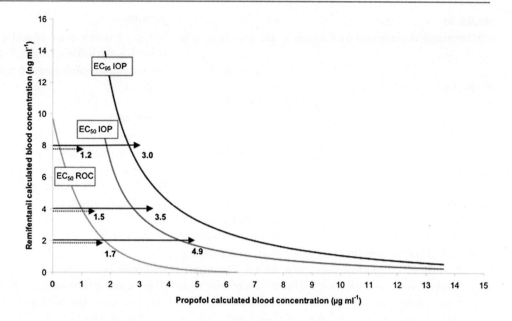

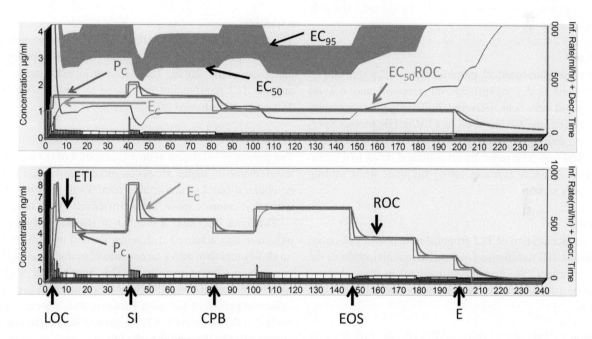

Fig. 23.12 Case study 4: anesthesia for cardiac surgery TCI propofol, TCI remifentanil and thoracic epidural. Plasma (C_p), effect-site concentration (C_e), effective concentration for 50 % (EC$_{50}$) and 95 % (EC$_{95}$) for lack of response to surgery, loss of consciousness (LOC), endotracheal intubation (ETI), surgical incision (SI), end of surgery (EOS), recovery of consciousness (ROC), extubation (E)

00:01:40

TCI remifentanil commenced target 3 ng/ml propofol, C_e is 0.3 μg/ml and the patient still has his eyes open. BP is 105/60, HR 60 and SpO$_2$ 100 %.

00:02:00

C_e remifentanil is 0.5 ng/ml and propofol 0.4 μg/ml; 2.3 ml (23 mg) propofol and 1 ml (20 μg) remifentanil have been delivered, again emphasising the importance of using a low

dead space and low compliance delivery system designed for TIVA. TCI propofol is increased to 1.5 μg/ml and remifentanil increased to 6 ng/ml.

00:03:00

C_e propofol is now 0.7 μg/ml and C_e remifentanil 2.5 ng/ml. The patient's eyes are closed but he opens them in response to verbal stimulation; BP is 90/60, HR 55 and SpO$_2$ 100 %.

00:03:30

Remifentanil is increased to 8 ng/ml as the patient is still conscious.

00:04:00

The patient has lost consciousness. C_e propofol is now 0.8 μg/ml and C_e remifentanil is 4 ng/ml: 4.1 ml propofol and 4.2 ml remifentanil have been delivered, 8 mg of vecuronium is given and bag mask ventilation is commenced.

00:05:00

TCI remifentanil is reduced to 5 ng/ml, BP 85/60, HR 55 and SpO_2 100 %. Again although the infusion rate of remifentanil is now zero, the C_e of remifentanil will continue to rise, while the C_p remains higher than the C_e. The adjustment is made now, as following intubation there will be a period with little stimulation, and so if we leave the TCI remifentanil at 8 ng/ml, the patient may suffer haemodynamic compromise as the C_e equilibrates towards 8 ng/ml.

00:07:00

The patient is intubated, C_e propofol is now 1.2 μg/ml and C_e remifentanil is 5.1 ng/ml; 5.8 ml propofol and 6.2 ml remifentanil have been delivered. Following the stimulation of intubation, the BP has risen to 110/70, HR 65 and SpO_2 99 %; a central line is inserted and the infusions moved to the central line. The remifentanil is titrated down to 4 ng/ml as there is very little stimulus during this phase while waiting for surgery to start.

00:36:00

Target concentration of TCI propofol is increased to 2 μg/ml and that of TCI remifentanil to 8 ng/ml in anticipation of the start of surgery. We do have an epidural in place, but we cannot be 100 % sure there will be zero stimulus from chest incision.

00:39:00

Skin incision. C_e propofol is now 1.2 μg/ml, with C_e remifentanil 5.1 ng/ml; there is no response to the surgical stimulus so the TCI targets for propofol and remifentanil are reduced to 1.5 μg/ml and 6 ng/ml, respectively.

1:19:10

Cardiopulmonary bypass (CPB) is established, the patient is cooled and the TCI propofol target concentration is reduced to 1 μg/ml; TCI target concentration remifentanil is reduced to 4 ng/ml until rewarming is commenced at which stage it is titrated back up to 6 ng/ml. An epidural infusion of 0.125 % bupivacaine with 0.6 μg/ml clonidine added is commenced at a rate of 8 ml/h.

2:25:00

Surgery has now finished and a single arterial graft has been placed on the left main stem. The TCI propofol target is 1 μg/ml and remifentanil target 6 ng/ml, but it is now reduced to 3 ng/ml.

02:40:00

Dressings have now been applied and the patient moved to a trolley awaiting transfer to the intensive care unit (ICU). The patient opens his eyes to verbal command but is comfortable and tolerant of the endotracheal tube and ventilation. The C_e remifentanil is 3.5 ng/ml and propofol 1 μg/ml. BP is 95/65, HR 70 and SpO_2 100 %. The patient is transferred to ICU.

03:05:00

The patient is now on ICU. He is sat up awake and comfortable and takes the occasional breath while on synchronised ventilation. The TCI remifentanil target is reduced to 2 ng/ml.

03:15:00

The patient is now self-ventilating on pressure support ventilation; gas exchange is good and the patient is cardiovascularly stable. The decision to extubate is made and the TCI remifentanil is reduced to 1 ng/ml, while the TCI propofol is turned off.

03:24:00

The patient is extubated at an EC propofol of 0.7 μg/ml and remifentanil 1.1 ng/ml. He is comfortable and stable and has an epidural block demonstrable from T3 to T8 when tested with ethyl chloride spray. The remifentanil TCI is turned off.

This case illustrates a number of issues; firstly a stable induction was achieved with a low dose of propofol titrated up slowly together with a larger dose of opioid, again titrated upwards in a stepwise fashion. This approach is rewarded with cardiovascular stability at the expense of a prolonged induction period of 4–5 min. However this is a price worth paying in the context of a 3–4 h operation in a patient with compromised myocardial perfusion.

The doses used for maintenance are titrated over the course of surgery to match the changes in surgical stimulus, although in this case with a functioning thoracic epidural the doses are lower than would be required without regional blockade. For the majority of the surgery, the C_e propofol is between 1 and 1.5 μg/ml and remifentanil between 4 and 6 ng/ml. Without a functioning epidural, one would expect to be in the range of 2–4 μg/ml propofol and 6–12 ng/ml remifentanil and perhaps briefly even higher during peak stimulation such as during sternotomy.

Figure 23.12 details the time course of the C_p and C_e of the two drugs; also illustrated is the EC_{50} and EC_{95} for the hypnotic/opioid combination as described by Vuyk and

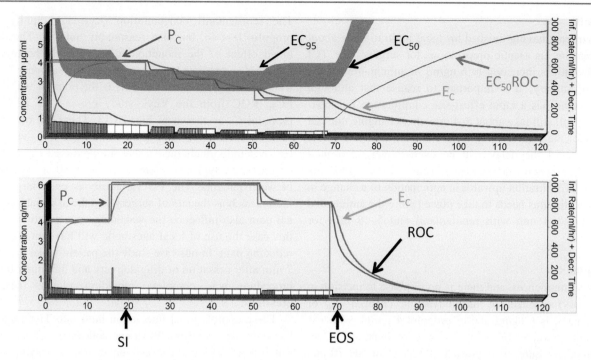

Fig. 23.13 Case study 5: anesthesia for septorhinoplasty co-induction with TCI propofol and TCI remifentanil. Target concentration (T_C), plasma concentration (C_p), effect-site concentration (C_e), surgical incision (SI), end of surgery (EOS), recovery of consciousness (ROC); in this case ROC 7 min after EOS and 3.5 min after dressings has been applied

colleagues [10]. This is represented by the grey band; the upper border is EC_{95} and lower border EC_{50}. It is clear that at all times during the surgery, the drug combination was actually below the EC_{50} described in this study. However in the Vuyk interaction model, no regional anesthesia was given nor additional analgesic supplements. Even so it is true to say that these doses are "sailing close to the wind". I would not consider such low doses, even with the regional technique in a paralysed patient. This subject had had one dose of vecuronium for endotracheal intubation and no further doses.

With regard to CPB, during initiation of bypass, the patient is hemodiluted by the acute administration of around 1.5 L of fluid containing no anesthetic drug. Thus we are hemodiluting by about one third of the blood volume. The natural response to this would be to think that we need to calculate a supplementary bolus dose of the anesthetic agents to return the plasma concentrations back to pre-CPB levels. However, if we consider that the Marsh model predicts that the central compartment volume is about 15 L for a 70 kg patient, then we realise that the hemodilution is much less severe than expected. Also the drug would move from the peripheral compartments to restore the concentration in the central compartment. With remifentanil the central compartment is smaller, around 5 L predicted by the Minto model, so the hemodilution will have more of an effect on the remifentanil concentration. However, both propofol and remifentanil are subject to a high degree of protein binding, and it is the free drug concentration that is more important than total. The addition of non-protein-containing fluid to the patient's blood volume has the effect of reducing this binding, thereby increasing the active free drug concentration. Hiraoka and colleagues [14] found that the fraction of unbound propofol in blood increased by twofold during cardiopulmonary bypass. The same group also reported that the total concentration of propofol in blood using doses of either 4 or 6 mg kg^{-1} h^{-1} remained unchanged after the initiation of CPB, when compared to pre-CPB plasma concentration values, in both groups. However, the fraction of unbound propofol in blood doubled during CPB [15]. This coupled with the fact that drug metabolism will fall during the hypothermic phase of bypass means that in practice the dose of both propofol and remifentanil should be reduced after the initiation of CPB particularly if the hypothermia is used.

Case Study 5

If we now return to the patient whose induction I detailed in case study 3, we can follow the rest of the case through surgery to emergence from anesthesia. The case was a co-induction with TCI propofol and TCI remifentanil in a 42-year-old male patient, scheduled for septorhinoplasty, whose weight was 65 kg and height 175 cm. We left the case at 2 min 48 s when our surgeon was injecting local anesthetic agent to the site of surgery with vital signs of BP 110/60, HR 70 and SpO$_2$ 99 %. Figure 23.13 details the drug concentration time course and clinical course for this case.

00:15:00

The surgeon, having finished his local infiltration, is about to complete his aseptic preparations for surgery. The TCI remifentanil is increased to 6 ng/ml in anticipation of the start of surgery. It is important to realise that although remifentanil has a rapid effect-site equilibration rate constant, it will still take about 3–4 min after changing the TCI target for the effect-site concentration to reach this value. For propofol the delay will be even longer, at around 10 min for an equivalent increase. Thus when using plasma control TCI, titration upwards in anticipation of a change in surgical stimulus needs to take place before the anticipated stimulus, 3–4 min with remifentanil and 5–10 min for propofol.

00:19:00

Surgery commences, and there is no response to incision in terms of movement or haemodynamic changes. C_e of remifentanil is 6 ng/ml and of propofol 4 µg/ml, which is above the predicted EC_{95} for this drug combination. In fact the blood pressure drifts down to 90/55, with HR 70 and SpO_2 99 over the next few min. In this case we are using relatively high opiate doses, which will allow a relatively low dose of hypnotic particularly towards the end of surgery. This will facilitate a rapid awakening taking advantage of the rapid offset of action seen with this drug. However, at these concentrations the patient is unlikely to breath and will require mechanical ventilation in this case via a LMA.

00:24:00

TCI propofol is reduced to 3.5 µg/ml, and over the course of the next 20 min, the TCI propofol is titrated down in 2 steps, allowing at least 10 min for effect-site equilibration, before making the next change. The C_e remifentanil is 6 ng/ml and propofol now 2.5 µg/ml, 45 min after the start of anesthesia. This is at the predicted EC_{50} for lower abdominal surgery and appears perfectly adequate in this case of body surface surgery with local anesthetic infiltration. There is no movement in response to surgery which is a useful sign in this patient, who has not been given any muscle relaxant.

00:52:00

The surgery is approaching completion. In anticipation the remifentanil is reduced to 5 ng/ml and the propofol to 2 µg/ml while keeping a close eye on the patient for any movement or signs of light anesthesia, such as tachycardia or hypertension.

00:70:00

Surgery is finished. The nose only has to be packed and dressings applied and both infusions are targeted to zero.

The remifentanil concentration decreases rapidly, the propofol less so, but also reasonably quickly. The combined effect of the reduction in C_e of both these drugs produces a predicted awakening time of around 5 min from cessation of infusions. This is the point at which the EC_{50} ROC from the Vuyk study crosses the declining propofol C_e as shown in Fig. 23.13. There are obviously several caveats to this prediction. The PK variation between individuals means that the predicted C_p may not be exact, as typically there is about a 30 % variability between patients. The PD variability is even larger and factors such as the site of surgery and the associated residual pain also influence the wakening concentration. As in this case the use of local anesthetic will have an effect by reducing pain. In our case study the patient woke up about 7 min after cessation of drug delivery and 3.5 min after the procedure was complete including placing surgical dressings.

The propofol/opioid interaction built into Tivatrainer is based on the study from Vuyk and colleagues. This interaction is defined for middle-aged female patients having lower abdominal surgery and no other analgesic drugs, so we must be careful in applying the data to other groups of patients having different surgeries. An interesting observation from Fig. 23.13 is that the EC_{50} ROC line rises sharply as the C_e of remifentanil falls. In fact if we follow this line as the C_e remifentanil approaches zero, the predicted propofol EC_{50} ROC approaches 6 µg/ml. Based on our propofol induction case studies, such a high awakening propofol C_e seems unreasonably high. However, we need to remember that this interaction is based on patients waking up with the surgical stimulus from a lower abdominal incision with no regional technique or additional opioid effect. This is a situation which we would hope would never occur in clinical practice. Also the data are being extrapolated to an extreme situation outside the clinical scenario from which they were derived, which is always problematic. In the cases studied by Vuyk and co-workers, the patients received supplementary bolus opiates as soon as they regained consciousness.

Table 23.4 gives a guide to the approximate required C_e combinations of propofol and remifentanil, for a variety of surgical procedures. However, as stated repeatedly, the intra-individual variability seen between patients means that any such "recipes" can only be a guide and dose always needs to be titrated to each individual subject. Some of these factors can be anticipated, for instance, elderly patients who tend to require less drug than younger individuals. The use of alcohol or other drugs tends to reduce subjects' susceptibility to anesthetic agents. An extreme example of this is opiate addicts, who require much larger opiate doses to achieve

Table 23.4 A guide to maintenance concentrations for remifentanil and propofol combined TIVA

Type of surgery	Without regional blockade		With regional blockade	
	Remifentanil (ng/ml)	Propofol (µg/ml)	Remifentanil (ng/ml)	Propofol (µg/ml)
Cardiac	6–12	2–4	5–8	1.5–3
Body surface	5–6	2–4	4–5	2–3
Minor general	5–6	2–4	4–5	2–3
Major general	6–12	3–5	5–7	3–4

Fig. 23.14 Intraoperative BIS recording showing a sharp fall during induction and a rapid rise during recovery

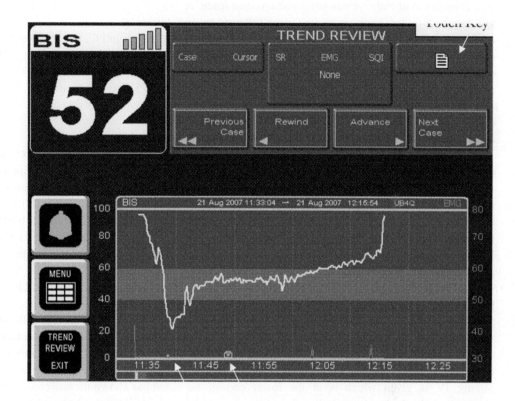

an adequate effect. Despite these general guidelines, individual patients still produce surprises, and not everyone is entirely honest about their personal drug use.

Our case studies and a number of publications show that there is a variation between individuals in their response to a given dose of anesthetic agent. This variability is related to both PK and PD differences. So we must always titrate our dose, but how do we assess the effect of the drug? If the patient is not paralysed, we can use movement in response to stimulation or if self-ventilating high respiratory rate as a signs of light anesthesia. However, if the patient has received muscle relaxants, we normally rely on haemodynamic responses and other autonomic signs as a guide to the depth of anesthesia. Over the last few decades, a number of "depth of anesthesia monitors" have been developed and marketed. Can we use these devices to guide dosing of anesthetic drugs? A full assessment of these devices is beyond the scope of this chapter. In general, these monitors use a moving average of processed EEG to calculate a single number or index, said to reflect hypnotic

drug effect. Figure 23.14 shows the intraoperative time course of the bispectral index (BIS) during a short general anesthetic. We see a fall in the value at induction of anesthesia and then a sharp rise associated with recovery of consciousness. Typically the number is developed from a database of cases on a probabilistic basis. Controversy exists as to the utility of such monitors in detecting light anesthesia and thus the potential for awareness. The influence of EMG activity on these indices is unclear, casting doubt on their validity in the very group of patients in which this information would be most beneficial [16]. Thus it is unwise to rely too heavily on such aids and rather to incorporate the information provided in the broad range of clinical information to the anaesthesiologist, particularly in unparalysed patients.

Case Study 6

The patient is a 53-year-old male with weight 110 kg and height 177 cm, scheduled for open large bowel resection for suspected tumour. The patient had a history of hypertension treated with candesartan and psoriasis with arthropathy treated with methotrexate and infliximab. Candesartan was omitted on the day of surgery by the surgical team. Admission Hb was 7.2 g/dl and the patient was transfused with 2 units of packed cells 2 days prior to surgery. Hb on the day of surgery was 10.1 g/dl and there was no evidence of coagulopathy on routine screening. A low thoracic epidural was placed prior to surgery at the T8–T9 level. There was good loss of resistance and the catheter passed easily with no blood or CSF seen on aspiration; 8 cm of catheter was left in the epidural space. A test dose of 5 ml levobupivacaine was given followed by an additional 5 ml when no response was seen 5 min after the initial dose. Ten minutes following the 2nd dose, loss of sensation to ice was detected at T8–L2, which was taken as evidence of an evolving block. The patient was taken to OR, and routine monitoring was established together with an arterial line and BIS monitoring, for which the electrode impedance was found to be acceptable.

00:00:00

BP was 150/90, HR 85, SaO_2 100 % and BIS 90–95. Preoxygenation was given over the previous 2 min.

Propofol TCI commenced at 4 µg/ml (weight entered into the propofol pump 100 kg) and remifentanil TCI 5 ng/ml. Dexamethasone 8 mg, ketorolac 30 mg and ketamine 30 mg are given as part of a multimodal approach to analgesia.

00:00:54

Loss of response to verbal command is seen, at a C_e remifentanil of 1.6 ng/ml and propofol 0.6 µg/ml. 107 mg of propofol and 48 µg of remifentanil have been infused. BP is 120/75, HR 80, SaO_2 99 % and BIS 55–60. Rocuronium 50 mg IV is given which is at the lower end of the recommended calculated weight-based dosing range, given the patients' high BMI.

00:02:26

C_e remifentanil is now 3.4 ng/ml and propofol 1.7 µg/ml. This was achieved with 143 mg propofol and 80 µg remifentanil. BP is 100/70, HR 80, SaO_2 99 % and BIS 40–45. The patient's jaw is relaxed and tracheal intubation is achieved. With this stimulus the BIS increases transiently to 55 before falling back to a value of 40–45. TCI propofol is reduced to 2.5 ng/ml and TCI remifentanil to 4 ng/ml, as there will now be a period without stimulation and despite both infusions running at 0 ml/h, the effect-site concentrations of both drugs will continue to rise, as the C_p is still higher than the current C_e.

00:20:00

The surgical team is now ready. BP is 95/60, HR 77, SaO_2 99 % and BIS 30–40. Propofol and remifentanil C_p and C_e have equilibrated at 2.5 µg/ml and 4 ng/ml, respectively; 33.2 ml (332) mg of propofol and 14.6 ml (292 µg) of remifentanil have been infused. The interaction data suggest that the combined drug effect is below the EC_{50}. In this case we have an epidural block in place, so without significant surgical stimulation, the patient should still have adequate anesthesia. However we can't be 100 % sure that we have a full effective epidural block for surgical incision, so to be safe we increase remifentanil to 6 ng/ml 5 min before the anticipated incision.

00:26:10

Remifentanil C_e has now reached 6 ng/ml. The drug combination is at EC_{50}, and there is no response to incision with reference to the BIS or haemodynamic status. BP is 98/60, HR 75, SaO_2 99 % and BIS 45–50. Remifentanil is reduced to 5 ng/ml.

01:15:00

Propofol and remifentanil C_p and C_e have equilibrated at 2.5 µg/ml and 5 ng/ml, respectively. At this point in surgery, the BP has increased progressively to 155/85 over the previous 15 min, HR is 90 and the BIS is 50. It appears plausible that the epidural block has started to recede and that the surgical stimulus is responsible for the hypertensive episode. The remifentanil TCI is increased to 6 ng/ml to achieve a rapid effect, and a supplementary dose of levobupivacaine is given. This increase in opiate dose and the epidural top-up have no effect of the hypertension. The BIS drops to 40, 15 min following these changes. The BIS electrode impedance is checked and found to be acceptable and the signal quality index is high. The patient has received no further muscle relaxant and so is not paralysed, but has shown no movement in response to surgical stimulus. It is now concluded that this hypertensive episode is not related to light anesthesia, but instead to the patients underlying hypertensive disease in combination with the omission of the candesartan. The hypertension was controlled over the course of surgery by a number of 5 mg aliquots of labetolol. The remifentanil TCI was reduced to 5 ng/ml.

The surgical procedure lasts almost 5 h; over the course of the surgery, the propofol is titrated (between 2 and 3.5 µg/ml) to keep the BIS in the range 40–55. No further muscle relaxant is given and the TCI remifentanil is left at 5 ng/ml until close to the end of the surgery. The epidural catheter is topped up with a total of 15 ml 0.5 % levobupivacaine in 3 further 5 ml aliquots at approximately 70 min intervals.

04:40:00

The abdomen is now closed and skin sutures are being applied; the C_p and C_e of propofol and remifentanil are 2 µg/ml and 4 ng/ml, respectively. The propofol and remifentanil TCI are reduced to 1.5 µg/ml and 3 ng/ml.

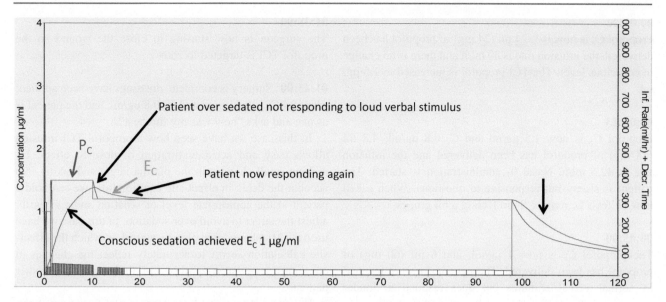

Fig. 23.15 Case study 7: anesthetist-controlled sedation with propofol TCI titrated to response. Effect-site concentration (C_e), plasma concentration (C_p), *white boxes* infusion rate ml/h

04:52:00

Surgery is now complete, the dressings are being applied and target concentrations of the infusions are set to zero. A total of 248 ml (2480 mg) of propofol and 195 ml (3.9 mg) have been infused.

04:58:10

.The patient takes a breath and opens his eyes in response to verbal stimulus. The C_e propofol is 1.2 µg/ml and remifentanil is 1.3 ng/ml. He is extubated and reports no abdominal pain but says his joints are stiff and a little sore, which responds to IV ketorolac 30 mg and paracetamol 1 g after 30 min.

In this case we have used a combined TIVA and regional analgesia regimen. The combination of the epidural block and the remifentanil infusion allowed us to keep the propofol dose to a minimum, to achieve a rapid awakening and a pain-free patient following a prolonged procedure. What this case also illustrates is the desirability of not routinely continuing neuromuscular blockade, when not required. This together with BIS monitoring allowed recognition of the fact that the hypertension seen in this case was not related to light anesthesia and resulted in the appropriate treatment rather than inappropriate deepening of anesthesia. In a paralysed patient without EEG monitoring, most anaesthesiologists would probably have deepened anesthesia, which would have resulted in a relative overdose and delayed recovery.

Sedation

Many surgical procedures can be performed under regional anesthesia. However, many patients are too anxious to tolerate surgeries under such circumstances and require anxiolysis or conscious sedation. Similarly some patients need sedation to tolerate diagnostic procedures such as MRI. Sedation with TCI propofol can be used to deliver highly titratable sedation in such cases.

Case Study 7 Anaesthesiologist-Controlled Sedation

The next scenario is of a 62-year-old male of weight 81 kg and height 178 cm. The patient has a history of angina pectoris and is on beta-blockers and an ACE inhibitor which was suspended the day before surgery. He has a spinal anesthetic injection (of 2.5 ml 0.5 % hyperbaric bupivacaine) and placement of an epidural catheter place in preparation for his total knee replacement, but has requested sedation as he does not want to hear the noise of the surgery. The timeline of the case is presented in Fig. 23.15 and Video 23.4.

00:00:00

The patient has a good regional block with loss of sensation to ethyl chloride spray from L1 to S1. BP is 95/60, HR 77 and SaO$_2$ 99 %. TCI propofol is started at a target concentration of 1 µg/ml. The patient is relaxed and alert.

00:00:22

Propofol C_p has reached the target of 1 µg/ml, but the C_e is only 0.1 µg/ml, 2 ml (20 mg) of propofol have been delivered and the infusion rate is 30 ml/h, but there is no discernible effect on the patient.

00:01:22

Propofol C_e is now 0.3, 24 ml (24 mg) of propofol has been delivered, the infusion rate is 30 ml/h and there is no change in conscious level. The TCI propofol is increased to 1.5 μg/ml.

00:03:23

Propofol C_p is now 1.5 μg/ml and C_e 0.8 μg/ml; 4.8 ml (48 mg) of propofol has been delivered and the infusion rate is 42.5 ml/h. Nasal 0_2 administration is started. The patient is sleepy but responsive to questions. When asked how he feels he replies "I am feeling a bit groggy".

00:05:00

The propofol C_e is now 1 μg/ml, and 6 ml (60 mg) of propofol has been delivered. The patient does not respond to normal verbal stimulus but does respond to louder vocalisation by raising his eyebrows and furrowing his brow. He is maintaining his own airway. BP is 95/60, HR 77 and SaO_2 99 %. This is just about the optimal state for this patient—maintaining his own airway, rousable, but unlikely to be concerned by the noise of surgery or indeed have any recall of events in the OR. Normally I would reduce the target to or just above the value in the effect site at this point to prevent over-sedation. However, in this case we have left the target at 1.5 to observe the effect in this patient.

00:10:00

The propofol C_e has risen to 1.4 μg/ml; a total of 9.2 ml (92 mg) of propofol has been delivered. Vital signs are BP 80/55, HR 77 and SaO_2 99 %. The patient, although self-ventilating and maintaining his airway, is now not responding to loud verbal or tactile stimulation and so is a little over-sedated. The propofol TCI is reduced to 1.2 μg/ml.

00:12:08

Propofol C_p is now 1.2 μg/ml and the C_e is 1.3 μg/ml. The patient responds to tactile and loud verbal stimuli by raising his eyebrows in an attempt to open his eyes. Vital signs are as follows: BP 80/55, HR 77 and SaO_2 99 %.

00:30:00

C_p and C_e have now equilibrated at 1.2 μg/ml, the surgeon is scrubbed, the patient has been positioned and surgery commences. There is no response to skin incision confirming the presence of an adequate spinal block.

01:00:02

Surgery is progressing well, there have been no further changes to the propofol TCI target, the patient is still responding to loud verbal stimulation and vital signs are stable.

01:38:00

The surgeon is now starting to close the wound so the propofol TCI is targeted to zero.

01:45:00 Surgery is complete, dressings have been applied; propofol C_p is 0.6 μg/ml and C_e 0.8 μg/ml, and the patient is awake and asks "how was my film test"?

In this case we have seen how a propofol TCI infusion allows easy and accurate titration of dose to effect. By making small changes in the plasma target and taking into account the delay in effect-site equilibration, we can hold a patient at the appropriate level of sedation and can easily adjust the target to avoid over-sedation. In this case we have used the Marsh model in plasma control, in which the effect-site calculation seems to accurately reflect the changes in conscious level seen in this and the majority of other patients.

However, if we consider another model for propofol, the Schnider model, which is also available for clinical practice, we see a different picture [17, 18]. Figure 23.16 shows the initial phase of the same patient with the Marsh calculated plasma and effect-site concentrations. Also displayed is the Schnider predicted concentrations given the same infusion regimen that was delivered to our patient. The smaller central compartment in the Schnider model (4.27 L fixed for all patients) results in a higher predicted plasma concentration associated with the two loading doses given by the TCI system at the start and when the TCI target is increased to 1.5 μg/ml. In fact this model calculates the peak plasma concentration to be over 4 μg/ml. Also the Schnider model has a "faster" K_{e0} and predicts a peak effect-site concentration of 2.4 μg/ml at 3 min 20 s. If we look at the clinical course in this patient at this point, he is sleepy but responding to questions. The Schnider model calculates that the effect-site concentration falls over the course of the next 6 min, so we should see a reduction in the sedative effect of propofol over this time. In fact we see just the opposite as the patient's conscious level drifts down, and he becomes unresponsive to stimulus. Of course this is only one patient and the inter-patient variability that we know exists may be responsible in this case. However, we have studied sedative doses of propofol in a group of 40 - un-premedicated patients. The time course of the effect-site prediction from both models was compared to the BIS and the OAAS score. In all cases both the BIS and the OAAS were more closely related to the time course of the Marsh, rather than the Schnider effect-site prediction [19]. Figure 23.17 summarises the data.

When physicians sedate patients, they rely on a subjective idea of how deeply sedated a patient needs to be. However, if control is given to the patient, they often self-administer less sedation than physicians do. This has the advantages of faster recovery, lower cost and better satisfaction. Patient-

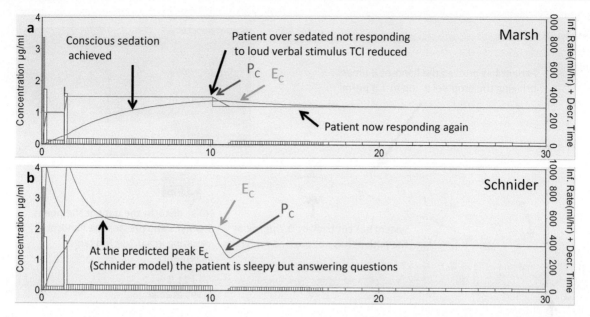

Fig. 23.16 Case study 7: re-simulated data propofol effect-site concentration (C_e) and plasma concentration (C_p) calculated for both **a** Marsh and **b** Schnider models, given the infusion regimen actually delivered; patient's clinical response also indicated. *White boxes* infusion rate ml/h

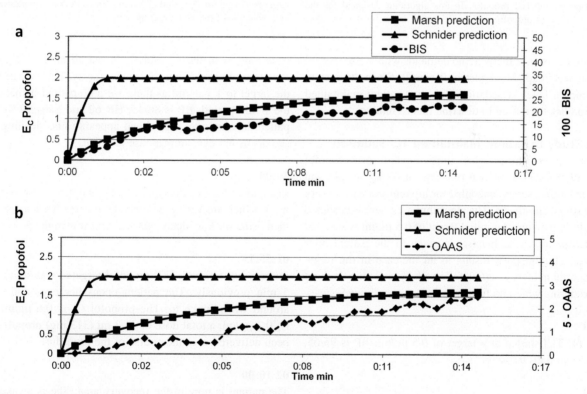

Fig. 23.17 Propofol effect-site concentration (C_e) calculated by the Marsh and Schnider models given the same infusion regimen and associated **a** BIS and **b** OAAS [19]

controlled sedation is dealt with elsewhere in this publication but I will briefly describe a case below. There have been a number of studies describing patient-controlled sedation, many using PCA pumps charged with propofol [20]. A more

sophisticated approach is to use a TCI device modified to interface with a handset, so that the patient can push a button to obtain an incremental increase in the target concentration, which is then maintained at the new level [21]. The system

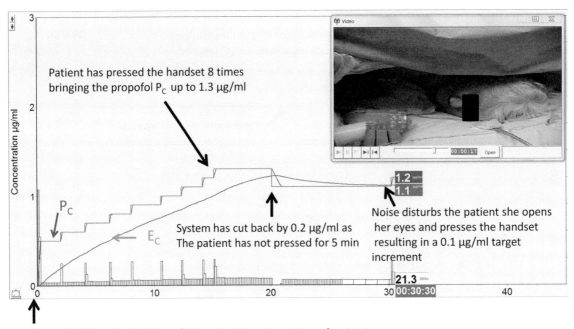

Propofol TCI started at 0.5 µg/ml handset given to patient after 2 min

Fig. 23.18 Case study 8: patient-maintained sedation (PMS) with patient-controlled TCI propofol. In this algorithm designed for the elderly, an initial propofol TCI of 0.5 µg/ml is set by the operator, control is then given to the patient and a button push increases the set target by 0.1 µg/ml. A period of 5 min with no button demands results in a reduction of the TCI target by 0.2 µg/ml

can also cut back if there are no demands within a set period (please see Chap. 21 [Anderson/Kenny]). Since the system maintains a level of sedation, the term patient-maintained sedation has been used to describe this technique.

Case Study 8: Patient-Maintained TCI Sedation

Figure 23.18 shows the time course of propofol concentrations in a 69-year-old lady of 69 kg weight and 168 cm height. She is scheduled for hip replacement surgery under spinal anesthesia. The algorithm used here is designed for elderly patients. An initial target of 0.5 µg/ml is selected by the operator. The handset is given to the patient after 2 min. A button push results in an increase in the target concentration of 0.1 µg/ml followed by a 2 min lockout period during which no further increases are allowed.

00:00

Propofol TCI started at a target of 0.5 µg/ml. BP is 95/65, HR 75 and SaO$_2$ 97 %.

02:00

The handset is given to the patient; she is instructed to press the button whenever she feels the need for more sedation.

25:00

The procedure is now underway. The patient has pressed the button on a number of occasions, and the system has increased the target as allowed by the lock out on eight

occasions, with the C_p and C_e increased up to 1.2 µg/ml. Five min after reaching this value, the system has cut back the target to 1.1 µg/ml as there were no patient demands in the 5 min period. BP is 86/45, HR 62 and SaO$_2$ 99 %. The patient has her eyes closed and appears to be sleeping, but she opens her eyes in response to voice.

30:00

The patient has her eyes closed, but then the power tools are used, which are very loud, and she presses her handset and then drifts back to sleep over the next few minutes.

01:55:15

Surgery has finished. TCI propofol targeted was set to zero 5 min previously. The patient opens her eyes and looks around when spoke to. The propofol C_p is 0.6 µg/ml and C_e 0.7 µg/ml; a total dose of 31.3 ml (313 mg) propofol has been delivered over the course of the procedure.

02:10:00

The patient is now in the recovery area. She is awake and alert, with a BP of 100/75, HR 70 and SaO$_2$ 99 %. She is pain-free and starting to move her feet. She has had 30 mg ketorolac and 1 g of paracetamol IV and is discharged to the ward, with regular oral analgesic medications prescribed.

The technique used here gives control of sedation to the individual who can best assess sedation requirements, that is the patient! There is a lot of interest in this area, and such automated drug delivery with both positive and negative feedback control has the potential to allow the use of propofol without supervision of an anaesthesiologist. However, it must be appreciated that propofol at sedative doses has no analgesic properties and is not suitable for procedures with significant pain and discomfort. Such devises will also require rigorous regulatory testing to prove efficacy and safety before being released for general use.

Conclusions

There are a number of potential advantages of intravenous anesthesia, and some procedures can only be completed with TIVA. Despite this, training in TIVA is suboptimal in many countries. TCI has some advantages over MCI. Some recent evidence suggests some potential benefits for patients, in terms of recovery profile and a reduced incidence of awareness. However, most of the advantages of TCI are in favour of the anaesthesiologist. The ease of dosing and titration afforded by TCI facilitates swift training of physicians who have previously had minimal experience with TIVA. Even novices can rapidly become competent in the use of TCI TIVA, once given the appropriate theoretical knowledge and practical hands-on training in OR, from an anaesthesiologist experienced in TCI.

A number of case studies have been presented which have illustrated different induction strategies and intraoperative dosing for maintenance of anesthesia with hypnotic/opiate combinations. Guidelines for approximate dosing for different types of surgeries have been given, but the interindividual variation between patients has been stressed, together with the need for titration. We have also described a case in which BIS monitoring proved to be useful. It may be that such "depth of anesthesia monitors" can aid our dosing in individual patients, helping to prevent over- and underdosing. However, such monitors are far from perfect; care must be taken to ensure the signal is clean and free from artefact. It may be that the influence of EMG on the derived index reduces the reliability of such monitors in paralysed patients. Finally, we have considered propofol dosing for sedation, including regimens for anaesthesiologist-controlled TCI sedation which affords a level of control not available with any other technique and patient-maintained sedation, which has the potential to deliver individualised dosing, dictated by the patient themselves.

References

1. Pandit JJ, Cook TM. Fifth National Audit Project of the Royal College of Anaesthetists in collaboration with the Association of Anaesthetists of Great Britain and Ireland: Accidental Awareness during General Anaesthesia in the United Kingdom and Ireland 2014. http://www.nationalauditprojects.org.uk/NAP5home.

2. Madhivathanan P, Kasivisvanathan R, Cohen A. Training in total intravenous anaesthesia: a regional survey. Anaesthesia. 2010;65 (5):540–2.

3. Leslie K, Clavisi O, Hargrove J. Target-controlled infusion versus manually-controlled infusion of propofol for general anaesthesia or sedation in adults. Cochrane Database Syst Rev. 2008;16(3): CD006059.

4. Mazzarella B, Melloni C, Montanini S, Novelli GP, Peduto VA, Santandrea E, Vincenti E, Zattoni J. Comparison of manual infusion of propofol and target-controlled infusion: effectiveness, safety and acceptability. Minerva Anestesiol. 1999;65(10):701–9.

5. Marsh B, White M, Morton N, Kenny GNC. Pharmacokinetic model driven infusion of propofol in children. Br J Anaesth. 1991;67:41–8.

6. Peacock JE, Lewis RP, Reilly CS, Nimmo WS. Effect of different rates of infusion of propofol for induction of anaesthesia in elderly patients. Br J Anaesth. 1990;65(3):346–52.

7. Dundee JW, Robinson FP, McCollum JS, Patterson CC. Sensitivity to propofol in the elderly. Anaesthesia. 1986;41(5):482–5.

8. Milne SE, Kenny GNC, Schraag S. Propofol sparing effect of remifentanil using closed-loop anaesthesia. Br J Anaesth. 2003;90 (5):623–9.

9. Tzabar Y, Brydon C, Gillies GW. Induction of anaesthesia with midazolam and a target controlled propofol infusion. Anaesthesia. 1996;53(6):1–86.

10. Vuyk J, Mertens MJ, Olofsen E, Burm AG, Bovill JG. Propofol anesthesia and rational opioid selection: determination of optimal EC50-EC95 propofol-opioid concentrations that assure adequate anesthesia and a rapid return of consciousness. Anesthesiology. 1997;87(6):1549–62.

11. Davidson JA, Macleod AD, Howie JC, White M, Kenny GN. Effective concentration 50 for propofol with and without 67% nitrous oxide. Acta Anaesthesiol Scand. 1993;37(5):458–64.

12. Mertens MJ, Engbers FH, Burm AG, Vuyk J. Predictive performance of computer-controlled infusion of remifentanil during propofol/remifentanil anaesthesia. Br J Anaesth. 2003;90(2):132–41.

13. Vuyk J, Lim T, Engbers FH, Burm AG, Vletter AA, Bovill JG. The pharmacodynamic interaction of propofol and alfentanil during lower abdominal surgery in women. Anesthesiology. 1995;83 (1):8–22.

14. Hiraoka H, Yamamoto K, Okano N, Morita T, Goto F, Horiuchi R. Changes in drug plasma concentrations of an extensively bound and highly extracted drug, propofol, in response to altered plasma binding. Clin Pharmacol Ther. 2004;75:324–30.

15. Takizawa E, Hiraoka H, Takizawa D, Goto F. Changes in the effect of propofol in response to altered plasma protein binding during normothermic cardiopulmonary bypass. Br J Anaesth. 2006;96:179–85.

16. Schuller PJ, Newell S, Strickland PA, Barry JJ. Response of bispectral index to neuromuscular block in awake volunteers. Br J Anesth. 2015;i95–i103.

17. Schnider TW, Minto CF, Shafer SL, Gambus PL, Andresen C, Goodale DB, Youngs EJ. The influence of method of administration and covariates on the pharmacokinetics of propofol in adult volunteers. Anesthesiology. 1998;88(5):1170–82.

18. Schnider TW, Minto CF, Shafer SL, Gambus PL, Andresen C, Goodale DB, Youngs EJ. The influence of age on propofol pharmacodynamics. Anesthesiology. 1999;90(6):1502–16.

19. Barakat A, Sutcliffe N, Schwab M. Effect site concentration during propofol TCI sedation: a comparison of sedation score with two pharmacokinetic models. Anaesthesia. 2007;(5):661–6.

20. Lu Y, Hao LX, Chen LX, Jin Z, Gong B. Systematic review and meta-analysis of patient-controlled sedation versus intravenous sedation for colonoscopy. Int J Clin Exp Med. 2015;8(11):19793–803.

21. Leitch JA, Sutcliffe N, Kenny GN. Patient-maintained sedation for oral surgery using a target-controlled infusion of propofol - a pilot study. Br Dent J. 2003;194(1):43–5.

Intravenous Anesthesia in Obese Patients

24

Pablo O. Sepúlveda V. and Luis Ignacio Cortínez

Introduction

Obesity has greatly increased in incidence in recent years, reaching epidemic proportions worldwide. Its growing prevalence means a larger number of obese patients will require sedation or anesthesia for different procedures, both inside and out of the operating room.

Administering anesthesia to an obese patient is usually a challenge for the anesthesiologist. Excess fat is commonly associated with technical difficulties such as with placing an intravenous line, surgical positioning and ventilation. In addition, different dosing strategies are required compared to normal weight subjects due to several physiological and pharmacological changes associated with obesity [1]. Understanding of these changes, and their impact on the administration of intravenous anesthetics, is crucial for successful intravenous anesthesia.

The scarcity of pharmacokinetic studies in the obese population, along with the huge variability within this group, means that current pharmacokinetic models, even those currently designed for the obese, might contain important errors in predictability which hinder the titration of anesthetics. In this chapter, we will revise the physiological changes associated with obesity, which impact the dosing of intravenous anesthetics and, based on current research, discuss different strategies for dose adjustment in this population.

Classification and Epidemiology of Obesity

According to the World Health Organization obesity is defined as the presence of excessive body fat, which increases the risk of various health problems. It is considered a chronic, complex, and multifactorial disease, in which there is an imbalance between energy intake and expenditure. The extent and severity of obesity is generally defined based on a Body Mass Index (BMI), calculated as total body weight in kilograms (kg) divided by height in meters squared. Patients can be classified as overweight or mildly obese if their BMI is between 25 and 29.9 kg/m^2, moderately to severely obese with a BMI of 30 to 39.9 kg/m^2 and morbidly obese if BMI is $\geq$40 kg/m^2. There are, however, more precise techniques of diagnosing and quantifying body fat such as impedance techniques and body densitometry [2].

According to official data from the World Health Organization, obesity has more than doubled worldwide since 1980. In 2014, 39 % of adults over 18 years old were overweight, and 13 % were obese. This problem has also affected children. It was reported in 2013 that over 42 million children under five were overweight. It is well known that obesity is associated with an increased incidence of chronic diseases such as: hypertension, diabetes mellitus, cholelithiasis, dyslipidemia, coronary heart disease, cancer, respiratory disease, psychiatric conditions, and osteoarticular problems [3]. All of which make this disease an important public health issue.

Physiological Changes and Their Importance in TIVA

Body Composition and Energy Expenditure Changes

The main body composition change in obese patients is an increase in body fat. Conversely, obesity can also be associated with a greater lean body mass, since stronger

24

P.O. Sepúlveda V., MD (✉)
Clinica Alemana de Santiago, Anestesia, Reanimación y Dolor, Vitacura 5951, Santiago 7580110, Chile
e-mail: pasevou@gmail.com

L.I. Cortínez, MD
Hospital Clinico Pontificia Universidad Catolica De Chile, Anesthesia, Marcoleta 377 Piso 4 Edificio Carlos Casanueva, Santiago, NA 8330024, Chile
e-mail: licorti@med.puc.cl

© Springer International Publishing AG 2017
A.R. Absalom, K.P. Mason (eds.), *Total Intravenous Anesthesia and Target Controlled Infusions*,
DOI 10.1007/978-3-319-47609-4_24

and larger muscles are necessary to support the load of additional adipose tissue. These changes must be considered in the dosage of anesthetics, as they are important in the distribution of drugs within the organism [1, 4]. Moreover, the basal metabolic demand increases with weight gain. This rise in metabolic demand is, nonetheless, lower than the increase in total body weight, because the metabolic rate of adipose tissue is very low compared to that of lean tissue [5, 6]. In other words, the resting metabolic rate per kg of total body weight is less in an obese patient, compared to a normal subject, yet similar if scaled to lean body weight [7].

Changes in body composition, as well as the physico-chemical properties of drugs, must be considered when administering intravenous anesthetics. Fat-soluble drugs present a greater volume of distribution and hence can accumulate, prolonging the time to recovery, especially after long continuous infusion schemes. In contrast, more water-soluble drugs have an increased distribution volume, mainly due to a greater lean mass (rather than because of additional fatty tissue). There is not a "one size fits all" dosing scheme for the obese, as it is thus necessary to determine specific body composition parameters, combined with an under-standing of individual drug properties. An example of this is remifentanil, because, despite being a fat-soluble drug, it does not accumulate in adipose tissue due to its high plasma and tissue metabolism.

Respiratory System Changes

The airway and respiratory system present important anatomic changes which impact the anesthetic management of the obese. Their fundamental importance is that obese patients are more susceptible to hypoxemia during the administration of anesthesia.

Obese patients have a greater neck circumference and an increased fatty infiltration of soft tissues (in the pharynx and peri-glottal area). These anatomic changes pose an increased risk of airway obstruction during natural sleep (obstructive sleep apnea) and this risk is increased during and after the administration of central nervous system depressants. Mor-bid obesity is therefore considered an independent risk factor for difficult ventilation [8]. Obesity is also associated with reduced thoracic compliance and lung volumes, mainly due to the effects of fatty deposits in the chest wall and increased intra-abdominal fat. The main changes in lung volumes are a reduced total lung capacity (TLC), expiratory reserve vol-ume (ERV), and functional residual capacity (FRC). These changes increase progressively with increasing BMI [9]. The diminished FRC and pulmonary compliance affect the ven-tilation perfusion ratio (V/Q), increasing the risk of hypox-emia in these patients. The supine position and surgery, especially thoracic or abdominal procedures, exacerbate these changes, and consequently the risk of perioperative

hypoxemia [10]. As a result, fine-tuning of dosage is critical in obese patients, to avoid the problems commonly associated with an overdose of central nervous system depressants such as opioids or hypnotics.

Cardiovascular Changes

Metabolic syndrome in obese patients is associated with a progressive deterioration of the cardiovascular system due to multiple contributing factors, such as excessive abdominal visceral fat, dyslipidemia, hypertension, insulin resistance, hyperglycemia, and a pro-thrombotic and pro-inflammatory state [11].

Increased secretion of pro-inflammatory peptides generated by excessive visceral fat, along with increased energy consumption (because of a greater lean mass), is associated with significant changes in the cardiovascular system, which include: increased blood volume, greater systolic volume, and a higher cardiac output [12]. While during initial stages of the disease cardiac ejection fraction is preserved, progressively left ventricular diastolic and sys-tolic dysfunction can occur. Furthermore, respiratory disorders in the obese can cause hypoxemia and hypercapnia which lead to pulmonary hypertension and consequently right ventricular failure [13]. Finally, concomitant diseases such as coronary atherosclerosis, type II diabetes, and hyper-tension can accelerate cardiovascular decline.

Overall, changes in the cardiovascular system have the greatest impact on the pharmacokinetics of drugs, both dur-ing their initial loading dose and distribution (increased blood volume and cardiac output) and during maintenance (increased blood flow to the liver and kidneys). It is impor-tant to emphasize that if scaled by kg of body weight, metabolic demand, blood volume, and cardiac output are actually lower in obese subjects. This is important in TIVA because if linear dosing formulas designed for non-obese patients are used, the result will be an overestimation of volumes and clearances, therefore leading to an overdose and side effects [1, 14].

Drug Metabolism and Excretion Changes

Obesity can significantly affect the excretion and metabo-lism of drugs, either increasing or diminishing these pro-cesses according to how the disease affects different systems and organs, such as the liver and kidneys [1, 4, 15].

The increase in cardiac output of the obese produces a greater perfusion of the liver and kidneys. This increased flow to the main excretory organs raises the absolute hepatic and renal clearance, especially during the early stages of the disease when no major structural damage of these organs has yet occurred [15]. However, as we previously mentioned, this increase is not proportional to body weight. If total body weight of the morbidly obese is used in the Cockcroft–Gault formula to estimate glomerular filtration rate (GFR), the result is an overestimation of GFR, and so it is advised to use lean body mass instead [16]. Similarly, the clearance of drugs which are highly dependent on hepatic blood flow, such as propofol, is similarly overestimated, if linearly scaled on a per kg base from normal weight subjects, and thus a better approach is the use of nonlinear allometric weight scales for this purpose [17, 18].

In chronic obesity, the initial rise in GFR entails an increase in blood pressure, hyperinsulinemia, and activation of the renin–angiotensin system, which can lead to a deterioration of renal function on account of irreversible glomerular structural damage [19]. In turn, diabetes mellitus and hypertension, two highly prevalent diseases in the obese, are themselves risk factors for renal disease [20].

In the liver, obesity is often associated with fatty liver disease [21] and hepatic fibrosis [22], which could impair its excretory and metabolic capacity. It has been reported that 87 % of patients undergoing bariatric surgery have abnormal liver histology, mainly fatty liver disease (83 %), nonalcoholic steatohepatitis (2.6 %), and cirrhosis (1.3 %). Furthermore, there is a correlation between the severity of liver damage and BMI [23]. Recent studies have shown an inverse correlation between the severity of fatty liver disease and intra-hepatic blood flow [24, 25]. As for liver enzyme activity, it has been reported that obesity can increase or decrease enzyme activity, depending on the enzymatic pathway involved, thus affecting drug metabolism in different ways [15].

Body Size and Dosage

Which Size Descriptor?

Total body weight (TBW) is the descriptor of body size most commonly used for drug dosing, however there are potentially more exact descriptors to adjust the dosage in the obese patient. Nonetheless, few studies have formally described volume changes and clearances of intravenous anesthetics in this population. Ideally pharmacokinetic models and dosing plans should be based on descriptors that reflect with greater precision the body composition changes of the obese that are relevant for each particular drug, according to their physical properties.

Body size descriptors used to adjust intravenous anesthetic doses in the obese patient:

1. Ideal body weight (IBW) [26]: Considers only height (HT) and gender in its estimation of weight. From a biological standpoint it seems unreasonable to adjust

doses without considering the impact of additional body weight (to which drugs may also re-distribute), and so its use is questionable in pharmacology [27].

$$IBW(kg) = 45.4 + 0.89(HT_{(CM)} - 152.4) \\ + 4.5(\text{if male})$$

2. Adjusted body weight (kg) [28]: Was derived to scale doses in the obese. It uses the ideal weight (IBW) and to a varying degree the amount of weight excess (TBW-IBW), which must be adjusted by a correcting factor (CF) based on the physical properties of the drug. In anesthesia it has been used to scale doses of propofol using a CF of 0.4 with good results [29, 30]. Its calculation is simple, and requires the weight, height, and gender of the patient.

$$ABW = IBW + CF(TBW - IBW)$$

3. Lean body weight (LBW): Is the difference between total body weight (TBW) and fat mass. Normally lean mass is between 70 % and 90 % of TBW. This ratio is altered in obesity due to excess fat. This descriptor has been recommended to adjust different doses of drugs in obese patients and non-obese [27]. Lean mass has a better correlation with metabolic processes than TBW, due to the lower contribution of fat to metabolic activity [27]. There are various formulas for calculating the lean mass, the most commonly used being those of James [31], and Hume [32]. Their calculation requires the weight, height, and gender of the patient.
James equation:

$$LBW_{(male)} = 1.10 \cdot TBW - 0.0128 \cdot BMI \cdot TBW$$

$$LBW_{(female)} = 1.07 \cdot TBW - 0.0148 \cdot BMI \cdot TBW$$

where the body mass index (BMI) is calculated as:

$$BMI = {}^{TBW(kg)}\!/_{Height(m)^2}$$

Hume equation:

$$LBW_{(male)} = 0.3281 \cdot TBW + 0.33929 \cdot H(cm) - 29.5336$$

$$LBW_{(female)} = 0.29569 \cdot TBW + 0.41813 \cdot H(cm) \\ - 43.2933$$

Using the James equation progressive weight gain entails an increase in lean mass until a BMI limit of 35 women and 42 men is reached. From then on the estimate of LBM starts to decrease until eventually reaching negative values, and so is inadequate in the morbidly obese (Fig. 24.1). Pharmacokinetic models such as the Schnider

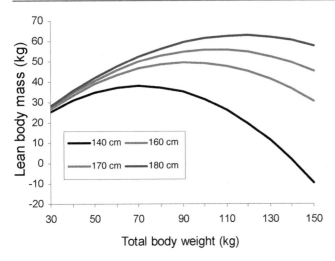

Fig. 24.1 Relationship between total body weight and lean body mass (LBM) of women according to James' equation for patients of different height

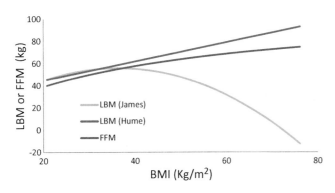

Fig. 24.2 Relationship between BMI and lean body mass (LBM) of women estimated by James and Hume equations and FFM (Janmahasatian Equation)

for propofol [33] and the Minto for Remifentanil [34] use this equation to calculate LBM as a covariate in some of its parameters, creating problems in the morbidly obese as discussed below.

4. Fat-free mass (FFM)

Fat-free mass (FFM) [2] considers muscles, bones, vital organs, and extracellular fluid. Unlike lean mass, it excludes lipid cell membranes, bone, and the central nervous system. Therefore FFM is very similar to lean mass and its main advantage is that it was derived from unbiased body mass measurements in people of a wide range of body weight (40–216 kg). The formula can be applied to the morbidly obese without the problems seen with the James equation (Fig. 24.2). FFM is determined using the weight (kg), height (m), and gender of the patient.

$$\mathrm{FFM} = \mathrm{WHS_{max}} \cdot \mathrm{H}^2 \cdot \left[\mathrm{TBW} \big/ _{(\mathrm{WHS_{50}} \cdot \mathrm{H}^2 + \mathrm{TBW})} \right]$$

For men, $\mathrm{WHS_{max}}$ is 42.92 kg/m^2 and $\mathrm{WHS_{50}}$ is 30.93 kg/m^2 and for women $\mathrm{WHS_{max}}$ is 37.99 kg/m^2 and $\mathrm{WHS_{50}}$ is 35.98 kg/m^2.

5. Normal fat mass (NFM)

NFM is an extension of the concept of ABW and predicted normal weight [34]. It incorporates an estimate of FFM plus a variable percentage (FFAT) of the estimated fat mass (TBW-FFM).

$$\mathrm{NFM(kg)} = \mathrm{FFM} + Ffat \cdot (\mathrm{TBW} - \mathrm{FFM})$$

The idea of NFM is to determine the value of *Ffat* that is most appropriate for the parameter being predicted. This will depend on the physical properties of the drug. If *Ffat* is estimated to be zero, then FFM alone is required to predict size while if *Ffat* is 1 then size is predicted by TBW.

Linear Body Weight Dosage Models

The larger body size of obese patients commonly causes a greater drug distribution volume and clearance. The magnitude of this rise is, however, variable depending on the characteristics of each drug [35]. Linear per kg dosing models assume that volumes and clearances increase proportionally to body weight. Commonly, pharmacokinetic models derived from normal weight patients use linear relationships between weight and model parameters [36–38]. Using these models in obese patients puts them at risk of overdose, mainly because the clearance of a drug does not increase linearly with weight [39]. The use of other size descriptors to scale down clearances, such as lean mass or normal fat mass (NFM), allows a better description of this nonlinear relationship [27]. In turn, allometric scaling models have been successfully used to describe changes in volumes and clearances of patients within a wide range of weight, as described below [17, 18, 40–42].

Allometry

Different organisms' characteristics and bodily functions can be scaled to body size by an exponential relationship to the power of a multiple of 1/4 [43]. Allometry describes this exponential relationship between size and function.

$$Y = aM^{\mathrm{PWR}}$$

where Y is the predicted biological characteristic, M is the mass of the body, a is an empirically derived constant, and PWR is the allometric exponent.

The growth of living beings, from single cell organisms to obese humans and elephants, can be described using allometric relationships. It is known, for example, that as living beings grow they do not remain isometric (same shape) because they would not be able to support their own weight—thus resulting in disproportional changes in body structure and composition. Allometry applies to many physiological, structural, and time related variables which follow the ¼ power law [43].

Allometry has been successfully used in pharmacology to adjust doses between different body sizes within species or between different species [44–46]. An allometric model based on theoretical principles scales volumes using a power of 1, clearances using a power of ¾, and half-times with a power of ¼, with respect to body size—no matter which body size descriptor is used, since that will depend on the physical properties of the drug [41, 47]. The basis of using a power of ¾ for clearances comes from its metabolic nature [43, 48]. There is strong evidence throughout a variety of species, including humans, that the basal metabolic rate can be adjusted according to body size using an allometric power of ¾ [43, 49]. Similarly, it is known that the metabolic rate of an organism is proportional to the energy produced by muscles, and can be scaled to body size using a power of ¾. In intravenous anesthesia there are many examples of the appropriateness of allometric relationships to describe the pharmacokinetic changes associated with growth in children [44–46] and obesity related size changes [17, 18, 41, 42, 47].

TIVA and TCI in the Obese Patient

Traditionally the administration of intravenous anesthesia using TCI in the obese has been done using dosing models derived from non-obese patients. The use of such models has proven inadequate in this population [41, 50]. Recently, however, there has been great interest in developing new PK and PD models that include obese patients. In this section we shall attempt to describe the pharmacokinetic changes associated with obesity, applied to frequently used intravenous anesthetics.

Opioids

Opioids are often used in general anesthesia to provide analgesia. Precise dosing in obese patients is crucial due to their greater susceptibility of developing respiratory complications. Nevertheless, the dose of opioids is often guided more by intuition than by scientific evidence. Furthermore, unlike the hypnotics, where there have been great advances in the monitoring of effect using EEG readings, to date there are no means to adequately monitor the effects of intra-operative opioid administration (see Chap. X on monitoring of the analgesic component of anesthesia).

Fentanyl

There are no pharmacokinetic models for fentanyl in the obese. Its pharmacokinetics are usually described using 3-compartment models, emphasizing its high lipid solubility (partition coefficient octanol-$H_2O = 813$), high volume of distribution (262 L), and relatively low clearance ($CL = 0.5$ L/min) [51]. These features cause long infusions, or repeated boluses of fentanyl to result in accumulation in peripheral tissues, especially fat tissue, potentially prolonging its duration of action [52]. Accumulation of this drug can be expected to increase in the obese due to the excess of fat mass. In turn, the increased cardiac output in these patients should result in increased clearances relative to normal weight patients. Shibutani et al. [53] evaluated the predictive ability of two pharmacokinetic models of fentanyl in obese and normal weight patients. In both models results showed a tendency to overestimate the concentrations of fentanyl in the obese. This is because the pharmacokinetic parameters of the models used were not scaled to weight and therefore were only representative of thin patients. In other words, the models did not consider the expected increase in volumes and clearances in these patients. In the same study, the authors were able to characterize the metabolic clearance and its relationship with weight, finding a nonlinear relationship. Based on their findings they suggest a standardized dose based on an empirical descriptor of body size called "pharmacokinetic mass."

Pharmacokinetic mass

$$= 52/\left[1 + \left(196.4e^{-0.025} \times TBW - 53.66/100\right)\right]$$

Figure 24.3 shows the relationship between weight and different size descriptors including pharmacokinetic mass. This figure suggests that, of the traditional size descriptors, the ABW with a correction factor of 0.4 (similar to that suggested for propofol) is the closest to the derived descriptor for this drug and could be a simple way of adjusting its dose.

Alfentanil

The pharmacokinetics of alfentanil are commonly described using a 3-compartment model [37]. Its pharmacokinetic characteristics include its relatively low lipid solubility (partition coefficient octanol-$H_2O = 145$), a volume of distribution of only 23 L and a slow clearance ($CL = 0.2$ L/min) [51].

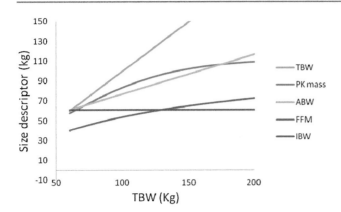

Fig. 24.3 Relationship between weight and different size descriptors including pharmacokinetic mass

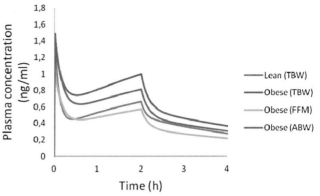

Fig. 24.4 Simulation of plasma concentration of sufentanil in a 70 kg (lean) and a 94 kg (obese) patient, both 170 cm tall. The dose of sufentanil administered is a 4 mcg/kg bolus, followed by a continuous infusion of 0.1 mcg/kg/min for 2 h. Obese patient schemes are based on actual weight (TBW), lean mass (FFM), or adjusted body weight, with a correcting factor of 0.4 (ABW)

Its lower lipid solubility compared to other opioids should lead to less accumulation in obese patients. There is only one PK model for this drug in obese patients, published by Pérus et al. [38], and this model was based on the study of only ten obese and six non-obese patients. In that study the authors found that the model of Maitre [37], derived from non-obese patients, underestimated alfentanil concentrations in obese patients—which could lead to an overdose. This error in estimation is attributed to the use of a lineal model based on weight to estimate volumes and clearances. Furthermore, based on the modeling analysis the authors describe an increase in alfentanil clearance in the obese, without any apparent effect on other parameters. With the scarce data available on this drug, definite recommendations cannot be made. It seems, however, reasonable to advise dosing of alfentanil using a descriptor of size such as lean mass (FFM) and not body weight.

Sufentanil

The pharmacokinetics of sufentanil are described using 2- and 3-compartment models. Its pharmacokinetic profile emphasizes its high lipid solubility (partition coefficient octanol-H_2O = 1778), high volume of distribution (541 L), and a relatively high clearance (CL = 1.2 L/min) [51, 54]. There are two models of sufentanil derived from an obese population [55, 56]. Unfortunately, due to limitations in their designs none of these studies is able to characterize the effect of body size as a continuous variable in volumes and clearances of the drug. Schwartz et al. [55] described the pharmacokinetics of sufentanil in eight obese and eight non-obese patients. The authors used a 2-compartment model to describe sufentanil PK and found a larger volume of distribution in obese (547 L) compared to non-obese (346 L) patients. With regard to clearance, they report slightly higher value of 1.99 (L/min) in obese compared with 1.78 (L/min) in the non-obese, however this difference was not statistically significant. Slepchenko et al. [56]

administered sufentanil by TCI in obese subjects using the non-obese model created by Gepts et al. [57]. The authors found an overall good performance, with a slight tendency to overestimate the drug concentration ("Median performance error" = −13 %). Although this result could be interpreted as a validation of this model in the obese, there remains a clear correlation between the degree of obesity and the amount of overestimation. That is, the error becomes more negative (more overestimation) with increasing weight, which could be explained because the model does not scale its parameters according to body size. Therefore, in heavier patients, there is a greater the risk of underdosing, because the model does not consider the expected increase in volumes and clearances of sufentanil as weight increase. Using the pharmacokinetic parameters reported by Schwartz et al. [55] in obese and non-obese patients, it is possible to simulate dosing using different size descriptors (Fig. 24.4). The figure shows that weight-based schemes result in higher concentrations in obese patients, and that dose normalization based on FFM or ABW would be preferable.

Remifentanil

The pharmacokinetics of remifentanil are characterized using 2- or 3-compartment models [14, 34, 58]. Its pharmacokinetic profile includes a moderate lipid solubility (partition coefficient octanol-H_2O = 17.9), low volume of distribution (20 L), and a rapid clearance (CL = 2.6 L/min). Egan et al. [14] described the pharmacokinetics of remifentanil after a large single bolus of approximately 10 mcg/kg (TBW) in 12 obese and 12 non-obese patients. In their results, the authors report higher concentrations and a longer duration of associated hemodynamic compromise in obese patients. Using a two-compartment model to describe

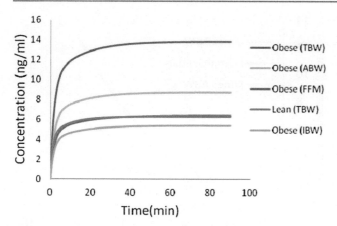

Fig. 24.5 Simulation of plasma concentration of remifentanil using the Egan model, in two patients—one 70 kg (lean) and the other 94 kg (obese), both 170 cm tall. The dose administered of remifentanil is 0.25 mcg/kg/min. Obese patient schemes are based on actual weight (TBW), lean mass (FFM), adjusted body weight, with a correcting factor of 0.4 (ABW) or ideal body weight (IBW)

Table 24.1 Pharmacokinetic parameters adjusted to LBM (James equation) in the Minto model for remifentanil

Parameter	Non-obese	Obese
$V1$ (L)	4.4	3.3
$V1$ (L)	8.8	7.2
CL (L/h)	144	128

Estimated parameters are shown for 40-year-old, 160 cm, male non-obese (65 kg) and obese (150 kg) subjects

the pharmacokinetics of the drug, the authors found no differences in volumes (L) and clearances (L/min) in both groups. It should be noted, however, that there was a tendency to a slight increase in volumes and clearances in obese patients, which was better correlated with the increase in lean mass than total body weight. This correlation explains overdose reported in obese patients when using a bolus scaled to weight. The model they designed suggests scaling of doses using lean mass. This is shown in Fig. 24.5 using the parameters reported by Egan et al. and different size descriptors.

Remifentanil TCI with the Minto PK Model in the Obese

The administration of remifentanil by TCI using the Minto model [34] is not recommended for the morbidly obese as this model was not derived from obese patients. As mentioned above, the James equation [31], used in this model to calculate lean mass, produces an underestimation of $V1$, $V2$, and CL in the morbidly obese (Table 24.1). If this model is used for TCI in patients with a BMI above a critical value (~35 in women and ~42 in men), the amount of drug administered will be progressively less than required. La Colla et al. [59] demonstrated that underestimation with the Minto model in the morbidly obese can be corrected by using the

Janmahasatian equation [2], instead of the James equation, for estimating FFM. This correction, nevertheless, has not been incorporated into commercially available TCI pumps. Alternatively, the use of a larger "fake height" to reduce error with the James equation has also been proposed by the same authors [59]. We believe that until there are adequate remifentanil TCI models implemented for use in obese patients, continuous infusions schemes based on FFM and adjusted according to clinical response should be preferred.

Propofol

Propofol is the hypnotic of choice for TIVA. Its pharmacokinetics are best described by three-compartment models [33, 36, 60–64]. Its pharmacokinetic profile features a high lipid solubility (partition coefficient octanol-H_2O = 6800), a high volume of distribution ($\approx$250 L), and rapid clearance ($\approx$1.8 L/min). Several studies have examined the pharmacokinetics of propofol in obese patients. Servin et al. [30] designed the first formal pharmacokinetic study of propofol in eight morbidly obese patients. The authors reported that the initial volume of distribution was not modified in obese patients, compared with the non-obese adults using data from another study. Furthermore, clearance and distribution volume at steady state were correlated to TBW. The authors suggested that maintenance schemes based on TBW should be the same as those for non-obese patients without an apparent risk for accumulation. The lack of a clear increase in the initial distribution volume might suggest adjusting the initial induction bolus to avoid overdosing and consequent hemodynamic repercussions. In line with this result Ingrande et al. [65] found that scaling the induction bolus of propofol to lean mass was more appropriate than TBW. In a study by our group [17] we studied 19 morbidly obese patients who received propofol and remifentanil based anesthesia. Plasma concentrations in these patients were analyzed, along with data from two other studies in morbidly obese patients [30] and healthy volunteers [33]. In total 51 subjects with a wide range of BMI (16–52 kg/m²) were included. In this study we found that a 3-compartment model, using TBW to allometrically scale volumes and clearances was superior to other size descriptors (FFM, LBM, NFM). Later studies [18, 66, 67] support the allometric relationship to TBW as a valid alternative for propofol dose adjustment in the obese. According to these new models the infusion rates of propofol during anesthetic maintenance (mg/kg/h) should be reduced nonlinearly with increasing body weight. Of the various models available, that developed by Eleveld et al. [18] deserves special mention, as it is derived from a large population of 660 individuals and 21 studies, to help estimate volumes and clearances, and the impact of other covariates besides body weight (such as age, sex, and gender).

Propofol TCI with the Marsh and Schnider Models in the Obese

Commercially available TCI pumps use the Marsh [36] and Schnider [33] propofol models which were derived from non-obese patients. When prospectively tested in obese patients both models have shown poor performance [68, 69]. Extrapolation of model predictions from a model derived from one population to another of different qualities (i.e., age, weight or disease) is not advisable since it carries the risk of important misspecifications and dosing errors.

The Marsh Model

The Marsh model scales all of its volumes and clearances to total body weight. Consequently, it delivers twice the dose in mg or mg/h, to a patient who weighs double that of another, without adjustment by other covariates. As mentioned above, it is evident that the clearance of a drug does not increase in proportion to body weight and thus this model will most likely administer an excess of drug with increasing magnitude according to degree of obesity. In turn, the central volume, a key parameter in the calculation of the initial bolus, will be overestimated in the obese patient generating a comparatively large bolus [69]. The use of the Marsh model for TCI in obese patients remains controversial [70]. Some studies suggest that, if used, anesthetic maintenance dose should be determined without weight correction [68, 71], whilst others recommend using ABW instead [29]. This last approach allows for a reduction in bolus size and maintenance dose, without the need to adjust the target concentration. We believe that using Marsh with ABW is a better alternative, nevertheless, due to model misspecifications from linear per kg assumptions, propofol administration should always be titrated using an EEG monitor to assure adequate anesthetic depth.

The Schnider Model

With the Schnider model errors are greater in the obese than the Marsh model [29]. One of the problems is caused by an underestimation of central volume, owing to the fact that it is fixed (not influenced by body size), which potentially leads to inadequate induction bolus doses. The biggest problem, however, is the overestimation of metabolic clearance. The latter is calculated by an equation including lean body mass (estimated by the James equation). As described above, lean mass is underestimated by the James equation in the severely obese, leading to an overestimation of clearance in this model. To avoid the risk of overdose, commercial TCI pumps block the use of this model upon reaching critical values of BMI. One way to address this problem is to use ABW, thereby artificially decreasing BMI and better estimate lean mass. Replacing the James equation with the Janmahasatian equation for estimating lean mass is not

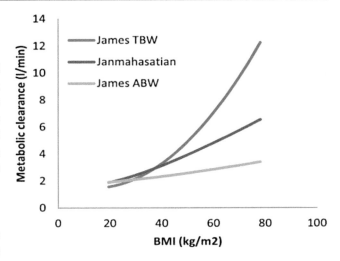

Fig. 24.6 Metabolic clearance of propofol estimated with the Schnider model using different approaches to calculate LBM. The *blue line* represents the original approach using James equation which results in the larger predictive errors

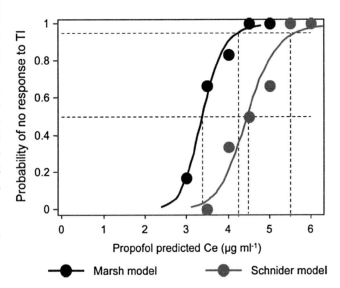

Fig. 24.7 Propofol predicted effect-site targets to induce general anesthesia in obese patients according to the model selected. Adequate hypnosis is BIS <60 up to 5 min after intubation

possible without altering the original model and proved ineffective in our study [29] (Fig. 24.6).

Marsh and Schnider Models at Induction

Echevarría et al. [72] studied the initial target concentration during induction of 66 obese patients using an effect site targeted TCI, with both the Marsh and Schnider models. All patients received fentanyl (3 mcg/kg), and the authors defined adequate hypnosis as BIS <60 up to 5 min after intubation. It was found that the effective target for 50 % of the patients was 4.5 mcg/ml using the Schnider model and 3.4 mcg/ml using the Marsh model (Fig. 24.7). These results are mainly explained by differences in the central volume, as previously discussed and therefore the magnitude of their difference will increase in heavier patients. It is our opinion that although these values can be used as a reference, the bottom line is that these models will behave very differently at induction and therefore initial target selection should be based on a good understanding of the model selected and patient characteristics.

Which Propofol Model for the Obese?

A recent study by Cortinez et al. [29] reviewed the performance of five propofol models in the morbidly obese, including those designed for use in obese [17, 18, 66] and non-obese patients t [33, 36]. Overall the Eleveld model performed the best, with an average absolute error of 27 % and a moderate tendency to underestimate the concentration of propofol of 18 % (both errors can be considered clinically acceptable [69, 70]). It is noteworthy that all models showed a tendency to overdose. This systematic error may be attributed to a pharmacokinetic interaction with remifentanil, which was administered in relatively high doses (0.36 ± 0.09 mg/kg TBW/min). In addition, in this study the effect time profile was characterized using a pharmacokinetic-pharmacodynamic model, by the means of a bispectral index (BIS) monitor of hypnosis. No obvious differences in the time profile of the BIS, nor in the concentration-BIS ratio when compared with other studies in non-obese patients was found, suggesting little influence of obesity on the hypnotic effect of propofol.

It is surprising that, having models specifically designed for obese patients, these have yet to be incorporated in commercial pumps. In Latin America Arcomed® (Arcomed_AG, Switzerland) pumps have incorporated the Cortínez model to administer propofol in obese patients. In contrast, other available pumps do not incorporate these new models. With the currently available TCI models we recommend the use of either the Marsh or the Schnider models with ABW. No matter what model is selected, it is recommended to titrate the concentration target aided by an anesthesia depth monitor.

Dexmedetomidine

Dexmedetomidine is a highly selective α-2 adrenergic agonist with sedative [73–75], and analgesic effects [74–76], and minimal respiratory changes [74–77]. In bariatric surgery dexmedetomidine is often administered as an anesthetic adjuvant, decreasing the consumption of opioids intra- and postoperatively [76, 77]. Dosage in this population is commonly done on the basis of schemes scaled by kg of weight, with recommendations to decrease the dose in obese patients [78]. Its pharmacokinetic profile includes a low lipid solubility (partition coefficient octanol-H_2O = 2.89) [79], volume of distribution of 120–150 L and clearance of 0.5–0.8 L/min [79–82]. Cortinez et al. [40] studied the pharmacokinetics of dexmedetomidine in obese and normal weight patients given two infusion schemes based on weight (0.25 mcg/kg/h; 0.5 mcg/kg/h). The study showed that dexmedetomidine dosing schemes using linear weight per kg produced higher concentrations of the drug in obese patients than in non-obese patients (Fig. 24.8).

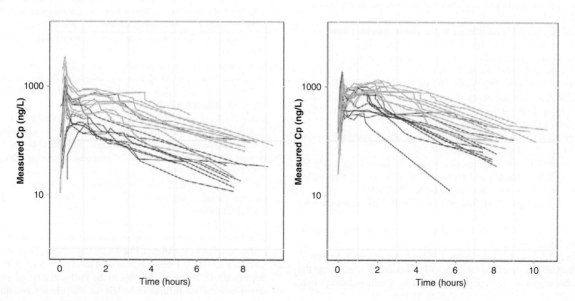

Fig. 24.8 Dexmedetomidine serum concentration time profiles according to the maintenance dose regime administered. *Left panel* (0.25 mcg/kg/h); *right panel* (0.5 mcg/kg/h). *Green lines* represent obese patients. *Blue lines* represent lean patients

Table 24.2 Estimated loading doses (LD) and maintenance infusion schemes (MD) at steady-state to obtain a dexmedetomidine plasma concentration of 700 ng/L in representative male and female patients of a wide range of body weights and composition

Gender	BMI (kg/m^2)	Height (m)	Weight (kg)	FFM (kg)	FAT (kg)	V1 (L/kg)	CL (L/h/kg)	LD (mcg/kg)	MD (mcg/kg/h)
Female	28	1.54	67	39.63	27.37	0.65	0.65	0.54	0.45
Female	36	1.79	115	60.79	54.21	0.58	0.45	0.47	0.31
Female	52	1.71	151	65.47	85.53	0.48	0.31	0.38	0.21
Male	28	1.54	67	48.59	18.41	0.80	0.79	0.65	0.55
Male	36	1.79	115	73.87	41.13	0.70	0.56	0.57	0.39
Male	52	1.71	151	78.49	72.51	0.57	0.38	0.45	0.26

Additionally, the pharmacokinetic profile of the drug was adequately described with a 2-compartment model, as in other previous studies [80–82]. The higher concentrations of dexmedetomidine attained in obese patients were explained by the lack of effect of fat mass on the estimated increases in volumes and clearances. Changes in these parameters were described using an allometric model, with FFM as a body size descriptor. Finally, excess fat was found to have a negative effect on clearance, potentially due to a concomitant hepatic impairment—a possibility that requires further research. The authors describe dose adjustments per kg of weight to illustrate the results of their model on the dosage of this population (Table 24.2).

References

1. Cheymol G. Effects of obesity on pharmacokinetics implications for drug therapy. Clin Pharmacokinet. 2000;39:215–31.
2. Janmahasatian S, Duffull SB, Ash S, Ward LC, Byrne NM, Green B. Quantification of lean bodyweight. Clin Pharmacokinet. 2005;44:1051–65.
3. Must A, Spadano J, Coakley EH, Field AE, Colditz G, Dietz WH. The disease burden associated with overweight and obesity. JAMA. 1999;282:1523–9.
4. Casati A, Putzu M. Anesthesia in the obese patient: pharmacokinetic considerations. J Clin Anesth. 2005;17:134–45.
5. Webb P. Energy expenditure and fat-free mass in men and women. Am J Clin Nutr. 1981;34:1816–26.
6. McNeill G, Rivers JP, Payne PR, de Britto JJ, Abel R. Basal metabolic rate of Indian men: no evidence of metabolic adaptation to a low plane of nutrition. Hum Nutr Clin Nutr. 1987;41:473–83.
7. Horgan GW, Stubbs J. Predicting basal metabolic rate in the obese is difficult. Eur J Clin Nutr. 2003;57:335–40.
8. Kheterpal S, Han R, Tremper KK, Shanks A, Tait AR, O'Reilly M, Ludwig TA. Incidence and predictors of difficult and impossible mask ventilation. Anesthesiology. 2006;105:885–91.
9. Jones RL, Nzekwu MM. The effects of body mass index on lung volumes. Chest. 2006;130:827–33.
10. Luce JM. Respiratory complications of obesity. Chest. 1980;78:626–31.
11. Despres JP, Lemieux I, Bergeron J, Pibarot P, Mathieu P, Larose E, Rodes-Cabau J, Bertrand OF, Poirier P. Abdominal obesity and the metabolic syndrome: contribution to global cardiometabolic risk. Arterioscler Thromb Vasc Biol. 2008;28:1039–49.
12. Wong C, Marwick TH. Obesity cardiomyopathy: pathogenesis and pathophysiology. Nat Clin Pract Cardiovasc Med. 2007;4:436–43.
13. Wong CY, O'Moore-Sullivan T, Leano R, Hukins C, Jenkins C, Marwick TH. Association of subclinical right ventricular dysfunction with obesity. J Am Coll Cardiol. 2006;47:611–6.
14. Egan TD, Huizinga B, Gupta SK, Jaarsma RL, Sperry RJ, Yee JB, Muir KT. Remifentanil pharmacokinetics in obese versus lean patients. Anesthesiology. 1998;89:562–73.
15. Brill MJ, Diepstraten J, van Rongen A, van Kralingen S, van den Anker JN, Knibbe CA. Impact of obesity on drug metabolism and elimination in adults and children. Clin Pharmacokinet. 2012;51:277–304.
16. Demirovic JA, Pai AB, Pai MP. Estimation of creatinine clearance in morbidly obese patients. Am J Health Syst Pharm. 2009;66:642–8.
17. Cortinez LI, Anderson BJ, Penna A, Olivares L, Munoz HR, Holford NH, Struys MM, Sepulveda P. Influence of obesity on propofol pharmacokinetics: derivation of a pharmacokinetic model. Br J Anaesth. 2010;105:448–56.
18. Eleveld DJ, Proost JH, Cortinez LI, Absalom AR, Struys MM. A general purpose pharmacokinetic model for propofol. Anesth Analg. 2014;118:1221–37.
19. Henegar JR, Bigler SA, Henegar LK, Tyagi SC, Hall JE. Functional and structural changes in the kidney in the early stages of obesity. J Am Soc Nephrol. 2001;12:1211–7.
20. Griffin KA, Kramer H, Bidani AK. Adverse renal consequences of obesity. Am J Physiol Renal Physiol. 2008;294:F685–96.
21. Adams JP, Murphy PG. Obesity in anaesthesia and intensive care. Br J Anaesth. 2000;85:91–108.
22. Moretto M, Kupski C, da Silva VD, Padoin AV, Mottin CC. Effect of bariatric surgery on liver fibrosis. Obes Surg. 2012;22:1044–9.
23. Moretto M, Kupski C, Mottin CC, Repetto G, Garcia Toneto M, Rizzolli J, Berleze D, de Souza Brito CL, Casagrande D, Colossi F. Hepatic steatosis in patients undergoing bariatric surgery and its relationship to body mass index and co-morbidities. Obes Surg. 2003;13:622–4.
24. Mohammadi A, Ghasemi-rad M, Zahedi H, Toldi G, Alinia T. Effect of severity of steatosis as assessed ultrasonographically on hepatic vascular indices in non-alcoholic fatty liver disease. Med Ultrason. 2011;13:200–6.
25. Balci A, Karazincir S, Sumbas H, Oter Y, Egilmez E, Inandi T. Effects of diffuse fatty infiltration of the liver on portal vein flow hemodynamics. J Clin Ultrasound. 2008;36:134–40.
26. Devine D. Case study number 25 gentamicin therapy. Drug Intell Clin Pharm. 1974;8:650–5.
27. Green B, Duffull SB. What is the best size descriptor to use for pharmacokinetic studies in the obese? Br J Clin Pharmacol. 2004;58:119–33.
28. Bauer LA, Edwards WA, Dellinger EP, Simonowitz DA. Influence of weight on aminoglycoside pharmacokinetics in normal weight and morbidly obese patients. Eur J Clin Pharmacol. 1983;24:643–7.
29. Cortinez LI, De la Fuente N, Eleveld DJ, Oliveros A, Crovari F, Sepulveda P, Ibacache M, Solari S. Performance of propofol target-controlled infusion models in the obese: pharmacokinetic and pharmacodynamic analysis. Anesth Analg. 2014;119:302–10.

30. Servin F, Farinotti R, Haberer JP, Desmonts JM. Propofol infusion for maintenance of anesthesia in morbidly obese patients receiving nitrous oxide. A clinical and pharmacokinetic study. Anesthesiology. 1993;78:657–65.

31. James WP. Research on obesity. London: Her Majesty's Stationary Office; 1976.

32. Hume R. Prediction of lean body mass from height and weight. J Clin Pathol. 1966;19:389–91.

33. Schnider TW, Minto CF, Gambus PL, Andresen C, Goodale DB, Shafer SL, Youngs EJ. The influence of method of administration and covariates on the pharmacokinetics of propofol in adult volunteers. Anesthesiology. 1998;88:1170–82.

34. Minto CF, Schnider TW, Egan TD, Youngs E, Lemmens HJ, Gambus PL, Billard V, Hoke JF, Moore KH, Hermann DJ, Muir KT, Mandema JW, Shafer SL. Influence of age and gender on the pharmacokinetics and pharmacodynamics of remifentanil. I. Model development. Anesthesiology. 1997;86:10–23.

35. Abernethy DR, Greenblatt DJ. Drug disposition in obese humans. An update. Clin Pharmacokinet. 1986;11:199–213.

36. Marsh BWM, Morton N, Kenny GN. Pharmacokinetic model driven infusion of propofol in children. Br J Anaesth. 1991;67:41–8.

37. Maitre PO, Vozeh S, Heykants J, Thomson DA, Stanski DR. Population pharmacokinetics of alfentanil: the average dose-plasma concentration relationship and interindividual variability in patients. Anesthesiology. 1987;66:3–12.

38. Perus O, Marsot A, Ramain E, Dahman M, Paci A, Raucoules-Aime M, Simon N. Performance of alfentanil target-controlled infusion in normal and morbidly obese female patients. Br J Anaesth. 2012;109:551–60.

39. Holford S, Allegaert K, Anderson BJ, Kukanich B, Sousa AB, Steinman A, Pypendop BH, Mehvar R, Giorgi M, Holford NH. -Parent-metabolite pharmacokinetic models for tramadol – tests of assumptions and predictions. J Pharmacol Clin Toxicol. 2014;2:1023.

40. Cortinez LI, Anderson BJ, Holford NH, Puga V, de la Fuente N, Auad H, Solari S, Allende FA, Ibacache M. Dexmedetomidine pharmacokinetics in the obese. Eur J Clin Pharmacol. 2015;71:1501–8.

41. Eleveld DJ, Proost JH, Absalom AR, Struys MM. Obesity and allometric scaling of pharmacokinetics. Clin Pharmacokinet. 2011;50:751–3. discussion 5–6.

42. Mahmood I. Prediction of clearance and volume of distribution in the obese from normal weight subjects: an allometric approach. Clin Pharmacokinet. 2012;51:527–42.

43. Savage VM, Gillooly JF, Woodruff WH, West GB, Allen AP, Enquist BJ, Brown JH. The predominance of quarter-power scaling in biology. Funct Ecol. 2004;18:257–82.

44. Anderson BJ, Holford NH. Mechanism-based concepts of size and maturity in pharmacokinetics. Annu Rev Pharmacol Toxicol. 2008;48:303–32.

45. Anderson BJ, Holford NH. Mechanistic basis of using body size and maturation to predict clearance in humans. Drug Metab Pharmacokinet. 2009;24:25–36.

46. Peeters MY, Allegaert K, Blusse van Oud-Alblas HJ, Cella M, Tibboel D, Danhof M, Knibbe CA. Prediction of propofol clearance in children from an allometric model developed in rats, children and adults versus a 0.75 fixed-exponent allometric model. Clin Pharmacokinet. 2010;49:269–75.

47. Cortinez LI, Anderson BJ, Holford NH. Dexmedetomidine pharmacokinetics in the obese. Eur J Clin Pharmacol. 2015;71:1501–8.

48. West GB, Brown JH, Enquist BJ. A general model for the origin of allometric scaling laws in biology. Science. 1997;276:122–6.

49. West GB, Brown JH. The origin of allometric scaling laws in biology from genomes to ecosystems: towards a quantitative unifying theory of biological structure and organization. J Exp Biol. 2005;208:1575–92.

50. Coetzee JF. Allometric or lean body mass scaling of propofol pharmacokinetics: towards simplifying parameter sets for target-controlled infusions. Clin Pharmacokinet. 2012;51:137–45.

51. Shafer SL, Varvel JR, Aziz N, Scott JC. Pharmacokinetics of fentanyl administered by computer-controlled infusion pump. Anesthesiology. 1990;73:1091–102.

52. Shafer SL, Varvel JR. Pharmacokinetics, pharmacodynamics, and rational opioid selection. Anesthesiology. 1991;74:53–63.

53. Shibutani K, Inchiosa Jr MA, Sawada K, Bairamian M. Accuracy of pharmacokinetic models for predicting plasma fentanyl concentrations in lean and obese surgical patients: derivation of dosing weight ("pharmacokinetic mass"). Anesthesiology. 2004;101:603–13.

54. Meuldermans WE, Hurkmans RM, Heykants JJ. Plasma protein binding and distribution of fentanyl, sufentanil, alfentanil and lofentanil in blood. Arch Int Pharmacodyn Ther. 1982;257:4–19.

55. Schwartz AE, Matteo RS, Ornstein E, Young WL, Myers KJ. Pharmacokinetics of sufentanil in obese patients. Anesth Analg. 1991;73:790–3.

56. Slepchenko G, Simon N, Goubaux B, Levron JC, Le Moing JP, Raucoules-Aime M. Performance of target-controlled sufentanil infusion in obese patients. Anesthesiology. 2003;98:65–73.

57. Gepts E, Shafer SL, Camu F, Stanski DR, Woestenborghs R, Van Peer A, Heykants JJ. Linearity of pharmacokinetics and model estimation of sufentanil. Anesthesiology. 1995;83:1194–204.

58. Egan TD, Lemmens HJ, Fiset P, Hermann DJ, Muir KT, Stanski DR, Shafer SL. The pharmacokinetics of the new short-acting opioid remifentanil (GI87084B) in healthy adult male volunteers. Anesthesiology. 1993;79:881–92.

59. La Colla L, Albertin A, La Colla G, Porta A, Aldegheri G, Di Candia D, Gigli F. Predictive performance of the 'Minto' remifentanil pharmacokinetic parameter set in morbidly obese patients ensuing from a new method for calculating lean body mass. Clin Pharmacokinet. 2010;49:131–9.

60. Coetzee JF, Glen JB, Wium CA, Boshoff L. Pharmacokinetic model selection for target controlled infusions of propofol. Assessment of three parameter sets. Anesthesiology. 1995;82:1328–45.

61. Kirkpatrick T, Cockshott ID, Douglas EJ, Nimmo WS. Pharmacokinetics of propofol (diprivan) in elderly patients. Br J Anaesth. 1988;60:146–50.

62. Landais A, Cockshott ID, Coppens MC, Cohn N, Richard MD, Saint-Maurice C. Pharmacokinetics of propofol as an induction agents in adults. Cah Anesthesiol. 1987;35:427–8.

63. Schüttler JIH. Population pharmacokinetics of propofol. Anesthesiology. 2000;92:727–38.

64. Shafer A, Doze VA, Shafer SL, White PF. Pharmacokinetics and pharmacodynamics of propofol infusions during general anesthesia. Anesthesiology. 1988;69:348–56.

65. Ingrande J, Brodsky JB, Lemmens HJ. Lean body weight scalar for the anesthetic induction dose of propofol in morbidly obese subjects. Anesth Analg. 2011;113:57–62.

66. van Kralingen S, van de Garde EM, van Dongen EP, Diepstraten J, Deneer VH, van Ramshorst B, Knibbe CA. Maintenance of anesthesia in morbidly obese patients using propofol with continuous BIS-monitoring: a comparison of propofol-remifentanil and propofol-epidural anesthesia. Acta Anaesthesiol Belg. 2011;62:73–82.

67. Diepstraten J, Chidambaran V, Sadhasivam S, Esslinger HR, Cox SL, Inge TH, Knibbe CA, Vinks AA. Propofol clearance in morbidly obese children and adolescents: influence of age and body size. Clin Pharmacokinet. 2012;51:543–51.

68. La Colla L, Albertin A, La Colla G, Ceriani V, Lodi T, Porta A, Aldegheri G, Mangano A, Khairallah I, Fermo I. No adjustment

vs. adjustment formula as input weight for propofol target-controlled infusion in morbidly obese patients. Eur J Anaesthesiol. 2009;26:362–9.

69. Absalom AR, Mani V, De Smet T, Struys MM. Pharmacokinetic models for propofol--defining and illuminating the devil in the detail. Br J Anaesth. 2009;103:26–37.

70. Coetzee JF. Total intravenous anaesthesia to obese patients: largely guesswork? Eur J Anaesthesiol. 2009;26:359–61.

71. Albertin A, Poli D, La Colla L, Gonfalini M, Turi S, Pasculli N, La Colla G, Bergonzi PC, Dedola E, Fermo I. Predictive performance of 'Servin's formula' during BIS-guided propofol-remifentanil target-controlled infusion in morbidly obese patients. Br J Anaesth. 2007;98:66–75.

72. Echevarria GC, Elgueta MF, Donoso MT, Bugedo DA, Cortinez LI, Munoz HR. The effective effect-site propofol concentration for induction and intubation with two pharmacokinetic models in morbidly obese patients using total body weight. Anesth Analg. 2012;115:823–9.

73. Belleville JP, Ward DS, Bloor BC, Maze M. Effects of intravenous dexmedetomidine in humans. I. Sedation, ventilation, and metabolic rate. Anesthesiology. 1992;77:1125–33.

74. Hall JE, Uhrich TD, Barney JA, Arain SR, Ebert TJ. Sedative, amnestic, and analgesic properties of small-dose dexmedetomidine infusions. Anesth Analg. 2000;90:699–705.

75. Ebert TJ, Hall JE, Barney JA, Uhrich TD, Colinco MD. The effects of increasing plasma concentrations of dexmedetomidine in humans. Anesthesiology. 2000;93:382–94.

76. Venn RM, Hell J, Grounds RM. Respiratory effects of dexmedetomidine in the surgical patient requiring intensive care. Crit Care. 2000;4:302–8.

77. Hsu YW, Cortinez LI, Robertson KM, Keifer JC, Sum-Ping ST, Moretti EW, Young CC, Wright DR, Macleod DB, Somma J. Dexmedetomidine pharmacodynamics: part I: crossover comparison of the respiratory effects of dexmedetomidine and remifentanil in healthy volunteers. Anesthesiology. 2004;101:1066–76.

78. Tufanogullari B, White PF, Peixoto MP, Kianpour D, Lacour T, Griffin J, Skrivanek G, Macaluso A, Shah M, Provost DA. Dexmedetomidine infusion during laparoscopic bariatric surgery: the effect on recovery outcome variables. Anesth Analg. 2008;106:1741–8.

79. Chrysostomou C, Schmitt CG. Dexmedetomidine: sedation, analgesia and beyond. Expert Opin Drug Metab Toxicol. 2008;4:619–27.

80. Talke P, Richardson CA, Scheinin M, Fisher DM. Postoperative pharmacokinetics and sympatholytic effects of dexmedetomidine. Anesth Analg. 1997;85:1136–42.

81. Venn RM, Karol MD, Grounds RM. Pharmacokinetics of dexmedetomidine infusions for sedation of postoperative patients requiring intensive caret. Br J Anaesth. 2002;88:669–75.

82. Iirola T, Ihmsen H, Laitio R, Kentala E, Aantaa R, Kurvinen JP, Scheinin M, Schwilden H, Schuttler J, Olkkola KT. Population pharmacokinetics of dexmedetomidine during long-term sedation in intensive care patients. Br J Anaesth. 2012;108:460–8.

Brian J. Anderson

The pharmacokinetics (PK), pharmacodynamics (PD) and side effect profile of most medications used in children differ from those in adults; these differences are most pronounced in neonates. PK are affected by maturation of organ function and body composition, altered protein binding, distinct disease spectrum, diverse behaviour and dissimilar receptor patterns [1]. The capacity of the end organ, such as the brain, heart or skeletal muscle, to respond to medications may also differ in children compared with adults (PD effects). Dose modification to achieve the desired clinical response and avoid toxicity is required for children. Dose calculations are based on knowledge of PK and PD [2].

Principles of PK and PD Modelling

The goal of pharmacologic treatment is a desired response, known as the target effect. An understanding of the concentration–response relationship (i.e. pharmacodynamics, PD) can be used to predict the target concentration required to achieve this target effect in a typical child [3]. Pharmacokinetic (PK) knowledge (e.g. clearance, volume) then determines the dose that will achieve the target concentration. Each child, however, is somewhat different, and there is variability associated with all parameters used in PK and PD equations (known as models). Covariate information (e.g. weight, age, pathology, drug interactions, pharmacogenomics) can be used to help predict the typical dose in a specific patient [2]. The Holy Grail of clinical pharmacology is the prediction of drug PK and PD in the individual patient [4], and this requires knowledge of the covariates that contribute to variability.

Anaesthesiologists are practising pharmacologists, and the use of total intravenous anaesthesia (TIVA) using propofol is a good example of 'pharmacology in action'. There is a defined target effect (e.g. bispectral index (BIS) 50–55), there is a target concentration of propofol known to achieve this (e.g. 3 mg/L), and the PK of propofol in children have been described. Advanced concepts in pharmacokinetic modelling and computer technology have led to sophisticated delivery systems that facilitate anaesthesia given by the intravenous route. Further advances involving feedback from receptor organs have been developed for children [5, 6]. - Target-controlled infusion (TCI) devices or 'smart pumps' may be directed at either plasma or effect site. These computerised pumps are a considerable advance over earlier manual techniques for children [7, 8] that targeted plasma alone. However, they require input of both pharmacokinetic and pharmacodynamic parameters, and a lack of robust PK–PD estimates and variability associated with parameter estimates limits the current accuracy of TCI in children under 5 years of age [9].

Compartment Modelling

If drug concentrations are measured several times within the first 15–30 min after IV administration as well as during a more prolonged period, more than one clearance is often present. This can be observed as a marked change in slope of a semilogarithmic graph of concentration versus time (Fig. 25.1). The number and nature of the compartments required to describe the clearance of a drug do not necessarily represent specific body fluids or tissues. When two first-order exponential equations are required to describe the clearance of drug from the circulation, the pharmacokinetics are described as first-order, two-compartment (e.g. central and peripheral compartments) that fit the following equation:

$$C(t) = Ae^{-\alpha t} + Be^{-\beta t} \qquad (25.1)$$

B.J. Anderson, MB ChB, PhD, FANZCA, FCICM (✉)
Anaesthesia and Intensive Care, Starship Children' Hospital, Park Road, Grafton, Auckland 1023, New Zealand
e-mail: briana@adhb.govt.nz

© Springer International Publishing AG 2017
A.R. Absalom, K.P. Mason (eds.), *Total Intravenous Anesthesia and Target Controlled Infusions*,
DOI 10.1007/978-3-319-47609-4_25

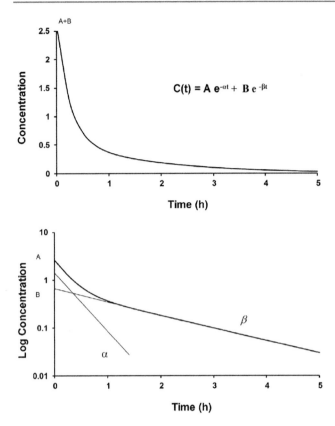

Fig. 25.1 A time–concentration profile of a two-compartment model (*upper panel*). This profile is shown in a semilogarithmic graph on the *lower panel*. The initial rapid decrease in serum concentration reflects distribution and elimination followed by a slower decrease due to elimination. Subtraction of the initial decrease in concentration due to elimination using the concentrations from the elimination line extrapolated back to time 0 at B produces the lower line with a steep slope = α (distribution rate constant)/2.303. The terminal elimination phase has a slope = β (elimination rate constant)/2.303

where concentration is C, t is time after the dose, A is the concentration at time 0 for the distribution rate represented by the broken line graph with the steepest slope, α is the rate constant for distribution, B is the concentration at time 0 for the terminal elimination rate, and β is the rate constant for terminal elimination. Rate constants indicate the rate of change in concentration and correspond to the slope of the line divided by 2.303 ($\log_e 10$) for logarithm concentration versus time.

Such two-compartment or biphasic kinetics are frequently observed after IV administration of drugs that rapidly distribute out of the central compartment (V_1) to a peripheral compartment (V_2) [10, 11]. In such situations, the initial rapid decrease in concentration is referred to as the α distribution phase and represents distribution to the peripheral (tissue) compartments in addition to drug elimination. The terminal (β) phase begins after the inflection point in the line when elimination starts to account for most of the change in drug concentration. To determine the

initial change in concentration due to distribution, the change in concentration due to elimination must be subtracted from the total change in concentration. The slope of the line representing the difference between these two rates is the rate constant for distribution.

These parameters (A, B, α, β) have little connection with the underlying physiology, and an alternative parameterisation is to use a central volume and three rate constants (k_{10}, k_{12}, k_{21}) that describe drug distribution between compartments. Another common method is to use two volumes (central, V_1; peripheral, V_2) and two clearances (CL, Q). Q is the inter-compartment clearance, and the volume of distribution at steady state (V_{ss}) is the sum of V_1 and V_2 (Fig. 25.2). Computers have made nonlinear regression techniques to directly estimate parameters easier through iterative techniques using least squares curve fitting. Models with two or more compartments are now commonly solved using differential equations rather than graphical techniques, e.g. for a two-compartment mammillary model comprising a central compartment with volume V_1 and concentration C_1 and a peripheral compartment (V_2, C_2) with drug input (ratein)

$$\frac{dC1}{dt} = \frac{(\text{ratein} + C2 \times Q) - C1 \times (Q + CL)}{V1} \quad (25.2)$$

$$\frac{dC2}{dt} = \frac{Q \times (C1 - C2)}{V2}. \quad (25.3)$$

A series of similar differential equations can be written and solved for models with more than two compartments.

Paediatric PK Parameter Sets

Most TCI techniques use propofol and remifentanil as the principle drugs for induction and maintenance of anaesthesia. Popular paediatric programmes used for propofol infusion targeting a plasma concentration are based on data from Marsh et al. [12] and Gepts et al. [13] (Diprifusor) and Kataria et al. [8] or Absalom et al. [14] (Paedfusor). Concentration can be predicted based on the reported parameters. These parameter sets are commonly termed 'models' and named after the author who reported them (e.g. 'Kataria model'). Parameter estimates (e.g. CL, Q, V_1 and V_2) are different for each parameter set (Table 25.1). Covariate influences that contribute variability such as severity of illness are often unaccounted for; the volume in the central compartment, for example, is increased in children after cardiac surgery [15]. Even weight or age, the commonest sources of variability [16], may be omitted from parameter estimates. Both the administration method

Fig. 25.2 A two-compartment model with an additional compartment used to describe concentration in the effect compartment. The effect compartment concentration is not the same as the blood or serum concentration and is not a real measurable concentration. It has negligible volume and contains negligible blood. A single first-order parameter (Keo) describes the equilibration rate between the central and effect compartments (see text for explanation)

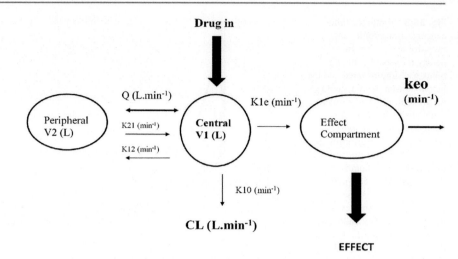

Table 25.1 Propofol parameter estimates for a 20 kg child

Parameter	Kataria [8]	Marsh [12, 13]	Paedfusor [14]	Short [284]	Schuttler [55]	Rigby-Jones [15]	Murat [285]	Saint-Maurice [286]	Coppens [287]
V_1 (L)	10.4	4.56	9.16	8.64	7.68	11.68	20.6	14.44	3.48
V_2 (L)	20.2	9.28	18.98	10.8	20.74	26.68	19.4	35.6	4.68
V_3 (L)	164	58.04	116.58	69.4	264.82	223.86	121.74	168	19.02
CL1 (L/min)	0.68	0.542	0.568	0.836	0.56	0.444	0.98	0.62	0.78
CL2 (L/min)	1.16	0.51	1.044	1.22	1.036	0.32	1.34	1.24	2.04
CL3 (L/min)	0.52	0.192	0.384	0.34	0.46	0.268	0.4	0.22	0.66

Performance of these models differed markedly during the different stages of propofol administration. Most models underestimated propofol concentration 1 min after the bolus dose, suggesting an overestimation of the initial volume of distribution. Not all models tested were within the accepted limits of performance (MDPE < 20 % and MDAPE < 30 %). The model derived by Short and colleagues performed best [18] in children 3–26 months. From Anderson BJ. Pharmacology of paediatric TIVA Rev Colomb Anestesiol 2013;41:205–14, with kind permission from the Colombian Society of Anesthesiology and Resuscitation. (Published with permission of the publisher. Original source: Anderson BJ. La farmacología de la anestesia total intravenosa en pediatría. Rev Colomb Anestesiol. 2013;41(3):205–214. Copyright © 2013 Sociedad Colombiana de Anestesiología y Reanimación. Publicado por Elsevier España, S. L. Todos los derechos reservados [730])

(intravenous bolus or infusion) [17] and the collection of venous blood for assay rather than arterial blood will have influence on PK parameter estimates in the early phase when movement of drug into the effect compartment is occurring. Time–concentration profiles (Fig. 25.3) and context-sensitive half-lives will differ depending on which parameter set is used [18].

Validation studies for these differing parameter sets are few. The Paedfusor has been examined [14] and reported to have a MDPE (median performance error, bias) of 4.1 % and a MDAPE (median absolute performance error, precision) of 9.7 % over the age range investigated (1–15 years). A later study suggested that all except Marsh performed acceptably in children 3–26 months [18]. Others have described a poor fit for Kataria, the most widely used model [19]. However, clearance (L h^{-1} kg^{-1}) decreases with age, and MPE is minimised at low CL and exaggerated at higher values. Evaluating models outside of the age range that they were determined from will increase bias and worsen precision.

Adult remifentanil PK parameters [20] continue to be used in TCI devices for all ages, despite an increasing knowledge about this drug in children [21]. There is an element of safety with this approach because both volume of distribution [22] and clearance (expressed as mL min^{-1} kg^{-1}) [23] decrease with age from adulthood and because the elimination half-life is small with a constant context-sensitive half-life. The larger volume of distribution results in lower peak concentrations after bolus; the higher clearance in children results in lower plasma concentration when infused at adult rates expressed as mg min^{-1} kg^{-1}. However, remifentanil PK can be described in all age groups by simple application of an allometric size model (see below) [23]. This standardised clearance of 2790 mL/min/70 kg^{-1} is similar to that reported by others in children [22, 24] and adults [20, 25]. The smaller the child, the greater the clearance when expressed as mL/min/kg. Owing to these enhanced clearance rates, smaller (younger) children will require higher remifentanil infusion rates than larger (older) children and adults to achieve equivalent blood concentrations.

Fig. 25.3 Simulated time–concentration profiles for propofol using differing parameter sets. A 3 mg kg^{-1} bolus was administered and the infusions were administered as for an adult (10-8-6 regimen) (Published with permission of the publisher. Original source: Anderson BJ. La farmacología de la anestesia total intravenosa en pediatría. Rev Colomb Anestesiol. 2013;41(3):205–214. Copyright © 2013 Sociedad Colombiana de Anestesiología y Reanimación. Publicado por Elsevier España, S.L. Todos los derechos reservados [730])

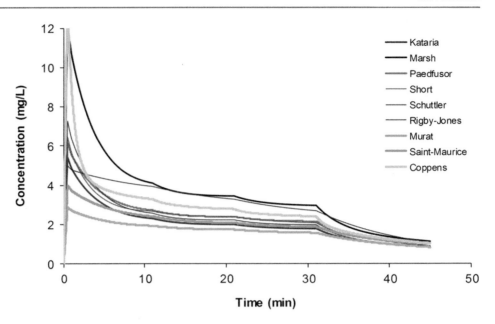

Half-Life

Half-life, the time for a drug concentration to decrease by one half, is a familiar parameter used to describe the kinetics of many drugs that demonstrate exponential decay. Half-life ($T_{1/2}$) helps describe this first-order kinetic process, because the same proportion or fraction of the drug is removed during equal periods of time.

$$T_{\frac{1}{2}} = LN(2)/k \qquad (25.4)$$

However, half-life is a poor parameter for a drug described using two compartments and may be poorly estimated in drugs with slow absorption after enteral dosing. Half-life does not predict dosing schedule, that is, predicted by effect duration [26]. Half-life is confounded by both clearance and volume; if the two are changing independently with age, the half-life may be the same in neonates as in adults even though clearance is immature in neonates.

A more useful concept for IV drugs used in anaesthesia is that of the context-sensitive half-time (CSHT) where 'context' refers to infusion duration. This is the time required for the plasma drug concentration to decline by 50 % after terminating infusion [27]. The CSHT is the same as the elimination half-life for a one-compartment model and does not change with infusion duration.

Context-sensitive half-time may be independent of infusion duration (e.g. remifentanil 2.5 min), moderately affected (propofol 12 min at 1 h, 38 min at 8 h in adults), or display marked prolongation (e.g. fentanyl 1 h at 24 min, 8 h at 280 min). This is due to return of drug to central from peripheral compartments after ceasing infusion. Peripheral compartment sizes and clearances differ in children from adults, and at termination of infusion more or less drug may remain in the

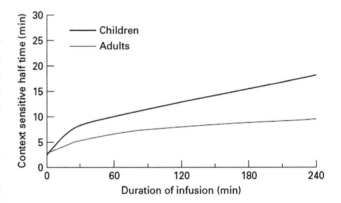

Fig. 25.4 The context-sensitive half-time for children and adults. From McFarlane CS, Anderson BJ, Short TG (Reproduced from: The use of propofol infusions in paediatric anaesthesia: a practical guide. Pediatr Anesth Paediatr Anaesth 1999; 9: 209–216 [7], with kind permission from John Wiley and Sons)

body for any given plasma concentration than in adults. The context-sensitive half-time for children given propofol, for example, is longer (Fig. 25.4) [7]. The context-sensitive half-time gives insight into the pharmacokinetics of a drug, but the parameter may not be clinically relevant; the percentage decrease in concentration required for recovery of drug effect is not necessarily 50 % (Fig. 25.5).

Zero-Order Kinetics

The elimination of some drugs occurs with loss of a constant amount per time, rather than a constant fraction per time. Such rates are termed zero order and because $e^0 = 1$. Zero-order (also known as Michaelis–Menten) kinetics may be designated saturation kinetics, because such processes

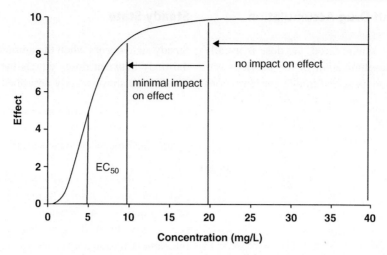

Fig. 25.5 The effect observed when the concentration decreases by 50 % depends on the shape of the concentration–response curve and where the initial concentration sits on that curve. In the example shown decreasing concentration from 40 mg L^{-1} to 20 mg L^{-1} will result in no effect change, while decreasing from 20 mg L^{-1} to 10 mg L^{-1} will have a minimal change. Impact will certainly be relevant when the concentration changes are around the EC$_{50}$. This scenario is commonly seen when a large dose of a neuromuscular blocking drug is administered. Dose determines duration of action (Reproduced from Anderson BJ, Holford NH. Tips and traps analyzing pediatric PK data. Pediatr Anesth 2011; 21: 222–37, with kind permission from John Wiley and Sons [26])

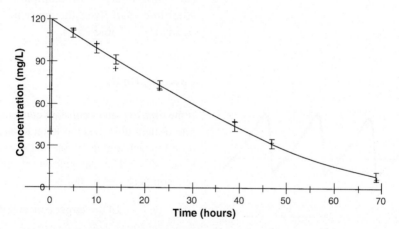

Fig. 25.6 Theophylline elimination in an infant given theophylline 80 mg/kg. Michaelis–Menten kinetics are exemplified by the straight line of the slope of elimination at concentrations above 35 mg/L (Reproduced from Anderson BJ, Holford NH, Woollard GA. Aspects of theophylline clearance in children. *Anaesth and Intensive Care* 1997; 25: 497–501, with the kind permission of the Australian Society of Anaesthetists [151])

occur when excess amounts of drug saturate the capacity of metabolic enzymes or transport systems. Ethyl alcohol is a classic example. In this situation, only a constant amount of drug is metabolised or transported per unit of time. If kinetics are zero order, a graph of serum concentration versus time is linear on linear–linear axes and is curved when graphed on linear–logarithmic (i.e. semilogarithmic) axes. Clearance is determined by the maximum rate of metabolism (V_{max}), the Michaelis–Menten constant (K_m) and the concentration (C):

$$CL = {V_{max}}/{K_m + C} \qquad (25.5)$$

Clinically, first-order elimination may become zero order after administration of excessive doses or prolonged infusions. Certain drugs administered to neonates (with immature clearance pathways) exhibit zero-order kinetics at therapeutic doses and may accumulate to excessive concentrations, including thiopentone, theophylline (Fig. 25.6), caffeine, diazepam, furosemide and phenytoin. Elimination may also be termed 'mixed order' (i.e. first order at low concentrations and zero order after enzymes are saturated at higher concentrations). For these drugs, a small increment in dose may cause disproportionately large increments in serum concentrations.

Repetitive Dosing and Drug Accumulation

When multiple doses are administered, the dose is usually repeated before complete elimination of the previous one (Fig. 25.7). In this situation, peak and trough concentrations increase until a steady-state concentration (C_{ss}) is reached. The average C_{ss} can be calculated as follows:

$$\text{Average } C_{ss} = \frac{1}{\text{CL}} \times \frac{f \times D}{\tau}$$
$$= \frac{1}{k \times V} \times \frac{f \times D}{\tau} \quad (25.6)$$

$$= \frac{1.44 \times T_{1/2}}{V} \times \frac{f \times D}{\tau} \quad (25.7)$$

In Eqs. (25.6) and (25.7), f is the fraction of the dose that is absorbed, D is the dose, τ is the dosing interval in the same units of time as the elimination half-life, k is the elimination rate constant, and 1.44 equals 1/Ln(2). The magnitude of the average C_{ss} is directly proportional to a ratio of $T_{1/2}/\tau$ and D.

Steady State

Steady state occurs when the amount of drug removed from the body between doses equals the rate of administration. This can be simplistically described as:

$$\text{rate in} = \text{rate out} \quad (25.8)$$

$$\text{amount/time} = \text{clearance} \times \text{targetconcentration} \quad (25.9)$$

Five half-lives are usually required for drug elimination and distribution among tissue and fluid compartments to reach equilibrium. When all tissues are at equilibrium (i.e. steady state), the peak and trough concentrations are the same after each dose. However, before this time, constant peak and trough concentrations after intermittent doses, or constant concentrations during drug infusions, do not prove that a steady state has been achieved because the drug may still be entering and leaving deep tissue compartments. During continuous infusion, the fraction of steady-state concentration that has been reached can be calculated in terms of multiples of the drug's half-life. After three half-lives, the concentration is 88 % of that at steady state (Table 25.2).

Loading Dose

If the time to reach a constant concentration by continuous or intermittent dosing is too long, a loading dose (LD) may be used to reach a greater constant concentration more quickly (Fig. 25.7). The calculation of the loading dose for a one-compartment model is:

$$\text{LD} = \text{target concentration} \times V$$

This is the principle underlying anaesthesia induction with propofol. Loading doses must be used cautiously, because they increase the likelihood of drug toxicity (e.g. hypotension with propofol).

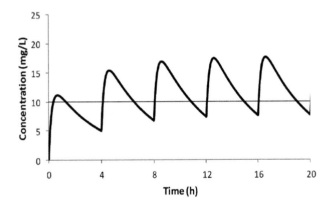

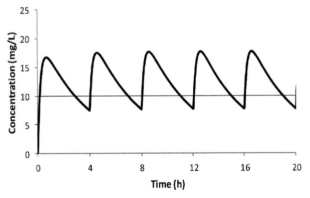

Fig. 25.7 Time–concentration profile for acetaminophen in a child given 250 mg 4 hourly (*upper panel*). The average C_{ss} of 10 mg/L is reached after three doses. The use of a loading dose rapidly achieves the target concentration (*lower panel*)

Table 25.2 Exponential decay and half-life

Half-lives elapsed	Fraction remaining	Percentage remaining	Percentage gone
0	1	100	0
1	1/2	50	50
2	1/4	25	75
3	1/8	12.5	87.5
4	1/16	6.25	93.75
5	1/32	3.125	96.875
6	1/64	1.156	98.844
n	$1/2^n$	$100/2^n$	$100 - 100/2^n$

Dose calculations using a one-compartment model are not applicable to those drugs that are characterised using multi-compartment models. The use of V_1 results in a loading dose too high, while the use of V_{ss} results in a loading dose too low. Too high a dose may cause transient toxicity, although slowing the rate of administration may prevent excessive concentrations during the distributive phase.

The time to peak effect (T_{peak}) is dependent on clearance and effect site equilibration half-time ($T_{1/2}\,k_{eo}$). At a submaximal dose, T_{peak} is independent of dose. At supramaximal doses, maximal effect will occur earlier than T_{peak} and persist for longer duration because of the shape of the sigmoid E_{max} response model. This is due to similar considerations described in time course of immediate effects. The T_{peak} concept has been used to calculate optimal initial bolus doses [28], because V_1 and V_{ss} poorly reflect the required scaling factor. A new parameter, the volume of distribution at the time of peak effect site concentration (V_{pe}), is used and is calculated.

$$V_{pe} = \frac{V_1}{\left(C_{peak}/C_0 \right)} \qquad (25.10)$$

C_0 is the theoretical plasma concentration at $t = 0$ after the bolus dose, and C_{peak} is the predicted effect site concentration at the time of peak effect site concentration. Loading dose can then be calculated as

$$LD = C_{peak} \times V_{pe} \qquad (25.11)$$

Population Modelling

The parameter estimates from the mathematical models used to analyse the data can be used to predict the time–concentration profiles of other doses. Attempts to predict what will happen in a further subject often become unstuck because a factor accounting for variability between subjects is missing. If the variability between patients is modelled, then it is possible to predict the magnitude of the difference between predictions and the observations in the next subject. There are three common approaches to modelling data collected from a group of subjects.

Naïve Pooled Data Approach
Time–concentration data are pooled together as if all doses and all observations pertain to a single subject. Samples are taken at the same time in each individual. No information is available on individual subject profiles or parameters. This approach may be satisfactory if data are extensive for each

subject and there is only minor between-subject variability, but may result in misrepresentation if data are few. Problems also arise interpreting results when data are missing from some subjects. No information can be gathered about the magnitude of between-subject variability and its causes.

Standard Two-Stage Approach
Individual profiles are analysed, and the individual structural parameters (e.g. V, CL) are then treated as variables and combined to achieve summary measures. Sampling times have greater flexibility but must be complete for each individual. If the estimates are not based on a similar number of measurements for each individual, or if the response in one individual is much more variable than another, some form of weighting is required. The between-subject variability can be estimated from the standard deviation of the individual estimates, but it is an overestimate of the true variability because each estimate also has variability due to imprecision of the estimate. It may be possible to identify covariates to explain some of the variability, but this does depend on having relatively good individual estimates of the parameters.

'True' Population Modelling
Population modelling using mixed-effects models [29, 30] has improved analysis and interpretation of PKPD data. Paediatric anaesthesiologists have embraced the population approach for investigating PK and PD. This approach provides a means to study variability in drug responses among individuals representative of those in whom the drug will be used clinically. Traditional approaches to interpretation of time–concentration profiles relied on 'rich' data from a small group of subjects. In contrast, mixed-effects models can be used to analyse 'sparse' (two to three samples) data from a large number of subjects. Sampling times are not crucial for population methods and can be fitted around clinical procedures or outpatient appointments. Sampling time bands rather than exact times are equally effective [31] and allow flexibility in children. Interpretation of truncated individual sets of data or missing data is also possible with this type of analysis, rendering it useful for paediatric studies. Population modelling also allows pooling of data across studies to provide a single robust PK analysis rather than comparing separate smaller studies that are complicated by different methods and analyses.

Mixed-effects models are 'mixed' because they describe the data using a mixture of fixed and random effects. Fixed effects predict the average influence of a covariate such as weight as an explanation of part of the between-subject variability in a parameter like clearance. Random effects describe the remaining variability between subjects that is not predictable from the fixed effect average. Explanatory covariates (e.g. age, size, renal function, sex, temperature) can be introduced that explain the predictable part of the between-individual variability. Nonlinear regression is performed by an iterative process to find the curve of best fit [32, 33].

Why Adult PK Parameters Do Not Work in Children

The use of adult parameter sets in TCI pumps for children results in concentrations lower than those observed in adults. A simple manual regimen for propofol infusion in adults [34] is of a bolus of 1 mg kg^{-1} followed by an infusion of 10 mg kg^{-1} h^{-1} (0–10 min), 8 mg kg^{-1} h^{-1} (10–20 min) and 6 mg kg^{-1} h^{-1} thereafter. Requirements for children, however, are greater. A loading dose of 3 mg kg^{-1} followed by an infusion rate of 15 mg kg^{-1} h^{-1} for the first 15 min, mg kg^{-1} h^{-1} from 15 to 30 min, 11 mg kg^{-1} h^{-1} from 30 to 60 min, 10 mg kg^{-1} h^{-1} from 1 to 2 h and 9 mg kg^{-1} h^{-1} from 2 to 4 h resulted in a steady-state target concentration of 3 mg L^{-1} in children 3–11 years [7]. Figure 25.3 shows that the adult 'Marsh model' predicts concentrations greater than all the paediatric model predictions, except that by Rigby-Jones et al. [15], unsurprising since the latter were derived from critically ill neonates! Increased requirements in children can be attributed to size factors. Decreased requirements in neonates are with consequent reduced clearance due to immature enzyme clearance systems. Organ dysfunction will also result in reduced requirements.

Major Paediatric PK Covariates

Growth and development are two major aspects of children not readily apparent in adults. How these factors interact is not necessarily easy to determine from observations because they are quite highly correlated. Drug elimination clearance, for example, may increase with weight, height, age, body surface area and creatinine clearance. One approach is to standardise for size before incorporating a factor for maturation [35].

Size

Clearance in children 1–2 years of age, expressed as L/h/kg, is commonly greater than that observed in older children and adolescents. This is a size effect and is not due to bigger livers or increased hepatic blood flow in that subpopulation. This 'artefact of size' disappears when allometric scaling is used to replot the same data. Allometry is a term used to describe the nonlinear relationship between size and function. This nonlinear relationship is expressed as

$$y = a \times \text{BodyMass}^{\text{PWR}} \quad (25.12)$$

where y is the variable of interest (e.g. basal metabolic rate), a is the allometric coefficient and PWR is the allometric exponent. The value of PWR has been the subject of much debate. Basal metabolic rate (BMR) is the commonest variable investigated, and camps advocating for a PWR value of 2/3 (i.e. body surface area) are at odds with those advocating a value of 3/4.

Support for a value of 3/4 comes from investigations that show the log of basal metabolic rate (BMR) plotted against the log of body weight produces a straight line with a slope of 3/4 in all species studied, including humans. Fractal geometry is used to mathematically explain this phenomenon. The 3/4 power law for metabolic rates was derived from a general model that describes how essential materials are transported through space-filled fractal networks of branching tubes [36]. A great many physiological, structural, and time-related variables scale predictably within and between species with weight (W) exponents (PWR) of 3/4, 1 and 1/4, respectively [37].

These exponents have applicability to pharmacokinetic parameters such as clearance (CL exponent of 3/4), volume (V exponent of 1), and half-time ($T_{1/2}$ exponent of 1/4) [37]. The factor for size (F_{size}) for total drug clearance may be expressed as

$$F_{\text{size}} = (W/70)^{3/4} \quad (25.13)$$

Clearance is a metabolic function, and while the process for drug clearance may differ between animals, the clearance of tramadol plotted against the log of body weight produces a straight line with a slope of 3/4 in all species studied (Fig. 25.8) [38].

Maintenance dose is determined by clearance. The difference in drug clearance between an adult and a child is predictable from weight using theory-based allometry:

$$\text{CL}_{\text{CHILD}} = \text{CL}_{\text{ADULT}} \times \left(\frac{\text{weight}_{\text{CHILD}}}{\text{weight}_{\text{ADULT}}} \right)^{3/4} \quad (25.14)$$

Allometric theory predicts maintenance dose per kg is higher in children. For example, remifentanil clearance is increased in neonates, infants and children when expressed as per kilogram [22]. However, remifentanil clearance in children 1 month–9 years is similar to adult rates when scaled using an allometric exponent of 3/4 [23]. Nonspecific blood esterases that metabolise remifentanil are mature at birth [39], and that is when clearance (L/h/kg) is highest.

Fig. 25.8 Weight-predicted tramadol total clearance (CLP total) compared to human allometric prediction using a 3/4 power exponent (*solid line*) (Reproduced From Holford S, Allgaert K, Anderson BJ, Kukanich B, Sousa AB, Steinman A, Pypendop BH, Mehvar M, Giorgi M, Holford NH. Parent-metabolite pharmacokinetic models for tramadol—tests of assumptions and predictions. J Pharmacol Clin Toxicol 2014;2(1):1023 [38], under a Creative Commons Attribution Licence. https://www. jscimedcentral.com/ Pharmacology/pharmacology-spidpharmacokinetics-1023.pdf)

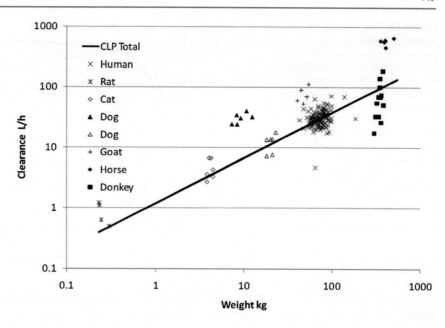

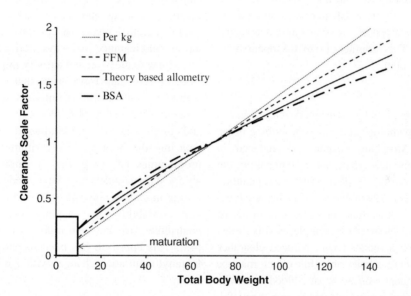

Fig. 25.9 Body size metrics used to describe clearance changes with weight for individuals of average height for weight. The clearance scale factor shows how clearance would differ with weight. A nonlinear relationship exists between weight and clearance using theory-based allometry. The per kg method increasingly overestimates clearance in adults and underestimates clearance in children. The BSA method overestimates clearance in children compared to theory-based allometry. Scaling with fat-free mass (FFM) lies between the per kg method and theory-based allometry. An additional function is required to describe maturation (Reproduced from Anderson BJ, Holford NH. Understanding dosing: children are small adults, neonates are immature children. Arch Dis Child 2013; 98: 737–44 [2] with kind permission of the BMJ Publishing Group)

Maturation

Unlike remifentanil clearance, allometry alone is insufficient to predict clearance in neonates and infants from adult estimates for most drugs (Fig. 25.9) [40, 41]. The addition of a model describing maturation is required. The sigmoid hyperbolic or Hill model [42] has been found useful for describing this maturation factor (MF).

$$MF = \frac{PMA^{Hill}}{TM_{50}^{Hill} + PMA^{Hill}} \qquad (25.15)$$

The TM_{50} describes the maturation half-time, while the Hill coefficient relates to the slope of this maturation profile. Maturation of clearance begins before birth, suggesting that postmenstrual age (PMA) would be a better predictor

Fig. 25.10 The clearance maturation profile of dexmedetomidine expressed using the per kilogram model and the allometric 3/4 power model. This maturation pattern is typical of many drugs cleared by the liver or kidneys (Data adapted from Potts AL, Anderson BJ, Warman GR, Lerman J, Diaz SM, Vilo S. Dexmedetomidine pharmacokinetics in pediatric intensive care—a pooled analysis. Pediatr Anesth 2009;19:1119–29 [624], with kind permission from John Wiley and Sons)

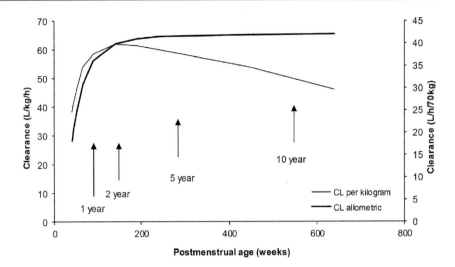

of drug elimination than postnatal age (PNA) [37]. Figure 25.10 shows the maturation profile for dexmedetomidine expressed as both the standard per kilogram model and using allometry. Clearance is immature in infancy. Clearance is greatest at 2 years of age, decreasing subsequently with age. This 'artefact of size' disappears with use of the allometric model.

Organ Function

Changes associated with normal growth and development can be distinguished from pathological changes describing organ function (OF) [35]. Morphine clearance is reduced in neonates because of immature glucuronide conjugation, but clearance was lower in critically ill neonates than healthier cohorts [43–45], possibly attributable to reduced hepatic function. The impact of organ function alteration may be concealed by another covariate. For example, positive pressure ventilation may be associated with reduced clearance rather than intensive care admission. This effect may be attributable to a consequent reduced hepatic blood flow with a drug that has perfusion-limited clearance (e.g. propofol, morphine).

Pharmacokinetic parameters (P) can be described in an individual as the product of size (F_{size}), maturation (MF) and organ function (OF) influences, where P_{std} is the value in a standard size adult without pathological changes in organ function [35]:

$$P = P_{std} \times F_{size} \times MF \times OF. \quad (25.16)$$

This methodology is increasingly used to describe clearance changes with age [46]. An understanding of these principles can be used to predict dose in children using target concentration methodology [2].

When maturation changes have not been described using real data, then an alternative method known as physiological-based pharmacokinetic (PBPK) models can be used to predict changes with age. Organ maturation, body composition and ontogeny of drug elimination pathways have marked effects on pharmacokinetic parameters in the first few years of life. PBPK models require detailed physiological data. Data on ontogeny of individual clearance pathways, derived from measurements of enzyme expression and activity in postmortem livers and from in vivo data from drugs that are cleared by similar pathways, are useful. Continued input of information concerning genetic, physiological, organ and tissue size and composition, protein binding, demographic and clinical data into the library and algorithms for PBPK modelling programmes has progressively improved their prediction ability. These models have been used to assist with first-time dosing in children [40, 41, 47]. The introduction of population variability in enzyme abundance and activity contributes to between-individual variability estimates [48]. This approach has been recently used to investigate fentanyl maturation changes with age in neonates [49].

Dosing in Obese Children

Volume (determining loading dose) and clearance (determining maintenance dose) of some drugs are known to be changed in obesity [50]. Although body fat has minimal metabolic activity, fat mass contributes to overall body size and may have an indirect influence on both metabolic and renal clearance. On the other hand, the volume of distribution of a drug depends on its physicochemical properties [51]. There are drugs whose apparent volume of distribution may be independent of fat mass (e.g. digoxin) or be extensively determined by it (e.g. diazepam). A number of size descriptors (Fig. 25.9) have been put forward for use in the obese patient, e.g. total body weight (TBW), lean body weight (LBW), ideal body weight (IBW), body mass index (BMI), fat-free mass (FFM) and normal fat mass (NFM).

These size descriptors invariably demonstrate nonlinear relationships between weight and clearance. The best size descriptor accounting for obesity remains unknown [52]. LBW is often advocated for use in obese, but that descriptor may not apply for all drugs. An infusion of propofol is commonly used for paediatric anaesthesia. Infusion rate is dependent on clearance, and an incorrect estimate of clearance may lead to inadequate anaesthesia and awareness. Propofol clearance in obese children [53] and adults [54] and nonobese adults and children [55, 56] is best predicted using TBW as the size descriptor with theory-based allometry.

However, TBW may be inappropriate for remifentanil where lean body weight appears to be a better size descriptor [57]. The use of normal fat mass (NFM) [58] with allometric scaling as a size descriptor may prove versatile [59–62]. That size descriptor uses the idea of fat-free mass (similar to LBW but excludes lipids in cell membranes, CNS and bone marrow) plus a 'bit more'. The 'bit more' will differ for each drug, and the maximum 'bit more' added to fat-free mass would equal TBW.

$$\text{FFM} = \text{WHS}_{max} \times \text{HT}^2 \times \left[\text{TBW} \Big/ \left(\text{WHS}_{50} \times \text{HT}^2 + \text{TBW}\right) \right] \quad (25.17)$$

where WHS_{max} is the maximum FFM for any given height (HT, m) and WHS_{50} is the TBW value when FFM is half of WHS_{max}. For men, WHS_{max} is 42.92 kg m^{-2} and WHS_{50} is 30.93 kg m^{-2}, and for women WHS_{max} is 37.99 kg m^{-2} and WHS_{50} is 35.98 kg m^{-2} [63].

$$\text{NFM} = \text{FFM} + F_{fat} \times (\text{TBW} - \text{FFM}) \quad (25.18)$$

The parameter F_{fat} is estimated and accounts for different contributions of fat mass. If F_{fat} is estimated to be zero, then FFM alone predicts size, while if F_{fat} is 1, then size is predicted by TBW. This parameter is drug specific and also specific to the PK parameter such as clearance or volume of distribution. It has a value of 0.211 for GFR which implies that 21 % of fat mass is a size driver for kidney function in addition to FFM [59]. Size based on NFM assumes that FFM is the primary determinant of size with an extra F_{fat} factor (which may be positive or negative) that determines how fat mass contributes to size. A negative value for F_{fat} might suggest organ dysfunction, not an uncommon scenario in the morbidly obese.

Pharmacodynamic Models

Pharmacokinetics is what the body does to the drug, while pharmacodynamics is what the drug does to the body. The precise boundary between these two processes is ill defined and often requires a link describing movement of drug from the plasma to the effect site and its target. Drugs may exert effect at nonspecific membrane sites, by interference with transport mechanisms, by enzyme inhibition or induction or by activation or inhibition of receptors.

Minimal Effective Concentration

The minimal effective analgesic concentration can sometimes be determined by titration of an analgesic to achieve satisfactory pain at rest or with stimulus. Blood assay for analgesic drug concentration at these times can be used to determine an effective concentration. Reassessment when pain recurs or after further analgesic administration improves accuracy of assessment. This technique has been used with to determine the minimal effective analgesic concentration for oxycodone [64].

Sigmoid E_{max} Model

A better understanding of drug effect is achieved if response over a broad concentration range is explored. The relation between drug concentration and effect may be described by the Hill equation (for sigmoid E_{max} model, see maturation model above) [42].

$$\text{Effect} = E_0 + \frac{(E_{max} \times \text{Ce}^N)}{\left(\text{EC}_{50}^N + \text{Ce}^N\right)} \quad (25.19)$$

where E_0 is the baseline response, E_{max} is the maximum effect change, Ce is the concentration in the effect compartment, EC_{50} is the concentration producing 50 % E_{max} and N is the Hill coefficient defining the steepness of the concentration–response curve (Fig. 25.11). Efficacy is the maximum response on a dose or concentration–response curve. EC_{50} can be considered a measure of potency relative to another drug provided N and E_{max} for the two drugs are the same. This model has been used to describe propofol [53, 65] and remifentanil [66] effect in children.

Quantal Effect Model

The potency of anaesthetic vapours may be expressed by minimal alveolar concentration (MAC), and this is the concentration at which 50 % of subjects move in response to a standard surgical stimulus. MAC appears at first sight to be similar to EC_{50} but is an expression of quantal response rather than magnitude of effect. There are two methods of estimating MAC. Responses can be recorded over the clinical dose range in a large number of subjects and logistic regression applied to estimate the relationship between dose and quantal effect; the

Fig. 25.11 The sigmoid E_{max} model is commonly used to describe the relationship between drug response and concentration. Changing the Hill coefficient dramatically alters the shape of the curve

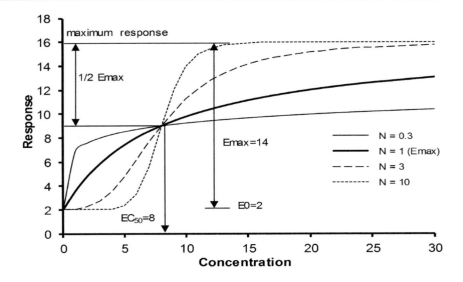

Fig. 25.12 Schematic of the 'up and down' method to estimate MAC. It involves a study of only one concentration in each subject, and, in a sequence of subjects, each receives a concentration depending upon the response of the previous subject

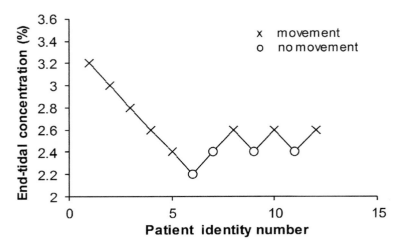

MAC can then be interpolated. Large numbers of subjects may not be available, and so an alternative is often used. The 'up and down' method described by Dixon [67, 68] estimates only the MAC rather than the entire sigmoid curve. It involves a study of only one concentration in each subject, and, in a sequence of subjects, each receives a concentration depending upon the response of the previous subject; the concentration is either increased if the previous subject did not respond or decreased if they did (Fig. 25.12). The MAC is usually calculated either as the mean concentration of equal numbers of responses and no responses or is the mean concentration of pairs of 'response–no response'.

This method has also been used for drugs other than inhalation vapours. In order to determine the dexmedetomidine dose that could be given as a rapid 5 s bolus to healthy children during TIVA without causing significant haemodynamic effects, children were given dexmedetomidine, starting at 0.3 mcg/kg with 0.1 mcg/kg intervals. The dose that had no haemodynamic response in half the subjects was 0.5 mcg/kg [69].

Logistic Regression Model

When the pharmacological effect is difficult to grade, then it may be useful to estimate the probability of achieving the effect as a function of plasma concentration. Effect measures such as movement/no movement or rousable/non-rousable are dichotomous. Logistic regression is commonly used to analyse such data, and the interpolated EC_{50} value refers to the probability of response. For example, an EC_{50} of 0.52 mg/L for arousal after ketamine sedation in children has been estimated using this technique [70].

Linking PK with PD

A simple situation in which drug effect is directly related to concentration does not mean that drug effects parallel the time course of concentration. This occurs only when the concentration is low in relation to EC_{50}. In this situation the half-life of the drug may correlate closely with the half

Fig. 25.13 The counterclockwise hysteresis loop observed after an orally administered drug is shown in the *upper panel*. Effect increases between 2 and 3.5 h even though serum concentration is decreasing. The *lower panel* shows that the time–concentration profile for an effect compartment is delayed compared to that in the serum

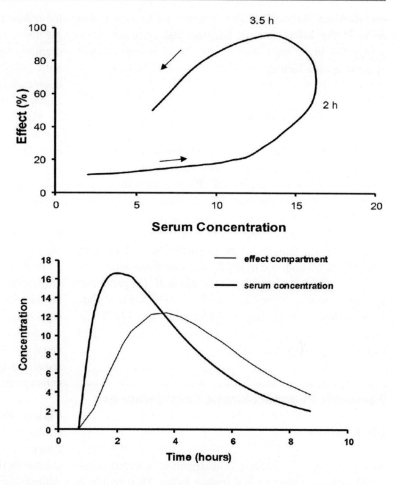

life of drug effect. Observed effects may not be directly related to serum concentration. Many drugs have a short half-life but a long duration of effect. This may be attributable to induced physiological changes (e.g. aspirin and platelet function) or may be due to the shape of the E_{max} model. If the initial concentration is very high in relation to the EC_{50}, then drug concentrations 5 half-lives later, when we might expect minimal concentration, may still exert considerable effect (Fig. 25.5). There may be a delay due to the transfer of the drug to effect site (NMBD), a lag time (diuretics), a physiological response (antipyresis), an active metabolite (propacetamol) or a synthesis of physiological substances (warfarin).

A plasma concentration–effect plot can form a hysteresis loop because of this delay in effect (Fig. 25.13). Hull et al. [71] and Sheiner et al. [72] introduced the effect compartment concept for muscle relaxants. A single first-order parameter ($T_{1/2}k_{eo}$) describes the equilibration half-time (Fig. 25.2).

$$T_{1/2}k_{eo} = \frac{Ln(2)}{k_{eo}} \qquad (25.20)$$

This mathematical trick assumes concentration in the central compartment is the same as that in the effect compartment at

equilibration but that a time delay exists before the drug reaches the effect compartment. The concentration in the effect compartment is used to describe the concentration–effect relationship [73].

Adult $T_{1/2}k_{eo}$ values are well described, e.g. morphine 16 min, fentanyl 5 min, alfentanil 1 min and propofol 3 min. This $T_{1/2}k_{eo}$ parameter is commonly incorporated into target-controlled infusion (TCI) pumps in order to achieve a rapid effect site concentration.

A $T_{1/2}k_{eo}$ for propofol in children determined by simultaneous PK–PD modelling is uncommonly described. An estimate of 1.2 min (95 %CI 0.85–2.1) has been reported in obese children [53]. We might expect a shorter $T_{1/2}k_{eo}$ with decreasing age based on size models [74] Faster half-times in children can be accounted for by considering physiologic time that scales to a power of 1/4 [75].

$$T_{1/2}k_{eo}\text{CHILD} = T_{1/2}k_{eo}\text{ADULT}$$
$$\times \left(\frac{WT}{70}\right)^{1/4} \qquad (25.21)$$

A decreasing $T_{1/2}k_{eo}$ with age (linked to weight) has been described for propofol in children [65]. Similar results have been demonstrated for sevoflurane and BIS [76]. If unrecognised, this will result in excessive dose in a young child if the effect site is targeted and peak effect is anticipated to be later than it actually is because it was determined in a teenager or adult.

What Is a PK–PD Model?

When both PK and PD data are collected simultaneously and parameters for both models are estimated together, then the model is described as 'integrated'. PK estimates should not be used in conjunction with PD estimates taken from a different data set without a few 'fudge factors'. T_{peak} methodology (Eqs. (25.10) and (25.11)) is commonly used to estimate $T_{1/2}k_{eo}$ that then links separate PK and PD data sets. Model dependence of the $T_{1/2}k_{eo}$ was demonstrated by an estimate of 1.7 min with the Kataria et al. [8] parameter set and 0.8 min with the Paedfusor® (Graseby Medical Ltd., Hertfordshire, United Kingdom) parameter set [14]. These estimates are similar to that estimated in obese children using PK–PD modelling [53].

Paediatric Pharmacokinetic Considerations

Distribution

At its simplest, the volume of distribution determines the initial dose of a drug. It is a scaling factor. Distribution is influenced by body composition, protein binding, haemodynamics (e.g. regional blood flow) and membrane permeability.

Body Composition

Total body water and extracellular fluid (ECF) [77] are increased in neonates, and reduction tends to follow postnatal age (PNA). Polar drugs such as the non-depolarising neuromuscular blocking drugs (NMBDs) and aminoglycosides distribute rapidly into the ECF, but enter cells more slowly. The initial dose of such drugs is consequently higher in the neonate compared to the infant, older child or adult.

The percentage of body weight contributed by fat is 3 % in a 1.5 kg premature neonate and 12 % in a term neonate; this proportion doubles by 4–5 months of age. 'Baby fat' is lost when infants start walking and protein mass increases (20 % in a term neonate, 50 % in an adult). These body component changes affect volumes of distribution of drugs. Volume of distribution influences initial dose estimates. Fentanyl has an increased volume of distribution in neonates. The volume of distribution at steady state is 5.9 (SD 1.5) L/kg in a neonate under 1 month of age compared to 1.6 (SD 0.3) L/kg in an adult [78]. This may contribute to

the reduced degree of respiratory depression seen after single doses as high as 10 mcg/kg in older term neonates. The dramatic increase in muscle bulk in children from 3 years until adolescence influences drug dose required for neuromuscular blockade. The ED_{95} of vecuronium, for example, is 47 SD 11 mcg/kg in neonates and infants, 81 SD 12 mcg/kg in children between 3 and 10 years of age and 55 SD 12 mcg/kg in patients aged 13 years or older [79]. Dose is greater than anticipated in neonates who have immaturity of the neuromuscular junction because the ECV is increased, but the duration of neuromuscular blockade is greater in neonates because of immature clearance pathways. The plasma concentration required in neonates to achieve the same level of neuromuscular block as in children or adults is 20–50 % less [80].

Reduction of propofol concentrations after induction is attributable to redistribution rather than rapid clearance because its pharmacokinetics is described using more than one compartment. Neonates have low body fat and muscle content, and so less propofol is apportioned to these tissues. Delayed awakening occurs because CNS concentration remains higher than that observed in older children as a consequence of reduced redistribution.

Plasma Proteins

Albumen and alpha-1 acid glycoprotein (AAG) concentrations (Fig. 25.14) are reduced in neonates but are similar to those in adults by 6 months, although between-patient variability is high (e.g. AAG 0.32–0.92 g/L) [81, 82]. Bupivacaine is bound to AAG. The recommended bolus epidural dose of bupivacaine in neonates is lower than in children (1.5–2 mg/kg vs. 2.5 mg/kg) because a greater proportion will be unbound drug and it is unbound drug that exerts effect. AAG is an acute-phase reactant that increases after surgical stress. This causes an increase in total plasma concentrations for low to intermediate extraction drugs such as bupivacaine [83]. The unbound concentration, however, will not change because clearance of the unbound drug is affected only by the intrinsic metabolising capacity of the liver. Any increase in unbound concentrations observed during long-term epidural is attributable to reduced clearance rather than AAG concentration [84, 85].

Plasma albumin concentrations are lowest in premature infants, and other foetal proteins such as alpha-fetoprotein (synthesised by the embryonic yolk sac, foetal gastrointestinal tract and liver that has 40 % homology with albumin) have reduced affinity for drugs. In addition, increased concentrations of free fatty acids and unconjugated bilirubin compete with acidic drugs for albumin binding sites. Neonates also have a tendency to manifest a metabolic acidosis that alters ionisation and binding properties of plasma proteins. Serum albumin concentrations approximate adult values by 5 months of age, and binding capacity approaches

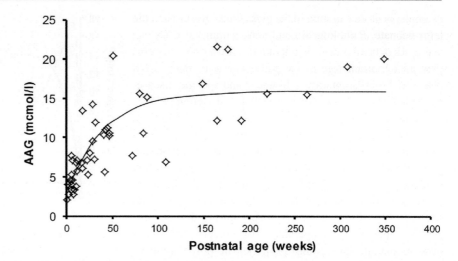

Fig. 25.14 Alpha-1 acid glycoprotein changes with age. Adapted from Booker P. Br J Anaesth 1996;76:365–8

adult values by 1 year of age. The induction dose of thiopentone is lower in neonates than older children. It is possible that this is related to decreased binding of thiopentone to plasma albumin; 13 % of the drug is unbound in newborns compared to 7 % in adults [86].

Regional Blood Flows

The initial phase of distribution after intravenous administration reflects regional blood flow. Consequently, the brain, heart and liver are the tissues first exposed to the drug. Drug is then redistributed to other relatively well-perfused tissues, such as the skeletal muscle. There is a much slower tertiary distribution to relatively underperfused tissues of the body that is noted with long-term drug infusions. These changes contribute to a shorter context-sensitive half-time in infants with quicker 'awakening' after sedative drugs; these infants have less fat and muscle bulk that the drug can redistribute to and later leach out from. Clearance, however, is typically reduced in neonates and contributes to the longer observed context-sensitive half-time.

Apart from the neonatal circulatory changes that occur at birth (e.g. secondary to functional closure of the ductus venosus and ductus arteriosus), there are differences in relative organ mass and regional blood flow change with growth and development during the first few months of life. Blood flow, relative to cardiac output, to the kidney and brain increases, while that to the liver decreases through the neonatal period [87]. Cerebral and hepatic mass as a proportion of body weight are much higher in the infant than in the adult [88].

Mean cerebral blood flow is highest in early childhood (70 mL/min/100 g) at about 3–8 years of age [89]. It is reduced before this age in neonates and later in adults, where flows are similar (50 mL/min/100 g) [90]. The highly lipophilic induction agents diffuse rapidly across the blood–brain barrier to achieve concentration equilibrium with brain tissue. Reduced cardiac output in neonates and reduced cerebral perfusion mean that the onset time after intravenous

induction is slower in neonates that in early childhood. Offset time is also delayed because redistribution to the well-perfused and deep, underperfused tissues is less.

Blood–Brain Barrier (BBB)

The BBB is an elaborate network of complex tight junctions between specialised endothelial cells that restricts the paracellular diffusion of hydrophilic molecules from the blood to the brain substance. Confusion over the importance of this barrier in the neonate exists, partly because of early studies comparing respiratory depression caused by the opioids, morphine and pethidine. Greater respiratory depression was evident in neonates after morphine given as an adult equipotent dose of pethidine [91]. This finding is consistent with pethidine, unlike morphine, being lipid soluble and therefore crossing the immature or mature BBB equally [91]. However, plasma opioid concentrations were not measured in that study, and the increased neonatal respiratory depression observed after morphine when given the same dose (mg/kg) as adults could be due to reduced volume of distribution of morphine in term neonates 1–4 days (1.3 L/kg) compared to those at 8–60 days (1.8 L/kg), 61–180 days (2.4 L/kg) and adults (2.8 L/kg) [43]. Consequently we might expect initial concentrations of morphine to be higher in neonates than in adults and consequent respiratory depression greater. Respiratory depression, as measured by carbon dioxide response curves or by arterial oxygen tension, is similar in children from 2 to 570 days of age at the same morphine concentration [92].

The BBB may have impact in other ways. There are specific transport systems selectively expressed in the barrier endothelial cell membranes that mediate the transport of nutrients into the CNS and of toxic metabolites out of the CNS. Small molecules access foetal and neonatal brains more readily than they do adult brains [93]. BBB function improves gradually throughout foetal brain development, possibly reaching maturity at term [93]. Kernicterus, for example, is more common in the premature neonate than the term neonate. Pathological conditions within the CNS can cause BBB breakdown, or alterations in transport systems play an important role in the pathogenesis of many CNS diseases. Proinflammatory substances and specific disease-associated proteins often mediate BBB dysfunction [94].

Fentanyl is actively transported across the BBB by a saturable ATP-dependent process, while ATP-binding cassette proteins such as P-glycoprotein actively pump out opioids such as fentanyl and morphine [95]. P-glycoprotein modulation significantly influences opioid brain distribution and onset time, magnitude and duration of analgesic response [96]. Modulation may occur during disease processes, increased temperature or other substances (e.g. verapamil, magnesium) [95]. Genetic polymorphisms affecting P-glycoprotein-related genes may explain some individual differences in CNS-active drug sensitivity [97].

Absorption

Absorption characteristics will impact on amount of drug available, maximum concentration, speed of onset of effect, duration of effect and time to offset of effect.

Enteral

The rate at which most drugs are absorbed when given by the oral route is slower in neonates than in older children because gastric emptying is delayed and normal adult rates may not be reached until 6–8 months [98–101]. Slow gastric emptying and reduced clearance may dictate both reduced doses and reduced frequency of administration (Fig. 25.15). This has been demonstrated for both cisapride [102] and acetaminophen [103].

Delayed gastric emptying and reduced clearance may dictate reduced doses and frequency of repeated drug administration. For example, a mean steady-state target paracetamol concentration greater than 10 mg/L at trough can be achieved by an oral dose of 25 mg/kg/day in preterm neonates at 30 weeks, 45 mg/kg/day at 34 weeks and 60 mg/kg/day at 40 weeks PMA [103]. Because gastric emptying is slow in preterm neonates, dosing may only be required twice a day [103].

Enteral administration through the rectum (e.g. thiopentone, methohexitone) takes approximately 8 min in children but is speedier for neonates undergoing cardiac catheter study or radiological sedation [104, 105].

Intramuscular

The intramuscular route is commonly frowned upon in children. It retains high bioavailability, but absorption is delayed compared to the intravenous route. Ketamine however remains popular, and peak concentrations are reached within

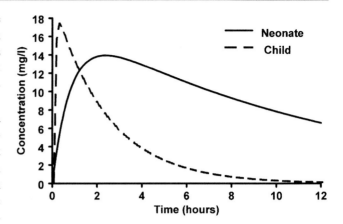

Fig. 25.15 Simulated mean predicted time–concentration profiles for a term neonate, a 1-year-old infant and a 5-year-old child given paracetamol elixir. The time to peak concentration is delayed in neonates due to slow gastric emptying and reduced clearance (Reproduced from Anderson BJ, van Lingen RA, Hansen TG, Lin YC, Holford NH. Acetaminophen developmental pharmacokinetics in premature neonates and infants: a pooled population analysis. Anesthesiology 2002; 96: 1336–45 [103], with kind permission of Wolters Kluwer Health)

10 min after 4 mg/kg [106]. Dexmedetomidine has a similar absorption profile [107, 108].

Nasal

Exploration of alternative delivery routes in young children has centred on the nasal passages [109]. Nasal diamorphine 0.1 mg/kg is used in the UK for forearm fracture pain in the emergency room [110–113]. It is rapidly absorbed as a nasal spray (0.1 mg/kg) in 0.2 mL sterile water, with peak morphine plasma concentrations (T_{peak}) occurring at 10 min [113]. Nasal S-ketamine 2 mg/kg results in peak plasma concentrations of 355 ng/mL within 18 min. Nasal fentanyl (150 mcg/mL) 1.5 mcg/kg given to children (3–17 years) for fracture pain resulted in good analgesia. Peak concentrations were at 13 min [114, 115]. Similar results are reported for nebulised fentanyl (4 mcg/kg) given through a standard nebuliser [116]. Flumazenil concentrations peak within a few minutes after nasal administration [117], while midazolam takes approximately 12 min [118]. Dexmedetomidine is somewhat slower and peak concentrations were not reached until 38 min [119]. Clonidine administered as nasal aerosol (3–8 mcg/kg) was not found to achieve adequate preoperative sedation within 30 min of administration [120], attributable to slow absorption (T_{peak} 1.5–3 h) [121]. There remain concerns that intranasal drugs may pass through the posterior nasopharynx or irritate the vocal cords [122].

Advances in aerosol delivery devices have improved dosing accuracy. Administration of ketorolac 15 mg (weight <50 kg) or 30 mg (weight >50 kg) by the intranasal route resulted in a rapid increase in plasma concentration (time to peak concentration was 52 SD 6 min) and may be a useful therapeutic alternative to IV injection. A target concentration of 0.37 mg/L in the effect compartment was achieved within 30 min and remained above that target for 10 h [123]. The nasal passages change with age, and so it would be unsurprising if absorption by that route did not also change with age.

Cutaneous

The larger relative skin surface area, increased cutaneous perfusion and thinner stratum corneum in neonates [124] increase absorption and exposure of topically applied drugs (corticosteroids, local anaesthetic creams, antiseptics). Neonates have a tendency to form methaemoglobin because they have reduced levels of methaemoglobin reductase and foetal haemoglobin is more readily oxidised compared to adult haemoglobin. This, combined with increased absorption through the neonatal epidermis, resulted in reluctance to use lidocaine–prilocaine cream for repeat use in this age group [125, 126].

Alveolar

Anaesthetic delivery to the alveoli is determined largely by alveolar ventilation and functional residual capacity (FRC). Neonates have increased alveolar ventilation. They also have a smaller FRC compared to adults because of increased chest wall compliance; this causes an increase in the speed of delivery. Pulmonary absorption is generally more rapid in infants and children than in adults [127]. The greater cardiac output and greater fraction of the cardiac output distributed to the vessel-rich tissue group (i.e. a clearance factor) and the lower tissue/blood solubility (i.e. a volume factor) also affect the more rapid wash-in of inhalational anaesthetics in the younger age group [128]. Solubility determines volume of distribution. An inhalational agent with a greater volume of distribution will take longer to reach a steady-state concentration when delivered at a constant rate. The solubility in blood of halothane, isoflurane, enflurane and methoxyflurane is 18 % less in neonates than in adults [129], attributable to altered serum albumin, globulin, cholesterol and triglyceride concentrations. The solubility of these same agents in the vessel-rich tissue group in neonates is approximately one half of those in adults [129]. The latter may be due to the greater water content and decreased protein and lipid concentration in neonatal tissues. Infants, with their decreased solubility would be expected to have a shorter time to reach a predetermined F_E/F_I ratio because of a smaller volume of distribution. Age has little effect on the solubility of the less soluble agents, nitrous oxide and sevoflurane [130].

Induction of anaesthesia may be slowed by right-to-left shunting of blood in neonates suffering cyanotic congenital cardiac disease or intrapulmonary conditions. This slowing is greatest with the least soluble anaesthetics. Left-to-right shunts usually have minimal impact on uptake because

cardiac output is increased so that systemic tissue perfusion is maintained at normal levels. The flow of mixed venous blood returning to the right heart ready for anaesthetic uptake is normal. If cardiac output is not increased, and peripheral perfusion is reduced, then there will be less anaesthetic uptake in the lung. Although alveolar anaesthetic partial pressure may be observed to rise rapidly, there is a slower rise in tissue partial pressure and anaesthetic effect is delayed.

Bioavailability

The oral bioavailability may be affected by interactions with food when feeding is frequent in the neonate (e.g. phenytoin [131]), by the use of adult formulations that are divided or altered for paediatric use (nizatidine [132]) and by lower cytochrome P450 enzyme activity in the intestine. The latter may cause an increased bioavailability of midazolam because CYP3A activity is reduced [133]. The use of adult vials for paediatric use may result in dose inaccuracy, causing a relative increase or decrease in assumed bioavailability [134].

Analgesic medications and delivery systems commonly used in adults may not be possible or practicable in children because they do not have behavioural maturity. Infants are unable to use patient-controlled analgesia devices. Dose accuracy is lost when buccal and sublingual administration is attempted because those routes require prolonged exposure to the mucosal surface. Infants find it difficult to hold drug in their mouth for the requisite retention time (particularly if taste is unfavourable), and this results in more swallowed drug or drug spat out than in adults [135]. If the drug has a high first-pass effect, then the lower relative bioavailability results in lower plasma concentrations. Although many analgesics are available in an oral liquid formulation, taste is a strong determinant of compliance and unpalatable preparations may be refused [136]. Taste preferences change with age.

First-pass effect impacts on bioavailability and contribution of active metabolites to effect. The oral bioavailability of clonidine is low ($F = 0.55$) in children 3–10 years. Consequently, higher oral doses of clonidine (per kg) are required when this formulation is used to achieve concentrations similar to those reported in adults [137]. Oral absorption is slow (absorption half-time 0.45 h) and peak concentrations not reached until 1 h. Similarly, oral ketamine needs to be given in doses of up to 10 mg/kg to achieve therapeutic effect in children 1–8 years suffering burns [138]. Not only was bioavailability reduced ($F = 0.45$) but absorption was also slow; absorption half-time was 59 min and had high between-subject variability in this cohort [138]. Analgesic effect, however, may be contributed by the increased concentration of the active metabolite norketamine.

The frequent passage of stools in the neonate may render suppository use ineffective. Variable absorption and bio-availability have resulted in respiratory arrest when repeat opioids are administered by the rectal route to children [139].

Metabolism and Excretion

Hepatic Metabolism

Hepatic metabolic reactions are categorised as phase I (non-synthetic) or phase II (synthetic). Phase I reactions include oxidation, reduction and hydrolysis, while phase II processes involve conjugation with other molecules, notably glucuronide, glycine and sulphate. These water-soluble metabolites are excreted by the kidneys.

Hepatic drug metabolism activity appears as early as 9–22 weeks' gestation when foetal liver enzyme activity may vary from 2 to 36 % of adult activity [140–142]. These pathways then develop at different rates. Microsomal enzyme activity can be classified into three groups: (1) mature at birth but decreasing with age (e.g. CYP3A7 responsible for methadone clearance in neonates [143]), (2) mature at birth and sustained through to adulthood (e.g. plasma esterases that clear remifentanil [39]) and (3) immature at birth [144].

Medications that are extensively metabolised by the liver or other organs (e.g. the intestines or lungs) are referred to as having high extraction ratios (perfusion-limited clearance, e.g. propranolol, morphine and midazolam). This extensive metabolism produces a first-pass effect in which a large proportion of an enteral dose is inactivated as it passes through the organ before reaching the systemic circulation. Other drugs with low intrinsic clearance (e.g. aspirin, diazepam) are known as having capacity-limited clearance.

Cytochromes P450: Phase I Reactions

Cytochromes P450 are heme-containing proteins that provide most of the phase I drug metabolism for lipophilic compounds in the body. The generally accepted nomenclature of the cytochrome P450 isozymes begins with CYP and groups enzymes with more than 36 % DNA homology into families designated with an Arabic number followed by alphanumeric letters for the subfamily of closely related proteins (>77 % homology) followed by a number for the specific enzyme gene, such as CYP3A4 [145–147]. Isozymes that are important in human drug metabolism are found in the *CYP1*, *CYP2* and *CYP3* gene families. Table 25.3 outlines the P450 isozymes and their common substrates. This table also outlines enzyme activity or enzyme concentration in the liver and changes with age; these are not the same as total clearance, which is determined by enzyme activity, hepatic size and blood flow. Clearance changes with age for many P450 enzyme processes remain poorly described. There are also both genetic and ethnic polymorphisms leading to clinically important differences in the capacity to metabolise drugs, and these differences can make individual drug responses in some cases unpredictable.

Developmental Changes of Specific Cytochromes

Cytochrome P4501A2 (CYP1A2) accounts for much of the metabolism of caffeine [148] and theophylline [149]; methylxanthines are frequently used to treat neonatal apnoea and bradycardia. They are effective because they have prolonged action in neonates. CYP1A2 activity is nearly absent in the foetal liver and remains minimal in the neonate. This limits *N-3-* and *N-7*-demethylation of caffeine in the neonatal period that prolongs elimination in preterm and term neonates. Elimination is through the immature renal system, and consequent clearance is reduced. An adult clearance rate is achieved within the first postnatal year (Table 25.4) [150]. A similar pharmacokinetic pattern of reduced metabolism at birth occurs with theophylline (Table 25.5) in which CYP1A2 catalyses 3-demethylation and 8-hydroxylation [151]. Both drugs illustrate Michaelis–Menten metabolism after overdose in neonates, resulting in prolonged toxic effects [150, 151].

Other P450 enzymes that are reduced or absent in the foetus include CYP2D6 and CYP2C9 [144, 152, 153]. CYP2D6, which is involved in the metabolism of β blockers, antiarrhythmics, antidepressants, antipsychotics, tramadol and codeine, is absent in the foetal liver and is eventually expressed postnatally [154–156]. In contrast to the slow maturation of CYP1A2 and CYP2D6, CYP2C9, which is responsible for the metabolism of non-steroidal anti-inflammatory drugs (NSAIDs), warfarin and phenytoin, has minimal activity antenatally and then develops rapidly postnatally [154, 157].

CYP3A is the most important cytochrome involved in drug metabolism, because of the broad range of drugs that it metabolises and because it comprises the majority of adult human liver cytochrome P450 (see Table 25.3). CYP3A is detectable during embryogenesis as early as 17 weeks, primarily in the form of CYP3A7, and reaches 75 % of adult activity by 30 weeks' gestation [158]. In vivo, CYP3A activity appears to be mature at birth; however, there is a poorly understood postnatal transition from the foetal CYP3A7 to the predominant adult isoform CYP3A4 [159]. This transition from CYP3A7 to 3A4 explains the similar clearance of methadone between neonates and adults (Fig. 25.16) [143]. Bupivacaine is metabolised by CYP3A4. This immature clearance of bupivacaine resulted in high plasma concentrations that caused seizures in

Table 25.3 Developmental patterns and activities for P450 enzymes in the neonate

Enzyme	Substrates	Inducers	Inhibitors	Developmental changes
CYP1A2	Acetaminophen, caffeine, theophylline, warfarin	Cigarette smoke, charcoal-broiled meat, omeprazole, cruciferous vegetables	α-Naphthoflavone	Not active to an appreciable extent in human foetal liver, but adult concentrations reached by 4 months of age
CYP2A6	Coumarin, nicotine	Barbiturates	Tranylcypromine	
CYP2C9	Diclofenac, phenytoin, torsemide, S-warfarin tolbutamide, ibuprofen	Rifampin	Sulfaphenazole, sulfinpyrazone	Low activity in neonate
CYP2C19	Phenytoin, diazepam, omeprazole, propranolol	Rifampin, phenobarbital	Tranylcypromine, cimetidine	Rapid maturation in the first week of life, with adult activity reached by 6 months of age
CYP2D6	Amitriptyline, captopril, codeine, dextromethorphan, fluoxetine, hydrocodone, ondansetron, propafenone, propranolol, timolol	None known	Fluoxetine, quinidine, cimetidine	Low to absent in foetal liver but uniformly present at 1 week of postnatal age. Poor activity (approximately 20 % of adult values) at 1 month of postnatal age
CYP3A4	Acetaminophen, alfentanil, amiodarone, budesonide, carbamazepine, diazepam, erythromycin, lidocaine, midazolam, nifedipine, omeprazole, cisapride, theophylline, verapamil, R-warfarin, oxycodone	Carbamazepine, dexamethasone, phenobarbital, phenytoin, rifampin	Azole antifungals, ethinyl estradiol, naringenin, troleandomycin, erythromycin	CYP3A4 has low activity in the first month of life, with approach towards adult levels by 6–12 months postnatally
CYP3A7	Dehydroepiandrosterone, ethinyl estradiol, various dihydropyrimidines	Carbamazepine, rifampin, dexamethasone, phenobarbital, phenytoin	Azole antifungals, erythromycin and cimetidine	CYP3A7 is functionally active in the foetus; approximately 30 to 75 % of adult levels of CYP3A4

Adapted from Leeder JS, Kearns GL: Pharmacogenetics in pediatrics: implications for practice. Pediatr Clin North Am 1997; 44:55–77 [731], with kind permission from Elsevier

Table 25.4 Maturation of caffeine clearance

Age	Weight (kg)	CL per kilogram (L h^{-1} kg^{-1})	CL allometric (L h^{-1} 70 kg^{-1})
Premature neonate	2	0.0041	0.118
Term neonate	3.5	0.004	0.132
3 months	6	0.091509	3.46
6 months	7.5	0.119719	4.8
1 year	10	0.126694	5.5
Adult	70	0.057–0.085	3.6–5.9

Reproduced from Anderson BJ, Gunn TR Holford NH, Johnson R Caffeine overdose in a premature infant: clinical course and pharmacokinetics *Anaesthesia and Intensive Care* 1999;29: 307–11 [150], with the kind permission of the Australian Society of Anaesthetists

Table 25.5 Maturation of theophylline clearance

Age	Weight (kg)	CL per kilogram (L h^{-1} kg^{-1})	CL allometric (L h^{-1} 70 kg^{-1})	V (L kg^{-1})
Neonate	3	20	0.38	0.86
Infant (4 months)	5	30–60	0.9–1.9	
Toddler (1 year)	10	90 (SD 18)	3.9 (SD 0.8)	0.63
Child (2 years)	12	76 (20)	3.4 (0.9)	
Child (7 years)	22	62 (20)	3.3 (1.0)	
Adolescent (13 years)	40	55 (18)	3.3 (1.0)	
Adult	70	40 (12)	2.8 (0.8)	0.5

Reproduced from Anderson BJ, Holford NH, Woollard GA. Aspects of theophylline clearance in children. *Anaesthesia and Intensive Care* 1997; 25: 497–501 [151], reproduced with the kind permission of the Australian Society of Anaesthetists

Fig. 25.16 The *upper panel* shows individual predicted methadone clearances, standardised to a 70 kg person, plotted against postmenstrual age. No relationship between age and standardised clearance was found. Individual predicted methadone peripheral compartment volume of distribution (V_2), standardised to a 70 kg person, is plotted against postmenstrual age in the *lower panel*. The *solid line* represents the nonlinear relation between V_2 and age (Reproduced from Ward RM, Drover DR, Hammer GB, Stemland CJ, Kern S, Tristani-Firouzi M, Lugo RA, Satterfield K, Anderson BJ. The pharmacokinetics of methadone and its metabolites in neonates, infants, and children. Pediatr Anesth 2014;24: 591–601 [143], with kind permission from John Wiley and Sons)

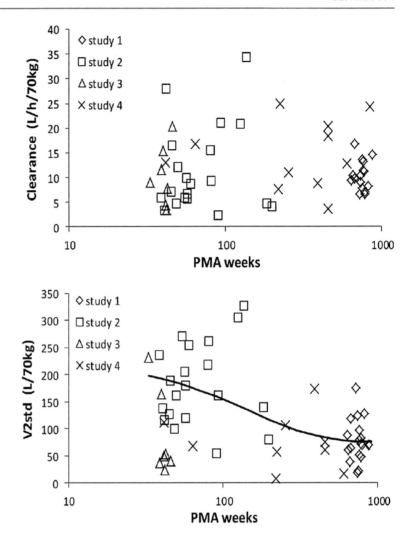

neonates given epidural infusion at rates greater than that at which it was metabolised [160].

Phase II Reactions

The other major route of hepatic drug metabolism, designated phase II reactions, involves synthetic or conjugation reactions that increase the hydrophilicity of molecules to facilitate renal elimination. The phase II enzymes include glucuronosyltransferase, sulphotransferase, *N*-acetyltransferase, glutathione *S*-transferase and methyl transferase.

Most conjugation reactions have limited activity during foetal development. One of the most familiar synthetic reactions in young infants involves conjugation by uridine diphosphoglucuronosyltransferases (UGT). This enzyme system (also responsible for bilirubin) has numerous isoforms that all mature at different rates. Failure to appreciate UGT immaturity at birth resulted in high concentrations of chloramphenicol and consequent fatal circulatory collapse in neonates [161, 162].

Morphine, acetaminophen and dexmedetomidine all undergo glucuronidation. Morphine clearance [163] increases with weight and postmenstrual age. The maturation of glucuronosyltransferase enzymes varies among isoforms, but, in general, adult activity is reached by 6–12 months of age. Some of the confusion relating to maturation rates is attributable to the use of the per kilogram size model. The use of allometry with a maturation model has assisted understanding. The time courses of maturation of drug metabolism (morphine [45], acetaminophen [164], dexmedetomidine [165] and GFR [59]) are strikingly similar (Fig. 25.17) with 50 % of size-adjusted adult values being reached between 8 and 12 weeks (TM_{50}) after full-term delivery. All three drugs are cleared predominantly by UGT that converts the parent compound into a water-soluble metabolite that is excreted by the kidneys. Glucuronidation is the major metabolic pathway of propofol metabolism, and this pathway is immature in neonates, although multiple cytochrome P450 isoenzymes, including CYP2B6, CYP2C9 or CYP2A6, also contribute to its metabolism and

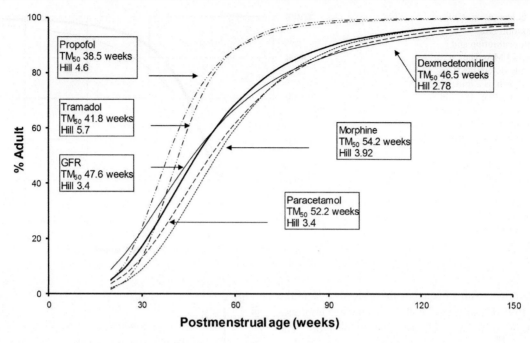

Fig. 25.17 Clearance maturation, expressed as a percentage of mature clearance, of drugs where glucuronide conjugation (paracetamol, morphine, dexmedetomidine) plays a major role. These profiles are closely aligned with glomerular filtration rate (GFR). In contrast, cytochrome P450 isoenzymes also contribute to propofol and tramadol metabolism and cause a faster maturation profile than expected from glucuronide conjugation alone. Maturation parameter estimates were taken from [45, 59, 156, 164, 165, 733]

Table 25.6 Developmental patterns for conjugation (phase II) reactions in the neonate

Enzymes	Selected substrates	Developmental patterns
Uridine diphosphoglucuronyltransferase (UGT)	Chloramphenicol, morphine, hydromorphone, acetaminophen, valproic acid, lorazepam, dexmedetomidine, naloxone	Ontogeny is isoform specific. In general, adult activity is achieved by 6–18 months of age. Induced by cigarette smoke and phenobarbital
Sulphotransferase	Bile acids, acetaminophen, cholesterol, polyethylene, glycols, chloramphenicol	Ontogeny seems to be more rapid than UGT; however, it is substrate specific
N-acetyltransferase	Hydralazine, procainamide, clonazepam, caffeine, sulfamethoxazole	Some foetal activity present by 16 weeks. Adult activity present by 1–3 years of age

Adapted from Leeder JS, Kearns GL: Pharmacogenetics in pediatrics: implications for practice. Pediatr Clin North Am 1997; 44:55–77 [731], with kind permission from Elsevier

cause a faster maturation profile than expected from glucuronide conjugation alone [166]. A phase I reaction (CYP2D6) is the major enzyme system tramadol, and clearance through this pathway is faster than those associated with UGT maturation. Table 25.6 outlines some typical phase II processes.

Alterations in Biotransformation

Transition from the intrauterine to the extrauterine environment is associated with major changes in blood flow. There may also be an environmental trigger for the expression of some metabolic enzyme activities resulting in a slight increase in maturation rate above that predicted by PMA at birth (Fig. 25.18) [26, 166]. Many biotransformation reactions, especially those involving certain forms of cytochrome P450, are inducible before birth through maternal exposure to drugs, cigarette smoke or other inducing agents. Postnatally, biotransformation reactions may be induced through drug exposure and may be slowed by hypoxia/asphyxia, organ damage and/or illness. Postnatal changes in hepatic blood flow, protein binding and/or biliary function may also alter drug elimination.

Genotypic Variations in Drug Metabolism; CYP2D6

Single nucleotide changes or polymorphisms (SNPs) in the DNA sequence in CYP enzymes may decrease or increase metabolic activity for a specific drug substrate [167]. Variability in the clinical response to codeine prompted investigations into genetic variants or polymorphisms of CYP2D6, the enzyme that converts codeine to its active metabolite, morphine [168]. This enzyme is mapped to chromosome 22 at 22q13.1. Over 55 polymorphisms of CYP2D6

Fig. 25.18 Change in glomerular filtration rate associated with maturation and birth at 40 weeks PMA. The maturation profile determined using PMA is shown as a thin line. The effect of adding PNA is shown as a thick line. Maturation is slower than anticipated before birth when PNA is unaccounted for, and there is a slight increase of clearance maturation after birth (Reproduced from Anderson BJ, Holford NH. Tips and traps analyzing pediatric PK data. Pediatr Anesth 2011; 21: 222–37 [25] with kind permission from John Wiley and Sons)

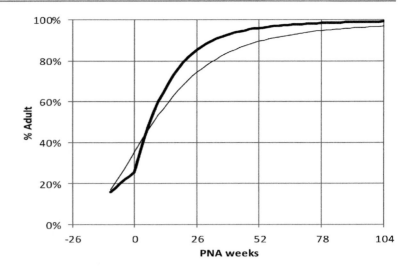

have been described with a frequency that exceeds 1 % of the population [169]. These include both functional and nonfunctional polymorphisms as well as gene duplication. The polymorphisms are numbered with *1 being the normal or wild allele (the * denotes an allele). The mutant alleles, *3, *4, *5, *6 and*9, for example, confer no CYP2D6 activity [169–171]. The latter polymorphisms account for more than 90 % of the poor metabolisers. Variants *2, *10 and 17 have modestly reduced activity and are referred as intermediate metabolisers. To further complicate the genetic pattern, multiple copies of the same genes [171] may be present in some individuals, resulting in bizarre phenotypes. The wide array of CYP2D6 polymorphisms of codeine may be summarised into three broad categories: poor metabolisers (negligible morphine produced [PM]), extensive metabolisers (normals [EM]) and ultra-extensive metabolisers (rapid and large amounts of morphine [UM]). Up to 10 % of whites and 30 % of Hong Kong Chinese are PM, rendering codeine an ineffective analgesic for these children. Alternately, 29 % of the Ethiopian and 1 % of Swedish, German and Chinese populations are UM. Children with the UM genotype who also have upregulated opioid receptors as a result of chronic intermittent nocturnal hypoxia may be particularly vulnerable to a mishap after a usual or subclinical dose of codeine [172].

Reduced metabolism through genetic polymorphisms leads to exaggerated effects when administered in conventional doses for many other drugs [167, 173]. Succinylcholine clearance through pseudocholinesterase is a well-known example [174]. Genotyping has become a routine part of the evaluation before treatment with methotrexate for detection of reduced activity of thiopurine methyltransferase that may be lethal with treatment with conventional dosages [175]. The drug irinotecan, used to treat cancer, has an active metabolite that is metabolised by a glucuronide (UGT1A1), a pathway similar to that involved in morphine clearance

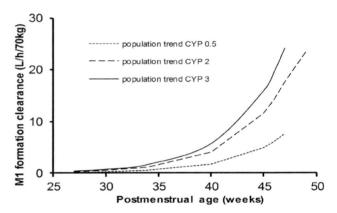

Fig. 25.19 Tramadol metabolite (M1) formation clearance (CYP2D6) increases with postmenstrual age. Rate of increase varies with genotype expression. Clearance is low in premature neonates, and genotype has minimal impact in early neonatal life (Adapted from Allegaert K, van den Anker JN, de Hoon JN, van Schaik RH, Debeer A, Tibboel D, Naulaers G, Anderson BJ. Covariates of tramadol disposition in the first months of life. Brit J Anaesth 2008;100:525–32 [178], with kind permission of Oxford University Press)

(UGT2B7). A variant allele UGT1A1*28 has been identified that is associated with severe neutropenia and diarrhoea. Genetic testing in patients to identify this allele (present in 10 % Caucasians) has been shown to be beneficial [176]. Specific SNPs of CYP2C9, CYP2C19, CYP2D6, CYP3A and uridine diphosphate-glucuronosyltransferase 1A1 (UGT1A1) account for a sufficient number of adverse pharmacologic outcomes to warrant future routine clinical testing [177].

Genotype may have little impact in the neonate when clearance is poor (Fig. 25.19) [178]. There is also evidence that possession of the genotype does not necessarily equate with phenotype. The clearance of tramadol by those with a low CYP2D6 genotype score was not reduced in all children studied (Fig. 25.20) [156].

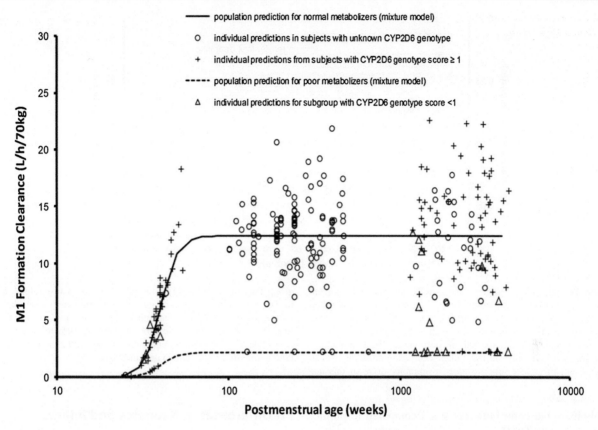

Fig. 25.20 Maturation of tramadol formation clearance (CLPM) to *O*-desmethyltramadol (M1 metabolite) labelled according to the availability of an individual *CYP2D6* genotype activity score. There is a distinct group of patients who are slow metabolisers identified by the phenotype (dashed line). Not all subjects with a low genotype *CYP2D6* activity ($n = 20$) are included in this slow metaboliser group. (From Allegaert K, Holford NHG, Anderson BJ, Holford S, Stuber F, Rochette A, Trocóniz IF, Beier H, de Hoon JN, Pedersen RS, Stamer U. Tramadol disposition throughout human life: a pooled pharmacokinetic study. Clin Parmacokinet 2015;54(2):167–78 [734], with kind permission from Springer)

Renal Excretion

Renal function in neonates and infants is less efficient than in adults due to the combination of incomplete glomerular development, low perfusion pressure and inadequate osmotic load to produce full countercurrent effects [179]. Preterm and term neonates have immature glomerular filtration and tubular function; both develop rapidly during the 6 months of life [59]. Glomerular filtration and tubular function are nearly mature by 20 weeks of postnatal age and fully mature by 2 years of age (Fig. 25.17) [59, 180]. Drugs eliminated primarily through the kidney, such as aminoglycoside antibiotics and milrinone, have reduced clearance in neonates and infants [181, 182].

In the presence of renal failure, one or two doses of drugs that are excreted via the kidneys often achieve and maintain prolonged therapeutic drug concentrations if there is no alternate pathway of excretion (e.g. caffeine or curare in the neonate). The PK and PD of the old muscle relaxant, curare, exemplify the complex interaction of increased *V*, smaller muscle mass and decreased rate of excretion due to immaturity of glomerular filtration. The initial dose of curare

needed to achieve neuromuscular blockade is similar in infants and adults [183]. In infants, however, this blockade is achieved at reduced serum concentrations compared with older children or adults, corresponding to differences in muscle mass. A larger *V* (total body water) accounts for the equivalent dose for each kilogram of body weight, and the reduced glomerular function in infants compared with older children or adults accounts in part for the longer duration of action [183].

Pulmonary Elimination

The factors determining anaesthetic absorption (alveolar ventilation, FRC, cardiac output, tissue/blood solubility) also contribute to elimination. We might anticipate more rapid washout in neonates than adults for any given duration of anaesthesia because there is less distribution to fat and muscle content. The greater decrease in cardiac output induced by halothane in neonates might be expected to speed elimination, but brain perfusion will also be reduced and this slows recovery. Halothane in particular and to a far lesser extent isoflurane and sevoflurane undergo hepatic

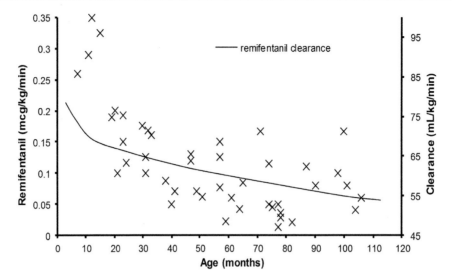

Fig. 25.21 The effect of age on the dose of remifentanil tolerated during spontaneous ventilation under anaesthesia in children undergoing strabismus surgery. Superimposed on this plot is estimated remifentanil clearance determined using an allometric model. There is a mismatch between clearance and infusion rate for those individuals still in infancy. The higher infusion rates recorded in those infants can be attributed to greater suppression of respiratory drive in this age group than the older children during the study; a respiratory rate of ten breaths per minute in an infant is disproportionately slow compared to the same rate in a 7-year-old child, suggesting excessive dose (Reproduced from Anderson BJ. Paediatric models for adult target-controlled infusion pumps. Pediatr Anesth 2010;20:223–32 [735], with kind permission from John Wiley and Sons)

metabolism, but contribution is small compared to pulmonary elimination [184].

Extrahepatic Routes of Metabolic Clearance

Many drugs undergo metabolic clearance at extrahepatic sites. Remifentanil and atracurium are degraded by nonspecific esterases in tissues and erythrocytes. Thus, plasma clearances of atracurium and remifentanil are independent of organ function and, when normalised for body weight, are somewhat greater in neonates and infants than in older children [23, 185]. This relationship is demonstrated for remifentanil in Fig. 25.21. Clearance determines infusion rate at steady state, and it can be seen that remifentanil infusion rates required achieving a target respiratory rate mirror clearance. Succinylcholine also exhibits a monophasic decline in weight-normalised dose requirements from birth that is predictable by the 3/4 power size model [186–188].

Paediatric Pharmacodynamic Considerations

Children's responses to drugs have much in common with the responses in adults [189]. The perception that drug effects differ in children arises because the drugs have not been adequately studied in paediatric populations who have size- and maturation-related effects as well as different diseases. Neonates and infant, however, often have altered pharmacodynamics.

PD Differences in Neonates and Infants

The minimal alveolar concentration (MAC) for almost all anaesthetic vapours is less in neonates than in infancy, which is in turn greater than that observed in children and adults [128]. MAC of isoflurane in preterm neonates less than 32 weeks gestation was 1.28 %, and MAC in neonates 32–37 weeks gestation was 1.41 % [190]. This value rose to 1.87 % by 6 months before decreasing again over childhood [190]. The cause of these differences is uncertain and may relate to maturation changes in cerebral blood flow, gamma-aminobutyric acid ($GABA_A$) receptor numbers or developmental shifts in the regulation of chloride transporters. Gamma-aminobutyric acid A receptor binding in human neonates is strikingly different from that in older children/adults [191].

Neonates have an increased sensitivity to the effects of neuromuscular blocking drugs [183]. The reason for this is unknown, but it is consistent with the observation that there is a threefold reduction in the release of acetylcholine from the infant rat phrenic nerve [192, 193]. The increased volume of distribution however means that a single NMBD dose is the same as the older child; reduced clearance prolongs duration.

The coagulation system [194, 195], including the fibrinolytic system at birth [196–199], is immature at birth. Consequently the target plasma concentration of antifibrinolytic drugs required to achieve similar effects as in adults is less in neonates. The concentration of epsilon aminocaproic acid

(EACA) required to inhibit fibrinolysis in adult plasma in vitro was originally described to be 130 mg/L in 1962 [200]. This has been confirmed as the effective concentration in adults by using thromboelastography [201]. However, neonates require a lower concentration of EACA (50 mg/L) to inhibit fibrinolysis [202]. Dose of EACA requires adjustment in neonates because of both immaturity of antifibrinolytic clearance pathways and coagulation cascade.

Cardiac calcium stores in the endoplasmic reticulum are reduced in the neonatal heart because of immaturity. Exogenous calcium has greater impact on contractility in this age group than in older children or adults. Catecholamine release and response to vasoactive drugs vary with age. These PD differences are based in part upon developmental changes in myocardial structure, cardiac innervation and adrenergic receptor function. Conversely neonates may suffer cardiac arrest if given the calcium antagonist, verapamil [203]. There are some data to suggest greater sensitivity to warfarin in children, but the mechanism is not determined [204]. Amide local anaesthetic agents induce shorter block duration and require a larger weight-scaled dose to achieve similar dermatomal levels when given by subarachnoid block to infants. This may be due, in part, to myelination, spacing of nodes of Ranvier and length of nerve exposed as well as size factors. There is an age-dependent expression of intestinal motilin receptors and the modulation of gastric antral contractions in neonates. Prokinetic agents may not be useful in very preterm infants, partially useful in older preterm infants and useful in full-term infants. Similarly, bronchodilators in infants are ineffective because of the paucity of bronchial smooth muscle that can cause bronchospasm.

The sensitivity of human neonates to most of the sedatives, hypnotics and narcotics is clinically well known and may in part be related to increased brain permeability (immature blood–brain barrier or damage to the blood–brain barrier), particularly in the premature neonate, for some medications [93, 205–208]. Regional blood flow and receptor density differences within the brain also contribute. Decreased protein binding, as in the neonate, results in a greater proportion of unbound drug that is available for passive diffusion. This may contribute to bupivacaine's propensity for seizures in neonates.

Measurement of PD Endpoints

Outcome measures are more difficult to assess in neonates and infants than in children or adults. Measurement techniques, disease and pathology differences, inhomogeneous groups, recruitment issues, ethical considerations and endpoint definition for establishing efficacy and safety confuse data interpretation [209].

Common effects measured include anaesthesia depth, pain and sedation and neuromuscular blockade. A common effect measure used to assess depth of anaesthesia is the electroencephalogram or a modification of detected EEG signals (spectral edge frequency, bispectral index, entropy). Physiological studies in adults and children indicate that EEG-derived anaesthesia depth monitors can provide an imprecise and drug-dependent measure of arousal. Although the outputs from these monitors do not closely represent any true physiological entity, they can be used as guides for anaesthesia and in so doing have improved outcomes in adults. In older children the physiology, anatomy and clinical observations indicate the performance of the monitors may be similar to that in adults. In infants their use cannot yet be supported in theory or in practice [210, 211]. During anaesthesia, the EEG in infants is fundamentally different from the EEG in older children; there remains a need for specific neonate-derived algorithms if EEG-derived anaesthesia depth monitors are to be used in neonates [212, 213].

The Children's Hospital of Wisconsin Sedation Scale [214] has been used to investigate ketamine in the emergency department [70]. However, despite the use of such scales in procedural pain or sedation studies, few behavioural scales have been adequately validated in this setting [215, 216]. Interobserver variability can be high [217]. More objective measures for pain such as pupillometry may improve scoring [218], but these measures also contain thorns to their execution [219]. Most scores are validated for the acute, procedural setting and perform less for subacute or chronic pain or stress.

PKPD Parameter Variability

There is considerable variability in any measured plasma concentration when identical doses are given to individuals. Typical values for population PK parameter variability are 50 % for compliance with medication regimens, 30 % for absorption, 10 % for tissue distribution, 50 % for metabolic elimination and 20 % for renal elimination [220]. The contribution of PD variability due to distribution from the blood to the site of action will depend largely on changes in perfusion of target tissue (5–60 %). Receptor sensitivity variability (5–50 %) and efficacy variability (30 %) also exist. The observed response may not be a direct consequence of drug–receptor binding, but rather through intermediate physiological mechanisms. A typical value for this variability is 30 % [220].

Size and age are the two major contributors to variability of PK parameters (Fig. 25.22) [16]. Genetic differences in drug metabolism, receptor binding and intracellular coupling to effector mechanisms contribute variability to PK and PD. We know much less about morphine PD and

Fig. 25.22 Size and maturation explain much of propofol variability. Plots show median and 90 % intervals (*solid and dashed lines*). The 90 % prediction intervals for observations (*lines with symbols*) and predictions (*lines*) with 95 % confidence intervals for prediction percentiles (*grey-shaded areas*) are shown. (Reproduced from Anderson BJ, Holford NHG. Tips and traps analyzing paediatric PK data. Pediatr Anesth 2011;21:222–37 [26], with kind permission from John Wiley and Sons)

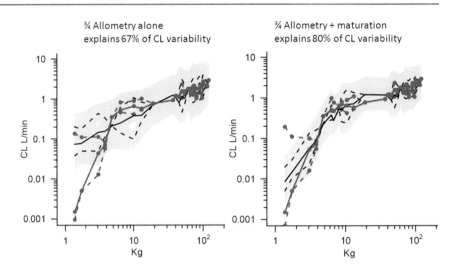

response variability than we know about PK [2], but genetic influences contribute to morphine PD variability [221].

Genetic, physiological and cultural differences exist between men and women [222–224]. Hormones possibly have influence on the higher levels of pain and decreased pain threshold experienced by women because these differences are less significant after the age of 40 years. PK differences are not apparent before puberty [225], although PD differences may exist from an early age. Pain differences exist between people of different races and ethnicities. The contribution to these differences due to culture, geography [226, 227] and genetics remains to be teased apart. The incidence of adverse effects after morphine is greater in Latino than non-Latino children. Neither differences in morphine or metabolite concentrations nor the genetic polymorphisms examined explained these findings [228]. Caucasian children had a higher incidence of opioid-related adverse effects but less pain than African American children [229]. The latter had higher morphine clearance, and although UGT2B7 genetic variations (2161C > T and 802C > T) were not associated with observed racial differences in morphine's clearance, the wild type of the UGT2B7 isozyme was more prevalent in African Americans [230].

The extremely anxious child may require a greater induction dose of propofol than less anxious children [231]. Increased circulating catecholamines may also contribute to perceived pain. Single nucleotide polymorphisms for the enzyme responsible for metabolising catecholamines (catechol-O-methyltransferase, COMT) have been described and distinct haplotypes categorised (low, average and high pain sensitivity). Haplotypes have also been associated with catecholamine synthesis (e.g. cofactor tetrahydrobiopterin (BH4) synthesis and metabolism) that is associated with chronic pain. BH4 blocking drugs may prove useful as a novel analgesic. In addition haplotypes for the B_2 adrenergic

receptor, based on eight single nucleotide polymorphisms, have been identified.

It is not surprising that inflammatory cytokines (interleukins, tumour necrosis factor) have impact on the pain response. The inflammatory response mediated after surgery has impact on pain [232]. Polymorphism in the interleukin-1 receptor antagonist gene is associated with serum interleukin-1 receptor antagonist concentrations and postoperative opioid consumption [233].

Morphine works through the μ-opioid receptor, a protein coded for by the OPRM1 gene on chromosome 6q24-q25. Polymorphisms of this gene (e.g. A118G) may increase this receptor's affinity for morphine and its metabolite morphine 6-glucuronide [234] although clinical impact continues to be debated [235, 236] A number of other genetic variations may also influence the μ-opioid receptor. The melanocortin-1 receptor that serves a role in skin pigmentation may influence morphine 6-glucuronide effects as well as the k-opioid receptor in females [237]. Signal transmission from opioid receptors requires involvement of ion channels (K, Na, Ca), and polymorphisms of these channels have also been noted to have an influence on pain sensitivity. Mutations in voltage-gated transient receptor potential channels have been identified and may modulate the effects of analgesics [238]. Efflux transporters like the P-glycoproteins are also associated with polymorphisms and may affect transport into or out of the brain [239].

Adverse Effects

Neonates and young children may suffer permanent effects resulting from a stimulus applied at a sensitive point in development. For example, congenital hypothyroidism, if untreated, causes lifelong phenotypic changes. The incidence of vaginal carcinoma is high in children of mothers treated with stilboestrol during pregnancy [240]. There are concerns that neonatal exposure to some anaesthetic agents (e.g. ketamine, midazolam) may cause widespread neuronal apoptosis and long-term memory deficits [241, 242].

Anaesthesia, analgesia or sedation generally involves examination of immediate adverse effects such as PONV, hypotension or respiratory depression. A dose–response curve for intravenous morphine and vomiting was investigated in children having day-stay tonsillectomy. Doses above 0.1 mg kg^{-1} were associated with a greater than 50 % incidence of vomiting [243]. These data are similar to those in children undergoing inguinal herniorrhaphy [244], suggesting that lower doses of morphine are associated with a decreased incidence of emesis after day-stay surgery and encourage the use of alternative analgesic drugs.

Therapeutic use of drugs balances beneficial effects against adverse effects. Adverse effects, however, may be simply consequent upon a poor understanding of pharmacokinetics. Propofol infusion dose in neonates, if based on adult dose (mg/kg/h), will overdose and cause hypotension; propofol infusion dose in 1–2-year-olds (where clearance is increased expressed as mg/kg/h) may underdose and result in awareness. Morphine dose in the very young was traditionally limited by fears of respiratory compromise; postoperative arterial oxygen desaturation continues to be reported with sedative drugs in neonates [245]. These are a result of poor PK understanding. However there are also PD differences. Premature neonates are more prone to apnoea. Sympathetic–parasympathetic tone is immature in neonates, and the use of propofol in neonates has recently been associated with profound hypotension [246], questioning our understanding of the dose–effect relationships of this common drug [247]. Such information allows informed dosing.

Drug Interactions

Drug interactions can increase or decrease response mediated through either PK or PD routes. Physical drug interactions may occur even before absorption or delivery, reducing bioavailability (e.g. direct chemical combinations). Drug interactions may involve either PK interactions, PD interactions or even both. A commonly used combination in which PK interactions exist is that of midazolam and propofol. When given together, these drugs reduce the clearance of one another, resulting in a 25 % increase in propofol concentrations and a 27 % increase in midazolam concentrations [248, 249]. They also both act on gamma-aminobutyric acid (GABA) cerebral receptors contributing to PD interactions as well. Clinically this results in a 25 %

reduction in required midazolam dose when given as bolus for short-term sedation with propofol in adults [248].

Pharmacokinetic Interactions

Interactions between co-administered drugs can affect all stages of PK processes (drug absorption, distribution, metabolism and elimination). A recent PK example is that of phenylephrine when administered orally with acetaminophen, typical of many over-the-counter preparations for upper respiratory tract infections [250]. This as yet unknown PK interaction results in nearly four times the normal maximum plasma concentration of phenylephrine, with changes to metabolism in the gut wall as one proposed mechanism [251].

PK interactions are often dealt with by including the effect of a second drug as a covariate on affected PK parameters such as those describing clearance (CL), volume of distribution (V) or bioavailability (F). The midazolam–propofol PK interaction has been investigated by adjusting midazolam CL and V using propofol plasma concentrations included in an exponential covariate model, i.e.

$$CL_{IND} = CL_{POP} \times exp^{(coc(C_{PROP}-Median\ C_{PROP}))} \quad (25.22)$$

where CL is clearance from the central compartment, for the population (CL_{POP}) and the individual (CL_{IND}). Here, the effect of plasma propofol concentration (C_{PROP}) on the CL parameter is estimated (the parameter 'cov') and scaled to the population median C_{PROP} (Median C_{PROP}).

Phenobarbitone induces a number of other pathways responsible for drug clearances, e.g. CYP1A2, CYP2C9, CYP2C19, CYP3A4 and UDP-glucuronosyltransferase (UGT) [252]. Ketamine in humans is metabolised mainly by CYP3A4. The steep concentration–response curve described for ketamine [70] means that small changes in the plasma concentration attributed to increased clearance can have dramatic impact on the degree of sedation (Fig. 25.23) [253]. Another example relates to the administration of drugs that interfere with the cytochrome isoforms that metabolise midazolam (CYP3A4). Examples of such drugs/foods are grapefruit juice, erythromycin, calcium channel blockers and protease inhibitors. The net effect is to prolong the duration of action of midazolam.

Pharmacodynamic Models

Pharmacodynamics (PD) describes the concentration–effect relationship. PD models are often linked to PK models by describing movement of drug from the plasma to the

Fig. 25.23 Simulation of plasma concentration and sedation score in a 6-year-old, 20 kg child given ketamine 2 mg kg^{-1} when clearance is doubled. The sedation score is graded from 0 to 5 where a score of 2 indicates the child arouses slowly to consciousness, with sustained painful stimulus, and a score of 3 indicates the child arouses with moderate tactile or loud verbal stimulus (Reproduced from Sumpter A, Anderson BJ. Phenobarbital and some anesthesia implications. Pediatr Anesth 2011; 21: 995–7 [736], with kind permission from John Wiley and Sons)

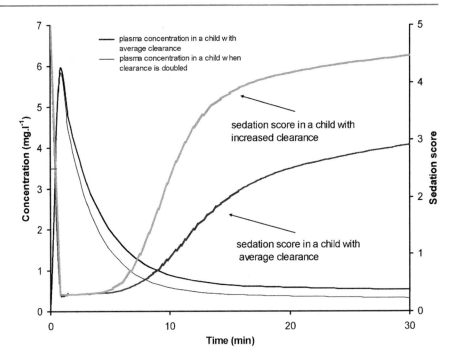

effect site and its target (e.g. use of the equilibration half-time $T_{1/2}k_{eo}$), and interactions may even occur at that level. An increase in the $T_{1/2}k_{eo}$ of d-tubocurarine with increasing inspired halothane concentrations has been demonstrated [254]. Halothane is a negative inotrope [255] and reduces skeletal muscle blood flow [256], so it seems reasonable to interpret changes in $T_{1/2}k_{eo}$ as due to changes in blood flow.

Traditional methods of evaluating PD interactions include using isoboles, shifts in dose (or concentration) response curves (Fig. 25.24a) or interaction indices based on parameters of potency derived from separate monotherapy and combination therapy analyses. For example, inhalation anaesthetic agents can also prolong duration of neuromuscular block, and this affect is agent specific. Sevoflurane potentiated vecuronium more than halothane; when compared to balanced anaesthesia, the dose requirements of vecuronium were reduced by approximately 60 % and 40 %, respectively [257]. Such methods provide an estimation of the magnitude of effect for dose or concentration combinations, but they do not inform us on the time course of that effect or its associated variability.

Drug effects can be described as a function of efficacy (e) and receptor occupation (i.e. the fraction of drug D bound to receptors R, [RD]), i.e.

$$E = f([RD] \cdot e) \qquad (25.23)$$

PD interactions occur through various mechanisms that disrupt or alter this relationship. For example, competitive antagonists reduce receptor availability by competing for occupancy at the same receptor site. Drugs that elicit an effect are called agonists, while those that do not are called antagonists, so the occupancy of some receptors by the antagonists results in less effect. In general, competitive antagonists shift the effect–concentration curve to the right by altering the C_{50}. The E_{MAX} equation can then be expressed as

$$\text{Effect} = E_0 + \frac{E_{MAX} \times Ce^{\gamma}}{\left(\left(C_{50}^{\gamma} \times \left[1 + \frac{A}{EA_{50}}\right]\right) + Ce^{\gamma}\right)} \qquad (25.24)$$

where A and EA_{50} represent ligand A concentration and potency. Noncompetitive antagonists shift the observed maximum effect (E_{MAX}) rather than the C_{50}.

$$\text{Effect} = E_0 + \frac{E_{MAX} \times \left(1 - \frac{A}{A + EA_{50}}\right) \times Ce^{\gamma}}{Ce^{\gamma} + C_{50}^{\gamma}} \qquad (25.25)$$

PD interactions are not restricted to same-site binding interactions; some proteins have multiple binding sites, and ligands binding at these sites can also alter the above relationship (i.e. through changes in protein conformation that lead to downstream changes or modulates agonist–receptor affinity).

Response Surface Models

A better way to investigate PD interactions is to use modelling and to take advantage of the benefits of population analyses. Models for monotherapy, derived using a population approach, can be combined and extended to incorporate PD interactions between two or more drugs.

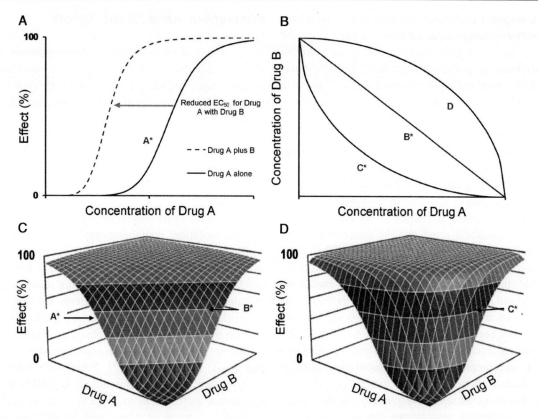

Fig. 25.24 Methods of investigating interactions. (**a**) Shift in response curve analyses involves plotting the concentration (or dose)–effect relationship for one drug alone and in the presence of steady-state concentrations of a second drug. (**b**) Isoboles are constructed using iso-effect lines with curves derived from observations assessed against the expected (or 'additive') response line (B*). Supra-additivity is depicted by curves bowing towards the plot origin (C*), while infra-additivity is shown with outward curves (D). Information from both methods is represented within response surfaces with isoboles displayed as horizontal planes and individual concentration–response curves as vertical slices (indicated by *arrows* on surfaces for A* single concentration–response curve drug A, B* additive isobole and C* supra-additive isobole). (**c**) Additive response surface for two drugs. (**d**) Synergistic response surface for two drugs, with synergy depicted through outward bowing of the surface (Reproduced from Hannam J, Anderson BJ. Pharmacodynamic interaction models in pediatric anesthesia. Pediatr Anesth 2015; 25:970–980 [737], with kind permission from John Wiley and Sons)

The 'response surface' models are an extension of empirical, single drug models that can be used to describe, and predict, the combined effects between two or more drugs. The name refers to the surface of response that is visualised by plotting effect versus two drug concentrations (on *x* and *y* axes). Synergy (supra-additivity) is depicted by outward bowing of the surface on the horizontal plane, while infra-additivity is depicted by inward bowing of the surface (Fig. 25.24c, d). Horizontal lines within the response surface hold equivalent information to that given by isoboles (Fig. 25.24b). Surface parameters are estimated using data points pertaining to all areas of the concentration and effect range for both drugs simultaneously (e.g. as opposed to considering individual concentration pairs or effect levels in isolation, as is done with isobolographic analyses). The magnitude of the interaction is quantified by an interaction parameter. This is initially fixed at a value denoting the simplest scenario: no interaction or 'additivity'. Resulting models can be used to characterise the type of interaction across the entire range of concentrations and effect levels and make predictions about effects for any ratio of the studied drugs.

Two equations are commonly used: those of Greco et al. [258] and Minto and Vuyk [259]. Greco equations have been used to describe additive effects for propofol, remifentanil and fentanyl on bispectral index response in children aged 1–16 years undergoing general surgery [65]. These authors reported C_{50} estimates of propofol 5.20 μg/mL, remifentanil 24.1 ng/mL and fentanyl 8.6 ng/mL and suggested a propofol and remifentanil pair of 2.3 μg/mL and 4.3 ng/mL, respectively, to maintain haemodynamic parameters and sedation scores within ranges suitable for surgery. The Greco model has also been used to describe loss of response to various noxious stimuli under propofol–remifentanil anaesthesia [260]. Synergistic surfaces for sedation and response to laryngoscopy were reported.

Minto equations have been used to assess synergy for hypnosis between three commonly combined drugs for anaesthesia: propofol, midazolam and alfentanil [261]. Computer simulations based on interactions at the effect site predicted that the maximally synergistic three-drug combination (midazolam, propofol and alfentanil) tripled the duration of effect compared with propofol alone. Response surfaces can describe anaesthetic interactions, even those between agonists, partial agonists, competitive antagonists and inverse agonists [261].

Synergism between propofol and alfentanil has been demonstrated using response surface methodology. Remifentanil alone had no appreciable effect on response to shaking and shouting or response to laryngoscopy, while propofol could ablate both responses. Modest remifentanil concentrations dramatically reduced the concentrations of propofol required to ablate both responses [262]. When comparing the different combinations of midazolam, propofol and alfentanil, the responses varied markedly at each endpoint assessed and could not be predicted from the responses of the individual agents [263]. Similar response surface methodology has been taken for investigation of the combined administration of sevoflurane and alfentanil [264] and remifentanil and propofol [265] on ventilation control. These combinations have a strikingly synergistic effect on respiration, resulting in severe respiratory depression in adults. These synergistic associations can be extended to paediatric sedation techniques. It is little wonder that the use of three or more sedating medications compared with 1 or 2 medications was strongly associated with adverse outcomes [266].

The ability of propofol to ablate response to noxious stimuli has been studied in children aged between 3 and 10 years undergoing oesophagogastroduodenoscopy [267]. The C_{50} for 50 % probability of no response was found to be reduced from a propofol concentration of 3.7 µg/mL to 2.8 µg/mL in the presence of 25 ng/kg/min remifentanil. The dose of remifentanil above this level did not result in large reductions in propofol requirements but did increase the risk of remifentanil-related respiratory depression.

'Ketofol' is a mixture of ketamine and propofol (1:1) that is finding a niche for procedural sedation in the emergency room [268]. Stable haemodynamics, analgesia and good recovery are reported [269]. The additive interaction for anaesthesia induction in adults has been reported [270]. These data have been used to simulate effect in children [271]. An optimal ratio of racemic ketamine to propofol of 1:5 for 30 min anaesthesia and 1:6.7 for 90 min anaesthesia was suggested (Fig. 25.25) [271]. The 'ideal mix' for sedation will depend on the duration of sedation and the degree of analgesia required. The context-sensitive half-time of ketamine increases with infusion duration, resulting in delayed recovery [272].

Intravenous Anaesthetic Agents

Intravenous anaesthetics are a heterogeneous group of sedative–hypnotic drugs that produce unconsciousness speedily when injected intravenously. Prompt awakening after a single dose of these agents occurs predominantly by redistribution.

Barbiturates

Propofol

Propofol is an isopropylphenol supplied as a 1, 2 or 10 % aqueous solution containing soybean oil, glycerol and purified egg phosphatide to improve solubility. Its use for induction and maintenance of anaesthesia is associated with rapid recovery. Although the package insert for propofol cautions against its use in all patients with 'egg allergy', the evidence for this is not convincing [273, 274]. Propofol also suppresses laryngeal and pharyngeal reflexes, thereby facilitating tracheal intubation and the insertion of a laryngeal mask airway [275–277]. Emergence delirium rarely occurs after propofol anaesthesia in children. Propofol reduces the incidence of nausea and vomiting when used as an induction agent or when used for the maintenance of anaesthesia [278]. In view of these advantages, propofol has replaced thiopental as the induction agent of choice.

Pharmacokinetics

Propofol clearance matures rapidly in the 6 months of life (Fig. 25.17) The shorter distribution half-time and more rapid plasma clearance of propofol are responsible for the faster and more clear-headed recovery following a single dose of this agent compared with thiopental [279]. The rapid elimination of propofol (plasma clearance up to ten times faster than thiopental in some adult studies) reduces the potential for accumulation, making the drug suitable for maintenance of anaesthesia. Induction and maintenance doses of propofol are higher in children than in adults because the volume of the central compartment is 50 % larger and the plasma clearance (per kilogram) 25 % faster in children [280, 281]. Average induction doses ($1.3 \times ED_{50}$) in infants and children and adults are 4, 3 and 2 mg/kg, respectively [282, 283]. Clearance is limited by the hepatic blood flow and is consequently reduced in children in low cardiac output states.

Clearance (per kilogram) is increased in children; consequently a higher infusion (expressed as L/h/kg) dose is required to achieve the same target concentration as adults [7, 34]. These increased requirements in children can be attributed to size factors. There are a number of paediatric parameter sets that can be used for propofol infusion

Fig. 25.25 The *upper panel* shows the probability of response during anaesthesia using a propofol/ketamine ratio of 5:1. The loading dose for induction of anaesthesia was 2.5 mg kg^{-1} propofol and 0.5 mg kg^{-1} of ketamine. Infusion rate was 67 % that suggested by McFarlan et al. [7]. The *lower panel* shows simulation results for a 90 min infusion. This panel also shows the probability of response as age increases from a 2-year-old (*thin black line*) to a 5-year-old (*bold black line*) and for a 10-year-old (*bold black hash line*) child (Reproduced from Coulter FL, Hannam JA, Anderson BJ. Ketofol dosing in anaesthesia. Pediatr Anesth 2014;24:806–12 [271], with kind permission from John Wiley and Sons)

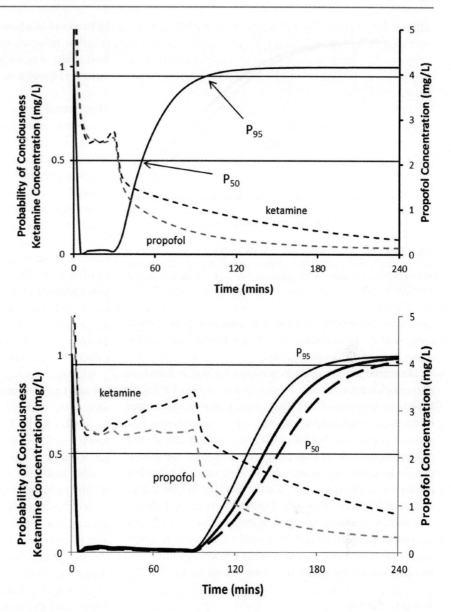

targeting a plasma concentration, e.g., Marsh et al. [12] and Gepts et al. [13], Kataria et al. [8], Short et al. [284], Rigby-Jones et al. [15], Schuttler and Ihmsen [55], Murat et al. [285], Saint-Maurice et al. [286], Coppens et al. [287] or Absalom et al. [14] (Table 25.1). Although parameter estimates are different for each author, most predict similar concentrations for the same infusion regimen (Fig. 25.3). Covariate influences such as severity of illness are unaccounted for; the volume in the central compartment, for example, is increased in children after cardiac surgery [15].

Pharmacodynamics

A propofol concentration of 2–3 mg/L is commonly sought for sedation, while 4–6 mg/L is used for anaesthesia. Both the loss and return of consciousness occur at similar target effect site propofol concentrations (2.0 SD 0.9 mg/L vs. 1.8

SD 0.7 mg/L) in adults [288], and a 'wake-up' concentration of 1.8 mg/L is described in children [289]. The relation between drug concentration and effect may be described by the Hill equation (Eq. (25.19)) [42]. Jeleazcov et al. [65] have described propofol pharmacodynamics in children 1–16 years using BIS where E_0 was estimated as 93.2, E_{max} −83.4, EC_{50} 5.2 mg L^{-1} and y 1.4. This relationship is very similar to that described in obese children [53]. The rate constant (k_{eo}) describing for the effect compartment was 0.6 min^{-1} ($T_{1/2}k_{eo}$ 1.15 min). Children possibly have a slightly lower sensitivity to propofol than adults (Fig. 25.26) [19], although this difference may be due to pharmacokinetic rather than pharmacodynamic factors [290]. The Kataria parameter set is known to underpredict concentration as age increases, consistent with allometric scaling. When this parameter set is used to estimate PD

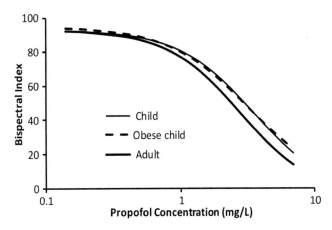

Fig. 25.26 Propofol concentration and its relationship with bispectral index in children and adults (Data from Coppens et al. Anesthesiology 2011;115:83–93 and Chidambaran et al Pediatr Anesth 2015;25:911–23)

parameters, it appears that the older children require lower concentration to maintain anaesthesia [291]; this is a PK effect and not a PD effect [292].

Decreased requirements in neonates are due to immature enzyme clearance systems. Propofol infusion rates for infants have been suggested [293]. Those regimens were determined by adapting an adult dosage scheme to the requirements of the younger population. Total number and time of administration of boluses and time to awakening were registered and used as criteria to adjust the dosage scheme. Predicted infusion rates are high (e.g. 24 mg kg^{-1} h^{-1} for the first 10 min in neonates) and should be used cautiously. Delayed awakening, hypotension and an increased incidence of bradycardia were reported in neonates and infants [293]. Propofol can cause profound hypotension in neonates, and pharmacokinetic–pharmacodynamic relationships in this age group remain elusive [247].

Adverse Effects

Pain on injection of propofol is a major problem occurring in up to 85 % of children [294]. It can be minimised by injecting into a large vein, injecting the solution slowly and administering at least 0.2 mg/kg of lidocaine immediately before, or with, propofol [295]. The vasodilator effects of propofol are greater than those of thiopental. Paediatric studies have consistently demonstrated a reduction in systolic and mean arterial pressures ranging from 5 to 30 % occurring in the first 5 min following injection of propofol [296–298]. Heart rate changes are variable in older children, but in one study, heart rate decreased significantly more in toddlers after propofol than after thiopental [296].

The use of propofol for prolonged sedation in paediatric intensive care units is associated with a rare syndrome comprising metabolic acidosis, heart failure, lipemia, rhabdomyolysis and death. The cause of this is unknown, but recent attention has focused on impairment of fatty acid oxidation

by propofol as a possible cause [299, 300]. The fact that this propofol infusion syndrome is more common in children than adults may be a reflection of the higher dose requirement for propofol in children [301].

Thiopental

Thiopental is an analogue of pentobarbital, in which the oxygen attached at C_2 of the barbituric acid ring is replaced by sulphur. This substitution confers high lipid solubility, which in conjunction with a high cerebral blood flow results in rapid penetration of the brain and hypnosis. Elimination occurs by oxidation in the liver to an inactive metabolite which is excreted by the kidney.

In the neonate, plasma protein binding of thiopental is reduced, so that the fraction of unbound drug is almost twice that found in older children and adults [302, 303]. In addition, clearance at 26 weeks PMA was 0.015 L/min/70 kg and increased to 0.119 L/min/70 kg by 42 weeks PMA (approximately 40 % of adult clearance at term [304]); however, as recovery depends mainly on redistribution, the effect of an induction dose is not significantly prolonged (Fig. 25.27).

Children aged 13–68 months given rectal thiopental (44 mg/kg) 45 min prior to surgery were either asleep or adequately sedated with plasma concentrations above 2.8 mg/L [305]. The ED_{50} sleep dose of intravenous thiopental varies with age [306, 307]. Doses of about $1.3 \times ED_{50}$ of thiopental are required to produce rapid, reliable induction of anaesthesia in all age groups; thus, healthy neonates require about 4–5 mg/kg, infants 7–8 mg/kg and children 5–6 mg/kg of thiopental for induction. The reduced requirement for thiopental in neonates compared with infants age 1–6 months may be explained by decreased plasma protein binding [302], greater penetration of the neonatal brain [206] or increased responsiveness of neonatal receptors [308]. The increased requirements for thiopental in infants and children compared with adults (average adult dose 4 mg/kg) remain unknown. A pharmacodynamic explanation attributable to increased cerebral $GABA_A$ receptor numbers or maturational differences in relative organ mass and regional blood flow may contribute. Blood flow, relative to cardiac output, to kidney and brain increases, while that to the liver decreases in early life. Cerebral and hepatic masses as a proportion of body weight are much higher in the young child than in the adult.

A few seconds of apnoea followed by a period of respiratory depression is common after an induction dose of thiopental. The hypotensive response in neonates given thiopental appears not as dramatic as that associated with propofol, although it still may occur with reversion to foetal circulation. Thiopental has little direct effect on vascular smooth muscle tone, although myocardial depression may occur with induction [296, 309] related to the dose given and the rate of injection. Other reported adverse effects include

Fig. 25.27 Simulated time–concentration profiles after an intravenous thiopentone bolus of 3 mg kg^{-1}. Predictions for a 25-week PMA and a 42-week PMA with neonate are shown alongside that of an adult (Reproduced from Larsson P, Anderson BJ, Norman E, Westrin P, Fellman V. Thiopentone elimination in newborn infants; exploring Michaelis Menten kinetics. Acta Anaesth Scand 2011; 55:444–51 [304], with kind permission from John Wiley and Sons)

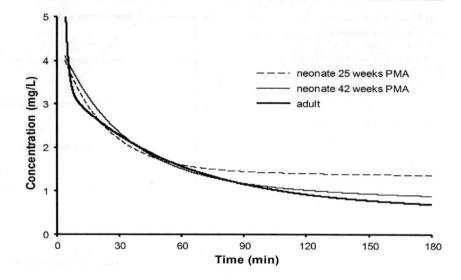

hiccups, coughing and laryngospasm. Extravasation of thiopental or intra-arterial injection can cause tissue injury, probably due to its extreme alkalinity.

Thiopental has also been used as a continuous infusion (2–4 mg/kg/h) to control intracranial hypertension. The elimination of thiopental after a continuous infusion may be markedly prolonged compared with that after a single bolus (11.7 vs. 6.1 h) [310]. These findings may in part be attributed to the underlying illness, intercurrent drug treatment and zero-order kinetics at higher concentrations (Michaelis constant 28.3 mg/L) [304, 311].

Ketamine

Ketamine is a derivative of phencyclidine that similarly antagonises the N-methyl-$_D$-aspartate (NMDA) receptor. Its action is related to central dissociation of the cerebral cortex, and it also causes cerebral excitation. Processed EEG monitoring devices do not work with ketamine sedation/anaesthesia [312].

Pharmacodynamics

Ketamine is available as a mixture of two enantiomers; the S(+)-enantiomer has four times the potency of the $R(-)$-enantiomer. S(+)-ketamine has approximately twice the potency of the racemate [313]. The metabolite norketamine has a potency that is one third that of its parent. Plasma concentrations associated with anaesthesia are approximately 3 μmcg/mL [272], hypnosis and amnesia during surgery are 0.8–4 cmg/mL and awakening usually occurs at concentrations less than 0.5 mcg/mL. Pain thresholds are increased at 0.1 mg/mL [314]. The concentration–response curve for ketamine sedation is steep [70, 315]. This means that small serum concentration changes will have dramatic

effect on the degree of sedation observed (Fig. 25.28) [70]. Ketamine is very lipid soluble with rapid distribution, and the onset of anaesthesia after IV ketamine is approximately 30 s. The $T_{1/2}k_{eo}$ was estimated ar 11 s [70].

Pharmacokinetics

Children require greater doses of ketamine (mg/kg) than adults because of greater clearance (L/h/kg); however, there is considerable patient-to-patient variability [316, 317]. Ketamine undergoes N-demethylation to norketamine; metabolised mainly by CYP3A4, although CYP2C9, CYP2B6 also has a role. Elimination of racemic ketamine is complicated by the $R(-)$-ketamine enantiomer, which inhibits the elimination of the S(+)-ketamine enantiomer [318]. Clearance in children is similar to adult rates (80 L/h/70 kg, i.e. liver blood flow) within the first 6 months of life, when corrected for size using allometric models [84]. Clearance in the neonate is reduced (26 L/h/70 kg) [319–321], while V_{ss} is increased in neonates (3.46 L/kg at birth, 1.18 L/kg at 4 years, 0.75 L/kg at adulthood [319]). This larger V_{ss} in neonates contributes to the observation that neonates require a fourfold greater dose than 6-year-old children to prevent gross motor movement [322]. The α-elimination half-life was 11 min and a β-elimination half-life was 2.5–3.0 h [323, 324]. S(+) ketamine clearance was found to be 35.8 mL kg^{-1} min^{-1} with 5 and 95 % confidence limits of 11.5 and 111.1 mL/kg/min, respectively, in adults [325]. Context-sensitive half-time increases dramatically with use between 1 and 2 h infusion causing delayed recovery (Fig. 25.29).

Ketamine has a high hepatic extraction ratio, and the relative bioavailability of oral, nasal and rectal formulations is 20–50 % [138, 326–328]. Children presenting for burns surgery had slow absorption (absorption half-time was 59 min) with high between-subject variability [138].

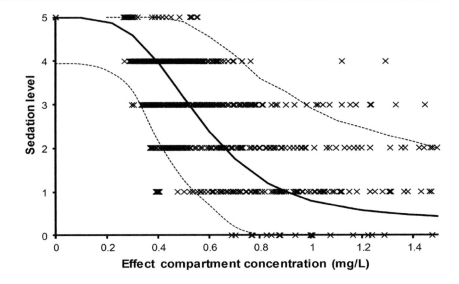

Fig. 25.28 The relationship between effect compartment concentration and level of sedation. The EC_{50} was 0.562 mg/ L. Categorical data are shown as crosses. The *dotted lines* demonstrate 90 % confidence intervals (Reproduced from Herd D, Anderson BJ, Keene NA, Holford NHG. Investigating the pharmacodynamics of ketamine in children. Pediatr Anesth 2008;18:36–42 [70], with kind permission from John Wiley and Sons)

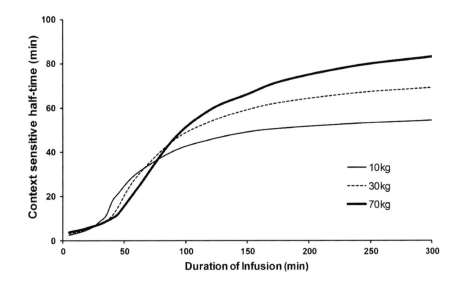

Fig. 25.29 Ketamine context-sensitive half-time following infusion at 3 mg/kg/h. The context-sensitive half-time in children was shorter than in adults after 1.5 h (Reproduced from Dallimore D, Anderson BJ, Short T, Herd DW. Ketamine anaesthesia in children— exploring infusion regimens. Pediatr Anesth 2008;18:708–14 [272], with kind permission from John Wiley and Sons)

Adverse Effects

The most common adverse reaction to ketamine anaesthesia is postoperative vomiting, which occurs in 33 % of children after doses used for anaesthesia [329]. Intraoperative and postoperative dreaming and hallucinations occur more commonly in older than in younger children [329]. The incidence of these latter adverse effects may be reduced when ketamine is supplemented with a benzodiazepine.

Atropine or another antisialagogue is commonly used to diminish the production of copious secretions that occur with ketamine. If an antisialagogue is not administered, there is a greater risk for laryngospasm [330], although guidelines for emergency departments suggest that supplementation with atropine or a benzodiazepine may not be necessary with lower doses [331–333]. Even small doses have the potential for apnoea or airway obstruction, particularly when combined with other sedating medications [334–336].

Ketamine increases heart rate, cardiac index and systemic blood pressure in adults [337]. In children, there is apparently no effect on pulmonary artery pressure provided that ventilation is controlled [338, 339]. Ketamine sedation has been shown to maintain peripheral vascular resistance, thus affecting intracardiac shunting less than propofol in children sedated for cardiac catheterisation [340]. Ketamine has negative inotropic effects in those who depend on vasopressors [341].

Ketamine may produce increases in intracranial pressure (ICP) as a result of cerebral vasodilation and may be contraindicated in children with intracranial hypertension. This concern regarding ICP has been challenged [342, 343]; control of respiration and consequent CO_2 ameliorate changes in ICP [344, 345]. A 30 % increase in IOP has also been noted; thus, ketamine may be potentially dangerous in the presence of a corneal laceration [346].

Animal studies have correlated ketamine treatment with increased neuronal apoptosis during rapid synaptogenesis after birth [347–349]. It is unclear whether these data can be extrapolated from animals to developing humans [350]. Similar observations in rodents have been made with isoflurane, nitrous oxide, benzodiazepines and other medications commonly used to provide sedation/analgesia and anaesthesia to infants.

Etomidate

Etomidate is a steroid-based hypnotic induction agent. It is metabolised principally by hepatic esterases. Concentrations associated with anaesthesia are 300–500 mcg/L. As with most induction agents, offset of effect is by redistribution; clearance is approximately 1000 mL/min/70 kg in children and adults.

Etomidate pharmacokinetics have been studied in children with a median age of 4 years (range 0.53–13.21 years) and weight 15.7 kg (7.5–52 kg). A three-compartment model found the most significant covariate was age, with increasing age having reduced size-adjusted CL, V_1 and V_3. The estimates of PK parameter (standardised to 70 kg adult) for a typical 4-year-old children were CL 1.50 L/min/70 kg, Q_2 1.95 L/min/70 kg, Q_3 1.23 L/min/70 kg, V_1 9.51 L/70 kg, V_2 11.0 L/70 kg and V_3 79.2 L/70 kg [351]. Similar to propofol, younger children require a larger etomidate bolus dose than older children to achieve equivalent plasma concentrations [351, 352].

Etomidate clearance is reduced in neonates and infants (postnatal age 0.3–11.7 months) with congenital heart disease. A two-compartment model with allometric scaling to a 70 kg adult revealed a CL 0.624 L/min/70 kg and Q 0.44 L/min/70 kg; central (V_1) and peripheral distribution volumes (V_2) were 9.47 L/70 kg and 22.8 L/70 kg, respectively. Interindividual variability was high (between 94 and 142 % for all parameters) attributable to maturation over the age span studied [353].

Etomidate is painful when administered intravenously. However, concerns regarding the risks of anaphylactoid reactions and suppression of adrenal function have resulted in most anaesthesiologists avoiding this induction agent in routine cases [354]. Novel etomidate derivatives without this adverse effect are under investigation [355]. Etomidate is very useful in children with head injury and those with an unstable cardiovascular status such as children with a cardiomyopathy because of the virtual absence of adverse effects on the haemodynamics or cardiac function [356, 357].

Opioids

Opioid agonists produce analgesia and respiratory depression by combining with μ- and κ-opioid receptors. The introduction of newer opioid drugs with short context-sensitive half-times has rekindled interest in the use of opioids to avoid the major cardiovascular effects of volatile agents.

Morphine

Brain uptake after intravenous dosing is slow due to poor lipid solubility and consequent slow passage across the blood–brain barrier. An equilibration half-time ($T_{1/2}k_{eo}$) of 16–23 min is reported for analgesia in adults [358–360]. Although a morphine concentration–response curve for analgesia has not been described for children [221], morphine may display similar pharmacodynamics for respiratory depression and analgesia [361]. An $T_{1/2}k_{eo}$ estimate for the morphine respiratory depressant effect was 16 min in a child [362], similar to that reported for analgesia. The EC_{50} for morphine's respiratory depressant effect of 10–18 ng/mL [360–363] is consistent with clinical observations for both analgesic concentrations (10–20 ng/mL) [364–366] and respiratory depression (hypercapnia in 46 % children with concentration >15 ng/mL) [92].

Empiric studies have taught us that a concentration range (10–20 mcg/L) has analgesic effect [364] without associated adverse effects such as the respiratory depression observed with higher concentrations [92] or postoperative nausea and vomiting reported with higher doses [243]. Fears of adverse effects, particularly respiratory depression, dictate that morphine dose is titrated to gain satisfactory analgesia [367, 368]. A regime such as a loading dose of 50 mcg/kg followed by 25 mcg/kg at 5 min intervals to control pain is a satisfactory method [369]. A smaller dose of 20 mcg/kg is used in neonates. The drug remains remarkably safe when used as an infusion in hospital practice. The overall incidence of serious harm was only 1:10 000 with opioid infusion techniques, and those predisposed to harm can be identified (e.g. young infants, those with neurodevelopmental, respiratory or cardiac comorbidities) [370, 371].

Infusion regimens are based on clearance. Conjugation with glucuronide (UGT2B7) produces both active (morphine-6-glucuronide) and inactive (morphine-3-glucuronide) metabolites, which are excreted by the kidneys [372]. Clearance increases from 3.2 L/h/70 kg at 24 weeks PMA to 19 L/h/70 kg at term, reaching adult values (80 L/h/70 kg) at 6–12 months (Fig. 25.17) [163, 372]. Oral bioavailability is approximately 35 %.

Fig. 25.30 Age-based infusion dosing for morphine with a target average steady-state concentration of 10 mcg/L in children not receiving positive pressure ventilation. The *dotted line* is the predictions based on age and typical weight for age. The *solid line* is the suggested practical infusion rate dose in mcg/kg/h at different postnatal ages. PNA years = (PMA weeks 40)/52. The *upper panel* shows dose related to postnatal age. The *lower panel* shows dose related to PMA (Reproduced from Anderson BJ, Holford NHG. Understanding dosing: children are small adults, neonates are immature children. Arch Dis Child 2013; 98: 737–44 [2], with kind permission from the BMJ Publishing Group)

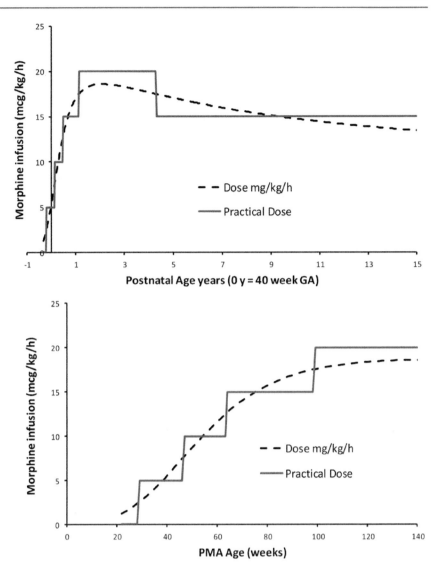

Infusion regimens that achieve a plasma concentration of 10 mcg/L can be predicted from clearance (Fig. 25.30). Morphine exhibits perfusion-limited clearance, and positive pressure ventilation, by reducing hepatic blood flow, also reduces clearance [163]. While hepatic failure may be an obvious cause for reduced clearance, it is little appreciated that renal failure may also reduce clearance by approximately 30 %. The kidney is also a major contributor to morphine–glucuronide conjugation [373–376]. Reduced morphine clearance has also been described in children with cancer [377, 378], following cardiac surgery [366], and in critically ill neonates requiring extracorporeal membrane oxygenation (ECMO) [44, 379], although contributions from hepatic failure, renal compromise or positive pressure ventilation towards these reduced clearances were not acknowledged.

Around 60 % of morphine is converted to morphine-3-glucuronide (M3G) and a further 6–10 % to morphine-6-glucuronide (M6G). M6G also has both analgesic and respiratory depressive effects. Animal data suggest that morphine and M6G act via distinct μ-receptor pathways and that an additive relationship exists between morphine and M6G for analgesic effects [380, 381]. The M6G $T_{1/2}k_{eo}$ for respiratory depression is within the 4–8 h range [362], similar to reported for delayed M6G analgesic effect [360]. The hypercapnoeic ventilator responses for both parent and metabolite are similar (EC_{50} 10–18 ng mL^{-1}) [360–363]. The response curve steepness (represented by the *Hill* parameter of 2.4) for morphine and M6G was also similar in a case study [362]; this has also been noted by others examining the hypercapnoeic ventilator [360] and pupillary responses to morphine and M6G [382]. Respiratory depression in a child with renal failure who was given morphine postoperatively was best described by additive morphine and M6G respiratory effects (Fig. 25.31).

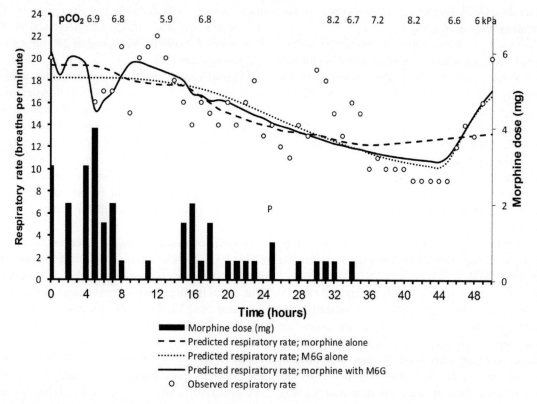

Fig. 25.31 Observed and predicted respiratory rate for a 12-year-old male child with end-stage renal failure given intravenous morphine via patient-controlled analgesia pump for postoperative pain. Predicted respiratory rates are for morphine only, M6G only and combined morphine–M6G effect. Observed partial pressure of CO_2 (κPa) is also given. Dialysis began at 45 h postoperatively (indicated by *arrow*) and continued for 3 h. (Reproduced from Hannam J, Anderson BJ. Contribution of morphine and morphine 6-glucuronide to respiratory depression in a child. Anaesth and Intens Care 2012;40:867–70 [362], with the kind permission of the Australian Society of Anaesthetists)

Fentanyl

Fentanyl is a synthetic opioid with lipid solubility about 600 times greater than that of morphine. High lipid solubility confers increased potency, rapid onset ($T_{1/2}k_{eo}$ 6.6 min in adults) and short duration of action. Fentanyl is a potent μ-receptor agonist with potency 100 times greater than that of morphine. A plasma concentration of 15–30 mcg/L is required to provide total intravenous anaesthesia (TIVA) in adults, whereas the EC_{50}, based on EEG evidence, is 10 mcg/L [383, 384]. After a dose of 1–2 μg/kg, the clinical effects of fentanyl are terminated by redistribution, and its duration of action is limited to 20–30 min. However, after repeated doses or a continuous infusion, progressive saturation of peripheral compartments will result in prolonged duration of action.

Fentanyl is metabolised by oxidative *N*-dealkylation (CYP3A4) into norfentanyl and hydroxylated fentanyl. Clearance in preterm neonates is markedly reduced ($T_{1/2}$ β is 17.7 h) contributing to prolonged respiratory depression in that population. The clearance of fentanyl is reduced to 70–80 % of adult values in term neonates and, when standardised using allometry, reaches adult values (approx. 50 L/h/70 kg) within the first 2 weeks of life [84]. Clearance of fentanyl in older infants (>3 months of age) and children is greater than in adults when expressed as per kilogram (30.6 mL/kg/min vs. 17.9 mL/kg/min, respectively) resulting in a reduced elimination half-time ($T_{1/2}$ β 68 min vs. 121 min, respectively). These age-related changes follow the expected pattern portrayed in Fig. 25.10. Fentanyl clearance may be impaired with decreased hepatic blood flow (e.g. from increased intra-abdominal pressure in neonatal omphalocele repair); a maldistribution of blood away from regions of concentrated cytochrome enzyme activity in the liver may also play a role [385]. Fentanyl's volume of distribution at steady state (V_{dss}) is ~5.9 L/kg in term neonates and decreases with age to 4.5 L/kg during infancy, 3.1 L/kg during childhood and 1.6 L/kg in adults [78].

Infants with cyanotic heart disease had reduced V_{ss} and greater plasma concentrations of fentanyl with infusion therapy [386]. These greater plasma concentrations resulted from a reduced clearance (34 L/h/70 kg) that was attributed to haemodynamic disturbance and consequent reduced hepatic blood flow [387]. Hypothermia has also been shown to reduce fentanyl clearance [388].

The infusion rates of fentanyl that are required to achieve a similar level of sedation/analgesia in critically ill children may vary as much as tenfold [389]. This variability in PK and PD strongly reinforces the need to titrate the dose to effect and to be prepared to provide postoperative ventilation support as needed. The context-sensitive half-time (CSHT) after a 1 h infusion of fentanyl is ~20 min, which increases to 270 min after an 8 h infusion in adults [27]. While the CSHT is reduced in children [390], there are no data in neonates. Children who receive a chronic infusion of fentanyl are at risk of rapidly developing tolerance to the opioid. On discontinuance of the infusion, these children may demonstrate signs of withdrawal. All long-term infusions should be tapered slowly over days rather than abruptly discontinuing the infusion [391, 392].

Chest wall and glottic rigidity have been reported after IV administration of all opioids, although most commonly after fentanyl [393, 394] One other concern is the rare association of increased vagal tone with bolus administration; bradycardia may have profound effects on the cardiac output of neonates. Additionally, fentanyl markedly depresses the baroreceptor reflex control of heart rate in neonates [395]. It is for these reasons that the combination of pancuronium and fentanyl became popular.

Remifentanil

Remifentanil is an ultrashort-acting synthetic opioid. Because of its ester linkage, it is susceptible to hydrolysis by nonspecific blood and tissue esterases. Its major metabolite is a carbolic acid compound with less than 0.3 % of the activity of the parent compound. Unlike other opioids, the duration of effect of remifentanil does not increase with increasing dose or duration of infusion, because its volume of distribution is small and its clearance is fast.

The target concentration may vary depending on the magnitude of desired effect. A remifentanil target of 2–3 mcg/L is adequate for laryngoscopy and 6–8 mcg/L for laparotomy, and 10–12 mcg/L might be sought to ablate the stress response associated with cardiac surgery [396]. Analgesic concentrations are 0.2–0.4 µg/L. Onset is rapid with a $T_{1/2}k_{eo}$ is 1.16 min in adults [20]. Remifentanil clearance can be described in all age groups by simple application of an allometric model [23]. A standardised clearance of 2790 mL/min/70 kg is similar to that reported by others in children and adults. The smaller the child, the greater the clearance when expressed as mL/min/kg (Fig. 25.21). Clearance decreases with increasing age, with rates of 90 mL/kg/min in infants <2 years of age, 60 mL/kg/min in children 2–12 years of age and 40 mL/kg/min in adults. The steady-

state volume of distribution was greatest in infants <2 months age (452 mL/kg) and decreased to 308 mL/kg in children 2 months–2 years and to 240 mL/kg in children >2 years of age [22].

Although covariate effects such as cardiac surgery appear to have a muted effect on PK, cardiopulmonary bypass (CPB) does have an impact. Remifentanil dosage adjustments are required during and after CPB due to marked changes in its volume of distribution [397]. Other PK changes during CPB are consistent with adult data in which a decreased metabolism occurred with a reduced temperature [398] and with reports of greater clearance after CPB (increased metabolism) compared with during CPB [24].

Respiratory depression is concentration dependent [399, 400]. Muscle rigidity remains a concern with bolus doses above 3 mcg/kg used for intubation in neonates [401]. The initial loading dose of remifentanil may cause hypotension and bradycardia [402] prompting some to target the plasma rather than effect site concentration when initiating infusion. This hypotensive response has been quantified in children undergoing cranioplasty surgery. A steady-state remifentanil concentration of 14 mcg/L would typically achieve a 30 % decrease in mean arterial blood pressure (Fig. 25.32). This concentration is twice that required for laparotomy, but is easily achieved with a bolus injection. The $T_{1/2}k_{eo}$ of 0.86 min for this haemodynamic effect [66] is less than remifentanil-induced spectral edge changes described in adults ($T_{1/2}k_{eo}$ = 1.34 min) [20, 403].

Adult remifentanil PK parameters [20] continue to be used in TCI devices for all ages, despite an increasing knowledge about this drug in children [21]. There is an element of safety with this approach because both volume of distribution [22] and clearance (expressed as mL min^{-1} kg^{-1}) [23] decrease with age throughout childhood and because the elimination half-time is small with a constant context-sensitive half-time. The larger volume of distribution results in lower peak concentrations after bolus; the higher clearance in children results in lower plasma concentration when infused at adult rates expressed as mg min^{-1} kg^{-1}. Owing to these enhanced clearance rates, smaller (younger) children will require higher remifentanil infusion rates than larger (older) children and adults to achieve equivalent blood concentrations.

The usual infusion dose of remifentanil is 0.1–0.5 µg/kg/min. The short elimination half-time frequently makes a loading dose unnecessary and facilitates control of the infusion. In a multicenter trial in full-term infants aged less than 2 months, remifentanil provided stable haemodynamic conditions with no new onset of postoperative apnoea [404]. Analgesic alternatives should be available for when the short-duration analgesic effect from remifentanil has dissipated. Reports of a rapid development

Fig. 25.32 The relationship between remifentanil concentration and mean arterial blood pressure (MAP) for a typical individual. A steady-state remifentanil concentration of 14 mcg/L would typically achieve a 30 % decrease in mean arterial blood pressure (Reproduced from Anderson BJ, Holford NHG. Leaving No Stone Unturned, Or Extracting Blood from Stone? Pediatr Anesth 2010;20:1–6 [403], with kind permission from John Wiley and Sons)

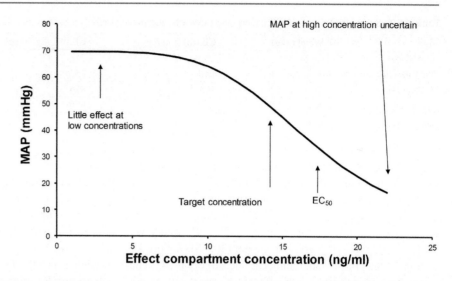

of μ-receptor tolerance with remifentanil use are conflicting. Activity at δ-opioid receptors may contribute [405].

Respiratory depression is concentration dependent [399, 400]. Muscle rigidity may occur when bolus doses above 3 μg/kg are used for intubation in neonates [401]. Remifentanil may cause hypotension and bradycardia at higher doses.

Alfentanil

Alfentanil (Alfenta) is a fentanyl analogue with reduced lipid solubility and smaller V compared with fentanyl [406, 407]. It has a rapid onset ($T_{1/2}k_{eo}$ 0.9 min in adults), a brief duration of action and one fourth the potency of fentanyl. A target plasma concentration of 400 ng/mL is used in anaesthesia. Metabolism is through oxidative N-dealkylation by CYP3A4 and O-dealkylation and then conjugation to end products that are excreted via the kidney [408].

Clearance in neonates (20–60 mL/min/70 kg) is one tenth that in adults (250–500 mL/min/70 kg) [74] with rapid maturation. In preterm neonates, the half-life is as long as 6–9 h [409, 410]. The V in children and adults is similar, but increased in preterm neonates (1.0 SD 0.39 vs. 0.48 SD 0.19 L/kg). Clearance is greater in children expressed as per kilogram (11.1 SD 3.9 mL/kg/min vs. 5.9 SD 1.6 mL/kg/min). As a result, the elimination half-life in children is less than adults (63 SD 24 vs. 95 SD 20 min) [411–414]. Clinical effects are prolonged in those with reduced hepatic blood flow (e.g. increased intra-abdominal pressure, vasopressor use, some forms of congenital heart disease) [415, 416]. Because less alfentanil is bound to $α_1$-acid glycoprotein in preterm infants (65 %) than in term infants (79 %), an increased fraction of alfentanil is available for biologic effect in the former [417].

The pharmacokinetics and pharmacodynamics of alfentanil have proven useful for the rapid control of analgesia and awakening from total intravenous anaesthesia [418, 419]. Alfentanil should be used with caution without neuromuscular blocking drugs in neonates because of the frequency of rigidity [420, 421].

Sufentanil

Sufentanil is a potent synthetic opioid that is similar to fentanyl and alfentanil. Sufentanil is five to ten times more potent than fentanyl, with a $T_{1/2}k_{eo}$ of 6.2 min in adults [422]. A concentration of 5–10 ng/mL is required for TIVA and 0.2–0.4 ng/mL for analgesia. Pharmacodynamic differences are suggested in neonates. The plasma concentration of sufentanil at the time of additional anaesthetic supplementation to suppress haemodynamic responses to surgical stimulation was 2.51 mcg/L in neonates, significantly greater than the concentrations of 1.58, 1.53 and 1.56 mcg/L observed in infants, children and adolescents, respectively [423].

The volume of distribution at steady state (V_{ss}) was 4.15 SD 1.0 L/kg in neonates, greater than the values of 2.73 SD 0.5 and 2.75 SD 0.5 L/kg observed in children and adolescents, respectively [423, 424]. Elimination of sufentanil has been suggested by O-demethylation and N-dealkylation in animal studies. Like fentanyl and alfentanil, the P450 CYP3A4 enzyme is responsible for N-dealkylation [425]. Clearance in neonates undergoing cardiovascular surgery (6.7 SD 6.1 mL/kg/min) is reduced compared with values of 18.1 SD 2.7, 16.9 SD 3.2 and 13.1 SD 3.6 mL/kg/min in infants, children and adolescents, respectively (Table 25.7) [423], consistent with rapid development of hepatic metabolic pathways. Clearance maturation standardised to a 70 kg person using allometry is similar to that of other drugs that depend on CYP3A4 for metabolism

Table 25.7 Sufentanil PK in children undergoing cardiovascular procedures

Age	Weight (kg)	CL (mL/min/kg)	CL (mL/kg/70 kg)	V (L/kg)	V (L/70 kg)
1–30 days	3.24	6.7	218	4.15	290.5
2–23 months	8.7	18.1	752	3.09	216.3
3–11 years	21.0	16.9	876	2.73	191.1
48–70 years	58.4	13.1	876	2.75	192.5

Data from Greeley WJ. Anesth Analg 1987; 66: 1067–72

(e.g. levobupivacaine, fentanyl, alfentanil) [426]. Similarly, clearance in infants (27.5 SD 9.3 mL kg^{-1} min^{-1}) was greater, expressed as per kilogram, than those in children (18.1 SD 10.7 mL kg^{-1} min^{-1}) in another study of children undergoing cardiovascular surgery [427]. Clearance in healthy children (2–8 years) was greater (30.5 SD 8.8 mL kg^{-1} min^{-1}) than those undergoing cardiac surgery [424]. The elimination of sufentanil is unaffected by renal failure but markedly altered by factors that influence hepatic blood flow (perfusion-limited clearance) [424]; cirrhosis has little effect on its elimination [428].

Reported adverse effects are similar to those described for other opioids, bradycardia, nausea and vomiting, chest wall rigidity and respiratory depression.

Intranasal sufentanil may have a role for premedication, procedural sedation and analgesia in children, although data in neonates are lacking [328, 429–431]. The dose of sufentanil that is most effective when administered intranasally is 2–3 mcg/kg [430, 432], although reduced dose can be used if combined with nasal ketamine [328]; this combination also reported fewer adverse effects.

Meperidine (Pethidine)

Meperidine is a weak opioid, primarily μ-receptor, agonist that has a potency of 1/10 that of morphine. The analgesic effects are detectable within 5 min of intravenous administration, and peak effect is reached within 10 min in adults [433, 434]. Meperidine is metabolised by N-demethylation to meperidinic acid and normeperidine. Meperidine clearance in infants and children is approximately 8–10 mL/min/kg [421, 435] Elimination in neonates is greatly reduced, and elimination half-time in neonates, who have received pethidine by placental transfer, may be two to seven times greater than that in adults [436]. The elimination half-life of meperidine in children after IV administration is approximately 3 SD 0.5 h with a variable half-life in neonates between 3.3 and 59.4 h. The V_{ss} in infants, 7.2 (3.3–11) L/kg [421], is greater than that in children 2–8 years of 2.8 SD 0.6 L/kg [435].

The principal current use of meperidine (pethidine, Demerol) in children is to stop postoperative shivering. Although its onset time is more rapid than morphine, there is a risk of seizures after repeated dosing due to accumulation of the metabolite normeperidine (norpethidine) [437]. Clinical use is decreasing as a consequence. The impression that meperidine causes less histamine release than morphine has been questioned [438]. Meperidine is no more effective for treating biliary or renal tract spasm than comparative μ-opioids [439]. The purported benefits of substituting meperidine for morphine in children who are hypovolemic or asthmatic are questionable.

Respiratory depression in infants after meperidine appears to be less than after morphine [91], probably a consequence of an increased V_{ss} in that age group. Meperidine was used for a number of years as a component of various 'lytic cocktails' that provided sedation. It was administered either rectally or orally. The safety of these admixtures especially in neonates is dubious, and use is now infrequent [266]. Meperidine's local anaesthetic properties have been found useful for epidural techniques [440].

Hydromorphone

Hydromorphone is a semisynthetic congener of morphine with a potency of around 5–7.5 times that of morphine [441]. Hydromorphone is metabolised to hydromorphone-3-glucuronide and also, to a lesser extent, to dihydroisomorphine and dihydromorphine [442]. Its bioavailability is about 55 % after nasal and oral administration and about 35 % after rectal administration (not recommended) [443–445]; there is high first-pass metabolism [446]. A clearance of 51.7 (range, 28.6–98.2) mL/min/kg is reported in children [447] with a half-life of 2.5 SD 0.9 h [443–445, 447].

Hydromorphone (Dilaudid) is commonly used when prolonged analgesia is required. Morphine is often changed to hydromorphone to reduce adverse effects or because of concern of accumulation of morphine metabolites, particularly in the presence of renal failure. Hydromorphone is commonly administered IV, orally, in the epidural space and more recently through the nasal mucosa [448, 449]. Hydromorphone is used for chronic cancer pain, and plasma concentrations of around 4.7 ng/mL (range 1.9–8.9 ng/mL) relieve mucositis in children given PCA devices [441, 447].

Oxycodone

Oxycodone is an analgesic with a minimal effective concentration of 25 mcg/L and a target concentration of 45–50 mcg/L for postoperative pain relief [64, 450]. Oxycodone (OxyContin) is another long-acting semisynthetic opioid that is usually administered orally and is available in a controlled-release formulation [451]. The relative bioavailability of intranasal, oral and rectal formulations was approximately 50 % that of intravenous in adults. The buccal and sublingual absorption of oxycodone is similar in young children [452]. The bioavailability after various routes IM is 68 %; buccal, 55 %; and orogastric, 37 % [453]. Oxycodone may also be administered rectally, with a similar bioavailability, although absorption can be slow [454]. The IV formulation of oxycodone significantly depresses respiration. Transmucosal deliver offers another route of administration [455]. Oxycodone (0.1 mg per kg) in children after ophthalmic surgery caused greater ventilatory depression than other opioids [456]. This respiratory depression was also evident in neonates breastfed by mothers treated with oxycodone. Maternal exposure to oxycodone during breastfeeding was associated with a 20.1 % rate of neonate CNS depression compared with 0.5 % in those given acetaminophen and 16.7 % in those given codeine [457].

As with many medications, interindividual variability in the elimination half-life of oxycodone in the neonates and infants is large [458, 459]. In children, the elimination half-life after IV, buccal, IM or orogastric administration is 2–3 h [460]. Oxycodone is metabolised mainly by CYP3A4 with a small contribution from CYP2D6 [461]. Mean values of drug clearance and volume of distribution (V_{ss}) were 15.2 (SD 4.2) mL/min/kg and 2.1 (SD 0.8) L/kg in children after ophthalmic surgery [456].

This opioid is commonly used to transition from patient-controlled analgesia and to treat chronic painful conditions.

Methadone

Methadone is a synthetic opioid with an analgesic potency similar to that of morphine but with a more rapid distribution and a slower elimination. Methadone is used as a maintenance drug in opioid-addicted adults to prevent withdrawal. Methadone might have beneficial effects because it is a long-acting synthetic opioid with a very high bioavailability (80 %) by the enteral route. It also has NMDA receptor antagonistic activity. Agonism of this receptor is associated with opioid tolerance and hyperalgesia. Methadone is a racemate and clinical effect is due to the R-methadone isomer. Methadone is 2.5–20 times more analgesic than morphine [462]. Methadone has high lipid solubility (octanol–water partition coefficient $LogP = 3.93$), similar to fentanyl ($LogP = 4.05$) and sufentanil ($LogP = 3.95$) [109], and such drugs rapidly distribute into fat tissues (including that in CNS).

The primary indication for methadone in children is to wean from long-term opioid infusions to prevent withdrawal [392, 463, 464] and to provide analgesia when other opioids have failed or have been associated with intolerable side effects [465, 466]. Intravenous methadone has been shown to be an effective analgesic for postoperative pain relief [467], and oral administration has been recommended as the first-line opioid for severe and persistent pain in children [468]. It seems also to be a safe enteral alternative for intravenous opioids in palliative paediatric oncological patients [469].

A minimum effective analgesic concentration of methadone in opioid-naïve adults is 0.058 mg/L [470], while no withdrawal symptoms were observed in neonates suffering opioid withdrawal if plasma concentrations of methadone were above 0.06 mg/L [471]. The racemate of methadone which is commonly used in paediatric and anaesthetic care is metabolised to EDDP (2-ethylidine-1,5-dimethyl-3,3-diphenylpyrrolidine) and EMDP (2-ethyl-5-methyl-3,3-diphenylpyrroline).

Methadone is cleared by the cytochrome P450-mixed oxidase (CYP3A4, CYP2B6 and CYP2D6) enzyme systems, all of which are immature at birth [144]. CYP3A7 may contribute to clearance in the neonate [158]. Foetal liver microsomes are reported to show extremely high CYP3A7 levels (311–158 pmol mg^{-1} protein), and there is significant expression through to 6 months postnatal age; the decrease in activity mirrors the rise of CYP3A4 activity [158]. Methadone has high lipid solubility [472] with a large volume of distribution of 6–7 L/kg in children and adults [473–475]. Pharmacokinetic parameters, standardised to a 70 kg adult using allometry, have been estimated using a three-compartment linear disposition model. Population parameter estimates (between-subject variability) were central volume (V_1) 21.5 (29 %) L 70 kg^{-1}, peripheral volumes of distribution V_2 75.1 (23 %) L 70 kg^{-1}, V_3 484 (8 %) L 70 kg^{-1}, clearance (CL) 9.45 (11 %) L h^{-1} 70 kg^{-1} and inter-compartment clearances Q2 325 (21 %) L h^{-1} 70 kg^{-1} and Q3 136 (14 %) L h^{-1} 70 kg^{-1}. EDDP formation clearance was 9.1 (11 %) L h^{-1} 70 kg^{-1}, formation clearance of EMDP from EDDP 7.4 (63 %) L h^{-1} 70 kg^{-1}, elimination clearance of EDDP 40.9 (26 %) L h^{-1} 70 kg^{-1} and the rate constant for intermediate compartments 2.17 (43 %)/h [143]. These parameter estimates in children and neonates are consistent with those reported by others in neonates [476], children [475], adolescents [477] and adults [478]. There was no clearance maturation with age (Fig. 25.16). Neonatal enantiomer clearances were also similar to those described in adults [143].

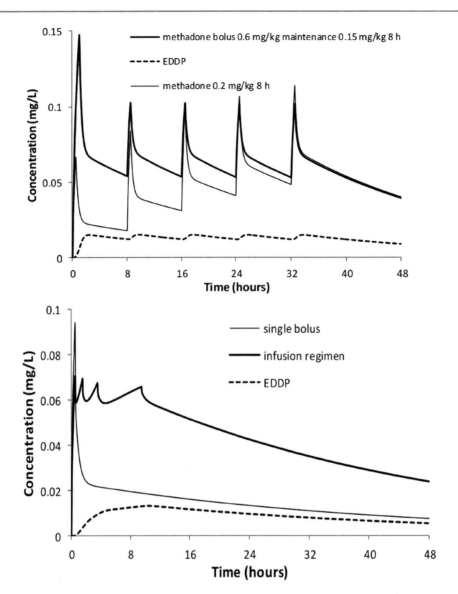

Fig. 25.33 The *upper panel* shows a simulation for a 3.5 kg neonate given a methadone loading dose of 0.6 mg kg^{-1} followed by a maintenance dose of 0.15 mg kg^{-1} 8 h. EDDP concentrations track parent drug concentrations. The methadone target concentration of 0.06 mg L^{-1} is achieved rapidly when compared to the neonate given 0.2 mg kg^{-1} 8 hourly without a loading dose. A single dose of methadone 0.2 mg kg^{-1} given for postoperative analgesia in a child is unlikely to achieve long duration of analgesia because concentrations are below 0.03 mg kg^{-1} within 1.5 h (*lower panel*). Infusion may be a better option. A regimen comprising methadone bolus 0.15 mg kg^{-1} followed by 0.15 mg kg^{-1} h^{-1} for 1 h, 0.075 mg kg^{-1} h^{-1} for 2 h and 0.025 mg kg^{-1} h^{-1} for 6 h maintains a concentration of 0.06 mg L^{-1}. EDDP concentrations after this infusion regimen are also shown. (Reproduced from Ward RM, Drover DR, Hammer GB, Stemland CJ, Kern S, Tristani-Firouzi M, Lugo RA, Satterfield K, Anderson BJ. The pharmacokinetics of methadone and its metabolites in neonates, Infants and children. Pediatr Anesth 2014;24: 591–601 [143], with kind permission from John Wiley and Sons)

A IV regimen of 0.2 mg kg^{-1} per 8 h in neonates achieves a target concentration of 0.06 mg L^{-1} within 36 h. Infusion, rather than intermittent dosing, should be considered if this target is to be achieved in older children after cardiac surgery. Analgesic response in adults on chronic methadone programmes suggests a steep concentration–response relationship for pain relief (Hill = 4.4 SD 3.8) with very rapid equilibration between plasma methadone concentrations and the sites mediating pain relief [479]. Consequently, the drug rapidly loses effect as concentrations fall below the EC$_{50}$. A single dose of 0.2 mg kg^{-1} will contribute little analgesia after a few hours. An infusion (Fig. 25.33) has been suggested for analgesia in teenagers after spinal instrumentation surgery [477], and consideration could be given to this technique after cardiac surgery in children.

Drug-induced prolongation of the QT interval is a recognised risk factor for ventricular arrhythmias. While methadone is known to prolong the QT interval, the effect of methadone on QTc is associated with chronic dosing in adults rather than an isolated dose, and it is the daily methadone dose that correlates positively with the QTc interval [480, 481].

Codeine

Codeine, or methylmorphine, is a morphine-like opioid with 1/10 the potency of morphine. It is mainly metabolised by glucuronidation, but minor pathways are N-demethylation to norcodeine (10–20 %) and O-demethylation (CYP2D6) to morphine (5–15 %) [170]. Although maturation of codeine clearance with age has not been reported, it is expected to follow that of morphine because glucuronidation is the major pathway, where maturation is mostly complete by 1 year of age [45].

Approximately 10 % of codeine is metabolised to morphine. As the affinity of codeine for opioid receptors is very low, the analgesic effect of codeine is mainly due to its metabolite, morphine [170]. Codeine is effectively a prodrug analgesic. There is little evidence for the broad belief that codeine causes fewer adverse effects, such as sedation and respiratory depression, compared with other opioids [170]. The continued use of this minor opium alkaloid for paediatric analgesia remains baffling and is subject to debate because it is a prodrug [482].

The primary routes for delivery of codeine are oral and IM. Intravenous codeine was used in the past, but serious life-threatening adverse effects including transient but severe cardiorespiratory depression [483–485] and seizures [486] led to proscription of this route of delivery.

Blood concentrations after oral codeine peak by 1 h. When given by the IM and rectal routes, peak blood concentrations are achieved rapidly, within 0.5 h, with the blood concentrations after the rectal route being less than after the IM route. The duration of action after these two routes of administration is 1–2 h.

The terminal elimination half-life is 3–3.5 h in adults. The neonatal half-life is longer due to immature clearance (e.g. 4.5 h), while that of an infant is shorter (e.g. 2.6 h) [168] attributable to size factors [74]. The pharmacokinetics of codeine are poorly described in children despite use over decades. A volume of distribution (V) of 3.6 L/kg and a clearance (CL) of 0.85 L/h have been described in adults, but there are few data detailing the developmental changes in children.

Recent reporting of mortality in children given codeine after adenotonsillectomy has raised questions about the use of this drug [482, 487, 488]. Deaths after codeine administration for postoperative tonsillectomy pain have been linked to ultrarapid metabolism of this drug [172, 489–491]. This has contributed to questioning the use of this drug in children after adenotonsillectomy [482, 487, 488] who have increased opioid sensitivity due to sleep apnoea [492]. Recent deaths in children administered codeine after adenotonsillectomy have led to further questioning whether this drug has a role on paediatric anaesthesia.

Codeine may be effective for pain control, although its limited conversion to morphine likely makes it suitable for only mild and moderate forms of pain. The limited conversion to morphine and fewer side effects of codeine made it popular for infants and young children, particularly when a single dose is involved. There is some evidence that codeine is associated with less nausea and vomiting than morphine [493]. Codeine is often used in combination with acetaminophen or NSAIDs. The addition of codeine to acetaminophen has been shown to improve postoperative pain relief in infants [494]. The analgesic effect of the combination of acetaminophen (10–15 mg/kg) and codeine (1–1.5 mg/kg) was comparable to that of ibuprofen (5–10 mg/kg) in children after tonsillectomy [495].

Evidence from children who are poor metabolisers suggested that codeine is a less reliable analgesic than morphine and that the analgesia did not correlate with the phenotype or morphine blood concentration [496]. In poor metabolisers, codeine confers little or no analgesia, although adverse effects persist [497]. In ultrarapid metabolisers on the other hand, large incidences of adverse effects might be expected including apnoea, because of large plasma morphine concentrations. Administration (especially of codeine preparations with an antihistamine and a decongestant) in the neonate may cause intoxication [498].

Naloxone

Naloxone, the N-alkyl derivative of oxymorphone, is used to antagonise opioid-induced respiratory depression. Unlike its predecessors nalorphine and levallorphan, naloxone is a pure opioid antagonist. Both the respiratory and analgesic effects mediated by μ-and κ-receptors are reversed by naloxone. In adults, the plasma clearance of naloxone is high, the volume of distribution low and the elimination half-time short ($T_{1/2}$ 1–1.5 h). There have been no pharmacokinetic studies in children, but neonates have prolonged elimination ($T_{1/2}$ 3 h), presumably due to their reduced clearance due to glucuronide conjugation [499].

Naloxone has a relatively short duration of action (30–45 min), and supplementary doses may be required to maintain antagonism after an initial dose 5–10 mcg/kg IV. The American Academy of Pediatrics simplified the naloxone dosing for infants and children up to 5 years of age, recommending 100 mcg/kg and for children older than 5 years (>20 kg), 2 mg naloxone for emergencies [500]. Severe opioid overdose may be treated by a continuous infusion of naloxone [501].

Nonopioid Analgesics

Acetaminophen (Tylenol, Paracetamol)

Acetaminophen is a mild analgesic, but lacks anti-inflammatory effects. Prostaglandin H_2 synthetase (PGHS) is the enzyme responsible for metabolism of arachidonic acid to the unstable prostaglandin H_2. The two major forms of this enzyme are the constitutive PGHS-1 (COX-1) and the inducible PGHS-2 (COX-2). PGHS comprises of two sites: a cyclooxygenase (COX) and a peroxidise (POX) site. The conversion of arachidonic acid to PGG_2, the precursor of the prostaglandins (Fig. 25.34), depends on a tyrosine-385 radical at the COX site. Acetaminophen acts as a reducing cosubstrate on the POX site. Alternatively, acetaminophen effects may be mediated by an active metabolite (*p*-aminophenol). *P*-aminophenol is conjugated with arachidonic acid by fatty acid amide hydrolase and exerts its effect through cannabinoid receptors [502].

Time delays of approximately 1 h between peak concentration and peak effect have been reported [503, 504]. An estimate of a maximum effect was 5.17 (the greatest possible pain relief (VAS 0–10) would equate to an E_{max} of 10) and an EC_{50} of 9.98 mg/L [505]. The equilibration half-time ($T_{1/2}k_{eo}$) of the analgesic effect compartment has been reported as 50–60 min [505, 506]. A target effect compartment concentration of 10 mg/L was associated with a pain reduction of 2.6/10 in both children and neonates [505, 507].

An intravenous formulation of acetaminophen is available and rapidly gaining popularity in anaesthesia practice. There are two intravenous paracetamol formulations available, and care must be taken with choice of formulation [508]. While one is an acetaminophen formulation, the other, propacetamol (*N*-acetylpara-aminophenoldiethyl aminoacetic ester), is a water-soluble prodrug of acetaminophen that can be administered intravenously over 15 min. It is rapidly hydroxylated into acetaminophen (1 g propacetamol = 0.5 g acetaminophen) [509]. The relative bioavailability of rectal to oral acetaminophen formulations (rectal/oral) is approximately 0.5 in children, but the relative bioavailability is greater in neonates and approaches unity [103].

The absorption half-time of acetaminophen from the duodenum is rapid in children ($T_{1/2}$abs 4.5 min) who were given acetaminophen as an elixir [510]. The absorption half-time in infants under the age of 3 months was delayed ($T_{1/2}$abs 16.6 min), consistent with delayed gastric emptying in young infants [103, 510]. Rectal absorption is slow and erratic with large variability. For example, absorption parameters for the triglyceride base were an absorption half-time ($T_{1/2}$abs) of 1.34 h (CV 90 %) with a lag time before absorption of 8 min (CV 31 %). The absorption half-time for rectal formulations was prolonged in infants less than 3 months (1.51 times greater) compared with those in older children [511].

Sulphate metabolism is the dominant route of elimination in neonates, while glucuronide conjugation (UGT1A6) is dominant in adults. A total body clearance of 0.74 L/h/70 kg at 28 weeks PMA and 4.9 (CV 38 %) L/h/70 kg in full-term neonates after enteral acetaminophen has been reported using an allometric 3/4 power model [511]. Clearance increases over the first year of life (Fig. 25.17) and reaches 80 % of that in older children (16 L/h/70 kg) by 6 months postnatal age [103, 164]. Similar clearance estimates are reported in neonates after intravenous formulations of acetaminophen [512–514]. The relative bioavailability of the oral formulation is 0.9.

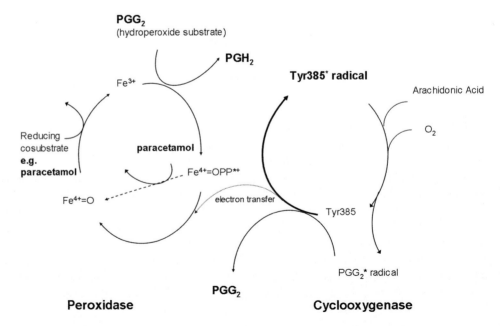

Fig. 25.34 Prostaglandin H_2 synthetase (PGHS) is the enzyme responsible for metabolism of arachidonic acid to the unstable prostaglandin H_2. Formation of tyrosine-385 radical (Tye385*) at the COX site is dependent on the reduction of a ferryl protoporphyrin IX radical cation ($Fe^{4+} = OPP^{*+}$) at the POX site. Acetaminophen is a reducing cosubstrate that partially reduces $Fe^{4+} = OPP^{*+}$, decreasing the amount available for regeneration of Tyr385*. (Reproduced from Anderson BJ. Paracetamol (acetaminophen) mechanisms of action. Pediatr Anesth 2008;18:915–21 [502], with kind permission from John Wiley and Sons)

The volume of distribution for acetaminophen is 49–70 L/70 kg. The volume of distribution decreases exponentially with a maturation half-life of 11.5 weeks from 109.7 L/70 kg at 28 weeks postconception to 72.9 L/70 kg by 60 weeks [103], reflective of foetal body composition and water distribution changes over the first few months of life.

The toxic metabolite of acetaminophen, N-acetyl-p-benzoquinone imine (NAPQI), is formed predominantly by the cytochrome P450 CYP2E1. This metabolite binds to intracellular hepatic macromolecules to produce cell necrosis and damage. Infants less than 90 days PNA have decreased expression of CYP2E1 activity in vitro compared with older infants, children and adults [515]. Neonates can produce hepatotoxic metabolites (e.g. NAPQI), but the reduced activity of cytochrome P450 in neonates may explain the rare occurrence of acetaminophen-induced hepatotoxicity in neonates. Hepatotoxicity is reported after single dose 250 mg/kg in children younger than 5 years of age [516] and after chronic dosing. The Rumack and Matthew [517] acetaminophen toxicity nomogram is widely used to guide management of acute acetaminophen overdose in adults and older children. Hepatotoxicity is dependent on the balance between the rate of NAPQI formation, the capacity of the safe elimination pathways of sulphate and glucuronide production and the initial content and maximal rate of synthesis of hepatic glutathione that mops up NAPQI. Significant hepatic and renal disease, malnutrition and dehydration may increase the propensity for toxicity. Medications that induce the NAPQI formation (e.g., phenobarbitone, phenytoin and rifampicin) may also increase the risk of hepatotoxicity. The influence of disease on acetaminophen toxicity is unknown. Hepatotoxicity causing death or requiring liver transplantation has been reported with doses above 75 mg/kg/day in children and 90 mg/kg/day in infants. It is possible that even these traditional regimens may cause hepatotoxicity if used for longer than 2–3 days [518].

Non-steroidal Anti-inflammatory Drugs

The non-steroidal anti-inflammatory drugs (NSAIDs) are a heterogeneous group of compounds that share common antipyretic, analgesic and anti-inflammatory effects. NSAIDs act by reducing prostaglandin biosynthesis through inhibition of cyclooxygenase (COX) site of the PGHS enzyme (Fig. 25.35).

The prostanoids produced by the COX-1 isoenzyme protect the gastric mucosa, regulate renal blood flow and induce platelet aggregation. NSAID-induced gastrointestinal toxicity, for example, is likely mediated through blockade of COX-1 activity, whereas the anti-inflammatory effects of NSAIDs are likely mediated primarily through inhibition of the inducible isoform, COX-2.

The NSAIDs are commonly used in children for antipyresis and analgesia. The anti-inflammatory properties of the NSAIDs have, in addition, been used in such diverse disorders as juvenile idiopathic arthritis, renal and biliary colic, dysmenorrhoea, Kawasaki disease and cystic fibrosis. The NSAIDs indomethacin and ibuprofen are also used to treat delayed closure of patent ductus arteriosus (PDA) in preterm infants.

Data from adults given ibuprofen after dental extraction suggest a similar E_{max} to that described for acetaminophen (1.54 of a scale 0–3) with an EC_{50} of 10.2 mg/L [519]. The equilibration half-time ($T_{1/2}k_{eo}$) of 28 min was less than the 53 min reported for acetaminophen [505]. In addition, the

Fig. 25.35 The conversion of arachidonic acid to PGG_2, the precursor of the prostaglandins is controlled by prostaglandin H_2 synthetase (PGHS). PGHS comprises of two sites: a cyclooxygenase (COX) site and a peroxidise (POX) site (From Anderson BJ. Paracetamol (acetaminophen) mechanisms of action. Pediatr Anesth 2008;18:915–21 [502], with kind permission from John Wiley and Sons)

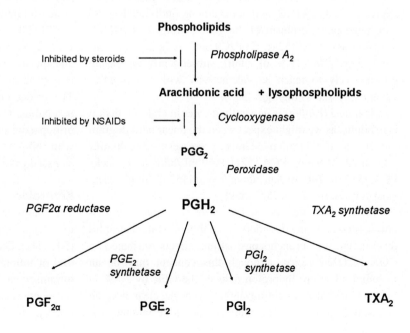

slope of the concentration–response curve was steeper than that for acetaminophen (Hill = 2 for ibuprofen, Hill = 1 for acetaminophen) indicating a more rapid onset of analgesia. Similar parameter estimates have been reported for diclofenac analgesia after adenotonsillectomy. The E_{max} was 4.9 (VAS 0–10) with an EC_{50} of 1.2 mg/L [520]. The equilibration half-time ($T_{1/2}k_{eo}$) of 14 min with a slope parameter (Hill) of 1 is again an indication of a more rapid onset of analgesia than paracetamol.

NSAIDs are rapidly absorbed in the gastrointestinal tract after oral administration in children. The relative bioavailability of oral preparations approaches unity. The rate and extent of absorption after rectal administration of NSAIDs such as ibuprofen, diclofenac, flurbiprofen, indomethacin and nimesulide are less than after the oral routes.

The apparent volume of distribution is small in adults (<0.2 L/kg) but larger in children. Preterm neonates (22–31 weeks gestational age) given intravenous ibuprofen had a volume of distribution of 0.62 (SD 0.04) L/kg [521]. There is a dramatic reduction in ibuprofen central volume after closure of the PDA in preterm neonates (0.244 vs. 0.171 L/kg) [522]. The NSAIDs, as a group, are weakly acidic, lipophilic and highly protein bound. The impact of altered protein binding is probably minimal with routine dosing because NSAIDs cleared by the liver have a low hepatic extraction ratio [523].

NSAIDs undergo extensive phase I and phase II enzyme biotransformation in the liver, with subsequent excretion into urine or bile. Renal elimination is not an important elimination pathway for the commonly used NSAIDs. Pharmacokinetic parameter variability is large, in part attributable to covariate effects of age, size and pharmacogenomics. Ibuprofen, for example, is metabolised by the CYP2C9 and CYP2C8 subfamily. Considerable variation exists in the expression of CYP2C activities among individuals, and functional polymorphism of the gene coding for CYP2C9 has been described [524]. CYP2C9 activity is low immediately after birth (21 % of adult), subsequently increasing progressively to reach a peak activity within 3 months, when expressed as mg/kg/h [525].

Clearance (L/h/kg) is generally greater in children than it is in adults, as we might expect when the linear per kilogram model is used. Ibuprofen clearance increases from 2.06 mL/h/kg at 22–31 weeks PCA [521], 9.49 mL/h/kg at 28 weeks PCA [522] to 140 mL/kg/min at 5 years [526]. Similar data exist for indomethacin [527–529].

NSAIDs have the potential to cause gastrointestinal irritation, blood clotting disorders, renal impairment, neutrophil dysfunction and bronchoconstriction; effects attributed to COX-1/COX-2 ratios, although this concept may be an oversimplification. Ibuprofen reduces the GFR by 20 % in preterm neonates, affecting aminoglycoside clearance, an effect that appears to be independent of gestational age

[530]. No significant difference in the change in cerebral blood volume, change in cerebral blood flow or tissue oxygenation index was found between administration of ibuprofen or placebo in neonates [531]. The risk of acute GI bleeding in children given short-term ibuprofen was estimated to be 7.2/100,000 (CI 2–18/100,000) [532, 533], a prevalence not different from children given acetaminophen. The incidence of clinically significant gastropathy in children with juvenile arthritis given NSAIDs is comparable to that in adults given long-term NSAIDs [534, 535], but the prevalence of gastroduodenal injury may be very much greater depending on the assessment criteria (e.g. abdominal pain, anaemia, endoscopy) applied. Aspirin or NSAID-exacerbated respiratory disease (ERD) is more a disorder of adults, but exacerbations in children and teenagers have been reported, particularly in the presence of chronic sinusitis [536]. These cases are countered by reports of beneficial reduction of asthma symptoms where ibuprofen was administered for antipyresis. Benefit is likely seen in younger children with mild episodic asthma and that aspirin ERD is a concern in one in three teenagers with severe asthma and coexistent nasal disease [537]. COX-2 inhibitors are reported as safe in NSAID-ERD [537].

The commonly used NSAIDs have reversible antiplatelet effects, which are attributable to the inhibition of thromboxane synthesis. Bleeding time is usually slightly increased, but remains within normal limits in children with normal coagulation systems. A Cochrane review has established that even after tonsillectomy, NSAIDs did not cause any increase in bleeding that required a return to theatre in children. There was significantly less nausea and vomiting with NSAIDs compared to alternative analgesics, suggesting their benefits outweigh their negative aspects [538]. Neonates given prophylactic ibuprofen to induce PDA closure did not have an increased frequency of intraventricular haemorrhage [539].

NSAIDs impair fracture healing in animal models. COX-2 activity plays an important role in bone healing, and the use of NSAIDs decreases osteogenic activity that may increase the incidence of nonunion after spinal surgery. The effect on osteogenic activity is dose-dependent and reversible. These effects are cause for concern after major orthopaedic surgery [540], but there was no risk of nonunion with NSAID exposure when high-quality studies were assessed [540].

Ketorolac

The analgesic properties of ketorolac are similar to those of low-dose morphine for post-tonsillectomy analgesia [541, 542]. Data from adult patients ($n = 522$) given a single oral or intramuscular administration of placebo or a single intramuscular dose of 10, 30, 60 or 90 mg ketorolac for postoperative pain relief after orthopaedic surgery revealed an E_{max} of 8.5/10, EC_{50} 0.37 mg L^{-1} and $T_{1/2}k_{eo}$ 24 min [543].

Table 25.8 Ketorolac age-related pharmacokinetic changes

Age (years)	Weight (kg)	V_{ss} (SD) (L/kg)	CL (SD) (L/min/kg)	CL_{std} (SD) (L/min/70 kg)
1–3	12	0.111 (0.025)	0.6 (0.2)	27.0 (9.0)
4–7	20	0.128 (0.047)	0.61 (0.22)	31.2 (11.3)
8–12	30	0.099 (0.014)	0.54 (0.15)	30.6 (8.5)
12–16	50	0.116 (0.040)	0.51 (0.12)	32.8 (7.7)
Adult [732]	70	0.11	0.3–0.55	21–38.5

V_{ss}, volume of distribution at steady state; CL_{std}, total body clearance standardised to a 70 kg person using an allometric 3/4 power model; weight is estimated. (Data are adapted from Dsida et al. Anesth Analg 2002;94:266–70)

Pharmacokinetics, standardised using allometry, are similar in adults and children (Table 25.8). The terminal elimination half-life in children 4–8 years of age is approximately 6 h [544]. Intranasal formulations have a bioavailability similar to IV, and PK parameter estimates are the same as those reported by others [123].

Pharmacokinetics may also be influenced by chronobiology [545], and many NSAIDs exhibit stereoselectivity [546, 547]. Ketorolac is supplied and administered as a racemic mixture that contains a 1:1 ratio of the $R(+)$ and $S(-)$ stereoisomers. Pharmacologic activity resides almost exclusively with the $S(-)$ stereoisomer [546, 548]. Clearance of the $S(-)$ enantiomer was four times that of the $R(+)$ enantiomer (6.2 vs. 1.4 mL min^{-1} kg^{-1}) in children 3–18 years [549]. Terminal half-life of $S(-)$-ketorolac was 40 % that of the $R(+)$ enantiomer (107 vs. 259 min), and the apparent volume of distribution of the $S(-)$ enantiomer was greater than that of the $R(+)$ form (0.82 vs. 0.50 L kg^{-1}). Recovery of $S(-)$-ketorolac glucuronide was 2.3 times that of the $R(+)$ enantiomer. Because of the greater clearance and shorter half-life of $S(-)$-ketorolac, pharmacokinetic predictions based on racemic assays may overestimate the duration of pharmacological effect [549].

One of the major concerns with ketorolac is the potential for postsurgical bleeding. The antiplatelet effect is reversible but remains a concern in children undergoing adenotonsillectomy. Most reports involved administration of the ketorolac during or at the beginning of the surgical procedure before haemostasis was achieved. Strom [550] has reported a dose–response relationship for this bleeding propensity; the risk associated with the drug was larger and clinically important when ketorolac was used in higher doses, in older subjects and for more than 5 days. Safety assessment showed no changes in renal or hepatic function tests, surgical drain output or continuous oximetry between groups given placebo 0.5 or 1 mg/kg at 6–18 h after surgery [546, 548]. Ketorolac can be used to treat pain after congenital heart surgery without an increased risk of bleeding complications [551]. Ketorolac has been safely used to provide analgesia for preterm and term neonates [552, 553]. Estimated PK parameters in infants (0.4–32 weeks PNA) using a two-compartment model were CL 67 mL/min/

70 kg, Q 11.5 mL/min, V_1 535 mL and V_2 322 mL [554]. The clearance values in these neonates and younger group of infants are surprisingly greater than that reported for older children and adults because metabolism is through hydroxylation and glucuronide conjugation [555], both of which are immature in infants.

One other concern is the report of sudden and profound bradycardia after rapid IV administration of ketorolac [556]. Although the mechanism of this response is unclear, ketorolac should be administered slowly when given intravenously.

Tramadol

Tramadol (Ultram) is a weak opioid with minimal effects on respiration and causes monoaminergic spinal cord inhibition of pain [557]. This formulation is structurally related to morphine and codeine. Two enantiomers provide analgesia; one is a mu-opioid receptor agonist, and the other inhibits neuronal reuptake of serotonin and inhibits norepinephrine uptake, thus producing 'multimodal antinociception'. It is primarily metabolised into O-desmethyltramadol (M1) by CYP2D6, with extensive polymorphism (see codeine) [178]. The active M1 metabolite has a mu-opioid affinity approximately 200 times greater than tramadol. Tramadol clearance increased from 25 weeks PMA (0.12 L/h/70 kg) to reach 90 % of the mature value (12.4 L/h/70 kg) by 52 weeks PMA (Fig. 25.20) [156, 558]. A target concentration of 300 mcg/L is proposed for effective analgesia [558]. Clearance in children is similar to that in adults, standardised using allometric models [156]. Tramadol has been shown to be effective for moderate to severe pain in a variety of paediatric populations and may offer some advantage for the treatment of pain after tonsillectomy in children with obstructive sleep apnoea [487, 559–561]. Tramadol (1.5–2 mg/kg) has been administered rectally with peak plasma concentrations occurring at approximately 2 h. The low incidence of respiratory depression and constipation, fewer controls on use and similar frequency of nausea and vomiting (10–40 %) compared to opioids make tramadol an attractive alternative [562].

Sedatives

Benzodiazepines

These drugs produce anxiolysis, amnesia and hypnosis. They are commonly used as adjuncts to both local and general anaesthesia. Benzodiazepines bind to $GABA_A$ receptors, resulting in increased cellular chloride entry. This renders these receptors resistant to excitation because they are hyperpolarised. Gamma-aminobutyric acid A receptor binding in human neonates is strikingly different from that in older children or adults and may contribute to age-related PD differences [191].

Midazolam

Midazolam is a water-soluble benzodiazepine that offers significant clinical advantages over diazepam. It is not painful when administered intravenously, and alternative routes are also available (intramuscular, orally, nasally, buccal and rectally). Midazolam offers a better pharmacokinetic profile than diazepam for neonates because the active metabolite has a half-life similar to the parent compound but with minimal clinical activity.

PKPD relationships have been described for intravenous midazolam in adults. When an EEG signal is used as an effect measure, the EC_{50} is 35–77 ng/mL, with a $T_{1/2}k_{eo}$ of 0.9–1.6 min described [563–565]. The $T_{1/2}k_{eo}$ is increased in the elderly and in low cardiac output states. PKPD relationships are more difficult to describe after oral midazolam because the active metabolite, 1-hydroxy metabolite (1-OHMDZ), has approximately half the activity of the parent drug [566].

Sedation in children is more difficult to quantify. No PKPD relationship was established in children 2 days–17 years who were given a midazolam infusion in intensive care. Midazolam dosing could, however, be effectively titrated to the desired level of sedation, assessed by the COMFORT scale [567]. Consistent with this finding, desirable sedation in children after cardiac surgery was achieved at mean serum concentrations between 0.1 and 0.5 mg/L [568–570]. Plasma concentrations of 0.3–0.4 mg/L are associated with anaesthesia in adults [571, 572]. A target concentration for sedation (rouses to command) in adults is 0.1 mg/L [573].

Midazolam is metabolised mainly by hepatic hydroxylation (CYP3A4) [153]. These hydroxy metabolites are glucuronidated and excreted in the urine. CYP3A7 is the dominant CYP3A enzyme in utero; it is expressed in the foetal liver and appears to have activity from as early as 50–60 days after conception (see methadone). CYP3A4 expression increases dramatically after the first week of life in term neonates, reaching 30–40 % of adult expression

by 1 month [426]. Midazolam has a hepatic extraction ratio in the intermediate range 0.3–0.7. Metabolic clearance depends on both liver perfusion and enzyme activity.

Clearance is reduced in neonates (0.8–2.2 mL/min/kg) [574–579], but increases rapidly after 39 weeks PMA [577] to reach 90 % mature clearance at 1 year of age. Mature CL was 523 (CV 32 %, 95 %CI 469, 597) mL/min/70 kg. The maturation half-time (TM_{50}) was 73.6 weeks PMA and the Hill coefficient 3 [580]. Central volume of distribution is related to weight (V_1 0.591 SD 0.065 L/kg), whereas peripheral volume of distribution remains constant (V_2 0.42 SD 0.11 L) in 187 neonates 0.7–5.2 kg [577]. It has been suggested that midazolam self-induces its own clearance [568]. The latter observation from infants after cardiac surgery likely results from the improved hepatic function after the insult of cardiopulmonary bypass. Neonates who require extracorporeal membrane oxygenation (ECMO) have an increase in V_{ss} during ECMO therapy (0.8 L/kg to 4.1 L/kg) caused by sequestration of midazolam by the circuitry, although clearance (1.4 SD 0.15 mL/min/kg) was unchanged [581].

Clearance may be reduced in the presence of pathology. A reduced clearance of midazolam has been reported after circulatory arrest for cardiac surgery [582]. Covariates such as renal failure, hepatic failure [570] and concomitant administration of CYP3A inhibitors [583] are important predictors of altered midazolam and metabolite pharmacokinetics in paediatric intensive care patients [567]. The clearance of midazolam was reduced by 30 % in neonates receiving sympathomimetic amines, probably as a consequence of the underlying compromised haemodynamics [577].

The desired clinical effects include anterograde amnesia (approximately 50 %) [584, 585] as well as sedation and anxiolysis before induction of anaesthesia or a medical procedure. Prolonged administration does lead to tolerance, dependency and benzodiazepine withdrawal [586]. Respiratory depression [587, 588], reduced pharyngeal muscle tone [589] and hypotension [590] are also well reported.

Diazepam

Diazepam is rapidly absorbed after oral administration, with peak plasma concentrations at 30–90 min; the absorption rate has been found to be more rapid in children than in adults [591, 592]. The greater fat solubility of diazepam compared to midazolam results in faster onset of effect (1.5 vs. 4.8 min) due to a more rapid transit into the CNS [565, 593–595]. It has been used extensively as a premedication, as an adjunct to balanced anaesthesia and for sedation, amnesia and control of seizures. Intramuscular administration is painful and results in irregular absorption

[596–598]. Rectal diazepam (0.2–0.5 mg/kg) is used for prehospital paediatric status epilepticus. The recommended IV dose is 0.1–0.2 mg/kg.

Diazepam undergoes oxidative metabolism by demethylation (CYP 2C19). Its active metabolite, desmethyldiazepam, has similar potency to the parent compound and with a half-life that is as long or longer than the parent compound [591, 599, 600]. Diazepam is highly plasma bound, with a serum half-life varying from 20 to 80 h in adults. Its half-life is reduced in younger adults and children (approximately 18 h) [601]. Studies in neonates who received diazepam transplacentally just before delivery demonstrate prolonged drug effects and serum half-lives (40–100 h), a result of immature hepatic excretory mechanisms [591, 602, 603].

Diazepam has capacity-limited clearance with low first-pass effect; hepatic disease may decrease the elimination of diazepam [604]. There was no relationship between diazepam plasma concentration and recall at induction in children [601], reflecting active metabolite effects. Diazepam has respiratory depressant effects that are quite variable, especially when combined with opioids. A major disadvantage when given intravenously is pain.

Flumazenil

Flumazenil (Romazicon) is a specific $GABA_A$ receptor competitive antagonist that reverses the effects of benzodiazepines. After a single IV dose, flumazenil shows limited protein binding (40 %) with an elimination half-life of approximately 1 h in adults owing primarily to rapid and extensive metabolism by hepatic carboxylesterases [605, 606]. In adults with severe liver disease, elimination of flumazenil is reduced [607]. In children (5–9 years), the elimination half-life after a single intravenous dose of 10 mcg/kg flumazenil followed by an infusion of 5 mcg/kg/min is 35 min [608]. Total plasma clearance was 20.6 SD 6.9 mL/min/kg and apparent volume of distribution at steady state 1.0 SD 0.2 L/kg. Nasal delivery has high bioavailability [117]. Oral flumazenil is also available, but its bioavailability is only 16 % owing to the first-pass effect in the liver [609].

In adults, a dose of 17 mcg/kg of flumazenil has antagonised benzodiazepine-induced sedation; studies in children have found doses of 24 mcg/kg to be clinically effective without evidence of re-sedation [608].

Alpha-2 Agonists

Dexmedetomidine

Dexmedetomidine is a pharmacologically selective α_2 agonist with sedative, anxiolytic and analgesic properties. Dexmedetomidine is a member of the same class of sedative/anxiolytic/analgesics as clonidine but differs from clonidine in that its affinity for α_2 compared with α_1 receptors is eightfold greater. In anaesthesia and intensive care, this agent is currently used as an IV sedative agent for procedural sedation and as an anaesthetic adjunct during surgery. It may also be administered by nasal, buccal, rectal and oral routes.

Sympathetic adrenoceptors are categorised as either α_1 or α_2 receptors, based on receptor selectivity. The latter are further subdivided into three subtypes: α_{2A}, α_{2B} and α_{2C} adrenoceptors according to ligand binding. The α_2 agonists such as dexmedetomidine bind all three receptor subtypes, although the common path for the effector response to dexmedetomidine is sympatholysis or suppression of the sympathetic nervous system. Depending on the specific receptor that is activated, α_2 agonists may cause hypotension, bradycardia, sedation, analgesia, attenuation of shivering and a number of other physiologic responses. Dexmedetomidine use in neonates and children has expanded to include prevention of emergence delirium, postoperative pain management, invasive and non-invasive procedural sedation and management of opioid withdrawal [610–618].

The α_2 adrenoceptors are located ubiquitously throughout the body. CNS manifestations of α_2 agonists include sedation and anxiolysis, both of which are mediated through the locus coeruleus. Sedation may also be mediated by α_2-agonist inhibition of the ascending norepinephrine pathways. Analgesia is mediated primarily via the spinal cord, although there is evidence that supraspinal and peripheral nerves may contribute to this effect as well. Cardiovascular manifestations of α_2 adrenoceptors include actions on the heart and on peripheral vasculature. The primary action of α_2 adrenoceptors on the heart is a chronotropic effect in which heart rate slows by blocking the cardioaccelerator nerves as well as by augmenting vagal activity. The α_2-agonist action on the autonomic ganglia includes decreasing sympathetic outflow, which leads to hypotension and bradycardia. Actions on the peripheral vasculature depend on the concentration of dexmedetomidine: vasodilatation is the result of sympatholysis, which occurs at low concentrations, and vasoconstriction is the result of direct action on smooth muscle vasculature at high concentrations (Fig. 25.36) [619, 620]. Other manifestations of α_2 adrenoceptors include inhibition of shivering as well as promoting diuresis, although the mechanisms by which these are affected remain elusive [621, 622].

A plasma concentration in excess of 0.6 mcg L^{-1} is estimated to produce satisfactory sedation in adult ICU patients [623], and similar target concentrations are estimated in children [624]. There was a 5 % incidence of hypertension in children presenting for sedation during radiological procedures; the incidence was greatest in those

Fig. 25.36 Composite E_{max} model, showing hyper- and hypotensive effect of dexmedetomidine on mean arterial blood pressure in children after cardiac surgery (**a**). The vasoconstrictor effect occurred with minimal time delay, while an equilibration half-time ($T_{1/2}k_{eo}$) of 9.66 min was estimated for the sympatholytic response. Combined hyper- and hypotensive effects of dexmedetomidine on mean arterial blood pressure are shown in (**b**). The *solid arrow* indicates the concentration at which the hypertensive effect begins; the *dashed arrow* indicates the concentration producing a 20 % increase in MAP from baseline (Reproduced from Potts AL, Anderson BJ, Holford NHG, Vu TC, Warman G. Dexmedetomidine haemodynamics in children after cardiac surgery. Pediatr Anesth 2010;20:425–33 [619], with kind permission from John Wiley and Sons)

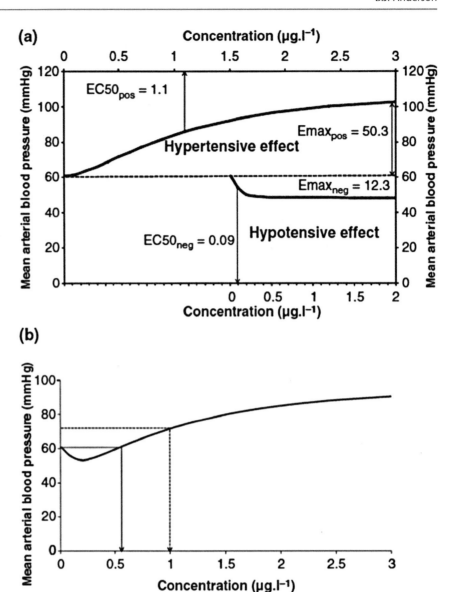

under 1 year of age and those who required an additional bolus dose to maintain sedation [625]. These cardiovascular effects of dexmedetomidine generate some concern. Dexmedetomidine decreases heart rate in a dose-dependent manner in children [626]. This effect is attributed to a centrally mediated sympathetic withdrawal, which results in unregulated cholinergic activity. Decreasing the dose of dexmedetomidine restores the heart rate to normal values. Administration of anticholinergics or other medications to increase the heart rate during dexmedetomidine-induced bradycardia have not usually been required. Less favourable results have been noted in the electrophysiology laboratory. Heart rate decreased, while arterial blood pressure increased significantly after 1 mcg/kg IV over 10 min followed by a 10 min continuous infusion of 0.7 mcg/kg/h. Sinus node function was significantly affected, and atrioventricular nodal function was also depressed. The use of

dexmedetomidine may not be desirable during electrophysiology study and may be associated with adverse effects in patients at risk for bradycardia or atrioventricular nodal block [627, 628]. It may have a role for the acute termination of reentrant supraventricular tachycardia [629, 630]. Ketamine, added to dexmedetomidine, mitigates sinus and atrioventricular nodal dysfunction [631].

Dexmedetomidine is metabolised in the liver by UGT1A4 and UGT2B10, aliphatic hydroxylation (CYP 2A6) and N-methylation. Population parameter estimates for a two-compartment model were clearance (CL) 42.1 (CV 30.9 %) L h^{-1} 70 kg^{-1}, central volume of distribution (V_1) 56.3 (61.3 %) L 70 kg^{-1}, inter-compartment clearance (Q) 78.3 (37.0 %) L h^{-1} 70 kg^{-1} and peripheral volume of distribution (V_2) 69.0 (47.0 %) L 70 kg^{-1}. Clearance increases from 18.2 L h^{-1} 70 kg^{-1} at birth in a full-term neonate to reach 84.5 % of the mature value by 1 year postnatal age (Figs. 25.11 and 25.18). Children given a dexmedetomidine infusion after cardiac surgery had reduced clearance (83.0 %) compared with a population given a bolus dose [624]. Similar parameter estimates with reduced clearance in children receiving dexmedetomidine infusion after cardiac surgery have been described by others [632]. Premature neonates (28–36 weeks) have further reduced clearance (5–11 L h^{-1} 70 kg^{-1}) and increased V_{ss} (189 L/70 kg) [633]. Parenteral delivery yielded similar kinetics to IV, buccal yielded an 82 % bioavailability and orogastric yielded only a 16 % bioavailability.

One of the major advantages of dexmedetomidine over other sedatives is its respiratory effects, which are minimal in adults and children [626]. Upper airway changes associated with increasing doses of dexmedetomidine (1–3 mcg/kg) in children with no OSA are small in magnitude and do not appear to be associated with clinical signs of airway obstruction [634]. Although similar upper airway changes were noted in children with known obstructive sleep apnoea given dexmedetomidine, airway support requirements were the same as in those given propofol 100 or 200 mcg/kg/min [635].

Dexmedetomidine provides a modest degree of analgesia, reducing the need for but not totally supplanting opioids and other analgesics [636]. Dexmedetomidine depresses sensory-evoked potentials, but, for the most part, the potentials are adequate for evaluations. Similarly, motor-evoked potentials are reduced in a dose-dependent manner during dexmedetomidine infusion but are measurable nonetheless. There are contrasting reports about the degree of evoked potential suppression, but most report successful spinal cord monitoring during scoliosis surgery [637–640]. Medications that attenuate the incidence of delirium after anaesthesia include dexmedetomidine and clonidine [641].

Clonidine

Clonidine is also commonly used in paediatric anaesthesia practice as a premedicant, as an adjunct to anaesthesia and analgesic agents, to reduce emergence delirium, as an antiemetic, for control of postoperative shivering, as supplement to regional blockade and for reduction of the stress response secondary to tracheal intubation and surgery [642]. Clonidine can be administered by the intravenous (IV), nasal, intramuscular, transdermal, oral, rectal and epidural routes [137, 643, 644].

The clonidine target concentration depends on the effect sought. A plasma clonidine concentration (range of 0.3–0.8 mcg/L) has been estimated as satisfactory for preoperative sedation in children 1–11 years [645]. Fifty percent of children achieve a modified Ramsay sedation score of 3 (appears asleep, purposeful responses to verbal commands at conversation level) at a concentration of 0.79 µg/L, and 90 % of children achieve this by 0.95 µg/L. The concentration required for 50 % of children to achieve a sedation scale of

4 (appears asleep, purposeful responses to verbal commands but at louder than usual conversation level or requiring light glabellar tap) or greater is slightly higher at 0.85 µg/L, and 90 % of children achieve this by 1.15 µg/L [646]. A BIS of less than 60 is associated with anaesthesia, and this is achieved with a concentration of 4 µg/L [647]. The target concentration for analgesia in adults is greater than that for sedation. Reduction of morphine use of up to 30 % is reported when clonidine is added to analgesic regimens [647, 648] with a plasma clonidine concentration of 1.5–2 mcg/L [649, 650]. The biphasic hypotensive/hypertensive blood pressure response, reported with dexmedetomidine [619], has also been demonstrated with clonidine. Falls in blood pressure were related to plasma concentration to 1.5–2 mcg/L, but at higher concentrations, the hypotensive effect was attenuated [651].

Approximately 50 % of clonidine is eliminated, unchanged by the kidney [651–653]. The exact amount of clonidine that undergoes hepatic biotransformation is uncertain, but has been reported to be between 40 and 60 % following IV administration [651–654]. The major metabolite of clonidine is p-hydroxyclonidine, formed by hydroxylation of the phenol ring which is present at <10 % of the concentration in the urine [652]. Cytochrome P450 2D6 is involved in this process.

Clearance estimates in children out of infancy are similar to those described in adults when standardised for size using allometric scaling (CL 12.8–16.7 L/h/70 kg). Population parameter estimates (between-subject variability) for a two-compartment model were clearance (CL) 14.6 (CV 35.1 %) L/h/70 kg, central volume of distribution (V_1) 62.5 (71.1 %) L/70 kg, inter-compartment clearance (Q) 157 (77.3 %) L/h/70 kg and peripheral volume of distribution (V_2) 119 (22.9 %) L/70 kg. Clearance at birth was 3.8 L/h/70 kg and matured with a half-time of 25.7 weeks to reach 82 % adult rate by 1 year of age (Fig. 25.37). Clearance in neonates is approximately one third that described in adults,

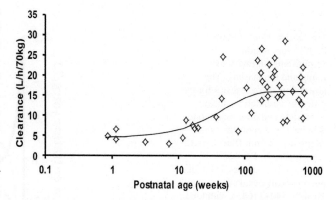

Fig. 25.37 Individual predicted clonidine clearances, standardised to a 70 kg person, from the NONMEM post hoc step, are plotted against postnatal age. The *solid line* represents the nonlinear relation between clearance and age (Reproduced from Potts AL, Larsson P, Eksborg S, Warman G, Lönnqvist P-A, Anderson BJ. Clonidine disposition in children: a population analysis. Pediatr Anesth 2007;17:924–33 [644], with kind permission from John Wiley and Sons)

consistent with immature elimination pathways [644]. The volumes of distribution, but not clearance, were increased after cardiac surgery (V_1 123 %, V_2 126 %). Context-sensitive half-times are shown in Table 25.9. There was a lag time of 2.3 (CV 73.2 %) min before absorption began in the rectum. The absorption half-life from the epidural space was slower than that from the rectum (0.98 CV 24.5 % h vs. 0.26 CV 32.3 % h). The relative bioavailability of epidural, nasal and rectal clonidine was unity ($F = 1$) [643, 644]. Oral bioavailability is reduced in children ($F = 0.55$) (Fig. 25.38) [137].

Neuromuscular Blocking Drugs

Neuromuscular Junction

Adult postjunctional acetylcholine receptors possess five subunits—two α, one β, δ and ϵ subunits. Preterm neonates (<31 weeks PMA) have a γ-subunit instead of an ϵ-subunit in their neuromuscular receptor [655]. Foetal receptors have a greater opening time than adult receptors, allowing more sodium to enter the cell with a consequent larger depolarising potential. Despite this larger depolarising potential, there are reduced acetylcholine stores in the terminal nerve endings [656]. Neonates have an increased sensitivity to NMBDs.

Neuromuscular transmission is immature in neonates and infants until the age of 2 months [657, 658]. Neonates deplete acetylcholine vesicle reserves more quickly than do infants >2 months old and in children [657] in response to tetanic nerve stimulation. Data from phrenic nerve–hemidiaphragm preparations from rats aged 11–28 days suggests this is due to a low quantal content of acetylcholine in neonatal endplate potentials [193]. Neonates display an increased sensitivity to NMBDs. An alternative proposal to explain this increased sensitivity is based on NMBD synergism observations [659, 660]. Neonates display poor synergism, and this has been explained on the basis that NMBDs occupy only one of the two α-subunit receptor sites in neonates as opposed to two in children and adults [660]. If this is true, then neonates may use NMBDs more efficiently than children.

Preterm infants tolerate respiratory loads poorly. The diaphragm in the preterm neonate contains only 10 % of the slowly contracting type I fibres. This proportion increases to 25 % at term and to 55 % by 2 years of age [661]. A similar maturation pattern has been observed for the intercostal muscles [661]. Type I fibres tend to be more sensitive to NMBDs than type II fibres, and consequently the diaphragmatic function in neonates may be better preserved and recover earlier than peripheral muscles [662–665].

NMBD volumes of distribution mirror changes in extracellular fluid (ECF) [77]. These are greatest in preterm neonates and decrease throughout gestation and postnatal life. Muscle contributes only 10 % of body weight in neonates and 33 % by the end of childhood. Increasing the muscle bulk contributes new acetylcholine receptors. This greater number of receptors requires a greater amount of drug to block activation of receptor ion channels.

Table 25.9 Steady-state concentration of tubocurarine for 50 % depression of twitch (C_{pss50}), steady-state volume of distribution (V_{ss}) and dose for 50 % depression of twitch (D_{50}) calculated from the other two parameters

	Cpss50 (mcg/mL)	V_{ss} (L/kg)	ED$_{50}$ (mcg/kg)
Neonates	0.18	0.74	155
Infants	0.27	0.52	158
Children	0.42	0.41	163
Adults	0.53	0.30	152

Data from Fisher et al. Anesthesiology 1982;57:203–8

Fig. 25.38 Concentration–time profiles for clonidine administered intravenously, orally and intranasally. The absorption characteristics for the different formulations dictate onset time and dose required to achieve target concentration (Reproduced from Blackburn L, Almenrader N, Larsson P, Anderson BJ. Intranasal clonidine pharmacokinetics. Pediatr Anesth 2014;24:340–2 [643], with kind permission from John Wiley and Sons)

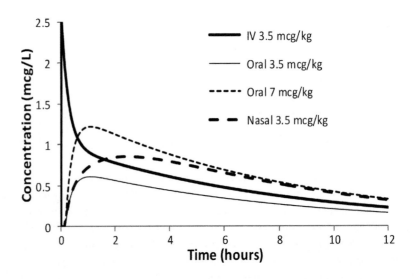

Fig. 25.39 Dose changes with age for vecuronium during balanced anaesthesia. ED_{50} is the dose that achieves 50 % of the maximum response, while ED_{95} is the dose that achieves 95 % of the maximum response (Data from Meretoja O. Anesth Analg 1988;67:21–6)

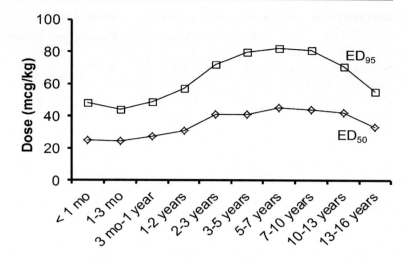

Table 25.10 Onset time of atracurium 0.3 mg/kg

Age group	Weight (kg)	Onset time (min)	Onset time std (min/70 kg)
Neonate <1 month	3.5	1.4	2.96
Infant <1 year	7	1.7	3.02
Child 3–10 years	25	2.3	2.97
Adult	70	2.8	2.8

Reproduced from Anderson BJ, McKee AD, Holford NH. Size, myths and the clinical pharmacokinetics of analgesia in paediatric patients. Clin Pharmacokinet 1997; 33: 313–327 [84], with kind permission from Springer

Pharmacodynamics

There is age-related variability in the dose required to achieve a predetermined level of neuromuscular blockade during balanced thiopental–N_2O–fentanyl anaesthesia. The ED_{95} of vecuronium is linked to muscle bulk: 47 SD 11 mcg/kg in neonates and infants, 81 SD 12 mcg/kg in children between 3 and 10 years of age and 55 SD 12 mcg/kg in patients aged 13 years or older (Fig. 25.39) [79]. Similar profiles have been reported for other NMBDs [664, 666–669]. The ED_{50} for rocuronium in infants 1–10 months was 0.63 mcg/mL compared to 1.2 mcg/mL in children and 0.95 mcg/mL in adults [670]. In addition, duration of neuromuscular blockade is greater in neonates than it is in children [671]. The reduced dose requirement in neonates is attributable to immaturity of the neuromuscular junction. The increased volume of distribution from an expanded ECF in neonates means a similar initial dose is given to neonates and teenagers. Investigation of concentration–response relationships is more revealing. The plasma concentration required in neonates to achieve the same level of neuromuscular block as in children or adults is 20–50 % less (Table 25.9) [80, 183, 672–674], consistent with immaturity of the neuromuscular junction. Plasma concentration requirements are reduced by volatile anaesthetic agents [675–677]. The use of halothane, isoflurane and sevoflurane in children 3–11 years resulted in lower rocuronium infusion requirements than the fentanyl–nitrous oxide. Rocuronium

requirement at 1 h from the commencement of anaesthesia was 16.7, 13.6, 13.1 and 8.4 mcg/kg/min for children receiving fentanyl–nitrous oxide, halothane, isoflurane and sevoflurane anaesthesia [678]. The EC50 of rocuronium was reduced from 2.32 mcg/mL with fentanyl–nitrous oxide anaesthesia to 1.41 mcg/mL with sevoflurane in children 3–11 years [679].

The onset time for NMBDs in neonates is faster than it is in older children than adults. Onset time (time to maximal effect) after vecuronium 70 mcg/kg was most rapid for infants (1.5 SD 0.6 min compared with that for children (2.4 SD 1.4 min) and adults (2.9 SD 0.2 min) [671]). These observations are similar to those reported for other intermediate- and long-acting NMBDs [662]. The more rapid onset of these drugs in neonates has been attributed to a greater cardiac output seen with the per kilogram model [662] and is consistent with allometric theory. Onset time, corrected using an exponent of 1/4 for time-related functions [75], is similar in all age groups (Table 25.10) [84].

The depolarising muscle relaxant, succinylcholine, is the only depolarising muscle relaxant in clinical use. Its structure resembles two molecules of acetylcholine joined back-to-back by an ester linkage. A unique combination of rapid onset and short duration of action make it especially useful for rapid sequence and emergency tracheal intubation.

Succinylcholine remains the NMBD with the more rapid onset. The onset time of a paralysing dose (1.0 mg/kg) of succinylcholine 1 mg/kg is 35–55 s in children and

Table 25.11 Age-related changes in the pharmacokinetics of tubocurarine

	Weight kg	CL mL/min/kg	CL surface area mL/min/m^2		CL allometric 3/4 mL/min/70 kg
(A) *Total body clearance*					
Neonate (1 day–2 months)	3.5	3.7 (2.1)	56 (32)		122 (70)
Infant (2 months–1 year)	7	3.3 (0.4)	59 (7)		130 (15)
Child (1–12 years)	22	4 (1.1)	110 (30)		210 (58)
Adult (12–30 years)	60	3 (0.8)	115 (31)		202 (54)
	Weight kg	V_{ss} L/kg	V_{ss} surface area L/m^2	V_{ss} allometric (power 1) L/70 kg	V_{ss} allometric (power 3/4) L/70 kg
(B) *Volume of distribution at steady state*					
Neonate	3.5	0.74 (0.33)	11 (5)	52 (23)	25 (11)
Infant	7	0.52 (0.22)	9 (4)	36 (15)	21 (9)
Child	22	0.41 (0.12)	11 (3)	29 (8)	22 (6)
Adult	60	0.3 (0.1)	12 (4)	21 (7)	20 (7)
	Chronological time (min)			Physiological time (min)		
	$T_{1/2\alpha}$	$T_{1/2\beta}$	$T_{1/2}k_{eo}$	$T_{1/2\alpha}$	$T_{1/2\beta}$	$T_{1/2}k_{eo}$
(C) *Half-times*						
Neonate	4.1 (2.2)	174 (60)	6.3 (3.5)	8.7 (4.7)	368 (127)	13.3 (7.4)
Infant	7.0 (4)	130 (54)	7.5 (3.5)	12.9 (7.4)	240 (100)	13.9 (6.5)
Child	6.7 (2.4)	90 (23)	7.9 (2.7)	8.9 (3.2)	120 (31)	10.6 (3.6)
Adult	7.9 (4.1)	89 (18)	6.8 (1.9)	8.2 (4.3)	93 (19)	7.1 (2.0)

Clearance (CL_{std}) and half-time ($T_{1/2\beta std}$, $T_{1/2\alpha}$) and volumes have been standardised to a 70 kg person using allometry
Data from Fisher et al. Anesthesiology 1982;57:203–8. Reproduced from Anderson BJ, Meakin GH. Scaling for size: some implications for paediatric anaesthesia dosing. Pediatr Anesth 2002;12;205–19 [74], with kind permission from John Wiley and Sons

Table 25.12 Pharmacokinetics of rocuronium in infants and children trials under sevoflurane (induction) and isoflurane/nitrous oxide (maintenance) anaesthesia

	CL (mL/kg/min)	CL_{std} (mL/min/70 kg)	V_{ss} (L/kg)	$T_{1/2\beta}$ (h)	$T_{1/2\beta std}$ (h/70 kg)
Neonates	0.31	10.26	0.42	1.1	2.33
28 days–3 months	0.30	10.86	0.31	0.9	1.74
3 months–2 years	0.33	14.20	0.23	0.8	1.30
2–11 years	0.35	18.94	0.18	0.7	0.91
11–17 years	0.29	19.53	0.18	0.8	0.83

Clearance has been standardised (CL_{std}) to a 70 kg person using allometry (Data from http://www.drugs.com/pro/rocuronium-bromide-injection.html)

adolescents. The onset time after 3 mg/kg in neonates is faster (30–40 s) [680]. Onset time is dependent on both age and dose; the younger the child and the greater the dose, the shorter the onset time. The onset times of equipotent doses of succinylcholine (0.9 min) and mivacurium (1.4 min) in infants (2–12 months) and children (1–12 years) are very similar [681]. Consequently an argument can be made for the use of larger dose of an intermediate-duration NMBD rather than succinylcholine for rapid sequence intubation. However, the use of increased dose of such drugs in the neonate will also prolong neuromuscular blockade. There is also potential for increased adverse effects (e.g. pain on injection, tachycardia). Phase II blockade may also develop with high or repeat succinylcholine dosing [682].

Succinylcholine may be given as an intramuscular injection for intubation in children [683]. There are few data available from neonates, but infant studies suggest that a dose of up to 5 mg/kg may be required to achieve satisfactory intubating conditions [684]. Onset to maximum blockade is slow (4 SD 6 min), and mean full recovery of T1

occurred in 15.6 SD 0.9 min after injection [684]. The slow onset time limits the usefulness of this technique. Intralingual or submental routes have also been used in children, but there are no neonatal data.

Pharmacokinetics

The clearance of *d*-tubocurarine, standardised to an allometric or surface area model, is reduced in neonates and infants compared with older children and adults (Table 25.11) [183]. These age-related clearance changes, standardised to a 70 kg person using allometry, follow age-related maturation of glomerular filtration in the kidney [59], which is the elimination route of *d*-tubocurarine. Total plasma clearances of other non-depolarising muscle relaxants cleared by renal (alcuronium) and/or hepatic pathways (pancuronium, pipecuronium, rocuronium and vecuronium) are all reduced in neonates [672, 673, 685–687]. Table 25.12 shows PK changes with age for rocuronium. In contrast, the clearances of atracurium and cisatracurium are neither renal nor hepatic-dependent bur rather depend on Hofmann elimination, ester hydrolysis and other unspecified pathways [688]. Clearance of these drugs is increased in neonates when expressed as per kilogram [185, 689, 690]. When clearance is standardised using allometric 3/4 power scaling, the clearances for atracurium and cisatracurium are similar throughout all age groups. The clearance of succinylcholine, expressed as per kilogram, also decreases as age increases [187, 188]. Succinylcholine is hydrolysed by butyrylcholinesterase. These observations are consistent with that observed for the clearance of remifentanil [23], which is also cleared by plasma esterases. These clearance pathways are mature at birth [39]. A deficiency of butyrylcholinesterase enzyme may result in prolonged block.

Conversion of d-tubocurarine half-times from chronological time to physiologic time is revealing (Tables 25.10 and 25.11). $T_{1/2}\alpha$ increases with age in chronological time, but in physiologic time it is the same at all ages, as we would expect from a distribution phase standardised by allometry. $T_{1/2}\beta$ decreases with age in physiologic time, consistent with reduced clearance related to volume in the very young. The $T_{1/2}k_{eo}$ is large in neonates and infants, reduced in children and further reduced in adults, possibly due to increased muscle bulk and concomitant increased muscle perfusion in older children and adults. The impact of halothane on prolonging $T_{1/2}k_{eo}$ of tubocurarine attributable to reduced muscle perfusion is reported in adults [254]. Similar results have been reported for rocuronium with sevoflurane anaesthesia in children. The $T_{1/2}k_{eo}$ increased from 2.9 min during fentanyl–nitrous oxide anaesthesia to 6.9 min when sevoflurane was administered [679].

Antagonism of Neuromuscular Blockade

Anticholinergics
Although edrophonium may establish a faster onset of effect, final recovery is invariably greater with neostigmine, which is why the latter is recommended for routine paediatric practice [691, 692]. The distribution volumes of neostigmine are similar in infants (2–10 months), children (1–6 years) and adults (V_{ss} 0.5 L/kg), whereas the elimination half-life is less in the paediatric patients [693]. Clearance decreases as age increases (13.6, 11.1, 9.6 mL/min/kg in infants, children and adults 29–48 years) [693] as we might expect from allometric scaling. The dose of neostigmine required to reverse d-tubocurarine blockade was 30–40 % less for infants and children than for adults (expressed as per kilogram) with duration of effect of neostigmine similar in both paediatric and adult patients. Other studies have confirmed that a train-of-four (TOF) ratio recovers to 0.7 in less than 10 min when a 90 % neuromuscular blockade from pancuronium is antagonised with neostigmine 30–40 mcg/kg in infants, children or adults [692, 694–696].

Neonates have the more rapid times to full recovery after neostigmine antagonism [692, 697]. For example, reversal of an atracurium-induced 90 % neuromuscular block in infants and children by neostigmine 50 mcg/kg was fastest in the youngest age group [691]. The time to a TOF ratio of 0.7 was 4 min in neonates and infants, 6 min in 2–10 years old children and 8 min in adolescents. These observations are consistent with allometric models for size [84].

Atropine
Atropine is commonly administered to manage the muscarinic effects of neostigmine. Atropine is metabolised in the liver by N-demethylation followed by conjugation with glucuronic acid [698]; both processes are immature in the neonate. Half the drug is also eliminated by the kidneys. An old technique to diagnose atropine poisoning was to put a drop of the victim's urine into the eye of a cat and observe for mydriasis! Clearance will be reduced in the neonatal age range because of an immaturity of renal and hepatic function. Allometric scaling of clearance in children less than 2 years of age was less than those older than 2 years of age (6.8 mL/min/kg, 270 mL/min/70 kg vs. 6.5 mL/min/kg, 330 mL/min/70 kg) [699]. The elimination half-life in healthy adults is 3 SD 0.9 h, while that in term neonates is four times this [699, 700].

Pharmacodynamic characterisation is similarly lacking in neonates. Atropine 0.1 mg is widely reported to be the minimum intravenous dose in neonates and young infants. The provenance of this recommendation is a single study in which two infants and three children suffered neither bradycardia nor sequelae after small serial doses of atropine [701]. The risk from adhering to this minimum dose is a relative overdose of atropine in very low birth weight and extremely premature infants. A dose of 5 mcg/kg intravenous atropine caused neither bradycardia nor asystole in young infants 4–6 months of age [702]. Systolic blood pressure did not change for any dose of atropine (5–40 mcg/kg) in a neonatal cohort [703].

Glycopyrrolate
Glycopyrrolate is a synthetic quaternary ammonium compound with potent anticholinergic properties. It offers some advantage over atropine and scopolamine because it minimally penetrates the blood–brain barrier and thus causes few CNS effects. Several studies have demonstrated that glycopyrrolate is superior to atropine because its anticholinergic effects are more prolonged, lasting several hours [704, 705]. Heart rate changes minimally after IV administration, causing fewer arrhythmias [706, 707]. In some children, gastric fluid volume and acidity are reduced after glycopyrrolate administration [708]. The drug remains popular for antagonising the parasympathomimetic effects of

neostigmine and is as effective as atropine for preventing the oculocardiac reflex [709].

There is poor absorption from the GI tract (10–25 %) [710]. Clearance in children aged less than 1 year ($n = 8$) was 1.01 (range 0.32–1.85) L/kg/h and V_{ss} 1.83 (range 0.70–3.87) L/kg, but there are no neonatal data. The renal system accounts for 85 % of elimination [704], and clearance is anticipated to be reduced in neonates because renal function is immature [59].

Sugammadex

Sugammadex is a new drug that reverses the NMB effects of rocuronium and, to a lesser extent, vecuronium. It has a cylinder-like cyclodextrin structure that irreversibly encapsulates rocuronium into its cavity. An early sugammadex study in children suggests that sugammadex 2 mg/kg reverses a rocuronium-induced moderate neuromuscular blockade in infants, children and adolescents [711]. The average time to recover a TOF ratio of 0.9 at the time of appearance of the second twitch response was 1.2, 1.1 and 1.2 min in children, adolescents and adults, respectively. Sugammadex is cleared through the renal system, and the elimination kinetics of rocuronium are known to be prolonged in renal failure [712]. Although GFR is immature in neonates, this is unlikely to be of consequence here. Sugammadex has been used in patients with end-stage renal failure [713, 714] with similar reversal characteristics as those with normal renal function.

Adverse Effects

Succinylcholine is the most pilloried NMBD despite its importance for rapid sequence intubation [715–717]. Its molecular structure resembles that of two acetylcholine molecules joined by an ester linkage. Consequently, stimulation of cholinergic autonomic receptors can be associated with cardiac arrhythmias, increased salivation and bronchial secretions. Muscle fasciculation is also associated with mild hyperkalaemia (0.2 nmol/L), increased intragastric and intraocular pressure, masseter spasm and skeletal muscle pains. Severe hyperkalaemia may occur in patients with burns, paraplegia, trauma or disuse atrophy. This may be associated with rhabdomyolysis and myoglobinaemia in those patients suffering neuromuscular disorders. These disorders are not always diagnosable in neonates. Congenital myotonic dystrophy, for example, may present with mild respiratory dysfunction or feeding difficulty in the neonate. The response to succinylcholine in these neonates, however, remains dramatic with sustained muscle contraction [718]. Succinylcholine is a trigger agent for malignant hyperthermia. Succinylcholine has a prolonged effect in children with butyrylcholinesterase deficiency. This is an inherited disease due to the presence of one or more abnormal genes (atypical, fluoride-resistant and silent genes) [719]. On the other hand, one genetic variant, the Cynthiana or Neitlich variant [720], represents an ultrarapid degradation of succinylcholine [721].

The non-depolarising NMBDs all have different adverse effects that are often used to therapeutic advantage. *d*-Tubocurarine may produce hypotension and bronchospasm after large doses and a rapid administration. Pancuronium confers sympathomimetic effects as a result of blocking the reuptake of noradrenaline; the resultant tachycardia may augment cardiac output during induction for cardiac surgery in neonates. Doses in excess of the ED_{95} of rocuronium have also proven popular for cardiac surgery to capitalise on its vagolytic activity that increases heart rate. Unfortunately, rocuronium also causes local pain when injected rapidly and may trigger anaphylaxis. Atracurium can liberate histamine precipitating bronchospasm and hypotension. These effects are attenuated with the isomer *cis*atracurium.

Antiemetics

Metoclopramide

Metoclopramide has been used in children for its antiemetic and gastric emptying properties [722]. The antiemetic properties result from its direct effects on the chemoreceptor trigger zone. Gastric emptying is a result of the antagonism of the neurotransmitter dopamine, which stimulates gastric smooth muscle activity [723]. Metoclopramide is less effective than 5-HT_3 inhibitors but does offer an alternative rescue medication [724]. As with many other medications cleared by sulphate and glucuronide conjugation (e.g. acetaminophen), the elimination half-life in neonates is prolonged compared with older children [725, 726]. Clearance in infants (0.9–5.6 months) was 0.67 SD 0.13 L/h/kg with V_{ss} 4.4 Sd 0.6 L/kg.

5-Hydroxytryptamine Type 3 Receptor (5-HT₃) Antagonists

This class of drugs includes ondansetron, granisetron, dolasetron and tropisetron. These agents have proven to be an effective preventive and therapeutic measure for postoperative nausea and vomiting (PONV). There is debate regarding which is the most effective, which has the better adverse effect profile, which lasts the longest, which is best combined with other agents and which costs too much (e.g. [727]). Ondansetron was the first in this class of serotonergic receptor antagonists that effectively reduced the incidence of nausea and vomiting in children [728].

Ondansetron clearance is by hydroxylation followed by glucuronide or sulphate conjugation in the liver. A mature clearance of 541 mL/min/70 kg is reported, but ondansetron CL was reduced by 31, 53 and 76 % for the typical 6-month-, 3-month-, and 1-month-old infant, respectively; clearance increased with a TM_{50} of 4 months. Simulations showed that an ondansetron dose of 0.1 mg/kg in children younger than 6 months produced exposure similar to a 0.15 mg/kg dose in older children [729].

References

1. Kearns GL, Abdel-Rahman SM, Alander SW, Blowey DL, Leeder JS, Kauffman RE. Developmental pharmacology—drug disposition, action, and therapy in infants and children. N Engl J Med. 2003;349(12):1157–67.
2. Anderson BJ, Holford NH. Understanding dosing: children are small adults, neonates are immature children. Arch Dis Child. 2013;98(9):737–44. doi:10.1136/archdischild-2013-303720.
3. Holford NHG. The target concentration approach to clinical drug development. Clin Pharmacokinet. 1995;29(5):287–91.
4. Benet LZ. A Holy Grail of clinical pharmacology: prediction of drug pharmacokinetics and pharmacodynamics in the individual patient. Clin Pharmacol Ther. 2009;86(2):133–4. doi:10.1038/clpt.2009.102.
5. West N, Dumont GA, van Heusden K, Petersen CL, Khosravi S, Soltesz K, Umedaly A, Reimer E, Ansermino JM. Robust closed-loop control of induction and maintenance of propofol anesthesia in children. Paediatr Anaesth. 2013;23(8):712–9. doi:10.1111/pan.12183.
6. Dumont GA, Ansermino JM. Closed-loop control of anesthesia: a primer for anesthesiologists. Anesth Analg. 2013;117(5):1130–8. doi:10.1213/ANE.0b013e3182973687.
7. McFarlan CS, Anderson BJ, Short TG. The use of propofol infusions in paediatric anaesthesia: a practical guide. Paediatr Anaesth. 1999;9(3):209–16.
8. Kataria BK, Ved SA, Nicodemus HF, Hoy GR, Lea D, Dubois MY, Mandema JW, Shafer SL. The pharmacokinetics of propofol in children using three different data analysis approaches. Anesthesiology. 1994;80(1):104–22.
9. van Heusden K, Ansermino JM, Soltesz K, Khosravi S, West N, Dumont GA. Quantification of the variability in response to propofol administration in children. IEEE Trans Biomed Eng. 2013;60(9):2521–9. doi:10.1109/tbme.2013.2259592.
10. Greenblatt DJ, Koch-Weser J. Clinical pharmacokinetics (second of two parts). N Engl J Med. 1975;293(19):964–70. doi:10.1056/NEJM197511062931905.
11. Greenblatt DJ, Kock-Weser J. Drug therapy. Clinical Pharmacokinetics (first of two parts). N Engl J Med. 1975;293(14):702–5. doi:10.1056/NEJM197510022931406.
12. Marsh B, White M, Morton N, Kenny GN. Pharmacokinetic model driven infusion of propofol in children. Br J Anaesth. 1991;67(1):41–8.
13. Gepts E, Camu F, Cockshott ID, Douglas EJ. Disposition of propofol administered as constant rate intravenous infusions in humans. Anesth Analg. 1987;66(12):1256–63.
14. Absalom A, Amutike D, Lal A, White M, Kenny GN. Accuracy of the 'Paedfusor' in children undergoing cardiac surgery or catheterization. Br J Anaesth. 2003;91(4):507–13.
15. Rigby-Jones AE, Nolan JA, Priston MJ, Wright PM, Sneyd JR, Wolf AR. Pharmacokinetics of propofol infusions in critically ill neonates, infants, and children in an intensive care unit. Anesthesiology. 2002;97(6):1393–400.
16. Anderson BJ. My child is unique; the pharmacokinetics are universal. Pediatr Anesth. 2012;22:530–8. doi:10.1111/j.1460-9592.2011.03788.x.
17. Minto C, Schnider T. Expanding clinical applications of population pharmacodynamic modelling. Br J Clin Pharmacol. 1998;46(4):321–33.
18. Sepulveda P, Cortinez LI, Saez C, Penna A, Solari S, Guerra I, Absalom AR. Performance evaluation of paediatric propofol pharmacokinetic models in healthy young children. Br J Anaesth. 2011;107(4):593–600. doi:10.1093/bja/aer198.
19. Rigouzzo A, Servin F, Constant I. Pharmacokinetic-pharmacodynamic modeling of propofol in children. Anesthesiology. 2010;113(2):343–52. doi:10.1097/ALN.0b013e3181e4f4ca.
20. Minto CF, Schnider TW, Egan TD, Youngs E, Lemmens HJ, Gambus PL, Billard V, Hoke JF, Moore KHP, Hermann DJ, Muir KT, Mandema JW, Shafer SL. Influence of age and gender on the pharmacokinetics and pharmacodynamics of remifentanil. Anesthesiology. 1997;86:10–23.
21. Marsh DF, Hodkinson B. Remifentanil in paediatric anaesthetic practice. Anaesthesia. 2009;64(3):301–8. doi:10.1111/j.1365-2044.2008.05731.x.
22. Ross AK, Davis PJ, Dear Gd GL, Ginsberg B, McGowan FX, Stiller RD, Henson LG, Huffman C, Muir KT. Pharmacokinetics of remifentanil in anesthetized pediatric patients undergoing elective surgery or diagnostic procedures. Anesth Analg. 2001;93(6):1393–401.
23. Rigby-Jones AE, Priston MJ, Sneyd JR, McCabe AP, Davis GI, Tooley MA, Thorne GC, Wolf AR. Remifentanil-midazolam sedation for paediatric patients receiving mechanical ventilation after cardiac surgery. Br J Anaesth. 2007;99(2):252–61.
24. Davis PJ, Wilson AS, Siewers RD, Pigula FA, Landsman IS. The effects of cardiopulmonary bypass on remifentanil kinetics in children undergoing atrial septal defect repair. Anesth Analg. 1999;89(4):904–8.
25. Egan TD. Remifentanil pharmacokinetics and pharmacodynamics. A preliminary appraisal. Clin Pharmacokinet. 1995;29(2):80–94.
26. Anderson BJ, Holford NH. Tips and traps analyzing pediatric PK data. Paediatr Anaesth. 2011;21(3):222–37. doi:10.1111/j.1460-9592.2011.03536.x.
27. Hughes MA, Glass PS, Jacobs JR. Context-sensitive half-time in multicompartment pharmacokinetic models for intravenous anesthetic drugs. Anesthesiology. 1992;76(3):334–41.
28. Wada DR, Drover DR, Lemmens HJ. Determination of the distribution volume that can be used to calculate the intravenous loading dose. Clin Pharmacokinet. 1998;35(1):1–7.
29. Anderson BJ, Allegaert K, Holford NH. Population clinical pharmacology of children: general principles. Eur J Pediatr. 2006;165(11):741–6.
30. Anderson BJ, Allegaert K, Holford NH. Population clinical pharmacology of children: modelling covariate effects. Eur J Pediatr. 2006;165(12):819–29.
31. Duffull S, Waterhouse T, Eccleston J. Some considerations on the design of population pharmacokinetic studies. J Pharmacokinet Pharmacodyn. 2005;32(3–4):441–57.
32. Peck CC, Sheiner LB, Nichols AI. The problem of choosing weights in nonlinear regression analysis of pharmacokinetic data. Drug Metab Rev. 1984;15(1 & 2):133–48.
33. Peck CC, Beal SL, Sheiner LB, Nichols AI. Extended least squares nonlinear regression: a possible solution to the "choice of weights" problem in analysis of individual pharmacokinetic parameters. J Pharmacokinet Biopharm. 1984;12(5):545–57.
34. Roberts FL, Dixon J, Lewis GT, Tackley RM, Prys Roberts C. Induction and maintenance of propofol anaesthesia. A manual infusion scheme. Anaesthesia. 1988;43(Suppl):14–7.
35. Tod M, Jullien V, Pons G. Facilitation of drug evaluation in children by population methods and modelling. Clin Pharmacokinet. 2008;47(4):231–43.

36. West GB, Brown JH, Enquist BJ. A general model for the origin of allometric scaling laws in biology. Science. 1997;276 (5309):122–6.

37. Anderson BJ, Holford NH. Mechanism-based concepts of size and maturity in pharmacokinetics. Annu Rev Pharmacol Toxicol. 2008;48:303–32.

38. Holford S, Allegaert K, Anderson BJ, Kukanich B, Sousa AB, Steinman A, Pypendop BH, Mehvar R, Giorgi M, Holford NH. - Parent-metabolite pharmacokinetic models for tramadol—tests of assumptions and predictions. J Pharmacol Clin Toxicol. 2014;2 (1):1023.

39. Welzing L, Ebenfeld S, Dlugay V, Wiesen MH, Roth B, Mueller C. Remifentanil degradation in umbilical cord blood of preterm infants. Anesthesiology. 2011;114(3):570–7. doi:10.1097/ALN. 0b013e318204e043.

40. Johnson TN. The problems in scaling adult drug doses to children. Arch Dis Child. 2008;93(3):207–11.

41. Edginton AN, Schmitt W, Voith B, Willmann S. A mechanistic approach for the scaling of clearance in children. Clin Pharmacokinet. 2006;45(7):683–704.

42. Hill AV. The possible effects of the aggregation of the molecules of haemoglobin on its dissociation curves. J Physiol. 1910;14:4–7.

43. Pokela ML, Olkkola KT, Seppala T, Koivisto M. Age-related morphine kinetics in infants. Dev Pharmacol Ther. 1993;20 (1–2):26–34.

44. Peters JW, Anderson BJ, Simons SH, Uges DR, Tibboel D. Morphine metabolite pharmacokinetics during venoarterial extra corporeal membrane oxygenation in neonates. Clin Pharmacokinet. 2006;45(7):705–14.

45. Anand KJ, Anderson BJ, Holford NH, Hall RW, Young T, Shephard B, Desai NS, Barton BA. Morphine pharmacokinetics and pharmacodynamics in preterm and term neonates: secondary results from the NEOPAIN trial. Br J Anaesth. 2008;101 (5):680–9.

46. Holford N, Heo YA, Anderson B. A pharmacokinetic standard for babies and adults. J Pharm Sci. 2013;102(9):2941–52. doi:10. 1002/jps.23574.

47. Johnson TN, Rostami-Hodjegan A, Tucker GT. Prediction of the clearance of eleven drugs and associated variability in neonates, infants and children. Clin Pharmacokinet. 2006;45(9):931–56.

48. Edginton AN, Theil FP, Schmitt W, Willmann S. Whole body physiologically-based pharmacokinetic models: their use in clinical drug development. Expert Opin Drug Metab Toxicol. 2008;4 (9):1143–52.

49. Encinas E, Calvo R, Lukas JC, Vozmediano V, Rodriguez M, Suarez E. A predictive pharmacokinetic/pharmacodynamic model of fentanyl for analgesia/sedation in neonates based on a semi-physiologic approach. Paediatr Drugs. 2013;15(3):247–57. doi:10.1007/s40272-013-0029-1.

50. Han PY, Duffull SB, Kirkpatrick CM, Green B. Dosing in obesity: a simple solution to a big problem. Clin Pharmacol Ther. 2007;82 (5):505–8.

51. Abernethy DR, Greenblatt DJ. Drug disposition in obese humans. An update. Clin Pharmacokinet. 1986;11(3):199–213.

52. Mulla H, Johnson TN. Dosing dilemmas in obese children. Arch Dis Child Educ Pract Ed. 2010;95(4):112–7. doi:10.1136/adc. 2009.163055.

53. Chidambaran V, Venkatasubramanian R, Sadhasivam S, Esslinger H, Cox S, Diepstraten J, Fukuda T, Inge T, Knibbe CA, Vinks AA. Population pharmacokinetic-pharmacodynamic modeling and dosing simulation of propofol maintenance anesthesia in severely obese adolescents. Paediatr Anaesth. 2015;25 (9):911–23. doi:10.1111/pan.12684.

54. Cortinez LI, Anderson BJ, Penna A, Olivares L, Munoz HR, Holford NH, Struys MM, Sepulveda P. Influence of obesity on propofol pharmacokinetics: derivation of a pharmacokinetic

model. Br J Anaesth. 2010;105(4):448–56. doi:10.1093/bja/ aeq195.

55. Schuttler J, Ihmsen H. Population pharmacokinetics of propofol: a multicenter study. Anesthesiology. 2000;92(3):727–38.

56. Diepstraten J, Chidambaran V, Sadhasivam S, Esslinger HR, Cox SL, Inge TH, Knibbe CA, Vinks AA. Propofol clearance in morbidly obese children and adolescents: influence of age and body size. Clin Pharmacokinet. 2012;51(8):543–51. doi:10.2165/ 11632940-000000000-00000.

57. Egan TD, Huizinga B, Gupta SK, Jaarsma RL, Sperry RJ, Yee JB, Muir KT. Remifentanil pharmacokinetics in obese versus lean patients. Anesthesiology. 1998;89(3):562–73.

58. Duffull SB, Dooley MJ, Green B, Poole SG, Kirkpatrick CM. A standard weight descriptor for dose adjustment in the obese patient. Clin Pharmacokinet. 2004;43(15):1167–78.

59. Rhodin MM, Anderson BJ, Peters AM, Coulthard MG, Wilkins B, Cole M, Chatelut E, Grubb A, Veal GJ, Keir MJ, Holford NH. Human renal function maturation: a quantitative description using weight and postmenstrual age. Pediatr Nephrol. 2009;24 (1):67–76. doi:10.1007/s00467-008-0997-5.

60. Allegaert K, Olkkola KT, Owens KH, Van de Velde M, de Maat MM, Anderson BJ. Covariates of intravenous paracetamol pharmacokinetics in adults. BMC Anesthesiol. 2014;14:77. doi:10. 1186/1471-2253-14-77.

61. Tham LS, Wang LZ, Soo RA, Lee HS, Lee SC, Goh BC, Holford NH. Does saturable formation of gemcitabine triphosphate occur in patients? Cancer Chemother Pharmacol. 2008;63(1):55–64. doi:10.1007/s00280-008-0707-9.

62. McCune JS, Bemer MJ, Barrett JS, Scott Baker K, Gamis AS, Holford NHG. Busulfan in infant to adult hematopoietic cell transplant recipients: a population pharmacokinetic model for initial and bayesian dose personalization. Clin Cancer Res. 2014;20(3):754–63. doi:10.1158/1078-0432.ccr-13-1960.

63. Janmahasatian S, Duffull SB, Ash S, Ward LC, Byrne NM, Green B. Quantification of lean bodyweight. Clin Pharmacokinet. 2005;44(10):1051–65.

64. Kokki M, Broms S, Eskelinen M, Rasanen I, Ojanpera I, Kokki H. Analgesic concentrations of oxycodone—a prospective clinical PK/PD study in patients with laparoscopic cholecystectomy. Basic Clin Pharmacol Toxicol. 2012;110(5):469–75. doi:10.1111/j. 1742-7843.2011.00839.x.

65. Jeleazcov C, Ihmsen H, Schmidt J, Ammon C, Schwilden H, Schuttler J, Fechner J. Pharmacodynamic modelling of the bispectral index response to propofol-based anaesthesia during general surgery in children. Br J Anaesth. 2008;100(4):509–16.

66. Standing JF, Hammer GB, Sam WJ, Drover DR. Pharmacokinetic-pharmacodynamic modeling of the hypotensive effect of remifentanil in infants undergoing cranioplasty. Paediatr Anaesth. 2011;20(1):7–18. doi:10.1111/j.1460-9592.2009.03174.x.

67. Dixon WJ. Efficient analysis of experimental observations. Annu Rev Pharmacol Toxicol. 1980;20:441–62.

68. Dixon WJ. Staircase bioassay: the up-and-down method. Neurosci Biobehav Rev. 1991;15(1):47–50.

69. Dawes J, Myers D, Gorges M, Zhou G, Ansermino JM, Montgomery CJ. Identifying a rapid bolus dose of dexmedetomidine (ED_{50}) with acceptable hemodynamic outcomes in children. Pediatr Anesth. 2014;24(12):1260–7. doi:10.1111/pan.12468.

70. Herd DW, Anderson BJ, Keene NA, Holford NH. Investigating the pharmacodynamics of ketamine in children. Paediatr Anaesth. 2008;18(1):36–42.

71. Hull CJ, Van Beem HB, McLeod K, Sibbald A, Watson MJ. A pharmacodynamic model for pancuronium. Br J Anaesth. 1978;50 (11):1113–23.

72. Sheiner LB, Stanski DR, Vozeh S, Miller RD, Ham J. Simultaneous modeling of pharmacokinetics and pharmacodynamics:

application to *D*-tubocurarine. Clin Pharmacol Ther. 1979;25 (3):358–71.

73. Holford NHG, Sheiner LB. Understanding the dose-effect relationship: clinical application of pharmacokinetic-pharmacodynamic models. Clin Pharmacokinet. 1981;6(6):429–53.

74. Anderson BJ, Meakin GH. Scaling for size: some implications for paediatric anaesthesia dosing. Paediatr Anaesth. 2002;12 (3):205–19.

75. West D, West BJ. Physiologic time: a hypothesis. Phys Life Rev. 2013;10(2):210–24. doi:10.1016/j.plrev.2013.04.006.

76. Cortinez LI, Troconiz IF, Fuentes R, Gambus P, Hsu YW, Altermatt F, Munoz HR. The influence of age on the dynamic relationship between end-tidal sevoflurane concentrations and bispectral index. Anesth Analg. 2008;107(5):1566–72. doi:10.1213/ane.0b013e318181f013.

77. Friis-Hansen B. Body water compartments in children: changes during growth and related changes in body composition. Pediatrics. 1961;28:169–81.

78. Johnson KL, Erickson JP, Holley FO, et al. Fentanyl pharmacokinetics in the paediatric population. Anesthesiology. 1984;61: A441.

79. Meretoja OA, Wirtavuori K, Neuvonen PJ. Age-dependence of the dose–response curve of vecuronium in pediatric patients during balanced anesthesia. Anesth Analg. 1988;67(1):21–6.

80. Fisher DM, Canfell PC, Spellman MJ, Miller RD. Pharmacokinetics and pharmacodynamics of atracurium in infants and children. Anesthesiology. 1990;73(1):33–7.

81. Luz G, Innerhofer P, Bachmann B, Frischhut B, Menardi G, Benzer A. Bupivacaine plasma concentrations during continuous epidural anesthesia in infants and children. Anesth Analg. 1996;82 (2):231–4.

82. Luz G, Wieser C, Innerhofer P, Frischhut B, Ulmer H, Benzer A. Free and total bupivacaine plasma concentrations after continuous epidural anaesthesia in infants and children. Paediatr Anaesth. 1998;8(6):473–8.

83. Erichsen CJ, Sjovall J, Kehlet H, Hedlund C, Arvidsson T. Pharmacokinetics and analgesic effect of ropivacaine during continuous epidural infusion for postoperative pain relief. Anesthesiology. 1996;84(4):834–42.

84. Anderson BJ, McKee AD, Holford NH. Size, myths and the clinical pharmacokinetics of analgesia in paediatric patients. Clin Pharmacokinet. 1997;33(5):313–27.

85. Calder A, Bell GT, Andersson M, Thomson AH, Watson DG, Morton NS. Pharmacokinetic profiles of epidural bupivacaine and ropivacaine following single-shot and continuous epidural use in young infants. Paediatr Anaesth. 2012;22(5):430–7. doi:10.1111/j.1460-9592.2011.03771.x.

86. Russo H, Bressolle F. Pharmacodynamics and pharmacokinetics of thiopental. Clin Pharmacokinet. 1998;35(2):95–134. doi:10.2165/00003088-199835020-00002.

87. Bjorkman S. Prediction of drug disposition in infants and children by means of physiologically based pharmacokinetic (PBPK) modelling: theophylline and midazolam as model drugs. Br J Clin Pharmacol. 2005;59(6):691–704.

88. Johnson TN, Tucker GT, Tanner MS, Rostami-Hodjegan A. Changes in liver volume from birth to adulthood: a meta-analysis. Liver Transpl. 2005;11(12):1481–93.

89. Schoning M, Hartig B. Age dependence of total cerebral blood flow volume from childhood to adulthood. J Cereb Blood Flow Metab. 1996;16(5):827–33. doi:10.1097/00004647-199609000-00007.

90. Chiron C, Raynaud C, Maziere B, Zilbovicius M, Laflamme L, Masure MC, Dulac O, Bourguignon M, Syrota A. Changes in regional cerebral blood flow during brain maturation in children and adolescents. J Nucl Med. 1992;33(5):696–703.

91. Way WL, Costley EC, Way EL. Respiratory sensitivity of the newborn infant to meperidine and morphine. Clin Pharmacol Ther. 1965;6:454–61.

92. Lynn AM, Nespeca MK, Opheim KE, Slattery JT. Respiratory effects of intravenous morphine infusions in neonates, infants, and children after cardiac surgery. Anesth Analg. 1993;77 (4):695–701.

93. Engelhardt B. Development of the blood–brain barrier. Cell Tissue Res. 2003;314(1):119–29. doi:10.1007/s00441-003-0751-z.

94. Persidsky Y, Ramirez SH, Haorah J, Kanmogne GD. Blood–brain barrier: structural components and function under physiologic and pathologic conditions. J Neuroimmune Pharmacol. 2006;1 (3):223–36. doi:10.1007/s11481-006-9025-3.

95. Henthorn TK, Liu Y, Mahapatro M, Ng KY. Active transport of fentanyl by the blood–brain barrier. J Pharmacol Exp Ther. 1999;289(2):1084–9.

96. Hamabe W, Maeda T, Kiguchi N, Yamamoto C, Tokuyama S, Kishioka S. Negative relationship between morphine analgesia and *P*-glycoprotein expression levels in the brain. J Pharm Sci. 2007;105(4):353–60.

97. Choudhuri S, Klaassen CD. Structure, function, expression, genomic organization, and single nucleotide polymorphisms of human ABCB1 (MDR1), ABCC (MRP), and ABCG2 (BCRP) efflux transporters. Int J Toxicol. 2006;25(4):231–59. doi:10.1080/10915810600746023.

98. Gupta M, Brans Y. Gastric retention in neonates. Pediatrics. 1978;62:26–9.

99. Grand RJ, Watkins JB, Torti FM. Development of the human intestinal tract: a review. Gastroenterology. 1976;70:790–810.

100. Liang J, Co E, Zhang M, Pineda J, Chen JD. Development of gastric slow waves in preterm infants measured by electrogastrography. Am J Physiol. 1998;274(3 Pt 1):G503–8.

101. Carlos MA, Babyn PS, Marcon MA, Moore AM. Changes in gastric emptying in early postnatal life. J Pediatr. 1997;130 (6):931–7.

102. Kearns GL, Robinson PK, Wilson JT, Wilson-Costello D, Knight GR, Ward RM, van den Anker JN. Cisapride disposition in neonates and infants: in vivo reflection of cytochrome P450 3A4 ontogeny. Clin Pharmacol Ther. 2003;74(4):312–25.

103. Anderson BJ, van Lingen RA, Hansen TG, Lin YC, Holford NH. Acetaminophen developmental pharmacokinetics in premature neonates and infants: a pooled population analysis. Anesthesiology. 2002;96(6):1336–45.

104. Pomeranz ES, Chudnofsky CR, Deegan TJ, Lozon MM, Mitchiner JC, Weber JE. Rectal methohexital sedation for computed tomography imaging of stable pediatric emergency department patients. Pediatrics. 2000;105(5):1110–4.

105. Burckart GJ, White 3rd TJ, Siegle RL, Jabbour JT, Ramey DR. Rectal thiopental versus an intramuscular cocktail for sedating children before computerized tomography. Am J Hosp Pharm. 1980;37(2):222–4.

106. Herd D, Anderson BJ. Lack of pharmacokinetic information in children leads clinicians to use experience and trial-and-error to determine how best to administer ketamine. Ann Emerg Med. 2007;49(6):824.e1. doi:10.1016/j.annemergmed.2006.11.036.

107. Mason KP, Lubisch N, Robinson F, Roskos R, Epstein MA. Intramuscular dexmedetomidine: an effective route of sedation preserves background activity for pediatric electroencephalograms. J Pediatr. 2012;161(5):927–32. doi:10.1016/j.jpeds.2012.05.011.

108. Mason KP, Lubisch NB, Robinson F, Roskos R. Intramuscular dexmedetomidine sedation for pediatric MRI and CT. AJR Am J Roentgenol. 2011;197(3):720–5. doi:10.2214/ajr.10.6134.

109. Grassin-Delyle S, Buenestado A, Naline E, Faisy C, Blouquit-Laye S, Couderc LJ, Le Guen M, Fischler M, Devillier P.

Intranasal drug delivery: an efficient and non-invasive route for systemic administration: focus on opioids. Pharmacol Ther. 2012;134(3):366–79. doi:10.1016/j.pharmthera.2012.03.003.

110. Hadley G, Maconochie I, Jackson A. A survey of intranasal medication use in the paediatric emergency setting in England and Wales. Emerg Med J. 2010;27(7):553–4. doi:10.1136/emj.2009.072538.

111. Kendall JM, Latter VS. Intranasal diamorphine as an alternative to intramuscular morphine: pharmacokinetic and pharmacodynamic aspects. Clin Pharmacokinet. 2003;42(6):501–13.

112. Kendall JM, Reeves BC, Latter VS. Multicentre randomised controlled trial of nasal diamorphine for analgesia in children and teenagers with clinical fractures. BMJ. 2001;322 (7281):261–5.

113. Kidd S, Brennan S, Stephen R, Minns R, Beattie T. Comparison of morphine concentration-time profiles following intravenous and intranasal diamorphine in children. Arch Dis Child. 2009;94 (12):974–8. doi:10.1136/adc.2008.140194.

114. Borland M, Jacobs I, King B, O'Brien D. A randomized controlled trial comparing intranasal fentanyl to intravenous morphine for managing acute pain in children in the emergency department. Ann Emerg Med. 2007;49(3):335–40. doi:10.1016/j.annemergmed.2006.06.016.

115. Borland M, Milsom S, Esson A. Equivalency of two concentrations of fentanyl administered by the intranasal route for acute analgesia in children in a paediatric emergency department: a randomized controlled trial. Emerg Med Australas. 2011;23(2):202–8. doi:10.1111/j.1742-6723.2011.01391.x.

116. Furyk JS, Grabowski WJ, Black LH. Nebulized fentanyl versus intravenous morphine in children with suspected limb fractures in the emergency department: a randomized controlled trial. Emerg Med Australas. 2009;21(3):203–9. doi:10.1111/j.1742-6723.2009.01183.x.

117. Scheepers LD, Montgomery CJ, Kinahan AM, Dunn GS, Bourne RA, McCormack JP. Plasma concentration of flumazenil following intranasal administration in children. Can J Anaesth. 2000;47 (2):120–4.

118. Rey E, Delaunay L, Pons G, Murat I, Richard MO, Saint-Maurice-C, Olive G. Pharmacokinetics of midazolam in children: comparative study of intranasal and intravenous administration. Eur J Clin Pharmacol. 1991;41(4):355–7.

119. Iirola T, Vilo S, Manner T, Aantaa R, Lahtinen M, Scheinin M, Olkkola KT. Bioavailability of dexmedetomidine after intranasal administration. Eur J Clin Pharmacol. 2011;67(8):825–31. doi:10.1007/s00228-011-1002-y.

120. Larsson P, Eksborg S, Lonnqvist PA. Onset time for pharmacologic premedication with clonidine as a nasal aerosol: a double-blind, placebo-controlled, randomized trial. Pediatr Anesth. 2012;22(9):877–83. doi:10.1111/j.1460-9592.2012.03877.x.

121. Almenrader N, Larsson P, Passariello M, Haiberger R, Pietropaoli P, Lonnqvist PA, Eksborg S. Absorption pharmacokinetics of clonidine nasal drops in children. Paediatr Anaesth. 2009;19(3):257–61. doi:10.1111/j.1460-9592.2008.02886.x.

122. Hippard HK, Govindan K, Friedman EM, Sulek M, Giannoni C, Larrier D, Minard CG, Watcha MF. Postoperative analgesic and behavioral effects of intranasal fentanyl, intravenous morphine, and intramuscular morphine in pediatric patients undergoing bilateral myringotomy and placement of ventilating tubes. Anesth Analg. 2012;115(2):356–63. doi:10.1213/ANE.0b013e31825afef3.

123. Drover DR, Hammer GB, Anderson BJ. The pharmacokinetics of ketorolac after single postoperative intranasal administration in adolescent patients. Anesth Analg. 2012;114(6):1270–6. doi:10.1213/ANE.0b013e31824f92c2.

124. Ginsberg G, Hattis D, Miller R, Sonawane B. Pediatric pharmacokinetic data: implications for environmental risk assessment for children. Pediatrics. 2004;113(4 Suppl):973–83.

125. Taddio A, Shennan AT, Stevens B, Leeder JS, Koren G. Safety of lidocaine-prilocaine cream in the treatment of preterm neonates. J Pediatr. 1995;127(6):1002–5.

126. Taddio A, Stevens B, Craig K, Rastogi P, Ben-David S, Shennan A, Mulligan P, Koren G. Efficacy and safety of lidocaine-prilocaine cream for pain during circumcision. N Engl J Med. 1997;336(17):1197–201.

127. Salanitre E, Rackow H. The pulmonary exchange of nitrous oxide and halothane in infants and children. Anesthesiology. 1969;30:388–94.

128. Lerman J. Pharmacology of inhalational anaesthetics in infants and children. Paediatr Anaesth. 1992;2:191–203.

129. Lerman J, Schmitt Bantel BI, Gregory GA, Willis MM, Eger EI. Effect of age on the solubility of volatile anesthetics in human tissues. Anesthesiology. 1986;65(3):307–11.

130. Malviya S, Lerman J. The blood/gas solubilities of sevoflurane, isoflurane, halothane, and serum constituent concentrations in neonates and adults. Anesthesiology. 1990;72(5):793–6.

131. Albani M, Wernicke I. Oral phenytoin in infancy: dose requirement, absorption, and elimination. Pediatr Pharmacol. 1983;3 (3–4):229–36.

132. Abdel-Rahman SM, Johnson FK, Connor JD, Staiano A, Dupont C, Tolia V, Winter H, Gauthier-Dubois G, Kearns GL. Developmental pharmacokinetics and pharmacodynamics of nizatidine. J Pediatr Gastroenterol Nutr. 2004;38(4):442–51.

133. de Wildt SN, Kearns GL, Hop WC, Murry DJ, Abdel-Rahman SM, van den Anker JN. Pharmacokinetics and metabolism of oral midazolam in preterm infants. Br J Clin Pharmacol. 2002;53 (4):390–2.

134. Allegaert K, Anderson BJ, Vrancken M, Debeer A, Desmet K, Tibboel D, Devlieger H. Impact of a paediatric vial on the magnitude of systematic medication errors in preterm neonates: amikacin as an example. Paediatr Perinat Drug Ther. 2006;7:59–63.

135. Karl HW, Rosenberger JL, Larach MG, Ruffle JM. Transmucosal administration of midazolam for premedication of pediatric patients. Comparison of the nasal and sublingual routes. Anesthesiology. 1993;78(5):885–91.

136. Herd DW, Salehi B. Palatability of two forms of paracetamol (acetaminophen) suspension: a randomised trial. Paed Perinatal Drug Ther. 2006;7:189–93.

137. Larsson P, Nordlinder A, Bergendahl HT, Lonnqvist PA, Eksborg S, Almenrader N, Anderson BJ. Oral bioavailability of clonidine in children. Pediatr Anesth. 2011;21(3):335–40. doi:10.1111/j.1460-9592.2010.03397.x.

138. Brunette KE, Anderson BJ, Thomas J, Wiesner L, Herd DW, Schulein S. Exploring the pharmacokinetics of oral ketamine in children undergoing burns procedures. Paediatr Anaesth. 2011;21 (6):653–62. doi:10.1111/j.1460-9592.2011.03548.x.

139. Gourlay GK, Boas RA. Fatal outcome with use of rectal morphine for postoperative pain control in an infant. BMJ. 1992;304 (6829):766–7.

140. Pelkonen O. Drug metabolism in the human fetal liver. Relationship to fetal age. Arch Int Pharmacodyn Ther. 1973;202(2):281–7.

141. Pelkonen O, Kaltiala EH, Larmi TK, Karki NT. Comparison of activities of drug-metabolizing enzymes in human fetal and adult livers. Clin Pharmacol Ther. 1973;14(5):840–6.

142. Pelkonen O, Karki NT. Drug metabolism in human fetal tissues. Life Sci. 1973;13:1163–80.

143. Ward RM, Drover DR, Hammer GB, Stemland CJ, Kern S, Tristani-Firouzi M, Lugo RA, Satterfield K, Anderson BJ. The pharmacokinetics of methadone and its metabolites in neonates,

infants, and children. Pediatr Anesth. 2014;24(6):591–601. doi:10.1111/pan.12385.

144. Hines RN. Developmental expression of drug metabolizing enzymes: impact on disposition in neonates and young children. Int J Pharm. 2013;452(1–2):3–7. doi:10.1016/j.ijpharm.2012.05.079.

145. Nebert DW, Adesnik M, Coon MJ, Estabrook RW, Gonzalez FJ, Guengerich FP, Gunsalus IC, Johnson EF, Kemper B, Levin W, et al. The P450 gene superfamily: recommended nomenclature. DNA. 1987;6(1):1–11.

146. Nebert DW, Gonzalez FJ. P450 genes: structure, evolution, and regulation. Annu Rev Biochem. 1987;56:945–93. doi:10.1146/annurev.bi.56.070187.004501.

147. Nebert DW, Jaiswal AK, Meyer UA, Gonzalez FJ. Human P-450 genes: evolution, regulation and possible role in carcinogenesis. Biochem Soc Trans. 1987;15(4):586–9.

148. Cazeneuve C, Pons G, Rey E, Treluyer JM, Cresteil T, Thiroux G, D'Athis P, Olive G. Biotransformation of caffeine in human liver microsomes from foetuses, neonates, infants and adults. Br J Clin Pharmacol. 1994;37(5):405–12.

149. Aranda JV, Sitar DS, Parsons WD, Loughnan PM, Neims AH. Pharmacokinetic aspects of theophylline in premature newborns. N Engl J Med. 1976;295(8):413–6.

150. Anderson BJ, Gunn TR, Holford NH, Johnson R. Caffeine overdose in a premature infant: clinical course and pharmacokinetics. Anaesth Intens Care. 1999;27(3):307–11.

151. Anderson BJ, Holford NH, Woollard GA. Aspects of theophylline clearance in children. Anaesth Intens Care. 1997;25(5):497–501.

152. Hines RN. Ontogeny of human hepatic cytochromes P450. J Biochem Mol Toxicol. 2007;21(4):169–75.

153. Hines RN, McCarver DG. The ontogeny of human drug-metabolizing enzymes: phase I oxidative enzymes. J Pharmacol Exp Ther. 2002;300(2):355–60.

154. Treluyer JM, Gueret G, Cheron G, Sonnier M, Cresteil T. Developmental expression of CYP2C and CYP2C-dependent activities in the human liver: in-vivo/in-vitro correlation and inducibility. Pharmacogenetics. 1997;7(6):441–52.

155. Treluyer JM, Jacqz-Aigrain E, Alvarez F, Cresteil T. Expression of CYP2D6 in developing human liver. Eur J Biochem. 1991;202 (2):583–8.

156. Allegaert K, Holford N, Anderson BJ, Holford S, Stuber F, Rochette A, Troconiz IF, Beier H, de Hoon JN, Pedersen RS, Stamer U. Tramadol and O-desmethyl tramadol clearance maturation and disposition in humans: a pooled pharmacokinetic study. Clin Pharmacokinet. 2014;54(2):167–78. doi:10.1007/s40262-014-0191-9.

157. Koukouritaki SB, Manro JR, Marsh SA, Stevens JC, Rettie AE, McCarver DG, Hines RN. Developmental expression of human hepatic CYP2C9 and CYP2C19. J Pharmacol Exp Ther. 2004;308 (3):965–74.

158. Stevens JC, Hines RN, Gu C, Koukouritaki SB, Manro JR, Tandler PJ, Zaya MJ. Developmental expression of the major human hepatic CYP3A enzymes. J Pharm Exp Ther. 2003;307 (2):573–82.

159. de Wildt SN, Kearns GL, Leeder JS, van den Anker JN. Cytochrome P450 3A: ontogeny and drug disposition. Clin Pharmacokinet. 1999;37(6):485–505.

160. Berde C. Convulsions associated with pediatric regional anesthesia. Anesth Analg. 1992;75:164–6.

161. Sutherland JM. Fatal cardiovascular collapse of infants receiving large amounts of chloramphenicol. Am J Dis Child. 1959;97:761–7.

162. Burns LE, Hodgman JE. Fatal circulatory collapse in premature infants receiving chloramphenicol. N Engl J Med. 1959;261:1318.

163. Holford NH, Ma SC, Anderson BJ. Prediction of morphine dose in humans. Pediatr Anesth. 2012;22(3):209–22. doi:10.1111/j.1460-9592.2011.03782.x.

164. Anderson BJ, Holford NH. Mechanistic basis of using body size and maturation to predict clearance in humans. Drug Metab Pharmacokinet. 2009;24(1):25–36.

165. Potts AL, Warman GR, Anderson BJ. Dexmedetomidine disposition in children: a population analysis. Paediatr Anaesth. 2008;18 (8):722–30.

166. Allegaert K, Peeters MY, Verbesselt R, Tibboel D, Naulaers G, de Hoon JN, Knibbe CA. Inter-individual variability in propofol pharmacokinetics in preterm and term neonates. Br J Anaesth. 2007;99(6):864–70.

167. Evans WE, Relling MV. Pharmacogenomics: translating functional genomics into rational therapeutics. Science. 1999;286 (5439):487–91.

168. Quiding H, Olsson GL, Boreus LO, Bondesson U. Infants and young children metabolise codeine to morphine. A study after single and repeated rectal administration. Br J Clin Pharmacol. 1992;33(1):45–9.

169. Palmer SN, Giesecke NM, Body SC, Shernan SK, Fox AA, Collard CD. Pharmacogenetics of anesthetic and analgesic agents. Anesthesiology. 2005;102(3):663–71.

170. Williams DG, Hatch DJ, Howard RF. Codeine phosphate in paediatric medicine. Br J Anaesth. 2001;86(3):413–21.

171. Eichelbaum M, Ingelman-Sundberg M, Evans WE. Pharmacogenomics and individualized drug therapy. Annu Rev Med. 2006;57:119–37.

172. Voronov P, Przybylo HJ, Jagannathan N. Apnea in a child after oral codeine: a genetic variant—an ultra-rapid metabolizer. Paediatr Anaesth. 2007;17(7):684–7. doi:10.1111/j.1460-9592.2006.02182.x.

173. Kearns GL. Pharmacogenetics and development: are infants and children at increased risk for adverse outcomes? Curr Opin Pediatr. 1995;7(2):220–33.

174. Fagerlund TH, Braaten O. No pain relief from codeine…? An introduction to pharmacogenomics. Acta Anaesthesiol Scand. 2001;45(2):140–9.

175. Relling MV, Hancock ML, Rivera GK, Sandlund JT, Ribeiro RC, Krynetski EY, Pui CH, Evans WE. Mercaptopurine therapy intolerance and heterozygosity at the thiopurine S-methyltransferase gene locus. J Natl Cancer Inst. 1999;91(23):2001–8.

176. Palomaki GE, Bradley LA, Douglas MP, Kolor K, Dotson WD. Can UGT1A1 genotyping reduce morbidity and mortality in patients with metastatic colorectal cancer treated with irinotecan? An evidence-based review. Genet Med. 2009;11 (1):21–34. doi:10.1097/GIM.0b013e31818efd77.

177. Andersson T, Flockhart DA, Goldstein DB, Huang SM, Kroetz DL, Milos PM, Ratain MJ, Thummel K. Drug-metabolizing enzymes: evidence for clinical utility of pharmacogenomic tests. Clin Pharmacol Ther. 2005;78(6):559–81. doi:10.1016/j.clpt.2005.08.013.

178. Allegaert K, van den Anker JN, de Hoon JN, van Schaik RH, Debeer A, Tibboel D, Naulaers G, Anderson BJ. Covariates of tramadol disposition in the first months of life. Br J Anaesth. 2008;100(4):525–32.

179. West JR, Smith HW, Chasis H. Glomerular filtration rate, effective renal blood flow, and maximal tubular excretory capacity in infancy. J Pediatr. 1948;32:10–8.

180. Fawer CL, Torrado A, Guignard JP. Maturation of renal function in full-term and premature neonates. Helv Paediatr Acta. 1979;34 (1):11–21.

181. Eichenwald HF, McCracken Jr GH. Antimicrobial therapy in infants and children. Part I Review of antimicrobial agents. J Pediatr. 1978;93(3):337–56.

182. Anderson BJ, Allegaert K, Van den Anker JN, Cossey V, Holford NH. Vancomycin pharmacokinetics in preterm neonates and the prediction of adult clearance. Br J Clin Pharmacol. 2007;63 (1):75–84.

183. Fisher DM, O'Keeffe C, Stanski DR, Cronnelly R, Miller RD, Gregory GA. Pharmacokinetics and pharmacodynamics of *d*-tubocurarine in infants, children, and adults. Anesthesiology. 1982;57(3):203–8.

184. Sawyer DC, Eger 2nd EI, Bahlman SH, Cullen BF, Impelman D. Concentration dependence of hepatic halothane metabolism. Anesthesiology. 1971;34(3):230–5.

185. Brandom BW, Stiller RL, Cook DR, Woelfel SK, Chakravorti S, Lai A. Pharmacokinetics of atracurium in anaesthetized infants and children. Br J Anaesth. 1986;58(11):1210–3.

186. Meakin G, McKiernan EP, Morris P, Baker RD. Dose–response curves for suxamethonium in neonates, infants and children. Br J Anaesth. 1989;62(6):655–8.

187. Cook DR, Wingard LB, Taylor FH. Pharmacokinetics of succinylcholine in infants, children, and adults. Clin Pharmacol Ther. 1976;20(4):493–8.

188. Goudsouzian NG, Liu LM. The neuromuscular response of infants to a continuous infusion of succinylcholine. Anesthesiology. 1984;60(2):97–101.

189. Stephenson T. How children's responses to drugs differ from adults. Br J Clin Pharmacol. 2005;59(6):670–3.

190. LeDez KM, Lerman J. The minimum alveolar concentration (MAC) of isoflurane in preterm neonates. Anesthesiology. 1987;67(3):301–7.

191. Chugani HT, Kumar A, Muzik O. GABA(A) receptor imaging with positron emission tomography in the human newborn: a unique binding pattern. Pediatr Neurol. 2013;48(6):459–62. doi:10.1016/j.pediatrneurol.2013.04.008.

192. Meakin G, Morton RH, Wareham AC. Age-dependent variation in response to tubocurarine in the isolated rat diaphragm. Br J Anaesth. 1992;68(2):161–3.

193. Wareham AC, Morton RH, Meakin GH. Low quantal content of the endplate potential reduces safety factor for neuromuscular transmission in the diaphragm of the newborn rat. Br J Anaesth. 1994;72(2):205–9.

194. Arnold PD. Coagulation and the surgical neonate. Paediatr Anaesth. 2014;24(1):89–97. doi:10.1111/pan.12296.

195. Guzzetta NA, Miller BE. Principles of hemostasis in children: models and maturation. Paediatr Anaesth. 2011;21(1):3–9. doi:10.1111/j.1460-9592.2010.03410.x.

196. Albisetti M. The fibrinolytic system in children. Semin Thromb Hemost. 2003;29(4):339–48. doi:10.1055/s-2003-42585.

197. Andrew M, Paes B, Milner R, Johnston M, Mitchell L, Tollefsen DM, Powers P. Development of the human coagulation system in the full-term infant. Blood. 1987;70(1):165–72.

198. Ries M, Easton RL, Longstaff C, Zenker M, Corran PH, Morris HR, Dell A, Gaffney PJ. Differences between neonates and adults in tissue-type-plasminogen activator (t-PA)-catalyzed plasminogen activation with various effectors and in carbohydrate sequences of fibrinogen chains. Thromb Res. 2001;103(3):173–84.

199. Ries M, Easton RL, Longstaff C, Zenker M, Morris HR, Dell A, Gaffney PJ. Differences between neonates and adults in carbohydrate sequences and reaction kinetics of plasmin and alpha(2)-antiplasmin. Thromb Res. 2002;105(3):247–56.

200. McNicol G, Fletcher A, Alkjaersig N, Sherry S. The absorption, distribution, and excretion of epsilon-aminocaproic acid following oral or intravenous administration to man. J Lab Clin. 1962;59:15–24.

201. Nielsen VG, Cankovic L, Steenwyk BL. Epsilon-aminocaproic acid inhibition of fibrinolysis in vitro: should the 'therapeutic' concentration be reconsidered? Blood Coagul Fibrinolysis. 2007;18(1):35–9. doi:10.1097/MBC.0b013e328010a359.

202. Yurka HG, Wissler RN, Zanghi CN, Liu X, Tu X, Eaton MP. The effective concentration of epsilon-aminocaproic Acid for inhibition of fibrinolysis in neonatal plasma in vitro.

Anesth Analg. 2010;111(1):180–4. doi:10.1213/ANE.0b013e3181e19cec.

203. Kirk CR, Gibbs JL, Thomas R, Radley-Smith R, Qureshi SA. Cardiovascular collapse after verapamil in supraventricular tachycardia. Arch Dis Child. 1987;62(12):1265–6.

204. Takahashi H, Ishikawa S, Nomoto S, Nishigaki Y, Ando F, Kashima T, Kimura S, Kanamori M, Echizen H. Developmental changes in pharmacokinetics and pharmacodynamics of warfarin enantiomers in Japanese children. Clin Pharmacol Ther. 2000;68(5):541–55.

205. Kupferberg HJ, Way EL. Pharmacologic basis for the increased sensitivity of the newborn rat to morphine. J Pharmacol Exp Ther. 1963;141:105–12.

206. Domek NS, Barlow CF, Roth LJ. An ontogenetic study of phenobarbital-C-14 in cat brain. J Pharmacol Exp Ther. 1960;130:285–93.

207. Arai T, Watanabe T, Nagaro T, Matsuo S. Blood–brain barrier impairment after cardiac resuscitation. Crit Care Med. 1981;9(6):444–8.

208. Hagberg H, Mallard C. Effect of inflammation on central nervous system development and vulnerability. Curr Opin Neurol. 2005;18(2):117–23.

209. Baber NS. Tripartite meeting. Paediatric regulatory guidelines: do they help in optimizing dose selection for children? Brit J Clin Pharmacol. 2005;59(6):660–2.

210. Davidson AJ. Measuring anesthesia in children using the EEG. Pediatr Anesthesia. 2006;16(4):374–87.

211. Davidson AJ, Huang GH, Rebmann CS, Ellery C. Performance of entropy and Bispectral Index as measures of anaesthesia effect in children of different ages. Br J Anaesth. 2005;95(5):674–9.

212. Davidson AJ, Sale SM, Wong C, McKeever S, Sheppard S, Chan Z, Williams C. The electroencephalograph during anesthesia and emergence in infants and children. Paediatr Anaesth. 2008;18(1):60–70.

213. Jeleazcov C, Schmidt J, Schmitz B, Becke K, Albrecht S. EEG variables as measures of arousal during propofol anaesthesia for general surgery in children: rational selection and age dependence. Br J Anaesth. 2007;99(6):845–54.

214. Hoffman GM, Nowakowski R, Troshynski TJ, Berens RJ, Weisman SJ. Risk reduction in pediatric procedural sedation by application of an American Academy of Pediatrics/American Society of Anesthesiologists process model. Pediatrics. 2002;109(2):236–43.

215. Crellin D, Sullivan TP, Babl FE, O'Sullivan R, Hutchinson A. Analysis of the validation of existing behavioral pain and distress scales for use in the procedural setting. Paediatr Anaesth. 2007;17(8):720–33.

216. von Baeyer CL, Spagrud LJ. Systematic review of observational (behavioral) measures of pain for children and adolescents aged 3 to 18 years. Pain. 2007;127(1–2):140–50.

217. Schade JG, Joyce BA, Gerkensmeyer J, Keck JF. Comparison of three preverbal scales for postoperative pain assessment in a diverse pediatric sample. J Pain Symptom Manage. 1996;12(6):348–59.

218. Connelly MA, Brown JT, Kearns GL, Anderson RA, St Peter SD, Neville KA. Pupillometry: a non-invasive technique for pain assessment in paediatric patients. Arch Dis Child. 2014;99(12):1125–31. doi:10.1136/archdischild-2014-306286.

219. Howard RF, Liossi C. Pain assessment in children. Arch Dis Child. 2014;99(12):1123–4. doi:10.1136/archdischild-2014-306432.

220. Holford NHG, Peck CC. Population pharmacodynamics and drug development. In: Boxtel CJ, Holford NHG, Danhof M, editors. The in vivo study of drug action. New York: Elsevier Science Publishers; 1992. p. 401–14.

221. Anderson BJ, van den Anker J. Why is there no morphine concentration-response curve for acute pain? Paediatr Anaesth. 2014;24(3):233–8. doi:10.1111/pan.12361.

222. Comer SD, Cooper ZD, Kowalczyk WJ, Sullivan MA, Evans SM, Bisaga AM, Vosburg SK. Evaluation of potential sex differences in the subjective and analgesic effects of morphine in normal, healthy volunteers. Psychopharmacology (Berl). 2010;208 (1):45–55. doi:10.1007/s00213-009-1703-4.

223. Djurendic-Brenesel M, Mimica-Dukic N, Pilija V, Tasic M. Gender-related differences in the pharmacokinetics of opiates. Forensic Sci Int. 2010;194(1–3):28–33. doi:10.1016/j.forsciint. 2009.10.003.

224. Sarton E, Romberg R, Dahan A. Gender differences in morphine pharmacokinetics and dynamics. Adv Exp Med Biol. 2003;523:71–80.

225. Schmitz AK, Vierhaus M, Lohaus A. Pain tolerance in children and adolescents: sex differences and psychosocial influences on pain threshold and endurance. Eur J Pain. 2013;17(1):124–31. doi:10.1002/j.1532-2149.2012.00169.x.

226. Rabbitts JA, Groenewald CB, Dietz NM, Morales C, Rasanen J. Perioperative opioid requirements are decreased in hypoxic children living at altitude. Pediatr Anesth. 2010;20(12):1078–83. doi:10.1111/j.1460-9592.2010.03453.x.

227. Rabbitts JA, Groenewald CB, Rasanen J. Geographic differences in perioperative opioid administration in children. Pediatr Anesth. 2012;22(7):676–81. doi:10.1111/j.1460-9592.2012. 03806.x.

228. Jimenez N, Anderson GD, Shen DD, Nielsen SS, Farin FM, Seidel K, Lynn AM. Is ethnicity associated with morphine's side effects in children? Morphine pharmacokinetics, analgesic response, and side effects in children having tonsillectomy. Pediatr Anesth. 2012;22(7):669–75. doi:10.1111/j.1460-9592. 2012.03844.x.

229. Sadhasivam S, Chidambaran V, Ngamprasertwong P, Esslinger HR, Prows C, Zhang X, Martin LJ, McAuliffe J. Race and unequal burden of perioperative pain and opioid related adverse effects in children. Pediatrics. 2012;129(5):832–8. doi:10.1542/peds.2011-2607.

230. Sadhasivam S, Krekels EH, Chidambaran V, Esslinger HR, Ngamprasertwong P, Zhang K, Fukuda T, Vinks AA. Morphine clearance in children: does race or genetics matter? J Opioid Manag. 2012;8(4):217–26. doi:10.5055/jom.2012.0119.

231. Rigby-Jones A, Sneyd JR. Cardiovascular changes after achieving constant effect site concentration of propofol. Anaesthesia. 2008;63(7):780. doi:10.1111/j.1365-2044.2008.05589_1.x.

232. Hutchinson MR, Coats BD, Lewis SS, Zhang Y, Sprunger DB, Rezvani N, Baker EM, Jekich BM, Wieseler JL, Somogyi AA, Martin D, Poole S, Judd CM, Maier SF, Watkins LR. Proinflammatory cytokines oppose opioid-induced acute and chronic analgesia. Brain Behav Immun. 2008;22(8):1178–89. doi:10.1016/j.bbi.2008.05.004.

233. Candiotti KA, Yang Z, Morris R, Yang J, Crescimone NA, Sanchez GC, Bird V, Leveillee R, Rodriguez Y, Liu H, Zhang YD, Bethea JR, Gitlin MC. Polymorphism in the interleukin-1 receptor antagonist gene is associated with serum interleukin-1 receptor antagonist concentrations and postoperative opioid consumption. Anesthesiology. 2011;114(5):1162–8. doi:10.1097/ ALN.0b013e318216e9cb.

234. Lotsch J, Geisslinger G. Relevance of frequent mu-opioid receptor polymorphisms for opioid activity in healthy volunteers. Pharmacogenomics J. 2006;6(3):200–10.

235. Walter C, Lotsch J. Meta-analysis of the relevance of the OPRM1 118A > G genetic variant for pain treatment. Pain. 2009;146 (3):270–5. doi:10.1016/j.pain.2009.07.013.

236. Ross JR, Rutter D, Welsh K, Joel SP, Goller K, Wells AU, Du Bois R, Riley J. Clinical response to morphine in cancer patients and genetic variation in candidate genes. Pharmacogenomics J. 2005;5(5):324–36. doi:10.1038/sj.tpj.6500327.

237. Liem EB, Joiner TV, Tsueda K, Sessler DI. Increased sensitivity to thermal pain and reduced subcutaneous lidocaine efficacy in redheads. Anesthesiology. 2005;102(3):509–14.

238. Lotsch J, Geisslinger G. Pharmacogenetics of new analgesics. Br J Pharmacol. 2011;163(3):447–60. doi:10.1111/j.1476-5381.2010. 01074.x.

239. Tournier N, Decleves X, Saubamea B, Scherrmann JM, Cisternino S. Opioid transport by ATP-binding cassette transporters at the blood–brain barrier: implications for neuropsychopharmacology. Curr Pharm Des. 2011;17(26):2829–42.

240. Linden G, Henderson BE. Genital-tract cancers in adolescents and young adults. N Engl J Med. 1972;286(14):760–1.

241. Fredriksson A, Archer T, Alm H, Gordh T, Eriksson P. Neurofunctional deficits and potentiated apoptosis by neonatal NMDA antagonist administration. Behav Brain Res. 2004;153 (2):367–76.

242. Wang C, Sadovova N, Fu X, Schmued L, Scallet A, Hanig J, Slikker W. The role of the N-methyl-D-aspartate receptor in ketamine-induced apoptosis in rat forebrain culture. Neuroscience. 2005;132(4):967–77.

243. Anderson BJ, Ralph CJ, Stewart AW, Barber C, Holford NH. The dose-effect relationship for morphine and vomiting after day-stay tonsillectomy in children. Anaesth Intens Care. 2000;28 (2):155–60.

244. Weinstein MS, Nicolson SC, Schreiner MS. A single dose of morphine sulfate increases the incidence of vomiting after outpatient inguinal surgery in children. Anesthesiology. 1994;81(3):572–7.

245. Ansermino M, Basu R, Vandebeek C, Montgomery C. Nonopioid additives to local anaesthetics for caudal blockade in children: a systematic review. Paediatr Anaesth. 2003;13(7):561–73.

246. Welzing L, Kribs A, Eifinger F, Huenseler C, Oberthuer A, Roth B. Propofol as an induction agent for endotracheal intubation can cause significant arterial hypotension in preterm neonates. Paediatr Anaesth. 2010;20(7):605–11. doi:10.1111/j.1460-9592. 2010.03330.x.

247. Lerman J, Heard C, Steward DJ. Neonatal tracheal intubation: an imbroglio unresolved. Paediatr Anaesth. 2010;20(7):585–90. doi:10.1111/j.1460-9592.2010.03356.x.

248. Lichtenbelt BJ, Olofsen E, Dahan A, van Kleef JW, Struys MM, Vuyk J. Propofol reduces the distribution and clearance of midazolam. Anesth Analg. 2010;110(6):1597–606. doi:10.1213/ ANE.0b013e3181da91bb.

249. Vuyk J, Lichtenbelt BJ, Olofsen E, van Kleef JW, Dahan A. Mixed-effects modeling of the influence of midazolam on propofol pharmacokinetics. Anesth Analg. 2009;108(5):1522–30. doi:10.1213/ane.0b013e31819e4058.

250. Atkinson HC, Stanescu I, Anderson BJ. Increased phenylephrine plasma levels with administration of acetaminophen. N Engl J Med. 2014;370(12):1171–2. doi:10.1056/NEJMc1313942.

251. Atkinson HC, Stanescu I, Salem II, Potts AL, Anderson BJ. Increased bioavailability of phenylephrine by co-administration of acetaminophen: results of four open-label, crossover pharmacokinetic trials in healthy volunteers. Eur J Clin Pharmacol. 2015;71(2):151–8. doi:10.1007/s00228-014-1788-5.

252. Strolin Benedetti M, Ruty B, Baltes E. Induction of endogenous pathways by antiepileptics and clinical implications. Fundam Clin Pharmacol. 2005;19(5):511–29. doi:10.1111/j.1472-8206.2005. 00341.x.

253. Eker HE, Yalcin Cok O, Aribogan A, Arslan G. Children on phenobarbital monotherapy requires more sedatives during MRI. Pediatr Anesth. 2011;10(10):998–1002. doi:10.1111/j.1460-9592. 2011.03606.x.

254. Stanski DR, Ham J, Miller RD, Sheiner LB. Pharmacokinetics and pharmacodynamics of d-tubocurarine during nitrous oxide-

narcotic and halothane anesthesia in man. Anesthesiology. 1979;51(3):235–41.

255. Prys-Roberts C, Lloyd JW, Fisher A, et al. Deliberate profound hypotension induced with halothane: studies of haemodynamics and pulmonary gas exchange. Br J Anaesth. 1974;46:105.

256. Pauca AL, Hopkins AM. Acute effects of halothane, nitrous oxide and thiopentone on upper limb blood flow. Br J Anaesth. 1972;43:326–33.

257. Taivainen T, Meretoja OA. The neuromuscular blocking effects of vecuronium during sevoflurane, halothane and balanced anaesthesia in children. Anaesthesia. 1995;50(12):1046–9.

258. Greco WR, Park HS, Rustum YM. Application of a new approach for the quantitation of drug synergism to the combination of cis-diamminedichloroplatinum and 1-beta-D-arabinofuranosyl-cytosine. Cancer Res. 1990;50(17):5318–27.

259. Minto C, Vuyk J. Response surface modelling of drug interactions. Adv Exp Med Biol. 2003;523:35–43.

260. Kern SE, Xie G, White JL, Egan TD. A response surface analysis of propofol-remifentanil pharmacodynamic interaction in volunteers. Anesthesiology. 2004;100(6):1373–81.

261. Minto CF, Schnider TW, Short TG, Gregg KM, Gentilini A, Shafer SL. Response surface model for anesthetic drug interactions. Anesthesiology. 2000;92(6):1603–16.

262. Bouillon TW, Bruhn J, Radulescu L, Andresen C, Shafer TJ, Cohane C, Shafer SL. Pharmacodynamic interaction between propofol and remifentanil regarding hypnosis, tolerance of laryngoscopy, bispectral index, and electroencephalographic approximate entropy. Anesthesiology. 2004;100(6):1353–72.

263. Short TG, Plummer JL, Chui PT. Hypnotic and anaesthetic interactions between midazolam, propofol and alfentanil. Br J Anaesth. 1992;69(2):162–7.

264. Dahan A, Nieuwenhuijs D, Olofsen E, Sarton E, Romberg R, Teppema L. Response surface modeling of alfentanil-sevoflurane interaction on cardiorespiratory control and bispectral index. Anesthesiology. 2001;94(6):982–91.

265. Nieuwenhuijs DJ, Olofsen E, Romberg RR, Sarton E, Ward D, Engbers F, Vuyk J, Mooren R, Teppema LJ, Dahan A. Response surface modeling of remifentanil-propofol interaction on cardiorespiratory control and bispectral index. Anesthesiology. 2003;98 (2):312–22.

266. Cote CJ, Karl HW, Notterman DA, Weinberg JA, McCloskey C. Adverse sedation events in pediatrics: analysis of medications used for sedation. Pediatrics. 2000;106(4):633–44.

267. Drover DR, Litalien C, Wellis V, Shafer SL, Hammer GB. Determination of the pharmacodynamic interaction of propofol and remifentanil during esophagogastroduodenoscopy in children. Anesthesiology. 2004;100(6):1382–6.

268. Coulter FL, Hannam JA, Anderson BJ. Ketofol dosing simulations for procedural sedation. Pediatr Emerg Care. 2014;30(9):621–30.

269. Andolfatto G, Abu-Laban RB, Zed PJ, Staniforth SM, Stackhouse S, Moadebi S, Willman E. Ketamine-propofol combination (ketofol) versus propofol alone for emergency department procedural sedation and analgesia: a randomized double-blind trial. Ann Emerg Med. 2012;59(6):504–512.e2. doi:10.1016/j.annemergmed.2012.01.017.

270. Hui TW, Short TG, Hong W, Suen T, Gin T, Plummer J. Additive interactions between propofol and ketamine when used for anesthesia induction in female patients. Anesthesiology. 1995;82 (3):641–8.

271. Coulter FL, Hannam JA, Anderson BJ. Ketofol simulations for dosing in pediatric anesthesia. Pediatr Anesth. 2014;24 (8):806–12. doi:10.1111/pan.12386.

272. Dallimore D, Anderson BJ, Short TG, Herd DW. Ketamine anesthesia in children—exploring infusion regimens. Paediatr Anaesth. 2008;18(8):708–14.

273. Murphy A, Campbell DE, Baines D, Mehr S. Allergic reactions to propofol in egg-allergic children. Anesth Analg. 2011;113 (1):140–4. doi:10.1213/ANE.0b013e31821b450f.

274. Molina-Infante J, Arias A, Vara-Brenes D, Prados-Manzano R, Gonzalez-Cervera J, Alvarado-Arenas M, Lucendo AJ. Propofol administration is safe in adult eosinophilic esophagitis patients sensitized to egg, soy, or peanut. Allergy. 2014;69(3):388–94. doi:10.1111/all.12360.

275. McKeating K, Bali IM, Dundee JW. The effects of thiopentone and propofol on upper airway integrity. Anaesthesia. 1988;43 (8):638–40.

276. Taha S, Siddik-Sayyid S, Alameddine M, Wakim C, Dahabra C, Moussa A, Khatib M, Baraka A. Propofol is superior to thiopental for intubation without muscle relaxants. Can J Anaes. 2005;52 (3):249–53. doi:10.1007/BF03016058.

277. Koh KF, Chen FG, Cheong KF, Esuvaranathan V. Laryngeal mask insertion using thiopental and low dose atracurium: a comparison with propofol. Can Anaesth Soc J. 1999;46(7):670–4. doi:10. 1007/BF03013956.

278. Lerman J, Johr M. Inhalational anesthesia vs total intravenous anesthesia (TIVA) for pediatric anesthesia. Paediatr Anaesth. 2009;19(5):521–34. doi:10.1111/j.1460-9592.2009.02962.x.

279. Sharples A, Shaw EA, Meakin G. Recovery times following induction of anaesthesia with propofol, methohexitone, enflurane or thiopentone in children. Paediatr Anaesth. 1994;4:101–4.

280. Jones RD, Chan K, Andrew LJ. Pharmacokinetics of propofol in children. Br J Anaesth. 1990;65(5):661–7.

281. Kirkpatrick T, Cockshott ID, Douglas EJ, Nimmo WS. Pharmacokinetics of propofol (diprivan) in elderly patients. Br J Anaesth. 1988;60(2):146–50.

282. Westrin P. The induction dose of propofol in infants 1–6 months of age and in children 10–16 years of age. Anesthesiology. 1991;74(3):455–8.

283. Naguib M, Samarkandi AH, Moniem MA, Mansour Eel D, Alshaer AA, Al-Ayyaf HA, Fadin A, Alharby SW. The effects of melatonin premedication on propofol and thiopental induction dose–response curves: a prospective, randomized, double-blind study. Anesth Analg. 2006;103(6):1448–52. doi:10.1213/01.ane. 0000244534.24216.3a.

284. Short TG, Aun CS, Tan P, Wong J, Tam YH, Oh TE. A prospective evaluation of pharmacokinetic model controlled infusion of propofol in paediatric patients. Br J Anaesth. 1994;72(3):302–6.

285. Murat I, Billard V, Vernois J, Zaouter M, Marsol P, Souron R, Farinotti R. Pharmacokinetics of propofol after a single dose in children aged 1–3 years with minor burns. Comparison of three data analysis approaches. Anesthesiology. 1996;84(3):526–32.

286. Saint-Maurice C, Cockshott ID, Douglas EJ, Richard MO, Harmey JL. Pharmacokinetics of propofol in young children after a single dose. Br J Anaesth. 1989;63(6):667–70.

287. Coppens MJ, Eleveld DJ, Proost JH, Marks LA, Van Bocxlaer JF, Vereecke H, Absalom AR, Struys MM. An evaluation of using population pharmacokinetic models to estimate pharmacodynamic parameters for propofol and bispectral index in children. Anesthesiology. 2011;115(1):83–93. doi:10.1097/ALN. 0b013e31821a8d80.

288. Iwakiri H, Nishihara N, Nagata O, Matsukawa T, Ozaki M, Sessler DI. Individual effect-site concentrations of propofol are similar at loss of consciousness and at awakening. Anesth Analg. 2005;100 (1):107–10. doi:10.1213/01.ANE.0000139358.15909.EA.

289. McCormack J, Mehta D, Peiris K, Dumont G, Fung P, Lim J, Ansermino JM. The effect of a target controlled infusion of propofol on predictability of recovery from anesthesia in children. Pediatr Anesth. 2010;20(1):56–62. doi:10.1111/j.1460-9592.2009.03196.x.

290. Rigouzzo A, Girault L, Louvet N, Servin F, De-Smet T, Piat V, Seeman R, Murat I, Constant I. The relationship between

bispectral index and propofol during target-controlled infusion anesthesia: a comparative study between children and young adults. Anesth Analg. 2008;106(4):1109–16. doi:10.1213/ane.0b013e318164f388.

291. Fuentes R, Cortinez I, Ibacache M, Concha M, Munoz H. Propofol concentration to induce general anesthesia in children aged 3–11 years with the Kataria effect-site model. Paediatr Anaesth. 2015;25(6):554–9. doi:10.1111/pan.12657.

292. Eleveld DJ, Absalom AR. Does it matter how you get from D (drug dose) to E (clinical effect)? Paediatr Anaesth. 2015;25(6):544–5. doi:10.1111/pan.12665.

293. Steur RJ, Perez RS, De Lange JJ. Dosage scheme for propofol in children under 3 years of age. Paediatr Anaesth. 2004;14(6):462–7. doi:10.1111/j.1460-9592.2004.01238.x.

294. Valtonen M, Iisalo E, Kanto J, Rosenberg P. Propofol as an induction agent in children: pain on injection and pharmacokinetics. Acta Anaesthesiol Scand. 1989;33(2):152–5.

295. Cameron E, Johnston G, Crofts S, Morton NS. The minimum effective dose of lignocaine to prevent injection pain due to propofol in children. Anaesthesia. 1992;47(7):604–6.

296. Aun CS, Sung RY, O'Meara ME, Short TG, Oh TE. Cardiovascular effects of i.v. induction in children: comparison between propofol and thiopentone. Br J Anaesth. 1993;70(6):647–53.

297. Wodey E, Chonow L, Beneux X, Azzis O, Bansard JY, Ecoffey C. Haemodynamic effects of propofol vs thiopental in infants: an echocardiographic study. Br J Anaesth. 1999;82(4):516–20.

298. Short SM, Aun CS. Haemodynamic effects of propofol in children. Anaesthesia. 1991;46(9):783–5.

299. Wolf AR, Potter F. Propofol infusion in children: when does an anesthetic tool become an intensive care liability? Paediatr Anaesth. 2004;14(6):435–8. doi:10.1111/j.1460-9592.2004.01332.x.

300. Wolf A, Weir P, Segar P, Stone J, Shield J. Impaired fatty acid oxidation in propofol infusion syndrome. Lancet. 2001;357(9256):606–7. doi:10.1016/S0140-6736(00)04064-2.

301. Crean P. Sedation and neuromuscular blockade in paediatric intensive care; practice in the United Kingdom and North America. Paediatr Anaesth. 2004;14(6):439–42. doi:10.1111/j.1460-9592.2004.01259.x.

302. Kingston HG, Kendrick A, Sommer KM, Olsen GD, Downes H. Binding of thiopental in neonatal serum. Anesthesiology. 1990;72(3):428–31.

303. Sorbo S, Hudson RJ, Loomis JC. The pharmacokinetics of thiopental in pediatric surgical patients. Anesthesiology. 1984;61(6):666–70.

304. Larsson P, Anderson BJ, Norman E, Westrin P, Fellman V. Thiopentone elimination in newborn infants: exploring Michaelis-Menten kinetics. Acta Anaesthesiol Scand. 2011;55(4):444–51. doi:10.1111/j.1399-6576.2010.02380.x.

305. Lindsay WA, Shepherd J. Plasma levels of thiopentone after premedication with rectal suppositories in young children. Br J Anaesth. 1969;41(11):977–84.

306. Jonmarker C, Westrin P, Larsson S, Werner O. Thiopental requirements for induction of anesthesia in children. Anesthesiology. 1987;67(1):104–7.

307. Westrin P, Jonmarker C, Werner O. Thiopental requirements for induction of anesthesia in neonates and in infants one to six months of age. Anesthesiology. 1989;71(3):344–6.

308. Fouts JR, Adamson RH. Drug metabolism in the newborn rabbit. Science. 1959;129(3353):897–8.

309. Tibballs J, Malbezin S. Cardiovascular responses to induction of anaesthesia with thiopentone and suxamethonium in infants and children. Anaesth Intens Care. 1988;16(3):278–84.

310. Russo H, Bressolle F, Duboin MP. Pharmacokinetics of high-dose thiopental in pediatric patients with increased intracranial pressure. Ther Drug Monit. 1997;19(1):63–70.

311. Turcant A, Delhumeau A, Premel-Cabic A, Granry JC, Cottineau C, Six P, Allain P. Thiopental pharmacokinetics under conditions of long-term infusion. Anesthesiology. 1985;63(1):50–4.

312. Sakai T, Singh H, Mi WD, Kudo T, Matsuki A. The effect of ketamine on clinical endpoints of hypnosis and EEG variables during propofol infusion. Acta Anaesthesiol Scand. 1999;43(2):212–6.

313. White PF, Schuttler J, Shafer A, Stanski DR, Horai Y, Trevor AJ. Comparative pharmacology of the ketamine isomers. Studies in volunteers. Br J Anaesth. 1985;57(2):197–203.

314. Grant IS, Nimmo WS, McNicol LR, Clements JA. Ketamine disposition in children and adults. Br J Anaesth. 1983;55(11):1107–11.

315. Schuttler J, Stanski DR, White PF, Trevor AJ, Horai Y, Verotta D, Sheiner LB. Pharmacodynamic modeling of the EEG effects of ketamine and its enantiomers in man. J Pharmacokinet Biopharm. 1987;15(3):241–53.

316. Reich DL, Silvay G. Ketamine: an update on the first twenty-five years of clinical experience. Can J Anaesth. 1989;36(2):186–97. doi:10.1007/bf03011442.

317. Herd D, Anderson BJ. Ketamine disposition in children presenting for procedural sedation and analgesia in a children's emergency department. Paediatr Anaesth. 2007;17(7):622–9.

318. Ihmsen H, Geisslinger G, Schuttler J. Stereoselective pharmacokinetics of ketamine: $R(-)$-ketamine inhibits the elimination of $S(+)$-ketamine. Clin Pharmacol Ther. 2001;70(5):431–8.

319. Cook RD, Davis PJ. Pediatric anesthesia pharmacology. In: Lake CL, editor. Pediatric cardiac anesthesia. 2nd ed. East Norwalk: Appleton & Lange; 1993. p. 134.

320. Hartvig P, Larsson E, Joachimsson PO. Postoperative analgesia and sedation following pediatric cardiac surgery using a constant infusion of ketamine. J Cardiothorac Vasc Anesth. 1993;7(2):148–53.

321. Chang T, Glazko AJ. Biotransformation and disposition of ketamine. Int Anesthesiol Clin. 1974;12(2):157–77.

322. Lockhart CH, Nelson WL. The relationship of ketamine requirement to age in pediatric patients. Anesthesiology. 1974;40(5):507–8.

323. Wieber J, Gugler R, Hengstmann JH, Dengler HJ. Pharmacokinetics of ketamine in man. Anaesthesist. 1975;24(6):260–3.

324. Herd DW, Anderson BJ, Holford NH. Modeling the norketamine metabolite in children and the implications for analgesia. Paediatr Anaesth. 2007;17(9):831–40.

325. White M, de Graaff P, Renshof B, van Kan E, Dzoljic M. Pharmacokinetics of S(+) ketamine derived from target controlled infusion. Br J Anaesth. 2006;96(3):330–4. doi:10.1093/bja/aei316.

326. Clements JA, Nimmo WS, Grant IS. Bioavailability, pharmacokinetics, and analgesic activity of ketamine in humans. J Pharm Sci. 1982;71(5):539–42.

327. Malinovsky JM, Servin F, Cozian A, Lepage JY, Pinaud M. Ketamine and norketamine plasma concentrations after i.v., nasal and rectal administration in children. Br J Anaesth. 1996;77(2):203–7.

328. Nielsen BN, Friis SM, Romsing J, Schmiegelow K, Anderson BJ, Ferreiros N, Labocha S, Henneberg SW. Intranasal sufentanil/ketamine analgesia in children. Paediatr Anaesth. 2014;24(2):170–80. doi:10.1111/pan.12268.

329. Hollister GR, Burn JM. Side effects of ketamine in pediatric anesthesia. Anesth Analg. 1974;53(2):264–7.

330. Gingrich BK. Difficulties encountered in a comparative study of orally administered midazolam and ketamine. Anesthesiology. 1994;80(6):1414–5.

331. Green SM, Roback MG, Kennedy RM, Krauss B. Clinical practice guideline for emergency department ketamine dissociative sedation: 2011 update. Ann Emerg Med. 2011;57(5):449–61. doi:10.1016/j.annemergmed.2010.11.030.

332. Green SM, Roback MG, Krauss B. Laryngospasm during emergency department ketamine sedation: a case–control study. Pediatr Emerg Care. 2010;26(11):798–802. doi:10.1097/PEC.0b013e3181fa8737.

333. Brown L, Christian-Kopp S, Sherwin TS, Khan A, Barcega B, Denmark TK, Moynihan JA, Kim GJ, Stewart G, Green SM. Adjunctive atropine is unnecessary during ketamine sedation in children. Acad Emerg Med. 2008;15(4):314–8. doi:10.1111/j.1553-2712.2008.00074.x.

334. Green SM, Rothrock SG. Transient apnea with intramuscular ketamine. Am J Emerg Med. 1997;15(4):440–1.

335. Greene CA, Gillette PC, Fyfe DA. Frequency of respiratory compromise after ketamine sedation for cardiac catheterization in patients less than 21 years of age. Am J Cardiol. 1991;68(10):1116–7.

336. Mitchell RK, Koury SI, Stone CK. Respiratory arrest after intramuscular ketamine in a 2-year-old child. Am J Emerg Med. 1996;14(6):580–1. doi:10.1016/S0735-6757(96)90105-9.

337. Tweed WA, Minuck M, Mymin D. Circulatory responses to ketamine anesthesia. Anesthesiology. 1972;37(6):613–9.

338. Hickey PR, Hansen DD, Cramolini GM, Vincent RN, Lang P. Pulmonary and systemic hemodynamic responses to ketamine in infants with normal and elevated pulmonary vascular resistance. Anesthesiology. 1985;62(3):287–93.

339. Williams GD, Maan H, Ramamoorthy C, Kamra K, Bratton SL, Bair E, Kuan CC, Hammer GB, Feinstein JA. Perioperative complications in children with pulmonary hypertension undergoing general anesthesia with ketamine. Pediatr Anesth. 2010;20(1):28–37. doi:10.1111/j.1460-9592.2009.03166.x.

340. Oklu E, Bulutcu FS, Yalcin Y, Ozbek U, Cakali E, Bayindir O. Which anesthetic agent alters the hemodynamic status during pediatric catheterization? Comparison of propofol versus ketamine. J Cardiothorac Vasc Anesth. 2003;17(6):686–90.

341. Christ G, Mundigler G, Merhaut C, Zehetgruber M, Kratochwill C, Heinz G, Siostrzonek P. Adverse cardiovascular effects of ketamine infusion in patients with catecholamine-dependent heart failure. Anaesth Intens Care. 1997;25(3):255–9.

342. Himmelseher S, Durieux ME. Revising a dogma: ketamine for patients with neurological injury? Anesth Analg. 2005;101(2):524–34.

343. Green SM, Andolfatto G, Krauss BS. Ketamine and intracranial pressure: no contraindication except hydrocephalus. Ann Emerg Med. 2015;65(1):52–4. doi:10.1016/j.annemergmed.2014.08.025.

344. Bourgoin A, Albanese J, Wereszczynski N, Charbit M, Vialet R, Martin C. Safety of sedation with ketamine in severe head injury patients: comparison with sufentanil. Crit Care Med. 2003;31(3):711–7. doi:10.1097/01.CCM.0000044505.24727.16.

345. Cohen L, Athaide V, Wickham ME, Doyle-Waters MM, Rose NG, Hohl CM. The effect of ketamine on intracranial and cerebral perfusion pressure and health outcomes: a systematic review. Ann Emerg Med. 2015;65(1):43–51.e42. doi:10.1016/j.annemergmed.2014.06.018.

346. Yoshikawa K, Murai Y. The effect of ketamine on intraocular pressure in children. Anesth Analg. 1971;50(2):199–202.

347. Davidson A, Flick RP. Neurodevelopmental implications of the use of sedation and analgesia in neonates. Clin Perinatol. 2013;40(3):559–73. doi:10.1016/j.clp.2013.05.009.

348. Lin EP, Soriano SG, Loepke AW. Anesthetic neurotoxicity. Anesthesiol Clin. 2014;32(1):133–55. doi:10.1016/j.anclin.2013.10.003.

349. Sinner B, Becke K, Engelhard K. General anaesthetics and the developing brain: an overview. Anaesthesia. 2014;69(9):1009–22. doi:10.1111/anae.12637.

350. Davidson AJ. Anesthesia and neurotoxicity to the developing brain: the clinical relevance. Paediatr Anaesth. 2011;21(7):716–21. doi:10.1111/j.1460-9592.2010.03506.x.

351. Lin L, Zhang JW, Huang Y, Bai J, Cai MH, Zhang MZ. Population pharmacokinetics of intravenous bolus etomidate in children over 6 months of age. Pediatr Anesth. 2012;22(4):318–26. doi:10.1111/j.1460-9592.2011.03696.x.

352. Sfez M, Le Mapihan Y, Levron JC, Gaillard JL, Rosemblatt JM, Le Moing JP. Comparison of the pharmacokinetics of etomidate in children and in adults. Ann Fr Anesth Reanim. 1990;9(2):127–31.

353. Su F, El-Komy MH, Hammer GB, Frymoyer A, Cohane CA, Drover DR. Population pharmacokinetics of etomidate in neonates and infants with congenital heart disease. Biopharm Drug Dispos. 2015;36(2):104–14. doi:10.1002/bdd.1924.

354. Wanscher M, Tonnesen E, Huttel M, Larsen K. Etomidate infusion and adrenocortical function. A study in elective surgery. Acta Anaesthesiol Scand. 1985;29(5):483–5.

355. Sneyd JR. Novel etomidate derivatives. Curr Pharm Des. 2012;18(38):6253–6.

356. Bramwell KJ, Haizlip J, Pribble C, VanDerHeyden TC, Witte M. The effect of etomidate on intracranial pressure and systemic blood pressure in pediatric patients with severe traumatic brain injury. Pediatr Emerg Care. 2006;22(2):90–3. doi:10.1097/01.pec.0000199563.64264.3a.

357. Sarkar M, Laussen PC, Zurakowski D, Shukla A, Kussman B, Odegard KC. Hemodynamic responses to etomidate on induction of anesthesia in pediatric patients. Anesth Analg. 2005;101(3):645–50. doi:10.1213/01.ane.0000166764.99863.b4.

358. Inturrisi CE, Colburn WA. Application of pharmacokinetic-pharmacodynamic modeling to analgesia. In: Foley KM, Inturrisi CE, editors. Advances in pain research and therapy. Opioid analgesics in the management of clinical pain. New York: Raven Press; 1986. p. 441–52.

359. Staahl C, Upton R, Foster DJ, Christrup LL, Kristensen K, Hansen SH, Arendt-Nielsen L, Drewes AM. Pharmacokinetic-pharmacodynamic modeling of morphine and oxycodone concentrations and analgesic effect in a multimodal experimental pain model. J Clin Pharmacol. 2008;48(5):619–31. doi:10.1177/0091270008314465.

360. van Dorp EL, Romberg R, Sarton E, Bovill JG, Dahan A. Morphine-6-glucuronide: morphine's successor for postoperative pain relief? Anesth Analg. 2006;102(6):1789–97.

361. Dahan A, Romberg R, Teppema L, Sarton E, Bijl H, Olofsen E. Simultaneous measurement and integrated analysis of analgesia and respiration after an intravenous morphine infusion. Anesthesiology. 2004;101(5):1201–9.

362. Hannam JA, Anderson BJ. Contribution of morphine and morphine-6-glucuronide to respiratory depression in a child. Anaesth Intensive Care. 2012;40(5):867–70.

363. Romberg R, Olofsen E, Sarton E, Teppema L, Dahan A. Pharmacodynamic effect of morphine-6-glucuronide versus morphine on hypoxic and hypercapnic breathing in healthy volunteers. Anesthesiology. 2003;99(4):788–98.

364. Bouwmeester NJ, van den Anker JN, Hop WC, Anand KJ, Tibboel D. Age- and therapy-related effects on morphine requirements and plasma concentrations of morphine and its metabolites in postoperative infants. Br J Anaesth. 2003;90(5):642–52.

365. Bray RJ, Beeton C, Hinton W, Seviour JA. Plasma morphine levels produced by continuous infusion in children. Anaesthesia. 1986;41(7):753–5.

366. Lynn AM, Opheim KE, Tyler DC. Morphine infusion after pediatric cardiac surgery. Crit Care Med. 1984;12(10):863–6.

367. Anderson BJ, Persson M, Anderson M. Rationalising intravenous morphine prescriptions in children. Acute Pain. 1999;2:59–67.

368. Aubrun F, Mazoit JX, Riou B. Postoperative intravenous morphine titration. Br J Anaesth. 2012;108(2):193–201. doi:10.1093/bja/aer458.

369. Bernard R, Salvi N, Gall O, Egan M, Treluyer JM, Carli PA, Orliaguet GA. MORPHIT: an observational study on morphine titration in the postanesthetic care unit in children. Paediatr Anaesth. 2014;24(3):303–8. doi:10.1111/pan.12286.

370. Morton NS, Errera A. APA national audit of pediatric opioid infusions. Paediatr Anaesth. 2010;20(2):119–25. doi:10.1111/j.1460-9592.2009.03187.x.

371. West N, Nilforushan V, Stinson J, Ansermino JM, Lauder G. Critical incidents related to opioid infusions in children: a five-year review and analysis. Can J Anaesth. 2014;61(4):312–21. doi:10.1007/s12630-013-0097-2.

372. Bouwmeester NJ, Anderson BJ, Tibboel D, Holford NH. Developmental pharmacokinetics of morphine and its metabolites in neonates, infants and young children. Br J Anaesth. 2004;92(2):208–17.

373. Osborne R, Joel S, Grebenik K, Trew D, Slevin M. The pharmacokinetics of morphine and morphine glucuronides in kidney failure. Clin Pharmacol Ther. 1993;54(2):158–67.

374. Miners JO, Knights KM, Houston JB, Mackenzie PI. In vitro-in vivo correlation for drugs and other compounds eliminated by glucuronidation in humans: pitfalls and promises. Biochem Pharmacol. 2006;71(11):1531–9. doi:10.1016/j.bcp.2005.12.019.

375. Wang J, Evans AM, Knights KM, Miners JO. Differential disposition of intra-renal generated and preformed glucuronides: studies with 4-methylumbelliferone and 4-methylumbelliferyl glucuronide in the filtering and nonfiltering isolated perfused rat kidney. J Pharm Pharmacol. 2011;63(4):507–14. doi:10.1111/j.2042-7158.2010.01244.x.

376. Knights KM, Rowland A, Miners JO. Renal drug metabolism in humans: the potential for drug-endobiotic interactions involving cytochrome P450 (CYP) and UDP-glucuronosyltransferase (UGT). Br J Clin Pharmacol. 2013;76(4):587–602. doi:10.1111/bcp.12086.

377. Nahata MC, Miser AW, Miser JS, Reuning RH. Variation in morphine pharmacokinetics in children with cancer. Dev Pharmacol Ther. 1985;8(3):182–8.

378. Nahata MC, Miser AW, Miser JS, Reuning RH. Analgesic plasma concentrations of morphine in children with terminal malignancy receiving a continuous subcutaneous infusion of morphine sulfate to control severe pain. Pain. 1984;18(2):109–14.

379. Peters JW, Anderson BJ, Simons SH, Uges DR, Tibboel D. Morphine pharmacokinetics during venoarterial extracorporeal membrane oxygenation in neonates. Intensive Care Med. 2005;31(2):257–63.

380. Bolan EA, Tallarida RJ, Pasternak GW. Synergy between mu opioid ligands: evidence for functional interactions among mu opioid receptor subtypes. J Pharmacol Exp Ther. 2002;303(2):557–62. doi:10.1124/jpet.102.035881.

381. Pasternak GW. Preclinical pharmacology and opioid combinations. Pain Med. 2012;13 Suppl 1:S4–11. doi:10.1111/j.1526-4637.2012.01335.x.

382. Lotsch J, Skarke C, Schmidt H, Grosch S, Geisslinger G. The transfer half-life of morphine-6-glucuronide from plasma to effect site assessed by pupil size measurement in healthy volunteers. Anesthesiology. 2001;95(6):1329–38.

383. Scott JC, Stanski DR. Decreased fentanyl and alfentanil dose requirements with age. A simultaneous pharmacokinetic and pharmacodynamic evaluation. J Pharmacol Exp Ther. 1987;240(1):159–66.

384. Wynands JE, Townsend GE, Wong P, Whalley DG, Srikant CB, Patel YC. Blood pressure response and plasma fentanyl concentrations during high- and very high-dose fentanyl anesthesia for coronary artery surgery. Anesth Analg. 1983;62(7):661–5.

385. Kuhls E, Gauntlett IS, Lau M, Brown R, Rudolph CD, Teitel DF, Fisher DM. Effect of increased intra-abdominal pressure on

386. Koren G, Goresky G, Crean P, Klein J, MacLeod SM. Pediatric fentanyl dosing based on pharmacokinetics during cardiac surgery. Anesth Analg. 1984;63(6):577–82.

387. Koren G, Goresky G, Crean P, Klein J, MacLeod SM. Unexpected alterations in fentanyl pharmacokinetics in children undergoing cardiac surgery: age related or disease related? Dev Pharmacol Ther. 1986;9(3):183–91.

388. Koren G, Barker C, Goresky G, Bohn D, Kent G, Klein J, MacLeod SM, Biggar WD. The influence of hypothermia on the disposition of fentanyl--human and animal studies. Eur J Clin Pharmacol. 1987;32(4):373–6.

389. Katz R, Kelly HW. Pharmacokinetics of continuous infusions of fentanyl in critically ill children. Crit Care Med. 1993;21(7):995–1000.

390. Ginsberg B, Howell S, Glass PS, Margolis JO, Ross AK, Dear GL, Shafer SL. Pharmacokinetic model-driven infusion of fentanyl in children. Anesthesiology. 1996;85(6):1268–75.

391. Katz R, Kelly HW, Hsi A. Prospective study on the occurrence of withdrawal in critically ill children who receive fentanyl by continuous infusion. Crit Care Med. 1994;22(5):763–7.

392. Suresh S, Anand KJS. Opioid tolerance in neonates: a state of the art review. Paediatr Anaesth. 2001;11:511–21.

393. Arandia HY, Patil VU. Glottic closure following large doses of fentanyl. Anesthesiology. 1987;66(4):574–5.

394. Sokoll MD, Hoyt JL, Gergis SD. Studies in muscle rigidity, nitrous oxide, and narcotic analgesic agents. Anesth Analg. 1972;51(1):16–20.

395. Murat I, Levron JC, Berg A, Saint-Maurice C. Effects of fentanyl on baroreceptor reflex control of heart rate in newborn infants. Anesthesiology. 1988;68(5):717–22.

396. Mani V, Morton NS. Overview of total intravenous anesthesia in children. Paediatr Anaesth. 2010;20(3):211–22. doi:10.1111/j.1460-9592.2009.03112.x.

397. Sam WJ, Hammer GB, Drover DR. Population pharmacokinetics of remifentanil in infants and children undergoing cardiac surgery. BMC Anesthesiol. 2009;9:5. doi:10.1186/1471-2253-9-5.

398. Michelsen LG, Holford NH, Lu W, Hoke JF, Hug CC, Bailey JM. The pharmacokinetics of remifentanil in patients undergoing coronary artery bypass grafting with cardiopulmonary bypass. Anesth Analg. 2001;93(5):1100–5.

399. Barker N, Lim J, Amari E, Malherbe S, Ansermino JM. Relationship between age and spontaneous ventilation during intravenous anesthesia in children. Paediatr Anaesth. 2007;17(10):948–55. doi:10.1111/j.1460-9592.2007.02301.x.

400. Litman RS. Conscious sedation with remifentanil during painful medical procedures. J Pain Symptom Manage. 2000;19(6):468–71.

401. Choong K, AlFaleh K, Doucette J, Gray S, Rich B, Verhey L, Paes B. Remifentanil for endotracheal intubation in neonates: a randomised controlled trial. Arch Dis Child. 2010;95(2):F80–4. doi:10.1136/adc.2009.167338.

402. Penido MG, Garra R, Sammartino M, Pereira e Silva Y. Remifentanil in neonatal intensive care and anaesthesia practice. Acta Paediatr. 2010;99(10):1454–63. doi:10.1111/j.1651-2227.2010.01868.x.

403. Anderson BJ, Holford NH. Leaving no stone unturned, or extracting blood from stone? Paediatr Anaesth. 2010;20(1):1–6. doi:10.1111/j.1460-9592.2009.03179.x.

404. Galinkin JL, Davis PJ, McGowan FX, Lynn AM, Rabb MF, Yaster M, Henson LG, Blum R, Hechtman D, Maxwell L, Szmuk P, Orr R, Krane EJ, Edwards S, Kurth CD. A randomized multicenter study of remifentanil compared with halothane in neonates and infants undergoing pyloromyotomy.

II Perioperative breathing patterns in neonates and infants with pyloric stenosis. Anesth Analg. 2001;93(6):1387–92.

405. Zhao M, Joo DT. Enhancement of spinal N-methyl-D-aspartate receptor function by remifentanil action at delta-opioid receptors as a mechanism for acute opioid-induced hyperalgesia or tolerance. Anesthesiology. 2008;109(2):308–17. doi:10.1097/ALN.0b013e31817f4c5d.

406. Scholz J, Steinfath M, Schulz M. Clinical pharmacokinetics of alfentanil, fentanyl and sufentanil. An update. Clin Pharmacokinet. 1996;31(4):275–92. doi:10.2165/00003088-199631040-00004.

407. Meuldermans W, Van Peer A, Hendrickx J, Woestenborghs R, Lauwers W, Heykants J, Vanden Bussche G, Van Craeyvelt H, Van der Aa P. Alfentanil pharmacokinetics and metabolism in humans. Anesthesiology. 1988;69(4):527–34.

408. Davis PJ, Cook DR. Clinical pharmacokinetics of the newer intravenous anaesthetic agents. Clin Pharmacokinet. 1986;11(1):18–35.

409. Marlow N, Weindling AM, Van Peer A, Heykants J. Alfentanil pharmacokinetics in preterm infants. Arch Dis Child. 1990;65(4 Spec No):349–51.

410. Killian A, Davis PJ, Stiller RL, Cicco R, Cook DR, Guthrie RD. Influence of gestational age on pharmacokinetics of alfentanil in neonates. Dev Pharmacol Ther. 1990;15(2):82–5.

411. Meistelman C, Saint-Maurice C, Lepaul M, Levron JC, Loose JP, MacGee K. A comparison of alfentanil pharmacokinetics in children and adults. Anesthesiology. 1987;66(1):13–6.

412. Roure P, Jean N, Leclerc AC, Cabanel N, Levron JC, Duvaldestin P. Pharmacokinetics of alfentanil in children undergoing surgery. Br J Anaesth. 1987;59(11):1437–40.

413. Goresky GV, Koren G, Sabourin MA, Sale JP, Strunin L. The pharmacokinetics of alfentanil in children. Anesthesiology. 1987;67(5):654–9.

414. Persson MP, Nilsson A, Hartvig P. Pharmacokinetics of alfentanil in total i.v. anaesthesia. Br J Anaesth. 1988;60(7):755–61.

415. Shafer A, Sung ML, White PF. Pharmacokinetics and pharmacodynamics of alfentanil infusions during general anesthesia. Anesth Analg. 1986;65(10):1021–8.

416. Chauvin M, Bonnet F, Montembault C, Levron JC, Viars P. The influence of hepatic plasma flow on alfentanil plasma concentration plateaus achieved with an infusion model in humans: measurement of alfentanil hepatic extraction coefficient. Anesth Analg. 1986;65(10):999–1003.

417. Wilson AS, Stiller RL, Davis PJ, Fedel G, Chakravorti S, Israel BA, McGowan Jr FX. Fentanyl and alfentanil plasma protein binding in preterm and term neonates. Anesth Analg. 1997;84(2):315–8.

418. Demirbilek S, Ganidagli S, Aksoy N, Becerik C, Baysal Z. The effects of remifentanil and alfentanil-based total intravenous anesthesia (TIVA) on the endocrine response to abdominal hysterectomy. J Clin Anesth. 2004;16(5):358–63. doi:10.1016/j.jclinane.2003.10.002.

419. Ganidagli S, Cengiz M, Baysal Z. Remifentanil vs alfentanil in the total intravenous anaesthesia for paediatric abdominal surgery. Paediatr Anaesth. 2003;13(8):695–700.

420. Saarenmaa E, Huttunen P, Leppaluoto J, Fellman V. Alfentanil as procedural pain relief in newborn infants. Arch Dis Child Fetal Neonatal Ed. 1996;75(2):F103–7.

421. Pokela ML, Olkkola KT, Koivisto M, Ryhanen P. Pharmacokinetics and pharmacodynamics of intravenous meperidine in neonates and infants. Clin Pharmacol Ther. 1992;52(4):342–9.

422. Hilberman M, Hyer D. Potency of sufentanil. Anesthesiology. 1986;64(5):665–8.

423. Greeley WJ, de Bruijn NP, Davis DP. Sufentanil pharmacokinetics in pediatric cardiovascular patients. Anesth Analg. 1987;66(11):1067–72.

424. Guay J, Gaudreault P, Tang A, Goulet B, Varin F. Pharmacokinetics of sufentanil in normal children. Can J Anaesth. 1992;39(1):14–20.

425. Tateishi T, Krivoruk Y, Ueng YF, Wood AJ, Guengerich FP, Wood M. Identification of human liver cytochrome P-450 3A4 as the enzyme responsible for fentanyl and sufentanil N-dealkylation. Anesth Analg. 1996;82(1):167–72.

426. Lacroix D, Sonnier M, Moncion A, Cheron G, Cresteil T. Expression of CYP3A in the human liver--evidence that the shift between CYP3A7 and CYP3A4 occurs immediately after birth. Eur J Biochem. 1997;247(2):625–34.

427. Davis PJ, Cook DR, Stiller RL, Davin-Robinson KA. Pharmacodynamics and pharmacokinetics of high-dose sufentanil in infants and children undergoing cardiac surgery. Anesth Analg. 1987;66(3):203–8.

428. Chauvin M, Ferrier C, Haberer JP, Spielvogel C, Lebrault C, Levron JC, Duvaldestin P. Sufentanil pharmacokinetics in patients with cirrhosis. Anesth Analg. 1989;68(1):1–4.

429. Helmers JH, Noorduin H, Van Peer A, Van Leeuwen L, Zuurmond WW. Comparison of intravenous and intranasal sufentanil absorption and sedation. Can J Anaesth. 1989;36(5):494–7. doi:10.1007/bf03005373.

430. Henderson JM, Brodsky DA, Fisher DM, Brett CM, Hertzka RE. Pre-induction of anesthesia in pediatric patients with nasally administered sufentanil. Anesthesiology. 1988;68(5):671–5.

431. Roelofse JA, Shipton EA, de la Harpe CJ, Blignaut RJ. Intranasal sufentanil/midazolam versus ketamine/midazolam for analgesia/sedation in the pediatric population prior to undergoing multiple dental extractions under general anesthesia: a prospective, double-blind, randomized comparison. Anesth Prog. 2004;51(4):114–21.

432. Zedie N, Amory DW, Wagner BK, O'Hara DA. Comparison of intranasal midazolam and sufentanil premedication in pediatric outpatients. Clin Pharmacol Ther. 1996;59(3):341–8.

433. Koren G, Maurice L. Pediatric uses of opioids. Pediatr Clin North Am. 1989;36(5):1141–56.

434. Jaffe JH, Martine WR. Opioid analgesics and antagonists. In: Goodman Gilman A, Rall TW, Nies AS, Taylor P, editors. The pharmacological basis of therapeutics. New York: Pergamon Press; 1990. p. 485–531.

435. Hamunen K, Maunuksela EL, Seppala T, Olkkola KT. Pharmacokinetics of i.v. and rectal pethidine in children undergoing ophthalmic surgery. Br J Anaesth. 1993;71(6):823–6.

436. Caldwell J, Wakile LA, Notarianni LJ, Smith RL, Correy GJ, Lieberman BA, Beard RW, Finnie MD, Snedden W. Maternal and neonatal disposition of pethidine in childbirth--a study using quantitative gas chromatography–mass spectrometry. Life Sci. 1978;22(7):589–96.

437. Hagmeyer KO, Mauro LS, Mauro VF. Meperidine-related seizures associated with patient-controlled analgesia pumps. Ann Pharmacother. 1993;27(1):29–32.

438. Flacke JW, Flacke WE, Bloor BC, Van Etten AP, Kripke BJ. Histamine release by four narcotics: a double-blind study in humans. Anesth Analg. 1987;66(8):723–30.

439. Latta KS, Ginsberg B, Barkin RL. Meperidine: a critical review. Am J Ther. 2002;9(1):53–68.

440. Ngan Kee WD. Intrathecal pethidine: pharmacology and clinical applications. Anaesth Intens Care. 1998;26(2):137–46.

441. Collins JJ, Geake J, Grier HE, Houck CS, Thaler HT, Weinstein HJ, Twum-Danso NY, Berde CB. Patient-controlled analgesia for mucositis pain in children: a three-period crossover study comparing morphine and hydromorphone. J Pediatr. 1996;129(5):722–8.

442. Hagen N, Thirlwell MP, Dhaliwal HS, Babul N, Harsanyi Z, Darke AC. Steady-state pharmacokinetics of hydromorphone and hydromorphone-3-glucuronide in cancer patients after immediate and controlled-release hydromorphone. J Clin Pharmacol. 1995;35(1):37–44.

443. Parab PV, Ritschel WA, Coyle DE, Gregg RV, Denson DD. Pharmacokinetics of hydromorphone after intravenous, peroral and rectal administration to human subjects. Biopharm Drug Dispos. 1988;9(2):187–99.

444. Ritschel WA, Parab PV, Denson DD, Coyle DE, Gregg RV. Absolute bioavailability of hydromorphone after peroral and rectal administration in humans: saliva/plasma ratio and clinical effects. J Clin Pharmacol. 1987;27(9):647–53.

445. Vallner JJ, Stewart JT, Kotzan JA, Kirsten EB, Honigberg IL. Pharmacokinetics and bioavailability of hydromorphone following intravenous and oral administration to human subjects. J Clin Pharmacol. 1981;21(4):152–6.

446. Volles DF, McGory R. Perspectives in pain management: pharmacokinetic considerations: pharmacokinetic considerations. Crit Care Clin. 1999;15(1):55–75.

447. Babul N, Darke AC, Hain R. Hydromorphone and metabolite pharmacokinetics in children. J Pain Symptom Manage. 1995;10 (5):335–7.

448. Wermeling DP, Clinch T, Rudy AC, Dreitlein D, Suner S, Lacouture PG. A multicenter, open-label, exploratory dose-ranging trial of intranasal hydromorphone for managing acute pain from traumatic injury. J Pain. 2010;11(1):24–31. doi:10.1016/j.jpain.2009.05.002.

449. Coda BA, Rudy AC, Archer SM, Wermeling DP. Pharmacokinetics and bioavailability of single-dose intranasal hydromorphone hydrochloride in healthy volunteers. Anesth Analg. 2003;97 (1):117–23.

450. Kokki M, Broms S, Eskelinen M, Neuvonen PJ, Halonen T, Kokki H. The analgesic concentration of oxycodone with co-administration of paracetamol—a dose-finding study in adult patients undergoing laparoscopic cholecystectomy. Basic Clin Pharmacol Toxicol. 2012;111(6):391–5. doi:10.1111/j.1742-7843.2012.00916.x.

451. Czarnecki ML, Jandrisevits MD, Theiler SC, Huth MM, Weisman SJ. Controlled-release oxycodone for the management of pediatric postoperative pain. J Pain Symptom Manage. 2004;27 (4):379–86.

452. Kokki H, Rasanen I, Lasalmi M, Lehtola S, Ranta VP, Vanamo K, Ojanpera I. Comparison of oxycodone pharmacokinetics after buccal and sublingual administration in children. Clin Pharmacokinet. 2006;45(7):745–54. doi:10.2165/00003088-200645070-00009.

453. Kokki H, Tuomilehto H, Karvinen M. Pharmacokinetics of ketoprofen following oral and intramuscular administration in young children. Eur J Clin Pharmacol. 2001;57(9):643–7.

454. Leow KP, Cramond T, Smith MT. Pharmacokinetics and pharmacodynamics of oxycodone when given intravenously and rectally to adult patients with cancer pain. Anesth Analg. 1995;80 (2):296–302.

455. Kokki H, Kokki M, Sjovall S. Oxycodone for the treatment of postoperative pain. Exp Opin Pharmacother. 2012;13(7):1045–58. doi:10.1517/14656566.2012.677823.

456. Olkkola KT, Hamunen K, Seppala T, Maunuksela EL. Pharmacokinetics and ventilatory effects of intravenous oxycodone in postoperative children. Br J Clin Pharmacol. 1994;38(1):71–6.

457. Lam J, Kelly L, Ciszkowski C, Landsmeer ML, Nauta M, Carleton BC, Hayden MR, Madadi P, Koren G. Central nervous system depression of neonates breastfed by mothers receiving oxycodone for postpartum analgesia. J Pediatr. 2012;160(1):33–7.e32. doi:10.1016/j.jpeds.2011.06.050.

458. Pokela ML, Anttila E, Seppala T, Olkkola KT. Marked variation in oxycodone pharmacokinetics in infants. Paediatr Anaesth. 2005;15(7):560–5.

459. El-Tahtawy A, Kokki H, Reidenberg BE. Population pharmacokinetics of oxycodone in children 6 months to 7 years old. J Clin Pharmacol. 2006;46(4):433–42.

460. Kokki H, Rasanen I, Reinikainen M, Suhonen P, Vanamo K, Ojanpera I. Pharmacokinetics of oxycodone after intravenous, buccal, intramuscular and gastric administration in children. Clin Pharmacokinet. 2004;43(9):613–22. doi:10.2165/00003088-200443090-00004.

461. Korjamo T, Tolonen A, Ranta VP, Turpeinen M, Kokki H. Metabolism of oxycodone in human hepatocytes from different age groups and prediction of hepatic plasma clearance. Front Pharmacol. 2011;2:87. doi:10.3389/fphar.2011.00087.

462. Sabatowski R, Kasper SM, Radbruch L. Patient-controlled analgesia with intravenous L-methadone in a child with cancer pain refractory to high-dose morphine. J Pain Sympt Manag. 2002;23 (1):3–5.

463. Suresh S, Anand KJ. Opioid tolerance in neonates: mechanisms, diagnosis, assessment, and management. Semin Perinatol. 1998;22(5):425–33.

464. Tobias JD. Tolerance, withdrawal, and physical dependency after long-term sedation and analgesia of children in the pediatric intensive care unit. Crit Care Med. 2000;28(6):2122–32.

465. Lugo RA, Satterfield KL, Kern SE. Pharmacokinetics of methadone. J Pain Palliat Care Pharmacother. 2005;19(4):13–24.

466. Robertson RC, Darsey E, Fortenberry JD, Pettignano R, Hartley G. Evaluation of an opiate-weaning protocol using methadone in pediatric intensive care unit patients. Pediatr Crit Care Med. 2000;1(2):119–23.

467. Berde CB, Beyer JE, Bournaki MC, Levin CR, Sethna NF. Comparison of morphine and methadone for prevention of postoperative pain in 3- to 7-year-old children. J Pediatr. 1991;119 (1 Pt 1):136–41.

468. Shir Y, Shenkman Z, Shavelson V, Davidson EM, Rosen G. Oral methadone for the treatment of severe pain in hospitalized children: a report of five cases. Clin J Pain. 1998;14(4):350–3.

469. Davies D, DeVlaming D, Haines C. Methadone analgesia for children with advanced cancer. Pediatr Blood Cancer. 2008;51 (3):393–7. doi:10.1002/pbc.21584.

470. Gourlay GK, Willis RJ, Wilson PR. Postoperative pain control with methadone: influence of supplementary methadone doses and blood concentration--response relationships. Anesthesiology. 1984;61(1):19–26.

471. Rosen TS, Pippenger CE. Pharmacologic observations on the neonatal withdrawal syndrome. J Pediatr. 1976;88(6):1044–8.

472. Berkowitz BA. The relationship of pharmacokinetics to pharmacological activity: morphine, methadone and naloxone. Clin Pharmacokinet. 1976;1(3):219–30.

473. Kaufmann JJ, Koski WS, Benson DN, Semo NM. Narcotic and narcotic antagonist pKa's and partition coefficients and their significance in clinical practice. Drug Alcohol Depend. 1975;1 (2):103–14.

474. Gourlay GK, Wilson PR, Glynn CJ. Pharmacodynamics and pharmacokinetics of methadone during the perioperative period. Anesthesiology. 1982;57(6):458–67.

475. Berde CB, Sethna NF, Holzman RS, Reidy RN, Gondek EJ. Pharmacokinetics of methadone in children and adolescents in the perioperative period. Anesthesiology. 1987;67(3A):A519.

476. Chana SK, Anand KJ. Can we use methadone for analgesia in neonates? Arch Dis Child Fetal Neonatal Ed. 2001;85(2):F79–81.

477. Stemland CJ, Witte J, Colquhoun DA, Durieux ME, Langman LJ, Balireddy R, Thammishetti S, Abel MF, Anderson BJ. The pharmacokinetics of methadone in adolescents undergoing posterior spinal fusion. Paediatr Anaesth. 2013;23(1):51–7. doi:10.1111/pan.12021.

478. Foster DJ, Somogyi AA, White JM, Bochner F. Population pharmacokinetics of (R)-, (S)- and rac-methadone in methadone maintenance patients. Br J Clin Pharmacol. 2004;57(6):742–55. doi:10.1111/j.1365-2125.2004.02079.x.

479. Inturrisi CE, Portenoy RK, Max MB, Colburn WA, Foley KM. - Pharmacokinetic-pharmacodynamic relationships of methadone infusions in patients with cancer pain. Clin Pharmacol Ther. 1990;47(5):565–77.

480. Krantz MJ, Kutinsky IB, Robertson AD, Mehler PS. Dose-related effects of methadone on QT prolongation in a series of patients with torsade de pointes. Pharmacotherapy. 2003;23(6):802–5.

481. Martell BA, Arnsten JH, Krantz MJ, Gourevitch MN. Impact of methadone treatment on cardiac repolarization and conduction in opioid users. Am J Cardiol. 2005;95(7):915–8. doi:10.1016/j.amjcard.2004.11.055.

482. Tremlett M, Anderson BJ, Wolf A. Pro-con debate: is codeine a drug that still has a useful role in pediatric practice? Paediatr Anaesth. 2010;20(2):183–94. doi:10.1111/j.1460-9592.2009.03234.x.

483. Cox RG. Hypoxaemia and hypotension after intravenous codeine phosphate. Can J Anaes. 1994;41(12):1211–3. doi:10.1007/BF03020664.

484. Parke TJ, Nandi PR, Bird KJ, Jewkes DA. Profound hypotension following intravenous codeine phosphate. Three case reports and some recommendations. Anaesthesia. 1992;47(10):852–4.

485. Shanahan EC, Marshall AG, Garrett CP. Adverse reactions to intravenous codeine phosphate in children. A report of three cases. Anaesthesia. 1983;38(1):40–3.

486. Zolezzi M, Al Mohaimeed SA. Seizures with intravenous codeine phosphate. Ann Pharmacother. 2001;35(10):1211–3.

487. Anderson BJ. Is it farewell to codeine? Arch Dis Child. 2013;98 (12):986–8. doi:10.1136/archdischild-2013-304974.

488. Tremlett MR. Wither codeine? Paediatr Anaesth. 2013;23 (8):677–83. doi:10.1111/pan.12190.

489. Kelly LE, Rieder M, van den Anker J, Malkin B, Ross C, Neely MN, Carleton B, Hayden MR, Madadi P, Koren G. More codeine fatalities after tonsillectomy in North American children. Pediatrics. 2012;129(5):e1343–7. doi:10.1542/peds.2011-2538.

490. Racoosin JA, Roberson DW, Pacanowski MA, Nielsen DR. New evidence about an old drug—risk with codeine after adenotonsillectomy. N Engl J Med. 2013;368(23):2155–7. doi:10.1056/NEJMp1302454.

491. Voelker R. Children's deaths linked with postsurgical codeine. JAMA. 2012;308(10):963. doi:10.1001/2012.jama.11525.

492. Waters KA, McBrien F, Stewart P, Hinder M, Wharton S. Effects of OSA, inhalational anesthesia, and fentanyl on the airway and ventilation of children. J Appl Physiol. 2002;92(5):1987–94. doi:10.1152/japplphysiol.00619.2001.

493. Semple D, Russell S, Doyle E, Aldridge LM. Comparison of morphine sulphate and codeine phosphate in children undergoing adenotonsillectomy. Paediatr Anaesth. 1999;9(2):135–8.

494. Tobias JD, Lowe S, Hersey S, Rasmussen GE, Werkhaven J. Analgesia after bilateral myringotomy and placement of pressure equalization tubes in children: acetaminophen versus acetaminophen with codeine. Anesth Analg. 1995;81(3):496–500.

495. St Charles CS, Matt BH, Hamilton MM, Katz BP. A comparison of ibuprofen versus acetaminophen with codeine in the young tonsillectomy patient. Otolaryngol Head Neck Surg. 1997;117 (1):76–82.

496. Persson K, Hammarlund-Udenaes M, Mortimer O, Rane A. The postoperative pharmacokinetics of codeine. Eur J Clin Pharmacol. 1992;42(6):663–6.

497. Eckhardt K, Li S, Ammon S, Schanzle G, Mikus G, Eichelbaum M. Same incidence of adverse drug events after codeine administration irrespective of the genetically determined differences in morphine formation. Pain. 1998;76(1–2):27–33.

498. Magnani B, Evans R. Codeine intoxication in the neonate. Pediatrics. 1999;104(6), e75.

499. Moreland TA, Brice JE, Walker CH, Parija AC. Naloxone pharmacokinetics in the newborn. Br J Clin Pharmacol. 1980;9 (6):609–12.

500. American Academy of Pediatrics Committee on Drugs: Naloxone dosage and route of administration for infants and children: addendum to emergency drug doses for infants and children. Pediatrics 1990;86(3):484–485.

501. Tenenbein M. Continuous naloxone infusion for opiate poisoning in infancy. J Pediatr. 1984;105(4):645–8.

502. Anderson BJ. Paracetamol (Acetaminophen): mechanisms of action. Paed Anaesth. 2008;18(10):915–21.

503. Gibb IA, Anderson BJ. Paracetamol (acetaminophen) pharmacodynamics; interpreting the plasma concentration. Arch Dis Child. 2008;93:241–7.

504. Murat I, Baujard C, Foussat C, Guyot E, Petel H, Rod B, Ricard C. Tolerance and analgesic efficacy of a new i.v. paracetamol solution in children after inguinal hernia repair. Paediatr Anaesth. 2005;15(8):663–70.

505. Anderson BJ, Woollard GA, Holford NH. Acetaminophen analgesia in children: placebo effect and pain resolution after tonsillectomy. Eur J Clin Pharmacol. 2001;57(8):559–69.

506. Shinoda S, Aoyama T, Aoyama Y, Tomioka S, Matsumoto Y, Ohe Y. Pharmacokinetics/pharmacodynamics of acetaminophen analgesia in Japanese patients with chronic pain. Biol Pharm Bull. 2007;30(1):157–61.

507. Allegaert K, Naulaers G, Vanhaesebrouck S, Anderson BJ. The paracetamol concentration-effect relation in neonates. Paediatr Anaesth. 2013;23(1):45–50. doi:10.1111/pan.12076.

508. Allegaert K, Murat I, Anderson BJ. Not all intravenous paracetamol formulations are created equal. Paediatr Anaesth. 2007;17 (8):811–2.

509. Anderson BJ, Pons G, Autret-Leca E, Allegaert K, Boccard E. Pediatric intravenous paracetamol (propacetamol) pharmacokinetics: a population analysis. Paediatr Anaesth. 2005;15 (4):282–92.

510. Anderson BJ, Pearce S, McGann JE, Newson AJ, Holford NH. Investigations using logistic regression models on the effect of the LMA on morphine induced vomiting after tonsillectomy. Paediatr Anaesth. 2000;10(6):633–8.

511. Anderson BJ, Woollard GA, Holford NH. A model for size and age changes in the pharmacokinetics of paracetamol in neonates, infants and children. Br J Clin Pharmacol. 2000;50 (2):125–34.

512. Allegaert K, Anderson BJ, Naulaers G, De Hoon J, Verbesselt R, Debeer A, Devlieger H, Tibboel D. Intravenous paracetamol (propacetamol) pharmacokinetics in term and preterm neonates. Eur J Clin Pharmacol. 2004;60(3):191–7.

513. Palmer GM, Atkins M, Anderson BJ, Smith KR, Culnane TJ, McNally CM, Perkins EJ, Chalkiadis GA, Hunt RW. I.-V. acetaminophen pharmacokinetics in neonates after multiple doses. Br J Anaesth. 2008;101(4):523–30.

514. Allegaert K, Palmer GM, Anderson BJ. The pharmacokinetics of intravenous paracetamol in neonates: size matters most. Arch Dis Child. 2011;96(6):575–80. doi:10.1136/adc.2010.204552.

515. Johnsrud EK, Koukouritaki SB, Divakaran K, Brunengraber LL, Hines RN, McCarver DG. Human hepatic CYP2E1 expression during development. J Pharmacol Exp Ther. 2003;307 (1):402–7.

516. Anderson BJ, Holford NHG, Armishaw JC, Aicken R. Predicting concentrations in children presenting with acetaminophen overdose. J Pediatrics. 1999;135:290–5.

517. Rumack BH, Matthew H. Acetaminophen poisoning and toxicity. Pediatrics. 1975;55:871–6.

518. Kearns GL, Leeder JS, Wasserman GS. Acetaminophen overdose with therapeutic intent. J Pediatr. 1998;132(1):5–8.

519. Li H, Mandema J, Wada R, Jayawardena S, Desjardins P, Doyle G, Kellstein D. Modeling the onset and offset of dental pain relief by ibuprofen. J Clin Pharmacol. 2012;52(1):89–101. doi:10.1177/0091270010389470.

520. Hannam JA, Anderson BJ, Mahadevan M, Holford NH. Postoperative analgesia using diclofenac and acetaminophen in children. Paediatr Anaesth. 2014;24(9):953–61. doi:10.1111/pan.12422.

521. Aranda JV, Varvarigou A, Beharry K, Bansal R, Bardin C, Modanlou H, Papageorgiou A, Chemtob S. Pharmacokinetics and protein binding of intravenous ibuprofen in the premature newborn infant. Acta Paediatr. 1997;86(3):289–93.

522. Van Overmeire B, Touw D, Schepens PJ, Kearns GL, van den Anker JN. Ibuprofen pharmacokinetics in preterm infants with patent ductus arteriosus. Clin Pharmacol Ther. 2001;70(4):336–43.

523. Benet LZ, Hoener BA. Changes in plasma protein binding have little clinical relevance. Clin Pharmacol Ther. 2002;71(3):115–21.

524. Hamman MA, Thompson GA, Hall SD. Regioselective and stereoselective metabolism of ibuprofen by human cytochrome P450 2C. Biochem Pharmacol. 1997;54(1):33–41.

525. Tanaka E. Clinically important pharmacokinetic drug-drug interactions: role of cytochrome P450 enzymes. J Clin Pharm Ther. 1998;23(6):403–16.

526. Scott CS, Retsch-Bogart GZ, Kustra RP, Graham KM, Glasscock BJ, Smith PC. The pharmacokinetics of ibuprofen suspension, chewable tablets, and tablets in children with cystic fibrosis. J Pediatr. 1999;134(1):58–63.

527. Wiest DB, Pinson JB, Gal PS, Brundage RC, Schall S, Ransom JL, Weaver RL, Purohit D, Brown Y. Population pharmacokinetics of intravenous indomethacin in neonates with symptomatic patent ductus arteriosus. Clin Pharmacol Ther. 1991;49(5):550–7.

528. Smyth JM, Collier PS, Darwish M, Millership JS, Halliday HL, Petersen S, McElnay JC. Intravenous indomethacin in preterm infants with symptomatic patent ductus arteriosus. A population pharmacokinetic study. Br J Clin Pharmacol. 2004;58(3):249–58.

529. Olkkola KT, Maunuksela EL, Korpela R. Pharmacokinetics of postoperative intravenous indomethacin in children. Pharmacol Toxicol. 1989;65(2):157–60.

530. Allegaert K, Cossey V, Debeer A, Langhendries JP, Van Overmeire B, de Hoon J, Devlieger H. The impact of ibuprofen on renal clearance in preterm infants is independent of the gestational age. Pediatr Nephrol. 2005;20(6):740–3.

531. Naulaers G, Delanghe G, Allegaert K, Debeer A, Cossey V, Vanhole C, Casaer P, Devlieger H, Van Overmeire B. Ibuprofen and cerebral oxygenation and circulation. Arch Dis Child Fetal Neonatal Ed. 2005;90(1):F75–6.

532. Lesko SM, Mitchell AA. An assessment of the safety of pediatric ibuprofen. A practitioner-based randomized clinical trial. JAMA. 1995;273(12):929–33.

533. Lesko SM, Mitchell AA. The safety of acetaminophen and ibuprofen among children younger than two years old. Pediatrics. 1999;104(4), e39.

534. Keenan GF, Giannini EH, Athreya BH. Clinically significant gastropathy associated with nonsteroidal antiinflammatory drug use in children with juvenile rheumatoid arthritis. J Rheumatol. 1995;22(6):1149–51.

535. Dowd JE, Cimaz R, Fink CW. Nonsteroidal antiinflammatory drug-induced gastroduodenal injury in children. Arthritis Rheum. 1995;38(9):1225–31.

536. Ameratunga R, Randall N, Dalziel S, Anderson BJ. Samter's triad in childhood: a warning for those prescribing NSAIDs. Paediatr Anaesth. 2013;23(8):757–9. doi:10.1111/pan.12216.

537. Palmer GM. A teenager with severe asthma exacerbation following ibuprofen. Anaesth Intensive Care. 2005;33(2):261–5.

538. Cardwell M, Siviter G, Smith A. Non-steroidal anti-inflammatory drugs and perioperative bleeding in paediatric tonsillectomy. Cochrane Database Syst Rev. 2005;2, CD003591.

539. Ment LR, Vohr BR, Makuch RW, Westerveld M, Katz KH, Schneider KC, Duncan CC, Ehrenkranz R, Oh W, Philip AG, Scott DT, Allan WC. Prevention of intraventricular hemorrhage by indomethacin in male preterm infants. J Pediatr. 2004;145(6):832–4.

540. Dodwell ER, Latorre JG, Parisini E, Zwettler E, Chandra D, Mulpuri K, Snyder B. NSAID exposure and risk of nonunion: a meta-analysis of case–control and cohort studies. Calcif Tissue Int. 2010;87(3):193–202. doi:10.1007/s00223-010-9379-7.

541. Kokki H. Nonsteroidal anti-inflammatory drugs for postoperative pain: a focus on children. Paediatr Drugs. 2003;5(2):103–23.

542. Watcha MF, Jones MB, Lagueruela RG, Schweiger C, White PF. Comparison of ketorolac and morphine as adjuvants during pediatric surgery. Anesthesiology. 1992;76(3):368–72.

543. Mandema JW, Stanski DR. Population pharmacodynamic model for ketorolac analgesia. Clin Pharmacol Ther. 1996;60(6):619–35.

544. Olkkola KT, Maunuksela EL. The pharmacokinetics of postoperative intravenous ketorolac tromethamine in children. Br J Clin Pharmacol. 1991;31(2):182–4.

545. Potts AL, Cheeseman JF, Warman GR. Circadian rhythms and their development in children: implications for pharmacokinetics and pharmacodynamics in anesthesia. Pediatr Anesth. 2011;21(3):238–46. doi:10.1111/j.1460-9592.2010.03343.x.

546. Lynn AM, Bradford H, Kantor ED, Seng KY, Salinger DH, Chen J, Ellenbogen RG, Vicini P, Anderson GD. Postoperative ketorolac tromethamine use in infants aged 6–18 months: the effect on morphine usage, safety assessment, and stereo-specific pharmacokinetics. Anesth Analg. 2007;104(5):1040–51. doi:10.1213/01.ane.0000260320.60867.6c.

547. Gregoire N, Gualano V, Geneteau A, Millerioux L, Brault M, Mignot A, Roze JC. Population pharmacokinetics of ibuprofen enantiomers in very premature neonates. J Clin Pharmacol. 2004;44(10):1114–24.

548. Lynn AM, Bradford H, Kantor ED, Andrew M, Vicini P, Anderson GD. Ketorolac tromethamine: stereo-specific pharmacokinetics and single-dose use in postoperative infants aged 2–6 months. Paediatr Anaesth. 2011;21(3):325–34. doi:10.1111/j.1460-9592.2010.03484.x.

549. Kauffman RE, Lieh-Lai MW, Uy HG, Aravind MK. Enantiomer-selective pharmacokinetics and metabolism of ketorolac in children. Clin Pharmacol Ther. 1999;65(4):382–8.

550. Strom BL, Berlin JA, Kinman JL, Spitz PW, Hennessy S, Feldman H, Kimmel S, Carson JL. Parenteral ketorolac and risk of gastrointestinal and operative site bleeding. A postmarketing surveillance study. JAMA. 1996;275(5):376–82.

551. Gupta A, Daggett C, Drant S, Rivero N, Lewis A. Prospective randomized trial of ketorolac after congenital heart surgery. J Cardiothorac Vasc Anesth. 2004;18(4):454–7.

552. Giannantonio C, Papacci P, Purcaro V, Cota F, Tesfagabir MG, Molle F, Lepore D, Baldascino A, Romagnoli C. Effectiveness of ketorolac tromethamine in prevention of severe retinopathy of prematurity. J Pediatr Ophthalmol Strabismus. 2011;48(4):247–51. doi:10.3928/01913913-20100920-01.

553. Papacci P, De Francisci G, Iacobucci T, Giannantonio C, De Carolis MP, Zecca E, Romagnoli C. Use of intravenous ketorolac in the neonate and premature babies. Paediatr Anaesth. 2004;14(6):487–92. doi:10.1111/j.1460-9592.2004.01250.x.

554. Zuppa AF, Mondick JT, Davis L, Cohen D. Population pharmacokinetics of ketorolac in neonates and young infants. Am J Ther. 2009;16(2):143–6. doi:10.1097/MJT.0b013e31818071df.

555. Brocks DR, Jamali F. Clinical pharmacokinetics of ketorolac tromethamine. Clin Pharmacokinet. 1992;23(6):415–27.

556. Foster PN, Williams JG. Bradycardia following intravenous ketorolac in children. Eur J Anaesthesiol. 1997;14(3):307–9.

557. Grond S, Sablotzki A. Clinical pharmacology of tramadol. Clin Pharmacokinet. 2004;43(13):879–923.

558. Allegaert K, Anderson BJ, Verbesselt R, Debeer A, de Hoon J, Devlieger H, Van Den Anker JN, Tibboel D. Tramadol disposition in the very young: an attempt to assess in vivo cytochrome P-450 2D6 activity. Br J Anaesth. 2005;95(2):231–9.

559. Engelhardt T, Steel E, Johnston G. Tramadol for pain relief in children undergoing tonsillectomy. A comparison with morphine. Paediatr Anaesth. 2002;12(9):834–5.

560. Umuroglu T, Eti Z, Ciftci H, Yilmaz Gogus F. Analgesia for adenotonsillectomy in children: a comparison of morphine, ketamine and tramadol. Paediatr Anaesth. 2004;14(7):568–73.

561. Hullett BJ, Chambers NA, Pascoe EM, Johnson C. Tramadol vs morphine during adenotonsillectomy for obstructive sleep apnea in children. Pediatr Anesth. 2006;16(6):648–53.

562. Allegaert K, Rochette A, Veyckemans F. Developmental pharmacology of tramadol during infancy: ontogeny, pharmacogenetics and elimination clearance. Paediatr Anaesth. 2011;21(3):266–73. doi:10.1111/j.1460-9592.2010.03389.x.

563. Mandema JW, Tuk B, van Steveninck AL, Breimer DD, Cohen AF, Danhof M. Pharmacokinetic-pharmacodynamic modeling of the central nervous system effects of midazolam and its main metabolite alpha-hydroxymidazolam in healthy volunteers. Clin Pharm Ther. 1992;51(6):715–28.

564. Greenblatt DJ, Ehrenberg BL, Gunderman J, Locniskar A, Scavone JM, Harmatz JS, Shader RI. Pharmacokinetic and electroencephalographic study of intravenous diazepam, midazolam, and placebo. Clin Pharm Ther. 1989;45(4):356–65.

565. Buhrer M, Maitre PO, Crevoisier C, Stanski DR. Electroencephalographic effects of benzodiazepines. II Pharmacodynamic modeling of the electroencephalographic effects of midazolam and diazepam. Clin Pharmacol Ther. 1990;48(5):555–67.

566. Johnson TN, Rostami-Hodjegan A, Goddard JM, Tanner MS, Tucker GT. Contribution of midazolam and its 1-hydroxy metabolite to preoperative sedation in children: a pharmacokinetic-pharmacodynamic analysis. Br J Anaesth. 2002;89(3):428–37.

567. de Wildt SN, de Hoog M, Vinks AA, van der Giesen E, van den Anker JN. Population pharmacokinetics and metabolism of midazolam in pediatric intensive care patients. Crit Care Med. 2003;31(7):1952–858.

568. Hartwig S, Roth B, Theisohn M. Clinical experience with continuous intravenous sedation using midazolam and fentanyl in the paediatric intensive care unit. Eur J Pediatr. 1991;150(11):784–8.

569. Lloyd-Thomas AR, Booker PD. Infusion of midazolam in paediatric patients after cardiac surgery. Br J Anaesth. 1986;58(10):1109–15.

570. Booker PD, Beechey A, Lloyd-Thomas AR. Sedation of children requiring artificial ventilation using an infusion of midazolam. Br J Anaesth. 1986;58(10):1104–8.

571. Persson P, Nilsson A, Hartvig P, Tamsen A. Pharmacokinetics of midazolam in total i.v. anaesthesia. Br J Anaesth. 1987;59(5):548–56.

572. Nilsson A, Tamsen A, Persson P. Midazolam-fentanyl anesthesia for major surgery. Plasma levels of midazolam during prolonged total intravenous anesthesia. Acta Anaesthiol Scand. 1986;30(1):66–9.

573. Allonen H, Ziegler G, Klotz U. Midazolam kinetics. Clin Pharm Ther. 1981;30(5):653–61.

574. Lee TC, Charles BG, Harte GJ, Gray PH, Steer PA, Flenady VJ. Population pharmacokinetic modeling in very premature infants receiving midazolam during mechanical ventilation: midazolam neonatal pharmacokinetics. Anesthesiology. 1999;90(2):451–7.

575. Harte GJ, Gray PH, Lee TC, Steer PA, Charles BG. Haemodynamic responses and population pharmacokinetics of midazolam following administration to ventilated, preterm neonates. J Paediatr Child Health. 1997;33(4):335–8.

576. de Wildt SN, Kearns GL, Hop WC, Murry DJ, Abdel-Rahman SM, van den Anker JN. Pharmacokinetics and metabolism of intravenous midazolam in preterm infants. Clin Pharm Ther. 2001;70(6):525–31.

577. Burtin P, Jacqz-Aigrain E, Girard P, Lenclen R, Magny JF, Betremieux P, Tehiry C, Desplanques L, Mussat P. Population pharmacokinetics of midazolam in neonates. Clin Pharm Ther. 1994;56(6 Pt 1):615–25.

578. Jacqz-Aigrain E, Daoud P, Burtin P, Maherzi S, Beaufils F. Pharmacokinetics of midazolam during continuous infusion in critically ill neonates. Eur J Clin Pharmacol. 1992;42(3):329–32.

579. Jacqz-Aigrain E, Wood C, Robieux I. Pharmacokinetics of midazolam in critically ill neonates. Eur J Clin Pharmacol. 1990;39(2):191–2.

580. Anderson BJ, Larsson P. A maturation model for midazolam clearance. Paediatr Anaesth. 2011;21(3):302–8. doi:10.1111/j.1460-9592.2010.03364.x.

581. Mulla H, McCormack P, Lawson G, Firmin RK, Upton DR. Pharmacokinetics of midazolam in neonates undergoing extracorporeal membrane oxygenation. Anesthesiology. 2003;99(2):275–82.

582. Mathews HM, Carson IW, Lyons SM, Orr IA, Collier PS, Howard PJ, Dundee JW. A pharmacokinetic study of midazolam in paediatric patients undergoing cardiac surgery. Br J Anaesth. 1988;61(3):302–7.

583. Hiller A, Olkkola KT, Isohanni P, Saarnivaara L. Unconsciousness associated with midazolam and erythromycin. Br J Anaesth. 1990;65(6):826–8.

584. Payne KA, Coetzee AR, Mattheyse FJ. Midazolam and amnesia in pediatric premedication. Acta Anaesthesiol Belg. 1991;42(2):101–5.

585. Twersky RS, Hartung J, Berger BJ, McClain J, Beaton C. Midazolam enhances anterograde but not retrograde amnesia in pediatric patients. Anesthesiology. 1993;78(1):51–5.

586. Tobias JD. Sedation and analgesia in the pediatric intensive care unit. Pediatr Ann. 2005;34(8):636–45.

587. Alexander CM, Gross JB. Sedative doses of midazolam depress hypoxic ventilatory responses in humans. Anesth Analg. 1988;67(4):377–82.

588. Yaster M, Nichols DG, Deshpande JK, Wetzel RC. Midazolam-fentanyl intravenous sedation in children: case report of respiratory arrest. Pediatrics. 1990;86(3):463–7.

589. Dhonneur G, Combes X, Leroux B, Duvaldestin P. Postoperative obstructive apnea. Anesth Analg. 1999;89(3):762–7.

590. Kensche M, Sander JW, Sisodiya SM. Significant hypotension following buccal midazolam administration. BMJ Case Rep. 2010. doi:10.1136/bcr.09.2010.3371

591. Mandelli M, Tognoni G, Garattini S. Clinical pharmacokinetics of diazepam. Clin Pharmacokinet. 1978;3(1):72–91.

592. Visudtibhan A, Chiemchanya S, Visudhiphan P, Kanjanarungsichai A, Kaojarern S, Pichaipat V. Serum diazepam levels after oral administration in children. J Med Assoc Thai. 2002;85 Suppl 4:S1065–70.

593. Buhrer M, Maitre PO, Hung O, Stanski DR. Electroencephalographic effects of benzodiazepines. I Choosing an electroencephalographic parameter to measure the effect of midazolam on the central nervous system. Clin Pharmacol Ther. 1990;48(5):544–54.

594. Mould DR, DeFeo TM, Reele S, Milla G, Limjuco R, Crews T, Choma N, Patel IH. Simultaneous modeling of the pharmacokinetics and pharmacodynamics of midazolam and diazepam. Clin Pharmacol Ther. 1995;58(1):35–43. doi:10.1016/0009-9236(95)90070-5.

595. Arendt RM, Greenblatt DJ, Liebisch DC, Luu MD, Paul SM. Determinants of benzodiazepine brain uptake: lipophilicity versus binding affinity. Psychopharmacology (Berl). 1987;93(1):72–6.

596. Gamble JA, Dundee JW, Assaf RA. Plasma diazepam levels after single dose oral and intramuscular administration. Anaesthesia. 1975;30(2):164–9.

597. Hillestad L, Hansen T, Melsom H. Diazepam metabolism in normal man. II Serum concentration and clinical effect after oral administration and cumulation. Clin Pharmacol Ther. 1974;16 (3):485–9.

598. Hillestad L, Hansen T, Melsom H, Drivenes A. Diazepam metabolism in normal man. I. Serum concentrations and clinical effects after intravenous, intramuscular, and oral administration. Clin Pharmacol Ther. 1974;16(3):479–84.

599. Meberg A, Langslet A, Bredesen JE, Lunde PK. Plasma concentration of diazepam and N-desmethyldiazepam in children after a single rectal or intramuscular dose of diazepam. Eur J Clin Pharmacol. 1978;14(4):273–6.

600. Kanto J. Plasma concentrations of diazepam and its metabolites after peroral, intramuscular, and rectal administration. Correlation between plasma concentration and sedatory effect of diazepam. Int J Clin Pharmacol Biopharm. 1975;12(4):427–32.

601. Fell D, Gough MB, Northan AA, Henderson CU. Diazepam premedication in children. Plasma levels and clinical effects. Anaesthesia. 1985;40(1):12–7.

602. Morselli PL, Principi N, Tognoni G, Reali E, Belvedere G, Standen SM, Sereni F. Diazepam elimination in premature and full term infants, and children. J Perinat Med. 1973;1 (2):133–41.

603. Peinemann F, Daldrup T. Severe and prolonged sedation in five neonates due to persistence of active diazepam metabolites. Eur J Pediatr. 2001;160(6):378–81.

604. Klotz U, Avant GR, Hoyumpa A, Schenker S, Wilkinson GR. The effects of age and liver disease on the disposition and elimination of diazepam in adult man. J Clin Invest. 1975;55(2):347–59. doi:10.1172/JCI107938.

605. Klotz U, Ziegler G, Reimann IW. Pharmacokinetics of the selective benzodiazepine antagonist Ro 15–1788 in man. Eur J Clin Pharmacol. 1984;27(1):115–7.

606. Klotz U, Kanto J. Pharmacokinetics and clinical use of flumazenil (Ro 15–1788). Clin Pharmacokinet. 1988;14(1):1–12. doi:10. 2165/00003088-198814010-00001.

607. Janssen U, Walker S, Maier K, von Gaisberg U, Klotz U. Flumazenil disposition and elimination in cirrhosis. Clin Pharmacol Ther. 1989;46(3):317–23.

608. Jones RD, Chan K, Roulson CJ, Brown AG, Smith ID, Mya GH. Pharmacokinetics of flumazenil and midazolam. Br J Anaesth. 1993;70(3):286–92.

609. Roncari G, Ziegler WH, Guentert TW. Pharmacokinetics of the new benzodiazepine antagonist Ro 15–1788 in man following intravenous and oral administration. Br J Clin Pharmacol. 1986;22(4):421–8.

610. Tobias JD. Controlled hypotension in children: a critical review of available agents. Paediatr Drugs. 2002;4(7):439–53.

611. Tobias JD, Berkenbosch JW. Sedation during mechanical ventilation in infants and children: dexmedetomidine versus midazolam. South Med J. 2004;97(5):451–5.

612. Nichols DP, Berkenbosch JW, Tobias JD. Rescue sedation with dexmedetomidine for diagnostic imaging: a preliminary report. Paediatr Anaesth. 2005;15(3):199–203.

613. Hammer GB, Philip BM, Schroeder AR, Rosen FS, Koltai PJ. Prolonged infusion of dexmedetomidine for sedation following tracheal resection. Paediatr Anaesth. 2005;15(7):616–20.

614. Tobias JD. Dexmedetomidine to treat opioid withdrawal in infants following prolonged sedation in the pediatric ICU. J Opioid Manag. 2006;2(4):201–5.

615. Ibacache ME, Munoz HR, Brandes V, Morales AL. Single-dose dexmedetomidine reduces agitation after sevoflurane anesthesia in children. Anesth Analg. 2004;98(1):60–3.

616. Walker J, Maccallum M, Fischer C, Kopcha R, Saylors R, McCall J. Sedation using dexmedetomidine in pediatric burn patients. J Burn Care Res. 2006;27(2):206–10. doi:10.1097/01.BCR. 0000200910.76019.CF.

617. Tobias JD. Dexmedetomidine: applications in pediatric critical care and pediatric anesthesiology. Pediatr Crit Care Med. 2007;8 (2):115–31. doi:10.1097/01.PCC.0000257100.31779.41.

618. Koroglu A, Teksan H, Sagir O, Yucel A, Toprak HI, Ersoy OM. A comparison of the sedative, hemodynamic, and respiratory effects of dexmedetomidine and propofol in children undergoing magnetic resonance imaging. Anesth Analg. 2006;103(1):63–7. doi:10.1213/01.ANE.0000219592.82598.AA.

619. Potts AL, Anderson BJ, Holford NH, Vu TC, Warman GR. Dexmedetomidine hemodynamics in children after cardiac surgery. Paediatr Anaesth. 2010;20(5):425–33. doi:10.1111/j. 1460-9592.2010.03285.x.

620. Ebert TJ, Hall JE, Barney JA, Uhrich TD, Colinco MD. The effects of increasing plasma concentrations of dexmedetomidine in humans. Anesthesiology. 2000;93(2):382–94.

621. Kamibayashi T, Maze M. Clinical uses of alpha2 -adrenergic agonists. Anesthesiology. 2000;93(5):1345–9.

622. Bhana N, Goa KL, McClellan KJ. Dexmedetomidine. Drugs. 2000;59(2):263–8.

623. Hsu YW, Cortinez LI, Robertson KM, Keifer JC, Sum-Ping ST, Moretti EW, Young CC, Wright DR, Macleod DB, Somma J. Dexmedetomidine pharmacodynamics: part I: crossover comparison of the respiratory effects of dexmedetomidine and remifentanil in healthy volunteers. Anesthesiology. 2004;101 (5):1066–76.

624. Potts AL, Anderson BJ, Warman GR, Lerman J, Diaz SM, Vilo S. Dexmedetomidine pharmacokinetics in pediatric intensive care--a pooled analysis. Pediatr Anaesth. 2009;19(11):1119–29. doi:10.1111/j.1460-9592.2009.03133.x.

625. Mason KP, Zurakowski D, Zgleszewski S, Prescilla R, Fontaine PJ, Dinardo JA. Incidence and predictors of hypertension during high-dose dexmedetomidine sedation for pediatric MRI. Paediatr Anaesth. 2010;20(6):516–23. doi:10.1111/j.1460-9592.2010. 03299.x.

626. Mason KP, Lerman J. Review article: dexmedetomidine in children: current knowledge and future applications. Anesth Analg. 2011;113(5):1129–42. doi:10.1213/ANE.0b013e31822b8629.

627. Hammer GB, Drover DR, Cao H, Jackson E, Williams GD, Ramamoorthy C, Van Hare GF, Niksch A, Dubin AM. The effects of dexmedetomidine on cardiac electrophysiology in children. Anesth Analg. 2008;106(1):79–83.

628. Tobias JD, Chrysostomou C. Dexmedetomidine: antiarrhythmic effects in the pediatric cardiac patient. Pediatr Cardiol. 2013;34 (4):779–85. doi:10.1007/s00246-013-0659-7.

629. Parent BA, Munoz R, Shiderly D, Chrysostomou C. Use of dexmedetomidine in sustained ventricular tachycardia. Anaesth Intensive Care. 2010;38(4):781.

630. Chrysostomou C, Morell VO, Wearden P, Sanchez-de-Toledo J, Jooste EH, Beerman L. Dexmedetomidine: therapeutic use for the termination of reentrant supraventricular tachycardia. Congenit Heart Dis. 2013;8(1):48–56. doi:10.1111/j.1747-0803.2012.00669.x.

631. Char D, Drover DR, Motonaga KS, Gupta S, Miyake CY, Dubin AM, Hammer GB. The effects of ketamine on dexmedetomidine-induced electrophysiologic changes in children. Paediatr Anaesth. 2013;23(10):898–905. doi:10.1111/pan.12143.

632. Su F, Nicolson SC, Gastonguay MR, Barrett JS, Adamson PC, Kang DS, Godinez RI, Zuppa AF. Population pharmacokinetics of dexmedetomidine in infants after open heart surgery. Anesth Analg. 2010;110(5):1383–92. doi:10.1213/ANE. 0b013e3181d783c8.

633. Chrysostomou C, Schulman SR, Herrera Castellanos M, Cofer BE, Mitra S, da Rocha MG, Wisemandle WA, Gramlich L.

A phase II/III, multicenter, safety, efficacy, and pharmacokinetic study of dexmedetomidine in preterm and term neonates. J Pediatr. 2014;164(2):276–282.e3. doi:10.1016/j.jpeds.2013.10.002.

634. Mahmoud M, Radhakrishman R, Gunter J, Sadhasivam S, Schapiro A, McAuliffe J, Kurth D, Wang Y, Nick TG, Donnelly LF. Effect of increasing depth of dexmedetomidine anesthesia on upper airway morphology in children. Paediatr Anaesth. 2010;20 (6):506–15. doi:10.1111/j.1460-9592.2010.03311.x.

635. Mahmoud M, Jung D, Salisbury S, McAuliffe J, Gunter J, Patio M, Donnelly LF, Fleck R. Effect of increasing depth of dexmedetomidine and propofol anesthesia on upper airway morphology in children and adolescents with obstructive sleep apnea. J Clin Anesth. 2013;25(7):529–41. doi:10.1016/j.jclinane.2013.04.011.

636. Olutoye OA, Glover CD, Diefenderfer JW, McGilberry M, Wyatt MM, Larrier DR, Friedman EM, Watcha MF. The effect of intraoperative dexmedetomidine on postoperative analgesia and sedation in pediatric patients undergoing tonsillectomy and adenoidectomy. Anesth Analg. 2010;111(2):490–5. doi:10.1213/ANE.0b013e3181e33429.

637. Tobias JD, Goble TJ, Bates G, Anderson JT, Hoernschemeyer DG. Effects of dexmedetomidine on intraoperative motor and somatosensory evoked potential monitoring during spinal surgery in adolescents. Paediatr Anaesth. 2008;18(11):1082–8. doi:10.1111/j.1460-9592.2008.02733.x.

638. Bala E, Sessler DI, Nair DR, McLain R, Dalton JE, Farag E. Motor and somatosensory evoked potentials are well maintained in patients given dexmedetomidine during spine surgery. Anesthesiology. 2008;109(3):417–25. doi:10.1097/ALN.0b013e318182a467.

639. Mahmoud M, Sadhasivam S, Salisbury S, Nick TG, Schnell B, Sestokas AK, Wiggins C, Samuels P, Kabalin T, McAuliffe J. Susceptibility of transcranial electric motor-evoked potentials to varying targeted blood levels of dexmedetomidine during spine surgery. Anesthesiology. 2010;112(6):1364–73. doi:10.1097/ALN.0b013e3181d74f55.

640. Anschel DJ, Aherne A, Soto RG, Carrion W, Hoegerl C, Nori P, Seidman PA. Successful intraoperative spinal cord monitoring during scoliosis surgery using a total intravenous anesthetic regimen including dexmedetomidine. J Clin Neurophysiol. 2008;25 (1):56–61. doi:10.1097/WNP.0b013e318163cca6.

641. Pickard A, Davies P, Birnie K, Beringer R. Systematic review and meta-analysis of the effect of intraoperative alpha(2)-adrenergic agonists on postoperative behaviour in children. Br J Anaesth. 2014;112(6):982–90. doi:10.1093/bja/aeu093.

642. Bergendahl H, Lonnqvist PA, Eksborg S. Clonidine in paediatric anaesthesia: review of the literature and comparison with benzodiazepines for premedication. Acta Anaesthesiol Scand. 2006;50(2):135–43.

643. Blackburn L, Almenrader N, Larsson P, Anderson BJ. Intranasal clonidine pharmacokinetics. Paediatr Anaesth. 2014;24(3):340–2. doi:10.1111/pan.12297.

644. Potts AL, Larsson P, Eksborg S, Warman G, Lonnqvist PA, Anderson BJ. Clonidine disposition in children; a population analysis. Pediatr Anesth. 2007;17(10):924–33. doi:10.1111/j.1460-9592.2007.02251.x.

645. Sumiya K, Homma M, Watanabe M, Baba Y, Inomata S, Kihara S, Toyooka H, Kohda Y. Sedation and plasma concentration of clonidine hydrochloride for pre-anesthetic medication in pediatric surgery. Biol Pharm Bull. 2003;26(4):421–3.

646. Klein RH, Alvarez-Jimenez R, Sukhai RN, Oostdijk W, Bakker B, Reeser HM, Ballieux BE, Hu P, Klaassen ES, Freijer J, Burggraaf J, Cohen AF, Wit JM. Pharmacokinetics and pharmacodynamics of orally administered clonidine: a model-based approach. Horm Res Paediatr. 2013;79(5):300–9. doi:10.1159/000350819.

647. Hall JE, Uhrich TD, Ebert TJ. Sedative, analgesic and cognitive effects of clonidine infusions in humans. Br J Anaesth. 2001;86 (1):5–11.

648. De Kock MF, Pichon G, Scholtes JL. Intraoperative clonidine enhances postoperative morphine patient-controlled analgesia. Can J Anaesth. 1992;39(6):537–44.

649. Bernard JM, Hommeril JL, Passuti N, Pinaud M. Postoperative analgesia by intravenous clonidine. Anesthesiology. 1991;75 (4):577–82.

650. Marinangeli F, Ciccozzi A, Donatelli F, Di Pietro A, Iovinelli G, Rawal N, Paladini A, Varrassi G. Clonidine for treatment of postoperative pain: a dose-finding study. Eur J Pain. 2002;6 (1):35–42.

651. Davies DS, Wing AM, Reid JL, Neill DM, Tippett P, Dollery CT. Pharmacokinetics and concentration-effect relationships of intervenous and oral clonidine. Clin Pharm Ther. 1977;21 (5):593–601.

652. Lowenthal DT, Matzek KM, MacGregor TR. Clinical pharmacokinetics of clonidine. Clin Pharmacokinet. 1988;14 (5):287–310.

653. Arndts D. New aspects of the clinical pharmacology of clonidine. Chest. 1983;83(2 Suppl):397–400.

654. Arndts D, Doevendans J, Kirsten R, Heintz B. New aspects of the pharmacokinetics and pharmacodynamics of clonidine in man. Eur J Clin Pharmacol. 1983;24(1):21–30.

655. Hesselmans LF, Jennekens FG, Van den Oord CJ, Veldman H, Vincent A. Development of innervation of skeletal muscle fibers in man: relation to acetylcholine receptors. Anat Rec. 1993;236 (3):553–62. doi:10.1002/ar.1092360315.

656. Jaramillo F, Schuetze SM. Kinetic difference between embryonic- and adult-type acetylcholine receptors in rat myotubes. J Physiol. 1988;396:267–96.

657. Goudsouzian NG. Maturation of neuromuscular transmission in the infant. Br J Anaesth. 1980;52(2):205–14.

658. Goudsouzian NG, Standaert FG. The infant and the myoneural junction. Anesth Analg. 1986;65(11):1208–17.

659. Meretoja OA, Brandom BW, Taivainen T, Jalkanen L. Synergism between atracurium and vecuronium in children. Br J Anaesth. 1993;71(3):440–2.

660. Meretoja OA, Taivainen T, Jalkanen L, Wirtavuori K. Synergism between atracurium and vecuronium in infants and children during nitrous oxide-oxygen-alfentanil anaesthesia. Br J Anaesth. 1994;73(5):605–7.

661. Keens TG, Bryan AC, Levison H, Ianuzzo CD. Developmental pattern of muscle fiber types in human ventilatory muscles. J Appl Physiol. 1978;44(6):909–13.

662. Meretoja OA. Neuromuscular blocking agents in paediatric patients: influence of age on the response. Anaesth Intens Care. 1990;18(4):440–8.

663. Donati F, Antzaka C, Bevan DR. Potency of pancuronium at the diaphragm and the adductor pollicis muscle in humans. Anesthesiology. 1986;65(1):1–5.

664. Laycock JR, Baxter MK, Bevan JC, Sangwan S, Donati F, Bevan DR. The potency of pancuronium at the adductor pollicis and diaphragm in infants and children. Anesthesiology. 1988;68 (6):908–11.

665. Laycock JR, Donati F, Smith CE, Bevan DR. Potency of atracurium and vecuronium at the diaphragm and the adductor pollicis muscle. Br J Anaesth. 1988;61(3):286–91.

666. Meakin G, Shaw EA, Baker RD, Morris P. Comparison of atracurium-induced neuromuscular blockade in neonates, infants and children. Br J Anaesth. 1988;60(2):171–5.

667. Basta SJ, Ali HH, Savarese JJ, Sunder N, Gionfriddo M, Cloutier G, Lineberry C, Cato AE. Clinical pharmacology of atracurium besylate (BW 33A): a new non-depolarizing muscle relaxant. Anesth Analg. 1982;61(9):723–9.

668. Woelfel SK, Brandom BW, McGowan Jr FX, Cook DR. Clinical pharmacology of mivacurium in pediatric patients less than off years old during nitrous oxide-halothane anesthesia. Anesth Analg. 1993;77(4):713–20.

669. Goudsouzian NG, Denman W, Schwartz A, Shorten G, Foster V, Samara B. Pharmacodynamic and hemodynamic effects of mivacurium in infants anesthetized with halothane and nitrous oxide. Anesthesiology. 1993;79(5):919–25.

670. Saldien V, Vermeyen KM, Wuyts FL. Target-controlled infusion of rocuronium in infants, children, and adults: a comparison of the pharmacokinetic and pharmacodynamic relationship. Anesth Analg. 2003;97(1):44–9.

671. Fisher DM, Miller RD. Neuromuscular effects of vecuronium (ORG NC45) in infants and children during N_2O, halothane anesthesia. Anesthesiology. 1983;58(6):519–23.

672. Fisher DM, Castagnoli K, Miller RD. Vecuronium kinetics and dynamics in anesthetized infants and children. Clin Pharm Ther. 1985;37(4):402–6.

673. Wierda JM, Meretoja OA, Taivainen T, Proost JH. Pharmacokinetics and pharmacokinetic-dynamic modelling of rocuronium in infants and children. Br J Anaesth. 1997;78(6):690–5.

674. Kalli I, Meretoja OA. Infusion of atracurium in neonates, infants and children. A study of dose requirements. Br J Anaesth. 1988;60 (6):651–4.

675. Alifimoff JK, Goudsouzian NG. Continuous infusion of mivacurium in children. Br J Anaesth. 1989;63(5):520–4.

676. Woelfel SK, Dong ML, Brandom BW, Sarner JB, Cook DR. Vecuronium infusion requirements in children during halothane-narcotic-nitrous oxide, isoflurane-narcotic-nitrous oxide, and narcotic-nitrous oxide anesthesia. Anesth Analg. 1991;73(1):33–8.

677. Brandom BW, Cook DR, Woelfel SK, Rudd GD, Fehr B, Lineberry CG. Atracurium infusion requirements in children during halothane, isoflurane, and narcotic anesthesia. Anesth Analg. 1985;64(5):471–6.

678. Woloszczuk-Gebicka B, Lapczynski T, Wierzejski W. The influence of halothane, isoflurane and sevoflurane on rocuronium infusion in children. Acta Anaesthesiol Scand. 2001;45(1):73–7.

679. Woloszczuk-Gebicka B, Wyska E, Grabowski T, Swierczewska A, Sawicka R. Pharmacokinetic-pharmacodynamic relationship of rocuronium under stable nitrous oxide-fentanyl or nitrous oxide-sevoflurane anesthesia in children. Paediatr Anaesth. 2006;16 (7):761–8. doi:10.1111/j.1460-9592.2005.01840.x.

680. Meakin G, Walker RW, Dearlove OR. Myotonic and neuromuscular blocking effects of increased doses of suxamethonium in infants and children. Br J Anaesth. 1990;65(6):816–8.

681. Cook DR, Gronert BJ, Woelfel SK. Comparison of the neuromuscular effects of mivacurium and suxamethonium in infants and children. Acta Anaesthesiol Scand. 1995;106:S35–40.

682. DeCook TH, Goudsouzian NG. Tachyphylaxis and phase II block development during infusion of succinylcholine in children. Anesth Analg. 1980;59(9):639–43.

683. Gronert BJ, Brandom BW. Neuromuscular blocking drugs in infants and children. Pediatr Clin N Am. 1994;41(1):73–91.

684. Sutherland GA, Bevan JC, Bevan DR. Neuromuscular blockade in infants following intramuscular succinylcholine in two or five per cent concentration. Can Anaesth Soc J. 1983;30(4):342–6.

685. Matteo RS, Lieberman IG, Salanitre E, McDaniel DD, Diaz J. Distribution, elimination, and action of d-tubocurarine in neonates, infants, children, and adults. Anesth Analg. 1984;63 (9):799–804.

686. Tassonyi E, Pittet JF, Schopfer CN, Rouge JC, Gemperle G, Wilder-Smith OH, Morel DR. Pharmacokinetics of pipecuronium in infants, children and adults. Eur J Drug Metab Pharmacokinet. 1995;20(3):203–8.

687. Meretoja OA, Erkola O. Pipecuronium revisited: dose–response and maintenance requirement in infants, children, and adults. J Clin Anesth. 1997;9(2):125–9. doi:10.1016/S0952-8180(96) 00235-8.

688. Fisher DM, Canfell PC, Fahey MR, Rosen JI, Rupp SM, Sheiner LB, Miller RD. Elimination of atracurium in humans: contribution of Hofmann elimination and ester hydrolysis versus organ-based elimination. Anesthesiology. 1986;65(1):6–12.

689. Imbeault K, Withington DE, Varin F. Pharmacokinetics and pharmacodynamics of a 0.1 mg/kg dose of cisatracurium besylate in children during N_2O/O_2/propofol anesthesia. Anesth Analg. 2006;102(3):738–43. doi:10.1213/01.ane.0000195342.29133.ce.

690. Reich DL, Hollinger I, Harrington DJ, Seiden HS, Chakravorti S, Cook DR. Comparison of cisatracurium and vecuronium by infusion in neonates and small infants after congenital heart surgery. Anesthesiology. 2004;101(5):1122–7.

691. Kirkegaard-Nielsen H, Meretoja OA, Wirtavuori K. Reversal of atracurium-induced neuromuscular block in paediatric patients. Acta Anaesth Scand. 1995;39(7):906–11.

692. Meakin G, Sweet PT, Bevan JC, Bevan DR. Neostigmine and edrophonium as antagonists of pancuronium in infants and children. Anesthesiology. 1983;59(4):316–21.

693. Fisher DM, Cronnelly R, Miller RD, Sharma M. The neuromuscular pharmacology of neostigmine in infants and children. Anesthesiology. 1983;59(3):220–5.

694. Meretoja OA, Taivainen T, Wirtavuori K. Cisatracurium during halothane and balanced anaesthesia in children. Paediatr Anaesth. 1996;6(5):373–8.

695. Meistelman C, Debaene B, D'Hollander A, Donati F, Saint-Maurice C. Importance of the level of paralysis recovery for a rapid antagonism of vecuronium with neostigmine in children during halothane anesthesia. Anesthesiology. 1988;69(1):97–9.

696. Debaene B, Meistelman C, d'Hollander A. Recovery from vecuronium neuromuscular blockade following neostigmine administration in infants, children, and adults during halothane anesthesia. Anesthesiology. 1989;71(6):840–4.

697. Bevan JC, Purday JP, Reimer EJ, Bevan DR. Reversal of doxacurium and pancuronium neuromuscular blockade with neostigmine in children. Can Anaesth Soc J. 1994;41(11):1074–80. doi:10.1007/BF03015657.

698. Hinderling PH, Gundert-Remy U, Schmidlin O. Integrated pharmacokinetics and pharmacodynamics of atropine in healthy humans. I: Pharmacokinetics. J Pharm Sci. 1985;74(7):703–10.

699. Virtanen R, Kanto J, Iisalo E, Iisalo EU, Salo M, Sjovall S. Pharmacokinetic studies on atropine with special reference to age. Acta Anaesthesiol Scand. 1982;26(4):297–300.

700. Pihlajamaki K, Kanto J, Aaltonen L, Iisalo E, Jaakkola P. Pharmacokinetics of atropine in children. Int J Clin Pharmacol Ther Toxicol. 1986;24(5):236–9.

701. Barrington KJ. The myth of a minimum dose for atropine. Pediatrics. 2011;127(4):783–4. doi:10.1542/peds.2010-1475.

702. Eisa L, Passi Y, Lerman J, Raczka M, Heard C. Do small doses of atropine (<0.1 mg) cause bradycardia in young children? Arch Dis Child. 2015;100(7):684–8. doi:10.1136/archdischild-2014-307868.

703. Palmisano BW, Setlock MA, Brown MP, Siker D, Tripuraneni R. Dose–response for atropine and heart rate in infants and children anesthetized with halothane and nitrous oxide. Anesthesiology. 1991;75(2):238–42.

704. Rautakorpi P, Ali-Melkkila T, Kaila T, Olkkola KT, Iisalo E, Kanto J. Pharmacokinetics of glycopyrrolate in children. J Clin Anesth. 1994;6(3):217–20.

705. Ali-Melkkila T, Kaila T, Kanto J. Glycopyrrolate: pharmacokinetics and some pharmacodynamic findings. Acta Anaesthesiol Scand. 1989;33(6):513–7.

706. Mirakhur RK, Dundee JW. Glycopyrrolate: pharmacology and clinical use. Anaesthesia. 1983;38(12):1195–204.

707. Mirakhur RK, Jones CJ. Atropine and glycopyrrolate: changes in cardiac rate and rhythm in conscious and anaesthetised children. Anaesth Intens Care. 1982;10(4):328–32.

708. Salem MR, Wong AY, Mani M, Bennett EJ, Toyama T. Premedicant drugs and gastric juice pH and volume in pediatric patients. Anesthesiology. 1976;44(3):216–9.

709. Meyers EF, Tomeldan SA. Glycopyrrolate compared with atropine in prevention of the oculocardiac reflex during eye-muscle surgery. Anesthesiology. 1979;51(4):350–2.

710. Rautakorpi P, Manner T, Ali-Melkkila T, Kaila T, Olkkola K, Kanto J. Pharmacokinetics and oral bioavailability of glycopyrrolate in children. Pharmacol Toxicol. 1998;83(3):132–4.

711. Plaud B, Meretoja O, Hofmockel R, Raft J, Stoddart PA, van Kuijk JH, Hermens Y, Mirakhur RK. Reversal of rocuronium-induced neuromuscular blockade with sugammadex in pediatric and adult surgical patients. Anesthesiology. 2009;110(2):284–94. doi:10.1097/ALN.0b013e318194caaa.

712. Robertson EN, Driessen JJ, Vogt M, De Boer H, Scheffer GJ. Pharmacodynamics of rocuronium 0.3 mg kg^{-1} in adult patients with and without renal failure. Eur J Anaesthesiol. 2005;22(12):929–32. doi:10.1017/S0265021505001584.

713. Staals LM, Snoeck MM, Driessen JJ, Flockton EA, Heeringa M, Hunter JM. Multicentre, parallel-group, comparative trial evaluating the efficacy and safety of sugammadex in patients with end-stage renal failure or normal renal function. Br J Anaesth. 2008;101(4):492–7. doi:10.1093/bja/aen216.

714. Staals LM, Snoeck MM, Driessen JJ, van Hamersvelt HW, Flockton EA, van den Heuvel MW, Hunter JM. Reduced clearance of rocuronium and sugammadex in patients with severe to end-stage renal failure: a pharmacokinetic study. Br J Anaesth. 2010;104(1):31–9. doi:10.1093/bja/aep340.

715. Morell RC, Berman JM, Royster RI, Petrozza PH, Kelly JS, Colonna DM. Revised label regarding use of succinylcholine in children and adolescents. Anesthesiology. 1994;80(1):242–5.

716. Badgwell JM, Hall SC, Lockhart C. Revised label regarding use of succinylcholine in children and adolescents. Anesthesiology. 1994;80(1):243–5.

717. Goudsouzian NG. Recent changes in the package insert for succinylcholine chloride: should this drug be contraindicated for routine use in children and adolescents? (Summary of the discussions of the anesthetic and life support drug advisory meeting of the Food and Drug Administration, FDA building, Rockville, MD, June 9, 1994). Anesth Analg. 1995;80 (1):207–8.

718. Anderson BJ, Brown TC. Anaesthesia for a child with congenital myotonic dystrophy. Anaesth Intens Care. 1989;17(3):351–4.

719. Galley HF, Mahdy A, Lowes DA. Pharmacogenetics and anesthesiologists. Pharmacogenomics. 2005;6(8):849–56. doi:10.2217/14622416.6.8.849.

720. Neitlich HW. Increased plasma cholinesterase activity and succinylcholine resistance: a genetic variant. J Clin Invest. 1966;45 (3):380–7. doi:10.1172/JCI105353.

721. Lockridge O. Genetic variants of human serum cholinesterase influence metabolism of the muscle relaxant succinylcholine. Pharmacol Ther. 1990;47(1):35–60.

722. Olsson GL, Hallen B. Pharmacological evacuation of the stomach with metoclopramide. Acta Anaesthesiol Scand. 1982;26 (5):417–20.

723. Albibi R, McCallum RW. Metoclopramide: pharmacology and clinical application. Ann Intern Med. 1983;98(1):86–95.

724. Kan KK, Rudd JA, Wai MK. Differential action of anti-emetic drugs on defecation and emesis induced by prostaglandin E2 in the ferret. Eur J Pharmacol. 2006;544(1–3):153–9. doi:10.1016/j.ejphar.2006.06.034.

725. Kearns GL, Butler HL, Lane JK, Carchman SH, Wright GJ. Metoclopramide pharmacokinetics and pharmacodynamics in infants with gastroesophageal reflux. J Pediatr Gastroenterol Nutr. 1988;7(6):823–9.

726. Kearns GL, van den Anker JN, Reed MD, Blumer JL. Pharmacokinetics of metoclopramide in neonates. J Clin Pharmacol. 1998;38(2):122–8.

727. Ho KY, Gan TJ. Pharmacology, pharmacogenetics, and clinical efficacy of 5-hydroxytryptamine type 3 receptor antagonists for postoperative nausea and vomiting. Curr Opin Anaesthesiol. 2006;19(6):606–11. doi:10.1097/01.aco.0000247340.61815.38.

728. Khalil SN, Roth AG, Cohen IT, Simhi E, Ansermino JM, Bolos ME, Cote CJ, Hannallah RS, Davis PJ, Brooks PB, Russo MW, Anschuetz GC, Blackburn LM. A double-blind comparison of intravenous ondansetron and placebo for preventing postoperative emesis in 1- to 24-month-old pediatric patients after surgery under general anesthesia. Anesth Analg. 2005;101(2):356–61. doi:10.1213/01.ANE.0000155261.27335.29.

729. Mondick JT, Johnson BM, Haberer LJ, Sale ME, Adamson PC, Cote CJ, Croop JM, Russo MW, Barrett JS, Hoke JF. Population pharmacokinetics of intravenous ondansetron in oncology and surgical patients aged 1–48 months. Eur J Clin Pharmacol. 2010;66(1):77–86. doi:10.1007/s00228-009-0730-8.

730. Anderson BJ. Pharmacology of paediatric TIVA. Rev Colomb Anestesiol. 2013;41:205–14.

731. Leeder JS, Kearns GL. Pharmacogenetics in pediatrics. Implications for practice. Pediatr Clin North Am. 1997;44(1):55–77.

732. Lotsch J, Kettenmann B, Renner B, Drover D, Brune K, Geisslinger G, Kobal G. Population pharmacokinetics of fast release oral diclofenac in healthy volunteers: relation to pharmacodynamics in an experimental pain model. Pharm Res. 2000;17(1):77–84.

733. Allegaert K, de Hoon J, Verbesselt R, Naulaers G, Murat I. Maturational pharmacokinetics of single intravenous bolus of propofol. Paediatr Anaesth. 2007;17(11):1028–34.

734. Allegaert K, Holford N, Anderson BJ, Holford S, Stuber F, Rochette A, Troconiz IF, Beier H, de Hoon JN, Pedersen RS, Stamer U. Tramadol and o-desmethyl tramadol clearance maturation and disposition in humans: a pooled pharmacokinetic study. Clin Pharmacokinet. 2015;54(2):167–78. doi:10.1007/s40262-014-0191-9.

735. Anderson BJ. Pediatric models for adult target-controlled infusion pumps. Paed Anaesth. 2010;20(3):223–32. doi:10.1111/j.1460-9592.2009.03072.x.

736. Sumpter A, Anderson BJ. Phenobarbital and some anesthesia implications. Pediatr Anesth. 2011;21:995–7.

737. Hannam JA, Anderson BJ. Pharmacodynamic interaction models in pediatric anesthesia. Paediatr Anaesth. 2015;25:970–80. doi:10.1111/pan.12735.

Clinical Pharmacology of Intravenous Sedation in Children

26

Oliver Bagshaw

Introduction

There are many situations in medicine where it is necessary to undertake procedures in children for therapeutic or diagnostic reasons. Often the former will involve some form of surgery or painful instrumentation, and will usually be undertaken with the aid of general anesthesia. If the procedure is diagnostic, minor, and relatively non-stimulating, then it may be possible to avoid general anesthesia and use sedation instead. There are also situations where anesthesia may be undesirable, unnecessary, or unavailable and the clinician has no option but to provide an alternative.

Sedation involves producing a state of depressed consciousness, improved co-operation, relative immobility, anxiolysis and amnesia, whilst minimizing side effects, such as depressed respiration, airway obstruction, hypotension, and reduced airway protective reflexes. The primary goal of sedation is always to provide the lightest level of hypnosis and analgesia by the safest means possible, thus minimizing adverse effects. With that in mind, any sedative regime should have a failure rate associated with it, because it is impossible to safely sedate all children in all situations, without straying into the realms of general anesthesia.

Over the years, a number of drugs have been used to provide sedation in children and various methods of delivery have been used. The focus of this chapter will be on drugs that can be administered by the intravenous route.

Definition

Several different definitions have been used to describe the level of sedation in patients. Traditionally it was described as either conscious sedation or deep sedation, but those definitions are no longer used, as the concept of conscious sedation does not exist in preschool children. The following are based on the guidelines for sedation in children produced by the American Academy of Pediatrics in the USA and National Institute of Clinical Excellence in the UK [1, 2].

Minimal Sedation

A drug-induced state during which patients are awake and calm, and respond normally to verbal commands. Although cognitive function and co-ordination may be impaired, ventilatory and cardiovascular functions are unaffected.

Moderate Sedation

Drug-induced depression of consciousness during which patients are sleepy but respond purposefully to verbal commands (known as conscious sedation in dentistry) or light tactile stimulation. No interventions are required to maintain a patent airway. Spontaneous ventilation is adequate. Cardiovascular function is usually maintained.

Deep Sedation

Drug-induced depression of consciousness during which patients are asleep and cannot easily be roused but do respond purposefully to repeated or painful stimulation (reflex withdrawal from a painful stimulus is not a purposeful response). The ability to maintain ventilatory function independently may be impaired. Patients may require

O. Bagshaw, MB ChB, FRCA(✉)
Department of Anaesthesia, Birmingham Children's Hospital,
Steelhouse Lane, Birmingham, West Midlands ZB4 6NH, UK
e-mail: oliver.bagshaw@bch.nhs.uk

© Springer International Publishing AG 2017
A.R. Absalom, K.P. Mason (eds.), *Total Intravenous Anesthesia and Target Controlled Infusions*,
DOI 10.1007/978-3-319-47609-4_26

assistance to maintain a patent airway. Spontaneous ventilation may be inadequate. Cardiovascular function is usually maintained

It is important to understand that sedation is a continuum from minimal sedation to general anesthesia, and that a patient may move from one level to another at any point during the sedation episode. Clearly, moving from a deep to light plane of sedation may have a negative impact on the success of the procedure, whereas excessive deepening of sedation may lead to significant, possibly serious, complications.

Indications

The indications for sedation are determined by the level of co-operation of the child (often related to age), the procedure, and a desire to avoid general anesthesia. The following are the indications for sedation in place of anesthesia:

- Diagnostic imaging
- Endoscopy
- Dental treatment
- Procedures such as suturing, fracture manipulation, lumbar puncture, and bone marrow

Cautions and Contraindications

Intravenous sedation is rarely completely contraindicated in a patient. However, there are a number of situations where extreme caution must be used. These are mainly situations in which the effects of sedation are likely to be exaggerated, or where the side effects may have more serious consequences. The following factors or conditions increase the risks associated with sedation:

- Age less than 1 year—particularly neonates or ex-premature infants less than 60 weeks post-menstrual age
- ASA status of 3 or above, congenital heart disease, critical illness or PICU admission, significant cardiac or respiratory compromise
- Significant neurological impairment or raised intracranial pressure
- Full stomach or risk thereof
- Risk of complete airway obstruction, including stridor, obstructive sleep apnea, and severe obesity

In all of these situations it is crucial that someone with the relevant seniority and experience assesses the patients and determines the safest course of action. That may involve

general anesthesia in a theater environment, rather than sedation in some other environment, such as the Ward or Emergency Department.

Sedation Endpoints

For any patient receiving sedation the aim is to achieve the following endpoints:

- Calm
- Asleep but arousable
- Not anxious
- Co-operative
- Not moving
- Pain-free
- Maintaining airway and ventilation
- Hemodynamically stable

In reality it may be impossible to achieve all of these endpoints every time you sedate a child or indeed throughout any single episode of sedation. However, the last two must be the clinician's priority to ensure the safety of the child, even if it is at the expense of succeeding with the procedure.

One of the advantages of sedation over anesthesia is that the key endpoints are easier to determine, therefore identification of any significant interindividual variability in terms of drug requirements is also easier to identify. This is important, as a major limitation of total intravenous anesthesia (TIVA) is the pharmacokinetic as well as the pharmacodynamic variability. In anesthesia, this may lead to patients being inadequately or excessively anesthetized, despite being administered what should be an appropriate amount of drug. The consequences are less significant for sedation, as generally the worst that will happen is that the patient will move or wake up. Indeed, for a technique to be regarded as safe, sedation must be carefully titrated to effect, to avoid inadvertent overdose.

Patient Preparation

Prior to administration of sedation to a child there need to be a number of considerations. These include:

- Relevant clinical history, including any underlying medical conditions, presence of intercurrent illness, and previous sedation episodes
- Clinical assessment of any physical risks of sedation to the child, such as ASA status, airway compromise, hemodynamic instability, or neurological impairment
- Starvation status
- Consent from the child and/or their carers

Pre-operative Fasting

The administration of minimal sedation, whereby patients remain responsive to verbal and tactile stimuli and maintain full protective airway reflexes, does not necessarily require the need for fasting, although the clinician needs to be aware that the patient may inadvertently enter a deeper stage of sedation during the procedure. Deeper levels of sedation may be associated with loss of airway protective reflexes and have the capacity to progress to a state of anesthesia. For these reasons it is prudent to fast all patients according to local guidelines for general anesthesia. However, a recent review suggests that the incidence of aspiration during episodes of sedation is low, irrespective of whether or not the patient is fasted [3].

Setup

As well as ensuring the patient is adequately starved for their procedure, it is important that other aspects of their preparation and setup are addressed prior to the administration of sedative drugs. These can be remembered by using the acronym **SOAPME**, which stands for the following:

Suction—working suction apparatus with an appropriate sized Yankeur connection

Oxygen—suitable quantity of oxygen for the procedure and more; delivery system, including flow meter, oxygen mask and/or nasal speculum for administering oxygen to the patient

Airway—a selection of airway devices, including Guedel airways, laryngeal mask airways and endotracheal tubes; age-appropriate facemasks, bag valve devices and functioning laryngoscopes

Pharmacy—other drugs that may be needed to support cardiopulmonary resuscitation or other emergencies such as anaphylaxis, as well as antidotes to an inadvertent sedation overdose

Monitoring—capability to measure oxygen saturation, heart rate, ECG, blood pressure, end-tidal carbon dioxide, respiratory rate

Equipment—special equipment such as a defibrillator, patient trolley, syringes, cannulae, needles and IV fluids, with appropriate giving set

As a general rule, it is better to be in a situation where you have the equipment available and the patient not need it, than not have the equipment available and the patient need it.

Monitoring

Full cardiorespiratory monitoring must be used in all cases where intravenous sedation is administered, as the effects of drugs may be unpredictable and over sedation may lead to a state of light anesthesia, with loss of airway patency. Clinical assessment would include continuous pulse oximetry, capnography, respiratory rate, ECG, and intermittent blood pressure measurement.

Administration

A number of different routes have been described for administering sedation in children. These are listed in Table 26.1, along with their advantages and disadvantages.

By far the commonest method used is by mouth, as this is often the most acceptable to the child and parents. However, intravenous administration offers the advantages of very rapid onset, titratability and repeatability, the option of continuous infusion and the possibility of fewer peaks and troughs in sedation. The main disadvantage is the need for vascular access, which may be challenging, particularly in the younger child. For the purposes of this chapter, the focus will be on intravenous sedation.

Table 26.1 Methods of sedative drug administration and their advantages and disadvantages

Route	Advantages	Disadvantages
Intravenous	Can be titrated and delivered continuously	Requires IV access, may have more side effects, may progress to anesthesia more easily
Oral	Simple, often most acceptable method to child, wide choice of drugs	Needs co-operation of child to take medication, slow onset, not titratable
Intranasal	Rapid onset, can be repeated	Unpleasant for the child, only effective for certain drugs
Intramuscular	Relatively rapid onset, better for uncooperative children	Painful, not titratable, absorption may be delayed in shock
Inhalational	Rapid onset and offset, readily titratable	Needs specialized drugs and equipment, may be unacceptable to younger children
Rectal	Very effective for certain drugs (barbiturates, chloral hydrate)	Slow onset, may not be acceptable to the child or parents

Measuring Level of Sedation

There are a number of different ways of assessing the level of sedation in patients. The simplest way is to make a clinical assessment based on the degree of hypnosis the patient exhibits and their response to verbal and tactile stimuli.

Alternative methods include more complex sedation scoring systems, which are mainly for situations of prolonged sedation such as on PICU, or when a less subjective method of assessment is necessary, such as during drug trials.

The primary purpose of a sedation scale is to provide a repeatable, objective assessment of the level of sedation. This allows the operator to recognize when the patient is becoming over-sedated and to avoid this from happening, thereby pre-empting serious complications.

Sedation Scoring Systems

A number of different scoring systems have been developed for both adults and children to assess the depth of sedation. In reality, the majority of patients do not need to have the depth of sedation scored, as a simple clinical assessment is sufficient. However, for documentation purposes, or to guide interventions, it may be useful to use a more defined assessment. The main disadvantage of any scoring system is that deeper levels of sedation inevitably require a degree of stimulation of the patient for assessment purposes, which may be counterproductive, negating the benefits of sedating the patient in the first place. Any scale or system that is used should be simple, consistent, and reproducible, both between observers and from episode to episode.

Scoring systems or scales can be divided into general scales/scores that can be used in both adults and children and specific pediatric scales/scores.

General Scoring Systems/Scales

Perhaps the two most commonly used sedation-scoring systems are the Ramsey scale and the Aldrete score.

Ramsay Scale

The Ramsay Sedation scale was the first scoring system to be used for sedated patients. It was developed in 1974 as an objective assessment of sedation in adult intensive care patients receiving an alphaxalone-alphadalone (Althesin) infusion [4]. It is intuitive, easy to remember, and can be used in any situation where patients are sedated, including PICU, procedural sedation, and imaging. Scores 1–3 apply to patients who are awake, whilst 4–6 apply to those who are asleep (Table 26.2).

Table 26.2 Ramsay scale for sedation

Sedation score	Clinical response
1	Fully awake
2	Drowsy but awakens spontaneously
3	Asleep but arouses and responds appropriately to simple verbal commands
4	Asleep, unresponsive to commands, but arouses to glabellar tap or loud verbal stimulus
5	Asleep and only responds to light glabellar tap and loud verbal stimulus
6	Asleep and unresponsive to light glabellar tap and loud verbal stimulus

Table 26.3 Aldrete sedation scale

Activity	
Voluntary movement of all limbs to command	2 points
Voluntary movement of 2 extremities to command	1 point
Unable to move	0 points
Respiration	
Breathe deeply and cough	2 points
Dyspnea, hypoventilation	1 point
Apneic	0 points
Circulation	
BP ± 20 mmHg of preanesthesia level	2 points
BP ± 20–50 mmHg of preanesthesia level	1 point
BP ± 50 mmHg of preanesthesia level	0 points
Consciousness	
Fully awake	2 points
Arousable	1 point
Unresponsive	0 points
Color	
Pink	2 points
Pale, blotchy	1 point
Cyanotic	0 points

Total score must be >8 at conclusion of monitoring

Aldrete Score

The Aldrete score was introduced into practice in 1970, as a postsurgical equivalent of the Apgar score [5]. Like the Apgar score, it contains 5 parameters to assess, and the total score can range from 0 to 10. Although it can be used as an assessment of the level of sedation, it was actually created for use in patients recovering from anesthesia. Patients are seldom significantly hypotensive, apneic, unresponsive and cyanotic, after sedation, and therefore this score has limited usefulness in this group, other than as an assessment of the level of recovery following treatment (Table 26.3).

The Observer's Assessment of Alertness/Sedation

The OAAS scale was originally developed in the 1990s to assess the level of sedation with midazolam in adults [6]. It used assessments of responsiveness, speech, facial expression, and eyes to produce a score between 1 and 5. Unlike the

Table 26.4 Original Observer's Assessment of Alertness/Sedation scale

Responsiveness	Speech	Facial Expression	Eyes	Score
Responds readily to name spoken in normal tone	Normal	Normal	Clear, no ptosis	5
Lethargic response to name spoken in normal tone	Mild slowing	Mild relaxation	Glazed or mild ptosis (<half the eye)	4
Responds only after name is called out loudly and/or repeatedly	Slurring or prominent slowing	Marked relaxation	Glazed and marked ptosis	3
Responds only after mild prodding or shaking	Few recognizable words	Marked relaxation	Glazed and marked ptosis	2
Does not response to mild prodding or shaking	Few recognizable words	Marked relaxation	Glazed and marked ptosis	1

Table 26.5 Modified Observer's Assessment of Alertness/Sedation scale

Responds readily to name spoken in normal tone	5
Lethargic response to name spoken in normal tone	4
Responds only after name is called loudly and/or repeatedly	3
Responds only after mild prodding or shaking	2
Does not respond to mild prodding or shaking	1

Table 26.6 University of Michigan Sedation scale

0	Awake and alert
1	Minimally sedated: Tired, sleepy, appropriate response to verbal conversation and/or sound
2	Moderately sedated: somnolent,/sleeping, easily aroused with light tactile stimulation or a simple verbal command
3	Deeply sedated: deep sleep, arousable with only significant physical stimulation
4	Unarousable

Ramsey scale, the OAAS score reduces as the level of sedation increases (Table 26.4).

The scale has subsequently been modified to make it simpler to use. In the modified version only the "responsiveness" category has been retained (Table 26.5).

As with other adult sedation scales, it has never been validated in the pediatric population.

Pediatric Scoring Systems

A number of sedation scales specific to pediatric patients have been developed over the years, for both research and clinical use.

University of Michigan Sedation Scale

This is a very simple scoring system, which has been shown to be reliable and valid for assessing depth of sedation in children [7]. It is similar to the Ramsay score, but based on a 5-point, rather than a 6-point scale (Table 26.6).

COMFORT Scale

The COMFORT scale was designed primarily for use in PICU to assess the depth of sedation in non-paralyzed patients undergoing mechanical ventilation [8]. It relies on assessment of a number of behavioral and physiological parameters. One of the limitations is that physiological parameters can be adversely influenced by critical illness or the use of sedative drugs, making the score less accurate when this is the case. Interestingly, validation studies have suggested that these are the source of greatest interindividual variability during assessment, rather than the behavioral parameters. Removal of the physiological variables from a subsequent version of the scale (COMFORT-behavior or B) has improved the accuracy [9, 10]. It requires assessment of seven different variables, level of consciousness, calmness/agitation, respiratory response, crying, physical movement, muscular tone and facial tension, on a scale of 1 to 5. The main limitation is that the respiratory assessment is designed for patients undergoing mechanical ventilation. Another limitation is that it may also be less useful in distinguishing distress due to pain from distress due to other factors, such as delirium or drug withdrawal.

Faces Legs Activity Cry Consolability Scale (FLACC)

There is potentially a significant overlap between assessment of sedation and pain depending on the procedure. There are several scales that specifically relate to the assessment of pain. One of these is FLACC, which stands for Facial expression, Leg movement, Activity, Cry and Consolability. It was developed for use in younger children, due to the inability to report in preverbal infants and the lack of reliability of self-reporting in preschool children [11]. The five categories score between 0 (no pain) and 2 (severe pain) in each, giving a maximum score of 10 (Table 26.7).

Clearly, it would be inappropriate to use a pure pain scale to assess level of sedation in the majority of patients, as untreated pain in any child is likely to produce both increased conscious level and movement; two situations we are trying to avoid by sedating the child in the first place. However, there may be some value in using FLACC during procedures where there is a significant painful stimulus, so that the analgesic component of the sedation is optimized.

Another commonly used pain scale is the Children's Hospital of Philadelphia pain scale (CHEOPS), which was developed in 1985 [12].

Table 26.7 Faces, Legs, Activity, Cry Consolability (FLACC) scale

Categories	Scoring		
	0	1	2
Face	No particular expression or smile; disinterested	Occasional grimace or frown, withdrawn	Frequent to constant frown, quivering chin, clenched jaw
Legs	Normal position or relaxed	Uneasy, restless, tense	Kicking or legs drawn up
Activity	Lying quietly, normal position, moves easily	Squirming, shifting back and forth, tense	Arched, rigid or jerking
Cry	No cry (awake or asleep)	Moans or whimpers; occasional complaint	Crying steadily, screams or sobs, frequent complaints
Consolability	Content, relaxed	Reassured by occasional touching, hugging or being talked to; distractible	Difficult to console or comfort

As previously mentioned, a big disadvantage of many sedation scales is that require some degree of stimulation of the patient in order to make the assessment. This is counter-intuitive, as one of the ways to ensure success with sedation is to minimize the degree of patient stimulation, be it move-ment, noise, pain or something as simple as a blood pressure cuff inflating and deflating. By regularly disturbing the patient in order to make an assessment of depth of sedation, the observer is likely to guarantee failure of the technique. Physiological data is useful, but safe parameters for different ages of patient and levels of sedation have never been deter-mined, so interventions can only be driven largely by proto-col or experience. Clearly, parameters such as oxygen saturation, heart rate, blood pressure, respiratory rate, and end-tidal carbon dioxide may all give an indication of when sedation has become excessive and complications are immi-nent, but in an ideal world it should be possible to pre-empt that by responding to changes in physiology as it happens.

Other considerations when using sedation scales are that there is no consensus amongst users as to which is the best, measured parameters may vary significantly between scales, validation may be limited to a small number of studies, and performance reliability may differ significantly between individuals.

Depth of Sedation Monitoring

An alternative to using a sedation scale or score is to use one of a number of the commercially available depth of anesthe-sia (DOA) monitors. These have been used in children to assess the level of sedation in several different environments, including the Operating Theater, PICU, and the ED. By far the most commonly studied monitor is the Bispectral Index (BIS). Several studies have used BIS monitoring to guide the administration of sedation [13–17]. However, studies in PICU patients comparing BIS with sedation scores such as Ramsay and COMFORT demonstrate moderate correlation only, with significant variation between patients [18–21].

Perhaps the best use of BIS is in distinguishing lighter levels of sedation from deeper levels in non-paralyzed patients, and for avoiding the patient lapsing into a state of general anesthesia, which has been described. In a study where propofol alone was administered for intrathecal che-motherapy and bone marrow aspirate, by a clinician blinded to the BIS value, the mean lowest BIS score was 29, with several patients achieving values of less than 20 [22]. Perhaps this was more a reflection of the inadequacy of the technique than of those who were using it, as there was no co-administration of an analgesic agent for what were stimulating interventions. A subsequent study demonstrated that a targeted BIS value of 45 was needed to provide ade-quate depth of sedation with propofol alone in children undergoing a range of painful procedures on PICU [15]. The mean dose of propofol administered to achieve this was more than 0.5 mg/kg/min (30 mg/kg/h). Given that the BIS range for general anesthesia is between 40 and 60, clearly most of these children were receiving anesthesia rather than deep sedation. A recent blinded study in the Emergency Department confirmed that nearly 80 % of patients were receiving general anesthesia rather than seda-tion, with a mean lowest BIS score of 43 [23]. Over 90 % of the sedating physicians underestimated the level of sedation.

As with assessments of depth of sedation, application of a monitor such as BIS may be quite stimulating for the patient. Ideally, the electrode should be attached before the start of sedative administration, so that the effect of stimulating the patient is minimized. However, some children will find this distressing, so that a balance needs to be found and will depend on the age of the child, the sedation being administered and the procedure being undertaken.

An alternative to the BIS monitor is the Narcotrend. The Narcotrend Index has been shown to correlate well with the depth of sedation in children undergoing upper GI endos-copy [24]. It also has the advantage that the sensor applica-tion is relatively non-stimulating and well tolerated by most children. Other systems that appear to correlate well with objective assessment of sedation are the Cerebral State Index and the A-line ARX [25].

The only hypnotic agent that does not show a good correlation between agent concentration and the output of the DOA monitors is ketamine, due to its excitatory effects on the EEG [17, 26]. There is also good evidence that in younger patients the BIS may be less accurate than in older children, due to differences in the underlying EEG pattern and it is certainly not indicated in patients less than 1 year of age [27].

Sedative Agents

A number of different drugs are currently used for sedation in children, either as a single agent or in combination with other drugs. The advantages of a single agent are that its effects are more predictable and controllable, and side effects are limited to those of one agent. Drug combinations can have the advantage of synergism, so that much lower doses of each agent can be used for a given effect. They may also combine effects, such as hypnosis, analgesia, and anxiolysis that no single agent can produce. The main disadvantages of combinations are the unpredictable response, increased risk of side effects, and potential for drug interactions. Table 26.8 lists the most commonly used agents for intravenous sedation, along with their advantages, disadvantages and the other drugs they are often used in combination with.

Single Agents

Propofol

Propofol or 2,6 di-isopropylphenol was first introduced into clinical practice in the late 1980s. It was marketed as having a faster recovery than thiopentone and less histamine release and chance of an allergic reaction. Propofol is formulated in soya and egg lecithin, but it can be safely used in soya and egg allergy patients, as they are allergic to the protein component of soya and egg, rather than the fat component. Patients in whom propofol should be avoided include those with mitochondrial disease, hereditary channelopathies, and acyl co-enzyme A dehydrogenase deficiency (MCADD and LCADD). The main side effects following administration are a dose-dependent reduction in respiratory rate, progressing to apnea, reduction in heart rate, vascular resistance and blood pressure, and extrapyramidal movements. Both onset and recovery are rapid; the latter due to redistribution. The half-life is about 30–60 min, making it an ideal agent for short-term sedation.

Mode of Administration

There are three main options when it comes to administering intravenous sedation to children. These are bolus dose, continuous intravenous infusion, or target-controlled infusion (TCI).

Bolus

The simplest method of administering propofol is by bolus injection. This has the advantage of not requiring any specific equipment. It is easy to titrate and repeated doses can be administered as required. The main disadvantage of bolus administration is that it leads to peaks and troughs in plasma concentration. This can exaggerate the side effects of propofol, such as respiratory depression and hypotension, although these

Table 26.8 Uses, advantages, and disadvantages of some of the most commonly used drugs in children

Drug	Class	Uses	Advs	Disadvs	Combination
Propofol	Phenol derivative	Induction anesthesia Procedural sedation	Short half-life Can be administered as mass rate infusion or TCI	Painful to inject No analgesic properties Can easily cause anesthesia effects	Opioids Ketamine Midazolam Alpha 2 agonists
Midazolam	Benzodiazepine	Procedural sedation	Anxiolysis Amnesia Can be antagonized	Some respiratory and CVS depression	Propofol Ketamine
Ketamine	Phencyclidine derivative	Procedural sedation	Immobilization Analgesia CVS stability	'Dissociative' state making sedation end points difficult to assess Hypersalivation Emergence phenomena Tachycardia & hypertension	Propofol Midazolam
Dexmedetomidine	Alpha 2 agonist	Procedural sedation	Airway and ventilation maintained Immobilization Reduced analgesia requirements	Hypotension Bradycardia Relatively long half-life	Propofol
Fentanyl	Synthetic opioid	Analgesia	Rapid onset Short duration Easily titratable CVS stability	Respiratory depression	Any hypnotic

will be short-lived. Also, the duration of sedation will be relatively short, requiring additional boluses. It is best for quick procedures, where variations in the depth of sedation are less important. An initial bolus of 0.5–1 mg/kg will produce an effect within 30 s and can be repeated as necessary. Larger doses (2–3 mg/kg) are likely to induce general anesthesia and almost invariably produce a period of apnea.

Clinical Example

A 6 m-old, 7.6 kg child, post-cardiac surgery, is scheduled for removal of a mediastinal chest drain. He is self-ventilating in wafting oxygen and analgesia is being provided by NCA morphine. A 20 mcg/kg bolus of morphine is administered from the NCA. After about 5 min, a propofol bolus of 5 mg (0.66 mg/kg) is given. The patient becomes only slightly sedated, so the bolus is repeated at the same dose. His conscious level reduces sufficiently for the drain to be removed successfully and the patient recovers quickly from the procedure.

The TivaTrainer© simulation in Fig. 26.1 demonstrates what happens to the plasma (red line) and effect-site (green line) concentration of propofol following the administration of the two boluses. The initial bolus leads to an effect-site concentration of just under 1 mcg/ml, which clearly isn't enough to produce significant sedation. The second bolus has a cumulative effect, resulting in a rapid rise in the effect-site concentration to about 1.5 mcg/ml. In combination with the morphine, this is sufficient for the patient to become lightly sedated, with minimal effect on HR, BP, RR, or oxygen saturations. As the procedure is likely to be painful, administration of propofol alone would not have been

appropriate and co-administration of an opioid is necessary. Care must be taken to ensure that the synergistic effect between propofol and opioids is considered when the drugs are given together. Patient movement would not have influenced the success of the procedure; so lighter levels of sedation can be tolerated and are advisable anyway in this case, given the underlying cardiac condition.

Continuous Infusion

For longer procedures, where repeated bolus doses might be required, it makes more sense to administer propofol as a continuous infusion, preferably a mass rate infusion, either mcg/kg/min or mg/kg/h. This helps smooth out some of the peaks and troughs in the level of sedation, as long as an initial bolus of propofol is given and an appropriate rate of infusion is administered. The pharmacokinetics of propofol is such that the infusion rate will need to be reduced over time, to maintain a stable plasma concentration, as redistribution to compartments V2 and V3 slows.

The main disadvantages of a manual infusion regime are as follows:

- Bolus administration is not incorporated, either at the beginning or when rapid changes in depth of sedation are required
- There may be no clear indication of the propofol dose being delivered if administered as a rate infusion (mls/h)

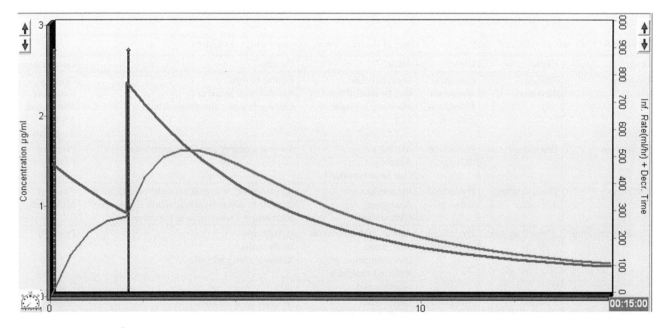

Fig. 26.1 TivaTrainer© simulation demonstrating the changes in plasma and effect-site concentration of propofol with the administration two bolus doses

- The estimated plasma propofol concentration being delivered is difficult to estimate, even for experts
- Frequent changes in the drug infusion rate are required to maintain a stable plasma propofol concentration
- It doesn't guarantee a stable plasma and therefore effect-site propofol concentration
- An increase in infusion rate without a bolus dose leads to a slow rise in plasma concentration
- Published regimens are often not based on valid pharmacokinetic data

Clinical Example

A nearly 3-year-old boy, estimated weight 12-kg, has been brought into ED. The history is that he fell out of first floor window onto concrete. He cried immediately and an ambulance was called. His GCS is 15 and he needs a CT of his head, c-spine, thorax, and abdomen, but is too awake and for uncooperative for scanning without either sedation or general anesthesia. ABC are stable and do not require intervention and there are no other indications for endotracheal intubation. The decision is made to sedate with propofol for the scan. He has an IV in situ and is given midazolam 2 mg and a further 1 mg to settle him. A propofol bolus is titrated up to 20 mg total (1.67 mg/kg) and an infusion commenced a 5 mg/kg/h (83 mcg/kg/min). This is increased to 7.5 mg/kg/h (125 mcg/kg/min) after about 5 min and he sedates nicely. He is transferred to scan in a lightly sedated state and the scan is successfully completed after about 45 min.

The TivaTrainer© simulation (Fig. 26.2) demonstrates how the relatively small bolus of propofol leads to a rapid rise in the effect-site concentration to just under 2 mcg/ml concentration. The infusion leads to a very gradual rise in the plasma and effect-site concentrations, so that by the end of the scan they are both about 2 mcg/ml. As with opioids, there is a significant synergistic effect between propofol and midazolam, which allows a lower dose of propofol to be administered. It is also unnecessary to produce anything other than a moderate state of sedation for a quick CT scan, particularly as the patient needs to be awake rapidly at the end, to facilitate neurological status assessment.

In situations where a mass rate infusion is being used, rather than TCI, it is useful to be able to estimate the target propofol concentration being delivered to the patient. Table 26.9 shows the target propofol concentration likely to be achieved following bolus administration and at different infusion rates.

Target-Controlled Infusion

The most pharmacokinetically complex, but also valid method of administering propofol is by target-controlled infusion (TCI). The propofol bolus and infusion rates are determined by PK information stored within the model, which has been previously derived from a population of patients by clinical studies. The pump constantly varies the rate of infusion of propofol to maintain an estimated plasma or effect-site concentration. Increases in the propofol concentration are achieved by the pump administering a bolus and increasing the infusion rate, whilst decreases lead to the

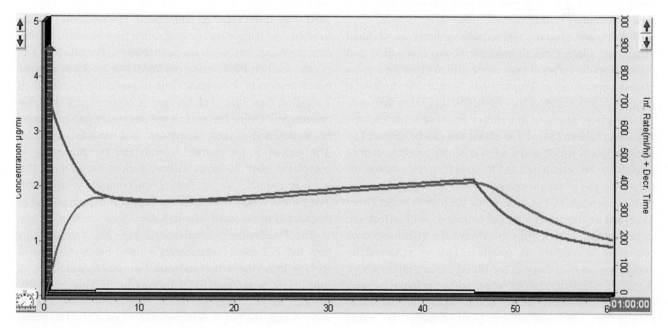

Fig. 26.2 TivaTrainer© simulation demonstrating the effect of a bolus dose of propofol followed by a continuous infusion on the plasma and effect-site concentration

Table 26.9 TivaTrainer simulation in a 25 kg, 8-year-old boy, using the Paedfusor model with a fast ke0 value (0.8). The propofol bolus used was 3 mg/kg

Estimated propofol target concentration (µg/ml)								
Propofol infusion rate (mg/kg/h)	Time (min)							
	Bolus	5	10	15	20	30	45	60
2	4.3	3.2	1.8	1.3	1.1	1.0	1.0	0.9
4	4.3	3.4	2.1	1.6	1.5	1.5	1.5	1.5
6	4.4	3.6	2.4	2.0	1.9	1.9	2.1	2.2
8	4.5	3.8	2.7	2.4	2.4	2.4	2.6	2.8
10	4.6	4.0	3.0	2.8	2.8	2.8	3.2	3.4

pump switching off the infusion for a period of time before restarting at a lower rate.

The first commercially available TCI systems incorporated the Diprifusor microprocessor which was programmed with the Marsh pharmacokinetic model for adults [28]. The age and weight limits for these pumps were set at 16 years and 30-kg, respectively, making it unsuitable for the majority of pediatric patients. Indeed, subsequent research has shown that use of the Marsh dataset leads to a significant overestimate of the plasma propofol concentration in children, due to children having a larger than predicted central compartment volume. More recently two pediatric models for propofol TCI administration have been developed: the Kataria [29] for children aged 3–16 years and the Paedfusor [30] for children aged 1–16 years. The Kataria model has two versions: a purely weight-based, and a weight-based, age-adjusted algorithm. The Paedfusor uses both age and weight. Both have been validated in children and have demonstrated that they reasonably accurately predict the plasma propofol concentration in steady-state conditions [31, 32].

The bigger central compartment volume in children means that a larger initial (induction) bolus is required, and higher propofol infusion rates are needed to maintain a given plasma concentration. Propofol has been shown to have a greater context-sensitive half-time (CSHT) [33] in the younger age group, resulting in a slower return of consciousness in young children [34]. To an extent this can be obviated by using adjuncts which allow a lower target concentration of propofol to be maintained and by switching the infusion off before the end of the procedure.

Modern adult TCI systems allow the user to target either the blood or the effect-site concentration. With effect-site targeting, the system aims to achieve the effect-site concentration as rapidly as possible. This is achieved by generating an overshoot in the blood concentration above the target effect-site concentration, when the initial target is set. The degree of overshoot required depends on the rate of blood-effect-site equilibration (k_eo). Clearly, it makes greater pharmacological sense to target the effect-site. However, unlike plasma concentration; effect-site

concentrations cannot be directly measured, and so effect-site targeting algorithms rely on estimates of the time course of the changes in effect-site concentration based on measurements of the clinical effect (usually an EEG measure). This means that effect-site targeting, although clinically acceptable, relies on several assumptions and estimates. The other problem of effect-site targeting is that it leads to much higher initial plasma concentrations of drugs, as the primary determinant of how fast the effect-site concentration is reached is the plasma concentration. In order to generate a rapid increase in effect-site concentration, the pumps deliver a large bolus of drug, which may not always be well tolerated by the patient or lead to an excessive depth of sedation. However, the estimated effect-site concentration may be a better predictor of when the patient will lose and regain consciousness, so may be more relevant when planning sedation. At present effect-site targeting has not been implemented in pediatric TCI systems, because the available models incorporate adult estimates of the k_eo. Recent studies in children suggest that the k_eo value increases as age decreases, therefore reducing the difference between plasma and effect-site concentrations during induction and emergence (hysteresis) [35, 36].

Clinical Example

A 5-year-old boy with severe combined immune deficiency had been admitted to the PICU post bone marrow transplant, with sepsis. His condition has improved and he had been extubated the previous day. Prior to discharge to the ward he develops sudden onset of weakness in his arms and legs. An urgent Neurology consult is requested and an immediate MRI scan of the spine recommended. The decision is taken to sedate the patient for the scan rather than anesthetize him, thus avoiding the need for reintubation. Propofol TCI is commenced on PICU using the Paedfusor model at a target concentration of 1 mcg/ml. This is gradually increased to 2 mcg/ml, then 3 mcg/ml. Oxygen is administered via nasal cannula at 2 l/min. The patient sedates nicely, but maintains his airway and oxygen saturations, and remains arousable. The patient is transferred to scan and the procedure is completed after 30 min, without patient movement. The scan is normal, so no further intervention is required. The patient wakes soon after the propofol is stopped and is discharged to the ward later that day.

The TivaTrainer© simulation in Fig. 26.3 demonstrates how the TCI model administers a small bolus of propofol (0.4 mg/kg) at the start of sedation, followed by a continuous infusion at 6 mg/kg/h (100 mcg/kg/min). This gradually reduces to 5.25 mg/kg/h (87.5 mcg/kg/min) by 5 min. After 5 min, the target is increased to 2 mcg/ml. The pump delivers another bolus of propofol (0.5 mg/kg) and the infusion rate is increased to 11 mg/kg/h (183 mcg/kg/min) to

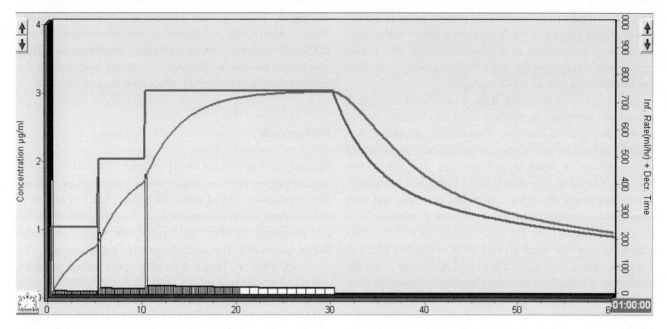

Fig. 26.3 TivaTrainer© simulation demonstrating how a propofol target-controlled infusion (TCI) administers changing infusion rates (shown by *black line* and *right-hand y* axis) and leads to a rapid change in both plasma (*red line*) and effect-site (*green line*) propofol concentrations to achieve the desired target concentration

maintain the higher target. Once more, this gradually reduces to about 10 mg/kg/h (167 mcg/kg/min) over 5 min. When the target is increased to 3 mcg/ml, a similar bolus of propofol is administered and the infusion rate increased up to 16 mg/kg/h (267 mcg/kg/min). Again, this gradually reduces for the duration of the procedure, until at the time of stopping the infusion; the rate is just under 11 mg/kg/h (183 mcg/kg/min). This produced a deep level of sedation, which is appropriate for MRI scanning, as it reduces the chances of the patient moving and sequences having to be repeated. However, given that the patient had demonstrated abnormal neurological symptoms, it was appropriate to gradually increase the level of sedation, to ensure no adverse consequences occurred as a result of altered sensitivity.

Safety

The Pediatric Sedation Research Consortium looked specifically at the incidence of adverse events with the administration of propofol for pediatric sedation outside the OR [37]. In their series of nearly 50,000 cases they demonstrated an overall incidence of 592 per 10,000 sedations, of which nearly 40 % were pulmonary in nature. No patient died, but two patients did require cardiopulmonary resuscitation. Unplanned airway interventions, including bag-mask ventilation, laryngeal mask insertion and intubation, were needed in 9.3 % of all patients. Other sedative agents were administered in 20 % of cases, most commonly opioids and midazolam.

Ketamine

Ketamine is a phencyclidine derivative, which has become a popular agent in pediatric anesthesia and sedation practice due to its hypnotic and analgesic properties, and the cardio-respiratory stability it confers. Unlike most other sedative agents, it acts mainly via antagonism of the excitatory NMDA receptor, although it is now thought to have effects on various other systems, including the HCN1, cholinergic, aminergic, and opioid systems.

Some TIVA practitioners use ketamine as an adjunct, although it is difficult to assess the added value over traditional analgesic agents and there is nothing in the literature to support this practice. Several studies have looked at the effect of low dose ketamine on postoperative analgesic requirements and a recent Cochrane review suggests that it is effective and may confer some advantage in terms of reducing hyperalgesia following remifentanil infusion [38].

The recommended intravenous dose for sedation ranges from 0.5 to 1 mg/kg. Unlike other sedative agents, ketamine produces a state of dissociation and immobilization, whereby the patient may appear to be conscious and awake, but in reality, does not respond purposefully to their environment or the people within it. This can make it difficult to titrate the drug and assess when the necessary dose has been delivered. Doses of 2 mg/kg or above will induce general anesthesia, so should be avoided if just sedation is required. Ketamine has the advantage of being just as effective when administered by the IM route, although larger doses (4–5 mg/kg) are needed and speed of onset is significantly slower (over 5 min). It also has a longer duration of action, which translates to a slower recovery. For longer procedures, a ketamine bolus can be followed by a continuous infusion at a rate of 0.5–2 mg/kg/h.

Side effects of ketamine include increased salivation, nausea and vomiting, nightmares and hallucinations, tachycardia, and muscle rigidity. Historically, ketamine was thought to produce an increase in intracranial pressure, but recent studies in head injured patients now refute this [39, 40]. The same is probably true of intraocular pressure, with lower doses (3 mg/kg) producing no effect and only large doses (6 mg/kg) leading to a modest increase [41]. Emergence phenomena are less common in children than adults, but may still occur in up to 10 % of children [42, 43]. They are more likely in the older child. Ketamine is not the ideal agent if sedation is necessary in order for the child to be immobile, such as during imaging studies, as occasional semi-purposeful movements are common, even when relatively large doses are administered. Hypersalivation may be attenuated by the co-administration of an anticholinergic agent, such as atropine or glycopyrrolate. They can be given either IV or IM, although the latter is more effective. Another disadvantage of ketamine is that, unlike opioids or benzodiazepines, there is no drug that will antagonize its effects if an accidental overdose occurs. Fortunately, it has a high therapeutic index, meaning that any accidental overdose is likely to be relatively well tolerated.

Ketamine can also be used in combination with other sedative drugs such as propofol or midazolam. The combination of propofol and ketamine ("ketofol") in a 1:1 ratio is being used in the Emergency Department with great success [44], although recent dosing simulation studies suggest a ratio of 1:3 for sedation and 1:5 for anesthesia may provide a better balance between analgesia and recovery [45, 46]. Ketofol is usually administered from a starting dose of 0.5 mg/kg of each drug and titrated to effect.

Although there has been much debate in the literature about the safety of non-anesthesiologists administering this combination to patients, there have now been several thousand reports of its use and the significant complication rate remains low, at less than 10 %. As with any technique, it depends on the inherent safety profile of the drugs being used, the experience of the operator administering them and the technique that has been devised to minimize risks to the patient.

Benzodiazepines

The benzodiazepines act at gamma-aminobutyric acid (GABA) receptors, potentiating GABA inhibitory effects. Apart from their sedative effects, they also induce anxiolysis, amnesia, and relaxation of skeletal muscle. Their primary site of action is the α1 subunit of the GABA-A receptor, which produces the hypnosis. They also act on the less widespread α2 subunit, primarily in the hippocampus and amygdala, producing anxiolysis.

Midazolam

Midazolam has an excellent pedigree as a sedative agent and remains a popular choice among sedation providers. It has relatively rapid onset of action, but has a slower time to peak effect compared with drugs such as propofol and ketamine. It also has a relatively high therapeutic index, providing the dose is carefully titrated and the recovery time is faster than for many other sedative agents. The clinical effect is more predictable in older children than in the younger age group. The latter often fight the effects of the drug or have a paradoxical excitatory reaction, and may require relatively higher doses to reach a satisfactory level of sedation. The dose needed for younger children may be up to 0.5 mg/kg, administered in aliquots of 0.05–0.1 mg/kg. Older children may need as little as 0.05–0.1 mg/kg in total to produce the same level of sedation. Due to the delay in reaching peak effect, further doses should only be administered every 5–10 min, to avoid over sedating the patient.

The main adverse effects associated with midazolam administration include paradoxical reactions, respiratory depression, and loss of airway reflexes. Some cardiovascular depression also occurs, primarily as a direct consequence of its effect on the CNS.

Midazolam remains a popular drug for premedication and co-administration at induction of anesthesia. The latter practice has been shown to reduce propofol requirements for induction, and the amnesic effect it confers may be desirable if lighter levels of sedation are used [47].

It can be administered by continuous infusion at a dose of 1–5 mcg/kg/min, if a longer duration of sedation is required. In reality, this is reserved for sedation on the PICU, as the risks of accumulation and relative overdose increase with increasing duration of infusion, due to an increase in the CSHT of the drug.

Diazepam

Diazepam has been largely superseded by midazolam for procedural sedation, due to its lack of water solubility, slower onset of action, longer duration of effect, longer half-life, and presence of active metabolites. However, in situations where midazolam is not available, it can be a useful alternative. The recommended IV dose is 0.25 mg/kg, repeated every 3 min, by careful titration, up to a maximum dose of 10 mg.

Lorazepam

Lorazepam has only a limited role in procedural sedation and is reserved mainly for the emergency treatment of seizures. It is used for sedation on PICU in the USA, either as repeated bolus doses or as a continuous infusion [48]. It has a long duration of action, making it less titratable and unsuitable for short duration or outpatient procedures. If used, a bolus dose of 0.05–0.1 mg/kg can be administered.

Flumazenil

Antagonism of benzodiazepines can be achieved through the administration of flumazenil. It is administered in a dose of 0.01–0.02 mg/kg and can be repeated as required. Care must be exercised if the patient has an underlying seizure disorder, is on long-term benzodiazepine treatment, or has ingested tricyclic antidepressants, as administration of flumazenil may precipitate seizures.

Barbiturates

Barbiturates act on GABA receptors and hyperpolarize the nerve cell membrane via chloride channels, eliciting first sedation and then anesthesia, in a dose-related manner. They have no analgesic properties and may even increase pain responses to noxious stimuli. They are neuroprotective by virtue of increasing metabolic rate and thus increasing ischemic tolerance time, by reducing intracranial pressure and by preventing or terminating seizures. Barbiturates have a relatively narrow therapeutic window and readily cause hypotension, hypoventilation, and apnea.

Historically, available agents have included pentobarbital, thiopental, and methohexital. Currently, only thiopental remains in routine clinical practice.

Thiopental

Thiopental was the favored agent for induction of anesthesia prior to the introduction of propofol into clinical practice. It can also be used as a sedative agent, with a rapid onset of action and initial short duration of action. It is particularly useful for the treatment of raised intracranial pressure or seizures, with an initial dose of 1–2 mg/kg, followed by a continuous infusion of 1–5 mg/kg/h. Prolonged administration by infusion leads to accumulation with a rapid increase in the CSHT from an initial value of 3–8 h, after an infusion of a few hours, up to 36 h after 4–8 days of infusion at 4 mg/kg/h [49].

α2 receptor Agonists

The α_2 receptor agonists were originally developed as antihypertensive agents, due to their centrally acting sympatholytic properties. However, it became clear that they also had widespread effects in the CNS, causing hypnosis, immobilization, muscle relaxation and analgesia, making them suitable agents for sedation in a variety of situations. All α_2 receptor agonists have some degree of activity at the α_1 receptor as well, although this varies from drug to drug.

Dexmedetomidine

Dexmedetomidine has replaced clonidine as the α_2 receptor agonist of choice for procedural sedation in children, as it is approximately eight times more specific to the receptor, with an α_2:α_1 ratio of 1600:1. When administered IV more than 90 % is protein bound. It has a relatively rapid redistribution half-life of 6–7 min, whilst the elimination half-life is approximately 2 h. At lower doses the metabolism follows, exponential or first order kinetics, whereas at higher doses it follows linear or zero order kinetics, meaning that a fixed amount of drug is eliminated per unit of time, irrespective of the blood concentration.

Sedation, anxiolysis, and analgesia occur in clinical doses, whilst there is minimal effect on respiratory function. The main side effects are bradycardia and hypotension, although transient hypertension may precede this, probably as a result of peripheral vasoconstriction mediated by a direct effect on vascular α_2C receptors. Treatment of bradycardia with anticholinergic drugs may cause severe hypertension. Dexmedetomidine may also cause depression of sinus and atrioventricular nodal function and is probably best avoided in patients with significant pre-existing bradycardia and those at risk of AV nodal block, or taking medications that depress AV nodal conduction [50].

Several indications for dexmedetomidine administration in relation to general anesthesia have been proposed. These include premedication, prevention of emergence delirium, treatment of shivering and reduction in postoperative opioid requirements [51, 52]. However, by far the biggest indication for dexmedetomidine use is as the main sedative agent for radiological imaging [53]. Comparison with existing commonly used agents such as midazolam or propofol is favorable [54, 55].

Various doses have been used, most commonly a loading dose of 1 mcg/kg with or without an infusion at 0.5 mcg/kg/h. Larger loading doses (2 mcg/kg) and higher infusion rates (2–3 mcg/kg/h) increase the success rates of procedural sedation above 90 %, but at the expense of increased hypotension and delayed recovery. Co-administration with other drugs such as propofol, midazolam, fentanyl, and ketamine may be beneficial for more invasive procedures and also increase the success rate in imaging [56].

Clonidine

Clonidine is a mixed α_1 and α_2 receptor agonist that has predominantly α_2 effects, in a ratio of 200:1. It was originally introduced as an antihypertensive agent, but has become established in pediatric practice for its sedative and analgesic properties. It can be administered orally, intravenously, or rectally. It has high bioavailability and metabolism occurs in the liver, with excretion of inactive metabolites by the kidneys. The half-life is prolonged at 12–33 h [57]. In infants, metabolism is further reduced and elimination can take up to three times as long as in adults [58].

The main indications for clonidine have been for premedication prior to anesthesia and as a sedative on the PICU. It may also have a role as a hypnotic-sparing agent when used in combination with other sedative agents, such as propofol. The intravenous dose of clonidine for sedation in PICU is 0.25–2 mcg/kg/h by continuous infusion, with or without an initial bolus dose of 0.5–1 mcg/kg. Some hemodynamically unstable children may not tolerate the bolus dose, in which case it can be omitted. There is very limited experience of clonidine for procedural sedation outside the PICU, other than as an adjunct in combination with other agents. During anesthesia, doses of 3–4 mcg/kg have been shown to reduce propofol requirements by 20–40% [59].

Opioids

Opioids are frequently used in combination with hypnotic agents for TIVA due to their analgesic and synergistic properties. Co-administration of potent synthetic opioids such as fentanyl, alfentanil, and remifentanil allows a significant reduction in propofol requirements for both sedation and anesthesia [60]. The opioids also have the advantage of blocking or attenuating any noxious stimuli.

Ideally the pharmacokinetic properties of the opioid should be reasonably similar to that of the hypnotic agent they are administered with, so that a balanced combination can be administered, which optimally reduce the required dosages and minimize any side effects. Thus, the shorter

acting synthetic opioids are better combined with propofol, whilst morphine is better combined with a drug such as midazolam.

Morphine

Morphine has a long and successful history as a sedative agent, particularly for short, painful procedures or longer-term sedation, such as on the PICU. It is often administered in combination with a hypnotic agent, although it does have some sedative properties of its own. Onset is relatively slow compared with some of the newer synthetic opioids, making it less titratable. It also has a relatively long duration of action, which may be a disadvantage if rapid recovery is desirable. However, in situations where a residual analgesic effect is needed, this is a significant advantage.

Side effects of morphine include those associated with any opioid, such as respiratory depression, apnea, reduced sensitivity to hypercapnea and hypoxia, and nausea and vomiting. Patients with renal failure and obstructive sleep apnea are particularly prone to respiratory depression [61]. Morphine can also cause histamine release, leading to flushing, vasodilatation, and hypotension. It also causes venodilatation, contributing to the decline in blood pressure often seen with administration. With that in mind, caution needs to be exercised if it is used in patients with untreated hypovolemia, as profound hypotension can result.

Fentanyl

Fentanyl is a lipophilic, synthetic opioid with potency approximately 100 times greater than morphine. Unlike morphine it has very little in the way of sedative properties, unless given in very high doses, so in most cases it is administered purely for its analgesic effect. It is also relatively cardiostable compared with morphine, producing little in the way of hypotension, even in large doses. Bradycardia can occur at higher doses, but is rarely troublesome enough to require intervention. The half-life of fentanyl is similar to morphine, at 3 h. The shorter clinical effect comes from rapid redistribution from the central compartment. However, the CSHT increases rapidly if fentanyl is administered by continuous infusion, due to accumulation in peripheral tissues.

The dose of fentanyl for analgesia in conscious patients ranges from 0.5 to 1 mcg/kg. Occasionally higher doses of up to 2–3 mcg/kg may be needed, if pain is a major component of the procedure. However, careful titration is necessary in these situations, to ensure an overdose is avoided.

The major side effect of fentanyl is respiratory depression, which can be rapid and profound, unless the dose is carefully titrated. There is also an increased risk of chest wall rigidity, with higher doses, but usually only with rapid administration and doses above 5 mcg/kg. This phenomenon has been described in neonates at standard doses of 1–2 mcg/kg, so extreme caution should be exercised in this age group [62]. Chest wall rigidity can often be overcome by the judicious use of CPAP. However, if that is not effective, then it can be antagonized by naloxone or reversed by the administration of a neuromuscular blocking agent [63, 64].

Alfentanil

Alfentanil remains an effective analgesic component of TIVA. It has a relatively fast onset, can be administered by bolus or infusion, and is readily titratable. It is less potent and lipophilic than fentanyl, and has a shorter half-life at less than 2 h. It is less likely to accumulate, due to the lower lipid solubility.

Alfentanil is often mixed in the propofol syringe for general anesthesia in a ratio of 1–1.5 mg of alfentanil to 500 mg propofol. The agents have similar pharmacokinetic characteristics, the combination is licensed and has been shown to be stable for up to 5 h [65].

Alfentanil has a longer CSHT than remifentanil. The half-time increases significantly from 10 to 45 min after a 2 h infusion, although this is still shorter than for morphine or fentanyl [66]. Propofol-alfentanil is a useful combination to use if spontaneous respiration needs to be maintained, although the propofol target may need to be set higher than if remifentanil is used. It may also lead to a more prolonged recovery and it is not recommend for procedures longer than 1 h in duration.

Alfentanil has been used for sedation on the PICU for a number of years. The shorter CSHT than morphine or fentanyl makes it more suitable for administration by continuous infusion in situations where rapid patient awakening is required, such as following head injury. Bolus doses of 0.07–0.15 mg/kg can be used, with or without a continuous infusion of 20–60 mcg/kg/min.

As with other opioids, alfentanil is probably most effective when used in combination with hypnotic agents, for stimulating procedures that have a significant pain component.

Remifentanil

Remifentanil has superseded alfentanil as the favored analgesic adjunct in TIVA. The high potency, fast onset and short (and context-insensitive) half-time of 2–3 min, mean that it can be safely and effectively used by infusion for prolonged periods of time. The synergism demonstrated between remifentanil and propofol also allows a significant reduction in the target concentration of propofol. Young children tend to be less sensitive to the effects of remifentanil, which means that larger doses can be administered to spontaneously breathing patients and that more is required to produce a given analgesic effect [67, 68].

As a rule of thumb, children less than 8 years or 25 kg in weight will require up to twice the dose of remifentanil to produce the same clinical effect as older children and adults. The reason for this is that clearance tends to be higher in the younger age group. Other PK parameters such as V_1 and the volume of distribution in steady state are very similar to adult values [69, 70]. The rapid offset of remifentanil means that adequate post procedure analgesia needs to be established prior to the infusion wearing off. With morphine, administration should be at least 40 min before the end of any painful procedure to allow time for it to bind to opioid receptors occupied by remifentanil [71].

Extreme care must be exercised if remifentanil is used for sedation in children, as it is less forgiving than other opioids and can cause profound respiratory depression and apnea. Ironically, infants outside the neonatal period and younger children are more resistant to this effect, due to their tolerance of higher doses, related to more rapid clearance of the drug [72].

Most studies that have looked at using remifentanil in combination with propofol for procedures are describing light general anesthesia, rather than deep sedation. There is also a high incidence of apnea associated with its use. For that reason, its use cannot be recommended outside the theater or intensive care environment, unless used by anesthesiologists [73].

Naloxone

Treatment of opioid overdose or antagonism of some side effects can be achieved by the administration of naloxone. The standard dose for reversal of respiratory depression is 10 mcg/kg, as a rapid bolus. Smaller bolus doses of 0.5 mcg/kg may be useful to treat other side effects such as itching, whilst being insufficient to significantly antagonize the analgesic effect. Very high doses (20–40 mcg/kg) have been used to rapidly reverse the chest rigidity associated with opioids [63].

Drug Combinations

Single-agent sedation has the advantage of predictable clinical effects, whilst side effects can be minimized. However, it may also limit the versatility of the technique, when differing properties are required. The ideal sedation agent should have the following properties:

- Fast acting
- Easy to titrate
- Predictable clinical effect
- Analgesic properties
- Amnesic properties
- Minimal effect on respiration
- Stable heart rate and blood pressure
- Wears off quickly
- No hangover effect
- No nausea and vomiting

No single intravenous sedative agent is able to provide these properties, but some drug combinations can come close. They have the advantage of being able to provide more of the positive effects of sedation, whilst minimizing some of the negative effects of the individual agents, as they are usually administered in lower doses. There is also the potential for synergism, whereby relatively smaller doses of each drug can be administered, but still produce the desired clinical effect.

When administering more than one drug, a number of factors need to be taken into consideration in order to determine the ideal combination. Table 26.10 indicates the different objectives of the drug combination and the types of drugs that might be used to achieve this.

Currently the most popular drug combinations are:

- Propofol and remifentanil
- Propofol and ketamine
- Propofol and midazolam

All have their pros and cons, and as with any drug administration, clinicians need to be aware of the appropriate doses and potential complications, which may vary significantly depending on the combination being used [74].

The main disadvantage of a propofol-remifentanil combination in the same syringe is that the drugs have different PK profiles. If a TCI system is being used, then only the propofol can be targeted directly, and a large bolus of remifentanil may be administered at the start, depending on the concentration in the mixture and the initial propofol target concentration set. Table 26.11 shows the varying amounts of remifentanil administered, with different mixtures and propofol target concentrations. Another consideration is the stability of the mixture. It has been shown that lower concentrations of remifentanil degrade over time, probably due to a pH effect on ester hydrolysis [75]. If the clinician is to use such a combination, then they have to be aware of these limitations.

Other combinations such as ketamine and midazolam, or propofol and dexmedetomidine, are used occasionally, but not commonly enough to warrant further discussion [76–79].

Conclusion

Sedation is increasingly being used in a number of situations in children, particularly where resources are limited or general anesthesia is not necessarily the best option. Irrespective of where the procedure is being undertaken, who is

Table 26.10 Sedative objectives and the ideal drug combination

Objective	Drug combination
Sedation + analgesia	Hypnotic + opioid or ketamine
Sedation + amnesia	Hypnotic + benzodiazepine
Sedation + immobilization	Hypnotic + alpha 2 receptor agonist

Table 26.11 The effect of differing remifentanil concentrations and propofol target concentrations on the dose and rate of remifentanil delivery

Propofol target concentration (µg/ml)	Remifentanil concentration in propofol (µg/ml)	Remifentanil bolus (µg/kg)	Time from start of sedation/anesthesia (min)					
			5	10	15	30	45	60
			Remifentanil infusion rate (µg/kg/min)					
1	5	0.22	0.04	0.04	0.03	0.03	0.02	0.02
	10	0.45	0.09	0.08	0.07	0.06	0.05	0.05
	20	0.9	0.17	0.15	0.14	0.11	0.1	0.09
2	5	0.47	0.09	0.08	0.07	0.06	0.05	0.05
	10	0.95	0.17	0.15	0.14	0.11	0.1	0.09
	20	1.9	0.35	0.31	0.28	0.22	0.2	0.18
3	5	0.72	0.13	0.12	0.1	0.08	0.07	0.07
	10	1.45	0.26	0.23	0.2	0.17	0.15	0.14
	20	2.9	0.52	0.46	0.41	0.33	0.3	0.28
4	5	0.95	0.17	0.15	0.14	0.11	0.1	0.09
	10	1.9	0.35	0.31	0.28	0.22	0.2	0.18
	20	3.8	0.7	0.62	0.55	0.45	0.4	0.37

These figures are derived from a TivaTrainer simulation in a 20-kg, 6-year-old boy, using the Paedfusor model undertaking it and the techniques that are being used, the priority must always be the safety of the child, and it is essential that systems are in place to provide the necessary education, training, equipment, and personnel for this to be the case. No child should ever be sedated for the sake of expediency and no child should ever be sedated without an adequate safety net being in place. The key to success is to ensure that in all cases, due consideration is given to the patient, the procedure, and the sedative agents required. Through national guidelines, ongoing pharmacological studies and reporting of adverse events, it should be possible to provide a sedation service for children that is both safe and effective, allowing a variety of procedures to be successfully undertaken with minimal risk to the child.

References

1. American Academy of Pediatrics, American Academy of Pediatric Dentistry, Cote CJ, Wilson S. Guidelines for monitoring and management of pediatric patients during and after sedation for diagnostic and therapeutic procedures: an update. Pediatrics. 2006;118:2587–602.
2. NHS National Institute for Health and Clinical Excellence. Sedation in children and young people. http://guidance.nice.org.uk/CG112
3. Beach ML, Cohen DM, Gallagher SM, Cravero JP. Major adverse events and relationship to nil per os status in pediatric sedation/anesthesia outside the operating room: a report of the pediatric sedation research consortium. Anesthesiology. 2016;124:80–8.
4. Ramsay MAE, Savege TM, Simpson BRJ, Goodwin R. Controlled sedation with alphaxalone-alphadolone. Br Med J. 1974;22:656–9.
5. Aldrete JA, Kroulik D. A postanesthetic recovery score. Anesth Analg. 1970;49:924–34.
6. Chernick DA, Gillings G, Laine H, et al. Validity and reliability of the Observer's: Assessment of Alertness/Sedation Scale: study with: intravenous midazolam. J Clin Psych. 1990;10:244–51.
7. Malviya S, Voepel-Lewis T, Tait AR, et al. Depth of sedation in children undergoing computed tomography: validity and reliability of the University of Michigan Sedation Scale (UMSS). Br J Anaesth. 2002;88:241–5.
8. Ambuel B, Hamlett K, Marx CM, et al. Assessing distress in pediatric intensive care environments: the COMFORT scale. J Pediatr Psych. 1992;17:95–109.
9. Ista E, van Dijk M, Tibboel D, et al. Assessment of sedation levels in pediatric intensive care patients can be improved by using the COMFORT "behavior" scale. Pediatr Crit Care Med. 2005;6:58–63.
10. Boerlage AA, Ista E, Duivenvoorden HJ, et al. The COMFORT behaviour scale detects clinically meaningful effects of analgesic and sedative treatment. Eur J Pain. 2015;19:473–9.
11. Merkel SI, Voepel-Lewis T, Shayevitz JR, et al. The FLACC: a behavioral scale for scoring postoperative pain in young children. Pediatr Nurs. 1997;23:293–7.
12. McGrath PJ, Johnson G, Goodman JT, et al. CHEOPS: a behavioral scale for rating postoperative pain in children. In: Fields HL, Dubner R, Cervero F, editors. Advances in pain research and therapy, vol. 9. New York: Raven Press; 1985. p. 395–402.
13. Tschiedel E, Müller O, Schara U, Felderhoff-Müser U, Dohna-Schwake C. Sedation monitoring during open muscle biopsy in children by Comfort Score and Bispectral Index – a prospective analysis. Paediatr Anaesth. 2015;25:265–71.
14. Dag C, Bezgin T, Özalp N, Gölcüklü Aydın G. Utility of bispectral index monitoring during deep sedation in pediatric dental patients. J Clin Pediatr Dent. 2014;39:68–73.
15. Powers KS, Nazarian EB, Tapyrik SA, Kohli SM, Yin H, van der Jagt EW, Sullivan JS, Rubenstein JS. Bispectral index as a guide for titration of propofol during procedural sedation among children. Pediatrics. 2005;115:1666–74.
16. Agrawal D, Feldman HA, Krauss B, Waltzman ML. Bispectral index monitoring quantifies depth of sedation during emergency department procedural sedation and analgesia in children. Ann Emerg Med. 2004;43:247–55.
17. McDermott NB, VanSickle T, Motas D, Friesen RH. Validation of the bispectral index monitor during conscious and deep sedation in children. Anesth Analg. 2003;97:39–43.
18. Crain N, Slonim A, Pollack M. Assessing sedation in the pediatric intensive care unit by using BIS and the COMFORT scale. Pediatr Crit Care Med. 2002;3:11–4.
19. Aneja R, Heard AMB, Fletcher JE, et al. Sedation monitoring of children by the Bispectral Index in the pediatric intensive care unit. Pediatr Crit Care Med. 2003;4:60–4.
20. Courtman SP, Wardurgh A, Petros AJ. Comparison of the bispectral index monitor with the Comfort score in assessing level of sedation of critically ill children. Intensive Care Med. 2003;29:2239–46.
21. Twite MD, Zuk J, Gralla J, Friesen RH. Correlation of the Bispectral Index Monitor with the COMFORT scale in the pediatric intensive care unit. Pediatr Crit Care Med. 2005;6:648–53.
22. Reeves ST, Havidich JE, Tobin DP. Conscious sedation of children with propofol is anything but conscious. Pediatrics. 2004;114:e74–6.
23. Gamble C, Gamble J, Seal R, Wright RB, Ali S. Bispectral analysis during procedural sedation in the pediatric emergency department. Pediatr Emerg Care. 2012;28:1003–8.
24. Weber F, Hollnberger H, Weber J. Electroencephalographic Narcotrend Index monitoring during procedural sedation and analgesia in children. Pediatr Anesth. 2008;18:823–30.
25. Disma N, Lauretta D, Palermo F, Sapienza D, Ingelmo PM, Astuto M. Level of sedation evaluation with Cerebral State Index and A-Line Arx in children undergoing diagnostic procedures. Paediatr Anaesth. 2007;17:445–51.
26. Malviya S, Voepel-Lewis T, Tait AR, et al. Effect of age and sedative agent on the accuracy of bispectral index in detecting depth of sedation in children. Pediatrics. 2007;120:e461–70.
27. Davidson AJ, McCann ME, Devavaram P, et al. The differences in the bispectral index between infants and children during emergence from anesthesia after circumcision surgery. Anesth Analg. 2001;93:326–30.
28. Marsh B, White M, Morton N, Kenny GN. Pharmacokinetic model driven infusion of propofol in children. Br J Anaesth. 1991;67:41–8.
29. Kataria BK, Ved SA, Nicodemus HF, Hoy GR, Lea D, Dubois MY, et al. The pharmacokinetics of propofol in children using three different data analysis approaches. Anesthesiology. 1994;80:104–22.
30. Absalom A, Kenny G. 'Paedfusor' pharmacokinetic data set. Br J Anaesth. 2005;95:110.
31. Absalom A, Amutike D, Lal A, White M, Kenny GN. Accuracy of the 'Paedfusor' in children undergoing cardiac surgery or catheterization. Br J Anaesth. 2003;91:507–13.
32. Engelhardt T, McCheyne AJ, Morton N, Karsli C, Luginbuehl I, Adeli K, Walsh W, Bissonnette B. Clinical adaptation of a pharmacokinetic model of Propofol plasma concentrations in children. Paediatr Anaesth. 2008;18:235–9.
33. Hughes MA, Glass PS, Jacobs JR. Context-sensitive half-time in multicompartment pharmacokinetic models for intravenous anesthetic drugs. Anesthesiology. 1992;76:334–41.

34. Steur RJ, Perez RSGM, De Lange JJ. Dosage scheme for propofol in children under 3 years of age. Pediatric Anesthesia. 2004;14:462–7.

35. Munoz HR, Cortinez LI, Ibacache ME, Altermatt FR. Estimation of the plasma effect site equilibration rate constant (ke0) of propofol in children using the time to peak effect. Anesthesiology. 2004;101:1269–74.

36. Jeleazcov C, Ihmsen H, Schmidt J, et al. Pharmacodynamic modelling of the bispectral index response to propofol-based anaesthesia during general surgery in children. Br J Anaest. 2008;100:509–16.

37. Cravero JP, Beach ML, Blike GT, et al. The incidence and nature of adverse events during pediatric sedation/anesthesia with propofol for procedures outside the operating room: a report from the Pediatric Sedation Research Consortium. Anesth Analg. 2009;108:795–804.

38. Bell RF, Dahl JB, Moore RA, Kalso E. Perioperative ketamine for acute postoperative pain. Cochrane Database Syst Rev. 2006;25, CD004603.

39. Bar-Joseph G, Guilburd Y, Tamir A, et al. Effectiveness of ketamine in decreasing intracranial pressure in children with intracranial hypertension; clinical article. J Neurosurg. 2009;4:40–6.

40. Chang LC, Raty SR, Ortiz J, Bailard NS, Mathew SJ. The emerging use of ketamine for anesthesia and sedation in traumatic brain injuries. CNS Neursci Ther. 2013;19:390–5.

41. Nagdeve NG, Yaddanapudi S, Pandav SS. The effect of different doses of ketamine on intraocular pressure in anesthetized children. J Pediatr Ophthal. 2006;43:219–23.

42. Cole JW, Murray DJ, McAllister JD, et al. Emergence behaviour in children: defining the incidence of excitement and agitation following anaesthesia. Paediatr Anaesth. 2002;12:442–7.

43. Wathen JE, Roback MG, Mackenzie T, et al. Does midazolam alter the clinical effects of intravenous ketamine sedation in children? A double-blind, randomized, controlled, emergency department trial. Ann Emerg Med. 2000;36:579–88.

44. Willman EV, Andolfatto G. A prospective evaluation of "ketofol" (ketamine/propofol combination) for procedural sedation and analgesia in the emergency department. Ann Emerg Med. 2007;49:31–6.

45. Coulter FL, Hannam JA, Anderson BJ. Ketofol simulations for dosing in pediatric anesthesia. Pediatr Anesth. 2014;24:806–12.

46. Coulter FL, Hannam JA, Anderson BJ. Ketofol dosing simulations for procedural sedation. Pediatr Emerg Care. 2014;30:621–30.

47. Ong LB, Plummer JL, Waldow WC, Owen H. Timing of midazolam and propofol administration for co-induction of anaesthesia. Anaesth Int Care. 2000;28:527–31.

48. Tobias JD, Rasmussen GE. Pain management and sedation in the pediatric intensive care unit. Pediatr Clin North Am. 1994;41:1261–92.

49. Turcant A, Delhumeau A, Premel-Cabic A, Granry JC, Cottineau C, Six P, Allain P. Thiopental pharmacokinetics under conditions of long-term infusion. Anesthesiology. 1985;63:50–4.

50. Hammer GB, Drover DR, Cao H, et al. The effects of dexmedetomidine on cardiac electrophysiology in children. Anesth Analg. 2008;106:79–83.

51. Mason KP, Lerman J. Dexmedetomidine in children: current knowledge and future applications. Anesth Analg. 2011;113:1129–42.

52. Mahmoud M, Mason KP. Dexmedetomidine: review, update, and future considerations of paediatric perioperative and periprocedural applications and limitations. Br J Anaesth. 2015;115:171–82.

53. Mason KP. Sedation trends in the 21st century: the transition to dexmedetomidine for radiological imaging studies. Paediatr Anaesth. 2010;20:265–72.

54. Koroglu A, Demirbilek S, Teksan H. Sedative, haemodynamic and respiratory effects of dexmedetomidine in children undergoing magnetic resonance imaging examination: preliminary results. Br J Anaesth. 2005;94:821–4.

55. Koroglu A, Teksan H, Sagr O. A comparison of the sedative, hemodynamic, and respiratory effects of dexmedetomidine and propofol in children undergoing magnetic resonance imaging. Anesth Analg. 2006;103:63–7.

56. Ulgey A, Aksu R, Bicer C, et al. Is the addition of dexmedetomidine to a ketamine-propofol combination in pediatric cardiac catheterization sedation useful? Pediatr Cardiol. 2012;33:770–4.

57. Basker S, Singh G, Jacob R. Clonidine in paediatrics – a review. Ind J Anaesth. 2009;53:270–80.

58. Al P, Larsson P, Eksborg S, et al. Clonidine disposition in children; a population analysis. Pediatr Anesth. 2007;17:924–33.

59. Fehr SB, Zalunardo MP, Seifert B et al. Clonidine decreases propofol requirements during anesthesia: effect on bispectral index. Br J Anaesth. 2001;86:627–32.

60. Vuyk J. Pharmacokinetic and pharmacodynamic interactions between opioids and propofol. J Clin Anesth. 1997;9:23S–6.

61. Niesters M, Overdyk F, Smith T. Opioid-induced respiratory depression in paediatrics: a review of case reports. Br J Anaesth. 2013;110:175–82.

62. Dewhirst E, Naguib A, Tobias JD. Chest wall rigidity in two infants after low-dose fentanyl administration. Pediatr Emerg Care. 2012;28:465–8.

63. Fahnenstich H, Steffan J, Kau N, et al. Fentanyl-induced chest wall rigidity and laryngospasm in preterm and term infants. Crit Care Med. 2000;28:836–9.

64. Eventov-Friedman S, Rozin I, Shinwell ES. Case of chest-wall rigidity in a preterm infant caused by prenatal fentanyl administration. J Perinatol. 2010;30:149–50.

65. Sim KM, Boey SK, Heng PW, et al. Total intravenous anaesthesia using 3-in-1 mixture of propofol, alfentanil and mivacurium. Ann Acad Med Singapore. 2000;29:182–8.

66. Ayres R. Update on TIVA. Pediatr Anest. 2004;14:374–9.

67. Barker N, Lim J, Amari E, Malherbe S, Ansermino JM. Relationship between age and spontaneous ventilation during intravenous anaesthesia in children. Pediatr Anesth. 2007;17:948–55.

68. Munoz HR, Cortinez LI, Ibacache ME, Altermatt FR. Remifentanil requirements during propofol administration to block the somatic response to skin incision in children and adults. Anesth Analg. 2007;104:77–80.

69. Rigby-Jones AE, Priston MJ, Sneyd JR, McCabe AP, Davis GI, Tooley MA, Thorne GC, Wolf AR. Remifentanil-midazolam sedation for paediatric patients receiving mechanical ventilation after cardiac surgery. Br J Anaest. 2007;99:252–61.

70. Minto CF, Schnider TW, Egan TD, Youngs E, Lemmens HJ, Gambus PL, Billard V, Hoke JF, Moore KH, Hermann DJ, Muir KT, Mandema JW, Shafer SL. Influence of age and gender on the pharmacokinetics and pharmacodynamics of remifentanil. I. Model development. Anesthesiology. 1997;86:10–23.

71. Munoz HR, Guerrero ME, Brandes V, Cortinez LI. The effect of morphine timing during remifentanil-anaesthesia on early recovery from anaesthesia and postoperative pain. Br J Anaesth. 2002;88:814–8.

72. Ansermino JM, Magruder W, Dosani M. Spontaneous respiration during intravenous anesthesia in children. Curr Opin Anaesthesiol. 2009;22:383–7.

73. Hirsh I, Lerner A, Shnaider I, Reuveni A, Pacht A, Segol O, Pizov R. Remifentanil versus fentanyl for esophagogastroduodenoscopy in children. J Pediatr Gastroenterol Nutr. 2010;51:618–21.

74. Seol TK, Lim JK, Yoo EK, et al. Propofol–ketamine or propofol–remifentanil for deep sedation and analgesia in pediatric patients

undergoing burn dressing changes: a randomized clinical trial. Paediatr Anaesth. 2015;25:560–6.

75. Stewart JT, Warren FW, Maddox FC, Viswanathan K, Fox JL. The stability of remifentanil hydrochloride and propofol mixtures in polypropylene syringes and polyvinylchloride bags at 22°–24°C. Anesth Analg 2000;90:1450–1

76. Parker RI, Mahan RA, Giugliano D, et al. Efficacy and safety of intravenous midazolam and ketamine as sedation for therapeutic and diagnostic procedures in children. Pediatrics. 1997;99:427–31.

77. Karapinar B, Yilmaz D, Demirag K, et al. Sedation with intravenous ketamine and midazolam for painful procedures in children. Pediatr Int. 2006;48:146–51.

78. Meyer S, Aliani S, Graf N, et al. Sedation with midazolam and ketamine for invasive procedures in children with malignancies and hematological disorders: a prospective study with reference to the sympathomimetic properties of ketamine. Pediatr Hematol Oncol. 2003;20:291–301.

79. Seigler RS, Avant MG, Gwyn DR, et al. A comparison of propofol and ketamine/midazolam for intravenous sedation of children. Pediatr Crit Care Med. 2001;2:20–3.

Sedation of the Critically Ill Child

Arno Brouwers*, Sanne Vaassen*, Gijs D. Vos, Jan N.M. Schieveld, and Piet L. Leroy

Introduction

Providing effective sedation and analgesia in infants and children admitted on a Pediatric Intensive Care Unit (PICU) is a cornerstone of daily patient care and probably one of the most challenging tasks that PICU professionals may face. The wide range in age, weight and body composition, underlying medical and neurological diseases, the usually high sensory stimulatory environment, the repetitive physical stimuli related to medical therapy (e.g., physical examination, invasive procedures, and interventions) and—most importantly—the scarcity of high quality evidence applicable for daily practice may all contribute to this difficulty.

An adequate sedation and analgesia policy should not only aim to achieve optimal patient-ventilator compliance but also need to include the prevention and treatment of pain, anxiety, delirium, sleep disorders, or other forms of discomfort. Undersedation is likely to result in patient anxiety, discomfort as well as patient-ventilator asynchrony and potentially dangerous adverse events such as unplanned extubation, displacement of catheters, or injury. Oversedation, on the other hand, may have substantial cardiorespiratory effects and may increase

both duration of mechanical ventilation and ICU length of stay [1]. In addition it may be associated with a higher risk of drug withdrawal, particularly in children treated with prolonged and/or high dosages of analgo-sedatives [2]. It has been suggested that sedation in pediatric intensive care patients is often suboptimal, in which oversedation occurs more common than undersedation [3]. Assessing the individual need for analgesia and sedation and careful tailoring analgo-sedative drugs are therefore of the utmost importance.

In this chapter we will present an overview of the most important drugs currently used for analgesia, sedation, or agitation in children (1 month–18 years old) admitted to the PICU. However, since a comprehensive comfort-directed policy goes far beyond pharmacological interventions only, we will discuss non-pharmacological strategies first. Indeed, in this chapter we strongly plead for a holistic comfort-directed policy, including both pharmacological interventions as well as non-pharmacological strategies such as sleep promotion, family-centered care, and environmental control. Next, several instruments, available for assessing comfort and/or pain, will be presented such as the COMFORT scale, COMFORT behavior scale, State Behavioral Scale, University of Michigan Sedation Scale (UMSS), and Ramsay score [4–6]. In three separate sections we specifically focus on particularly challenging clinical problems related to ICU sedation, i.e. the management of, respectively, refractory agitation, drug withdrawal, and delirium. This is followed by general considerations on possible strategies for daily analgo-sedative management of critically ill children admitted to the PICU including a proposed treatment algorithm. We conclude this chapter with procedural sedation and palliative or terminal sedation on the PICU.

A major limitation of this chapter is the absence of high quality randomized controlled trials and standardized, up to date and evidence-based guidelines on this topic [7]. In this

*both first authors have contributed equally to this chapter

A. Brouwers*, MD • S. Vaassen*, MD • G.D. Vos, MD, PhD •
P.L. Leroy, MD, MSc, PhD (✉)
Pediatric Intensive Care Unit, Department of Pediatrics, Maastricht University Medical Centre, Maastricht, The Netherlands
e-mail: p.leroy@mumc.nl

J.N.M. Schieveld, MD, PhD
Division Child- and Adolescent Psychiatry, Department Psychiatry and Neuro-Psychology, Maastricht University Medical Centre, Maastricht, The Netherlands

The Mutsaersstichting, Venlo, The Netherlands

The Koraalgroep, Sittard, The Netherlands

© Springer International Publishing AG 2017
A.R. Absalom, K.P. Mason (eds.), *Total Intravenous Anesthesia and Target Controlled Infusions*,
DOI 10.1007/978-3-319-47609-4_27

narrative review we therefore aim to present the current state of the art regarding analgesia and sedation on a pediatric intensive care unit. A critical, semi-systematic study of the recent literature up to March 2016 was performed. Literature on neonates was largely excluded. In addition, recent insights and guidelines from adult intensive care literature were used wherever needed to answer clinical dilemmas for which insufficient pediatric evidence was found. All findings were discussed in inter-professional meetings and agreement on best practices was sought. Unreferenced statements should be considered as the personal professional opinion of the authors.

Non-pharmacological Comfort-Directed Strategies on a PICU

Critical illness and critical care are associated with pain, anxiety, and a multitude of distresses. Furthermore, prolonged immobility and optimal compliance with therapy (e.g., ventilation) are often crucial for both healing and patient safety (e.g., prevention of unplanned extubation; accidental removal of indwelling catheters or accidental falls). Consequently, controlling pain, anxiety and cooperation among critically ill children is a key priority in daily PICU care. This goal is usually achieved by the administration of sedative and analgesic drugs. Although sedation regimens have been used extensively across intensive care units, the data are lacking as to the best drugs, dosing, regimens, and short- and long-term safety profiles for use in the pediatric population [7, 8]. Substantially less evidence is available on the effect of non-pharmacological strategies (NPS) for comfort management on a pediatric ICU. Nevertheless, human, psychological as well as scientific considerations warrant the use of NPS as a cornerstone of a comprehensive comfort-directed policy. Within this perspective Maslow's construct [9] on fundamental human needs is relevant to consider. Maslow proposes 5 levels of needs that must be satisfied to promote healthy well-being (Fig. 27.1). In order to achieve optimal procedural care we should not only focus on assuring physical and physiological integrity (i.e., maintaining patient safety) but pay equal attention to the 4 higher order needs as well: Patients (and their parents) should feel safe (i.e., being free from fear; level 2), feel surrounded by and belonging to loving, caring people, including empathic professionals (level 3), feel respectfully treated as individuals and feel self-confident that they can achieve the goal (level 4) and finally, feel that they can control and decide autonomously (level 5). Real (i.e., non-pretending!) child- or family-centered (procedural) care could be defined as care that includes all levels of needs. Using the prism of Maslow's hierarchy for reconsidering traditional medical care processes is

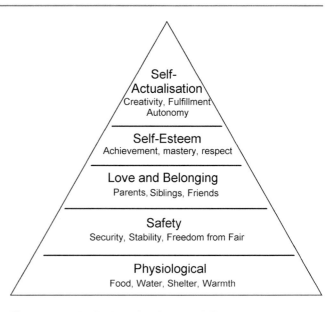

Fig. 27.1 Maslow's hierarchy of needs (1943)

increasingly considered as a new standard of care, particularly for ICU patients [10, 11].

Furthermore, both the growing concern on potential long-term neurological adverse effects of prolonged sedation as well as the modern trend to minimize (or interrupt regularly) sedation, to avoid longstanding immobilization and to use new sedatives with a clearly lighter sedation profile (e.g., dexmedetomidine) result in a growing interest in NPS. Finally, some preliminary evidence suggests that the reduction of environmental stimuli and stress by use of NPS may improve healing and decrease the need for sedation [12, 13].

A recent qualitative survey among family members and nurses on an adult ICU showed that the top four non-pharmacological interventions found to be useful, relevant, and feasible were music therapy and distraction (cognitive-behavioral category), simple massage (physical category), and family presence facilitation (emotional support category) [14]. The potential advantages of healing environmental interventions have been described in an adult ICU [15]. Currently, no similar research on PICUs is available. Despite this limited evidence we believe that at least four relevant strategies can be identified as essential for a policy directed towards optimal comfort experience. Definitely more research is needed to explore the effects of these strategies on patient comfort.

Careful Identification and Treatment of Underlying Causes of Anxiety, Agitation, and Insomnia

Distress in pediatric patients is rarely a spontaneous behavior but rather the result of an underlying problem. At first, potentially (life) threatening causes need to be excluded, such as hypoxemia, imminent respiratory or circulatory failure, and hypoglycemia. Also delirium and (sub-optimally managed) pain need to be excluded systematically. "Fighting-the-ventilator" can often be reduced by carefully tailoring a support ventilatory mode (including optimal trigger-function, inspiratory times, and airway pressures) according to the individual child's respiratory needs. Finally hunger, cold, bladder retention, constipation, malpositioning (e.g., infants may prefer a prone position), fear for medical procedures and lack of age-appropriate comfort may all contribute to distress.

Child Centered Care

Verbal and non-verbal communication should be adapted to the child's (developmental) age. Whereas young infants may benefit from gentle and tactile interaction while reducing exposure to ambient stimuli (e.g., by swaddling) within a warm "shelter," older children may prefer more control and sufficient sight on toys, television, or tablets. Guided imagery, storytelling, age-adapted music, presence of parents and siblings at any time and even animal-assisted therapy are all reasonable interventions to optimize feelings of comfort and normalize the ICU experience [16].

Family-Centered Care

Family-centered care (FCC) is increasingly considered to be a key component of high quality health care for children and their parents/caretakers. FCC can be characterized by health care practices that are respectful of and responsive to individual patient and family preferences, needs, and values. In FCC a major role of health care providers is to enable and empower patients and their family members to play an active role in healthcare decision-making and treatment. When done well and consistently, FCC can lead to safer, more personalized and effective care, improved health care experiences and patient outcomes, and more responsive organizations [17]. Although no research has been published on the effects of FCC on children's experiences during their stay on a PICU, it is very likely that an FCC approach will result in patient comfort management that better meets with individual needs. Furthermore, involving parents and siblings in daily care may result in more confidence and collaboration.

Environmental Control

Traditionally, ICUs are process-focused departments designed and constructed to proceed efficiently within a setting of high workload and complex technical support.

Lightning conditions are usually bright and uninterrupted in order to optimize patient observation and interventions. Furthermore, sensitive alarm settings of all kind of technical devices result in many auditory stimuli, not to mention the inter-professional communication as a substantial source of noise. Excellent evidence exists on the negative effects of this type of busy environment on feelings of comfort, incidence of delirium and agitation, and need for sedation [15, 18].

In a well-intended attempt to camouflage the medical atmosphere, child friendly gadgets, bright colors, cartoons, comic characters or art may be added to the interior design of patient rooms. Although no systematic research whatsoever exists within this specific field, there are several reasons to question the effectiveness of this common practice. The most important criticism to this design lies in its usually static character that limits individualized modifications according to the (developmental) age and individual characteristics or needs of a child. Comic characters that are popular in one age group or gender may be meaningless or even frightening or childish in another. It has been shown that children's emotional associations with colors are determined by age and gender [19]. Furthermore, a recent study on the stress-reducing effects of art in pediatric health care indicated that children may be less in tune with art and possibly more affected by social support, e.g. parental care [20]. In a recent qualitative study, parents of children with autism spectrum disorder indicated that "autism-friendly" modifications to the built environment (being: quiet and/or sensory rooms, warm colors, no fluorescent lights) would result in less stressful visits [21].

In the last decade there is a growing interest in the effects of the physical, built environment on patient safety, caring processes and staff efficiency but also on the general well-being and healing in patients [22, 23]. This has resulted in fascinating new design objectives for patient facilities [24], including the creation of highly innovative healing environments for children's hospitals and pediatric units [25, 26]. Design considerations for children's health and emergency services have been published and include family-centered approach, separation from adult patients, privacy and acoustic control, a child and family friendly environment and provision of play and entertainment [27]. A quieter environment, one that includes familiar persons, dotted with windows and natural light, creates a space that makes people feel balanced and reassured.

Clinical Pharmacology of Intravenous Analgesics and Sedatives

In this section the most important drugs currently used for analgesia and sedation in children (1 month–18 years old) admitted to the PICU will be discussed. Despite their

Table 27.1 Loading and maintenance dosages for the most import iv drugs currently used for analgesia and sedation in critically ill children

	Loading dose	Maintenance dose	T½	Dependency and withdrawal	
Morphine	50–100 µg/kg	5–40 (−100) µg/kg/h	2–3 h	++	++
Fentanyl	0.5–2 µg/kg	0.5–5 µg/kg/h	3–4 h	++	++
Remifentanil	0.5–1 µg/kg	0.1–2 µg/kg/min	3–10 min	++	++
Midazolam	50–100 µg/kg	50–400 (−1000) µg/kg/h	3–11 h	++	++
Lorazepam	20–40 µg/kg	20–100 µg/kg/h	8–15 h	++	++
Dexmedetomidine	0.05–1 µg/kg (10–20 min)	0.05–0.7 (−2) µg/kg/h	2–2 ½ h	+/−	+
Clonidine	1–3 µg/kg	0.25–3 µg/kg/h	5–25 h	+/−	+/−
Propofol	1–3 mg/kg	1–4 mg/kg/h (max 48 h)	30–60 min	−	−
Ketamine	1–2 mg/kg	5–60 µg/kg/min	2–4 h	−	−

widespread use evidence-based dosages of most drugs are scarce. Furthermore these dosages are usually not supported by pharmacokinetic or pharmacodynamics models. Applying such models could enhance tailoring of dosages to the individual patient and prevent for instance both under- and over-dosing [28]. Table 27.1 summarizes the most commonly used analgo-sedative drugs with their doses used in a PICU.

Opioids

Pain is one of the key factors of discomfort and agitation in critically ill children. Opioids are therefore one of the most prescribed drugs in the pediatric ICU. There are several opioids currently in use. All opioids have mainly analgesic effects, relieving visceral, somatic, and neuropathic pain. In higher dosages they also offer sedation and anxiolysis. The analgesic effect is mainly the result of binding to µ-receptors and k-receptors, and (for some synthetic opioids) to δ-receptors. It is thought that the main side effects are caused through binding to other receptors [29].

Several natural and synthetic opioids are available for clinical use in pediatric patients. Morphine is the only natural opioid currently used and fentanyl and remifentanil are the most used synthetic opioids in this population. Sufentanil is mainly used outside the ICU in operating rooms. Other opioids such as codeine, oxycodone, methadone, and meperidine are usually used for analgesia outside the ICU and therefore not included in this overview. Morphine and fentanyl are currently the most used opioid analgesics in critically ill children [30, 31]. Morphine may offer advantages over fentanyl because it induces less tolerance in general and causes less withdrawal symptoms in neonates [32, 33]. As far as we know no studies are available comparing morphine with fentanyl for analgesia in critically ill children.

The main advantage of opioids is the strong analgesic effects and the relatively large therapeutic window. Given their relatively limited sedative effects, opioids are rarely indicated when pain can reasonably be excluded.

Opioids can be administered either by intermittent boluses or by continuous infusion. In children with severe vaso-occlusive disease, continuous infusion of morphine provided better analgesia than intermittent opioid therapy [34]. A randomized double-blind clinical trial comparing the efficacy of 10 mcg/kg/h morphine (continuous intravenous infusion) with that of 30 mcg/kg morphine every 3 h (bolus intravenous injection) in 181 young children aged 0–3 years, admitted on a PICU following major abdominal or thoracic surgery showed no differences in reducing postoperative pain. However, in children >1 year old continuous infusion turned out to be favorable [35]. Adding paracetamol and/or nonsteroidal anti-inflammatory drugs (NSAIDs) to the pain treatment reduces opioid requirements and may also reduce adverse effects [36]. Therefore the use of opioids should always be accompanied by either paracetamol or an NSAID.

Side Effects

The most important side effect of all opioids is respiratory depression, caused by direct inhibitory effects on the brainstem respiratory centers. This effect is dose-dependent and may occur before consciousness is impaired. The decrease in minute volume is primarily due to a decreased respiratory rate, while tidal volume remains usually intact. Opioids also cause a diminished sense and reaction to CO_2 levels. As a consequence, fatal accidents related to morphine toxicity use are nearly always due to respiratory arrest. Newborn infants, patients with pre-existing respiratory problems (e.g., chronic respiratory failure) and recurrent hypoxic events (e.g., obstructive sleep apnea syndrome) have a higher risk of opioid associated respiratory depression[37]. In critically ill children on mechanical ventilation, however, the respiratory depressive effects may in fact be advantageous, as they may enhance patient-ventilator synchrony. Morphine can also cause hypotension, which is especially important in hemodynamically instable or cardiac patients.

Opioids are also particularly known for their gastro-intestinal side effects such as the prolongation of gastric emptying time and the reduction of pro-pulsatile activity in the small and large intestines. These mechanisms explain the most important gastro-intestinal adverse effects. Nausea and vomiting may be associated with the use of any opioid, although it is mostly seen in ambulatory patients while it seems to be only a minor problem in ventilated (not-moving) patients. A far more important problem for the PICU patient is constipation, which occurs in 40–95 % of patients treated with opioids. The best way to treat this is by starting laxatives early in the course of opioid administration. Enemas may be an effective alternative.

Pruritus is another common problem with opioids, especially with morphine, causing potential additional discomfort. Since this effect is at least partially caused by histamine release anti-histamines may be a reasonable choice [29]. Also opioid-induced disinhibition of itch-specific neurons in the spinal dorsal horn may play a role [38]. Lowering the dose is usually an effective strategy. Sometimes the pruritus leads to agitation in such extent that switching to a synthetic opioid seems to be the best choice [39].

Another common problem with especially continuous administration of opioids is the occurrence of a retention bladder caused by an inhibitory effect on voiding reflexes and increasing the external sphincter tone with resultant increase in bladder volume [29]. Especially in young children this can be a problem because they cannot properly convey where they feel pain, which can cause a delay in treating a retention bladder. When thought of, it is easily resolved by inserting a urinary catheter.

Tolerance and withdrawal are also very common with opioids. Dependency can even occur after only a few days of opioid use [29, 39]. A large prospective study has shown that prolonged opioid exposure leads to a significant increase in dose. An opioid exposure of 7 or 14 days, for instance, requires doubling of the daily opioid dose in 16 and 20 % of patients, respectively. This doubling occurred in 43 % of those receiving opioids for 14 days or more. Doubling of the opioid dose was furthermore more likely to occur in the case of co-therapy with benzodiazepines and less likely to occur if morphine was used as the primary opioid [32]. Besides a lower tendency to deliver tolerance morphine also has a significantly lower prevalence of developing withdrawal symptoms in neonates compared to fentanyl [33].

Withdrawal symptoms after cessation can consist of a hyper alert state, hyperalgesia, hyperthermia, and diarrhea [29]. Withdrawal symptoms can be prevented by gradually tapering the intravenous dose or by switching to a long-acting oral opioid (e.g., methadone) [39]. This will be further discussed in the section withdrawal in this chapter.

Finally, neuro-apoptosis has come under growing attention as a possible relevant adverse effect of opioids. Recent animal studies have shown that, especially in the developing brain, neuro-apoptosis occurs with long-term opioid infusion [40–42]. Evidence from research in humans remains limited, however. A follow-up study of critically ill neonates treated with continuously administered morphine infusion of 10 µg/kg/h demonstrated, however, that it didn't harm general functioning and may even have a positive influence on executive functions at the age of 8–9 years [43]. In children with meningococcal septic shock the use of opioids during admission was associated with long-term adverse neuropsychological outcome independent of severity of illness scores. These results are limited, however, by the fact that it concerns a retrospective cohort study [44].

Morphine

Morphine is a water-soluble molecule whose low-lipid-solubility accounts for its slow penetrance into the brain causing its delayed onset of clinical effect [29]. Peak effect occurs 20 min after administration. The duration of action is about 2 h following a single iv loading dose of 100 µg/kg. Maintenance dosages up to 60 µg/kg/h are safe to use but usually a dose within the range of 10–30 µg/kg/h is sufficient in most postoperative patients with pain [45].

Morphine undergoes extensive hepatic and extra-hepatic glucuronidation. Metabolites are excreted primarily in the urine. Only one of the metabolites of morphine is active, namely morphine-6-glucuronide. Accumulation of this active metabolite in renal disease may cause prolonged opioid effects. Neonates have a slower metabolization and excretion and it is thought that they form more morphine-3-glucuronide. This metabolite is thought to cause anti-analgesic effects. Towards the age of one month metabolization is similar compared to adults [45]. It is well known that glomerular filtration rate and tubular secretion are reduced in neonates and therefore dose reduction might be necessary to prevent excessive accumulation. This of course is also true for patients with renal impairment in general.

Fentanyl

Fentanyl is one of the most currently used synthetic opioids. It is the second most used analgesic after morphine and is about 100 times more potent compared to morphine. It has a relatively short half-life of about 3–4 h. Especially in neonates it is the drug of first choice when IV analgesia is needed. This is mainly due to the difference in metabolization compared to morphine. Fentanyl undergoes hepatic metabolization and is then renally excreted, and it has no known active metabolites. A disadvantage of fentanyl is the fact that it is stored in peripheral tissue, which can lead to accumulation with repeated doses and continuous infusion. This can lead to a prolonged half-life up to 21 h.

Because of the relatively short half-life time a bolus is not necessary in every increase in maintenance dose. But boluses are often used before handling the patient or before painful interventions. Bolus dosages of 1–2 µg/kg/h are usually sufficient. Fentanyl is usually dosed at 0.5–5 µg/kg/h, but dosages up to 10 µg/kg/h are proven to be safe [45]. One of the main complications, both in non-ventilated and in ventilated patients is chest wall rigidity, especially after fast infusion of a bolus and in younger children especially neonates [39]. Therefore it is recommended to give boluses by slow infusion up to 10 min. Fentanyl associated acute chest wall rigidity can be successfully treated with instant antagonizing drugs (naloxone (10–40 µg/kg IV) or with direct administration of a neuromuscular blocking agent.

Remifentanil

Remifentanil is a synthetic opioid that is relatively new, but upcoming in pediatric ICUs. It is a strong opioid agonist, and it is comparable to fentanyl in potency but ultra-short acting with an onset time of 1–3 min. It has a half-life time of 3–10 min, which makes it ideal for weaning a patient from mechanical ventilation. Remifentanil is usually dosed at 0.1–2 µg/kg/min. Most experience is with short-term, procedure-related analgesia, which is usually achieved by repeated administration of small bolus dosages (up to 1 µg/kg) up to a desired analgesic effect is reached [46]. There is very limited evidence on the use of remifentanil as a continuous IV infusion for analgesia in critically ill children [47].

Remifentanil is metabolized by plasma esterases into minimally active metabolites resulting in a very short duration of action (even after repeated or prolonged administration) and an elimination that is independent of hepatic metabolism or renal excretion.

Conclusions

Opioids are drugs with strong analgesic effects making them very useful for analgesia in critically ill children but should be accompanied by either paracetamol or an NSAID to reduce the dose of the opioid. The side effects are mostly preventable or easily treatable. Therefore it is a good choice as the primary drug in critically ill children to provide analgesia when (severe) pain is involved. Morphine should be used with some care in neonates because of different metabolization and fentanyl seems to be the better choice in these patients. With all opioids there is a high risk of dependency and withdrawal after cessation, and therefore slow tapering or converting to oral administration of methadone is necessary. There is some evidence that opioids cause neuro-apoptosis in long-term sedation, especially in the developing brain. At this moment evidence is still conflicting and therefore there is no reason to change current practice.

Benzodiazepines

Benzodiazepines are the most used sedatives in critically ill children. Midazolam and secondly lorazepam are the preferred benzodiazepines for sedation in mechanically ventilated children accounting for, respectively, 82–97 % and 1–16 % of used benzodiazepines. Diazepam is very rarely used for sedation in this patient category [48]. No studies in the pediatric population directly compared lorazepam and midazolam for sedation in the intensive care unit.

Benzodiazepines mainly bind with χ-aminobutyric acid A receptor (GABA-A receptors). GABA is the most important inhibitory neurotransmitter in the CNS. Binding to the GABA-receptors causes a hyperpolarization of neurons, leading to a decreased sensitivity to excitatory neurotransmitters and, consequently, to CNS depression. The clinical effects of benzodiazepines on the central nervous system are dose-dependent, resulting in a progressive increase of sedative effects: anxiolysis, moderate sedation, deep sedation, full loss of consciousness (coma), and eventually death [29, 49]. Next to sedative effects, benzodiazepines have also amnesic and anti-epileptic properties.

One of the advantages of benzodiazepines compared to many other sedatives such as propofol or dexmedetomidine is that it provides a pronounced stability because of long plasma half-life time. In long-term sedation it can provide stability making the child less at risk for accidental extubation and catheter removal [50, 51]. On the other hand, the long plasma half-life time may impede short-term awakening that may be desirable in particular patient categories (e.g., patients with traumatic brain injury and need for repeated neurological assessment; postoperative patients with expected early extubation) [52].

Midazolam is metabolized by cytochrome P450 (CYP) enzymes and by glucuronide conjugation whereas lorazepam directly undergoes glucuronide conjugation. Midazolam and lorazepam thus have different routes of metabolization [53]. This difference may be relevant when CYP450 activity could be altered due to pharmaco-genetic variability, disease conditions or interactive co-medication. Since the metabolites of midazolam are also active sedative agents, impaired excretion may lead to oversedation, especially in long-term sedation and renal failure [54]. Other drugs which can inhibit CYP enzymes (e.g., macrolide antibiotics, certain antiviral drugs, antifungal drugs (itraconazole, ketoconazole) and grapefruit juice) can cause significant interactions leading to stronger effects of midazolam due to its reduced clearance. It has also been shown that increased disease severity reduces midazolam clearance in critically ill children by inflammation mediated CYP3A downregulation and by organ failure in itself [55].

Side Effects

The most important side effects of benzodiazepines in children are respiratory depression and apnea, which will be aggravated when combined with opioid analgesics. Furthermore benzodiazepines may cause vasodilatation leading to hypotension, especially in neonates and after fast infusion of midazolam [29, 31]. These effects may be more pronounced in hemodynamically instable patients or hypovolemic patients. Both midazolam and lorazepam are also associated with mild gastro-intestinal side effects such as nausea and vomiting [29]. Some children are known to react paradoxically to midazolam with agitation and restlessness needing conversion to other sedatives [56, 57].

Although benzodiazepines are efficient in providing sedation, anxiolysis and amnesia they carry several important disadvantages. In adults the use of benzodiazepines has been associated with an increased risk of development of delirium [58, 59]. Benzodiazepines also impose a high risk for the development of withdrawal symptoms especially after prolonged administration and/or use of high dosages [60, 61]. Some researchers claim that withdrawal symptoms can occur even after only 3 days of use [61]. Abrupt cessation is therefore not recommended. In case of necessity of abrupt cessation it is possible to switch to oral lorazepam, to prevent withdrawal from both lorazepam and midazolam [62]. Withdrawal will be further discussed in another section of this chapter.

In adults it has been shown that the use of benzodiazepines for ICU sedation is associated with a prolonged length of hospital stay and longer duration of mechanical ventilation compared to non-benzodiazepine sedation regimens [63].

Finally, benzodiazepines have been associated with neuro-apoptosis in the developing brain, especially when they are used for an extended period of time [41, 42, 64]. The clinical consequences, however, still have to be established.

Midazolam

Midazolam is more lipid soluble compared to lorazepam, resulting in a quicker onset of sedation and a larger distribution volume [54]. It has a slightly shorter half-life time compared to lorazepam. Elimination half-life time is 3–11 h, depending on individual clearance characteristics and duration of administration [54].

In most children dosages of 50–300 µg/kg/h are sufficient to reach adequate sedation. There is some evidence that it might not even be beneficial to administer higher doses than 300 µg/kg/h for the purpose of sedation [65, 66]. In patients with status epilepticus dosages up to 1600 µg/kg/h are used for a limited duration of time [67]. Because of long plasma half-life time a bolus of 50–100 µg/kg should be given whenever maintenance doses are increased.

Lorazepam

Lorazepam is twice as potent compared to midazolam [68]. As mentioned before it has a slightly longer plasma half-life time. Elimination half-life time is 8–15 h [54]. In most children dosages of 20–100 µg/kg/h are sufficient. Because of the long plasma half-life time a bolus of 20–40 µg/kg is recommended in order to reach a steady state [39].

Conclusions

Benzodiazepines are suitable drugs for sedation with strong sedative effects. As they have no analgesic effects whatsoever they should always be combined with adequate analgesia whenever pain is involved. Because the plasma half-life time may substantially increase following continuous administration benzodiazepines may not be the best choice in patients who are expected to only need sedation for a short period of time. Benzodiazepine use is an independent predictor of prolonged mechanical ventilation and length of hospital stay.

NMDA-Receptor Antagonist: Ketamine

Ketamine is a phencyclidine derivative and its main action is antagonizing NMDA-receptors in the brain. It has sedative, dissociative, and analgesic effects. Ketamine is a racemic mixture of an active (S) and a (practically) inactive (R) enantiomer. The R-enantiomer, however, interferes with the clearance of the S-enantiomer. The S-isomer alone (available for clinical use in some European countries as S-Ketamine or Esketamine) has less side effects, a faster recovery and more or less twice the potency compared to the racemic compound. Dosages of S-ketamine are therefore about 50 % of those published for racemic Ketamine.

Because of the high hydrophobic chemical characteristics ketamine preferentially moves into highly perfused and lipophilic tissues such as the brain and spinal cord and therefore has a large volume of distribution. This causes the rapid onset of action, even after a single loading dose. Subsequently, blood levels fall rapidly, resulting in drug redistribution out of the CNS back into the blood and other tissues. This accounts for the short time of action, and this occurs a lot faster than metabolization [29].

Metabolization occurs in the liver by forming norketamine, which has reduced CNS activity. Norketamine is then further metabolized and excreted in urine and bile. Ketamine is rapidly cleared making it suitable for continuous infusion.

Clinical Uses

There is hardly any evidence supporting the use of ketamine for prolonged sedation in pediatric ICU patients. However, it has been used in doses ranging from 5 to 60 µg/kg/min for the sedation of children who respond poorly to the opioid-benzodiazepine combination [69, 70].

Because of its secondary sympathomimetic, bronchodilating effects, Ketamine has been recommended for use in children presenting with severe asthma [71]. A limited number of case reports have reported beneficial effects on bronchoconstriction following ketamine administration, including non-intubated children [72]. A recent Cochrane review, however, showed the limited evidence for routine use in severe asthma and the absent evidence for a beneficial effect in intubated asthma patients [73].

More recently, low-dose peri-operative ketamine administration has been shown in a meta-analysis to decrease postoperative pain intensity and non-opioid analgesic requirement. However, ketamine failed to exhibit a postoperative opioid-sparing effect [74].

One of the main advantages of ketamine over many other sedatives is its little effect on the respiratory drive. Induction doses of ketamine might have a minor effect on respiratory minute volume, but the risk of respiratory depression or apnea is much less compared to many other sedatives. Furthermore retention of protective pharyngeal and laryngeal reflexes makes it a popular drug for procedural analgosedation.

Unlike many other sedatives, ketamine typically increases hearth rate, mean arterial pressure and cardiac output. These effects are most likely mediated by inhibition of catecholamine reuptake. Therefore it seems to be a good choice in patients at risk for hypotension [70]. However, in patients with pronounced circulatory failure and thus relatively depleted of catecholamines (e.g., septic shock) ketamine may cause deep hypotension and cardiac arrest [75].

Side Effects

One of the main reasons why ketamine is not much used for sedation in critically ill patients is the risk of hallucinations and delirium. These side effects seem to occur less frequently in children (about 10 % of cases), although no systematic research has been done within this perspective. There is some limited evidence, but no proof, that these effects are counteracted by simultaneous use of a benzodiazepine [39, 76].

Furthermore ketamine increases salivation and mucus production, which can be a very unwanted effect in mechanically ventilated patients.

It is often mentioned that ketamine causes increased intracranial pressure thereby making it unusable in traumatic brain injury. A recent systematic review, however, suggests that ketamine does not adversely affect intracranial or cerebral perfusion pressures compared with other intravenous agents. This study, however, only studied ketamine as an inductive agent and is further limited by the lack of large, randomized trials addressing this topic [77].

Ketamine also seems to cause neuro-apoptosis in long-term use [64]. As with many other sedatives there is no clear evidence of the neurodevelopmental consequences.

Conclusions

Ketamine is a strong sedative and analgesic drug that can be used for continuous sedation in critically ill children. It is a very attractive drug in short-term sedation and procedural sedation because it does not cause respiratory depression and has a very short half-life time. It also seems to be a safe choice in patients with cardiovascular instability but should not be used in patients with pronounced circulatory failure. The main side effects of delirium and hallucinations seem to be of less importance in children compared to adults, but it does occur in children as well which can be a reason to discontinue ketamine or add a benzodiazepine to the sedation regiment.

Alpha-2-Receptor Agonists

Alpha-2-receptor agonists are among the newer used sedatives in pediatric ICUs. They have a range of effects including sedation, analgesia, and anxiolysis. Clonidine has been used for hypertension for many years and was discovered to also be effective for withdrawal symptoms. Later on its sedative properties became more apparent. Dexmedetomidine is more recently discovered as a highly selective alpha-2-receptor agonist with even less side effects compared to clonidine. The selectivity ratio of alpha-2 compared to alpha-1 stimulation is 1620:1 for dexmedetomidine compared to 220:1 for clonidine [78]. The main sedative actions of both agents are achieved by stimulation of alpha-2-receptors in the central nervous system, especially in the locus ceruleus and the dorsal horn of the spinal cord [79]. Currently, dexmedetomidine is not yet approved for prolonged use in pediatric patients. Nevertheless, there is growing evidence that long-term use for sedation in pediatric ICU patients is safe and effective [79, 80].

One of the typical characteristics of alpha-2-receptor agonists is that they generate sedation without limiting patient interaction. Particularly for dexmedetomidine this typical effect has been described as "generating natural sleep" [81, 82]. This means that all non-pharmacological means of providing comfort are even more important to reach effective sedation with dexmedetomidine alone. Compared to Propofol and midazolam, the use of dexmedetomidine has been shown to maintain patient interactivity, resulting in a better opportunity for patients to communicate their needs. Alpha-2-receptor agonists may be less suitable when a painful or otherwise unpleasant stimulus is present [80].

A particular advantage of alpha-2 receptor agonists is the absence of respiratory depressant effects [83]. The combination of these advantages over many other sedatives are thought to be the explanation for the reduction in days of mechanical ventilation and length of hospital stay, proven in adults when alpha-2-agonists are compared to benzodiazepines or propofol [83–85]. Also in children the use of dexmedetomidine is associated with a shorter duration of mechanical ventilation when compared with the use of fentanyl in postoperative pediatric cardiac surgical patients [86]. Besides all of these advantages, alpha-2 receptor agonists seem to give a decreased risk of both delirium and oversedation, compared to traditional sedatives [83].

Elimination is through both hepatic metabolism to inactive metabolites and direct renal excretion [29, 87].

Alpha-2-agonists provide analgesia and sedation and are therefore a good alternative to other sedatives but can also be used as an adjuvant especially in addition or replacement of benzodiazepines [79, 88]. Studies directly comparing dexmedetomidine to midazolam are rare. The prospective study by Tobias et al. shows that at a dose of 0.25 μgr/kg/h dexmedetomidine was approximately equivalent to midazolam at 0.22 mg/kg/h. At higher infusion rates of 0.5 μgr/kg/h it provides more effective sedation as demonstrated by a need for fewer doses of morphine as well as better sedation scores [89]. A retrospective study by Whalen et al. didn't notice a significant difference in the dosing of opiates or benzodiazepines after starting dexmedetomidine. This study is, however, biased by the retrospective nature of it [79]. For clonidine it has been shown that it can be used as an alternative for midazolam as a primary sedative agent [87, 90]. In ventilated newborns clonidine reduced fentanyl and midazolam demand with deeper levels of analgesia and sedation without substantial side effects. This effect was not seen in older children [91]. More and larger randomized controlled trials investigating the additive effect of dexmedetomidine and clonidine and/or the direct comparison

with benzodiazepines are therefore urgently needed. Also studies comparing clonidine with dexmedetomidine are lacking.

Therefore, the exact place of these drugs for sedation of critically ill children, including their optimal and maximum dosages, still has to be determined.

Side Effects

Alpha-2-agonists are, like other sedatives, associated with tolerance and, consequently, withdrawal following discontinuation [79, 92]. The main side effects of alpha-2-agonists are, in accordance with stimulating Θ-receptors, of cardiovascular origin. The major side effects therefore are bradycardia and hypotension. Because of the higher alpha-2-selectivity, dexmedetomidine has less cardiovascular effects than clonidine.

Hypertension is described as well, which is thought to be due to alpha-1 agonistic and peripheral alpha-2B agonistic effects, leading to peripheral vasoconstriction [93]. This hypertension is described after intravenous start of clonidine, which then subdues shortly after [29]. It is also described when higher doses of dexmedetomidine are used. Lowering the dose may be indicated to reverse this effect. Dexmedetomidine administration has been shown to be safe in children with (congenital) heart disease. In this category of patients its use has been associated with decrease of opioid and benzodiazepine requirement and also a decreased need for inotropic support [94]. Similar findings have been observed in children with heart failure [95]. However, we believe that alpha-2-agonists need to be used cautiously in patients at risk for bradycardia, hypotension, and hypertension and that bolus dosages should be avoided especially in the latter patient categories.

Clonidine

Intravenous dosages for clonidine range from 0.25 up to 3 mcg/kg/h [83, 87]. Some studies describe a loading dose of 1–3 μg/kg [83, 87]. Others state that a loading dose is not indicated as continuous infusion will achieve sedation goals quickly and loading dose may provoke hypotension and/or bradycardia.

Oral clonidine is used for withdrawal symptoms after long-term use of opioids, benzodiazepines as well as alpha-2-receptor agonists. In addition, clonidine has independent local effects on tubular function which promote both diuresis and natriuresis (http://www.journalslibrary.nihr.ac.uk/hta/volume-18/back-section-2.html-ref1-bib37). In adults the peripheral α_1 effects can cause hypertension and vasoconstriction in overdose, but this appears to be far less common in children [87].

Dexmedetomidine

Dexmedetomidine is a new generation alpha-2-receptor agonist with a high Θ_2-selectivity. It has potent sedative and modest analgesic properties.

Usually dexmedetomidine is administered intravenously at a dose ranging from 0.2 to 0.7 µg/kg/h. Several studies have demonstrated that dosages up to 2 µg/kg/h are safe and sometimes necessary to achieve sufficient sedation scores [96]. Higher dosages may lead to hypertension as one case report suggests [97]. Some studies propose a slow-loading dose of 0.05–1 µg/kg in 10–20 min to achieve sedation earlier [79, 96]. As with clonidine giving a loading dose may provoke hypotension and/or bradycardia.

In contrast to most other sedatives, which have been associated with neuro-apoptosis, dexmedetomidine might have a neuro-protective effect [98–100]. The clinical significance of this suggestion, however, still needs to be elucidated.

Conclusions

Alpha-2-agonists are a relatively novel group of sedatives, but with great potency. They provide sedation combined with moderate analgesia. They can be used as a sole sedative or as an adjuvant, which may lead to lower dosages of the primary used sedative. The most relevant side effects are bradycardia and hypotension, and therefore they should be used with care in hemodynamically unstable patients.

Propofol

Propofol is a short-acting, lipophilic intravenous anesthetic. Propofol causes global CNS depression, presumably through agonism of $GABA_A$ receptors and perhaps reduced glutamatergic activity through NMDA-receptor blockade. Propofol has no analgesic effects. Propofol is metabolized in the liver by conjugation to sulfate and glucuronide and further metabolized to less active metabolites that are renally excreted. Since hepatic clearance exceeds hepatic blood flow, biological availability following oral ingestion is zero. Clearance is decreased in neonates with a high risk of accumulation and therefore lower doses are advised.

One advantage of propofol over many other sedatives is the low risk of dependency and tolerance. Therefore propofol does not need to be weaned off slowly.

Side Effects

Although propofol is one of the most administered sedatives in adult ICUs, its clinical use in children is limited. This is because of the risk of propofol infusion syndrome (PRIS), which is more common in children compared to adults. PRIS is a potentially life threatening complication, seen with prolonged and/or high dose propofol infusion. It's characterized by metabolic acidosis, hyperlipidemia, rhabdomyolysis, and eventually bradyarrhythmias and asystole. Many case reports describe the fatal ends in children with PRIS, and only a few reports on survivors are found [101]. Especially young children, children with head injury and children with an underlying mitochondrial dysfunction seem to have a high risk for PRIS. Especially the characteristically irreversible fatal course once PRIS has become symptomatic makes that pediatric ICUs are rather reluctant using propofol for long-term sedation. If used, dosages of 1–4 mg/kg/h seem to be sufficient for sedation in critically ill children. For anesthesia dosages up to 18 mg/kg/h are proven to be safe. Usually a loading dose of 1–3 mg/kg is used to reach adequate sedation within minutes.

Most guidelines recommend infusion for a maximum of 48 h and a maximum of 4 mg/kg/h to avoid PRIS [102]. Appropriate monitoring by frequently measuring lactate and creatine kinase levels is still warranted under these circumstances [103].

One of the major common side effects of propofol is hypotension, which is dose-dependent and caused by vasodilation and possibly mild depression of myocardial contractility. Therefore propofol should be used with caution in hemodynamically unstable patients. Furthermore propofol has a risk of respiratory depression, a side effect which is also dose-dependent.

There is some evidence that propofol also causes neuro-apoptosis when used in a critical period of brain development [64]. As with many other sedatives there is currently no certainty regarding the neurodevelopmental consequences.

Conclusions

Propofol is a widely used sedative in adult ICUs, but its use is limited in pediatric patients mainly because of the risk of developing the potentially fatal complication PRIS. Therefore it should not be used for long-term sedation in critically ill children. On the other hand, propofol seems to be a good choice for short-term or postoperative sedation, when the child is likely to be weaned off mechanical ventilation within 24 h. It also is an excellent choice for procedural sedation in children undergoing deep-sedation for medical procedures, including non-intubated patients.

Monitoring Depth of Sedation and Analgesia

Undersedation as well as oversedation can be harmful to the patient and need to be avoided. In order to tailor sedative drugs according to the individual optimal sedation level, the careful assessment of the sedation level in each individual patient at any time of ICU management is extremely important. Different tools are available for assessing the quality and depth of sedation in pediatric ICU patients. In this chapter we will discuss the most commonly applied tools: the COMFORT scale, the COMFORT behavior scale, the State behavioral scale, and the Ramsay scale [48].

The COMFORT scale was developed as a nonintrusive measure for assessing distress in children admitted to pediatric intensive care units. Eight dimensions of behavioral and/or physiologic distress were selected based upon a literature review and survey of PICU nurses [5]. After the introduction of this scale Marx et al. found that adequacy of sedation is measured more consistently by observers using the COMFORT scale than by intensivist global assessment [104].

An important drawback of this scoring system is the fact that it incorporates the physiologic parameters hearth rate and blood pressure which can be influenced by many more factors than distress alone. This has been confirmed by the study of Ista et al. who showed that physiologic variables do not correlate well with the behavioral items of the COMFORT scale. For this reason an abbreviated COMFORT scale restricted to behavior items was developed named the COMFORT behavior scale. It has proven a reliable alternative to the original COMFORT scale [105]. A recent study has shown that the COMFORT behavior scale detects treatment-related changes in pain or distress intensity. This implies that it can effectively guide both analgesic and sedation treatment in critically ill children [4]. The advantage of both the COMFORT and the COMFORT behavior scales is that it is suitable for the assessment of both pain and non-pain related distress in critically ill children. Furthermore they are age independent.

The state behavioral scale was developed to assess sedation and agitation in young (6 weeks to 6 years) pediatric patients on mechanical ventilation [106]. Its main drawback therefore is that it is only suitable for this age group.

The Ramsey scale was originally developed to determine the level of sedation in adult patients admitted to the ICU [107]. It classifies the consciousness into six categories. Although it's widely used in adults, it has not been validated in children. The same holds true for the Richmond agitation sedation scale (RASS) [108].

In conclusion the COMFORT and COMFORT behavior scale seem to be the most suitable tools for assessing sedation because they have been extensively investigated and assess both pain and non-pain related distress. When using other scoring systems for sedation it is therefore of the utmost importance to assess pain in addition because the scoring systems only assess sedation. In paralyzed children assessing sedation levels is very difficult. In this patient category the PICU modified comfort sedation scale for muscle relaxed patients can be used [109]. For an extensive evaluation of instruments for scoring pain, non-pain related distress and adequacy of analgesia and sedation in ventilated children we refer to the recent review of Dorfman et al. [110].

When assessing comfort of children admitted to an intensive care unit it is very important to consider that pediatric delirium is a frequent occurring phenomenon. Therefore besides assessing the level of sedation and pain it is important to incorporate delirium screening into daily practice. This item is discussed separately in this chapter.

Titrating the depth of sedation thus will ideally prevent both under and oversedation. The question is, however, whether it also will lead to a reduction in duration of mechanical ventilation and/or length of stay. Reports on this subject are contradictory. A recent large trial among children undergoing mechanical ventilation for acute respiratory failure in which the use of a sedation protocol was compared with usual care did not reduce the duration of mechanical ventilation [111]. Another study showed that implementing a sedation protocol for mechanically ventilated children reduced the duration of sedation but only tended to reduce the duration of mechanically ventilation [30]. Reduction of the cumulative dose of benzodiazepines is also shown by another study in which a nurse-driven pediatric analgesia and sedation protocol was studied. In this study also a reduction in the occurrence of withdrawal symptoms was observed [112].

Delirium in the Critically Ill Child

In the last few years there has been a growing awareness of the clinical importance of pediatric delirium (PD) in critically ill children [7, 48, 113]. The prevalence in this patient category (i.e., critically ill children) ranges from 11 to 21 % [114–116].

Delirium is a neuro-cognitive disorder due to a somatic illness or its treatment and is characterized by loss of attention, interests, appetite, emotional irritability, tiredness, and increased need of sleep. According to DSM-5 (American Psychiatric Association, 2013) the four essential features of delirium are:

- A disturbance of attention or awareness
- This disturbance is accompanied by changes in cognition that cannot be better accounted for by another pre-existing neuro-cognitive disorder (e.g., mental retardation)

- The condition develops in a short period of time, hours or days, and often fluctuates during the day, typically worsening in the evening
- There are indications from the patients' history, examination or laboratory results that the disturbance is probably the result of a medical condition or its treatment [117].

This definition officially has a fifth criterion, which has been criticized because of the requirement to exclude cases of reduced level of arousal ("coma") without specifying how this has to be done [118]. ICD-10 defines delirium as an etiologically nonspecific organic cerebral syndrome characterized by concurrent disturbances of consciousness and attention, perception, thinking, memory, psychomotor behavior, emotion, and the sleep–wake schedule. The duration is variable and the degree of severity ranges from mild to very severe [119].

Delirium has three subtypes: hyperactive (acute agitation, anxiety, hallucinations, delusions), hypoactive (apathy, empty gaze, and formal thought and speech disturbances), and mixed [120].

There are many important reasons for the systematical assessment of PD in the pediatric intensive care unit:

- Delirium is "acute brain failure," and as the brain also is the director of the autonomic- and endocrine systems the consequences may be severe leading to increased morbidity and mortality.
- A hyperactive delirium is accompanied by various risks, such as pulling out IV lines and catheters, auto-extubation, stepping or falling out of bed, etc.
- It is stressful for the patient who may experience terrifying hallucinations or delusions (sometimes without amnesia) that may lead to a post-traumatic stress disorder (PTSD) and
- It can also be very stressful for the child's family and clinical staff. Up to 25 % of parents of children who have been in a pediatric ICU may develop PTSD [121].

In general, critically ill children with delirium have a higher resilience (and better prognosis) than adults. The negative neuro-cognitive effects of delirium in adults and the elderly are well known, but we do not know yet whether this is also true for children.

The acute occurrence of a disturbance of cognition, emotions, consciousness, or behavioral disturbances in a critically ill child should raise the suspicion of PD. Nurses and physicians may find it difficult to assess symptoms of delirium, including cognitive changes, especially in pre-verbal, critically ill, and mechanically ventilated children. In these children, other aspects, such as behavioral characteristics and non-verbal interactions between parent and child, should be considered.

Answering the following questions based on one of the delirium screening tools (CAPD) can be helpful in raising the possibility of delirium [122]:

- Does the child make eye contact?
- Are the child's actions purposeful?
- Is the child aware of its surroundings?
- Does the child communicate needs and wants?
- Is the child restless?
- Is the child inconsolable?
- Is the child underactive (moves very little while awake)?
- Does the child take a long time to respond to interactions?

The diagnosis of delirium in children older than 5 years with normal development is based on DSM-5 or ICD-10 criteria. Accurately diagnosing pediatric delirium requires using a reliable, valid, and clinically suitable bedside tool that may also serve for screening and to guide treatment such as the Pediatric Anesthesia Emergence Delirium Scale (PAED), the pediatric Confusion Assessment Method for ICU (PCAM-ICU), the Cornell Assessment Pediatric Delirium tool (CAPD), and the Sophia Observation Withdrawal Symptoms-Pediatric Delirium scale (SOS-PD) [115, 122–129].

It must be emphasized that the right diagnosis and treatment of PD cannot be made merely on the basis of observational screening tools. It is mandatory to evaluate all other differential diagnostic explanations. The underlying somatic differential diagnosis of conditions potentially leading to delirium is described in the section refractory agitation in this chapter—see below.

The differential diagnosis of particularly hypoactive delirium, given its high prevalence and frequently disappointing response to treatment deserves particular attention:

- Withdrawal of medication
- Underlying intoxication with psychotropics and/or a neuroleptic-induced "deficit" syndrome due to sensitivity to antipsychotics
- Non-convulsive status epilepticus, major depressive disorder, and/or catatonic inhibition.

Many risk factors for delirium have been identified. These can be classified as relating to the patient, iatrogenic, and environmental (e.g., hospital ward, pediatric ICU). Medical conditions (especially Infections) often predispose for PD. Iatrogenic factors include mechanical ventilation, medication such as corticosteroids and vaso-active medication, withdrawal of medication, restraints, sleep disturbance, painful procedures, catheters and IV lines, and psychosocial deprivation from the primary caretakers and family. Minimizing these factors is a logical and important approach [130].

Table 27.2 Recommended dosages of intravenous haloperidol for hyperactive PD

Age (years)	Weight (kg)	Maximum loading dose IV	Average maintenance dose IV	Maximum dose IV
0–1	3.5–10	• 0.05 mg in 30 min	• 0.01–0.05 mg/kg/day, divided into 2–3 doses	• Unknown
1–3	10–15	• 0.15 mg in 30 min	• 0.025 mg/kg/day divided into 2–3 doses	• Unknown
3–18	>15 kg	• 0.25–0.5 mg in 30 min	• 0.05 mg/kg/day divided into 2–3 doses	• Unknown in children younger than 16 years of age • In children 16 years of age or older, 5 mg/day; divided into 2–4 doses

Table 27.3 Recommended doses of haloperidol or risperidone orally (po) for hyperactive pediatric delirium

Weight (kg)	Loading dose (mg) (po)	Average maintenance dose (po)	Maximum dose (po)
<45	• 0.02 mg/kg	• 0.01–0.08 mg/kg/day divided into 2 doses	• 4 mg/day
>45	• 0.5–1 mg	• 0.01–0.08 mg/kg/day divided into 2 doses	• 6 mg/day • Dosages >6 mg are not studied

Oral doses of haloperidol and risperidone are equal

Non-pharmacological Treatment

Parents can have a major role in the prevention, detection, and treatment of delirium. With implementing family-centered care as described earlier in this chapter one seeks to create a soothing environment for the child in order to prevent or mitigate the onset of delirium and to optimize the child's chances of recovery.

Symptoms associated with delirium, such as acute onset of delusions or hallucinations may come as a complete surprise, something the family has never encountered before, and can be very frightening for both child and parents. This may lead to parents not recognizing their child's behavior, becoming afraid that neurological damage has occurred or that their child is going to die [131]. Not knowing how to cope with these behaviors makes parents insecure and anxious; this in turn can influence the child, causing a vicious circle and the delirium to worsen. A soothing stimulation of all the five senses of the child with PD is advocated. The constant presence of one parent during the hospitalization, hearing parents' voices, readily visible photographs of parents or other well-known family members, and favorite toys decrease the severity of delirium [131–133].

Pharmacological Treatment

Medication may be considered to treat the acute hyperactive PD symptoms. Pharmacokinetics in children is different from adults. The same antipsychotics (typical antipsychotics such as haloperidol, and atypical antipsychotics, such as risperidone) are used in children as in adults. Studies on the pharmacological treatment of PD are scarce and have serious methodological flaws [134]. There are indications that haloperidol and risperidone, quetiapine, and olanzapine are effective for hyperactive PD [115, 131].

Haloperidol is mostly given intravenously; risperidone is only available for oral administration. The recommended average dosages, acquired especially in the first 24 h of trial and error treatment of the PD are summarized in Tables 27.2 and 27.3.

Adverse effects are extrapyramidal symptoms, such as dystonia (torticollis, trismus), oculogyric crisis, akathisia, and hyperpyrexia. Extrapyramidal symptoms are seen frequently, particularly if antipsychotics are increased rapidly. Therefore "Start low and go slow" and trying first to find a therapeutic effect in the first 24 h are important principles.

However, it can take 24–48 h before an adequate response is achieved. To cover this time-window of ongoing agitation the short-term addition of levomepromazine (also known as methotrimeprazine) has been successfully described as in the case of refractory agitation.

Recognizing and treating these possible adverse events is important. Treatment consists in reducing the dose of antipsychotics and in case of acute dystonia administration of an anticholinergic drug such as biperiden (2.5–5 mg iv in 15 min) [135].

In adult patients lengthening of the QTc interval is known [136]. A meta-analysis in children showed that none of the investigated antipsychotics showed a significant increase in QTc time. Therefore the risk of QTc prolongation seems low in children. However both medication and other patient factors have to be taken into account when choosing treatment and an ECG should be made if indicated [137].

Hypoactive delirium in all its characteristics (apathy-lethargy-drowsiness and formal thought and speech disorders) is generally non-responsive to any neuro-psychiatric drug.

In conclusion PD in critical illness is a common, but until recently neglected, clinical issue of great importance. Non-pharmacological interventions and the role and position of the parents are of utmost relevance. Haloperidol (p.o. or i. v.) and risperidone (only available po) can both be used for treatment of hyperactive PD. Hypoactive PD is generally not responsive to drug therapy.

Refractory Agitation in Critically Ill Children

Refractory agitation (RA) can be defined as a neuro-psychiatric disorder characterized by (extreme) anxiety, which is non-responsive to conventional sedative treatment. The level of agitation/anxiety can be monitored by using, e.g. the COMFORT behavior scale which has been previously described. RA most frequently occurs in the context of hyperactive delirium. RA is just as delirium assumed to always be due to, or occurring in the context of, an underlying somatic disorder, its treatments and/or its terminations. Nevertheless in 10 % of cases of PD no identifiable cause can be found.

The differential diagnosis (DD) of an acute emotional-behavioral disturbance in a critical ill patient is clearly presented in two short algorithmic papers [138, 139]. The specific underlying somatic DD for RA is given by the famous and apt acronym I WATCH DEATH, in which each of the capitals represents an important cause (e.g., Infection, Withdrawal, etc.) [140]. Only if agitation persists after adequate treatment of the underlying disease, possible other causes of discomfort, ongoing anxiety, and treating an existing delirium one finally can speak of RA.

In the case of RA there are three treatment options: (1) patience; (2) rescue sedation; (3) electro convulsive therapy (ECT).

1. Treatment efficacy of hyperactive delirium can take some time before the administration of an antipsychotic drug has resulted in a therapeutic effect. This time delay is depending on the route of administration (orally vs. intravenously), the resorption, distribution, and receptor binding, possible interactions with other drugs, and the cytochrome P450 status of the patient. Sometimes this delay is undesirable and even dangerous. After all, the agitated and "non- responding" patient can pull out lines, auto extubate, fight the ventilator, and suffer terribly from hallucinations and delusions, leading also to a post-traumatic stress disorder, including horrible flash backs. The most important but very difficult question to answer is how long to be patient?
2. In case of RA rescue sedative medication is usually indicated, especially when there exists an urgent need to bridge—safely but effectively—the time gap between the start of the antipsychotic medication and its antipsychotic effect. We prefer to use levomepromazine (aka nozinan/ methotrimeprazine) [141]. This is an aliphatic phenothiazine that is very well known in acute psychiatry and especially in severe mental illness. It has weak antipsychotic, strong analgesic, and very strong sedative effects. It also has potential anticholinergic side effects which usually are not significant. In critically ill children it is used depending on weight and agitation level—with an initial IV loading dose of 1 to 3 mg (administering slowly in 30 min). Following doses are in function of responses and side effects up to 1 mg/kg/24 h intravenously. Another sedative that can be used as rescue medication is pentobarbital. It is a very effective sedative, which may represent an adjunctive sedative but can also serve as a substitute for the other sedatives. Its use, however, is associated with potentially serious side effects mainly cardiovascular depression. Used dosages range from 1 to 5 mg/kg/h [142, 143].
3. Refractory cases of major psychiatric disorders frequently also respond well to ECT treatment: e.g., refractory: (lethal) catatonia, mood disorder; melancholia (psychotic depression); pernicious psychosis. There are also data emerging of successful ECT for refractory delirium/ RA as well [144]. The procedure is well known, is easy to perform also in a PICU surrounding, and takes no more than approximately 15 min. The most important side effects are temporarily short-term memory problems. Confirmation studies for this specific indication and context are urgently needed, but this seems a very promising alternative.

In conclusion RA is a common, clinically important and often complicated issue, which can be very hard to manage.

Sedation and Analgesia of the Critically Ill Child: General Considerations and Proposed Treatment Algorithm

A recently performed survey among member societies of the world federation of pediatric intensive and critical care societies has shown that the most commonly used sedation regimen used in critically ill children is the combination of opioids with benzodiazepines [48]. This is in line with published guidelines on sedation and analgesia management in critically ill children [45, 145].

Despite the widespread use of the abovementioned sedatives and analgesics updated evidence-based guidelines addressing this topic in children are lacking in contrast to the literature of adult patients in the intensive care unit [7, 54, 146]. For the pediatric cardiac intensive care patients a consensus statement has been published as well. It doesn't, however, give a uniform treatment algorithm but states that post cardiac surgery patients require an individualized both sedative and analgesic strategy [147].

In general, with the currently available data in mind the combination of benzodiazepines with opiates seems to be a good choice to start with in all ventilated critically ill children.

We strongly plead, however, for a policy combining these pharmacological interventions with continuous careful identification and treatment of underlying causes of anxiety, agitation, and insomnia in a family-centered way with special attention for environmental control (Fig. 27.1). These measures have been discussed previously in this chapter.

With respect to the pharmacological treatment the combinations midazolam/fentanyl or midazolam/morphine seem the best choices based on the available literature. For analgesia fentanyl is the preferred opioid among many pediatric intensivists followed by morphine [48].

Morphine, however, may be a better choice compared to fentanyl because of a slower development of tolerance and less withdrawal symptoms. In the case of insufficient sedation and/or analgesia dexmedetomidine seems to be the best candidate to add to midazolam if this doesn't provide adequate sedation in a dose of 300 µg/kg/h. It might even be the most appropriate sedative to start with to possibly reduce the abovementioned negative effects of benzodiazepines and thereby reducing both length of stay and mechanical ventilation duration. As mentioned before randomized trials addressing this question are, however, lacking in children.

Morphine, fentanyl, and midazolam are usually administered as a continuous maintenance infusion. An alternative to reduce the negative effects of sedatives and analgesics such as prolongation of the period of mechanical ventilation and development of withdrawal by reducing the bioaccumulation of these products is daily sedation interruption. This encompasses the suspension of sedatives and sometimes analgesics, usually in the morning, during which time the patient is closely observed for signs of discomfort or agitation. If the patient stays comfortable based on frequently assessing of both sedation and pain restarting sedative drugs are not recommended. If discomfort appears the sedative(s) are usually restarted at 50% of the previous dose. A meta-analysis including nine trials performed in adult ICU patients did not find strong evidence that daily interruption of sedation alters the duration of mechanical ventilation, mortality, length of ICU or hospital stay, adverse event rates, drug consumption, or quality of life compared to sedation strategies that do not include daily interruption of sedation [148]. Daily sedation interruption or a light target level of sedation is, however, still recommended in mechanically ventilated adult ICU patients [54].

In children however, some trials showed that daily interruption led to earlier extubation and shorter length of stay [149, 150]. Another multicenter randomized controlled trial, however, showed that daily sedation interruption in addition to protocolized sedation didn't lead to earlier extubation but was associated with increased mortality. No causal relationship with the intervention could be found, however [151].

Bioaccumulation of both sedatives and analgesics can also be limited by regular switching between different sedatives and analgesics. Trials on this topic are, however, lacking.

During the last few years the topic of neuro-apoptosis became a subject of much speculation and research. Several animal studies have since then reported apoptosis after exposure to different anesthetic and sedative drugs. The theory is that synaptogenesis is disrupted and causes apoptotic death of cells that would otherwise develop into functioning neurons. The period of peak vulnerability coincides with the developmental period of rapid synaptogenesis which is known as the brain growth spurt [41]. In humans this period extends from about mid-gestation to several years after birth. There is evidence that heavy sedation, prolonged use of sedatives, and combining different sedatives have a negative impact on neuronal cell development [41, 42]. So far research has focused mainly on animal models, which cannot be easily translated to human effects. There is very little known about equivalent doses of sedation medication or the comparable period of brain development when animal models are used to investigate these effects on neuronal cells [152]. The research and evidence in neonates and pediatric patients is very limited. Therefore we cannot give any advice for the current practice regarding this topic. But since it is a very important issue, we will present the available evidence.

Anesthetic drugs as well as drugs that interact with GABA-receptors or NMDA-receptors, such as benzodiazepines, esketamine, and propofol, might lead to neuro-apoptosis in neonatal animal models [41, 42, 64]. Recent literature also shows that neuro-apoptosis might occur with long-term opioid infusion as well [40–42]. But there is hardly any evidence that the neuro-apoptotic effects may effect neurodevelopmental outcome, which might be due to the fact that the medication effects are irrelevant compared to other negative factors such as deprived stimulation and environment [152]. In contrast, animal studies have shown that dexmedetomidine is not associated with neuro-apoptotic effects, and there might even be a neuro-protective effect [98–100].

Furthermore it is known that stressful and painful experiences may lead to neurodevelopmental problems and hyperalgesia later in life [153, 154]. It has also been shown that administering morphine to neonates might even have a protective effect on executive functions [43]. All in all, there is still conflicting evidence, and results so far are not a suitable basis for definitive conclusions or decision making with respect to which sedative is preferred in critically ill children regarding this aspect. However, this does support our statement that one should always seek the optimum level of sedation and analgesia to prevent over and undersedation and try to minimize polypharmacy whenever possible.

In the case of inadequate sedation or perhaps even refractory agitation despite the use of benzodiazepines in combination with dexmedetomidine and opioids in adequate dosages there are several options to provide adequate comfort for the patient. First, as mentioned before other causes of discomfort and pain such as urine retention, constipation, itching, hunger or thirst, lying on a IV line, delirium, etc.

have to be ruled out. Secondly one has to question whether tolerance, especially for opioids could play a role and if so the dosage of the opioids should be raised in combination with giving a bolus.

If the abovementioned causes and tolerance have been ruled out adjustments to the sedation regime come into place. A first option is to replace a sedative by another, for example, switching midazolam or dexmedetomidine to ketamine. If possible adding sedatives instead of replacing them should in our opinion be avoided to further prevent polypharmacy. Another option is to add rescue medication temporarily to the treatment. In our experience levomepromazine is a good choice for this purpose. Another option is adding pentobarbital to the sedative treatment either as a substitute or to replace the other sedatives (Fig. 27.2).

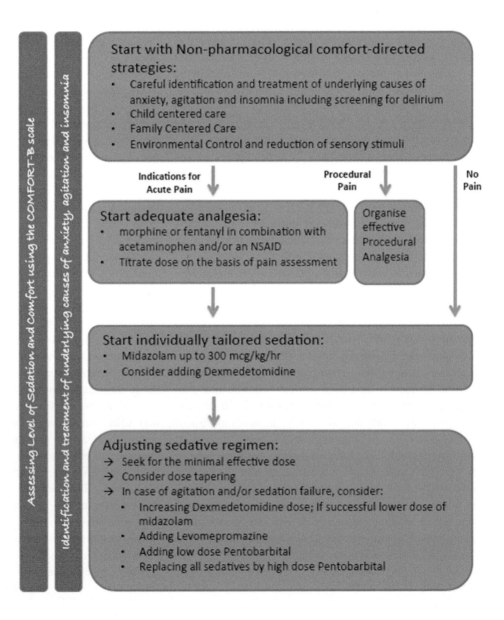

Fig. 27.2 Sedation and analgesia of the critically ill child—proposed treatment algorithm

Withdrawal

Withdrawal symptoms can develop after administering sedative and/or analgesic drugs in the pediatric intensive care unit. The signs and symptoms of sedative/analgesic agent withdrawal include central nervous system activation such as irritability, increased wakefulness, yawning, hyper tonicity, delirium, and gastro-intestinal tract disturbances such as vomiting and diarrhea. Hypertension and tachycardia can also be presenting symptoms [155]. Withdrawal is mainly described in association with the use of benzodiazepines and opioids because these are the most commonly used sedatives and analgesics and occurs in 35–50 % of critically ill children [60, 61, 156, 157]. Withdrawal syndrome is, however, also described in children sedated with dexmedetomidine in up to 30 % of children [79, 92]. Longer duration of use and high dosing are risk factors for the development of withdrawal symptoms in children but they can develop already after only 3 days of administration [2, 61].

Therefore withdrawal syndrome should be considered in every patient after three or more days of sedation with opioids, benzodiazepines, and/or alpha-2-receptor agonists in which this medication is tapered.

Various screening tools for withdrawal syndrome in critically ill children are available. Most commonly used are the Sophia Observation withdrawal symptoms scale (SOS) and the withdrawal assessment tool-1 (WAT-1) [158–160].

From the above it can be concluded that withdrawal can be prevented or treated by slow tapering of dosages of the sedative and/or analgesic agents. Another option is converting the IV agent to an oral equivalent which can be subsequently tapered. Midazolam can be substituted by oral administration of lorazepam and IV opioids can be substituted by oral administration of methadone. For converting intravenous midazolam to oral lorazepam the total daily dose of midazolam is divided by 12 and this daily dose of lorazepam is divided into 4 doses. After the second oral dose of lorazepam the intravenous midazolam infusion is decreased by 50% and after the third dose is further reduced by another 50 %. After the fourth dose, the intravenous midazolam infusion is discontinued [155]. In the case of fentanyl the total daily dose of methadone is equal to three times the total daily dose of fentanyl divided into 2 doses. After the second oral dose of methadone, the intravenous fentanyl infusion is decreased by 50 % and after the third dose further decreased by 50%. After the fourth oral dose, the intravenous fentanyl infusion is discontinued [161]. The conversion of intravenous morphine to methadone is straightforward. The daily dose of methadone should equal the total daily dose of morphine. The further tapering of morphine is similar to the tapering of fentanyl. For dexmedetomidine after prolonged infusions it has been proposed that slow tapering via the intravenous route (0.1 μg/kg/h. every 12–24 h) or switching to an orally equivalent dose of clonidine would prevent withdrawal syndrome [92].

Procedural Sedation and Analgesia on the PICU

During their stay on the ICU children often need to undergo medical procedures that require controlled immobility (e.g., imaging) and/or are (very) painful. For these short procedural episodes the maintenance continuous sedation and analgesia will often be insufficient to guarantee procedural success and comfort. Therefore additional procedural sedation and/or analgesia (PSA) will be indicated. PSA has been defined as the specific use of sedative, analgesic, or dissociative drugs to relieve anxiety and pain associated with diagnostic and therapeutic procedures, while maintaining spontaneous ventilation and minimally disturbing basic vital conditions [162]. For a comprehensive overview of the topic, in general, we refer to many recently published guidelines and reviews[163]. In this chapter we will, however, formulate some general recommendations for effective and safe PSA in a PICU population.

PSA, in general, covers a large spectrum of sedatives and involves a wide range of sedation levels, efficacy and associated risks. PSA provided in a context of limited training, competence or safety precautions is associated with a greater likelihood of potentially fatal complications [164, 165]. PSA by the untrained also bares the risk of ineffective sedation, possibly leading to unsuccessful and/or uncomfortable procedures. For a PICU population, however, it can be expected that competent professionals are always involved in patient management, including procedure-related care. In addition, in recent years, there has been a shift in the philosophy regarding PSA given, firstly, the increasing recognition of the negative aspects and consequences of procedural discomfort and pain [166] and, secondly, the fact that appropriately trained (so-called) non-anesthesiology professionals can be entrusted to deliver high quality PSA, including the use of titratable intravenous anesthetics (e.g., Propofol) in non-intubated patients [167–170]. In fact, pediatric intensivists have been prominent in organizing hospital-wide sedation services outside the boundaries of the PICU as well [171]. The use of carefully titrated doses of Propofol by well-trained professionals and the implementation of advanced safety-settings (including easily accessible capnography devices [172, 173]) have enhanced the quality of PSA to a highly safe and effective practice [174].

From a practical point of view, in defining effective PSA a distinction must be made between procedural analgesia and procedural sedation. Whenever pain is involved, additional analgesic therapy must be considered. For blood sampling and peripheral intravascular access, topical anesthesia (e.g., EMLA cream or a similar product) should always be used and applied sufficient time preceding the intended procedure. For EMLA the optimal application time precedes the actual procedure with 1–2 h [175]. For deeper vascular access (e.g., central venous catheterization) and limited surgical procedures (e.g., chest tube placement) local infiltration of anesthetics (e.g., lidocaine) should be standard of care. As the infiltration of the acid (lido)caines will cause a burning pain sensation, the drug needs to be buffered with bicarbonate. An effective but pain-free dilution is a 10 ml syringe containing 9 ml lidocaine (1 % or 2 %) and 1 ml NaHCO3 8,4 % [176]. For procedures where local/topical anesthesia is unlikely to be sufficient more powerful analgesia is required. Short-acting synthetic opioids (e.g., fentanyl, remifentanil) are the drugs of choice because of their quick onset of effect and short half-life time. As such they will provide sufficient analgesia for the usually short but intensive pain sensation related to most procedures. For extended procedures (e.g., extensive wound care; burn wound dressing) repeated doses may be needed. In the absence of an IV access intranasal administration may be an effective alternative for acute pain and (combined with procedural sedation) for pronounced procedural pain [177, 178]. Ketamine has also been used for PSA. Especially the broad range of therapeutic effects (including sedation, analgesia, and amnesia) and the limited effects on respiratory drive and airway control make it an interesting choice for PSA in non-intubated patients. The secondary sympathico-mimetic effects of Ketamine make it an attractive option for PSA in hemodynamically unstable patients who need to undergo an invasive procedure (e.g., central venous line placement in a patient with circulatory failure). However, catastrophic circulatory collapse following a single dose of IV ketamine has been reported in patients with septic shock [75]. Emergence delirium and/or agitation has been frequently reported following ketamine-based PSA. Occurrence seems to be unrelated with patient age and not to be influenced by the co-administration of anticholinergics or benzodiazepines [179]. Although the emergence reactions following a single ketamine-PSA experience seem to be rather benign [180], it is our own clinical impression that in repeated procedures (e.g., extensive wound care requiring multiple procedures over an extended period of time) patients may experience the emergence phenomena as highly distressing and frightening.

For procedural sedation only, Propofol, either as (repeated) single IV boluses or a short-time continuous infusion (5–15 mg/kg/h) is an excellent choice for an individually titrated sedation.

Using IV opioids and/or powerful sedatives may result in hemodynamic instability in patients with (imminent) circulatory failure and respiratory compromise in non-intubated patients. Therefore all precautions to monitor and manage these potential adverse events must be taken prior to the start of the procedure.

Palliative Sedation in Pediatrics

In children with acute or chronic conditions, which are incurable medical treatment might be withhold or withdrawn in the absence of any quality of life. These children and their families are entitled to custom palliative care. Sometimes analgesics and/or sedatives are needed to prevent or reduce suffering and to control refractory symptoms such as pain, anxiety, distress, nausea, and dyspnea. This is where palliative sedation comes into palliative care. The definition of palliative sedation, also called terminal sedation, according to the British Encyclopedia is "the palliative practice of relieving distress in a terminally ill person in the last hours or days of a dying patient's life, usually by means of a continuous intravenous or subcutaneous infusion of a sedative drug." In this section we will further discuss the options for palliative sedation without discussing the ethical dilemmas of palliative sedation [181–183].

The practical implementation and management of palliative sedation in general, and particularly in children, varies across cultural differences, and therefore by countries and even within countries. It is also depending on the legal issues [183–188]. Therefore it is impossible to reach a worldwide protocol for palliative sedation, and even to come to a national protocol is almost impossible.

Regarding the choice of palliative sedation several items are important such as the place where the sedation takes place (home, hospital, or at the ICU), sedatives and pain medication already prescribed, access to medication and most importantly the nature and severity of the refractory symptoms. In children receiving palliative sedation at home the preferable route of drug administration is subcutaneous. Drugs that might be given subcutaneously are midazolam, morphine, levomepromazine and dexmedetomidine. In children having an intravenous access the preferable route of administration is intravenous. In the hospital and especially in the pediatric intensive care unit the route of drug administration in most children will be intravenous, but also in this setting subcutaneous infusion may have a place to prevent the insertion of a new intravenous catheter.

It is important to make a distinction between refractory symptoms and pain or delirium. Before increasing sedation pain relief has to be started or increased in case there are symptoms of pain. In case of symptoms of delirium, as described earlier in this chapter, haloperidol might be given.

Midazolam is the most used drug in palliative sedation in both adults and children [185, 189]. Midazolam can be given intravenously and subcutaneously with a bolus of 0.05 up to 0.1 mg/kg. The initial maintenance dose is 0.01 up to 0.05 mg/kg/h, which can be increased stepwise every 2–4 h with 50 % of the actual dose. At a dose of 0.5 mg/kg/h adding levomepromazine might be considered or a switch to another sedative drug, for instance propofol. The disadvantage of a switch to propofol is the need for an intravenous access, especially when the child is getting palliative sedation at home. In children the combination of midazolam and morphine is also widely used [189].

Levomepromazine is a phenothiazine derivative with antipsychotic, analgesic, and sedative action. Therefore it is a useful drug for palliative sedation, especially because it can be given subcutaneously [185, 189]. The initial dose is 0.025 mg/kg/h with a maximum dose of 0.2 mg/kg/h.

Propofol is mentioned in studies as a sedative drug of last resort in case that the effect of other drugs to relieve refractory symptoms is insufficient. Propofol can only be given intravenously. The effect is fast and titration by initial boluses of 1–2 mg/kg until a good palliative result is reached can be done in a short period of time. In the literature initial doses range from 0.6 to 2.0 mg/kg/h, and maintenance doses from 0.6 to 6 mg/kg/h [190–192]. With these doses in most patients the results of the treatment were rated as "good" or "very good." The before mentioned doses are used in adults. In children higher doses are mentioned up to 7.8 mg/kg/h [193]. In children the chance on propofol infusion syndrome is higher than in adults and a maximum dose of 4 mg/kg/h is recommended for sedation in the intensive care unit. However, in cases of palliative sedation higher doses are sometimes needed for a satisfactory palliative result.

Dexmedetomidine can be given both subcutaneously and intravenously. The use of dexmedetomidine in the sedation on the pediatric intensive care and the prevention of drug withdrawal following prolonged sedation has been the subject in several publications, however there are limited publications on dexmedetomidine in palliative sedation [194–196]. Since dexmedetomidine can be given subcutaneously it might be of use in palliative sedation at home. The initial intravenous dose is 0.7 μg/kg/h, which might also be the subcutaneous dose. Loading doses should be avoided because of the risk of developing hypotension. The dose can be titrated up to 1.4 μg/kg/h. Studies have, however, documented no significant side effects in doses up to 2.5 μg/kg/h. After each step of titration at least 1 h is needed to reach a new stabile level of sedation.

Morphine is not stated in literature for sedative purpose but the continuation of opioids for the relieve of pain is widely recommended. Opioids are less effective in palliative sedation since their sedative effect is weak and especially in adults delirium is a frequently reported side effect. In children morphine is more frequently used in palliative sedation. First of all this might be because in young children the symptoms of discomfort and pain are more difficult to differentiate. Also delirium is less frequently seen in children as a side effect of opioids. Morphine can also be given both intravenously and subcutaneously in palliative sedation. The initial bolus of morphine is 0.04 mg/kg, followed by a continuous infusion of 0.025 mg/kg/h up to 0.25 mg/kg/h.

In children receiving palliative sedation at home and are not already treated with sedatives before the start of palliative sedation, we suggest to start with continuous subcutaneous infusion with midazolam and morphine. When the refractory symptoms are not adequately relieved levomepromazine can be added, also subcutaneously. As an alternative, dexmedetomidine can be chosen. In the case of refractory symptoms, propofol can be started intravenously. After the start of propofol, midazolam can be stopped.

References

1. Kollef MH, Levy NT, Ahrens TS, Schaiff R, Prentice D, Sherman G. The use of continuous i.v. sedation is associated with prolongation of mechanical ventilation. Chest. 1998;114 (2):541–8.
2. Ista E, van Dijk M, Gamel C, Tibboel D, de Hoog M. Withdrawal symptoms in critically ill children after long-term administration of sedatives and/or analgesics: a first evaluation. Crit Care Med. 2008;36(8):2427–32.
3. Vet NJ, Ista E, de Wildt SN, van Dijk M, Tibboel D, de Hoog M. Optimal sedation in pediatric intensive care patients: a systematic review. Intensive Care Med. 2013;39(9):1524–34.
4. Boerlage AA, Ista E, Duivenvoorden HJ, de Wildt SN, Tibboel D, van Dijk M. The COMFORT behaviour scale detects clinically meaningful effects of analgesic and sedative treatment. Eur J Pain. 2015;19(4):473–9.
5. Ambuel B, Hamlett KW, Marx CM, Blumer JL. Assessing distress in pediatric intensive care environments: the COMFORT scale. J Pediatr Psychol. 1992;17(1):95–109.
6. Lamas A, Lopez-Herce J. Monitoring sedation in the critically ill child. Anaesthesia. 2010;65(5):516–24.
7. Schieveld JN, Brouwers AG, Schieveld BR. On the lack of standardized essential PICU guidelines*. Crit Care Med. 2014;42(7):1724–5.
8. Zalieckas J, Weldon C. Sedation and analgesia in the ICU. Semin Pediatr Surg. 2015;24(1):37–46.
9. Maslow A. A theory of human motivation. Psychol Rev. 1943;50:370–98.
10. Jackson JC, Santoro MJ, Ely TM, Boehm L, Kiehl AL, Anderson LS, et al. Improving patient care through the prism of psychology: application of Maslow's hierarchy to sedation, delirium, and early mobility in the intensive care unit. J Crit Care. 2014;29(3):438–44.
11. Polmear C. Letter to the editor re: Jackson et al. Improving patient care through the prism of psychology: application of Maslow's hierarchy to sedation, delirium and early mobility in the intensive care unit. J Crit Care. 2015;30(1):209.

12. Evans D. The effectiveness of music as an intervention for hospital patients: a systematic review. J Adv Nurs. 2002;37(1):8–18.

13. Koschwanez H, Vurnek M, Weinman J, Tarlton J, Whiting C, Amirapu S, et al. Stress-related changes to immune cells in the skin prior to wounding may impair subsequent healing. Brain Behav Immun. 2015;50:47–51.

14. Gelinas C, Arbour C, Michaud C, Robar L, Cote J. Patients and ICU nurses' perspectives of non-pharmacological interventions for pain management. Nurs Crit Care. 2013;18(6):307–18.

15. Zborowsky T, Hellmich LB. Impact of place on people and process: the integration of research on the built environment in the planning and design of critical care areas. Crit Care Nurs Q. 2011;34(4):268–81.

16. Vos GD, van Os J, Leroy PL, Schieveld JN. Pets or meds: how to tackle misery in a paediatric intensive care unit. Intensive Care Med. 2007;33(8):1492–3.

17. Committee On Hospital C, Institute For P, Family-Centered C. Patient- and family-centered care and the pediatrician's role. Pediatrics. 2012;129(2):394–404.

18. Dijkstra K. Understanding healing environments: effects of physical environmental stimuli on patients' health and well-being. Thesis, University of Twente, The Netherlands, 2009

19. Boyatzis CJ, Varghese R. Children's emotional associations with colors. J Genet Psychol. 1994;155(1):77–85.

20. Eisen SL, Ulrich RS, Shepley MM, Varni JW, Sherman S. The stress-reducing effects of art in pediatric health care: art preferences of healthy children and hospitalized children. J Child Health Care. 2008;12(3):173–90.

21. Davignon MN, Friedlaender E, Cronholm PF, Paciotti B, Levy SE. Parent and provider perspectives on procedural care for children with autism spectrum disorders. J Dev Behav Pediatr. 2014;35(3):207–15.

22. Sternberg E. Healing spaces. Cambridge, Massachusetts, London: The Belknap Press of Harvard University Press; 2009.

23. Huisman E, Morales E, van Hoof J, Kort HSM. Healing environment: a review of the impact of physical environmental factors on users. Build Environ. 2012;58:70–80.

24. Ruthven D, Ferenc J. A new vision of care. A smarter patient room. Design team creates a view into the future. Health Facil Manag. 2014;27(2):11–3.

25. Silvis JK. Children's hospital design grows up. HealthCare Design [Internet]. 2013. Available from: http://www.healthcaredesignmagazine.com/article/childrens-hospital-design-grows.

26. Komiske B. Designing the world's best children's hospitals. 2nd ed. Mulgrave: Images Publishing Group Pty Ltd; 2013.

27. Design Considerations and Summary of Evidence: children's emergency, inpatient and ambulatory health services 2010. Available from: http://www.health.qld.gov.au/qhpolicy/docs/gdl/qh-gdl-374-6.pdf.

28. Krekels EH, Tibboel D, de Wildt SN, Ceelie I, Dahan A, van Dijk M, et al. Evidence-based morphine dosing for postoperative neonates and infants. Clin Pharmacokinet. 2014;53(6):553–63.

29. Brunton LL, Chabner BA, Knollmann BC. Goodman & Gilman's The pharmacological basis of therapeutics. 12th ed. New York: Mc Graw Hill Medical; 2011. p. 482–97.

30. Deeter KH, King MA, Ridling D, Irby GL, Lynn AM, Zimmerman JJ. Successful implementation of a pediatric sedation protocol for mechanically ventilated patients. Crit Care Med. 2011;39 (4):683–8.

31. Hartman ME, McCrory DC, Schulman SR. Efficacy of sedation regimens to facilitate mechanical ventilation in the pediatric intensive care unit: a systematic review. Pediatr Crit Care Med. 2009;10(2):246–55.

32. Anand KJ, Clark AE, Willson DF, Berger J, Meert KL, Zimmerman JJ, et al. Opioid analgesia in mechanically ventilated children: results from the multicenter Measuring Opioid Tolerance Induced by Fentanyl study. Pediatr Crit Care Med. 2013;14 (1):27–36.

33. Franck LS, Vilardi J, Durand D, Powers R. Opioid withdrawal in neonates after continuous infusions of morphine or fentanyl during extracorporeal membrane oxygenation. Am J Crit Care. 1998;7(5):364–9.

34. Robieux IC, Kellner JD, Coppes MJ, Shaw D, Brown E, Good C, et al. Analgesia in children with sickle cell crisis: comparison of intermittent opioids vs. continuous intravenous infusion of morphine and placebo-controlled study of oxygen inhalation. Pediatr Hematol Oncol. 1992;9(4):317–26.

35. van Dijk M, Bouwmeester NJ, Duivenvoorden HJ, Koot HM, Tibboel D, Passchier J, et al. Efficacy of continuous versus intermittent morphine administration after major surgery in 0-3-year-old infants; a double-blind randomized controlled trial. Pain. 2002;98(3):305–13.

36. Wong I, St John-Green C, Walker SM. Opioid-sparing effects of perioperative paracetamol and nonsteroidal anti-inflammatory drugs (NSAIDs) in children. Paediatr Anaesth. 2013;23(6):475–95.

37. Brown KA, Laferriere A, Lakheeram I, Moss IR. Recurrent hypoxemia in children is associated with increased analgesic sensitivity to opiates. Anesthesiology. 2006;105(4):665–9.

38. Schmelz M. Itch--mediators and mechanisms. J Dermatol Sci. 2002;28(2):91–6.

39. Johnson PN, Miller JL, Hagemann TM. Sedation and analgesia in critically ill children. AACN Adv Crit Care. 2012;23(4):415–34. quiz 35-6.

40. Attarian S, Tran LC, Moore A, Stanton G, Meyer E, Moore RP. The neurodevelopmental impact of neonatal morphine administration. Brain Sci. 2014;4(2):321–34.

41. Creeley CE, Olney JW. The young: neuroapoptosis induced by anesthetics and what to do about it. Anesth Analg. 2010;110 (2):442–8.

42. Loepke AW. Developmental neurotoxicity of sedatives and anesthetics: a concern for neonatal and pediatric critical care medicine? Pediatr Crit Care Med. 2010;11(2):217–26.

43. de Graaf J, van Lingen RA, Valkenburg AJ, Weisglas-Kuperus N, Groot Jebbink L, Wijnberg-Williams B, et al. Does neonatal morphine use affect neuropsychological outcomes at 8 to 9 years of age? Pain. 2013;154(3):449–58.

44. van Zellem L, Utens EM, de Wildt SN, Vet NJ, Tibboel D, Buysse C. Analgesia-sedation in PICU and neurological outcome: a secondary analysis of long-term neuropsychological follow-up in meningococcal septic shock survivors*. Pediatr Crit Care Med. 2014;15(3):189–96.

45. Playfor S, Jenkins I, Boyles C, Choonara I, Davies G, Haywood T, et al. Consensus guidelines on sedation and analgesia in critically ill children. Intensive Care Med. 2006;32(8):1125–36.

46. Welzing L, Oberthuer A, Junghaenel S, Harnischmacher U, Stutzer H, Roth B. Remifentanil/midazolam versus fentanyl/midazolam for analgesia and sedation of mechanically ventilated neonates and young infants: a randomized controlled trial. Intensive Care Med. 2012;38(6):1017–24.

47. Rigby-Jones AE, Priston MJ, Sneyd JR, McCabe AP, Davis GI, Tooley MA, et al. Remifentanil-midazolam sedation for paediatric patients receiving mechanical ventilation after cardiac surgery. Br J Anaesth. 2007;99(2):252–61.

48. Kudchadkar SR, Yaster M, Punjabi NM. Sedation, sleep promotion, and delirium screening practices in the care of mechanically ventilated children: a wake-up call for the pediatric critical care community*. Crit Care Med. 2014;42(7):1592–600.

49. Blumer JL. Clinical pharmacology of midazolam in infants and children. Clin Pharmacokinet. 1998;35(1):37–47.

50. Grant MJ, Scoppettuolo LA, Wypij D, Curley MA. Prospective evaluation of sedation-related adverse events in pediatric patients

ventilated for acute respiratory failure. Crit Care Med. 2012;40 (4):1317–23.

51. Lucas da Silva PS, de Carvalho WB. Unplanned extubation in pediatric critically ill patients: a systematic review and best practice recommendations. Pediatr Crit Care Med. 2010;11(2):287–94.

52. Roberts DJ, Haroon B, Hall RI. Sedation for critically ill or injured adults in the intensive care unit: a shifting paradigm. Drugs. 2012;72(14):1881–916.

53. Olkkola KT, Ahonen J. Midazolam and other benzodiazepines. Handb Exp Pharmacol. 2008;182:335–60.

54. Barr J, Fraser GL, Puntillo K, Ely EW, Gelinas C, Dasta JF, et al. Clinical practice guidelines for the management of pain, agitation, and delirium in adult patients in the intensive care unit. Crit Care Med. 2013;41(1):263–306.

55. Vet NJ, Brussee JM, de Hoog M, Mooij MG, Verlaat CW, Jerchel IS, et al. Inflammation and organ failure severely affect midazolam clearance in critically ill children. Am J Respir Crit Care Med. 2016;194(1):58–66.

56. Golparvar M, Saghaei M, Sajedi P, Razavi SS. Paradoxical reaction following intravenous midazolam premedication in pediatric patients – a randomized placebo controlled trial of ketamine for rapid tranquilization. Paediatr Anaesth. 2004;14 (11):924–30.

57. Gutierrez MA, Roper JM, Hahn P. Paradoxical reactions to benzodiazepines. Am J Nurs. 2001;101(7):34–9. quiz 9-40.

58. Mehta S, Cook D, Devlin JW, Skrobik Y, Meade M, Fergusson D, et al. Prevalence, risk factors, and outcomes of delirium in mechanically ventilated adults. Crit Care Med. 2015;43 (3):557–66.

59. Pandharipande P, Shintani A, Peterson J, Pun BT, Wilkinson GR, Dittus RS, et al. Lorazepam is an independent risk factor for transitioning to delirium in intensive care unit patients. Anesthesiology. 2006;104(1):21–6.

60. Fernandez-Carrion F, Gaboli M, Gonzalez-Celador R, Gomez de Quero-Masia P, Fernandez-de Miguel S, Murga-Herrera V, et al. Withdrawal syndrome in the pediatric intensive care unit. Incidence and risk factors. Med Intensiva. 2013;37(2):67–74.

61. Amigoni A, Vettore E, Brugnolaro V, Brugnaro L, Gaffo D, Masola M, et al. High doses of benzodiazepine predict analgesic and sedative drug withdrawal syndrome in paediatric intensive care patients. Acta Paediatr. 2014;103(12):e538–43.

62. Darnell C, Steiner J, Szmuk P, Sheeran P. Withdrawal from multiple sedative agent therapy in an infant: is dexmedetomidine the cause or the cure? Pediatr Crit Care Med. 2010;11(1):e1–3.

63. Fraser GL, Devlin JW, Worby CP, Alhazzani W, Barr J, Dasta JF, et al. Benzodiazepine versus nonbenzodiazepine-based sedation for mechanically ventilated, critically ill adults: a systematic review and meta-analysis of randomized trials. Crit Care Med. 2013;41(9 Suppl 1):S30–8.

64. Fredriksson A, Ponten E, Gordh T, Eriksson P. Neonatal exposure to a combination of N-methyl-D-aspartate and gamma-aminobutyric acid type A receptor anesthetic agents potentiates apoptotic neurodegeneration and persistent behavioral deficits. Anesthesiology. 2007;107(3):427–36.

65. de Wildt SN, de Hoog M, Vinks AA, van der Giesen E, van den Anker JN. Population pharmacokinetics and metabolism of midazolam in pediatric intensive care patients. Crit Care Med. 2003;31(7):1952–8.

66. Ince I, de Wildt SN, Wang C, Peeters MY, Burggraaf J, Jacqz-Aigrain E, et al. A novel maturation function for clearance of the cytochrome P450 3A substrate midazolam from preterm neonates to adults. Clin Pharmacokinet. 2013;52(7):555–65.

67. Tasker RC, Vitali SH. Continuous infusion, general anesthesia and other intensive care treatment for uncontrolled status epilepticus. Curr Opin Pediatr. 2014;26(6):682–9.

68. Barr J, Zomorodi K, Bertaccini EJ, Shafer SL, Geller E. A double-blind, randomized comparison of i.v. lorazepam versus midazolam for sedation of ICU patients via a pharmacologic model. Anesthesiology. 2001;95(2):286–98.

69. Tobias JD, Martin LD, Wetzel RC. Ketamine by continuous infusion for sedation in the pediatric intensive care unit. Crit Care Med. 1990;18(8):819–21.

70. Miller AC, Jamin CT, Elamin EM. Continuous intravenous infusion of ketamine for maintenance sedation. Minerva Anestesiol. 2011;77(8):812–20.

71. Koninckx M, Buysse C, de Hoog M. Management of status asthmaticus in children. Paediatr Respir Rev. 2013;14(2):78–85.

72. Denmark TK, Crane HA, Brown L. Ketamine to avoid mechanical ventilation in severe pediatric asthma. J Emerg Med. 2006;30 (2):163–6.

73. Jat KR, Chawla D. Ketamine for management of acute exacerbations of asthma in children. Cochrane Database Syst Rev. 2012;11, CD009293.

74. Dahmani S, Michelet D, Abback PS, Wood C, Brasher C, Nivoche Y, et al. Ketamine for perioperative pain management in children: a meta-analysis of published studies. Paediatr Anaesth. 2011;21(6):636–52.

75. Dewhirst E, Frazier WJ, Leder M, Fraser DD, Tobias JD. Cardiac arrest following ketamine administration for rapid sequence intubation. J Intensive Care Med. 2013;28(6):375–9.

76. Tobias JD. Sedation and analgesia in paediatric intensive care units: a guide to drug selection and use. Paediatr Drugs. 1999;1 (2):109–26.

77. Cohen L, Athaide V, Wickham ME, Doyle-Waters MM, Rose NG, Hohl CM. The effect of ketamine on intracranial and cerebral perfusion pressure and health outcomes: a systematic review. Ann Emerg Med. 2015;65(1):43–51. e2.

78. Virtanen R. Pharmacological profiles of medetomidine and its antagonist, atipamezole. Acta Veterinaria Scand Suppl. 1989;85:29–37.

79. Whalen LD, Di Gennaro JL, Irby GA, Yanay O, Zimmerman JJ. Long-term dexmedetomidine use and safety profile among critically ill children and neonates. Pediatr Crit Care Med. 2014;15(8):706–14.

80. Reiter PD, Pietras M, Dobyns EL. Prolonged dexmedetomidine infusions in critically ill infants and children. Indian Pediatr. 2009;46(9):767–73.

81. Huupponen E, Maksimow A, Lapinlampi P, Sarkela M, Saastamoinen A, Snapir A, et al. Electroencephalogram spindle activity during dexmedetomidine sedation and physiological sleep. Acta Anaesthesiol Scand. 2008;52(2):289–94.

82. Mason KP, O'Mahony E, Zurakowski D, Libenson MH. Effects of dexmedetomidine sedation on the EEG in children. Paediatr Anaesth. 2009;19(12):1175–83.

83. Chen K, Lu Z, Xin YC, Cai Y, Chen Y, Pan SM. Alpha-2 agonists for long-term sedation during mechanical ventilation in critically ill patients. Cochrane Database Syst Rev. 2015;1:Cd010269.

84. Riker RR, Shehabi Y, Bokesch PM, Ceraso D, Wisemandle W, Koura F, et al. Dexmedetomidine vs midazolam for sedation of critically ill patients: a randomized trial. JAMA. 2009;301 (5):489–99.

85. Constantin JM, Momon A, Mantz J, Payen JF, De Jonghe B, Perbet S, et al. Efficacy and safety of sedation with dexmedetomidine in critical care patients: a meta-analysis of randomized controlled trials. Anaest Crit Care Pain Med. 2016;35(1):7–15.

86. Prasad SR, Simha PP, Jagadeesh AM. Comparative study between dexmedetomidine and fentanyl for sedation during mechanical ventilation in post-operative paediatric cardiac surgical patients. Indian J Anaesth. 2012;56(6):547–52.

87. Wolf A, McKay A, Spowart C, Granville H, Boland A, Petrou S, et al. Prospective multicentre randomised, double-blind,

equivalence study comparing clonidine and midazolam as intravenous sedative agents in critically ill children: the SLEEPS (Safety profiLe, Efficacy and Equivalence in Paediatric intensive care Sedation) study. Health Technol Assessment. (Winchester, England). 2014;18(71):1–212.

88. Hayden JC, Breatnach C, Doherty DR, Healy M, Howlett MM, Gallagher PJ, et al. Efficacy of alpha2-Agonists for Sedation in Pediatric Critical Care: a Systematic Review. Pediatr Crit Care Med. 2016;17(2):e66–75.

89. Tobias JD, Berkenbosch JW. Sedation during mechanical ventilation in infants and children: dexmedetomidine versus midazolam. South Med J. 2004;97(5):451–5.

90. Kleiber N, de Wildt SN, Cortina G, Clifford M, Ducruet T, Tibboel D, et al. Clonidine as a first-line sedative agent after neonatal cardiac surgery: retrospective Cohort study. Pediatr Crit Care Med. 2016.

91. Hunseler C, Balling G, Rohlig C, Blickheuser R, Trieschmann U, Lieser U, et al. Continuous infusion of clonidine in ventilated newborns and infants: a randomized controlled trial. Pediatr Crit Care Med. 2014;15(6):511–22.

92. Tobias JD. Dexmedetomidine: are tolerance and withdrawal going to be an issue with long-term infusions? Pediatr Crit Care Med. 2010;11(1):158–60.

93. Tobias JD. Dexmedetomidine: applications in pediatric critical care and pediatric anesthesiology. Pediatr Crit Care Med. 2007;8 (2):115–31.

94. Gupta P, Whiteside W, Sabati A, Tesoro TM, Gossett JM, Tobias JD, et al. Safety and efficacy of prolonged dexmedetomidine use in critically ill children with heart disease*. Pediatr Crit Care Med. 2012;13(6):660–6.

95. Lam F, Ransom C, Gossett JM, Kelkhoff A, Seib PM, Schmitz ML, et al. Safety and efficacy of dexmedetomidine in children with heart failure. Pediatr Cardiol. 2013;34(4):835–41.

96. Walker J, Maccallum M, Fischer C, Kopcha R, Saylors R, McCall J. Sedation using dexmedetomidine in pediatric burn patients. J Burn Care Res. 2006;27(2):206–10.

97. Erkonen G, Lamb F, Tobias JD. High-dose dexmedetomidine-induced hypertension in a child with traumatic brain injury. Neurocrit Care. 2008;9(3):366–9.

98. Sanders RD, Sun P, Patel S, Li M, Maze M, Ma D. Dexmedetomidine provides cortical neuroprotection: impact on anaesthetic-induced neuroapoptosis in the rat developing brain. Acta Anaesthesiol Scand. 2010;54(6):710–6.

99. Sanders RD, Xu J, Shu Y, Januszewski A, Halder S, Fidalgo A, et al. Dexmedetomidine attenuates isoflurane-induced neurocognitive impairment in neonatal rats. Anesthesiology. 2009;110(5):1077–85.

100. Tachibana K, Hashimoto T, Kato R, Uchida Y, Ito R, Takita K, et al. Neonatal administration with dexmedetomidine does not impair the rat hippocampal synaptic plasticity later in adulthood. Paediatr Anaesth. 2012;22(7):713–9.

101. Bray RJ. Propofol infusion syndrome in children. Paediatr Anaesth. 1998;8(6):491–9.

102. Bray RJ. Propofol-infusion syndrome in children. Lancet. 1999;353(9169):2074–5.

103. Koriyama H, Duff JP, Guerra GG, Chan AW. Is propofol a friend or a foe of the pediatric intensivist? Description of propofol use in a PICU*. Pediatr Crit Care Med. 2014;15(2):e66–71.

104. Marx CM, Smith PG, Lowrie LH, Hamlett KW, Ambuel B, Yamashita TS, et al. Optimal sedation of mechanically ventilated pediatric critical care patients. Crit Care Med. 1994;22 (1):163–70.

105. Ista E, van Dijk M, Tibboel D, de Hoog M. Assessment of sedation levels in pediatric intensive care patients can be improved by using the COMFORT "behavior" scale. Pediatr Crit Care Med. 2005;6(1):58–63.

106. Curley MA, Harris SK, Fraser KA, Johnson RA, Arnold JH. State Behavioral Scale: a sedation assessment instrument for infants and young children supported on mechanical ventilation. Pediatr Crit Care Med. 2006;7(2):107–14.

107. Ramsay MA, Savege TM, Simpson BR, Goodwin R. Controlled sedation with alphaxalone-alphadolone. Br Med J. 1974;2 (5920):656–9.

108. Sessler CN, Gosnell MS, Grap MJ, Brophy GM, O'Neal PV, Keane KA, et al. The Richmond Agitation-Sedation Scale: validity and reliability in adult intensive care unit patients. Am J Respir Crit Care Med. 2002;166(10):1338–44.

109. Razmus I, Clarke K, Naufel K. Development of a sedation scale for the mechanically ventilated muscle relaxed pediatric critical care patient. Pediatr Intensive Care Nurs. 2003;4(1):7–11.

110. Dorfman TL, Sumamo Schellenberg E, Rempel GR, Scott SD, Hartling L. An evaluation of instruments for scoring physiological and behavioral cues of pain, non-pain related distress, and adequacy of analgesia and sedation in pediatric mechanically ventilated patients: A systematic review. Int J Nurs Stud. 2014;51(4):654–76.

111. Curley MA, Wypij D, Watson RS, Grant MJ, Asaro LA, Cheifetz IM, et al. Protocolized sedation vs usual care in pediatric patients mechanically ventilated for acute respiratory failure: a randomized clinical trial. JAMA. 2015;313 (4):379–89.

112. Neunhoeffer F, Kumpf M, Renk H, Hanelt M, Berneck N, Bosk A, et al. Nurse-driven pediatric analgesia and sedation protocol reduces withdrawal symptoms in critically ill medical pediatric patients. Paediatr Anaesth. 2015;25(8):786–94.

113. Schieveld JN, Janssen NJ. Delirium in the pediatric patient: on the growing awareness of its clinical interdisciplinary importance. JAMA Pediatr. 2014;168(7):595–6.

114. Silver G, Traube C, Gerber LM, Sun X, Kearney J, Patel A, et al. Pediatric delirium and associated risk factors: a single-center prospective observational study. Pediatr Crit Care Med. 2015;16 (4):303–9.

115. Traube C, Silver G, Kearney J, Patel A, Atkinson TM, Yoon MJ, et al. Cornell Assessment of Pediatric Delirium: a valid, rapid, observational tool for screening delirium in the PICU*. Crit Care Med. 2014;42(3):656–63.

116. Stamper MJ, Hawks SJ, Taicher BM, Bonta J, Brandon DH. Identifying pediatric emergence delirium by using the PAED Scale: a quality improvement project. AORN J. 2014;99 (4):480–94.

117. American Psychiatric Association, editor. Diagnostic and statistical manual of mental disorders. 5th ed. Arlington: American Psychiatric Publishing; 2013. p. 596.

118. European delirium association, American delirium society. The DSM-5 criteria, level of arousal and delirium diagnosis: inclusiveness is safer. BMC Med. 2014;12:141.

119. WHO. Mental and behavioural disorders 2015. Available from: http://apps.who.int/classifications/icd10/browse/2015/en#/F00-F09.

120. Hermus IP, Willems SJ, Bogman AC, Brabers L, Schieveld JN. "Delirium" is no delirium: on type specifying and drug response. Crit Care Med. 2015;43(12):e589.

121. Colville G, Pierce C. Patterns of post-traumatic stress symptoms in families after paediatric intensive care. Intensive Care Med. 2012;38(9):1523–31.

122. Silver G, Traube C, Kearney J, Kelly D, Yoon MJ, Nash Moyal W, et al. Detecting pediatric delirium: development of a rapid observational assessment tool. Intensive Care Med. 2012;38 (6):1025–31.

123. Sikich N, Lerman J. Development and psychometric evaluation of the pediatric anesthesia emergence delirium scale. Anesthesiology. 2004;100(5):1138–45.

124. Smith HA, Boyd J, Fuchs DC, Melvin K, Berry P, Shintani A, et al. Diagnosing delirium in critically ill children: validity and reliability of the Pediatric Confusion Assessment Method for the Intensive Care Unit. Crit Care Med. 2011;39(1):150–7.
125. van Dijk M, Knoester H, van Beusekom BS, Ista E. Screening pediatric delirium with an adapted version of the Sophia Observation withdrawal Symptoms scale (SOS). Intensive Care Med. 2012;38(3):531–2.
126. Smith HA, Gangopadhyay M, Goben CM, Jacobowski NL, Chestnut MH, Savage S, et al. The preschool confusion assessment method for the ICU: valid and reliable delirium monitoring for critically ill infants and children. Crit Care Med. 2016;44 (3):592–600.
127. Schieveld JN, Hermus IP, Oomen JW. Delirium in preschool children: diagnostic challenge, piece of cake, or both? Crit Care Med. 2016;44(3):646–7.
128. Groves A, Traube C, Silver G. Detection and management of delirium in the neonatal unit: a case series. Pediatrics. 2016;137 (3):1–4.
129. Brahmbhatt K, Whitgob E. Diagnosis and management of delirium in critically ill infants: case report and review. Pediatrics. 2016;137(3):1–5.
130. Marcantonio ER, Flacker JM, Wright RJ, Resnick NM. Reducing delirium after hip fracture: a randomized trial. J Am Geriatr Soc. 2001;49(5):516–22.
131. Schieveld JN, Leroy PL, van Os J, Nicolai J, Vos GD, Leentjens AF. Pediatric delirium in critical illness: phenomenology, clinical correlates and treatment response in 40 cases in the pediatric intensive care unit. Intensive Care Med. 2007;33(6):1033–40.
132. Kim SJ, Oh YJ, Kim KJ, Kwak YL, Na S. The effect of recorded maternal voice on perioperative anxiety and emergence in children. Anaesth Intensive Care. 2010;38(6):1064–9.
133. Hatherill S, Flisher AJ, Nassen R. Delirium among children and adolescents in an urban sub-Saharan African setting. J Psychosom Res. 2010;69(2):187–92.
134. Daoud A, Duff JP, Joffe AR. Diagnostic accuracy of delirium diagnosis in pediatric intensive care: a systematic review. Crit Care. 2014;18(5):489.
135. Kanburoglu MK, Derinoz O, Cizmeci MN, Havali C. Is acute dystonia an emergency? Sometimes, it really is! Pediatr Emerg Care. 2013;29(3):380–2.
136. Meyer-Massetti C, Cheng CM, Sharpe BA, Meier CR, Guglielmo BJ. The FDA extended warning for intravenous haloperidol and torsades de pointes: how should institutions respond? J Hosp Med. 2010;5(4):E8–16.
137. Jensen KG, Juul K, Fink-Jensen A, Correll CU, Pagsberg AK. Corrected QT changes during antipsychotic treatment of children and adolescents: a systematic review and meta-analysis of clinical trials. J Am Acad Child Adolesc Psychiatry. 2015;54 (1):25–36.
138. Schieveld JN, van der Valk JA, Smeets I, Berghmans E, Wassenberg R, Leroy PL, et al. Diagnostic considerations regarding pediatric delirium: a review and a proposal for an algorithm for pediatric intensive care units. Intensive Care Med. 2009;35 (11):1843–9.
139. Esseveld MM, Leroy PL, Leue C, Strik J, Tijssen M, van de Riet EH, et al. Catatonia and refractory agitation in an updated flow chart for the evaluation of emotional-behavioral disturbances in severely ill children. Intensive Care Med. 2013;39(3):528–9.
140. Hales RE, Yudofsky SC. Textbook of psychiatry. 2nd ed. Washington, DC: The American Psychiatric Press; 1992. p. 291–310.
141. van der Zwaan S, Blankespoor RJ, Wolters AM, Creten C, Leroy PL, Schieveld JN. Additional use of methotrimeprazine for treating refractory agitation in pediatric patients. Intensive Care Med. 2012;38(1):175–6.

142. Tobias JD, Deshpande JK, Pietsch JB, Wheeler TJ, Gregory DF. Pentobarbital sedation for patients in the pediatric intensive care unit. South Med J. 1995;88(3):290–4.
143. Yanay O, Brogan TV, Martin LD. Continuous pentobarbital infusion in children is associated with high rates of complications. J Crit Care. 2004;19(3):174–8.
144. Nielsen RM, Olsen KS, Lauritsen AO, Boesen HC. Electroconvulsive therapy as a treatment for protracted refractory delirium in the intensive care unit–five cases and a review. J Crit Care. 2014;29(5):881 e1–6.
145. Keogh SJ, Long DA, Horn DV. Practice guidelines for sedation and analgesia management of critically ill children: a pilot study evaluating guideline impact and feasibility in the PICU. BMJ Open. 2015;5(3), e006428.
146. Baron R, Binder A, Biniek R, Braune S, Buerkle H, Dall P, et al. Evidence and consensus based guideline for the management of delirium, analgesia, and sedation in intensive care medicine. Revision 2015 (DAS-Guideline 2015) – short version. German Med Sci. 2015;13:Doc19.
147. Lucas SS, Nasr VG, Ng AJ, Joe C, Bond M, DiNardo JA. Pediatric Cardiac Intensive Care Society 2014 consensus statement: pharmacotherapies in cardiac critical care: sedation, analgesia and muscle relaxant. Pediatr Crit Care Med. 2016;17(3 Suppl 1): S3–15.
148. Burry L, Rose L, McCullagh IJ, Fergusson DA, Ferguson ND, Mehta S. Daily sedation interruption versus no daily sedation interruption for critically ill adult patients requiring invasive mechanical ventilation. Cochrane Database Syst Rev. 2014;7, CD009176.
149. Verlaat CW, Heesen GP, Vet NJ, de Hoog M, van der Hoeven JG, Kox M, et al. Randomized controlled trial of daily interruption of sedatives in critically ill children. Paediatr Anaesth. 2014;24 (2):151–6.
150. Gupta K, Gupta VK, Jayashree M, Singhi S. Randomized controlled trial of interrupted versus continuous sedative infusions in ventilated children. Pediatr Crit Care Med. 2012;13(2):131–5.
151. Vet NJ, de Wildt SN, Verlaat CW, Knibbe CA, Mooij MG, van Woensel JB, et al. A randomized controlled trial of daily sedation interruption in critically ill children. Intensive Care Med. 2016;42 (2):233–44.
152. Davidson A, Flick RP. Neurodevelopmental implications of the use of sedation and analgesia in neonates. Clin Perinatol. 2013;40 (3):559–73.
153. Weisman SJ, Bernstein B, Schechter NL. Consequences of inadequate analgesia during painful procedures in children. Arch Pediatr Adolesc Med. 1998;152(2):147–9.
154. Wintgens A, Boileau B, Robaey P. Posttraumatic stress symptoms and medical procedures in children. Can J Psychiatry. 1997;42 (6):611–6.
155. Tobias JD. Tolerance, withdrawal, and physical dependency after long-term sedation and analgesia of children in the pediatric intensive care unit. Crit Care Med. 2000;28(6):2122–32.
156. Fonsmark L, Rasmussen YH, Carl P. Occurrence of withdrawal in critically ill sedated children. Crit Care Med. 1999;27(1):196–9.
157. Anand KJ, Willson DF, Berger J, Harrison R, Meert KL, Zimmerman J, et al. Tolerance and withdrawal from prolonged opioid use in critically ill children. Pediatrics. 2010;125(5): e1208–25.
158. Ista E, de Hoog M, Tibboel D, Duivenvoorden HJ, van Dijk M. Psychometric evaluation of the Sophia Observation withdrawal symptoms scale in critically ill children. Pediatr Crit Care Med. 2013;14(8):761–9.
159. Ista E, van Dijk M, de Hoog M, Tibboel D, Duivenvoorden HJ. Construction of the Sophia Observation withdrawal Symptoms-scale (SOS) for critically ill children. Intensive Care Med. 2009;35(6):1075–81.

160. Franck LS, Scoppettuolo LA, Wypij D, Curley MA. Validity and generalizability of the Withdrawal Assessment Tool-1 (WAT-1) for monitoring iatrogenic withdrawal syndrome in pediatric patients. Pain. 2012;153(1):142–8.

161. Siddappa R, Fletcher JE, Heard AM, Kielma D, Cimino M, Heard CM. Methadone dosage for prevention of opioid withdrawal in children. Paediatr Anaesth. 2003;13(9):805–10.

162. Krauss B, Green SM. Procedural sedation and analgesia in children. Lancet. 2006;367(9512):766–80.

163. Mason KP. Pediatric sedation outside of the operating room: a multispecialty international collaboration. 2nd ed. New York: Springer; 2015.

164. Cote CJ, Notterman DA, Karl HW, Weinberg JA, McCloskey C. Adverse sedation events in pediatrics: a critical incident analysis of contributing factors. Pediatrics. 2000;105(4 Pt 1):805–14.

165. Barbi E, Petaros P, Badina L, Pahor T, Giuseppin I, Biasotto E, et al. Deep sedation with propofol for upper gastrointestinal endoscopy in children, administered by specially trained pediatricians: a prospective case series with emphasis on side effects. Endoscopy. 2006;38(4):368–75.

166. Cravero JP, Cote CJ. Raising the bar for pediatric sedation studies and trials. Paediatr Anaesth. 2015;25(1):2–4.

167. Couloures KG, Beach M, Cravero JP, Monroe KK, Hertzog JH. Impact of provider specialty on pediatric procedural sedation complication rates. Pediatrics. 2011;127(5):e1154–60.

168. Cravero JP. Risk and safety of pediatric sedation/anesthesia for procedures outside the operating room. Curr Opin Anaesthesiol. 2009;22(4):509–13.

169. Cravero JP, Beach ML, Blike GT, Gallagher SM, Hertzog JH. The incidence and nature of adverse events during pediatric sedation/anesthesia with propofol for procedures outside the operating room: a report from the Pediatric Sedation Research Consortium. Anesth Analg. 2009;108(3):795–804.

170. Monroe KK, Beach M, Reindel R, Badwan L, Couloures KG, Hertzog JH, et al. Analysis of procedural sedation provided by pediatricians. Pediatr Int. 2013;55(1):17–23.

171. Vespasiano M, Finkelstein M, Kurachek S. Propofol sedation: intensivists' experience with 7304 cases in a children's hospital. Pediatrics. 2007;120(6):e1411–7.

172. Anderson JL, Junkins E, Pribble C, Guenther E. Capnography and depth of sedation during propofol sedation in children. Ann Emerg Med. 2007;49(1):9–13.

173. Krauss B, Hess DR. Capnography for procedural sedation and analgesia in the emergency department. Ann Emerg Med. 2007;50(2):172–81.

174. Chiaretti A, Benini F, Pierri F, Vecchiato K, Ronfani L, Agosto C, et al. Safety and efficacy of propofol administered by paediatricians during procedural sedation in children. Acta Paediatr. 2013

175. Baxter AL, Ewing PH, Young GB, Ware A, Evans N, Manworren RC. EMLA application exceeding two hours improves pediatric emergency department venipuncture success. Adv Emerg Nurs J. 2013;35(1):67–75.

176. Davies RJ. Buffering the pain of local anaesthetics: a systematic review. Emergency medicine. Emerg Med (Fremantle, WA). 2003;15(1):81–8.

177. Seith RW, Theophilos T, Babl FE. Intranasal fentanyl and high-concentration inhaled nitrous oxide for procedural sedation: a prospective observational pilot study of adverse events and depth of sedation. Acad Emerg Med. 2012;19(1):31–6.

178. Murphy A, O'Sullivan R, Wakai A, Grant TS, Barrett MJ, Cronin J, et al. Intranasal fentanyl for the management of acute pain in children. Cochrane Database Syst Rev (Online). 2014;10: CD009942.

179. Green SM, Roback MG, Krauss B, Brown L, McGlone RG, Agrawal D, et al. Predictors of emesis and recovery agitation with emergency department ketamine sedation: an individual-patient data meta-analysis of 8,282 children. Ann Emerg Med. 2009;54(2):171–80 e1-4.

180. Treston G, Bell A, Cardwell R, Fincher G, Chand D, Cashion G. What is the nature of the emergence phenomenon when using intravenous or intramuscular ketamine for paediatric procedural sedation? Emerg Med Australasia. 2009;21(4):315–22.

181. Leeuwenburgh-Pronk WG, Miller-Smith L, Forman V, Lantos JD, Tibboel D, Buysse C. Are we allowed to discontinue medical treatment in this child? Pediatrics. 2015;135(3):545–9.

182. Morrison W, Kang T. Judging the quality of mercy: drawing a line between palliation and euthanasia. Pediatrics. 2014;133 Suppl 1: S31–6.

183. Clement de Cley S, Friedel M, Verhagen AA, Lantos JD, Carter BS. Please do whatever it takes to end our daughter's suffering! Pediatrics. 2016;137(1):1–6.

184. Kiman R, Wuiloud AC, Requena ML. End of life care sedation for children. Curr Opin Support Palliat Care. 2011;5(3):285–90.

185. Schildmann EK, Schildmann J, Kiesewetter I. Medication and monitoring in palliative sedation therapy: a systematic review and quality assessment of published guidelines. J Pain Symptom Manag. 2015;49(4):734–46.

186. Kovacs J, Casey N, Weixler D. Palliative sedation in pediatric oncology. Wien Med Wochenschr. 2008;158(23-24):659–63.

187. Postovsky S, Moaed B, Krivoy E, Ofir R, Ben Arush MW. Practice of palliative sedation in children with brain tumors and sarcomas at the end of life. Pediatr Hematol Oncol. 2007;24 (6):409–15.

188. Vallero SG, Lijoi S, Bertin D, Pittana LS, Bellini S, Rossi F, et al. End-of-life care in pediatric neuro-oncology. Pediatr Blood Cancer. 2014;61(11):2004–11.

189. Korzeniewska-Eksterowicz A, Przyslo L, Fendler W, Stolarska M, Mlynarski W. Palliative sedation at home for terminally ill children with cancer. J Pain Symptom Manag. 2014;48(5):968–74.

190. Lundstrom S, Zachrisson U, Furst CJ. When nothing helps: propofol as sedative and antiemetic in palliative cancer care. J Pain Symptom Manag. 2005;30(6):570–7.

191. McWilliams K, Keeley PW, Waterhouse ET. Propofol for terminal sedation in palliative care: a systematic review. J Palliat Med. 2010;13(1):73–6.

192. Tobias JD. Propofol sedation for terminal care in a pediatric patient. Clin Pediatr (Phila). 1997;36(5):291–3.

193. Anghelescu DL, Hamilton H, Faughnan LG, Johnson LM, Baker JN. Pediatric palliative sedation therapy with propofol: recommendations based on experience in children with terminal cancer. J Palliat Med. 2012;15(10):1082–90.

194. Tobias JD. Subcutaneous dexmedetomidine infusions to treat or prevent drug withdrawal in infants and children. J Opioid Manag. 2008;4(4):187–91.

195. Prommer E. Review article: dexmedetomidine: does it have potential in palliative medicine? Am J Hosp Palliat Care. 2011;28(4):276–83.

196. Hohl CM, Stenekes S, Harlos MS, Shepherd E, McClement S, Chochinov HM. Methotrimeprazine for the management of end-of-life symptoms in infants and children. J Palliat Care. 2013;29 (3):178–85.

TCI and TIVA for Neurosurgery: Considerations and Techniques

28

Massimo Lamperti and Fazil Ashiq

The main goals of neurosurgical anesthesia are to provide the patient with an adequate anesthetic that provides a stable hemodynamics, reduces cerebral metabolism, avoids intracranial hypertension, avoids interference with intraoperative neuromonitoring, and allows rapid emergence from anesthesia for neurological examination [1]. Volatile anesthetics combined with synthetic opioids have been used in the past years for neurosurgical procedures because these combinations allow for rapid recovery and prompt neurological assessment [2, 3]. However, volatile anesthetics have been shown to affect cerebral autoregulation [4] and intracranial pressure (ICP) [2, 5], which can make the surgery more difficult and dangerous, increasing the risk of ischemic cerebral insults.

The modern use of total intravenous anesthesia (TIVA) began in the late 1970s with the introduction of propofol which was then combined with synthetic opioids [6–8] to provide general anesthesia (GA) during cranial procedures and spine surgery. Propofol, barbiturates (thiopental), and etomidate have minimal effect on or even decrease ICP [9]. A clear advantage of this new anesthetic technique was the fast recovery and a reduction in postoperative side effects as nausea and vomiting when compared to inhalational anesthetics [10].

It is important to understand how the normal brain and nervous system are affected during general anesthesia to avoid overdosing anesthetic drugs causing an intraoperative impairment of cerebral autoregulation and postoperative adverse events such as delirium and delayed awakening.

In specific conditions such as in patients with acute brain injuries (traumatic brain injury, subarachnoid hemorrhage,

intraparenchymal hemorrhage) and acute spine trauma, one of the major goals is to avoid secondary neuronal injuries caused by administration of anesthetics (and their consequences such as hypotension) if our patients should have to undergo emergent neurosurgical procedures. For these reasons, it is essential to have continuous monitoring of the depth of anesthesia and where appropriate of the spinal pathways during the intraoperative period [11, 12].

More recently, target-controlled infusion (TCI) of intravenous anesthetics has been introduced during neurosurgical procedures. The use of these new anesthetic techniques associated with an accurate depth of anesthesia monitoring represents an open field of research in terms of recovery and outcome.

Neurophysiology of the Brain During Anesthesia

Assessment of Consciousness During General Anesthesia

Loss of consciousness is an essential element of general anesthesia (GA) [13], but anesthesiologists have no reliable ways to be certain that a patient is unconscious. In practice, responsiveness to verbal commands is the standard method to assess the level of consciousness [14]. However, the level of consciousness cannot be reliably assessed in patients who are paralyzed by neuromuscular blocking agents [15]. The standards for assessing if patients are adequately anesthetized include indirect measures of brain state—such as changes in heart rate and blood pressure, which reflect sympathetic activity, and muscle tone—along with estimated blood and brain concentrations of intravenous anesthetics, presumed pharmacodynamic effects thereof, and, for inhaled anesthetics, the exhaled anesthetic agent concentrations.

M. Lamperti, MD (✉) • F. Ashiq, MD
Anesthesiology Institute, Cleveland Clinic Abu Dhabi (CCAD),
Swing Wing L7, Al Maryah Island, P O Box# 112412,
Abu Dhabi, United Arab Emirates
e-mail: LamperM@clevelandclinicabudhabi.ae;
AshiqF@clevelandclinicabudhabi.ae

© Springer International Publishing AG 2017
A.R. Absalom, K.P. Mason (eds.), *Total Intravenous Anesthesia and Target Controlled Infusions*,
DOI 10.1007/978-3-319-47609-4_28

The electroencephalogram (EEG), which measures scalp electrical potentials generated by cortical postsynaptic currents [16], has long been considered the most feasible approach for tracking brain states under GA. Despite attempts to characterize EEG morphology under GA [17, 18], reading the EEG has not become part of routine anesthesiology practice. A variety of EEG patterns are known to arise during GA maintained by both GABA-A receptor-specific and ether-derived anesthetics. These EEG patterns include increases in frontal EEG power [19, 20], a shift in EEG power toward lower frequencies (alpha from 8 to 12 Hz and delta 0–4 Hz) [21], changes in coherence [22, 23], and burst suppression and isoelectricity [24].

The relationship between these or other EEG patterns and the loss and recovery of consciousness remain poorly understood. In particular, it has been difficult to identify specific EEG signatures that are associated with the point of loss of consciousness (LOC), because most anesthesia-related EEG data come from clinical settings in which GA induction is performed rapidly, causing the crucial transition from consciousness to unconsciousness within 30–60 s [25]. Compounding this rapid LOC is the problem of measuring level of consciousness. The most common approach is to ask patients to respond to a verbal or physical stimulus and rate the quality of responses on a 0–5 numerical scale [26]. This highly subjective assessment usually is repeated on a time scale of minutes [27] and resolves poorly the time point at which consciousness is lost or regained. EEG signatures that predict return of consciousness have been difficult to establish for similar reasons. Purdon and colleagues studied the relationship between EEG activity and the LOC and recovery of consciousness (ROC) [28] recording high-density EEGs while administering increasing and decreasing doses of propofol to healthy volunteers who were executing an auditory-response task used to assess conscious behavior. They used a propofol TCI from 0 to 5 μg/ml and then decreased the target-effect site concentration to 0 μg/ml. They found that LOC was marked simultaneously by an increase in low-frequency EEG power (<1 Hz), the loss of spatially coherent occipital alpha oscillations (8–12 Hz), and the appearance of spatially coherent frontal alpha oscillations. These dynamics reversed with recovery of consciousness. The low-frequency phase modulated alpha amplitude in two distinct patterns. During profound unconsciousness, alpha amplitudes were maximal at low-frequency peaks, whereas during the transition into and out of unconsciousness, alpha amplitudes were maximal at low-frequency nadirs. This latter phase–amplitude relationship predicted recovery of consciousness. Their findings can be used to track transitions into and out of unconsciousness.

Commercially available monitors for bispectral analysis are unable to detect these modulation patterns most likely because the broad range of frequencies that are pooled together (0.5–47 Hz) cancels out phase information.

In some neurosurgical patients, these neurophysiological monitoring techniques are not always possible or are only partially possible (e.g., when a full EEG montage cannot be used) when the underlying brain tissue can be altered because of an inflammatory process or a tumor. Nonetheless, it is surprising how much reliable information concerning the depth of anesthesia is still found in the EEG.

The situation appears to be more promising with regard to sensory-evoked potentials, in particular auditory-evoked potentials (AEPs). AEPs are obtained by giving a series of very brief tones via headphones to a normal subject and then recording and averaging the resulting electrical potential over the scalp. The middle latency response (MLR) lasts from 10 ms to about 100 ms following stimulus onset, arises from the auditory cortex, and resembles three to five cycles of a 40 Hz wave [29]. Later responses such as the P300 wave peaking at 300 ms can be greatly enhanced with selective attention [30]. Madler and colleagues studied the effect of various anesthetics on the 40 Hz oscillations in the MLR [31]. For patients anesthetized with Pentothal or propofol, the 30–40 Hz oscillations shifted to lower frequencies (10Hz or less) or even disappeared. Nonspecific gas anesthetics such as isoflurane or enflurane are associated with a concentration-dependent reduction in the oscillatory frequency of the AEPs. However, these 30–40 Hz oscillations were not abolished by receptor-specific agents, such as fentanyl, ketamine, or various benzodiazepines. The same authors conclude that as long as 30–40 Hz oscillations are present, the patient is still to some extent conscious. The above results become more significant when seen in the light of other reports [31] of stimulus-induced 40–60 Hz oscillations in the neuronal discharge of neurons in the visual cortex of the anesthetized and the awake cat.

Anesthetic Drugs and Models Used for Intravenous Anesthesia in Neurosurgery

Anesthetic Drugs

The use of intravenous agents for induction and maintenance of general anesthesia during neurosurgical procedures is becoming more popular than in the past when the use of TIVA was not supported by sufficient evidence and accurate pharmacokinetic models (and the necessary computer power) were not available to guide or even control the administration of intravenous drugs [3].

Propofol shares with volatile anesthetics the important attribute of depressing cerebral metabolic rate [32], but, in common with other intravenous agents, it causes cerebral vasoconstriction in proportion to the suppression of metabolic rate [33]. Propofol has clear advantages as it is able to maintain stable the cerebral blood volume hence preserving autoregulation and vascular reactivity [34]. In a randomized prospective study of neurosurgical patients undergoing craniotomy for cerebral tumors with propofol, the patients presented lower ICP, less cerebral swelling at the opening of the dura, and higher CPP than those anesthetized with volatile anesthetics [35]. There are still some conflicting results on the effect of propofol on CBF as in healthy subjects it has been demonstrated to significantly reduce both CBF and jugular venous oxygen saturation when compared to sevoflurane, especially when associated with hypocapnia [36] although recent data show that increases in propofol concentrations do not affect jugular venous bulb oxygen saturations within the dose range used clinically [37].

Remifentanil can be considered a valuable component of neuroanesthetic pharmacology. When it was compared with fentanyl in a randomized, multiinstitutional, double-blinded, prospective trial [38], it was found to be a reasonable alternative to fentanyl during elective supratentorial craniotomy for space-occupying lesions. The frequency of adverse events, hemodynamic profiles, and median recovery times were generally similar between groups. However, 7 of 32 patients in the fentanyl group required naloxone to recover from anesthesia compared with no patients in the remifentanil group. More recently, another randomized controlled trial [39] compared remifentanil and fentanyl when used in patients undergoing surgical procedures to remove intracranial space-occupying lesions. Remifentanil was given according to manufacturer recommendations. Fentanyl was given according to the usual practice of the anesthesiologist. The study demonstrated no differences between opioid groups for the frequency of responses to intubation, pinhead holder placement, skin incision, or closure of the surgical wound. Adverse event frequencies were similar between groups. Times to follow verbal commands and tracheal extubation were more rapid for remifentanil. The percentage of patients with a normal recovery score at 10 min after surgery was higher when remifentanil was used. The study demonstrated a lesser need for opioid use when remifentanil was associated with isoflurane leading to a faster recovery from anesthesia. The association of propofol–remifentanil has shown a reduced risk of coughing during emergence [40], and this is desirable after neurosurgical and neurointerventional procedures, where coughing can precipitously increase the ICP.

The use of sufentanil–propofol TIVA was compared to remifentanil–propofol [41], and both regimens had similar results in terms of postoperative nausea and vomiting, shivering, and respiratory depression. The sufentanil–propofol regimen had a better outcome in terms of reduced supplemental postoperative analgesic requirements and better postoperative cognitive recovery than in the remifentanil–propofol group.

Dexmedetomidine (DEX) has been introduced to clinical anesthesia for its sympatholytic, sedative, anesthetic sparing and hemodynamic stabilizing properties without significant respiratory depression. Its role during general anesthesia for neurosurgical procedures has been validated as an adjunct to other agents to decrease the intraoperative opioid dose requirements [42]. Animal and human studies [43, 44] have shown that DEX causes a reduction in CBF and cerebral metabolism rate of oxygen ($CMRO_2$) and suggest a careful control during its administration to avoid hazardous hypotension and a reduction in the cerebral autoregulation. Its role as an intravenous anesthetic agent has been studied as an adjunct to local anesthesia during awake anesthesia [45] or as an adjunct to TIVA techniques including remifentanil [43] during which it decreased allowed analgesic requirements and improved hemodynamic stability. A possible disadvantage could be related to its prolonged sedative effect when used as an adjunct to propofol although this has not been demonstrated in clinical studies. Anesthesiologists must remain alert to the main complications occurring after neurosurgical procedures, which can also occur after TIVA administration, and include postoperative hypertension, shivering, and postoperative nausea and vomiting (PONV) [46]. Careful intraoperative management and choice of drugs and techniques may help reduce the incidence of these complications.

Anesthetic Techniques

Induction of anesthesia with anesthetic agents and opioids administered by manual injection can cause significant depression of the mean arterial pressure, apneic episodes, and chest wall rigidity. The introduction of TCI according to pharmacokinetic models facilitates smoother induction, with smaller doses, and slower infusion rates, than with manually administered and controlled infusions, and this may attenuate the reduction of mean blood pressure on induction.

The two main pharmacokinetic models used for TCI of propofol in neurosurgery are the Marsh model and the Schnider model [47]. The Schnider model requires the user to input age, height, gender, and total body weight during start-up of the TCI pump. The pump calculates the lean body mass for that patient and calculates doses and infusion rates accordingly. It is be more suitable in the elderly who have a lower lean body mass and provides smaller doses of propofol for induction and maintenance of a constant plasma concentration than in younger patients. The induction dose is small compared with that for manual administration (often

<50 %). Actual plasma levels are difficult to predict as neurosurgical patients are often taking enzyme-inducing anticonvulsants that can influence drug metabolism and thus the achieved plasma concentration. Final levels chosen on the TCI pump therefore may vary widely.

Induction of anesthesia with propofol can be achieved by titrating the dosage by 0.5–1 µg ml^{-1} up to reach loss of consciousness then maintaining the dosage between 3 and 4 µg ml^{-1} or starting at 4.5 µg ml^{-1} and increasing up to 7 µg ml^{-1} if required. Monitoring of depth of anesthesia is essential when using TCI, to facilitate titration of the target concentration according to a combination of depth of anesthesia and the hemodynamic response, to avoid excessively deep levels of anesthesia such as that associated with prolonged periods of burst suppression. A new model has been recently suggested in obese patients to improve the performance of the Marsh and Schnider models [48]

The most commonly used pharmacokinetic model for remifentanil in neuroanesthesia is the Minto model, which is a three-compartment pharmacokinetic model specific for remifentanil. This model was produced from a study of pharmacokinetics of remifentanil in a heterogeneous population of healthy adults [49]. As with propofol infusions, if blood targeting is used and rapid onset of anesthesia is required, then the blood concentration should be set to a level higher than the desired and likely therapeutic effect site concentration. After induction, target concentration has to be adjusted accordingly to blunt responses to placement of the Mayfield head holder and subsequent surgical stimuli. Typical target concentrations for remifentanil during induction and intubation are initially set at around 4–7 ng ml^{-1}. This could be soon reduced after intubation depending on the patients' clinical response. In the absence of muscle relaxants, target concentrations below 3 ng/ml are not advisable, as coughing and movement are more likely, even with reasonable propofol doses. Target remifentanil concentrations up to 10–15 ng/ml may be required during neurosurgical procedures involving cranial nerve stimulation or extensive craniotomies, but anesthesiologists should bear in mind that these high concentrations may be associated with acute tolerance or hyperalgesia. In any case, a careful neuromonitoring assessment with pEEG monitors should be performed to avoid excessive sedation and prolonged periods of burst suppression rate.

Propofol and remifentanil show synergistic interactions. Partly this is caused by pharmacokinetic interactions (remifentanil causes a 41 % decrease in apparent volume of distribution of propofol), but the drugs also have strongly synergistic pharmacodynamic interactions.

The pharmacokinetic model used for TCI administration of sufentanil infusion is the Gepts model with a target concentration at effect site of 0.5 ng ml^{-1}. When used in combination with propofol, it provides similar intraoperative hemodynamics, awakening and extubation times to propofol–remifentanil but with delayed cognitive recovery [50].

Older pharmacokinetic models for DEX (Dyck and Talke) tended to underpredict the plasma concentration at higher concentrations. Hannivoort has recently published a new combined PK model for DEX [51]

Monitoring the Brain and Spinal Cord During Intravenous Anesthesia

Electrophysiological monitoring is applied during cranial and spine surgery for monitoring and for mapping. Monitoring is used to detect early changes in the transmission of the applied or recorded signal that can predict damage to the nervous tissue, whereas mapping is used to guide surgical excision treatment during epilepsy surgery and excision of tumors in important speech or motor function areas.

Electrocorticography (ECoG) is frequently used for brain mapping during epileptic foci resection. When this is performed under general anesthesia, propofol dosage should be carefully titrated (to 1.8–2.0 µg ml^{-1}) to minimize the effect on the EEG, and an association with remifentanil (up to 10–15 ng ml^{-1}) is useful to avoid hypertension during dura opening and foci removal.

Another field of application of TCI is during deep-brain stimulation (DBS) a procedure increasingly used in treatment of Parkinson's disease, dystonia, and certain psychiatric disorders such a depression and obsessive–compulsive disorders. An awake technique is often preferred in many institutions although in some patients there is the need for general anesthesia or monitored anesthesia care to avoid severe movements caused by the "off-drug state" in these patients. Propofol and remifentanil are commonly used for electrode insertion for conscious sedation [52]. An alternative is a low-dose infusion (0.3–0.6 µg/kg/h) of dexmedetomidine, which has the advantages that its non-GABA-mediated mechanism of action has minimal effects on microelectrode recordings, and is associated with hemodynamic stability and analgesic properties.

EEG is usually monitored during craniotomy for cerebral aneurysm clipping, during carotid endarterectomy, cardiopulmonary bypass, extracranial–intracranial bypass procedures, and pharmacological depression of the brain for "cerebral protection." The EEG reflects the metabolic activity of the brain, and any factors adversely affecting the cerebral brain activity including anesthetics can impair the EEG activity. The use of TCI allows a constant level of anesthetic effect which can help to avoid misinterpretation of EEG depression caused by boluses or rapid changes in anesthetic level from true physiologic/pathologic insults to the cortex. A closed-loop communication between anesthesiologist, neurophysiologist, and neurosurgeon can guide the level of anesthesia during the critical phases of a complex surgery.

During spine surgery, somatosensory-evoked potentials (SSEP) have been introduced for neurological investigation and monitoring of the integrity of the neural pathways during surgical procedures. This technique allows an online surveillance and early diagnosis of spinal cord dysfunction and aims to provide warning signals before any irreversible damage has occurred. Owing to the sensitivity and specificity of SSEP monitoring, the incidence of postoperative paraplegia can be significantly reduced [53, 54]. TCI allows the determination of the amount of administered propofol and the estimation of the plasma propofol concentration. This allows long-duration, stable anesthesia and the possibility of comparable anesthesia. The intraoperative within-case variability of SSEP is of relevance in performing neuromonitoring during surgery. It is of importance to determine the range of SSEP variability, which can be expected due to specific protocols of anesthesia [55].

Motor-evoked potentials (MEP) are usually monitored to assess the motor pathways and avoid the need for a wake-up test. A report of paraplegia, despite normal MEP obtained by direct stimulation of the spinal cord, suggests that MEP should be measured using transcranial stimulation of the motor cortex (tcMEP). However, tcMEP recordings are markedly affected by anesthetics and a TCI infusion of propofol–remifentanil allowed recording and interpretation of tcMEP signals [56].

Auditory and visual-evoked potentials (VEP) are not commonly used during intraoperative neuromonitoring. The use of propofol strongly affects the amplitude of VEP and makes the use of these parameters during anesthesia for neurosurgical procedures unreliable [57].

Intravenous Anesthesia in Neurosurgery

Intravenous Anesthesia in Cranial Surgery

The ideal anesthetic agent for neurosurgery must allow for an uneventful induction, cardiovascular stability, little or no interference with cerebral autoregulation, and little effect on brain function to allow for electrophysiological monitoring, decreased ICP, brain relaxation, neuroprotection, reactivity to carbon dioxide, and rapid emergence to permit neurological evaluation.

The inhalational versus intravenous method of anesthesia debate to determine which method satisfies most of the required characteristics is still ongoing [58–60]. Total intravenous anesthesia has gained widespread popularity among anesthetists providing anesthesia for patients undergoing neurosurgery for intracranial tumors.

Intravenous agents have beneficial effects on cerebral blood flow (CBF) and autoregulation by decreasing the CBF by causing cerebral vasoconstriction as well as by reducing the cerebral metabolic rate. This effect is seen most with propofol and barbiturates and least with etomidate [61, 62]. Opioids have minimal effects on CBF. About 15 % of the cerebral blood volume (CBV) is in the arterial cerebral circulation, while about 15 % is within the venous sinuses. Intravenous agents like propofol decrease the CBV [63, 64]. This decrease in CBV, though small, can result in a decrease in ICP.

The combined use of inhalational as well as intravenous agents can have beneficial effects on ICP and may better preserve CPP [35].The prolonged use of intravenous agents will result in cerebral vasoconstriction and may result in cerebral hypoperfusion and ischemia. Opioids have minimal effects on ICP [38]. The cerebral metabolic oxygen rate ($CMRO_2$) is reduced by intravenous agents and can lead to decreased CBF, CBV, and ICP making it useful in patients with raised ICP. Propofol-maintained anesthesia when compared to volatile-maintained anesthesia was associated with lower mean ICP values and higher CPP values [65].

In the last decade, many studies have addressed the intravenous versus the volatile anesthesia method, and no significant differences were found between the study groups in terms of emergence times and early complications such as pain, postoperative nausea and vomiting, shivering, and seizures [59, 66, 67]. It is reasonable to speculate that delivering individualized anesthesia using target-controlled infusion of intravenous anesthetic drugs with depth of anesthesia monitoring might have resulted in improved recovery profiles for this group of patients [68–72].

A total intravenous anesthesia technique is the technique choice among many neuroanesthetists on the basis of an appraisal of the differences between propofol and potent inhalational agents on the cerebral vessels, CBF, and metabolism ($CMRO_2$) [73]. The CBF-$CMRO_2$ coupling is better maintained with propofol, whereas with volatile agents, their direct vasodilatory effects result in a loss of this coupling a doses >1 MAC, causing unnecessary increases in CBF, coupled with increases in ICP.

Intravenous Anesthesia in Functional Neurosurgery

Functional neurosurgery is concerned with the surgical management of conditions where the central nervous system (brain and spinal cord) physiology is altered without a gross anatomical or structural anomaly [74, 75]. The results are produced by interrupting or modifying malfunctional pathways and thus altering their physiology. The goal is to provide symptomatic relief to patients with movement disorders, chronic pain, and psychiatric disorders [76, 77].

The most common and well recognized of the movement disorders is Parkinson's disease (PD). The advent of computer-guided stereotactic surgery and deep-brain stimulation (DBS) fostered a renewed interest in the surgical management of PD. Deep-brain stimulators are implantable devices that consist of electrodes placed at the target brain structures connected by wires to a remotely placed module.

The anesthetic goals are to keep the patient responsive and cooperative for very long period of time, maintain stable hemodynamics, and minimize respiratory depression. DBS is a three-part procedure; the patient need only be responsive and cooperative during the second part. This has led to the use of the asleep–awake–asleep technique in which general anesthesia is provided for the first and third part [78–80].

The use of propofol with or without remifentanil offers rapid kinetics and easy titration. Oversedation, respiratory depression, and loss of patient cooperation can be overcome to a great extent with the use of brain function monitors [81, 82].

Dexmedetomidine has also been advocated for sedation during awake craniotomy. It produces a unique form of sedation due to its subcortical mode of action and allows the patient to transition easily between quiet sleep and cooperative wakefulness [83].

Intravenous Anesthesia in Vascular Neurosurgery

The agents used for induction and maintenance of general anesthesia should reflect the goals of anesthesia for any patient with an intracranial lesion. This includes the possibility of impaired autoregulation in and around hypervascular tumors, hemodynamic instability, and possible increase in ICP. There is no definite consensus between balanced anesthesia with inhalational agents and total IV anesthesia [84].

Intravenous Anesthesia in Pediatric Neurosurgery

The use of TCI in children is not very popular. Children have a larger central volume of distribution and a rapid clearance in comparison with adults. In the 1990s, the accuracy of TCI propofol using Marsh model in 20 children was studied and found to be associated with a significant overestimation in blood concentrations. Consistent findings from several groups found pharmacokinetics of propofol differs between

adults and children. Later models like the Paedfusor model performed better than the Marsh model [85]. Currently there are no large randomized trials to establish their efficiency. There have been several reports of metabolic acidosis, lipemia, and fatty liver infiltration with the use of prolonged propofol infusion in intensive care.

Future of Intravenous Anesthesia in Neurosurgical Procedures and Postoperative Neurocritical Care

The pharmacokinetic models estimated concentrations in the plasma or at effect site, but there is wide variation within and between patients. A large degree of interindividual variability is likely due to the pharmacogenomics of the patient, age, and the pharmacodynamic influence of neurological conditions. The new pharmacokinetic models for delivering general anesthesia during neurosurgical procedures should be driven by a closed-loop communication between the infusion pumps and depth of anesthesia in terms of suppression rate and spectrogram. In this way, it will be possible to optimally titrate sedative and hypnotic administration to avoid oversedation but also awareness.

A further improvement would be to extend the use of TCI not only to the perioperative period but to the ICU staying especially in patients with prolonged need for sedation or in the acute phase of primary brain insult.

There is a need for further confirmatory studies that will clearly demonstrate the safety and efficacy of TCI compared to inhalational anesthesia although the current literature provides some evidence of a better hemodynamic stability and enhanced recovery.

Conclusions

Total intravenous anesthesia delivered by TCI has been widely applied during neurosurgical procedures as it allows a better titration of the drugs and an improved interpretation of the neuromonitoring data. Depth of anesthesia monitoring is a fundamental tool for guidance of accurate titration of the dosage of drugs during TIVA and TCI for neurosurgical procedures.

References

1. Talke P, Caldwell J, Brown R, et al. A comparison of three anesthetic techniques in patients undergoing craniotomy for supratentorial intracranial surgery. Anesth Analg. 2002;95:430–5.
2. Magni G, Baisi F, La Rosa I, et al. No difference in emergence time and early cognitive function between sevoflurane-fentanyl and propofol-remifentanil in patients undergoing craniotomy for

supratentorial intracranial surgery. J Neurosurg Anesthesiol. 2005;17:134–8.

3. Todd M, Warner D, Sokoll M, et al. A prospective, comparative trial of three anesthetics for elective supratentorial craniotomy. Propofol/fentanyl, isoflurane/nitrous oxide, and fentanyl/nitrous oxide. Anesthesiology. 1993;78:1005–20.

4. Matta BF, Heath KJ, Tipping K. Direct cerebral vasodilatory effects of sevoflurane and isoflurane. Anesthesiology. 1999;91:677–80.

5. Strebel S, Lam A, Matta B, et al. Dynamic and static cerebral autoregulation during isoflurane, desflurane, and propofol anesthesia. Anesthesiology. 1995;83:66–76.

6. Kay B, Stephenson D. ICI 35868 (Diprivan): a new intravenous anaesthetic. A comparison with Althesin. Anaesthesia. 1980;35:1182–7.

7. Kay B, Rolly G. ICI 35868, a new intravenous induction agent. Acta Anaesthesiol Belg. 1977;28:303–16.

8. Walmsley A, McLeod B, Ponte J. The new formulation of ICI 35868 (propofol) as the main agent for minor surgical procedures. Eur J Anaesthesiol. 1986;3:19–26.

9. Ravussin P, Guinard J, Ralley F, et al. Effect of propofol on cerebrospinal fluid pressure and cerebral perfusion pressure in patients undergoing craniotomy. Anaesthesia. 1988;43 (Suppl):37–41.

10. Hans P, Bonhomme V. Why we still use intravenous drugs as the basic regimen for neurosurgical anaesthesia. Curr Opin Anaesthesiol. 2006;19:498–503.

11. Wiedemayer H, Sandalcioglu I, Armbruster W, et al. False negative findings in introperative SEP monitoring: analysis of 658 consecutive neurosurgical cases and review of published reports. J Neurol Neurosurg Psychiatry. 2004;75:280–6.

12. Hans P, Bonhomme V, Born J, et al. Target-controlled infusion of propofol and remifentanil combined with bispectral index monitoring for awake craniotomy. Anaesthesia. 2000;55:255–9.

13. Kissin I. General anesthetic action: an obsolete notion? Anesth Analg. 1993;76:215–8.

14. Posner J, Saper C, Schiff N, et al. Plum and Posner's diagnosis of stupor and coma. 4th ed. Philadelphia: Oxford University Press; 2007. p. 5–7.

15. Heier T, Steen P. Awareness in anaesthesia: incidence, consequences and prevention. Acta Anaesthesiol Scand. 1996;40:1073–86.

16. Niedermeyer E, Lopes da Silva F. Electroencephalography: basic principles, clinical applications, and related fields. 5th ed. Philadelphia: Lippincott Williams & Wilkins; 2005. p. xiii, 1309.

17. Gibbs F, Gibbs E, Lennox W. Effect on the electroencephalogram of certain drugs which influence nervous activity. Arch Intern Med. 1937;60:154–69.

18. Clark D, Rosner BS. Neurophysiologic effects of general anesthetics. I. The electroencephalogram and sensory evoked responses in man. Anesthesiology. 1973;38:564–82.

19. Gugino L, Chabot R, Prichepet L, et al. Quantitative EEG changes associated with loss and return of consciousness in healthy adult volunteers anesthetized with propofol or sevoflurane. Br J Anaesth. 2001;87:421–8.

20. Feshchenko V, Veselis R, Reinsel R. Propofol-induced alpha rhythm. Neuropsychobiology. 2004;50:257–66.

21. Rampil IJ, Matteo RS. Changes in EEG spectral edge frequency correlate with the hemodynamic response to laryngoscopy and intubation. Anesthesiology. 1987;67:139–42.

22. John E, Prichep L, Kox W, et al. Invariant reversible QEEG effects of anesthetics. Conscious Cogn. 2001;10:165–83.

23. Supp G, Siegel M, Hipp J, et al. Cortical hypersynchrony predicts breakdown of sensory processing during loss of consciousness. Curr Biol. 2011;21:1988–93.

24. Jäntti V, Yli-Hankala A, Baer G, et al. Slow potentials of EEG burst suppression pattern during anaesthesia. Acta Anaesthesiol Scand. 1993;37:121–3.

25. Brown E, Lydic R, Schiff ND. General anesthesia, sleep, and coma. N Engl J Med. 2010;363:2638–50.

26. Chernik D, Gillings D, Laine H, et al. Validity and reliability of the Observer's Assessment of Alertness/Sedation Scale: study with intravenous midazolam. J Clin Psychopharmacol. 1990;10:244–51.

27. Kearse LA, Rosow C, Zaslavsky A, et al. Bispectral analysis of the electroencephalogram predicts conscious processing of information during propofol sedation and hypnosis. Anesthesiology. 1998;88:25–34.

28. Purdon P, Pierce E, Mukamel E, et al. Electroencephalogram signatures of loss and recovery of consciousness from propofol. Proc Natl Acad Sci. 2013;110:E1142–51.

29. Galambos R, Makeig S, Talmachoff P. A 40-Hz auditory potential recorded from the human scalp. Proc Natl Acad Sci U S A. 1981;78:2643–7.

30. Hillyard S. Electrophysiology of human selective attention. Trends Neurosci. 1985;8:400–5.

31. Madler C, Keller I, Scwender D, et al. Sensory information processing during general anaesthesia:effect of isoflurane on auditory evoked neuronal oscillations. Br J Anaesth. 1991;66:81–7.

32. Alkire M, Haier R, Barker S, et al. Cerebral metabolism during propofol anesthesia in humans studied with positron emission tomography. Anesthesiology. 1995;53:393–403.

33. Eng C, Lam A, Mayberg T, et al. The influence of propofol with and without nitrous oxide on cerebral blood flow velocity and CO_2 reactivity in humans. Anesthesiology. 1992;53:872–9.

34. Conti A, Iacopino D, Fodale V, et al. Cerebral haemodynamic changes during propofol-remifentanil or sevoflurane anaesthesia: transcranial Doppler study under bispectral index monitoring. Br J Anaesth. 2006;97:333–9.

35. Petersen KD, Landsfeldt U, Cold G, et al. Intracranial pressure and cerebral haemodynamics in patients with cerebral tumours: a randomised prospective study of patients subjected to craniotomy in propofol–fentanyl, isoflurane–fentanyl, or sevoflurane–fentanyl anaesthesia. Anesthesiology. 2003;98:329–36.

36. Kawano Y, Kawaguchi M, Inoue S, et al. Jugular bulb oxygen saturation under propofol or sevoflurane/nitrous oxide anaesthesia during deliberate mild hypothermia in neurosurgical patients. J Neurosurg Anesthesiol. 2004;16:6–10.

37. Iwata M, Kawaguchi M, Inoue S, et al. The effects of increasing concentrations of propofol on jugular venous bulb oxygen saturation in neurosurgical patients under normothermic and mildly hypothermic conditions. Anesthesiology. 2006;104:33–8.

38. Guy J, Hindman B, Baker K, et al. Comparison of remifentanil and fentanyl in patients undergoing craniotomy for supratentorial space-occupying lesions. Anesthesiology. 1997;86:514–24.

39. Balakrishnan G, Raudzens P, Samra S, et al. A comparison of remifentanil and fentanyl in patients undergoing surgery for intracranial mass lesions. Anesth Analg. 2000;91:163–9.

40. Holrieder M, Tiefenthaler W, Klaus H, et al. Effect of total intravenous anaesthesia and balanced anaesthesia on the frequency of coughing during emergence from the anaesthesia. Br J Anaesth. 2007;99:587–91.

41. Martorano P, Aloj F, Baietta S, et al. Sufentanil-propofol vs remifentanil-propofol during total intravenous anesthesia for neurosurgery. A multicentre study. Minerva Anestesiol. 2008;74:233–43.

42. Tanskanen P, Kyttä J, Randell T, et al. Dexmedetomidine as an anaesthetic adjuvant in patients undergoing intracranial tumour surgery: a double-blind, randomized and placebo-controlled study. Br J Anaesth. 2006;97:658–65.

43. Karlsson B, Forsman M, Roald O, et al. Effect of dexmedetomidine, a selective and potent alpha agonist, on cerebral blood flow and

oxygen consumption during halothane anesthesia in dogs. Anesth Analg. 1990;71:125–9.

44. Drummond J, Dao A, Roth D, et al. Effect of dexmedetomidine on cerebral blood flow velocity, cerebral metabolic rate, and carbon dioxide response in normal humans. Anesthesiology. 2008;108:225–3.

45. Mack P, Perrine K, Kobylarz E, et al. Dexmedetomidine and neurocognitive testing in awake craniotomy. J Neurosurg Anaesthesiol. 2004;16:20–5.

46. Gunes Y, Gunduz M, Ozcengiz D, et al. Dexmedetomidine-remifentanil or propofol-remifentanil anesthesia in patients undergoing intracranial surgery. Neurosurger Quart. 2005;15:122–6.

47. Schnider T, Minto C, Gambus P, et al. The influence of method of administration and covariances on the pharmacokinetics of propofol in adult volunteers. Anesthesiology. 1998;88:1170–82.

48. Cortínez L, De la Fuente N, Eleveld D, et al. Performance of propofol target-controlled infusion models in the obese: pharmacokinetic and pharmacodynamic analysis. Anesth Analg. 2014;119:302–10.

49. Minto C, Schnider T, Shafer S. Pharmacokinetics and pharmacodynamics of remifentanil. II. Model application. Anesthesiology. 1997;86:24–33.

50. Bilotta F, Caramia R, Paolon F, et al. Early postoperative cognitive recovery after remifentanil–propofol or sufentanil–propofol anaesthesia for supratentorial craniotomy: a randomized trial. Eur J Anaesth. 2006;24:122–7.

51. Hannivoort L, Eleveld D, Proost J, et al. Development of an optimized pharmacokinetic model of dexmedetomidine using target-controlled infusion in healthy volunteers. Anesthesiology. 2015;123:357–67.

52. Keifer J, Dentchev D, Little K, et al. A retrospective analysis of a remifentanil/propofol general anesthetic for craniotomy before awake functional brain mapping. Anesth Analg. 2005;101:502–8.

53. Epstein N, Danto J, Nardi D. Evaluation of intraoperative somatosensory-evoked potential monitoring during 100 cervical operations. Spine. 1993;18:737–47.

54. Chatrian G, Berger M, Wirch A. Discrepancy between intraoperative SSEP's and postoperative function. Case report. J Neurosurg. 1988;69:450–4.

55. Strahm C, Min K, Boos N. Reliability of perioperative SSEP recordings in spine surgery. Spinal Cord. 2003;41:483–9.

56. Nathan N, Tabaraud F, Lacroix F. Influence of propofol concentrations on multipulse transcranial motor evoked potentials. Br J Anaesth. 2003;91:493–7.

57. Hamaguchi K, Nakagawa I, Hidaka S. Effect of propofol on visual evoked potentials during neurosurgery. Masui. 2005;54:998–1002.

58. Hans P, Bonhomme V, et al. Why we still use intravenous drugs as the basic regimen for neurosurgical anesthesia? Curr Opin Anesthesiol. 2006;19:498–503.

59. Engelhard K, Werner C, et al. Inhalational or intravenous anesthetics for craniotomies? Pro inhalational. Curr Opin Anesthesiol. 2006;19:504–8.

60. Citerio G, Franzosi M, Latini R, et al. Anesthesiological strategies in elective craniotomy :randomized equivalence, open trial- the NeuroMorfeo trial. Trials. 2009;10:19.

61. Petersen K, Landsfeldt U, Cold G, et al. ICP is lower during propofol anesthesia compared to isoflurane and sevoflurane. Acta Neurochir Suppl. 2002;81:89–91.

62. Roberts I. Barbiturates for acute traumatic brain injury. Cochrane Database Syst Rev. 2000, CD000033.

63. Kaisti KK, Langsjo J, Aalto S, et al. Effects of sevoflurane, propofol and adjunct nitrous oxide on regional cerebral blood flow, oxygen consumption and blood volume in humans. Anesthesiology. 2003;99:603–13.

64. Lorenz IH, Kolbitsch C, Hormann C, et al. Subanaesthetic concentration of sevoflurane increases regional cerebral blood flow more, but regional blood volume less than subanaesthetic concentration of isoflurane in human volunteers. J Neurosurg Anesthesiol Scand. 2001;13:288–95.

65. Chui J, Mariappan R, Mehta J, et al. Comparison of propofol and volatile agents for maintenance of anesthesia during elective craniotomy procedures: systematic review and meta-analysis. Can J Anaesth. 2014;61:347–56.

66. Lauta E, Abbinante C, Del Gaudio A, et al. Emergence times are similar with sevoflurane and total intravenous anesthesia: results of a multicenter RCT of patients scheduled for elective supratentorial craniotomy. J Neurosurg Anesthesiol. 2010;22:110–8.

67. Magni G, La Rosa I, Gimignani S, et al. Early postoperative complications after intracranial surgery, comparison between total intravenous and balanced anesthesia. J Neurosurg Anesthesiol. 2007;19:229–34.

68. Boztuğ N, Bigat Z, Akyuz M, Demir S, Ertok E. Does using bispectral index (BIS) during craniotomy affect the quality of recovery? J Neurosurg Anesthesiol. 2006;18:1–4.

69. De Castro V, Godet G, Mencia G, et al. Target controlled infusion for remifentanil in vascular patients improves hemodynamics and decreases remifentanil requirements. Anesth Analg. 2003;96:33–8.

70. Ferreira DA, Nunes CS, Antunes L, et al. Practical aspects of the use of target controlled infusion with remifentanil in neurosurgical patients: predicted cerebral concentrations at intubation, incision and extubation. Acta Anesthesiol Belgica. 2006;57:265–70.

71. Lobo F, Beiras A, et al. Propofol and remifentanil effect-site concentrations estimated by pharmacokinetic simulation and bispectral index monitoring during craniotomy with intraoperative awakening for brain tumor resection. J Neurosurg Anesthesiol. 2007;19:183–9.

72. Russell D. Intravenous anesthesia: manual infusion schemes versus TCI systems. Anesthesia. 1998;53 Suppl 1:42–5.

73. Cole CD, Gottfried ON, Gupta D, et al. Total intravenous anesthesia: advantages for intracranial surgery. Neurosurgery. 2007;61 Suppl 2:369–77.

74. Miocinovic S, Somayajula S, Chitnis S, et al. History, applications and mechanisms of deep brain stimulation. JAMA Neurol. 2013;70:163–71.

75. Speelman JD, Bosch D, et al. Resurgence of functional neurosurgery for Parkinson's disease: a historical perspective. Mov Disord. 1998;13:582–8.

76. Hu W, Klassen B, Stead M, et al. Surgery for movement disorders. J Neurosurg Sci. 2011;55:305–17.

77. Diering SL, Bell W, et al. Functional neurosurgery for psychiatric disorders: a historical perspective. Stereotact Funct Neurosurg. 1991;57:175–94.

78. Poon CC, Irwin M, et al. Anesthesia for deep brain stimulation and in patients with implanted neurostimulator devices. Br J Anaesthesia. 2009;103:152–65.

79. Venkatraghavan L, Manninen P, Mak P, et al. Anesthesia for functional neurosurgery:review of complications. J Neurosurg Anesthesiol. 2006;18:64–7.

80. Gebhard R, Berry J, Maggio W, et al. The successful use of regional anesthesia to prevent involuntary movements in patient undergoing awake craniotomy. Anesth Analg. 2000;91(5):1230–1.

81. Berkenstadt H, Perel A, Hadani M, et al. Monitored anesthesia care using remifentanil and propofol for awake craniotomy. J Neurosurg Anesthesiol. 2001;13:246–9.

82. Hans P, Bonhomme V, Born J, et al. Target controlled infusion of propofol and remifentanil combined with spectral index monitoring for awake craniotomy. Anesthesia. 2000;55:255–9.

83. Souter M, Rozet I, Ojemann J, et al. Dexmedetomidine sedation during awake craniotomy for seizure resection: effects on electrocorticography. J Neurosurg Anesthesiol. 2007;19:38–44.

84. Duffis E, Gandhi C, Prestigiacomo C, et al. Society for Neurointerventional Surgery. Head, neck and brain tumor embolization guidelines. J Neurointerv Surg. 2012;4:251–5.

85. Absalom A, Amutike D, Lal A, et al. Accuracy of the 'Paedfusor' in children undergoing cardiac surgery or catheterization. Br J Anaesth. 2003;91:507–13.

TCI in Special Patients Groups: The Elderly and Obese

Frederique S. Servin

Introduction

A generally recognized benefit of target-controlled infusion (TCI) systems is that they provide the anesthetist with a convenient and precise way to titrate intravenous drugs (currently propofol, remifentanil, and sufentanil in commercially available devices) according to the patient's needs. This is of course particularly important in special patients groups when the usual dosing schemes may not apply. However, the use of a TCI system does not modify the drug's intrinsic pharmacology, and the accuracy of the system depends widely on how well the pharmacokinetic (PK) model implemented in the device matches the characteristics of the patient receiving the infusion. This chapter will describe the way that TCI may be used in specific, special populations such as the elderly or obese patients: populations frequently presenting for surgery and in whom precautions should be taken when applying pharmacokinetic models since their characteristics may be outside of the ranges of the covariates of the population in whom the model(s) were developed.

The Elderly Patient

One of the main characteristics associated with aging is the loss of functional tissues which are progressively replaced by fibrosis [1]. As a consequence, the ability to respond to a surgical challenge is reduced, even if basal functions may be preserved for a long time. Among the features particularly important to the anesthetist are cardiovascular changes such as hypovolemia, functional beta-blockade, reduction in local blood flow, and stiffening of arteries leading to wide changes

in blood pressure (peaks and valleys anesthesia) [2]. Silent regurgitation in the postanesthesia care unit (PACU) leading to aspiration of gastric fluid is best avoided by a rapid painless clear-headed recovery.

In this context, TCI is an interesting option, since it has the potential to confer good intraoperative control and to allow efficient administration of propofol and opioids, enabling the patient to benefit from the quality of recovery associated with propofol anesthesia.

However, the changes associated with aging modify both the pharmacokinetics and the pharmacodynamics of anesthetic drugs, and it is important to understand how this may impact TCI and how, if need be, the anesthetist may circumvent those difficulties to ensure a smooth anesthetic course.

Main Pharmacokinetic Changes

Distribution

In the elderly, a reduction in lean body mass and total body water and an increase in fat modify drug distribution [3]. These changes are more significant in males than in females. The volume of distribution at steady state of highly lipid-soluble drugs is markedly increased in aged individuals, which lowers their plasma concentration (resulting from a given dose) and delays their elimination [4]. On the contrary, less lipid-soluble drugs have a smaller volume of distribution in the elderly and may have a higher rate of elimination in this population.

The so-called greater sensitivity of aged patients to the action of many drugs can in some cases be related to a reduction in the initial volume of distribution or in the initial distribution clearance [5]. In elderly patients compared with younger ones, the same dose will generate a markedly higher plasma concentration and thus a greater pharmacological effect. This is typically the case with propofol [6].

F.S. Servin, MD, PhD(✉)
APHP HUPNVS Hôpital Bichat, Anesthesia and Intensive Care,
46, rue Henri Huchard, Paris 75018, France
e-mail: frederique.servin@aphp.fr

© Springer International Publishing AG 2017
A.R. Absalom, K.P. Mason (eds.), *Total Intravenous Anesthesia and Target Controlled Infusions*,
DOI 10.1007/978-3-319-47609-4_29

Plasma albumin concentration tends to decrease with age, and even if the albumin plasma concentration remains normal, structural protein changes may lead to a reduced efficiency of albumin binding sites [7]. At the same time, many chronically administered drugs that are seemingly not dangerous may compete with the anesthetic agents on those sites and thus increase their unbound fraction (i.e., nonsteroidal anti-inflammatory drugs—NSAIDs). On the contrary, the concentration of alpha1-acid glycoprotein (which binds basic drugs such as the opioids) is increased in many situations, such as inflammation or cancer, which are frequently present in the elderly. The increase in the free fraction of propofol (bound up to 98 % to albumin) will not alter its clearance, which is nonrestrictive, but may increase its access to the receptor sites and consequently the pharmacodynamic effect of the administered dose.

Elimination

Hepatic Metabolism

Up to about 50 years of age, the liver represents a fairly constant fraction of total body weight (around 2.5 %). After 50 years of age, this proportion is progressively reduced to reach only 1.6 % at 90 years. Liver blood flow also decreases with age, by about 0.3–1.5 % per year. Thus, at 65 years, the liver blood flow has decreased by an average of 40 % of its value at 25 years [8]. The elimination clearance of drugs with high extraction ratios (such as etomidate, ketamine, flumazenil, morphine, fentanyl, sufentanil, naloxone, lidocaine, etc.) is thereby reduced in the aged population.

Hepatic drug metabolism is achieved through two major processes: phase I (oxidation, reduction, hydrolysis) and phase II (acetylation, conjugation) reactions. Phase I reactions are mainly carried out by microsomal monooxygenases which include the P450 cytochromes (CYP450). Most studies agree that the liver metabolizing capacities are not modified by aging when phase II reactions are activated. For example, the intrinsic clearance of conjugated agents is not modified, but their elimination clearance will usually be reduced because it depends on hepatic blood flow.

Changes over time in phase I reactions are more controversial. Age does not appear as an independent covariate for the mean clearance value, but increases the interindividual variability of this parameter [9].

Propofol and remifentanil are currently the two drugs most often administered by TCI. Propofol clearance depends on hepatic metabolism. It undergoes phase II reactions and the clearance is close to the hepatic blood flow and nonrestrictive. Propofol also has extrahepatic sites of metabolism [10]. As a consequence, propofol clearance is more or less independent of age, and age is not a significant covariate of elimination clearance in Schnider's PK model [11]. This model confirms that propofol administration by TCI is independent of age during maintenance of anesthesia, when the dose to maintain a given concentration directly depends on clearance and clearance only.

Conversely, remifentanil clearance is independent of hepatic metabolism since this drug is eliminated by tissues esterases. However, as during aging functional tissues are progressively replaced by fibrosis, remifentanil clearance is reduced in the elderly [12].

Renal Excretion

Aging and associated diseases impair glomerular filtration rate [13]. A reduced creatinine synthesis may lead to low plasma creatinine levels even in the presence of renal dysfunction. Thus, glomerular filtration rate should always be estimated in this population (the Modification of Diet in Renal Disease, or MDRD formula, is better than the Cockcroft–Gault formula [14]). Most anesthetic agents are lipid soluble, thus they are filtered by the glomeruli and immediately undergo a complete tubular reabsorption which precludes their renal elimination. The kidney will excrete only their more hydrosoluble metabolites. Some metabolites (such as morphine-6-glucuronide) are pharmacologically active, and their retention may prolong the pharmacological effect of the native compound due to decreased renal function.

Neither propofol nor remifentanil has active metabolites, and so their metabolism is unaffected by impaired renal function.

Transfer to the Effect Site

The site of action of the opioids and hypnotics is not in the blood, but at sites in the central nervous system, loosely termed the "effect site." By observation of differences between the time course of effect of various drugs and the evolution of their plasma concentrations over time, modeling techniques can be used to estimate an "effect-site concentration." This is closely related to the time course of effect and can be calculated from the plasma concentration via a transfer rate constant and can, for example, be used to predict the time to peak effect following bolus administration of a drug. Frequently, in the elderly, the transfer rate of anesthetic drugs from the plasma to the biophase (where the drugs exert their molecular effects) is slower than that found in younger adults. This may explain a delayed onset and a delayed recovery even for drugs for which the pharmacokinetics are not modified by aging.

Main Pharmacodynamic Changes in the Elderly

The central nervous system is the target of nearly all anesthetic agents, and consequently all changes over time in this system will directly influence the handling of anesthetic drugs in the elderly population.

From a pharmacological point of view, the sensitivity of the elderly brain to the action of propofol is indeed increased, but not as much as might appear if the same dose is given to an aged individual and a younger one (vide supra, initial distribution) [15]. Conversely, the elderly are very sensitive to the action of opioids, and so it is more important to titrate remifentanil to age than to total body weight [12]. Thus, during TCI in the elderly, provided the PK model implemented in the device is adequate, the propofol target should be slightly reduced, whereas a larger modification of the target concentration of remifentanil (or sufentanil or alfentanil) should be made.

Propofol TCI

Propofol is currently the most popular hypnotic agent for induction as well as for maintenance of anesthesia. Nevertheless, in the aged population, its use has been limited by its hemodynamic effects. As early as 1986, it was observed that in the elderly the dose necessary to obtain loss of consciousness was lower and the incidence of apnea and hypotension increased [16].

Age-related changes in propofol pharmacokinetics include alterations in initial distribution (decreased initial volume and/or impaired rapid intercompartment clearance) leading to higher plasma concentration and an increased effect from the same induction dose and a nonsignificant reduction in elimination clearance mainly due to a decrease in hepatic blood flow buffered by extrahepatic metabolism [17]. On the contrary, propofol elimination is not delayed in the elderly (vide supra). When administering propofol as a target-controlled infusion for induction and maintenance of anesthesia, which improves its safety profile in this population [18], it is important to ascertain that the model implemented in the TCI device includes age as a covariate. Two pharmacokinetic models are currently recommended for propofol TCI in the adult patient. One of them, the so-called Marsh model, includes only total body weight as a covariate [19]. Consequently, for the same target concentration, it will administer the same dose whatever the patient's age. This is the reason why, in the regulatory recommendations to users, Diprifusor™ (a device which incorporates the Marsh PK model) use was limited to patient's under 55 years old. Conversely, the Schnider model was developed from a study involving a group of subjects that included elderly patients, and in this model,

age is a covariate for both the rapid redistribution compartment (sometimes also called the shallow peripheral volume) and the corresponding distribution clearance [17]. As a consequence for the same set target concentration, the use of the Schnider model will result in a smaller dose in elderly patients. Therefore, the Schnider model is recommended in the elderly, whereas the Marsh model is not. It should be mentioned that the influence of age is most significant during the induction of anesthesia or after any significant increase in target concentration, since these actions result in delivery of a bolus (or rapid infusion) of propofol. After a bolus or rapid infusion, plasma propofol concentrations will decline more slowly in the elderly because of the reduced rate of rapid redistribution clearance. Thus, when compelled to use the Marsh model in elderly patients (i.e., when using a Diprifusor™ device), induction should start at a very low target concentration to reduce the dose, and the target concentration should thereafter be titrated upward with great caution.

Pharmacodynamic studies have shown that the concentration–effect relationship was only moderately modified in the elderly, whereas the transfer time to the effect site remains unchanged [15]. Thus, provided an adequate PK model has been selected, the propofol target need only be slightly reduced in the elderly.

Propofol is a potent vasodilator and numerous publications have outlined the risk of hypotension when using this drug in elderly patients [20], in whom the hemodynamic effect is also delayed [15]. Thus, for the same hypnotic effect, the hemodynamic effect will be increased and delayed in the elderly when compared with young subjects. It is therefore particularly important to titrate propofol to effect in order to give only the required dose and no more. TCI may help to improve the accuracy of titration [18]. As far as drug interactions are concerned, the addition of opioids to propofol for induction of anesthesia does not allow any significant reduction in the propofol dose, but does potentate the drop in systolic blood pressure (SBP) and may lead to major hypotension in the absence of adrenergic stimuli [21].

Remifentanil TCI

When remifentanil was first administered to elderly patients with manually controlled infusions, major hemodynamic effects were observed, so much so that its use was not recommended in this population. This was due to a poor knowledge of both the pharmacokinetics and the pharmacodynamics of this drug in the aged patient. Then, the influence of aging on remifentanil behavior was described in detail by Minto et al. [12] who published a PK/PD model based on a population which included individuals aged more than 80 years.

Remifentanil pharmacokinetics in elderly individuals is characterized by a decreased initial volume of distribution (reduced by about 25 % from age 20 to age 80), resulting in higher initial plasma concentrations following the same bolus dose. Concurrently, remifentanil clearance, which is independent of hepatic function and renal blood flow but depends on the number and efficiency of tissue esterases, is decreased by about 30 % from age 20 to 80 years.

The transfer rate from the effect site, k_e0, is reduced with increasing age, hinting at a delayed onset of action. Moreover, the central nervous system is more sensitive to the effect of remifentanil: the concentration required to induce 50 % of EEG depression (CE_{50}) is halved in 80-year-old patients when compared with that in young adults.

Whatever his or her lean body mass, an 80-year-old patient will require approximately half the dose of a 20-year-old to reach the same EEG peak effect. This end point will be delayed in the elderly (approximately 1 min at 20 years and 2 min at 80 years). This adjustment in the initial bolus dose is due to pharmacodynamic changes (decreased CE_{50}). The adjustment in bolus dose for age is far more important than the adjustment in bolus dose for body weight.

The infusion rate required to maintain a constant EEG effect in an 80-year-old person is approximately one-third of that required in a 20-year-old. Again, the adjustment for age is far more important than the adjustment for body weight. This reduction in infusion rate is based on both pharmacokinetic (decreased clearance with age) and pharmacodynamic considerations (decreased CE_{50} with age).

Thus, owing to its titratability and absence of prolonged effects, remifentanil appears to be a very useful drug in elderly patients, provided its dosage is carefully titrated to effect. This can optimally be achieved through a target-controlled remifentanil infusion [22]. A recently recommended use of remifentanil TCI in the elderly is for conscious sedation, where easy titration may help prevent excessive respiratory depression and, if it does occur, may assist with rapid management of it [23].

The time required for remifentanil concentrations to decrease by 50 % (the so-called context-sensitive half time) or even the time taken for the concentrations to decrease by 80 % following prolonged infusions is rapid and little affected by age or duration of infusion. However, although the decrement time is rapid in all age groups, the interindividual variability is increased in the elderly [12].

Sufentanil TCI

The influence of age on sufentanil pharmacokinetics has mainly been described in two studies, both of which concluded that sufentanil pharmacokinetic parameters were not affected by aging, with the exception of a reduced initial volume of distribution leading to a higher plasma peak concentration in elderly patients [24, 25]. Thus, the Gepts pharmacokinetic model currently implemented in TCI devices can be used in elderly patients. Even if we lack data on the pharmacodynamics of sufentanil in the elderly, it seems reasonable to extrapolate those from fentanyl, alfentanil, and morphine and conclude that sufentanil target should be reduced by 50 % in this population.

The Obese Patient

Patients are said to be overweight or obese if they have abnormal or excessive fat accumulation. In many countries, including developing ones, obesity is growing into an epidemic and a major health problem, so much so that as early as 2001 the US Department of Health and Human Services issued a plan of action against this condition, "The Surgeon General's Call to Action to Prevent and Decrease Overweight and Obesity."

A crude measure of obesity is body mass index (BMI), a person's weight (in kilograms) divided by the square of his or her height (in meters). A person with a BMI of 30 or more is generally considered obese. A person with a BMI equal to or more than 25 is considered overweight. The average patient currently presenting for bariatric surgery has a BMI around 50, and patients with BMIs over 70 are not uncommon.

Thus, any anesthesiologist will have to treat obese patients either for bariatric surgery, or for any other surgical condition, including emergencies. In this context, in order to facilitate rational and appropriate care of those patients, all anesthesiologists should have an appropriate understanding of the pathophysiological changes associated with obesity and of the specific problems and challenges associated with the anesthetic care of such patients.

Main Pharmacokinetic Changes in the Obese

Distribution

Obesity is associated with an inflammatory state [26]. Acid $\alpha 1$-glycoprotein (AAG) concentration may double in obese patients when compared to normal-weight controls [27]. As a consequence, the active free fraction of weakly basic drugs such as fentanyl and congeners may be markedly lowered, thus reducing their efficiency.

Increase in fat tissue mass is obviously a major factor increasing the volume of distribution in obese patients. But obesity is also associated with increases in blood volume and in the size of many organs (e.g., liver or kidneys) [28]. Consequently, the volume of the central compartment is usually increased, as is the volume of distribution at steady state, even in drugs that do not readily penetrate fat. Lean body mass (LBM), which also includes muscle mass, is also greater in obese patients, particularly in those who are still mobile [29]. Thus, to reach the same concentration and therefore the same clinical effect, the doses of most drugs need to be increased. Of course, the drugs that are readily distributed into fat need more dosage adjustments than those that remain in the extracellular spaces, since fat body mass (FBM) is much more increased than LBM [30]. One must nevertheless keep in mind that adjusting hydrophilic drug dosage according to ideal body weight in morbidly obese patients may lead to underdosing.

Elimination

Hepatic Metabolism

Obesity is associated with increased cardiac output, blood volume, and organ blood flow, but functional hepatic blood flow remains mostly unchanged despite the increase in liver size, possibly due to fatty infiltration of the liver which may impair liver function even if commonly performed liver function test results remain normal[31]. The clearance of phase I metabolized drugs is usually unchanged, as well as that of acetylated drugs, despite an increased activity of some P450 cytochromes. Conversely, the elimination clearance of many conjugated drugs increases in parallel with total body weight, possibly through extrahepatic conjugation pathways [32].

Renal Elimination

Obese patients have larger kidneys than normal-weight controls [33]. The glomerular filtration rate is increased as is tubular excretion, which may be proportionally even greater [34]. As a consequence, the elimination of drugs excreted through the kidney is enhanced.

Main Pharmacodynamic Changes in the Obese

There is very little information in the literature on pharmacodynamic changes in obese patients. This condition does not seem to influence the concentration–effect relationship for hypnotic drugs [35, 36] or muscle relaxants. Some studies on human pain thresholds have yielded contradictory results, some claiming increased, and others reduced pain sensitivity in the obese [37–39]. Pain threshold appears increased in obese rats [38]. It seems that even nondiabetic obese patients display a subclinical involvement of different diameter sensory fibers, mimicking a subclinical peripheral neuropathy related to metabolic alterations such as hyperinsulinemia [40].

TCI in the Obese Patient: Estimation of the Lean Body Mass

At the end of the 1990s, when both the Schnider model for propofol [11] and the Minto model for remifentanil [12] were developed, the current obesity epidemic had not reached its full magnitude. As a result, even though PK models, developed from two-stage modeling processes, existed for propofol [36] and remifentanil [41] use in the obese, the clinical use of TCI was at its early stages. No morbidly obese patients were included in the study populations from which the Schnider and Minto models were developed, and for both these PK models, lean body mass (LBM) was a significant covariate. Thus, during the use of these models, LBM had to be estimated for every patient, and so an LBM calculation formula was associated with the models. At that time several formulas were available to calculate LBM [42, 43], and their performance in normal-weight patients was more or less similar (see Fig. 29.1). The most recently published at that time, albeit in a rather confidential medium, was chosen [43]. This so-called James formula included in its calculation both total body weight (TBW) in kilograms and height (H) in cm and was different for men and women:

Men: LBM = $1.1 \times$ TBW $- 128 \times$ (TBW/H)^2
Women: LBM = $1.07 \times$ TBW $- 148 \times$ (TBW/H)^2

Unfortunately, in this formula, if the weight increases without a change in the height, the calculated LBM reaches a maximum and then decreases and may even reach negative values (see Fig. 29.1). As a consequence, this formula was totally inadequate to describe LBM in obese patients (whose

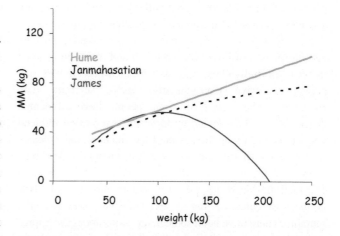

Fig. 29.1 Evolution as a function of total body weight of the LBM calculated with, respectively, Hume, James, and Janmahasatian formulas

LBM in reality does increase with TBW). Solutions had to be proposed for TCI use in this population. The first safety measure has been to limit the use of TCI to patients whose weight was in the increasing part of the James LBM curve (namely, less than BMI 35) when using models that included LBM as a covariate. Thus, devices implementing the Schnider and Minto models will not allow TCI propofol or remifentanil administration to patients with higher weight values. A few years ago, a new formula to calculate LBM in all patients including the morbidly obese was published [29]. A solution to the problem might be to replace the James LBM formula with another, such as the Janmahasatian formula. However, this would require prospective revalidation of the models, which has not been done so far. In the current situation, the required approach is different depending on the drug.

Propofol TCI in the Obese Patient

Currently, two models are routinely implemented in TCI devices (vide supra).The Marsh model, having only TBW as a covariate, is unaffected by the problem of the James formula. The Schnider model, on the contrary, uses this formula to calculate LBM, which is a significant covariate for elimination clearance, in such a way that when the calculated LBM is less than 59 kg with a TBW over 77 kg, the calculated clearance actually increases exponentially and out of proportion with reality. As a consequence, when this model and formula are applied as published by a TCI system, the amount of drug administered to compensate for this supposed increased clearance is also increased, and in morbidly obese patients, the Schnider model administers excessive propofol doses. It is therefore not recommended in this population.

What of the Marsh model? Most obese patients presenting for surgery, specifically bariatric surgery, are younger than 60 years of age. Consequently, there is no age issue with the Marsh model in this population. The amount of propofol required to reach and maintain a given target in morbidly obese patients with the Marsh model may appear excessive. Consequently, despite scientific data suggesting otherwise [36], some people have advocated "tricking" the TCI device by inputting a modified reduced weight on starting up the device. La Colla et al. have clearly demonstrated that this attitude was not justified [44]. Thus, propofol TCI may be used in morbidly obese patients provided the Marsh PK model is chosen and the real TBW is used to calculate the doses. However, one problem remains. There have been some discussions about the appropriate dose for propofol induction of anesthesia in morbidly obese patients [45]. While the use of ideal body weight obviously leads to insufficient induction doses, some believe that the use of TBW may convey a risk of excessive doses with hemodynamic consequences. For example, few would consider administering a 2 mg/kg induction dose considered a standard dose in normal patients to a patient weighing 175 kg. TCI may help in that the initial bolus dose is always smaller than the recommended bolus doses in manual control. Thus, if using the Marsh model in a morbidly obese patient, with the TBW entered as the weight, then it may be important to keep this discussion in mind and perhaps use a lower target concentration during induction and thereafter titrate the target upward according to the clinical response of the patient.

Remifentanil TCI

Remifentanil has a very small volume of distribution that is nearly independent of body mass index. This drug will thereby not accumulate in obese patients. Its dosage should therefore not be based upon total body weight and hence the importance of the estimation of the LBM in remifentanil PK models. In the Minto model, LBM is a significant covariate for both the volumes of distribution and the elimination clearance. With regard to elimination clearance, an important difference with regard to the Schnider model is that when the calculated LBM decreases below 55 kg, the calculated elimination clearance also decreases. As a consequence, the Minto model actually underdoses the morbidly obese patient, which is not ideal but nevertheless safer than overdosing in that it allows upward titration without hemodynamic consequences.

What is the magnitude of this underdosing? For a given target concentration, it is possible to recalculate from the infusion rates given by the TCI pump the predicted concentration in a given morbidly obese patient using a LBM is estimated by the Janmahasatian formula [29] (Fig. 29.2). As expected, the underdosage increases with increasing BMI. However, if the LBM is not allowed to decrease by fixing it to its maximum as estimated by the James formula, it appears that in patients with a BMI up to 50, the bias is less than 20 % (Fig. 29.2) which is clinically safe and acceptable. For manually controlled infusions, the remifentanil infusion rate must not be calculated according to total body weight. However, it is unlikely that the clinician will be willing and able to calculate the LBM of the patient (which in the obese is quite different from the ideal body weight) in the OR. Thus, to use remifentanil in morbidly obese patients up to a BMI of 50, it is probably best to use TCI and program the device with the highest weight it will accept (which depends on height) and increase the target concentration as needed.

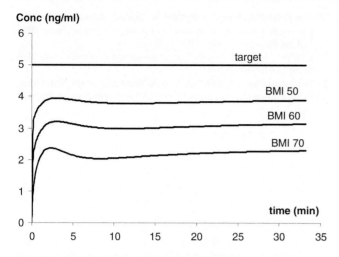

Fig. 29.2 Evolution of remifentanil predicted concentrations in morbidly obese patients with a BMI of 50, 60, and 70 when the Minto model is applied unrestrictively with the James formula. To perform the simulations, the LBM of the patients were calculated using Janmahasatian formula

Sufentanil TCI

The most recently published PK model for sufentanil does not include body weight as a significant covariate [46]. Interestingly, it performed well when used for sufentanil TCI in morbidly obese patients despite a slight overestimation of plasma sufentanil concentrations specifically for patients with body mass indices greater than 40 [47]. The authors concluded that this pharmacokinetic parameter set, derived from a normal-weight population, accurately predicted plasma sufentanil concentrations in morbidly obese patients.

So, to summarize, in morbidly obese patients, propofol TCI may be used with the Marsh model, sufentanil TCI may be used with the Gepts model, and the use of the Minto model for remifentanil is safe provided the device is programmed with the maximum accepted weight by the device, and the clinician is aware of the fact that this technique will yield blood concentrations significantly lower than the set target concentration.

Other Pharmacokinetic Approaches: The Allometric Model

Allometry, dating back to the end of the nineteenth century, is the study of the relationship of body size to a number of physiological parameters such as heart rate, life span, or skeleton structure, usually in different species (i.e., in mammals from mice to elephants). The relationship between

the two studied parameters follows a power law, $y = Cx^{\alpha}$, where α is the scaling exponent of the law.

Allometry was first proposed in anesthetic pharmacology to derive pharmacokinetic pediatric models [48]. Obese patients were also a good model to try to use allometric scaling to accurately estimate pharmacokinetics as a function of body size. Cortinez et al. recently demonstrated the value of allometry to describe the evolution of propofol clearance in morbidly obese patients [35]. They used a model developed by Eleveld et al. [49], which uses allometric scaling and was not restricted to obese patients but also included children and elderly patients. This model needs to be prospectively validated, but may be a future approach to adequately address the problem of propofol TCI in some special patients groups.

Conclusion

The examples of the use of TCI in special patient groups both demonstrate its value in titrating drug effect when the usual dosing schemes do not apply and the importance of an adequate knowledge of the pharmacokinetic models implemented in the device and of their covariates. The best way to benefit from ease of titration facilitated by TCI, and adapt the dosing scheme to the patient's needs as much as possible, is to titrate the target concentration according to the output of cortical EEG-based monitors of the anesthetic state and estimation of the reactivity to adrenergic stimuli. In this way titration will be according to individually measured parameters of clinical effect, as opposed to predicted concentrations.

References

1. Novak LP. Aging, total body potassium, fat-free mass, and cell mass in males and females between ages 18 and 85 years. J Gerontol. 1972;27(4):438–43.
2. Lakatta EG. Age-associated cardiovascular changes in health: impact on cardiovascular disease in older persons. Heart Fail Rev. 2002;7(1):29–49.
3. Hughes VA, Frontera WR, Roubenoff R, Evans WJ, Singh MA. Longitudinal changes in body composition in older men and women: role of body weight change and physical activity. Am J Clin Nutr. 2002;76(2):473–81.
4. Klotz U, Avant G, Hoyumpa A, Schenker S, Wilkinson G. The effect of age and liver disease on the disposition and elimination of diazepam in adult man. J Clin Invest. 1975;55:347–59.
5. Homer TD, Stanski DR. The effect of increasing age on thiopental disposition and anesthetic requirement. Anesthesiology. 1985;62 (6):714–24.
6. Kirkpatrick T, Cockshott ID, Douglas EJ, Nimmo WS. Pharmacokinetics of propofol (diprivan) in elderly patients. Br J Anaesth. 1988;60(2):146–50.
7. Wallace S, Whiting B. Factors affecting drug binding in plasma of elderly patients. Br J Clin Pharmacol. 1976;3(2):327–30.

8. Wynne HA, Cope LH, Mutch E, Rawlins MD, Woodhouse KW, James OF. The effect of age upon liver volume and apparent liver blood flow in healthy man. Hepatology. 1989;9(2):297–301.

9. Schmucker DL. Liver function and phase I drug metabolism in the elderly: a paradox. Drugs Aging. 2001;18(11):837–51.

10. Veroli P, O'Kelly B, Bertrand F, Trouvin JH, Farinotti R, Ecoffey C. Extrahepatic metabolism of propofol in man during the anhepatic phase of orthotopic liver transplantation. Br J Anaesth. 1992;68(2):183–6.

11. Schnider TW, Minto CF, Gambus PL, Andresen C, Goodale DB, Shafer SL, et al. The influence of method of administration and covariates on the pharmacokinetics of propofol in adult volunteers. Anesthesiology. 1998;88(5):1170–82.

12. Minto CF, Schnider TW, Shafer SL. Pharmacokinetics and pharmacodynamics of remifentanil. II Model application. Anesthesiology. 1997;86:24–33.

13. Fehrman-Ekholm I, Skeppholm L. Renal function in the elderly (>70 years old) measured by means of iohexol clearance, serum creatinine, serum urea and estimated clearance. Scand J Urol Nephrol. 2004;38(1):73–7.

14. Musso CG, Alvarez-Gregori J, Jauregui J, Macias-Nunez JF. Glomerular filtration rate equations: a comprehensive review. Int Urol Nephrol. 2016;48:1105–10.

15. Kazama T, Ikeda K, Morita K, Kikura M, Doi M, Ikeda T, et al. Comparison of the effect-site k(eO)s of propofol for blood pressure and EEG bispectral index in elderly and younger patients. Anesthesiology. 1999;90(6):1517–27.

16. Dundee JW, Robinson FP, McCollum JS, Patterson CC. Sensitivity to propofol in the elderly. Anaesthesia. 1986;41(5):482–5.

17. Schnider TW, Minto CF, Shafer SL, Gambus PL, Andresen C, Goodale DB, et al. The influence of age on propofol pharmacodynamics. Anesthesiology. 1999;90(6):1502–16.

18. Passot S, Servin F, Pascal J, Charret F, Auboyer C, Molliex S. A comparison of target- and manually-controlled infusion propofol, and etomidate/desflurane anesthesia in elderly patients undergoing hip fracture surgery. Anesth Analg. 2005;100:1338–42.

19. Marsh B, White M, Morton N, Kenny GN. Pharmacokinetic model driven infusion of propofol in children. Br J Anaesth. 1991;67(1):41–8.

20. Peacock JE, Lewis RP, Reilly CS, Nimmo WS. Effect of different rates of infusion of propofol for induction of anaesthesia in elderly patients. Br J Anaesth. 1990;65:346–52.

21. Billard V, Moulla F, Bourgain JL, Megnigbeto A, Stanski DR. Hemodynamic response to induction and intubation. Propofol/fentanyl interaction. Anesthesiology. 1994;81(6):1384–93.

22. De Castro V, Godet G, Mencia G, Raux M, Coriat P. Target-controlled infusion for remifentanil in vascular patients improves hemodynamics and decreases remifentanil requirement. Anesth Analg. 2003;96(1):33–8.

23. Yamamoto M, Meguro K, Mouillet G, Bergoend E, Monin JL, Lim P, et al. Effect of local anesthetic management with conscious sedation in patients undergoing transcatheter aortic valve implantation. Am J Cardiol. 2013;111(1):94–9.

24. Helmers JH, van Leeuwen L, Zuurmond WW. Sufentanil pharmacokinetics in young adult and elderly surgical patients. Eur J Anaesthiol. 1994;11(3):181–5.

25. Matteo RS, Schwartz AE, Ornstein E, Young WL, Chang WJ. Pharmacokinetics of sufentanil in the elderly surgical patient. Can J Anaesth. 1990;37(8):852–6.

26. Wellen KE, Hotamisligil GS. Obesity-induced inflammatory changes in adipose tissue. J Clin Invest. 2003;112(12):1785–8.

27. Zini R, Riant P, Barre J, Tillement JP. Disease-induced variations in plasma protein levels. Implications for drug dosage regimens (Part I). Clin Pharmacokinet. 1990;19(2):147–59.

28. Kjellberg J, Reizenstein P. Body composition in obesity. Acta Med Scand. 1970;188:161–9.

29. Janmahasatian S, Duffull SB, Ash S, Ward LC, Byrne NM, Green B. Quantification of lean bodyweight. Clin Pharmacokinet. 2005;44(10):1051–65.

30. Cheymol G. Clinical pharmacokinetics of drugs in obesity. An update. Clin Pharmacokinet. 1993;25(2):103–14.

31. Adler M, Schaffner F. Fatty liver hepatitis and cirrhosis in obese patients. Am J Med. 1979;67:811–6.

32. Abernethy D, Greenblatt D, Divoll M, Shader R. Enhanced glucuronide conjugation of drugs in obesity: studies of lorazepam, oxazepam and acetaminophen. J Lab Clin Med. 1983;101:873–80.

33. Naeye R, Rood E. The size and number of cells in visceral organs in human obesity. Am J Clin Pathol. 1970;54:215–53.

34. Stockholm KH, Biochner-Mortensen J, Hoilund-Carlsen PF. Increased glomerular filtration rate and adrenocortical function in obese women. Int J Obes. 1980;4:57–63.

35. Cortinez LI, De la Fuente N, Eleveld DJ, Oliveros A, Crovari F, Sepulveda P, et al. Performance of propofol target-controlled infusion models in the obese: pharmacokinetic and pharmacodynamic analysis. Anesth Analg. 2014;119(2):302–10.

36. Servin F, Farinotti R, Haberer JP, Desmonts JM. Propofol infusion for maintenance of anesthesia in morbidly obese patients receiving nitrous oxide. A clinical and pharmacokinetic study. Anesthesiology. 1993;78(4):657–65.

37. McKendall MJ, Haier RJ. Pain sensitivity and obesity. Psychiatry Res. 1983;8(2):119–25.

38. Ramzan I, Wong BK, Corcoran GB. Pain sensitivity in dietary-induced obese rats. Physiol Behav. 1993;54(3):433–5.

39. Zahorska-Markiewicz B, Kucio C, Pyszkowska J. Obesity and pain. Hum Nutr Clin Nutr. 1983;37(4):307–10.

40. Miscio G, Guastamacchia G, Brunani A, Priano L, Baudo S, Mauro A. Obesity and peripheral neuropathy risk: a dangerous liaison. J Peripher Nerv Syst. 2005;10(4):354–8.

41. Egan TD, Huizinga B, Gupta SK, Jaarsma RL, Sperry RJ, Yee JB, et al. Remifentanil pharmacokinetics in obese versus lean patients. Anesthesiology. 1998;89(3):562–73.

42. Hume R. Prediction of lean body mass from height and weight. J Clin Pathol. 1966;19:389–91.

43. James WPT. Research on obesity. London: Her Majesty's Stationary Office; 1976.

44. La Colla L, Albertin A, La Colla G, Ceriani V, Lodi T, Porta A, et al. No adjustment vs. adjustment formula as input weight for propofol target-controlled infusion in morbidly obese patients. Eur J Anaesthesiol. 2009;26(5):362–9.

45. Ingrande J, Brodsky JB, Lemmens HJ. Lean body weight scalar for the anesthetic induction dose of propofol in morbidly obese subjects. Anesth Analg. 2011;113(1):57–62.

46. Gepts E, Shafer SL, Camu F, Stanski DR, Woestenborghs R, Van Peer A, et al. Linearity of pharmacokinetics and model estimation of sufentanil. Anesthesiology. 1995;83(6):1194–204.

47. Slepchenko G, Simon N, Goubaux B, Levron JC, Le Moing JP, Raucoules-Aime M. Performance of target-controlled sufentanil infusion in obese patients. Anesthesiology. 2003;98(1):65–73.

48. Anderson BJ. Pediatric models for adult target-controlled infusion pumps. Paediatr Anaesth. 2010;20(3):223–32.

49. Eleveld DJ, Proost JH, Cortinez LI, Absalom AR, Struys MM. A general purpose pharmacokinetic model for propofol. Anesth ANalg. 2014;118(6):1221–37.

TIVA for Cardiac Surgery

30

Stefan Schraag

Introduction

Over the last few decades, cardiac surgery, like most surgical specialties, has developed into a modern, multifaceted specialty that covers many areas of cardiovascular disease and keeps evolving by adapting new techniques that are driven by advances in biotechnology, engineering, and imaging. Contemporary cardiac surgery is characterized by a patient population that is aging and present with more and more complex medical problems. On the other hand, there is a drive to enhance the perioperative process, improve recovery, and reduce hospital length of stay. Finally, the clear distinction of care domains between cardiac surgery and interventional cardiology is narrowing and beginning to overlap. Modern cardiac surgery has widened its remit and now includes, beyond traditional open-heart surgery, mechanical assist devices, semi-invasive valve interventions (TAVR, MitraClips), and resynchronization procedures.

As in many other specialties, anesthesia had to follow this development and adapt its services and continue to provide excellence in this enriched perioperative cardiac portfolio. As a result, cardiac anesthesia is now perceived as an equally broader specialty compared to 20 years ago, where the main focus was on cardiopulmonary bypass. The choice of anesthetic agents and techniques in cardiac surgery has always been the ultimate test of how widely the anesthetic community would adopt this technique on a broader scale. Safe and efficient anesthesia was always going to be a reassurance for use in other specialties. However, safety and efficacy, let alone effects on long-term outcome, were never described clearly enough and only beginning to emerge in recent years, although overall mortality after cardiac surgery

has decreased over the last few decades. This process has been partially offset by changes in the patient population toward more complex disease and significant comorbidity as mentioned earlier [1]. Perioperative morbidity has therefore remained roughly the same and remains a relevant burden to health-care providers. Attempts to identify independent risk factors for cardiac surgery are complex and include patient factors as expressed in the EuroSCORE or Parsonnet score, surgical technique, and the presence or absence of systematic goal-directed protocols [2]. The contribution of anesthesia, however, is largely unknown.

With the availability of newer and shorter-acting intravenous and volatile anesthetic agents, cardiac anesthesia has fundamentally shifted from a high-dose opioid/narcotic technique in recent years to a more balanced, synergistic approach. This shifted paradigm has also led to an emphasis on early tracheal extubation, with application of multimodal analgesia including local anesthetic techniques, resulting in the establishment of safe and effective fast-track protocols [3, 4]. Hence, modern anesthesia techniques for cardiac surgery need to offer qualities that go beyond safety alone.

Early Foundations of Intravenous Anesthesia in Cardiac Surgery

The development of modern anesthesiology has occurred concurrently with significant developments in anesthetic pharmacology, mainly in Europe and North America. The introduction of neuroleptanalgesia, the combination of a potent phenoperidine-type opioid with a neuroleptic and later with a long-acting benzodiazepine, provided the initial basis for the concept of stress-free anesthesia and surgery [5], becoming the preferred option for cardiac surgery. Further refinement in the pharmacology of two opioids, the fentanyl congeners alfentanil and sufentanil, by Dr. Paul Janssen in the 1970s and 1980s, improved the spectrum of applications of IV techniques beyond cardiac anesthesia.

S. Schraag, MD, PhD, FRCA, FFICM(✉)
Department of Anaesthesia and Perioperative Medicine, Golden Jubilee National Hospital, Agamemnon Street Clydebank, Scotland G81 4DY, Scotland, UK
e-mail: stefanschraag@btinternet.com

© Springer International Publishing AG 2017
A.R. Absalom, K.P. Mason (eds.), *Total Intravenous Anesthesia and Target Controlled Infusions*,
DOI 10.1007/978-3-319-47609-4_30

After the rather disappointing appearance (and subsequent disappearance) of the steroid-based agents althesin, pregnanolone, and etomidate, the development of propofol [6] and the establishment of comprehensive pharmacokinetic (PK) knowledge as the basis of drug delivery [7] eventually led many European clinicians to adopt the technique of total intravenous anesthesia (TIVA) [8, 9]. This was enhanced by the availability of smart infusion pumps allowing target-controlled infusion (TCI) of most IV anesthetic agents suitable for TIVA based on their PK models [10–12]. With the advent of propofol TCI, most countries established formal training courses on IV pharmacology assisted by academic institutions and leading researchers. In 1996, remifentanil, an even faster and better titratable opioid, was introduced into clinical practice. Supplementation with remifentanil allowed more rapid intraoperative adaptation to surgery and enhancement of recovery in cardiac patients [13]. Although this drug was initially not well understood in terms of dose requirements, leading to excessive dosing at times, the knowledge gained from PK simulations and applications of TCI has since improved drug delivery and made remifentanil a popular component for TIVA [12].

It became apparent that using TCI allowed more precise titration of TIVA to clinical effect, leading to a reduction of the side effects seen with the at times cumbersome manual infusion regimes [14, 15]. Together with propofol's favorable effects in reducing postoperative nausea and vomiting and possibly postoperative pain [16, 17], a patient's well-being is enhanced after TIVA compared with volatile-based techniques [18, 19].

Pharmacology of Cardiopulmonary Bypass

Hemodynamic Effects of Propofol

Most physiological studies on the effects of IV anesthetic agents during cardiopulmonary bypass (CPB) originate from the 1980s and early 1990s, and only a few new pharmacokinetic studies have been added since that time [20]. Traditionally, the hemodynamic effects of an intravenous bolus induction dose of either thiopentone, etomidate, Althesin, or propofol were compared by the immediate or delayed effects on blood pressure, heart rate, and cardiac output [21–24]. In those days, the method of ascertaining equipotency of induction doses was not standardized, and the pharmacokinetic and pharmacodynamics of each drug were of little consideration as concepts of concentration-related effect and distribution were only emerging. It was, however, noticed that propofol may have a more pronounced cardio-depressant effect compared to its forerunners.

This was soon put into perspective by further research on the exact mechanism of action of propofol on the cardiovascular system. It became apparent that propofol has little to no direct inotropic effect on the heart but seems to act as a vasodilator via Ca^{++}-antagonist-like effects on the arterial and more so on the venous vasculature reducing pre- and afterload [25, 26]. Assessment of cardiovascular effects by transesophageal echocardiography (TEE) showed that propofol, in comparison to thiopentone, had little effect on inotropy as measured by fractional shortening and performed similarly to etomidate [27]. Also with TEE, the difference between propofol and desflurane on splanchnic circulation and hepatic blood flow was studied. In a clinical experiment, it could be demonstrated that due to its vasodilatory effects, TIVA with propofol could maintain a significantly higher hepatic blood flow and oxygen delivery compared to desflurane anesthesia [28]. A more recent investigation studying EEG-controlled intravenous induction providing equipotency of the surrogate measure of effect demonstrated that propofol use, as compared with etomidate, resulted in less hypertension and tachycardia at and after intubation, but in more hypotension [29] (Fig. 30.1). Probably the most interesting feature of the hemodynamic effects induced by propofol is the fact that the maximal degree of hemodynamic depression for a given dose seems to happen well after its hypnotic or anesthetic effect has peaked, assuming a contribution by the sympathetic nervous system. This led to the publication of a hemodynamic effect-site constant [30]. Putting all these physiological observations together, it would appear prudent to offset the hemodynamic effects of propofol by judiciously titrating fluid to increase pre-load in order to offset vasodilatation and thus retain cardiac output. This is exactly what was reported clinically by Bell at al. [31]. Even when systemic hemodynamic variables are unchanged in the presence of a high propofol concentration, a lack of fluid equilibrium may result in impaired microcirculation as studied with sublingual polarization spectral imaging [32].

Cardiopulmonary Bypass and TIVA

In the context of cardiac anesthesia and surgery, propofol has been found to be a mild vasodilator [33] and to reduce oxygen consumption during hypothermic CPB [34]. Unlike the volatile agents, propofol retains myocardial contractility at clinically relevant concentrations [35] and does not alter the arrhythmogenic myocardial threshold, stabilizing Ca^{++} homeostasis [36]. As a potent scavenger of oxygen free radicals [37], propofol also attenuates ischemia-reperfusion injury, which helps to reduce oxidative stress during the intra- and postoperative phase [38].

Fig. 30.1 Time course of percent change in mean arterial pressure, cardiac index, systemic vascular resistance, heart rate, and absolute bispectral index values. *MAP* mean arterial pressure, *CI* cardiac index, *SVRI* systemic vascular resistance index, *HR* heart rate, *BIS* bispectral index. *$P<0.05$ between the groups. †$P<0.05$ with respect to baseline. (Reprinted from [29] with permission from Oxford University Press)

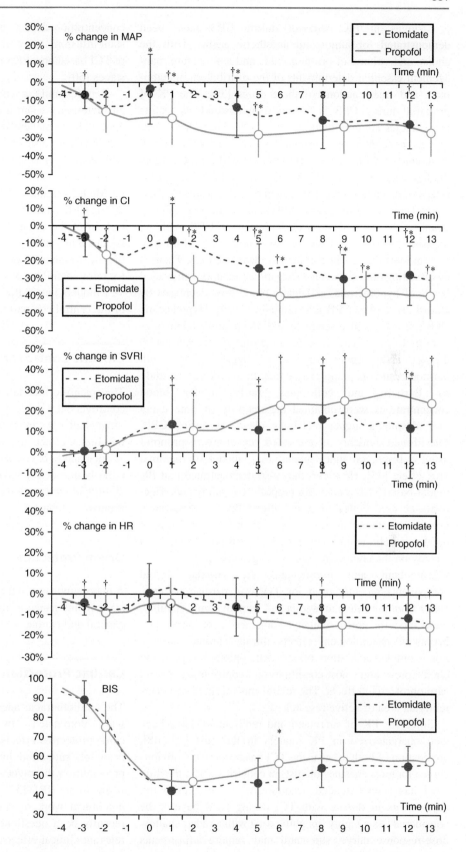

Changes in PK behavior during CPB have been demonstrated for almost all anesthetic agents, with the choice and volume of priming fluids and temperature management essential determinants of the distribution, metabolism, and free fractions of these drugs [39]. The PK of propofol during CPB is not fully understood, as results from studies are conflicting. Early studies have shown that the total concentration of propofol is likely to decrease when commencing CPB due to hemodilution and an increase in the free fraction [40] or remain unchanged [41]. Pre-bypass steady-state values are reestablished during rewarming. Bailey and colleagues undertook a PK analysis and were able to quantify this step change of initiation of CPB with an increase of the size of the central compartment from 6 to 15 l and an increase in elimination clearance [42]. There is an offsetting effect of reduced hepatic extraction with graded levels of hypothermia, as hepatic blood flow decreases by almost 20 % after CPB is instituted [43, 44]. Hypothermic CPB (32–34 °C) also seems to alter the pharmacodynamics of propofol, with a higher central nervous system sensitivity during and immediately after bypass than with normothermic off-pump procedures. In a more recent study by Barbosa and colleagues, fairly similar blood concentrations were obtained the majority of time using TCI, despite a higher metabolic clearance during CPB. They found evidence of enhanced sensitivity to propofol using a bispectral index-guided E_{max} model of maximal drug effect [45]. However, they also demonstrated that PK model-based TCI systems for propofol can safely and effectively be used both during and after CPB. In comparison, volatile anesthetic agents show even larger variations in uptake and elimination when used on CPB [46] and depend heavily on the choice and use of oxygenators [47].

Sufentanil and remifentanil are popular opioid components recently used for TIVA in cardiac patients. Apart from providing analgesia and hemodynamic stability, these modern, potent fentanyl congeners contribute other beneficial physiological effects during cardiac surgery. For example, activation of the delta-opioid receptor can elicit pre- and post-conditioning, contributing direct cardioprotective effects. The role of this mechanism is currently an area of active research.

Since the PK of sufentanil and remifentanil have been well characterized in PK models in the past [12, 48], application of both drugs using TCI has become the obvious choice for most anesthesiologists in countries where the drug label has been extended accordingly. As with propofol, adjustments in dosing with TCI during CPB have to be considered. As a highly lipophilic drug with a rather shallow dose-response curve, sufentanil may require adjustments during CPB based less on changes of clearance and calculated compartments than on higher unbound concentrations [49]. Although there is a 17 % reduction in sufentanil concentration during initiation of CPB when using a constant infusion, this effect is short-lived, and the performance of TCI based on a PK model is little affected during the later stages [50].

Remifentanil, in contrast, shows slightly different PK characteristics when used during CPB. This potent opioid, with a high metabolic clearance and tissue distribution, exhibits a significantly increased volume of distribution with institution of CPB. This increased volume of distribution remains increased even after the end of CPB, as noted by Michelsen and colleagues [51]. The PK of remifentanil during CPB is best described with a two-compartment model instead of the usual three-compartment model description. Again, elimination clearance seems to be reduced proportionally to the level of hypothermia. As metabolic clearance for remifentanil is constant and nearly infinite, the benefit of TCI models lies in the calculated loading and maintenance of the central compartment over time.

Current Controversies

The scientific foundation for some current and proposed is controversial. Gathering evidence for these topics faced the same challenges in translating basic research into meaningful clinical effects that are faced by those working in neuroscience and behavioral science. A particularly controversial issue is that of the balance of evidence with regard to the ability of intravenous or volatile anesthetic agents to improve outcome.

Organ Protection

A major emphasis in the conduct of modern cardiac anesthesia is maintenance of the integrity of end organ function in general and cardiac and brain protection in particular.

Cardiac Protection and Preconditioning

The cardiothoracic anesthesia literature of the last decade was dominated by publications advocating the cardioprotective effects of volatile agents over TIVA with propofol, supported by evidence that the volatile agents precondition the myocardium or minimize ischemia-reperfusion injury (IRI) [52]. These results, which are either from preclinical work or studies of secondary outcomes, have recently been questioned in terms of their translational to relevant clinical effects [53–56].

The concept of pharmacological interventions as a protective strategy during cardiopulmonary bypass is based on established experimental findings. It has been shown that repeated episodes of brief myocardial ischemia protect the heart against a subsequent more prolonged ischemic insult [57]. The molecular mechanism of this endogenous protective response to ischemia-reperfusion injury (IRI) triggers various signaling pathways involving reactive oxygen species (ROS) and a process that stabilizes mitochondrial membranes leading to decreased activity of mitochondrial permeability transition pores (mPTP) [58]. From this relatively universal concept, potential pharmacological protective interventions have been suggested and derived [59]. In particular, it seemed to be feasible to demonstrate evidence in the laboratory setting that volatile anesthetics provide protection before (preconditioning) and after (postconditioning) myocardial ischemia [60, 61]. Based on these, preliminary clinical studies found evidence of reduced biomarkers of myocardial injury when volatile agents were used before, during, and after cardiopulmonary bypass, as compared with TIVA based on propofol [62, 63]. Claims of improved patient outcome in terms of survival or clinical myocardial events remained inconsistent. De Hert who initially reported a significant reduced troponin T release with sevoflurane compared to propofol could not demonstrate this in a follow-up clinical trial [53, 64]. Although the study was not powered for this secondary endpoint, the authors of the latter study showed an apparent advantage in one-year survival in the sevoflurane group against TIVA propofol. Unfortunately, this statistically questionable result was included in a highly quoted meta-analysis and was the pivotal study in it shifting the odds ratio of influence on mortality slightly in favor of halogenated agents [65]. Other authors of another meta-analysis were more cautious in their interpretation of the literature [66]. Nevertheless, the American College of Cardiology Foundation/American Heart Association still recommend a "volatile-based anesthetic" for CABG surgery procedures in their current guideline dating from 2011 [67].

However, recently, larger clinical studies could not convincingly demonstrate clinical benefits in either myocardial damage or outcome with volatile agents compared to TIVA both in cardiac and noncardiac patient populations of high risk. Lurati Buse et al. studied 385 high-risk noncardiac surgical patients and could not demonstrate a reduction in either cardiac biomarkers or major adverse events at 1 year [55]. This was confirmed in a Scandinavian study in vascular surgery patients [54]. In a randomized multicenter study from Italy in 200 high-risk CABG and valve patients, Landoni et al. reported no impact of the choice of volatile versus TIVA-based techniques on a composite endpoint of death, ICU stay, and 30-day and 1-year mortality [68]. Flier et al. concluded from their study in CABG patients that the clinical relevance of volatile cardioprotection is questionable since significant effects may only be detected in very homogenous groups [69]. A recent proof-of-concept study

demonstrated only a reduction of inflammatory markers with cardio-specific sevoflurane exposure, but there was a lack of attenuation of release of markers of myocardial cell damage [70]. Similarly, other strategies of cardioprotection, in particular remote ischemic preconditioning (RIPC), have obtained negative clinical effects despite proof in principal in animal experiments [71–74]. The claim that propofol itself antagonizes or inhibits a potential organ-protective effect by RIPC is not substantive. In fact, no single study proves this hypothesis. One small study suggested that RIPC in 14 patients, as compared to propofol anesthesia in 19 controls, mildly reduced the area under the receiver-operator-characteristic curve at 72 h for the result of a troponin I assay [75]. This phase I study is however too small to allow a definite conclusion [76]. More importantly, while a recent meta-analysis of 15 randomized trials confirmed that RIPC was cardioprotective, it also showed that the use of volatile anesthetics with RIPC attenuated this cardioprotective effect [77].

We need to bear in mind though that propofol itself, as part of TIVA techniques, is a potent scavenger of ROS and thus may influence the degree of myocardial injury and inflammatory response in a different way [78]. Corcoran et al. could demonstrate a beneficial effect of propofol infusion on neutrophil function, lipid peroxidation, and inflammatory response immediately after cross-clamp release and reperfusion in patients with impaired ventricular function. The data show no difference of reduced biomarkers of myocardial injury in TIVA patients compared to those in the isoflurane group [37]. This may cause clinical interference in confirming isolated volatile effects but more likely provide synergistic protection in its own right [79].

Maybe more importantly, the opioids that are part of modern TIVA techniques are also important factors influencing cardioprotection. Opioids have been shown to confer acute and delayed cardioprotection via opioid receptors, effects similar to ischemic pre- and postconditioning [80, 81]. Remifentanil, in particular, was studied extensively both experimentally and clinically in terms of its cardioprotective effects. Using a rat model of ischemia-reperfusion injury, Zhang et al. demonstrated that remifentanil preconditioning reduces the size of myocardial infarction after lethal ischemia to a similar extent as ischemic preconditioning [82]. Further studies have accumulated evidence on the complexity of opioid-induced cardioprotection via various receptor subtypes that include effects on the oxidative and nitrosative stress balance in the myocardium [83] with remifentanil preconditioning also providing a second window of protection in a delayed fashion [84]. Clinical studies have in part confirmed these assumptions and also suggest a dose-dependent protective effect of remifentanil on markers of myocardial injury [85–87]. A meta-analysis examining the use of remifentanil versus other opioids showed a reduction in troponin release, time of mechanical ventilation, and length of hospital stay in patients undergoing cardiac surgery [88].

Due to the complex molecular pathways of cardioprotection and the likely influence of genotype and other patient factors on these pathways [71], clinical studies so far have overall provided less than convincing proof that a particular anesthetic agent can consistently be associated with a better outcome after cardiac surgery. As risk prediction for cardiac surgery shifts toward biomarker screening alongside scoring individual patients' risk factors [89], the likelihood that the presence or absence of one particular intervention within the highly complex perioperative process of cardiac surgery will consistently affect mortality still remains highly speculative.

Neuroprotection and Postoperative Cognitive Deficit (POCD)

A more tangible outcome after cardiac surgery is the possible effects of anesthesia on the integrity of brain function and, in particular, its impact on neurocognitive outcome after CPB [90]. Although stroke is still considered a rare complication after CPB, various degrees of cognitive dysfunction and decline are rather common and may last longer compared with noncardiac surgery [91]. Conflicting evidence exists as to whether intravenous or volatile agents are implicated in the development of POCD [92]. There is evidence, however, that volatile agents impair peripheral and cerebral microcirculation which may have an indirect contribution to cognitive decline [93]. Based on experimental research, there is now a possible association between exposure to volatile anesthetic agents and the formation of neurofibrillary tangles and amyloid plaques in patients with Alzheimer disease [94, 95]. In contrast, propofol has been shown to elicit direct neuroprotection by attenuating inflammatory responses during CPB [37], by scavenging hydroxyl radicals formed by brain injury [96], and by reducing the infarct size after experimental ischemia-reperfusion (neuroapoptosis challenge) in the brain [97].

Practical Aspects of TIVA in Cardiac Surgery

The practical aspects of TIVA for the cardiac surgical patient include adequate but safe titration during induction, consideration of anesthetic requirements and drug interaction during CPB and rewarming, and the smooth transition from intraoperative opioids to postoperative analgesia. As in other specialties, there is no one recipe that fits all patients but a few important points should be discussed here.

Firstly, the availability of TCI has allowed us to titrate small incremental changes in drug concentration with a much higher margin of safety compared to manual infusions [98]. This applies particularly for the induction process. As with any frail, old, or otherwise vulnerable patient, we would allow the propofol infusion to be titrated in small increments from around 2–2.5 µg/ml target concentration when using the Marsh pharmacokinetic model. A slightly higher initial target concentration of 3.0–4.0 is advised when the Schnider model is used in effect-site control as explained elsewhere in this book (see Chap. 11 on Propofol PK/PD). Dependent on individual choice, the concomitant opioid infusion should have achieved satisfactory levels when endotracheal intubation is performed; for remifentanil TCI, this is in the range of 3.0–4.0 ng/ml.

Secondly, brain function monitoring is essential during cardiac surgery. Not only does a form of processed EEG inform a judgment of the individual response to various levels of anesthetic drugs, it also gives good feedback on nonspecific factors influencing cortical cerebral depression such as cooling and its reversal. The bispectral index (BIS), for example, has the potential to indicate and identify vulnerable patients with a risk of a poorer outcome [99]. Combining EEG monitoring with surrogate measures of cerebral perfusion and oxygen supply, such as near-infrared spectroscopy, facilitates a comprehensive assessment of the patient's brain function and can be established to aid prognostication of possible postoperative cognitive impairment [100, 101].

Finally, attention should be drawn to the importance of formulating good plans for a smooth and safe transition to recovery, extubation, and step-down analgesia for the cardiac patient. Although so-called fast-track protocols or enhanced recovery after surgery (ERAS) programs have been successfully reported independent of the opioid used [3, 4], remifentanil is most predictably suited to establish fast recovery, in particular when used as TCI [102]. A very effective way to facilitate early weaning cardiac patients postoperatively from opioids is by supplementing intravenous or oral analgesia with effective local anesthetic techniques, namely, sternal infiltration or high thoracic epidural analgesia (HTEA). HTEA has been successfully used in cardiac patients and has been shown to reduce the incidence of atrial fibrillation and chest infections [103] and to improve overall outcome and reduce mortality [104]. Concerns about a higher risk of epidural hematoma have materialized in larger cohort studies [105].

Table 30.1 provides a graphical flowchart on how TIVA is typically used in our institution and gives a practical example on how TIVA in cardiac surgery can be managed within a protocol of multimodal analgesia for ERAS.

Table 30.1 Practical guide for TIVA in the cardiac surgical patient: BIS-guided perioperative titration of target concentration for propofol (Marsh model, plasma-control) and remifentanil (Minto model, plasma-control) for the transition from intraoperative to postoperative phase in an ERAS program together with adjuvant agents (according to protocols at the Golden Jubilee National Hospital).

Drug	Premedication	Induction	Sternotomy	CPB	Rewarming	Transfer	Recovery	Extubation
Propofol TCI (µg/ml)		2.0–2.5	2.8–3.5	2.0–2.5	2.5–2.8	1.0–1.5	0.5–0.8	0
Remifentanil TCI (ng/ml)		3.5–4.0	5.0–6.0	4.5–5.0	5.0–5.5	3.0–3.5	2.0–2.5	1.0–1.5
Ketamine (µg/kg/min)		2.5	2.5	2.5	2.5	2.5	2.5	0
Fentanyl (mg)		0.5						
Temazepam (mg)	10							
Gabapentin (mg)	600							
Dexamethasone (mg)		8						

Conclusion

TIVA has a variety of characteristics that make it a sensible alternative to the use of volatile agents [106]. The availability of TCI in most parts of the world has made TIVA an economically viable technique that allows precise titration to clinical effect in high-risk patients. The benefits of TIVA include organ protection, patient well-being, and enhanced recovery after cardiac surgery, especially when propofol is combined with remifentanil, which also contributes to cardioprotection. There is great potential to improve neurocognitive outcomes in cardiac surgical patients as well. It remains to be seen though if early claims of improved brain protection, that currently merely hinge on experimental research, improve outcomes with TIVA versus inhaled anesthetics and can be demonstrated in prospective and well-powered clinical studies. Until then, intravenous anesthetic techniques with TCI propofol and short-acting opioids like remifentanil are safe and effective and remain the preferred choice for many cardiac anesthetists.

References

1. Ferguson T, Hammill B, Peterson E, et al. A decade of change-risk profiles and outcomes for isolated coronary artery bypass grafting procedures, 1990–1999: A report from the STS National Database Committee and the Duke Clinical Research Institute. Ann Thorac Surg. 2002;73:480–9.
2. Aya HD, Cecconi M, Hamilton M, et al. Goal-directed therapy in cardiac surgery: a systematic review and meta-analysis. Br J Anaesth. 2013;110:510–7.
3. Svircevic V, Nierich AP, Moons KGM, et al. Fast track anesthesia and cardiac surgery: a retrospective cohort study of 7989 patients. Anesth Analg. 2009;108:727–33.
4. Ender J, Borger MA, Scholz M, et al. Cardiac surgery fast-track treatment in a postanesthetic care unit: Six-month results of the Leipzig fast track concept. Anesthesiology. 2008;109:61–6.
5. DeCastro J, Mundeleer P, Bauduin T. Critical evaluation of ventilation and acid-base balance during neuroleptanalgesia. Ann Anaesthesiol Fr. 1964;5:425–36.
6. Glen JB, Hunter SC. Pharmacology of an emulsion formulation of ICI35868. Br J Anaesth. 1984;56:617–26.
7. Krueger-Thiemer E. Continuous intravenous infusion and multi-compartment accumulation. Eur J Pharmacol. 1968;4:317–34.
8. Dundee JW, Robinson FP, McCollum JSC, et al. Sensitivity to propofol in the elderly. Anaesthesia. 1986;41:482–5.
9. Schwilden H, Stoeckel H, Schuttler J, et al. Pharmacological models and their use in clinical anaesthesia. Eur J Anaesthesiol. 1986;3:175–208.
10. Marsh B, White M, Morton N, et al. Pharmacokinetic model driven infusion of propofol in children. Br J Anaesth. 1991;67:41–8.
11. Schnider TW, Minto CF, Gambus PL, et al. The influence of method of administration and covariates on the pharmacokinetics of propofol in adult volunteers. Anesthesiology. 1998;88:1170–82.
12. Minto CF, Schnider TW, Egan TD, et al. Influence of age and gender on the pharmacokinetics and pharmacodynamics of remifentanil. I. Model development. Anesthesiology. 1997;86:12–23.
13. Muellejans B, Matthey T, Schlopp J, et al. Sedation in the intensive care unit with remifentanil/propofol versus midazolam/fentanyl: a randomized open-label pharmacoeconomic trial. Crit Care. 2006;10:R91.
14. Leslie K, Clavisi O, Hargrove J. Target-controlled infusion versus manually-controlled infusion of propofol for general anaesthesia in adults. Cochrane Database Syst Rev. 2007. doi:10.1002/14651858.CD006059.pub2.
15. De Castro V, Godet G, Mancia G, et al. Target-controlled infusion for remifentanil in vascular patients improves hemodynamics and decreases remifentanil requirements. Anesth Analg. 2003;96:33–8.
16. Cheng S, Yeh J, Flood P. Anesthesia matters: patients anesthetized with propofol have less postoperative pain than those anesthetized with isoflurane. Anesth Analg. 2008;106:264–9.
17. Bandschapp O, Filitz J, Ihmsen H, et al. Analgesic and antihyperalgesic properties of propofol in a human pain model. Anesthesiology. 2010;113:421–8.
18. Hofer CK, Zollinger A, Buechi S, et al. Patient well-being after general anaesthesia: a prospective, randomized, controlled multicenter trial comparing intravenous and inhalational anaesthesia. Br J Anaesth. 2003;91:631–7.
19. Royse CF, Chung F, Newman S, et al. Predictors of patient satisfaction with anaesthesia and surgical care: a cohort study using the quality of recovery scale. Eur J Anaesthesiol. 2013;30:106–10.
20. Goodchild CS, Serrao JM. Propofol-induced cardiovascular depression: science and art. Br J Anaesth. 2015;115:641–2.
21. Lippmann M, Paicius R, Gingerich S, et al. A controlled study of the haemodynamic effects of propofol vs thiopental during anesthesia induction. Anesth Analg. 1986;65:S89.
22. Grounds TM, Twigley AJ, Carli F, et al. The haemodynamics of intravenous induction. Comparison of the effects of thiopentone and propofol. Anaesthesia. 1985;40:735–40.

23. Monk CR, Coates DP, Prys-Roberts C, et al. Haemodynamic effects of a prolonged infusion of propofol as a supplement to nitrous oxide anaesthesia. Br J Anaesth. 1987;59:954–60.

24. Sear JW, Prys-Roberst C. Dose-related haemodynamic effects of continuous infusion of Althesin in man. Br J Anaesth. 1979;51:867–73.

25. Bentley GN, Gent JP, Goodchild CS. Vascular effects of propofol: smooth muscle relaxation in isolated veins and arteries. J Pharm Pharmacol. 1989;41:797–8.

26. Goodchild CS. Serrao JM.: Cardiovascular effects of propofol in the anaesthetized dog. Br J Anaesth. 1989;63:87–92.

27. Gauss A, Heinrich H, Wilder-Smith OH. Echocardiographic assessment of the haemodynamic effects of propofol: a comparison with etomidate and thiopentone. Anaesthesia. 1991;46:99–105.

28. Meierhenrich R, Gauss A, Muehling B, et al. The effect of propofol and desflurane on human hepatic blood flow: a pilot study. Anaesthesia. 2010;65:1085–93.

29. Moller Petrun A, Kamenik M. Bispectral index-guided induction of general anaesthesia in patients undergoing major abdominal surgery using propofol or etomidate: a double-blind, randomized, clinical trial. Br J Anaesth. 2013;110:388–96.

30. Kazama T, Ikeda K, Morita K, et al. Comparison of the effect site Ke0s of propofol for blood pressure and EEG bispectral index in elderly and younger patients. Anesthesiology. 1999;90:1517–27.

31. Bell MD, Goodchild CS. Hypertrophic obstructive cardiomyopathy in combination with prolapsing valve. Anaesthesia for surgical correction with propofol. Anaesthesia. 1989;44:409–11.

32. Koch M, DeBacker D, Vincent JL, et al. Effects of propofol on human microcirculation. Br J Anaesth. 2008;101:473–8.

33. Pensado A, Molins N, Alvarez J. Effects of propofol on mean arterial pressure and systemic vascular resistance during cardiopulmonary bypass. Acta Anaesthesiol Scand. 1993;37:498–501.

34. Laycock GJA, Alston RP. Propofol and hypothermic cardiopulmonary bypass: vasodilatation and enhanced protection? Anaesthesia. 1992;47:382–7.

35. Sprung J, Ogletree-Hughes ML, McConnel BK, et al. The effects of propofol on the contractility of failing and non-failing human heart muscles. Anesth Analg. 2001;93:550.

36. Kanaya N, Gable B, Murray PA, et al. Propofol increases phosphorylation of troponin I and myosin light chain 2 via protein kinase C activation in cardiomyocytes. Anesthesiology. 2003;98:1363.

37. Corcoran TB, Engel A, Sakamoto H, et al. The effects of propofol on neutrophil function, lipid peroxidation and inflammatory response during elective coronary artery bypass grafting in patients with impaired ventricular function. Br J Anaesth. 2006;97:825–31.

38. Ko SH, Yu CW, Lee SK, et al. Propofol attenuates ischemia-reperfusion injury in the isolated rat heart. Anesth Analg. 1997;85:719.

39. Gedney JA, Gosh S. Pharmacokinetics of analgesics, sedatives and anaesthetic agents during cardiopulmonary bypass. Br J Anaesth. 1995;75:344–51.

40. Russell GN, Wright EL, Fox MA, et al. Propofol-fentanyl anaesthesia for coronary artery surgery and cardiopulmonary bypass. Anaesthesia. 1989;44:205–8.

41. Massey NJA, Sherry KM, Oldroyd S, et al. Pharmacokinetics of an infusion of propofol during cardiac surgery. Br J Anaesth. 1990;65:475–9.

42. Bailey JM, Mora CT, Shafer SL. Pharmacokinetics of propofol in adult patients undergoing coronary revascularization. Anesthesiology. 1996;84:1288–97.

43. Hampton WW, Townsend MC, Schirmer WJ, et al. Effective hepatic blood flow during cardiopulmonary bypass. Arch Surg. 1989;124:458–9.

44. Leslie K, Sessler DI, Bjorksten AR, et al. Mild hypothermia alters propofol pharmacokinetics and increases the duration of action of atracurium. Anesth Analg. 1995;80:1007–14.

45. Barbosa RAG, Jorge Santos SRC, White PF, et al. Effects of cardiopulmonary bypass on propofol pharmacokinetics and bispectral index during coronary surgery. Clinics. 2009;64:215–21.

46. Wiesenack C, Wiesner G, Keyl C, et al. In vivo uptake and elimination of isoflurane by different membrane oxygenators during cardiopulmonary bypass. Anesthesiology. 2002;97:133–8.

47. Philipp A, Wiesenack C, Behr R, et al. High risk of awareness during cardiopulmonary bypass with isoflurane administration via diffusion membrane oxygenators. Perfusion. 2002;17:175–8.

48. Gepts E, Shafer SL, Camu F, et al. Linearity of pharmacokinetics and model estimation of sufentanil. Anesthesiology. 1995;83:1194–204.

49. Jeleazcov C, Saari TI, Ihmsen H, et al. Changes in total and unbound concentrations of sufentanil during target controlled infusion for cardiac surgery with cardiopulmonary bypass. Br J Anaesth. 2012;109:698–706.

50. Hudson RJ, Thomson IR, Jassai R. Effects of cardiopulmonary bypass on sufentanil pharmacokinetics in patients undergoing coronary artery bypass surgery. Anesthesiology. 2004;101:862–71.

51. Michelsen LG, Holford NHG, Lu W, et al. The pharmacokinetics of remifentanil in patients undergoing coronary bypass grafting with cardiopulmonary bypass. Anesth Analg. 2001;93:1100–5.

52. Zaugg M, Lucchinetti E, Spahn DR, et al. Volatile anaesthetics mimic cardiac preconditioning by priming the activation of mitochondrial K(ATP) channels via multiple signalling pathways. Anesthesiology. 2002;97:4–14.

53. DeHert S, Vlasselaers D, Barbé R, et al. A comparison of volatile and non-volatile agents for cardioprotection during on-pump cardiac surgery. Anaesthesia. 2009;64:953–60.

54. Lindholm EE, Aune E, Noren CB, et al. The anesthesia in abdominal surgery (ABSENT) trial. Anesthesiology. 2013;119:802–12.

55. Lorati Buse GAL, Schumacher P, Seeberger E, et al. Randomized comparison of sevoflurane versus propofol to reduce perioperative myocardial ischemia in patients undergoing non-cardiac surgery. Circulation. 2012;126:2696–704.

56. Heusch G. Cardioprotection: chances and challenges of its translation to the clinic. Lancet. 2013;12:166–75.

57. Murry CE, Jennings RB, Reimer KA. Preconditioning with ischemia: a delay of lethal cell injury in ischemic myocardium. Circulation. 1986;74:1124–36.

58. Brooks MJ, Andrews DT. Molecular mechanisms of ischemic preconditioning: translation into patient outcomes. Future Cardiol. 2013;9:549–68.

59. Wu L, Zhao H, Wang T, et al. Cellular signaling pathways and molecular mechanisms involving inhalational anesthetics-induced organoprotection. J Anesth. 2014;28:740–58.

60. Zaugg M, Lucchinetti E, Uecker M, et al. Anaesthetics and cardiac preconditioning. Part I. Signaling and cytoprotective mechanisms. Br J Anaesth. 2003;91:551–65.

61. Kojima A, Kitigawa H, Omatsu-Kanbe M, et al. Sevoflurane protects ventricular myocytes against oxidative stress-induced cellular Ca^{2+} overload and hypercontracture. Anesthesiology. 2013;119:606–20.

62. De Hert SG, Van der Linden PJ, Cromheecke S, et al. Cardioprotective properties of sevoflurane in patients undergoing coronary surgery with cardiopulmonary bypass are related to the modalities of its administration. Anesthesiology. 2004;101:299–310.

63. Garcia C, Julier K, Bestmann L, et al. Preconditioning with sevoflurane decreases PECAM-1 expression and improves one-year cardiovascular outcome in coronary artery bypass graft surgery. Br J Anaesth. 2005;94:159–65.

64. De Hert SG, Van der Linden PJ, Cromheecke S, et al. Choice of primary anesthetic regimen can influence intensive care unit length of stay after coronary surgery with cardiopulmonary bypass. Anesthesiology. 2004;101:9–20.

65. Landoni G, Greco T, Biondi-Zoccai G, et al. Anaesthetic drugs and survival: a Bayesian network meta-analysis of randomized trials in cardiac surgery. Br J Anaesth. 2013;111:886–96.

66. Symons JA, Myles PS. Myocardial protection with volatile anaesthetic agents during coronary artery bypass surgery: a meta-analysis. Br J Anaesth. 2006;97:127–36.

67. Hillis DL, Smith PK, Anderson JL, et al. ACCF/AHA guideline for coronary artery bypass graft surgery: a report of the American College of Cardiology Foundation/American Heart Association Task Force on Practice Guidelines. Circulation. 2011;124: e652–735.

68. Landoni G, Guarracino F, Cariello C, Franco A, Baldassarri R, Borghi G, Covello RD, Gerli C, Crivellari M, Zangrillo A. Volatile compared with total intravenous anaesthesia in patients undergoing high-risk cardiac surgery: a randomized multicentre study. Br J Anaesth. 2014;113:955–63.

69. Flier S, Post J, Conception AN, et al. Influence of propofol-opioid vs isoflurane-opioid anaesthesia on postoperative troponin release in patients undergoing coronary artery bypass grafting. Br J Anaesth. 2010;105:122–30.

70. Kortekaas FA, van der Baan A, Aarts LPHJ, et al. Cardiospecific sevoflurane treatment quenches inflammation but does not attenuate myocardial cell damage markers: a proof-of-concept study in patients undergoing mitral valve repair. Br J Anaesth. 2013;112:1005–14.

71. Lucchinetti E, Bestmann L, Fest J, et al. Remote ischemic preconditioning applied during isoflurane inhalation provides no benefit to the myocardium of patients undergoing on-pump coronary artery bypass graft surgery: lack of synergy or evidence of antagonism in cardioprotection? Anesthesiology. 2012;116:296–310.

72. Zhang B, Zhou J, Li H, et al. Remote ischemic preconditioning does not improve the clinical outcomes in patients undergoing coronary artery bypass grafting: a meta-analysis of randomized controlled trials. Int J Cardiol. 2014;172:e36–8.

73. Hausenloy DJ, Candilio L, Evans R, et al. Remote ischemic preconditioning and outcome of cardiac surgery. N Engl J Med. 2015;373:1408–17.

74. Meybohm P, Bein B, Brosteanu O, et al. A multicenter trial of remote ischemic preconditioning for heart surgery. N Engl J Med. 2015;373:1397–407.

75. Kottenberg E, Thielmann M, Bergmann L, et al. Protection by remote ischemic preconditioning during coronary artery bypass graft surgery with isoflurane but not propofol – a clinical trial. Acta Anaesthesiol Scand. 2012;56:30–8.

76. Meybohm P, Hasenclever D, Zacharowski K. Remote ischemic preconditioning and cardiac surgery. N Engl J Med. 2016;374:491.

77. Zhou C, Liu Y, Yao Y, et al. Beta-blockers and volatile anesthetics may attenuate cardioprotection by remore preconditioning in adult cardiac surgery: a meta-analysis of 15 randomized trials. J Cardiothorac Vasc Anesth. 2013;27:305–11.

78. Kottenberg E, Musiolik J, Thielmann M, et al. Interference of propofol with signal transducer and activator of transcription 5 activation and cardioprotection by remote ischemic preconditioning during coronary artery bypass grafting. J Thorac Cardiovasc Surg. 2014;147:376–82.

79. Huang Z, Zhong X, Irwin MG, et al. Synergy of isoflurane preconditioning and propofol postconditioning reduces myocardial reperfusion injury in patients. Clin Sci. 2011;121:57–69.

80. Irwin MG, Wong GTC. Remifentanil and opioid-induced cardioprotection. J Cardiothorac Vasc Anesth. 2015;29:S23–6.

81. Schultz JJ, Hsu AK, Gross GJ. Ischemic preconditioning is mediated by a peripheral opioid receptor mechanism in the intact rat heart. J Mol Cell Cardiol. 1997;29:1355–62.

82. Zhang Y, Irwin MG, Wong TM. Remifentanil preconditioning protects against ischemic injury in the intact rat heart. Anesthesiology. 2004;101:918–23.

83. Mei B, Wang T, Wang Y, et al. High-dose remifentanil increases myocardial oxidative stress and compromises remifentanil infarct-sparing effects in rats. Eur J Pharmacol. 2013;718:484–92.

84. Yu CK, Li YH, Wong GT, et al. Remifentanil preconditioning confers delayed cardioprotection in the rat. Br J Anaesth. 2007;99:632–8.

85. Wong GT, Huang Z, Ji S, Irwin MG. Remifentanil reduces the release of biochemical markers of myocardial damage after coronary artery bypass surgery: a randomized trial. J Cardiothorac Vasc Anesth. 2010;24:790–6.

86. Myles PS, Hunt JO, Fletcher H, et al. Remifentanil, fentanyl, and cardiac surgery: a double-blinded, randomized, controlled trial of costs and outcomes. Anesth Analg. 2002;95:805–12.

87. Howie MB, Cheng D, Newman MF, et al. A randomized double-blinded multicenter comparison of remifentanil versus fentanyl when combined with isoflurane/propofol for early extubation in coronary artery bypass surgery. Anesth Analg. 2001;92:1084–93.

88. Greco M, Landoni G, Biondi-Zoccai G, et al. Remifentanil in cardiac surgery: a meta-analysis of randomized controlled trials. J Cardiothorac Vasc Anesth. 2012;26:110–6.

89. Holm J, Vidlund M, Vanky F, et al. EuroSCORE2 and N-terminal pro-B-type natriuretic peptide for risk evaluation: an observational longitudinal study in patients undergoing coronary artery bypass graft surgery. Br J Anaesth. 2014;113:75–82.

90. Van Harten AE, Scheeren TW, Absalom AR, et al. A review of post-operative cognitive dysfunction and neuroinflammation associated with cardiac surgery and anesthesia. Anaesthesia. 2011;66:280–93.

91. Newman MF, Kirchner JL, Phillips-Bute B, et al. Longitudinal assessment of neurocognitive function after coronary-artery bypass surgery. N Engl J Med. 2001;344:395–402.

92. Royse CF, Andrews DT, Newman SN, et al. The influence of propofol or desflurane on postoperative cognitive dysfunction in patients undergoing coronary artery bypass surgery. Anaesthesia. 2011;66:455–64.

93. Bentov I, Reed MJ. Anesthesia, microcirculation, and wound repair in aging. Anesthesiology. 2014;120:760–72.

94. Yamamoto N, Arima H, Sugiura T, et al. Propofol and thiopental suppress amyloid fibril formation and GM1 ganglioside expression through the γ-aminobutyric acid A receptor. Anesthesiology. 2013;118:1408–16.

95. Lobo FA, P Saraiva A. Playing games with the brain: the possible link between anesthesia and Alzheimer's disease revisited. Rev Esp Anestesiol Reanim. 2014. doi:10.1016/j.redar.2014.07.008.

96. Kobayashi K, Yoshino F, Takahashi SS, et al. Direct assessments of the antioxidant effects of propofol medium chain triglyceride/long chain triglyceride on the brain of stroke-prone spontaneously hypertensive rats using electron spin resonance spectroscopy. Anesthesiology. 2008;109:426–35.

97. Gelb AW, Bayona NA, Wilson JX, et al. Propofol anesthesia compared to awake reduces infarct size in rats. Anesthesiology. 2002;96:1183–90.

98. Schnider TW, Minto CF, Struys MM, Absalom AR. The safety of target-controlled infusions. Anesth Analg. 2016;122:79–85.

99. Short TG, Leslie K, Campbell D, et al. A pilot study for a prospective, randomized, double-blind trial of the influence of

anesthetic depth on long-term outcome. Anesth Analg. 2014;118:981–6.

100. Heringlake M, Garbers C, Käbler JH, et al. Postoperative cerebral oxygen saturation and clinical outcome in cardiac surgery. Anesthesiology. 2011;114:58–69.

101. Slater GP, Guarino T, Stack J, et al. Cerebral oxygen desaturation predicts cognitive decline and longer hospital stay after cardiac surgery. Ann Thorac Surg. 2009;87:36–44.

102. Le Guen M, Liu N, Bourgeois E, et al. Automated sedation outperforms manual administration of propofol and remifentanil in critically ill patients with deep sedation: a randomized phase II trial. Intensive Care Med. 2013;39:454–62.

103. Scott NB, Turfrey DJ, Ray DA, et al. A prospective randomized study of the potential benefits of thoracic epidural anesthesia and analgesia in patients undergoing coronary artery bypass grafting. Anesth Analg. 2001;93:528–35.

104. Landoni G, Isella F, Greco M, et al. Benefits and risks of epidural analgesia in cardiac surgery. Br J Anaesth. 2015;115:25–32.

105. Bracco D, Hemmerling T. Epidural analgesia in cardiac surgery: an updated risk assessment. Heart Surg Forum. 2007;10:E334–7.

106. Schraag S. The current role of total intravenous anesthesia in cardiac surgery: total intravenous anesthesia and cardiopulmonary bypass. J Cardiothorac Vasc Anesth. 2015;29:S27–30.

TIVA/TCI in Veterinary Practice

Thierry Beths

Introduction

Once they have graduated, veterinarians are permitted to provide anesthesia to any patient of almost if not all species (except humans). In general practice, due to the lack of health insurance and the resulting higher health cost, anesthesia is induced, maintained and monitored by nurses, trained or not, under the supervision of a veterinarian who might concurrently be performing a surgical procedure. Consequently, the veterinary practitioner is looking for the cheapest and easiest way to provide anesthesia to their patients and, in most general practices, this will be through the use of inhalants (i.e. isoflurane, sevoflurane). Therefore, Total Intravenous Anesthesia (TIVA) or any other form of drug infusion will be last on their list of anesthetic choices due to the apparent difficulty of use, time and cost constraints. In teaching institutions or in specialised centres (emergency clinic, referral centres), dedicated and/or specialised veterinary anesthetists and anesthesia nurses will be in charge of providing anesthesia. Consequently, the use of a drug infusion to provide muscle relaxation and/or analgesia will be part of the routine, with or without intravenous based hypnotic anesthesia (as opposed to inhalant).

Specialisation in anesthesia is possible in veterinary medicine. It can be achieved by undertaking a rotating internship (or equivalent experience) followed by a 3 year residency program in an approved clinic at the end of which, if his/her credentials are accepted, the resident will be eligible to sit the board exam of either the American (ACVAA—American College of Veterinary Anesthesia and Analgesia), European (ECVAA—European College of Veterinary Anesthesia and Analgesia) or Australian (ANZCVS—Australian and New Zealand College of Veterinary Scientists) colleges. The specialist in veterinary anesthesia will most likely work in academia, a referee centre and sometimes in the industrial sectors. Some may become a consultant for general practitioners and drug companies, but very few will work in general practice.

In veterinary medicine, TIVA, which involves providing anesthesia using intravenous agents only, is a well-known form of anesthesia. In most of the developed countries, veterinarians will provide anesthesia using inhalants and TIVA will only be used for those specific cases where the technique might bring some advantage to the patient (i.e. raised intracranial pressure, bronchoscopy, preservation of the hypoxic pulmonary vasoconstriction reflex). On the other hand, a TIVA technique will be preferentially chosen in remote areas where inhalation is not practical or available (i.e. equine field anesthesia). In shelter medicine and during humanitarian work in countries in need or following disasters, TIVA will be the technique of choice for providing general anesthesia. The different reasons for this include: short surgical procedures not needing prolonged anesthesia; the number of surgeries to be done and the hectic nature of the environment; the higher risk and technical difficulties associated with anesthesia machines and accessories such as O_2 cylinders and vaporisers; finally, shelter medicine has a mobile aspect attached to it which makes it very difficult to move around bulky equipment [1].

Balanced anesthesia is a technique where a hypnotic agent (inhalant or intravenous) is administered concurrently with other drugs (sometimes referred to as adjuvants) to deliver more analgesia, muscle relaxation and cardiovascular stability in order to decrease the amount of hypnotic used and associated side effects [2]. This technique of co-infusion of agents during intravenous or inhalation anesthesia has been used for quite some time in small animal medicine (dogs and cats). While in equine medicine, the advantages of co-infusion have only recently been emphasized and the technique is now becoming more commonly used [3].

T. Beths, MRCVS, PhD, Cert VA, CVA, CVPP (✉)
U-Vet – University of Melbourne, Veterinary Anesthesiology,
250 Princes Highway, Werribee, VIC CODE3030, Australia
e-mail: thierry.beths@unimelb.edu.au

© Springer International Publishing AG 2017
A.R. Absalom, K.P. Mason (eds.), *Total Intravenous Anesthesia and Target Controlled Infusions*,
DOI 10.1007/978-3-319-47609-4_31

In veterinary medicine, when the hypnotic is an inhalant, the technique of using co-infusion to achieve balanced anesthesia is also referred to as Partial Intravenous Anesthesia or PIVA as opposed to TIVA where the hypnotic as well as the other agents are all provided intravenously [3].

The distribution of intravenously infused drugs in the body of an animal is governed by the general principles of pharmacokinetics (PK). Unfortunately for veterinary anesthetists, for any given drug those PK parameters will vary between species and sometimes even between breeds in the same species. An example is the slower propofol clearance observed in greyhound dogs by comparison with other breeds of dogs and beagle dogs in particular [4]. The PK for most of the intravenous agents used in TIVA (or PIVA), have been developed in the targeted species, facilitating the adaptation of infusion protocols per species (Tables 31.1, 31.2 and 31.3). In some cases, those infusion protocols have not been developed through actual scientific research, but were instead either simply extrapolated from similar species (i.e. from the horse for the donkey) or were developed from clinical experience [53].

Ideal drugs for intravenous anesthesia and analgesia should have a rapid onset of action, quick metabolism, and elimination time. Amongst the important PK parameters that veterinarians need to be familiar with, is the context sensitive half-time of elimination (CSHT). This parameter highlights the fact that the elimination half time of a drug during an infusion may be dynamic and may vary with the duration of the infusion, the context. Very little information exists in veterinary medicine about the CSHT of the drugs used for infusion. In addition, like any other PK parameters in veterinary medicine it will also vary between species. For example CSHT for fentanyl in humans increases substantially after 2–3 h of infusion, while this has not been observed in dogs and cats where a steady state is reached after 2–4 and 6 h of infusion, respectively [54–58].

In addition to PK knowledge of the drugs, the (specialist) veterinary anesthetist must be aware of the pharmacodynamic (PD) differences that can exist between species for any given agent. In some cases, drugs which are considered safe for infusion in some species may have dramatic and even lethal effects in others. For example, lidocaine infusion may induce cardiovascular depression in the isoflurane anesthetized cat [59]. Still in the cat, propofol is suspected to be responsible of Heinz Body formation anaemia when infused daily for 2–3 consecutive days [60].

The total intravenous techniques used to maintain anesthesia in animals are not different in principle from those described for human (see Chaps. 6 and 25). Repeated bolus dose administration (intermittent administration) is the simplest technique and the most commonly used for short procedures such as skin biopsies, ultrasound or X-ray in small animals (dogs and cats), and field castration in the horse. When providing continuous infusion, the easiest method involves a fluid bag containing the hypnotic mixture and a giving set attached to an intravenous catheter. With this system, the flow rate can be adjusted varying the diameter of the infusion set using a regulating clamp (Fig. 31.1). The infusion rate can be calculated from knowledge of the volume of each drop of fluid. This methodology is commonly used for "field" anesthesia in the horse (Figs. 31.2 and 31.3). The veterinarian must remember that as the fluid disappears from the infusion bag, the infusion rate will reduce and will therefore need frequent re-adjusting. Although this method provides a more consistent level of anesthesia by comparison with intermittent administration, it has a high potential for miscalculation and overdose, mainly in smaller patient (i.e. cats) and burettes or micro drips are advised for use in those cases. The use of infusion pumps and syringe drivers brings more safety and precision to the continuous infusion. These devices have seen their technology and safety as well as their affordability increase over the last few decades and their use has therefore become more and more common in the veterinary world.

While most of the veterinarians doing TIVA use recipes or published infusion rates (Table 31.2), veterinary anesthesia is seeing the development of pharmacokinetic-dependent infusion techniques to allow specific drug plasma concentrations to be reached. Although most of those PK dependent techniques are mainly used in teaching and referee centres for research purposes, their use has been described in a few clinical cases. Research groups have developed stepped infusion systems for different agents such as for medetomidine or dexmedetomidine in the dog [35] or ketamine in the horse [22]. Stepped infusion systems consist of a group of well-defined different infusion rates which are started at specific times and have been developed so that a desired plasma concentration is reached rapidly and with little accumulation or hangover. This system unfortunately is very rigid and does not allow for target plasma concentration changes. Therefore, the Target Controlled Infusion (TCI) system has been introduced where a computer programmed with the PK of a specific drug for a determined species drives the infusion. The TCI system will maintain a stable desired drug plasma target concentration while adapting the infusion rate to compensate for accumulation. Some TCI systems have been developed in veterinary medicine, but, they have not yet found their way into clinical anesthesia. This is mostly due to the limited availability of hardware and software and due to the paucity of evaluation of population pharmacokinetics. Different drugs have been studied and their PK parameters identified for use in TCI system for different species: propofol in the dog, and ketamine and detomidine (an α_2-adrenoceptor agonist licenced in the horse) in the equine patient [61–63].

Table 31.1 Pharmacokinetics parameters in commonly used intravenous anaesthetics in different species

Drugs	Species	Elimination half-life	Volume of distribution	Total systemic clearance	Comments	References
Propofol	Dogs	322 min	6.5 L/kg	50.1 mg/kg/min	No premed, no co-infusion Beagle dogs	[5]a
		486.2 min	3.38 L/kg	34.4 mg/kg/min	Premedication medetomidine 10 µg/kg, IM Mixed breed dogs	Hall et al. [6]a
		85.3 min	3.27 L/kg	53.35 mg/kg/min	Co-infusion Fentanyl 0.1–0.5 µg/kg/min) LD 2 µg/kg, IV Greyhound dogs	Hughes and Nolan [7]a
		53 min	6.6 L/kg	34 mg/kg/min	No premed, no co-infusion Greyhound dogs	Cockshott et al. [8]a
		74 min	2.46 L/kg	40 mg/kg/min	No premed, no co-infusion Greyhound dogs	Mandsager et al. [9]a
	Cats	527.7 min	6.83 L/kg	17.2 mg/kg/min	No premed, no co-infusion	[10]b bolus
	Ponies	453 min	7.737 L/kg	11.5 mg/kg/min	Co induction Propofol/Ketamine 2 mg/kg each, IV (Ketofol) Co-infusion Propofol/Ketamine 0.17 mg/kg/min each, IV (ketofol)	Zonca et al. [11]a
		69 min	0.89 L/kg	33.1 mg/kg/min	Premed detomidine 20 µg/kg, IV Induction with ketamine 2.2 mg/kg IV Co-infusion ketamine 50 µg/kg/min, IV	Nolan et al. [12]a
	Sheep	56.6	1.037 L/kg	85.4 mg/kg/min	Premed acepromazine/papaveretum No co-infusion	[13]a
		50.3 min	1.515 L/kg	128 mg/kg/min	Same premed as above Ketamine co-induction 1 mg/kg Ketamine co-infusion VRI	
	Swine		1.42–2.72 L/kg	23–32.8 mg/kg/min	Isoflurane anesthetized pigs	Egan et al. [14]a
Alfaxalone	Dogs	24 min	2.4 L/kg	59.4 mg/kg/min	Alfaxalone 2 mg/kg IV bolus; no premed Beagle dogs	[15]b
		34.3 min	2.4 L/kg	48.5 mg/kg/min	Alfaxalone 2 mg/kg IV bolus; no premed Greyhound dogs	[16]b
		42.1 min	2.3 L/kg	36.9 mg/kg/min	Same as above with acepromazine and morphine, 0.03 and 0.3 mg/kg, respectively, IM	
Alfaxalone	Cats	45.2 min	1.8 L/kg	25.1 mg/kg/min	Alfaxalone 5 mg/kg, IV bolus	[17]b
		76.6 min	2.1 L/kg	14.8 mg/kg/min	Alfaxalone 25 mg/kg IV, bolus	[18]b
	Horses	33.4 min	1.6 L/kg	37.1 mg/kg/min	Alfaxalone 1 mg/kg IV with GGE 35 mg/kg, IV Premed acepromazine/xylazine 0.03/1 mg/kg, IV	[18]b
	Neonatal foals	22.8 min	0.6 L/kg	19.9 mg/kg/min	Alfaxalone 3 mg/kg, IV bolus Premed butorphanol 0.05 mg/kg, IV	[19]b

(continued)

Table 31.1 (continued)

Drugs	Species	Elimination half-life	Volume of distribution	Total systemic clearance	Comments	References
Ketamine	Dogs	61 min	1.95 L/kg	39.5 mg/kg/min	Ketamine 15 mg/kg, IV, bolus	Kaka and Hayton [20][b]
	Cats	78.7 min	2.12 L/kg	21.33 mg/kg/min	Ketamine 25 mg/kg, IV, bolus	[21]
	Horses	67.4 min	1.03 L/kg	0.076 mg/kg/min	Ketamine 0.08–0.025 mg/kg/min (stepped infusion) Conscious horses for IV analgesia	[22][a]
		42 min	1.63 L/kg	26.6 mg/kg/min	Xylazine premed; Ketamine 2.2 mg/kg, IV, bolus	Kaka et al. [23][b]
		66 min	2.72 L/kg	31.1 mg/kg/min	Xylazine premed 1.1 mg/kg, IV Induction ketamine 2.2 mg/kg, IV; halothane anaesthesia	Waterman et al. [24][b]
		90 min	1.43 L/kg	23.9 mg/kg/min	Premed detomidine 20 µg/kg, IV Induction with ketamine 2.2 mg/kg IV Co-infusion ketamine 50 µg/kg/min, IV	Nolan et al. 1996 [12][a]
	Ponies	15 min	0.012 L/kg	0.6 mg/kg/min	Ketamine 0.02 mg/mg/min, LD 0.6 mg/kg, IV Conscious horses for IV analgesia	[25][a] PK values for
S-Ketamine		7.8 min	0.013 L/kg	1 mg/kg/min	S-Ketamine 0.01 mg/kg/min, LD 0.3 mg/kg, IV Conscious horses for IV analgesia	S-ketamine only

LD loading dose

[a]Infusion

[b]Bolus only

Table 31.2 Examples of infusion protocols for analgesic adjuncts in different species

Drugs	Species	Loading dose IV	Infusion rate IV	Comments	Reference
α₂ adrenoceptor agonists					
Xylazine	Horse		0.035–0.07 mg/kg/min	With ketamine 0.09–0.15 mg/kg/min	[26]
	Horse	1.1 mg/kg	1–1.5 mL/kg/h	GKX triple drip with 0.5 mg/mL of xylazine, 1 mg/mL ketamine and 50 mg/mL guaifenesin	[27]
Medetomidine	Horse	0.007 mg/kg	0.0035 mg/kg/h	With propofol 0.01–0.11 mg/kg/min	[28]
	Dog/cat		0.001–0.002 mg/kg/h		[19]
Dexmedetomidine	Dog/cat		0.0005–0.001 mg/kg/h		[29]
	Horse	0.0035 mg/kg	0.0001–0.000175 µg/kg/h		[30]
Ketamine	Dog/cat	0.2–0.5 mg/kg	5–20 µg/kg/min	The author usually uses 5–10 µg/kg/min to limit possible side effect resulting from ketamine infusion	[29]
	Horse		40–50 µg/kg/min	With propofol 0.12–0.16 mg/kg min	[31, 32]
Opioids					
Morphine	Dog		0.1–0.2 mg/kg/h		[29]
	Horse	0.05–0.15 mg/kg	0.03–0.1 mg/kg/h	With or without anaesthesia	[30, 33, 34]
Fentanyl	Dog	0.005 mg/kg	0.2–0.5 µg/kg/min	With propofol 0.1–0.3 mg/kg/min	[29]
	Feline	0.001 mg/kg	0.1 µg/kg/min	With propofol 0.1–0.3 mg/kg/min	
Remifentanil	Dog/cat		0.2–0.6 µg/kg/min	With propofol 0.3–0.5 mg/kg/min	
	Feline		0.2–0.3 µg/kg/min	With propofol 0.3 mg/kg/min	
Miscellaneous					
Lignocaine	Dog	2–4 mg/kg	25–80 mic/kg/min		[29]
	Horse	1.5–5 mg/kg	0.025–0.1 µg/kg/min		[2]

For more information, the author refers the reader to more specific veterinary anaesthesia textbook
GKX Guaifenesin Ketamine and Xylazine mixture (triple drip)

The ketamine TCI system for the horse is still in development and a team from Switzerland has recently determined and validated a set of PK parameters in ponies [63]. A few years earlier, in 2006, Knobloch et al., developed a physiologically based pharmacokinetic (PKPB) model for ketamine in ponies targeting low dose of ketamine (S-ketamine 1 µg/mL) to provide analgesia [64]. The models provided reliable prediction of plasma level of R- and S-ketamine. In the dog, a TCI system for propofol (Figs. 31.4 and 31.5) was developed and validated by Beths et al. in 2001 and has since been used in different clinical settings such as neurosurgery [61, 65]; cardiac surgery in a patient with ductus arteriosus [66]; and neutering procedures [67, 68]. In addition, combinations with other agents have been studied: remifentanil, medetomidine and dexmedetomidine [35, 67, 69]. Furthermore, Beths in 2008 and Beier et al., in 2009, looked at the influence of medetomidine and dexmedetomidine, and remifentanil infusion, respectively, on the minimum propofol target concentration needed to stop reaction to supramaximal stimulation in dogs (Table 31.4) [35, 67, 69].

To decrease the dose of drugs used and therefore reduce their potential side effects, anesthetists balance their anesthesia by combining different agents. Doing so, they manage to not only decrease the amount of drug used, but also give a more stable anesthesia with muscle relaxation, analgesia,

hypnosis and cardiorespiratory function that are improved. The most commonly used agents in addition to the hypnotics to balance anesthesia are the α₂-adrenoceptor agonists, ketamine, the opioids and lidocaine, to name a few (Table 31.2).

The α₂-adrenoceptor agonists provide in most species a reliable dose-dependent analgesia, muscle relaxation and sedation. They are therefore ideal agents for balanced anesthesia and are the most widely used sedatives in veterinary anesthesia. Unfortunately their cardiovascular effects, characterised by an increase in blood pressure and systemic vascular resistance with reduced heart rate and cardiac output, are limitations to their use. While xylazine, romifidine and detomidine are most commonly used in the equine patient, medetomidine and its active enantiomer dexmedetomidine are used in dogs and cats. The sparing effect of the α₂-adrenoceptor agonists has been shown on inhalant as well as IV agents such as propofol [35, 77].

Xylazine was synthesize in Germany in 1962 for use in human as an antihypertensive. It was the first α₂-adrenoceptor used in veterinary medicine. Although its use is also licenced in dogs and in cats, it is mostly used in cattle and horses. Romifidine is licenced in horses and has a higher potency than xylazine. Detomidine and medetomidine are more potent than Romifidine. While detomidine is licenced for use in horses, medetomidine is licenced for use in dogs and cats.

Table 31.3 Examples of infusion protocols for the most common intravenous hypnotics used for TIVA in veterinary medicine

Drugs	Species	Premedication	Induction IV	Infusion rate, IV	Comments	References
Propofol	Dogs	As required	Propofol 2–6 mg/kg	Propofol 0.1–0.5 mg/kg/min	Dose rate will vary depending on analgesia and procedure	[29]
	Dogs	Acepromazine 0.03 mg/kg, IM Methadone 0.2 mg/kg, IM	Target of 3 µg/mL	Target 2.7–3.4 µg/mL Dexmedetomidine plasma target of 0.85 ng/mL	TCI propofol Stepped infusion	[35]
	Cats	As required	Propofol 4–8 mg/kg	Propofol 0.12–0.5 mg/kg/min	Dose rate will vary depending on analgesia and procedure	[29]
	Horses	Detomidine	Propofol 2 mg/kg	Propofol 0.18 mg/kg/min	VRI	[36]
	Horses	Xylazine 1 mg/kg, IV Midazolam 0.05 mg/kg, IV	Propofol 3 mg/kg Poor quality	Propofol 0.16 mg/kg/min Ketamine 3 mg/kg/h	VRI CRI	[32]
	Horses	Medetomidine 0.007 mg/kg, IV	Ketamine 2 mg/kg	Propofol 0.1 mg/kg/min Medetomidine 3.5 µg/kg/h	VRI CRI	[28]
	Horses	Medetomidine 0.005 mg/kg, IV	Ketamine 2.5 mg/kg Midazolam 0.04 mg/kg	Propofol 0.14 mg/kg/min Ketamine 1 mg/kg/h Medetomidine 1.25 µg/kg/h	VRI CRI CRI	[37]
	Calves		Propofol 5 mg/kg	Propofol 0.6–0.6 mg/kg/min	VRI	[38]
	Goats		Propofol 2.5–6 mg/kg	Propofol 0.2–0.6 mg/kg/min	VRI	[25, 39, 40]
Alfaxalone	Dogs	As required	Alfaxalone 2–3 mg/kg	Alfaxalone 0.07–0.15 mg/kg/min	VRI	[41, 42]
	Cats	As required	Alfaxalone 1.7–5 mg/kg	Alfaxalone 0.11–0.18 mg/kg/min	VRI	Datasheet [43–45]
	Horses	Acepromazine 0.03 mg/kg, IV Medetomidine 0.007 mg/kg, IV	Guaiphenesin 35 mg/kg Alfaxalone 1 mg/kg	Alfaxalone 2 mg/kg/h Medetomidine 5 µg/kg/h	Colt castration	[46]
	Sheep		Alfaxalone 2 mg/kg	10 mg/kg/h		[47]
	Swine	Alfaxalone 4 mg/kg, IM Medetomidine 0.04 mg/kg, IM Butorphanol 0.4 mg/kg, IM	Alfaxalone 1.2 mg/kg	0.08 mg/kg/min	VRI Placement of epidural catheter	[48]
	Green Vervet monkeys	Ketamine 5 mg/kg, IM	Alfaxalone 0.4–1.2 mg/kg	0.15 mg/kg/min	VRI Imaging study	[49, 50]
Ketamine	Dogs			2–20 µg/kg/min	CRI to provide analgesia in order to reduce anaesthetic requirements	[29]
	Cats			0.15–0.46 µg/kg/min	CRI to provide analgesia in order to reduce anaesthetic requirements	[29, 51, 52]
	Horses	α_2 agonist	Ketamine Diazepam		Triple drip with GGE and α_2-adrenoceptor agonist	See main text

Medetomidine is a racemic mixture composed of dexmedetomidine, the active enantiomer and levomedetomidine the inactive one. While dexmedetomidine has been available in human medicine for a long time, it is only in the last decade that it became available to veterinarians. One of the advantages of this class of drugs is that their effect can be reversed with the use of α_2-antagonists such as yohimbine and atipamezole. The former was developed to reverse the effects of xylazine in particular (dogs, cats, ruminants and exotic species), and the latter is used primarily to reverse the effects of medetomidine or dexmedetomidine in dogs, cats and several exotic species. The reversal agents are usually used to speed up the recovery and/or in an emergency situation. While their use is frequent in exotic species and with wild

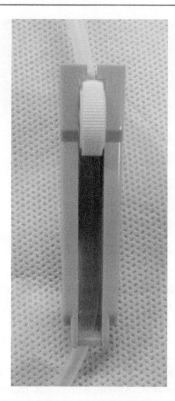

Fig. 31.1 Regulating clamp used to modify fluid rate through a giving set

animals where prolonged recumbency may be associated with higher morbidity and mortality, in equine and small animal practices, veterinarians tend not to reverse it allowing the patient to recover slowly and calmly from the anesthesia. In fact, in horses, following inhalation anesthesia, it is recommended to give the horse a sedative, usually an α_2-adrenoceptor agonist, while it is still anesthetised in the recovery box, to smoothen the recovery and to avoid any excitation which could result in self-induced wound or worse, limb fracture. Figure 31.6 shows some important phases of anesthesia in a horse, including recovery. When using a reversal agent, the analgesic effect of the α_2-adrenoceptor agonists will be reversed and veterinarians must therefore ensure that analgesia is well under control using other agents such as opioids or local anesthetics.

Ketamine is a dissociative agent which is used clinically to provide immobilization or anesthesia (wild animals, horses). In addition to its hypnotic effect, it also provides analgesia and is mostly used at low rate infusion for this effect in different species including dogs, cats and horses. NMDA antagonism is believed to be the most likely molecular mechanism responsible for most of ketamine's clinical properties [78]. Through its NMDA antagonistic properties, ketamine is known as an antihyperalgesic agent that decreases wind-up and may provide pain relief in patients suffering from chronic pain. Infusion schemes have been developed in small animals as well as horses and its sparing

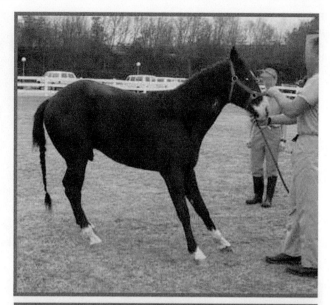

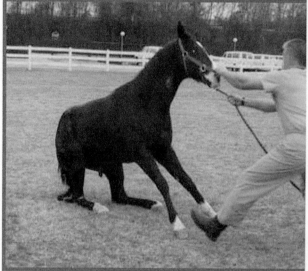

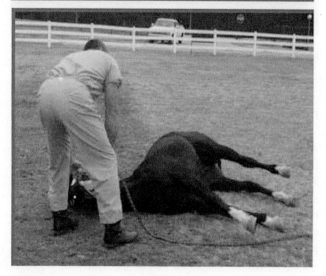

Fig. 31.2 Equine field anaesthesia—induction of anesthesia

Fig. 31.3 Equine field anesthesia—maintenance of anaesthesia using a triple drip based protocol

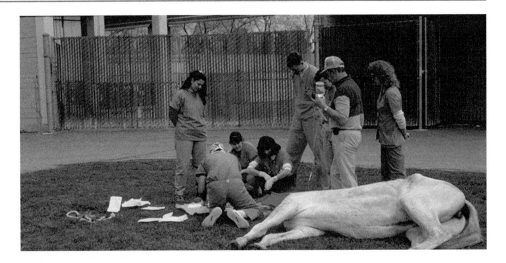

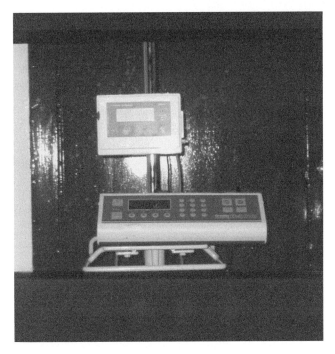

Fig. 31.4 TCI for propofol in the dog—first version

effects have been well documented with inhalant as well as IV agents in different species (Table 31.2) [29, 31, 32, 34].

The opioids are known for their analgesic effects. Although agents characterised by short onset and short duration time such as fentanyl or remifentanil are more appropriate for constant rate infusion (CRI), longer acting agent such as morphine or methadone have also been used in veterinary medicine (Table 31.1) [2, 29, 30, 33, 34]. Etorphine, a potent mu-opioid agonist (about 3000 times the potency of morphine), is mostly used for the restraint and the capture of wild animals. Its use as an infusion to maintain a patient under general anesthesia has been described in the elephant (Fig. 31.7) [79].

Lidocaine is a sodium channel blocker local anesthetic that has been used intravenously to provide analgesia systemically. Its analgesic and anti-inflammatory effects are mediated, among others, by blockade of Na channels, inhibition of glycine receptors, inhibition of NMDA and neurokinin (NK) receptors, promotion of and the release of endogenous opioids. Although it is not recommended for infusion in the cat where severe cardiovascular depression has been observed when used as an infusion [59], it has been successfully used peri-and postoperatively in different species, including dogs and horses [2, 29].

Hypnotic Agents

Propofol

The properties of propofol differentiate it from other intravenous agents. A rapid onset of action, short duration due to high biotransformation, rapid redistribution and an apparent lack of accumulation made it the ideal agent for induction and maintenance of anesthesia in human as well as veterinary medicine.

It is a substituted isopropyl phenol which is insoluble in water and was first formulated with Cremophor EL (1977). Pain associated with injection as well as complement mediated adverse reactions to the Cremophor resulted in radical changes in its formulation [80]. Since 1986, it is formulated in an oil in water emulsion containing 1 % propofol, 10 % soybean oil, 2.25 % glycerol, and 1.2 % purified egg lecithin.

Although this formulation (macro emulsion) is the most popular in human and veterinary medicine, pain on injection has still been reported in humans [81–83] as well as in dogs and cats [84, 85]. In addition, its lack of preservative allows for fungal and bacterial growths leading to a very short shelf life of about 12 h after which time any used vials and tubings

Fig. 31.5 TCI for propofol in the dog—second version

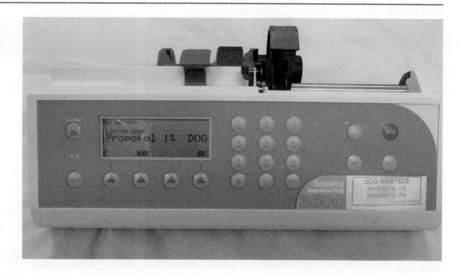

Table 31.4 Examples of minimum infusion rates (MIR) for propofol in different species

Species	Premedication	Induction IV	MIR IV	Comments	References
Dogs	Acepromazine, IM Methadone, IM	Propofol TCI Target 3 µg/mL	Propofol TCI, mCp 3.3 (±1.04) µg/mL	Co-infusion Dexmedetomidine, Measured Plasma concentration of 0.83 ng/mL	[35][a]
			Propofol TCI, mCP 6.2 (±1.35) µg/mL	No co-infusion	
	None	Propofol 6 mg/kg	0.51 (±0.08) mg/kg/min	No co-infusion	[70][a]
			0.42 (±0.08) mg/kg/min	Co-infusion Lidocaine 0.25 mg/kg min CRI (LD 1.5 mg/kg)	
			0.31 (±0.074) mg/kg/min	Co-infusion Lidocaine 0.25 mg/kg/min, CRI (LD 1.5 mg/kg) Ketamine 0.1 mg/kg/min, CRI (1 mg/kg)	
	None	Propofol 6 mg/kg	0.76 (±0.1) mg/kg/min	No co-infusion	[71][a]
		Propofol 5 mg/kg Ketamine 2 mg/kg	0.6 (±0.1) mg/kg/min	Co-infusion Ketamine 0.0025 mg/kg/min	
		Propofol 4 mg/kg Ketamine 3 mg/kg	0.41 (±0.1) mg/kg/min	Co-infusion Ketamine 0.05 mg/kg/min	
Cats	None	Propofol 0.05–0.1 mg/kg/min	0.21 (±0.02) mg/kg/min	No co-infusion	[51][b]
			0.14 (±0.01) mg/kg/min	Co-infusion Ketamine 0.023 mg/kg/min	
			0.14 (±0.01) mg/kg/min	Co-infusion Ketamine 0.046 mg/kg/min	
Horses	Medetomidine 0.007 mg/kg, IV	Propofol 2 mg/kg	0.06–0.1 mg/kg/min	Co-infusion Medetomidine 0.0035 mg/kg/h	[72, 73][a]
	Xylazine 1 mg/kg, IV	Propofol 3 mg/kg	0.1 (±0.02) or mCp 5.3 (±1.4) µg/mL	None	[74][a]
	None	Propofol 7 mg/kg	0.2 (±0.03) or mCp 17.5 (±4.0) µg/mL	None	[75][a]
Rabbit	None	Propofol 1 mg/kg/min	0.64–1.19 mg/kg/min	None	[76][c]

LD loading dose, *mCp* measured plasma concentration
[a]Electric stimulation
[b]Toe pinching
[c]Tail clamping

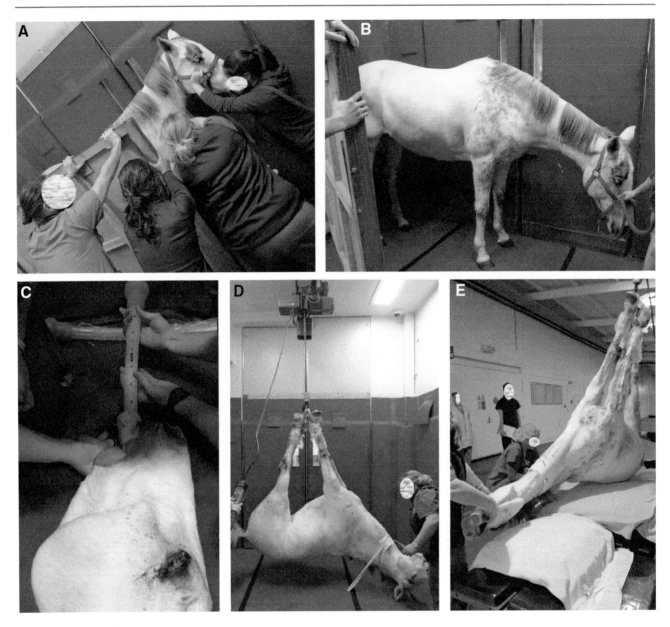

Fig. 31.6 (continued)

(infusion) should be discarded (Label Diprivan® 451094 F/ Issued: February 2014). To increase the shelf life of propofol and possibly decrease pain on administration, other formulations have been developed and tested such as a nano droplet formulation and a propofol containing 2 % benzyl alcohol preservative [10, 86]. Amongst the formulations developed to decrease the pain, the most successful one is fospropofol which is a prodrug of propofol. Unfortunately, PK studies in the dog and the rabbit have shown longer onset and duration of action when compared with the macro emulsion [76, 87].

Pharmacokinetics

In terms of pharmacokinetics, propofol's rapid distribution and clearance are mostly responsible for its clinical success and make it the drug of choice for maintenance of anesthesia. In most species (but not cats) propofol does not seem to clinically accumulate after multiple injections or prolonged infusion resulting in rapid recoveries of relatively good quality. Following a single bolus IV administration, propofol rapidly reaches the brain and induces anesthesia. Then it will redistribute to other tissues, leaving the brain and terminating the anesthesia. In most species

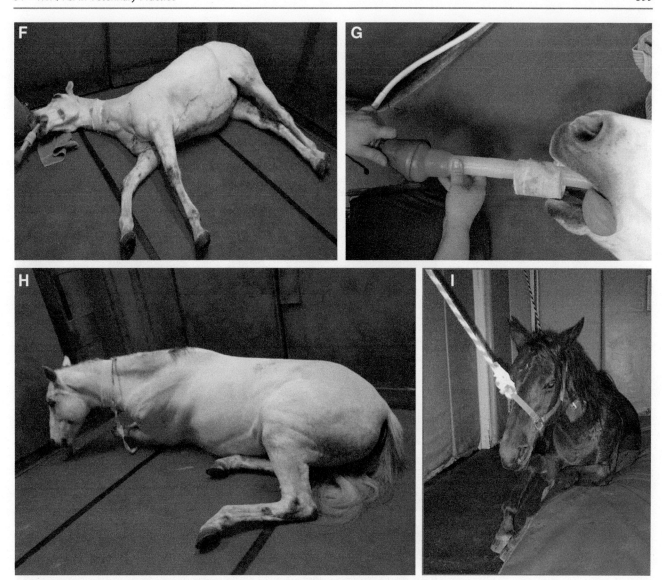

Fig. 31.6 Illustration of some important phases of equine anesthesiaEquine anaesthesiaphases of. (**a**) Sedation horse placed between a wall and a mobile panel to minimize lateral movement during induction; (**b**) induction of anaesthesia; (**c**) blind endotracheal intubation; (**d**) lifting of a horse under anaesthesia from the induction box to the surgery table; (**e**) placement of the horse on the surgery table; (**f**) horse recovering from anesthesia in a padded (wall and floor) recovery box; (**g**) same horse as previous, recovering from an anesthesia, still intubated and breathing 100 % O_2 through a demand valve; (**h**) unassisted recovery; (**i**) assisted recovery

(but not cats) propofol is extensively and rapidly metabolised by the liver, resulting in the production of water soluble sulphide and glucuronide metabolites which will be excreted by the kidneys [88–90]. Propofol's clearance from the plasma far exceeds the hepatic blood flow, which marks the importance of the peripheral tissue uptake as well as the possibility of extra hepatic metabolism (lung, kidney). The latter was confirmed when metabolites of propofol were still detected during the anhepatic phase of orthotopic liver transplantation in man [90]. Although lungs and kidneys have been suggested as possible sites for the extra hepatic metabolism, it is still debated and recent studies have confirmed the importance of the role of the kidneys over the lungs in the extra hepatic propofol clearance [91–95].

Pharmacodynamics

Regarding the central nervous system (CNS), cerebral blood flow (CBF) regulation is not impaired by propofol administration while cerebral metabolic rate (CMR) is decreased which may protect neuronal function in compromised patients [96–98]. The decrease in CMR will also result in vasoconstriction, decreasing ICP (intracranial pressure). Therefore the use of propofol has been advised in humans as well as in dogs with intracranial diseases [99–103].

The cardiovascular (CV) effects of propofol are a dose dependant decrease in myocardial contractility and a decrease in systemic vascular resistance (SVR). The resulting decrease in blood pressure from baseline (no hypotension per se) does not usually trigger a

Fig. 31.7 Elephant undergoing tooth surgery and maintained anesthetized with etorphine infusion. The patient was intubated (Murphy style endotracheal tube ID = 30). The patient was breathing 100 % O₂ and was ventilated (Intermittent Positive Pressure Ventilation) using a demand valve

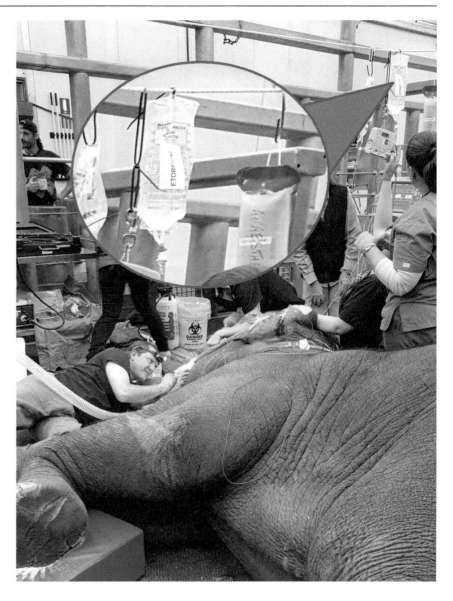

compensatory increase in heart rate as observed with other agents such as thiopental. It has been speculated that in fact propofol resets the baroreceptor reflex set point [104].

Respiratory depression is an important side-effect of propofol and it will dose dependently decrease tidal volume and/or respiratory rate leading to apnea [84, 105]. The incidence of the latter is not only dose dependant, but also administration rate dependant [105]. The ventilatory response to hypoxemia and hypercarbia are decreased with propofol administration and this may be exacerbated with co-administration of opioids [18, 106, 107]. To avoid or limit the respiratory depression, it is advised to administer propofol slowly to effect [84, 108, 109].

It is a great muscle relaxant although myoclonic movements and muscle twitching as well as opisthotonos have been reported during anesthesia in the dog [84, 110–112]. The incidence of these reactions is greatly decreased with the use of preanesthetic tranquillisers, sedatives or opioids.

Propofol lacks analgesic properties, and therefore needs to be co-administered with analgesic agents such as opioids.

Propofol is licenced in dogs and cats but its use has also been reported in other species, either as an induction agent or for TIVA [5, 13, 113–117].

Propofol TIVA in Different Species (Table 31.3)

Canine

Although propofol may depress the CV system through myocardial depression and arteriolar and venous vasodilation, in healthy patient, hemodynamic stability is usually well maintained with a lower blood pressure than baseline and decrease in cardiac output but with minimal changes in heart rate [118, 119]. To avoid higher infusion rates to compensate for propofol's lack of analgesia, analgesic agents (opioids, ketamine) are usually administered in the premedication (bolus) and/or the maintenance (bolus or more commonly as co-infusion period) phase of anesthesia. Although the aim is to decrease the propofol requirements and therefore the associated cardiovascular depression, in the healthy dog, the addition of potent opioids such as remifentanil during the maintenance period shows, in addition to the propofol sparing effect, a decrease in the heart rate (HR), stroke volume (SV) and cardiac output (CO) while still maintaining good arterial blood pressure [118, 120]. To limit those CV effects observed with opioid infusion, ketamine infusion has also been used during propofol based anesthesia: a combination sometimes referred to as Ketofol [119, 121]. Ketamine holds a particular place amongst anesthetic agents as it maintains or increases CO in the healthy patient as a result of increased sympathetic tone [122]. In a recent study in healthy beagle dogs, the combination resulted in a decrease of the amount of propofol used with an increase in HR and arterial blood pressure [119].

In the healthy dog, the main side-effect resulting from propofol administration is respiratory depression which tends to be exacerbated with the addition of opioids as well as ketamine and consequently the anesthetists must be ready to provide assisted ventilation [118, 119].

A recent retrospective study looking at myoclonus in dogs anesthetised with propofol TIVA reported a 1.2 % incidence [123]. This is much lower than the previously described incidences: 21 % [124], 7.5 % [111] or 46.1 % [125]. The difference may result from the fact that in the most recent study, myoclonus was precisely defined as involuntary muscle contractions which did not cease following bolus administration of propofol, and due to their intensity made continuation of anesthesia difficult without further treatment [123]. Any uncoordinated movements, tremor, paddling (running like movement) that could be explained by a lack of hypnosis or analgesia or were present during the awakening phase were not counted. For example, in the Hall and Chambers study [124] the dogs did not receive any analgesia in the premedication or during the procedure and therefore the observed movements could have been attributed to insufficient anesthesia and/or analgesia [124].

Pain on injection has been described in the dog and the incidence varies between 1 and 7.5 % [84, 85]. In a recent study (2012), Michou et al. reported a 3 % incidence with the macro emulsion compared with a 20 % incidence with a new lipid free formulation (propoClear®, Pfizer Animal Health, UK) [126]. Similar results with the lipid free emulsion were reported by Minghella in 2010 [127].

In a recent study, the induction and maintenance doses in unpremedicated animals were respectively 5.3 ± 1.1 and 0.6 ± 0.1 mg/kg [119]. In this study dogs were not undergoing any surgery and anesthesia was maintained for 60 min while the infusion rate was altered up or down following clinical assessment including ocular reflexes, jaw tone, swallowing reflexes and presence or absence of limb withdrawal following toe pinching. The authors did not observe any effect on the HR or the SpO_2 and PaO_2 by comparison to baseline while mean arterial blood pressure (MAP) was lower than baseline, but hypotensive events (MAP < 60 mmHg) were not reported by the authors (lowest MAP observed at was 78 ± 7 mmHg at time 40 min). Five of the ten dogs of the study had short (15 min) apneic events. The time to extubation was 9.4 min and the recovery quality was scored as smooth or with some paddling of short duration. Other infusion protocols are provided in Table 31.3.

The minimum infusion rate (MIR) and the minimum target concentration (TCI) for propofol necessary to block a response to a supramaximal stimulation (tetanic twitch) in 50 % of dogs has been determined with different co-infusions including dexmedetomidine, lidocaine and ketamine [35, 70, 61] (Table 31.4).

Feline

The CV and respiratory effects are very similar to those observed in the dog. The addition of analgesic agents such as potent opioids (fentanyl, alfentanil or sufentanil) in healthy un-premedicated cats undergoing ovariohysterectomy and maintained under anesthesia with propofol TIVA had similar effects as in dogs with a decrease in HR and arterial blood pressure as well as a respiratory depression (decrease respiratory rate, increase in $EtCO_2$) [128]. On the other hand, Padilla and colleagues show that, in acepromazine premedicated cats also undergoing neutering procedures and receiving either remifentanil or alfentanil infusion in addition to propofol TIVA, HR and arterial blood pressure were equal or increased by comparison with baseline while ventilatory parameters were well maintained [129]. In earlier studies, it has been reported that HR and systolic arterial blood pressure (SAP) could increase in cats secondary to sympathetic activation in consequence to the administration of high doses of ultrashort acting opioids [130, 131]. While we cannot comment on the infusion rate for remifentanil, the alfentanil infusion rate was higher in the Padilla's study at 0.5 versus 0.08 μg/kg/min and could have been responsible for the different CV parameters in that study. An additional explanation could be that as the cats underwent ovariohysterectomy in both studies, it is still possible that the surgical stimulation was different enough to have caused the observed difference.

In injured cats, cardiorespiratory variables were compared between propofol/fentanyl and isoflurane/fentanyl anesthesia. A higher requirement for respiratory system support through IPPV was found in the propofol group than in the isoflurane group (9/11 vs 1/11), but CV parameters such as arterial blood pressures in particular were better maintained in the propofol group [132].

In 2015, Campagna et al. reported that, in medetomidine premedicated cats undergoing ovariohysterectomy under propofol TIVA, 80 % of their patients required controlled ventilation [44]. In an earlier study in cats premedicated with morphine and medetomidine, undergoing neutering procedure, Beths et al. did not report post induction apnea or patients requiring controlled ventilation [49]. In the latter study, propofol based anesthesia was induced with less propofol (0.25 vs. 11.7 mg/kg). Although the propofol maintenance infusion rate was higher in the Beths et al. study (0.339 vs. 0.178 mg/kg/min), the recovery times were shorter (33.4 vs. 57 min). This was certainly the result of a shorter duration of anesthesia in the Beths et al. study (26.1 vs. 74 min) and the fact that it has been shown, in cats, that recovery time increases with longer propofol infusion time [133]. This is not really a surprise since we know that the PK of propofol in that species has a longer elimination half time which could result from slower metabolism. In humans, about 60 % of propofol metabolism is via glucuronidation through the glucuronyl transferase enzyme [134]. In the cat, the gene responsible for that enzyme has been classified as a pseudogene and is very likely non-functional [135]. Also in humans, a proportion of propofol undergoes phase one metabolism involving cytochrome P450 (CYP) microsomal enzyme followed by glucuronidation. While the specific enzyme has been identified in humans (CYP2B6) and in dogs (CYP2B11), this has not yet been done in the cat [136–138]. Moreover, Beths in 2008 did not observe much propofol related CYP activity in feline hepatic microsomal preparations by comparison to dogs and rats (Fig. 31.8) (unpublished data).

In addition to this slower metabolism, the use of propofol for TIVA in the cat is still controversial. In a study in 1989, Andress et al. reported, following repeated daily administration of propofol, oxidative injuries to feline red blood cells (Heinz Body formation) as well as facial oedema, generalized malaise, anorexia and diarrhoea [60]. Recovery times were also increased following the second consecutive day of administration. A study performed 12 years later, in cats repeatedly anesthetised with propofol and undergoing radiotherapy, did not report any relevant hematologic changes [142]. While recovery times were not recorded, it was believed that they were not increased. The authors reported similar quality of recovery in all cases without any of the side-effects reported in the Andress study (anorexia and malaises).

The MIR for propofol necessary to block a response to a supramaximal stimulation (tetanic twitch) in 50 % of cats has been determined with two different ketamine co-infusions (Table 31.4) [51].

Equine

Due to the lack of analgesic effect of propofol, the doses required to produce surgical anesthesia are such that while the CV function is more or less well maintained, respiratory depression is of concern and oxygen support is recommended as well as positive pressure ventilation [5, 31, 36, 143, 144].

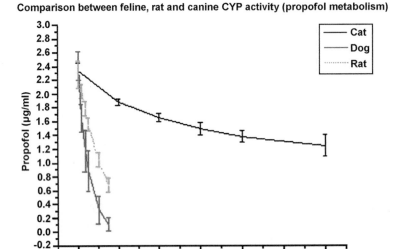

Comparison between feline, rat and canine CYP activity (propofol metabolism)

Fig. 31.8 Degradation of propofol concentrations (2.5 μg/mL) over time in rat, dog and cat hepatic microsomes. At each time, the mean value of two propofol determinations (HPLC) was calculated. Each point is the mean (± SD) propofol concentration from microsomes of six rats, dogs or cats. The incubation times in rats and dog were 0, 5, 10, 15 30 and 45 min while in cats the incubation times were 0, 1,2 3, 4 and 6 h. Isolation of the microsomes followed the methods described by Rutten et al. [139] and Correia [140]. Propofol was extracted from the microsomes and was analysed by HPLC with fluorescence following the method described by Plummer [141]

As far as the author is aware, propofol is the only IV anesthetic which, thanks to its pharmacokinetic quality, is sufficiently non-cumulative to be used in the equine patient for procedures lasting longer than 2 h [73, 145]. Although the induction of anesthesia with propofol may be of poor quality, recoveries are usually good and smooth [116, 146]. In unpremedicated horses, a 4 mg/kg IV dose of propofol is necessary to induce anesthesia [116]. As propofol exists as a 1 % solution, that brings the volume of propofol for induction of anesthesia for a 500 kg horse to about 2000 mg or about 200 mL, which is a big and expensive volume. This and the unreliable quality of induction necessitate combinations of different drugs with propofol such as xylazine or detomidine but with little improvement in the quality of induction [26, 36, 116]. The best results so far seems to have been obtained with the addition of guaiphenesin (GGE), an IV centrally acting muscle relaxant (74–100 mg/kg), or ketamine in the induction protocol or medetomidine in the premedication [37, 73, 147, 148]. Other authors have even recommended anaesthetising horses using a ketamine based protocol followed once anesthesia is induced, by a bolus of propofol and propofol TIVA [28, 31].

In two different studies, following premedication with medetomidine (7 µg/kg IV) and induction of anesthesia with propofol IV 2 mg/kg, anesthesia was maintained up to 4 h at an infusion rate between 0.07–0.11 mg/kg/min and 3.5 µg/kg/h for propofol and medetomidine, respectively [72, 73]. In both cases, although all the horses were breathing spontaneously, the rhythm was irregular in the majority of the horses, no apnea was noticed and $PaCO_2$ did not change significantly, while hypoxemia was recorded in some ponies with PaO_2 values as low as 35 mmHg [72]. In terms of CV parameters, those were relatively well maintained with a few cases of mild hypotension recorded in some ponies with the lowest value recorded for SAP of 78 mmHg [73]. Recoveries were smooth and of good quality with fewer attempts at standing and better overall recovery score when atipamezole (specific (dex)medetomidine reversal agent) was not used. The recovery time varied between 20 and 38 min between the two studies and was not significantly affected by the addition of atipamezole.

In a similar study to the previous one the replacement of propofol with ketamine to induce anesthesia allowed for better induction quality with more difficult intubation and very similar cardiopulmonary parameters. Following 4 h of anesthesia, the mean recovery time was of 31.1 min with a quality scored of good to excellent [149].

The addition of diazepam (0.02 mg/kg, IV) to the previous protocol in 50 client owned horses undergoing different surgeries, provided excellent induction and endotracheal intubation conditions [28]. With a similar medetomidine CRI, but a propofol variable rate infusion (VRI) (0.098–0.108 mg/kg/min) CV parameters were well maintained (no vasopressor agents required) but still 23 horses needed IPPV. While the anesthesia time varied between 46 and 225 min, the recoveries were reported as been uneventful with a mean recovery time of 42.2 min.

When adding GGE (100 mg/kg) to a similar protocol (medetomidine 5 µg/kg and propofol 3 mg/kg, IV) to induce anesthesia in seven horses, Oku et al. recorded better quality of anesthesia and considered 3 µg/kg/min of medetomidine and 1 mg/kg/min of propofol as the minimum infusion rate (MIR) required to maintain anesthesia in horses undergoing castration [148]. Spontaneous breathing was maintained but one horse was apneic at 10 and 15 min and two others at 35 min after receiving a bolus of propofol. Cardiovascular parameters were well maintained and recoveries were of fair (five horses) good (one horse) and excellent (one horse) quality. The number of attempts at standing varied from one to five, with a mean recovery time of about 44 min.

Similarly to other species (dogs and cats), co-infusion of ketamine (20–50 µg/kg/min) allows for a decrease of propofol infusion rate while maintaining good cardiopulmonary parameters [31, 32, 150].

In Flaherty's study, the protocol consisted of detomidine (20 µg/kg IV) premedication followed by induction with ketamine 2.2 mg/kg IV and maintenance of anesthesia with ketamine 40 µg/kg/min and propofol 0.12 mg/kg/min (preceded with a 0.5 mg/kg, IV) in four ponies [31]. Following a propofol infusion lasting 65 min (ketamine 60 min) the recovery was of good quality and lasted about 27.2 min.

Ohta's et al., premedicated horses with 1 mg/kg of xylazine, but used a propofol based IV induction (3 mg/kg) with midazolam (0.05 mg/kg) which resulted in unacceptable induction conditions with some horses paddling [32]. Thereafter, they maintained anesthesia with a ketamine and propofol infusion rate of 50 µg/kg/min and 0.16 mg/kg min, respectively. Ketamine was stopped 20 min before the estimated end of the surgery. While propofol was stopped 112–140 min after the start of the infusion, recoveries were of good quality and lasted about 70 (±23) minutes.

Ketamine (2 mg/kg) and diazepam (0.03 mg/kg) IV were used to induce acepromazine (0.03 mg/kg, IV) and detomidine (0.015 mg/kg, IV) premedicated horses [150]. Induction of anesthesia was then followed by a propofol bolus of 0.3 mg/kg and anesthesia was maintained with infusions of propofol (0.16 mg/kg/min) and ketamine (20–40 µg/kg/min). The ketamine infusion was started at a rate of 40 µg/kg/min and was decreased by 10 µg/kg/min every 20 min. It was terminated 30 min before the estimated end of anesthesia. After a mean anesthesia time of 59 ± 17 min, recovery time was 34 ± 7 min and of good quality.

The addition of medetomidine infusion to ketamine/propofol anesthesia was studied by Umar et al. [37, 144,

151]. The basic protocol was the same between the three studies: premedication with medetomidine 5 µg/kg, IV followed by induction of anesthesia with midazolam 0.04 mg/kg and ketamine 2.5 mg/kg IV. To maintain anesthesia, ketamine at 1 mg/kg/h and medetomidine 1.25 µg/kg/h was added to a propofol VRI of 0.14 mg/kg/min (2006 and 2007 studies) and 0.17–0.13 mg/kg/min (2015 study). In all the studies the CV parameters were very well maintained. In the first study (2006), apnea was observed in all horses (six) after the propofol loading dose and therefore IPPV was initiated in this study as well as the following two studies. Once IPPV was started, no respiratory issues were observed in any of the studies. Duration of anesthesia was 115 ± 17 min, 4 h and 175 ± 14 min in the 2006, 2007 and 2015 study, respectively. Recovery quality was good in all the studies, with a time to standing of $62 \pm 10, 98 \pm 21$ and 74 ± 28 min, respectively.

The MIR for propofol necessary to block a response to a supramaximal stimulation (tetanic twitch) in 50 % of horses have been determined with different premedication (xylazine, medetomidine and no drug) and co-infusion protocols (no drug and medetomidine) (Table 31.4) [73, 74, 145].

Ruminants

Very little information is available on the use of propofol based TIVA in cattle. In 2015, Deschk et al. reported the use of propofol in unsedated calves (6–12 months old) for induction (5 mg/kg IV) and maintenance (0.6 and 0.8 mg/kg/min for 60 min) of anesthesia [38]. The calves were allowed to breathe room air. Recoveries were uneventful. No apnea was noticed at any time while some muscle tremors were observed in three out of eight calves at a propofol infusion rate of 0.6 mg/kg/min but in only one out of eight at a propofol infusion rate of 0.8 mg/kg/min. The arterial pressures decreased in both groups but to a greater extent in the 0.8 mg/kg/min group which also had a bigger decrease in SVRI (systemic vascular resistance index). Cardiac index (CI) increased in the 0.8 mg/kg/min group while staying constant in the 0.6 mg/kg/min group.

Propofol anesthesia (2.5–6 mg/kg, IV) has been induced in goats either alone or following a premedication [40]. Maintenance of anesthesia varied with the level of sedation resulting from the premedication (0.2–0.6 mg/kg/min). When compared to fentanyl premedication (0.02 mg/kg) and co-infusion (0.02 mg/kg/h), midazolam premedication (0.3 mg/kg) and co-infusion (0.3 mg/kg/h) resulted in a smoother recovery following a 90 min propofol anesthesia (12–18 mg/kg/h) [39]. In both cases, cardiopulmonary parameters were well maintained. When ketamine is used as a co-infusion (0.03 mg/kg/min) in propofol anesthetised goats (0.3 mg/kg/min) following midazolam premedication (0.4 mg/kg IV) and ketamine (3 mg/kg, IV)/propofol (1 mg/kg, IV) induction, the authors reported stable cardiopulmonary parameters and recoveries of good to excellent quality [25].

Swine

In pigs propofol is often combined with a potent short acting opioid such as fentanyl [152]. Schoffmann et al. [153] reported the use of propofol for induction (1 mg/kg IV) and maintenance of anesthesia (8 mg/kg/h) with co-infusion of fentanyl (35 µg/kg/h) in midazolam (0.5 mg/kg, IM), ketamine (10 mg/kg IM) and butorphanol (0.5 mg/kg, IM) premedicated piglets [153]. They reported very stable mean blood pressure and heart rates for 300 min of anesthesia time. There is no information on the recovery times or quality as it was a non-recovery surgery.

Miscellaneous

Propofol-ketamine in the donkey [154]: Following xylazine premedication (1 mg/kg, IV) and induction of anesthesia with ketamine (1.5 mg/kg, IV) and propofol (0.5 mg/kg, IV), anesthesia was maintained for 1 h in eight healthy donkeys with a CRI of propofol (0.15 mg/kg/min) and ketamine (0.05 mg/kg/min). The donkeys were placed in lateral recumbency following induction of anesthesia, their tracheas were intubated and they were allowed to breathe room air. While all the donkeys had PaO_2 values between 47 and 93 mmHg, ventilation was well maintained ($PaCO_2$ between 38 and 51 mmHg). Heart rate and mean blood pressure stayed in acceptable ranges. Recovery was uneventful and the donkeys were standing 29 ± 9 min following cessation of the CRI's.

Propofol (3.7 mg/kg, IV) was used to induce anesthesia in a medetomidine (25 µg/kg, IM) and diazepam (0.38 mg/kg, IM) premedicated King penguin with a history of seizures who was undergoing brain MRI (Figs. 31.9 and 31.10) [38]. Anesthesia was maintained for 138 min with propofol at a rate of 0.1–0.3 mg/kg/min. IPPV was continued from the start of anesthesia until the end with 100 % O_2. Spontaneous breathing was recorded 10 min after the end of the infusion and extubation was achieved 15 min later when the penguin started lifting his head and moving his wings. Recovery was smooth without any excitation or adverse behaviour.

The MIR for propofol necessary to block a response to a supramaximal stimulation (tail clamping) in 50 % of rabbits has been determined (Table 31.4) [76].

Alfaxalone

Alfaxalone is a neuroactive steroid which has been used in veterinary medicine since the early 1970s. At that time, the poorly water soluble agent was combined with a weak anesthetic alfadolone and formulated in Cremophor EL

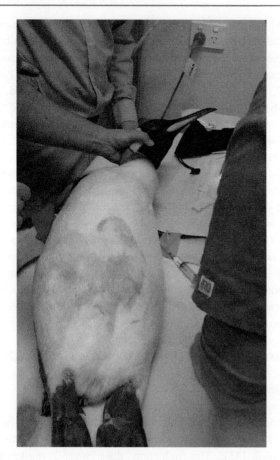

Fig. 31.9 Induction of anaesthesia of a King Penguin with propofol prior the MRI examination under propofol TIVA

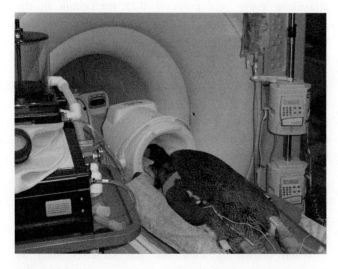

Fig. 31.10 King penguin undergoing MRI examination and anesthetized with propofol TIVA (variable rate infusion). The patient had an endotracheal tube and was connected to an anesthesia machine with a universal F breathing system (FiO$_2$ = 1.0)

[155]. The latter was responsible for hyperaemia in cats, and histamine release with anaphylactic reactions in dogs [156]. The formulation was characterised by rapid onset and offset of action, no irritating effects on the blood vessels, and minimum CV and respiratory effects with a high therapeutic index [157–159]. Athesin (human formulation) or Saffan (veterinary formulation) were removed from the market in the middle of the 1980s [160]. Recently, Jurox, an Australian drug company reintroduced alfaxalone, without the alfadolone and this time, formulated in a non-cremophor vehicle, 2-hydroxypropyl-β-cyclodextrin (Alfaxan CD®). This drug has now been approved in dogs and cats in Australia, Canada, and Europe and more recently in the USA. This new formulation is not associated with histamine release and has been evaluated in other species (sheep, horses).

Meanwhile, in humans, alfaxalone in sulfobutyl-ether-β-cyclodextrin has been developed by another Australian company, Dawbridge Pharmaceuticals Pty Ltd (Malver, Victoria, Australia) [160]. Following comparison of the new formulation with propofol in rats, the authors concluded that the new formulation had a similar onset and offset timing as propofol, and a higher therapeutic index. The new formulation recently went through phase 1c trials and showed very promising result in humans with a fast onset and short duration of anesthesia similar to propofol, but with less reported CV depression and no pain on injection [161].

From now on, all the following information regarding alfaxalone will concern the new veterinary formulation, Alfaxan CD®, unless specified otherwise. This formulation does not contain a preservative and therefore supports micro-organism growth, but not as readily as does propofol and any solution remaining after withdrawal should be discarded [162].

Its mechanism of action is similar to thiopental or propofol and results from its interaction with the GABA$_A$ receptors and yields a state of anesthesia and provides good muscle relaxation.

Pharmacokinetics

Alfaxalone shares some PK advantages with propofol such as fast onset and short duration of action attributable to the fact that both are rapidly redistributed and metabolized [15, 16, 163].

The pharmacokinetics of alfaxalone have been determined in different species such as dogs, cats and horses (Table 31.1) and has been determined to be non-linear (in the dog and the cat), meaning that with increasing doses, plasma concentration and the area under the plasma concentration-time curve (AUC) increase out of proportion to the change in doses [16, 17]. In the cat, Whittem et al. [17] reported that despite the non-linear kinetic of alfaxalone, at clinical dose rates, no accumulation of the agent or its effects were observed [17]. Alfaxalone undergoes both phase I (cytochrome P450 metabolism) and phase II (conjugation dependent) hepatic metabolism. While both dogs and cats seem to produce the same five metabolites following phase I (allopregnatrione, 3β-alfaxalone, 20-hydroxy-3β-alfaxalone, 20-hydroxyalfaxalone and 2α-hydroxyalfaxalone), dogs predominantly produce alfaxalone glucuronide in phase 2 whereas cats also produce alfaxalone sulphate [164]. Unlike propofol, it seems that breed has little effect on alfaxalone PK as the PK parameters observed in un-premedicated greyhounds were very similar to those observed in un-premedicated beagles [15, 16]. In contrast, acepromazine/morphine premedicated greyhounds saw their anesthesia time, following a bolus of alfaxalone, increased by a factor of 5. A decrease in perfusion due to acepromazine was thought to be the reason of the observed decrease in clearance, but this could not be substantiated [16].

In a study looking at PK in male and female dogs, it seems that although the agent is derived from the hormone progesterone, there was no gender effect in the PK and therefore it could be administered at the same dose to either sex [15].

Pharmacodynamics

Although we do not know the effects of Alfaxan CD® itself on cerebral hemodynamic and metabolism, it is very likely that the effect will be similar to those observed with the previous alfaxalone-alfadolone formulation: a dose-dependent decrease in cerebral blood flow (CBF) and cerebral metabolic rate oxygen ($CMRO_2$) [165–158]. When maintaining anesthesia in cats via a CRI of the former CT 1341 formulation, Baldy-Moulinier and Besset-Lehmann reported a dose dependent decrease in CBF and intracranial pressure (ICP) as well as concurrent vasoconstriction [165]. Those attributes in relation to the cerebral hemodynamic and metabolism supported the use of the new formulation with remifentanil CRI in a dog undergoing craniotomy for tumour resection [164].

At clinical doses in different species, the CV parameters remain quite stable. When given at clinically relevant doses in dogs (2 mg/kg, IV) and in cats (5 mg/kg, IV), the CV parameters were reported to stay stable [169, 170]. With increasing doses, the studied CV parameters deviated from normal, but these changes differed between species. In the cat, when doses of up to 10 times the clinical dose (50 mg/kg) were administered IV, HR, CO and ABP decrease while in the dog a tenfold clinical dose (20 mg/kg) administration resulted in an increase of HR while ABP decreased [169, 170].

Although possibly more pronounced in dogs than in cats, a dose dependant respiratory depression is observed in both species, with a decrease in respiratory rate leading to apnea, decreased tidal volume, minute volume and PaO_2 [169, 170]. In both species hypercarbia is also noticed. As for the CV effect, at clinical doses the effects are mild and manageable. And as for propofol, titration to effect at induction will reduce the risk of respiratory depression and post induction apnea [43, 171].

To the author's knowledge there are no known contra-indications for the use of alfaxalone but, as it demonstrates dose-dependant pharmacokinetics and undergoes hepatic metabolism, the author would advise caution for its use as an infusion in patients with liver damage. In both dogs and cats dose-dependant mild CV depression has been observed after induction of anesthesia with alfaxalone. Therefore the authors advise caution when used in hemodynamically compromised patient and propose dose-titration to effect as a means of decreasing those CV side-effects.

Alfaxalone TIVA in Different Species (Table 31.2)

Canine

Following acepromazine (0.02 mg/kg, IV) and hydromorphone (0.05 mg/kg, IV) premedication, anesthesia was induced and maintained either with alfaxalone or propofol [41]. The induction dose was 2 mg/kg for alfaxalone and 4 mg/kg for propofol. Both doses were administered over 60 s. Anesthesia was then maintained for 120 min with alfaxalone 0.07 mg/kg/min for the alfaxalone group and propofol 0.25 mg/kg/min in the propofol group. Between the two groups, systemic and pulmonary artery pressures, HR, CO and CI, stroke volume (SV) and stroke volume index (SVI), and SVR did not vary significantly and were well maintained compared to baseline. Although no significant changes were observed between groups for parameters such as respiratory rate, arterial pH, PaO_2, or $PaCO_2$, in both groups, respiratory depression was evident with low respiratory rate, increased $EtCO_2$, decreased pH (respiratory acidosis). Post induction apnea was observed in one dog in each group and lasted 210 s in the alfaxalone vs. 82 s in the propofol group. Time from end of CRI to standing was 52 ± 10 and 62 ± 18 min for alfaxalone and propofol respectively. The quality of recovery was good in both groups.

When comparing their use for surgeries such as ovariohysterectomy, following acepromazine (0.01 mg/kg IM) and morphine (0.4 mg/kg IM) premedication, induction and maintenance of anesthesia with propofol (5.8 ± 0.3 mg/kg and 0.37 ± 0.09 mg/kg/min, respectively) and alfaxalone (1.9 ± 0.07 mg/kg and 0.11 ± 0.01 mg/kg/min, respectively) showed similar results with no difference between groups in the measured cardiopulmonary parameters [42].

Table 31.5 Examples of minimum infusion rates (MIR) for Alfaxalone in different species

Species	Premedication	Induction IV	MIR IV	Comments	References
Cats	Acepromazine 0.1 mg/kg, IM Butorphanol, 0.2, IM	Alfaxalone 2.57 (±0.4) mg/kg	0.19 (±0.02) mg/kg/min	Ovariohysterectomy	[45]
	Medetomidine 0.02, IM Butorphanol, 0.2, IM	Alfaxalone 1.87 (±0.5) mg/kg	0.18 (±0.02) mg/kg/min		
Goats		Alfaxalone 3 mg/kg	0.16 (0.14–0.18) mg/kg/min	None	[180][a]
	Fentanyl 0.005, IV	Alfaxalone 2 mg/kg	0.11 (0.11–0.14) mg/kg/min	Co-infusion Fentanyl 0.005 mg/kg/h	[181][a]
	Fentanyl 0.015, IV		0.05 (0.017–0.11) mg/kg/min	Co-infusion Fentanyl 0.015 mg/kg/h	
	Fentanyl 0.03, IV		0.017 (0.017–0.08) mg/kg/min	Co-infusion Fentanyl 0.03 mg/kg/h	
	Midazolam 0.1, IV	Alfaxalone 2.3 mg/kg	0.11 (0.11–0.14) mg/kg/min	Co-infusion Midazolam 0.1 mg/kg/h	[181][a]
	Midazolam 0.3, IV	Alfaxalone 2 mg/kg	0.11 (0.08–0.11) mg/kg/min	Co-infusion Midazolam 0.3 mg/kg/h	
	Midazolam 0.9, IV	Alfaxalone 2 mg/kg	0.048 (0.016–0.08) mg/kg/min	Co-infusion Midazolam 0.9 mg/kg/h	

[a]Clamping proximal part of one digit of the hoof

While HR and blood pressures were well maintained in both groups, hypoventilation was observed while maintaining good oxygenation (dogs breathed 100 % O_2 through an appropriate breathing system). Therefore, as a conclusion, the authors suggested that ventilatory support should be considered when those protocols were used in bitches undergoing neutering procedure.

When replacing acepromazine (0.05 mg/kg) with the α_2-adrenoceptor agonist dexmedetomidine (10 μg/kg, IM) in a buprenorphine (20 μg/kg, IM) based premedication in dogs undergoing similar procedures, the alfaxalone infusion rate was reduced from 0.11 with acepromazine to 0.08 mg/kg/min in dexmedetomidine group [172]. The difference resulted most probably from the analgesic properties of the α_2-adrenoceptor agonist [173, 174]. Similarly to the previous study, the authors reported very good CV parameters while apnea and hypoventilation were commonly observed. After 2 h of anesthesia, recoveries were of short duration (about 10 min) in both groups, but of better quality in the acepromazine group which could be due to the longer lasting sedative properties of that agent.

Alfaxalone has been studied in both juvenile (12 weeks of age) dogs and cats and shown to provide acceptable anesthesia [175, 176]. Most recently, it has demonstrated favourable characteristics including improved neonatal APGAR scores when used for induction of anesthesia for canine caesarean section by comparison with propofol [177]. Both agents have similar puppy survival rates. When compared to alfaxalone induction followed by isoflurane anesthesia, alfaxalone TIVA in un-premedicated female dogs undergoing caesarean section resulted in longer recovery of poorer quality [178]. Unfortunately, in this study the alfaxalone CRI was predefined not tailored to the patients' requirements and therefore, boluses of alfaxalone were required to be administered to maintain anesthesia. As alfaxalone clearance is dose dependant (non-linear kinetics) and as incremental bolus administration results in higher peak plasma concentration, it is very likely that the lengthy recovery was due to an "excessive" dose of alfaxalone. Similarly the poorer recovery quality observed in the alfaxalone group may have also resulted from the high dose of alfaxalone as this agent has been reported to increase noise sensitivity in dog, leading to poor recoveries [179]. Although the alfaxalone TIVA resulted in a lower APGAR score than isoflurane, puppies' survival was the same in both groups.

The MIR for alfaxalone necessary to maintain anesthesia in female dogs undergoing ovariohysterectomy has been determined with two different butorphanol based premedication protocols (acepromazine vs. medetomidine) (Table 31.5) [45].

Feline

In medetomidine (20 μg/kg, IM) and morphine (0.3 mg/kg, IM) premedicated cats (10 male and 24 female) undergoing neutering procedure, the reported alfaxalone induction and maintenance doses were 1.7 (0.3–3) mg/kg and 0.18 (0.06–0.25) mg/kg/min [43]. None of the cats became apneic and respiratory and heart rates were well maintained. Hypotensive episodes of short duration and responding to fluid therapy and decrease of alfaxalone infusion rate were reported in 20 cats (59 %). The anesthesia time was longer in female cats than in male cats (126.5 ± 24.7 vs. 39.6 ± 21.6 min) resulting in a higher maintenance dose been administered to the female cats (about 22 vs. 7 mg/kg). This might have resulted in the longer recovery time (time to first head tilt) also observed in the female cats (49 vs. 27 min). Alfaxalone PK, as in the dog, is described as being non-linear and dose-dependant recovery times have been describes in other studies [170, 182]. The quality of the recovery was good in 31 cats while noise induced excitation of short duration (10–20 min) was reported in three cats. This side-effect was previously reported in cats with the former alfaxalone-alfadolone formulation [158, 183].

In a study in female cats undergoing neutering procedure, Schwarz et al. [45] compared acepromazine and medetomidine (both with butorphanol) premedication in alfaxalone TIVA [45]. While the induction dose was lower in the medetomidine group (1.87 ± 0.5 vs. 2.57 ± 0.41 mg/kg), the infusion rates were very similar between the two groups (around 0.18 mg/kg/min). Although those results are very similar to the previous study, the authors reported inadequate quality of anesthesia and the need for alfaxalone boluses during the procedure. This difference was possibly due to the use of butorphanol (a partial µ agonist opioid) which has been shown to provide very little analgesia in the cats recovering from neutering surgery by comparison to a full agonist opioid such as methadone [184]. Cardiopulmonary data were similar to the previous study. They reported neither apneic events nor respiratory depression. Some myoclonus, mostly of the hind limbs, was reported during the recovery period which lasted about 60 min (time to first head tilt).

When comparing alfaxalone and propofol TIVA in dexmedetomidine (15 µg/kg, IM) and morphine (0.3 mg/kg, IM) premedicated female cats undergoing neutering procedures, no cardiopulmonary difference (HR and arterial blood pressure), $EtCO_2$, SpO_2, RR)) were noted between the two groups [49]. No cats required ventilatory support. Neither hypotensive nor apneic events were reported. Following approximatively 26 min of anesthesia, recovery quality was very good in both groups with a non-significant longer time to reach sternal position with alfaxalone (35 vs 47 min).

In a later study, comparing the same two hypnotic agents in medetomidine (10 µg/kg, IM) and meloxicam (0.3 mg/kg, IM) premedicated female cats undergoing neutering procedure, Campagna et al. also reported very good CV parameters in both groups with no hypotension [44]. With regards to respiration, the authors reported significantly better maintained respiratory function in the alfaxalone group where the $EtCO_2$ over time was kept lower and where only 2/10 cats (vs. 8/10) needed ventilatory support. The possible difference between those two last studies with regards to the reported respiratory effects could come from the fact that in Campagna et al.'s study, the induction doses were five (propofol) to ten (alfaxalone) times higher than in Beths et al.'s study.

Equine

The pharmacokinetic of alfaxalone in the adult horses and neonatal foals have been previously determined following a single IV bolus (Table 31.1) [18, 19].

So far, only three studies report the clinical use of alfaxalone TIVA in the horse [46, 185, 186]. As TIVA is mostly used in field anesthesia and as castration is the most common surgery done in the field conditions, those three studies are on horses undergoing field castration.

Following romifidine (an α_2-adrenoceptor agonist at 100 µg/kg, IV) and butorphanol (50 µg/kg, IV) premedication, anesthesia was induced with diazepam (0.05 mg/kg, IV) and alfaxalone (1 mg/kg, IV) and maintained with incremental IV dose(s) of alfaxalone (0.2 mg/kg) as required [186]. Induction and maintenance of anesthesia as well as recovery were scored good to excellent. Horses were standing 34 ± 9 min following induction. Although HR did not change following induction of anesthesia, a slight increase in RR was recorded. Of the 17 ponies undergoing castration surgery, one needed four increments while nine needed one.

When compared to ketamine in a similar setting (romifidine/butorphanol premedication and diazepam co-induction), alfaxalone shows shorter induction time (18 ± 4 vs. 30 ± 6 s) but needed to be topped up more frequently than ketamine (4/21 vs. 7/20 ponies) [185]. While both HR and RR increase following ketamine induction, no changes were observed with alfaxalone. There was no clinical difference in terms of recovery times and quality.

Infusion of alfaxalone (2 mg/kg/h) and medetomidine (5 µg/kg/h) has been describes in 11 colts undergoing castration surgery [46]. Anesthesia was maintained for about 45 min with this regimen following acepromazine (0.03 mg/kg, IV) and medetomidine (7 µg/kg/min) premedication and induction of anesthesia with guaiphenesin (35 mg/kg, IV) and alfaxalone (1 mg/kg, IV). Quality of induction and recovery were good to excellent, with only one attempt to stand and a time from end of infusion to standing of 37 ± 13.5 min. Horses were spontaneously breathing O_2 enriched air and cardiopulmonary data were clinically acceptable with no apneic and/or hypotensive events been recorded.

Ruminant

While no information exist on the use of alfaxalone in cattle, a study in un-premedicated sheep induced with alfaxalone 2 mg/kg IV and maintained anesthetised with a CRI of alfaxalone at 10 mg/kg/h, reported clinically acceptable hemodynamic results (HR and ABP) with mild respiratory depression (decreased RR, increased $PaCO_2$, decreased pH) [47]. Following 72.5 min of anesthesia, recovery was of good quality and about 22 min long. In 2015, Ndwanna et al. determined the MIR of alfaxalone in sheep [180]. In the same year, Dzikiti et al. determined the MIR of alfaxalone in sheep with either a fentanyl or a midazolam co-infusion (Table 31.5) [181, 187].

Swine

Although alfaxalone based TIVA has not yet been reported in pigs, the author's group has submitted for publication a study on the use of alfaxalone TIVA in the pig [48].

In this study, 12 pigs were anesthetised for about 51.5 min for epidural catheter placement as part of another study. Premedication consisted of 4 mg/kg of alfaxalone, medetomidine 40 µg/kg and butorphanol 0.4 mg/kg IM. Twenty to forty minutes later anesthesia was induced with alfaxalone (1.2 mg/kg, IV) and maintained with alfaxalone at a rate of 0.08 mg/kg/min. Induction of anesthesia was smooth and endotracheal intubation was very easy in all pigs. The cardiorespiratory variables (HR, NIBP, RR, and SPO$_2$) remained within normal limits for all animals throughout anesthesia. No pigs developed hypotension or apnea.

Miscellaneous

Induction and maintenance of anesthesia with alfaxalone (0.8 ± 0.4 mg/kg, IV and 0.15 ± 0.02 mg/kg/min, IV, respectively) in ten green vervet monkeys (3.1–6.4 kg) has been describes [50]. The monkeys underwent X-ray and ultrasound studies. Following 73 ± 13 min of anesthesia, recoveries were uneventful and time to standing from the end of infusion was 32.7 ± 12.1 min. HR values were unchanged from pre-induction values while hypotensive event were recorded in six monkeys and responded to fluid therapy and lowering depth of anesthesia. Although RR was decreased from pre-induction values, no apneic events were observed.

More recently, a study describes the use of alfaxalone TIVA (similar rate as in the previous study) in alfaxalone (2 mg/kg, IM) and medetomidine (15 µg/kg, IM) premedicated cynomolgus monkeys [188]. Those monkeys underwent MRI examination and were anesthetised for about 117 min. At the end of the anesthesia, atipamezole (50 µg/kg, IM) was administered and the monkeys were able to stand about 20 min after the end of the CRI. Mean arterial blood pressure, HR and RR were at or below the lower limits of the normal range.

Ketamine

Ketamine is a dissociative agent derived from phencyclidine, and results in a change of awareness by dissociation of the thalamocortical and limbic systems where the thalamic and limbic system seem to be stimulated while cortical activity is depressed or disconnected from any incoming signals [189, 190]. The depression of the thalamocortical and limbic systems results from NMDA antagonism via the phencyclidine binding site. This prevents the excitatory neurotransmitter glycine from binding, causing a cataleptic state where the patient does not respond to external stimuli but does not look asleep either.

Dissociative anesthesia is characterised by: analgesia, light sleep, amnesia, catatonia/catalepsy, poor muscle relaxation, hypersensitivity to noise; active cranial nerves reflexes (palpebral, corneal, gag, nystagmus) [189].

Ketamine exists in most of the preparations as a racemic mixture while a purified S-ketamine formulation is available in some countries. The S isomer offers some advantage over the racemic mixture such as quicker metabolism, more intense analgesia, less delirium emergence [191].

The pH of the racemic mixture is usually low (3.5–5.5) and pain at injection during IM administration has been reported [189].

Ketamine is very lipophilic and rapidly crosses the blood brain barrier. It has a relatively short onset (about 1 min) and duration of action (15–20 min).

Pharmacokinetics

In most species (except cats) ketamine undergoes demethylation through hepatic microsomal enzymes into the active metabolite, norketamine which has about 10–30 % of the anesthetic potency of ketamine. After repeated doses or long infusion of ketamine, accumulation of norketamine contributes to a prolonged recovery and hangover. After hydroxylation and conjugation, norketamine becomes water soluble and is excreted by the kidneys [192]. In cats, although almost all the parent compound is excreted through the kidneys unchanged, some ketamine is bio-transformed into norketamine that is directly excreted through the kidneys [21]. Caution should therefore be taken when using ketamine in animals with liver and/or renal dysfunction as prolonged activity and anesthetic time may result.

Recovery following one injection results mainly from redistribution and metabolism. Unfortunately, with repeated administrations or infusion, the agent tends to accumulate as the redistribution sites become saturated and the recovery becomes more dependant on metabolism and excretion. In cats, as there is no metabolism, redistribution and excretion are the main pathways for blood ketamine level to decrease [29].

Pharmacodynamics

The delirium emergence, bronchodilation and sympathomimetic actions observed with ketamine is believed to be a product of its antagonistic effect at the muscarinic receptors, or to be a direct stimulating effect of the drug on the sympathetic system [193].

Ketamine increases cerebral blood flow which with the observed increase in blood pressure will result in increase in ICP. Caution is therefore advised when using ketamine in patients with increased risk of abnormal ICP. This effect can be attenuated by maintaining in normocapnia and/or co-administering drugs such as the benzodiazepines. In addition, due to increased EEG activity observed with ketamine, it is usually advised not to use ketamine in patients with a history of seizures.

Abnormal behaviours have been reported in the recovery period, ranging from ataxia, hyper-reflexivity, increased motor activity to frank hyperexcitability where the animals are hyperresponsive to noise, light and handling [29]. The incidence or intensity of those reactions can be decreased by the addition of benzodiazepines and/or α_2 adrenoceptor agonists [192].

Ketamine has a direct negative inotropic effect on the myocardium partly through its Ca channel blocking effect. These effects are usually overcome by the centrally mediated ketamine stimulation of the sympathetic system. Therefore, increases in ABP, CO, HR are more commonly observed following its administration. Although the ketamine effect very likely originates from increased sympathetic nervous system outflow, ketamine also inhibits noradrenaline reuptake at the postganglionic sympathetic nerve endings, increasing plasma catecholamine [122, 194]. Consequently, the administration of ketamine in a critically ill patient where the catecholamine stores and the sympathetic compensatory mechanism are exhausted may unveil ketamine's negative inotropic effects.

With regards to the respiratory system the administration of ketamine usually results in bronchodilation and a maintained ventilatory response to hypoxia and hypercarbia. Apneustic breathing has been reported where a pause appears after the inspiratory time of the breathing cycle. Minute ventilation and CO_2 level are usually stable. Please note that although pharyngeal and laryngeal reflexes are maintained, they are usually uncoordinated and endotracheal intubation to secure the airways is strongly advised.

Ketamine is known for its analgesic effect, even at sub anesthetic doses, which has resulted in many protocols having been developed where the infusion rate of the agent is below anesthetic levels (i.e. 2–20 μg/kg/min) [189]. Although some of its analgesic effect is possibly due to activity on opioid receptors, it is believed that most of its effect is through its activity as an NMDA receptor antagonist at the level of the dorsal horn limiting central sensitization and wind-up [29, 195].

Ketamine TIVA in Different Species (Table 31.2)

Canine

Ketamine is used at a low infusion rate (5–10 μg/kg/min) to provide analgesia during inhalation and TIVA (propofol or alfaxalone) anesthesia [189, 196–199].

Due to possible accumulation over time and associated rough recoveries, ketamine is not commonly used as the main hypnotic agent for TIVA in dogs. Still, different ketamine based TIVA protocols have been describes using different combinations aiming to alleviate the poor muscle relaxation usually observed with ketamine anesthesia [200]. These include: guaiphenesin (GGE) and xylazine [201]; medetomidine premedication [202, 203]; propofol co-administration [119, 204]; midazolam xylazine/medetomidine co-administration [205].

In all those studies, the quality of anesthesia was of good quality and the measured CV functions were well maintained while some respiratory depression was observed. The quality of recovery was only reported as good in two studies [119, 205]. Fdo et al. used midazolam infusion as previously describes in a human study with ketamine based TIVA where recovery was also graded as good and better than following halothane N_2O anesthesia [206]. In addition to midazolam, Fdo et al. used an α_2-adrenoceptor agonist xylazine or medetomidine for premedication and co-administration. Those agents are known to provide good muscle relaxation and are usually recommended while using ketamine based anesthesia [189]. Although medetomidine was also used in Hellebrekers (2 studies) and Selikar's studies, it was only used in the premedication. As the anesthesia in those three studies lasted longer than 60 min, this may have led to having little to no medetomidine left in those dogs at the time of the awakening, resulting in rougher recoveries being reported.

Cats

In 1991, Brown et al. describes the use of ketamine as part of a GGE/xylazine combination for a 6 h anesthesia in the cat [207]. The recorded CV and respiratory parameters stayed within the normal ranges and the cats were back in sternal recumbency exhibiting voluntary movement in just over 2 h following cessation of the infusion.

As in dogs, ketamine based TIVA is seldom used in cats due to accumulation as well as the poor recovery quality. It is therefore most commonly used at lower doses for its analgesic and sparing effects as well its possible sympathomimetic effects [51]. Studies in humans have shown that the CV and respiratory depressing effects of IV drugs such as propofol could be offset by the addition of ketamine [208, 209]. In a study looking at the minimum infusion rate (MIR) of propofol in cats when ketamine was added, Ilkiw et al. [51] showed that the addition of ketamine (0.23 or 0.46 μg/kg/min) allowed a decrease of the propofol infusion rate for a number of end points such as response to toe pinch, tetanic stimulation or tail clamp [51]. In addition, CV and respiratory functions were very well maintained. In a similar study, Ilkiw and Pascoe showed (2003) that the addition of ketamine (0.23 μg/kg/min) and the resulting decrease in propofol infusion rate did not change measurements such as MAP, CVP, SI, CI, SVRI, O_2 delivery index, O_2 consumption, PvO_2, pH or arterial blood $PaCO_2$, base deficit by comparison to propofol alone [210]. However, the application of noxious stimulation for MIR determination resulted in an increase of the HR and PaO_2 in the propofol alone group. Ravasio et al. [52] reported the use of "ketofol', an extemporaneous combination of a low dose of ketamine and propofol in the same syringe (1:1 ratio) [52]. Following an induction dose of the mixture at 2 mg/kg of each drug, and a maintenance infusion rate set at 10 mg/kg/h each, with or without dexmedetomidine premedication (0.003 mg/kg, IM), cats underwent neutering surgery. Following a 25 min infusion, cats were extubated sooner (7 vs 29 min) in the group without dexmedetomidine and also had a lower sedation score for the first hour post-surgery. With or without the premedication with dexmedetomidine, all cardiopulmonary parameters were well within normal ranges, with HR and SpO_2 being lower and MAP been higher in the dexmedetomidine group. All the cats breathed spontaneously.

Equine

Ketamine is the most commonly used IV agent with the equine patient not only to induce general anesthesia but also to maintain general anesthesia when a TIVA based technique is needed (i.e. field anesthesia) [211].

Due to the risk of accumulation, it is usually advised not to keep the patients under ketamine TIVA for longer than 90 min as longer anesthesia has been associated with longer and rougher recoveries [145].

TIVA techniques in equine anesthesia are principally used for surgical procedures in the field where anesthesia machine are impractical [212]. Greene and co-workers first describes a combination of ketamine (1 mg/mL), xylazine (0.5 mg/mL) and guaiphenesin (GGE) 5 % (1 L) [27]. This became the so called "triple drip" or GKX which is given at a rate of 1.5 mL/kg/h. Since then, modifications of the original triple drip have been made by either changing the α_2-adrenoceptor agonist to detomidine (GKD) or to romifidine (GKR) [213, 214]. To increase the time of infusion and as the GGE is the main cumulative agent, people have increased the dose of xylazine to 1 mg/mL and the ketamine to 2 mg/mL.

Although the above combinations can be used to induce anesthesia after a premedication with an α_2-adrenoceptor agonist, it is not advised. This is to avoid using too much GGE before the start of the procedure and therefore limiting the infusion time to maintain anesthesia. It is instead more common to use an induction protocol such as ketamine and diazepam and then start the triple drip. The triple drip is considered a safe way to anesthetise horses and is characterised by smooth recoveries, with the horse going into sternal recumbency, followed later on by standing. While the CV function is well maintained, the respiratory function although of good quality at the beginning of the anesthesia tends to decrease with anesthesia of 45 min or longer. It is therefore advised to allow the patient to be breathing an oxygen-enriched gas mixture and to be intubated [215]. The combination including an α_2-adrenoceptor agonist will result in copious amounts of urine being produced which may be of concern when working in hot weather conditions [215].

Other ketamine based TIVA regimens have been describes such as the MKX where the GGE is replaced by another muscle relaxant agent, midazolam (0.05 mg/mL) [216]. The main finding from that study was a prolonged ataxia observed in the recovery period and therefore the authors proposed a reduction of the midazolam concentration to minimize the observed side-effect.

Combinations of xylazine (2–4 mg/kg/h) and ketamine (5–7 mg/kg/h) have been evaluated by Mama et al. in 2005. Oxygen supplementation was advised with that protocol [217].

Yamashita et al. in 2007 reported the use of a mixture of midazolam (01.8 mg/mL) ketamine (40 mg/mL) and medetomidine (0.1 mg/mL) to maintain anesthesia in medetomidine premedicated (5 μg/kg, IV) horses undergoing castration [218]. Following induction of anesthesia with midazolam (0.04 mg/kg, IV) and ketamine (2 mg/kg, IV), general anesthesia was maintained with the mixture at a rate of about 0.09 mL/kg/h. Following 38 (±8) minutes of infusion, recoveries of satisfactory (3/9) to good (6/9) qualities lasted about 33 (±13) minutes. In the same study, five horses were anesthetised using the same protocol, but with an infusion rate of 1 mL/kg/h, for 1 h without a surgical procedure being performed so that the cardiopulmonary effects could be assessed. It was concluded that although there was mild cardiopulmonary depression, MKM-TIVA provided clinically acceptable general anesthesia. Oxygen supplementation was advised as hypoxemia was observed during the study with PaO_2 values of around 50–60 mmHg.

Recently, the use of S-ketamine (2.5 mg/kg, IV) along with diazepam (0.05 mg/kg, IV) was describes to induce general anesthesia in horses premedicated with romifidine (0.1 mg/kg, IV) and L-methadone (0.05 mg/kg, IV) and undergoing field castration [219]. It was concluded that although the inductions and recoveries were of good qualities, the duration of the surgical anesthesia following one single injection tended to be insufficient to complete surgical castration and that general anesthesia could therefore be maintained by an additional doses of S-Ketamine of 1 mg/kg, IV, at 10–15 min, without impairing the quality and duration of the recoveries.

More information about the use of ketamine TIVA in equine patients can be found in more specialized literature [145, 211, 215].

Ruminant

Similarly to horses, the triple drip mixture has been used successfully in cattle, sheep, and even lamas [220]. Although the concentration of ketamine in the mixture will be similar to that in horses (1–2 mg/mL), xylazine is often reduced to 0.1 and even to 0.05 mg/mL for prolonged anesthesia due to the risk of accumulation and the increased sensitivity to this agent observed in ruminants. In all cases, the GGE concentration is 50 mg/mL. The reported infusions of mixtures of 0.1 mg/mL of xylazine, 1–2 mg/mL of ketamine in GGE 50 mg/mL are as follow: 1.5–2.5 mL/kg/h in calves, 2 mL/kg/h in adult cattle, 2–2.6 mL/kg/h in sheep and 1.2–2.4 mL/kg/h in lama [220].

Swine

A triple drip combination of ketamine (1–2 mg/mL), xylazine (1 mg/mL) in GGE (50 mg/mL) has been used in pigs at rates of about 2.2 mL/kg/h for anesthesia up to 2 h [221, 222]. Recoveries although of good qualities are prolonged (30–45 min) and yohimbine (a xylazine specific reversal agent (0.06–1 mg/kg)) could be administered to shorten the recovery, but with the potential consequence of diminishing post-operative analgesia.

Miscellaneous

A triple drip protocol using 0.5 mg/mL of xylazine, 2 mg/mL of ketamine and 50 mg/mL of GGE at a 2 mL/kg/h rate has been used to maintain anesthesia for 1 h in the spontaneously breathing donkey [154]. Although hypoxemia (oxygen supplementation was not provided) was observed, no other cardiorespiratory or metabolic changes were observed. Recoveries took on average 32 min with some epiphora and salivation with good quality score in all the donkeys (7/8) but one who only scored acceptable. This protocol still needs to be evaluated for surgical conditions.

Conclusion

Veterinary anesthetists are very familiar with drug infusions either as a means to maintain a patient under general anesthesia (TIVA) and/or to provide extra analgesia, sedation or muscle relaxation (co-infusion, balanced anesthesia, PIVA).

The actual use of TIVA or PIVA techniques to help maintain a patient under general anesthesia will depend upon factors such as the veterinarian's qualification (general practitioner vs. specialist in anesthesia), the veterinarian's practice (equine vs. dogs and cats vs. wildlife) and the veterinarian's location (general practice, referee centre, outdoor, third world country, disaster zone).

In human anesthesia, the development of PK dependant infusion systems such as the TCI for propofol revolutionised TIVA by making propofol an IV agent as simple to administer and as rapid to titrate as an inhalational anesthesia.

Although TCI systems have been developed for propofol in the dog or detomidine and ketamine in the horses, the use of this technology stayed mostly at the research level. Beside the lack of enough knowledge/availability of population pharmacokinetics for individual target agents, the actual cost associated with the infusion of drugs such as propofol and even more alfaxalone to maintain anesthesia is very likely to be the main reason if not the only factor responsible for this lack of movement to the clinical world. It is important to remember that in veterinary medicine, the health cost are not supported by health insurance and therefore veterinarians need to be very cautious with their charges, keeping their clients happy while still making a living. Using propofol or alfaxalone instead of isoflurane to maintain a dog under general anesthesia would increase the cost to the small animal (dogs and cats) veterinarian by a factor of 4 and 8, respectively while in horses, the factor would be of about 12 and 24, respectively. Therefore, as most of the veterinarians in practice will be using inhalation anesthesia to maintain their patient anesthetised, it is very unlikely that the TCI system or similar system will become popular soon.

Another very interesting evolution in human anesthesia was the linking of the TCI system with monitors of depth of anesthesia such as the BIS (Bispectral Index) resulting in a "closed loop anesthesia" or CLAN [223–226]. As far as the author is aware, such a system has not yet been tested in animal even so BIS monitoring has been used in dogs and other species with more or less some success [75, 227–235].

Drug companies are still looking for the "ideal" IV agent. While some are developing completely new agents, others are revisiting old agents and making them more TIVA friendly [236]. This revamping of old drugs involved techniques such as: isolation of active enantiomers (dexmedetomidine, s-ketamine, l bupivacaine); replacement of less suitable excipient (Cremophor EL with cyclodextrin for alfaxalone); transforming an agent into a prodrug to make it more water soluble (fospropofol). More information can be found elsewhere in the literature [236, 237].

Will TIVA supersede inhalational anesthesia in human anesthesia? It is difficult to predict, but some seems to think it will, or at least in some specific areas such as paediatric

[238]. Although this seems very unlikely to happen in veterinary medicine in the near future, veterinarians will have no choice but to follow their human colleagues if those decided to go "full" TIVA as drug companies would not find the veterinary market economically viable to keep producing the inhalant agents.

References

1. Looney AL. Anesthesia and pain management of shelter populations. In: Grimm KA, Lamont LA, Tranquilli W, et al., editors. Veterinary anesthesia and analgesia the fifth edition of Lumb and Jones. 5th ed. Oxford: Wiley; 2015. p. 731–9.

2. Valverde A. Balanced anesthesia and constant-rate infusions in horses. Vet Clin North Am Equine Pract. 2013;29:89–122.

3. White K. Total and partial intravenous anesthesia of horses. In Pract. 2015;37:189–98.

4. Court MH, Hay-Kraus BL, Hill DW, et al. Propofol hydroxylation by dog liver microsomes: assay development and dog breed differences. Drug Metab Dispos. 1999;27:1293–9.

5. Nolan AM, Hall LW. Total intravenous anesthesia in the horse with propofol. Equine Vet J. 1985;17:394–8.

6. Hall LW, Lagerwij E, Noaln AM, et al. Effect of medetomidine on the pharmacokinetics of propofol in dogs. Am J Vet Res. 1994;55(1):116–20.

7. Hughes JM, Nolan AM. Total intravenous anesthesia in greyhounds: pharmacokinetics of propofol and fentanyl: a preliminary study. Vet Surg. 1999;28(6):513–24.

8. Cockshott ID, Douglas EJ, Plummer GF, et al. The pharmacokinetics of propofol in laboratory animals. Xenobiotica. 1992;22(3):369–75.

9. Mandsager RE, Clarke CR, Shawley RW, et al. Effects of chloramphenicol on infusion pharmacokinetics of propofol in greyhounds. Am J Vet Res. 1995;56(1):95–9.

10. Cleale RM, Muir WW, Waselau AC, et al. Pharmacokinetic and pharmacodynamic evaluation of propofol administered to cats in a novel, aqueous, nano-droplet formulation or as an oil-in-water macroemulsion. J Vet Pharmacol Ther. 2009;32:436–45.

11. Zonca A, Ravasio G, Gallo M, et al. Pharmacokinetics of ketamine and propofol combination administered as ketofol via continuous infusion in cats. J Vet Pharmacol Ther. 2012;35(6):580–7.

12. Nolan AM, Reid J, Welsh E, et al. Simultaneous infusions of propofol and ketamine in ponies premedicated with detomidine: a pharmacokinetic study. Res Vet Sci. 1996;60(3):262–6.

13. Correia D, Nolan AM, Reid J. Pharmacokinetics of propofol infusions, either alone or with ketamine, in sheep premedicated with acepromazine and papaveretum. Res Vet Sci. 1996;60:213–7.

14. Egan TD, Kem SE, Johnson KB, et al. The pharmacokinetics and pharmacodynamics of propofol in a modified cyclodextrin formulation (Captisol) versus propofol in a lipid formulation (Diprivan): an electroencephalographic and hemodynamic study in a porcine model. Anesth Analg. 2003;97(1):72–9.

15. Ferre PJ, Pasloske K, Whittem T, et al. Plasma pharmacokinetics of alfaxalone in dogs after an intravenous bolus of Alfaxan-CD RTU. Vet Anaesth Analg. 2006;33:229–36.

16. Pasloske K, Sauer B, Perkins N, et al. Plasma pharmacokinetics of alfaxalone in both premedicated and unpremedicated Greyhound dogs after single, intravenous administration of Alfaxan at a clinical dose. J Vet Pharmacol Ther. 2009;32:510–3.

17. Whittem T, Pasloske KS, Heit MC, et al. The pharmacokinetics and pharmacodynamics of alfaxalone in cats after single and multiple intravenous administration of Alfaxan at clinical and supraclinical doses. J Vet Pharmacol Ther. 2008;31:571–9.

18. Goodwin WA, Keates HL, Pasloske K, et al. The pharmacokinetics and pharmacodynamics of the injectable anesthetic alfaxalone in the horse. Vet Anaesth Analg. 2011;38:431–8.

19. Goodwin W, Keates H, Pasloske K, et al. Plasma pharmacokinetics and pharmacodynamics of alfaxalone in neonatal foals after an intravenous bolus of alfaxalone following premedication with butorphanol tartrate. Vet Anaesth Analg. 2012;39:503–10.

20. Kaka JS, Hayton WL. Pharmacokinetics of ketamine and two metabolites in the dog. J Pharmacokinet Biopharm. 1980;8(2):193–202.

21. Hanna RM, Borchard RE, Schmidt SL. Pharmacokinetics of ketamine HCl and metabolite I in the cat: a comparison of i.v., i.m., and rectal administration. J Vet Pharmacol Ther. 1988;11:84–93.

22. Lankveld DP, Driessen B, Soma LR, et al. Pharmacodynamic effects and pharmacokinetic profile of a long-term continuous rate infusion of racemic ketamine in healthy conscious horses. J Vet Pharmacol Ther. 2006;29:477–88.

23. Kaka JS, Klavano PA, Hayton WL. Pharmacokinetics of ketamine in the horse. Am J Vet Res. 1979;40(7):978–81.

24. Waterman AE, Roberson SA, Lane JG. Pharmacokinetics of intravenously administered ketamine in the horse. Res Vet Sci. 1987;42(2):162–6.

25. Larenza MP, Bergadano A, Iff I, et al. Comparison of the cardiopulmonary effects of anesthesia maintained by continuous infusion of ketamine and propofol with anesthesia maintained by inhalation of sevoflurane in goats undergoing magnetic resonance imaging. Am J Vet Res. 2005;66:2135–41.

26. Mama KR, Steffey EP, Pascoe PJ. Evaluation of propofol for general anesthesia in premedicated horses. Am J Vet Res. 1996;57:512–6.

27. Greene SA, Thurmon JC, Tranquilli WJ, et al. Cardiopulmonary effects of continuous intravenous infusion of guaifenesin, ketamine, and xylazine in ponies. Am J Vet Res. 1986;47:2364–7.

28. Bettschart-Wolfensberger R, Kalchofner K, Neges K, et al. Total intravenous anesthesia in horses using medetomidine and propofol. Vet Anaesth Analg. 2005;32:348–54.

29. Kastner SBR. Intravenous anesthetics. In: Seymour C, Duke T, editors. BSAVA manual of canine and feline anesthesia and analgesia. 2nd ed. Gloucester: BSAVA; 2007. p. 133–49.

30. Gozalo-Marcilla M, Gasthuys F, Schauvliege S. Partial intravenous anesthesia in the horse: a review of intravenous agents used to supplement equine inhalation anesthesia. Part 2: opioids and alpha-2 adrenoceptor agonists. Vet Anaesth Analg. 2015;42:1–16.

31. Flaherty D, Reid J, Welsh E, et al. A pharmacodynamic study of propofol or propofol and ketamine infusions in ponies undergoing surgery. Res Vet Sci. 1997;62:179–84.

32. Ohta M, Oku K, Mukai K, et al. Propofol-ketamine anesthesia for internal fixation of fractures in racehorses. J Vet Med Sci. 2004;66:1433–6.

33. Solano AM, Valverde A, Desrochers A, et al. Behavioural and cardiorespiratory effects of a constant rate infusion of medetomidine and morphine for sedation during standing laparoscopy in horses. Equine Vet J. 2009;41:153–9.

34. Villalba M, Santiago I, Gomez de Segura IA. Effects of constant rate infusion of lidocaine and ketamine, with or without morphine, on isoflurane MAC in horses. Equine Vet J. 2011;43:721–6.

35. Beths, T. Pharmacodynamic and pharmacokinetic properties of medetomidine and dexmedetomidine infusions in dogs anesthetised with propofol administered by TCI. In: Total intravenous anesthesia in dogs: development of a target controlled infusion (TCI) scheme for propofol. PhD. Glasgow: University of Glasgow; 2008. p. 114–67.

36. Matthews NS, Hartsfield SM, Hague B, et al. Detomidine-propofol anesthesia for abdominal surgery in horses. Vet Surg. 1999;28:196–201.

37. Umar MA, Yamashita K, Kushiro T, et al. Evaluation of total intravenous anesthesia with propofol or ketamine-medetomidine-propofol combination in horses. J Am Vet Med Assoc. 2006;228:1221–7.

38. Deschk M, Wagatsuma JT, Araujo MA, et al. Continuous infusion of propofol in calves: bispectral index and hemodynamic effects. Vet Anaesth Analg. 2016;43:309–15.

39. Dzikiti BT, Stegmann FG, Dzikiti LN, et al. Total intravenous anesthesia (TIVA) with propofol-fentanyl and propofol-midazolam combinations in spontaneously-breathing goats. Vet Anaesth Analg. 2010;37:519–25.

40. Dzikiti TB, Stegmann GF, Hellebrekers LJ, et al. Sedative and cardiopulmonary effects of acepromazine, midazolam, butorphanol, acepromazine-butorphanol and midazolam-butorphanol on propofol anesthesia in goats. J S Afr Vet Assoc. 2009;80:10–6.

41. Ambros B, Duke-Novakovski T, Pasloske KS. Comparison of the anesthetic efficacy and cardiopulmonary effects of continuous rate infusions of alfaxalone-2-hydroxypropyl-beta-cyclodextrin and propofol in dogs. Am J Vet Res. 2008;69:1391–8.

42. Suarez MA, Dzikiti BT, Stegmann FG, et al. Comparison of alfaxalone and propofol administered as total intravenous anesthesia for ovariohysterectomy in dogs. Vet Anaesth Analg. 2012;39:236–44.

43. Beths T, Touzot-Jourde G, Musk G, et al. Clinical evaluation of alfaxalone to induce and maintain anesthesia in cats undergoing neutering procedures. J Feline Med Surg. 2014;16:609–15.

44. Campagna I, Schwarz A, Keller S, et al. Comparison of the effects of propofol or alfaxalone for anesthesia induction and maintenance on respiration in cats. Vet Anaesth Analg. 2015;42:484–92.

45. Schwarz A, Kalchofner K, Palm J, et al. Minimum infusion rate of alfaxalone for total intravenous anesthesia after sedation with acepromazine or medetomidine in cats undergoing ovariohysterectomy. Vet Anaesth Analg. 2014;41:480–90.

46. Goodwin WA, Keates HL, Pearson M, et al. Alfaxalone and medetomidine intravenous infusion to maintain anesthesia in colts undergoing field castration. Equine Vet J. 2013;45:315–9.

47. Moll X, Santos L, Garcia F, et al. The effects on cardio-respiratory and acid-base variables of a constant rate infusion of alfaxalone-HPCD in sheep. Vet J. 2013;196:209–12.

48. Bigby SE, Carter JE, Bauquier S, et al. Use of propofol for induction and maintenance of anesthesia in a King Penguin (Aptenodytes patagonicus) undergoing magnetic resonance imaging. J Avian Med Surg. 2016;30(3):237–42

49. Beths T, McNally E, Freeman M, et al. Total intravenous anesthesia (TIVA) in cats: comparison between propofol intralipid and alfaxalone in hydroxypropyl-beta-cyclodextrin to induce and maintain anesthesia in feral female cats undergoing spay procedures. In: 11th World Congress of Veterinary Anaesthesiology, Cape Town, South Africa, 2012.

50. Beths T, Taylor J, Beierschmitt A, et al. Total intravenous anesthesia (TIVA): evaluation of alfaxalone in hydroxypropyl-beta-cyclodextrin to induce and maintain anesthesia in a group of vervet monkeys undergoing an ultrasound study. In: Proceedings of the 11th World Congress of Veterinary Anaesthesiology, 2012.

51. Ilkiw JE, Pascoe PJ, Tripp LD. Effect of variable-dose propofol alone and in combination with two fixed doses of ketamine for total intravenous anesthesia in cats. Am J Vet Res. 2003;64:907–12.

52. Ravasio G, Gallo M, Beccaglia M, et al. Evaluation of a ketamine-propofol drug combination with or without dexmedetomidine for intravenous anesthesia in cats undergoing ovariectomy. J Am Vet Med Assoc. 2012;241:1307–13.

53. Matthews NS, van Loon JPAM. Anesthesia and analgesia of the donkey and the mule. Equine Vet Educ. 2013;25:47–51.

54. Iizuka T, Nishimura R. Context-sensitive half-time of fentanyl in dogs. J Vet Med Sci. 2015;77:615–7.

55. Murphy MR, Hug Jr CC, McClain DA. Dose-independant pharmacokinetics of fentanyl. Anesthesiology. 1983;59:537–40.

56. Pypendop BH. Context-sensitive half-times of fentanyl, alfentanil, sufentanil and remifentanil in cats anesthetized with isoflurane obtained by pharmacokinetic simulation. In: 11th World Congress of Veterinary Anaesthesiology, Cape Town, 2013.

57. Sano T, Nishimura R, Kanazawa H, et al. Pharmacokinetics of fentanyl after single intravenous injection and constant rate infusion in dogs. Vet Anaesth Analg. 2006;33:266–73.

58. Scott JC, Stanski DR. Decreased fentanyl and alfentanil dose requirements with age. A simultaneous pharmacokinetic and pharmacodynamic evaluation. J Pharmacol Exp Ther. 1987;240:159–66.

59. Pypendop BH, Ilkiw JE. Assessment of the hemodynamic effects of lidocaine administered IV in isoflurane-anesthetized cats. Am J Vet Res. 2005;66:661–8.

60. Andress JL, Day TK, Day D. The effects of consecutive day propofol anesthesia on feline red blood cells. Vet Surg. 1995;24:277–82.

61. Beths T, Glen JB, Reid J, et al. Evaluation and optimisation of a target-controlled infusion system for administering propofol to dogs as part of a total intravenous anesthetic technique during dental surgery. Vet Rec. 2001;148:198–203.

62. Daunt DA, Dunlop CI, Chapman PL, et al. Cardiopulmonary and behavioral responses to computer-driven infusion of detomidine in standing horses. Am J Vet Res. 1993;54:2075–82.

63. Levionnois OL, Mevissen M, Thormann W, et al. Assessing the efficiency of a pharmacokinetic-based algorithm for target-controlled infusion of ketamine in ponies. Res Vet Sci. 2010;88:512–8.

64. Knobloch M, Portier CJ, Levionnois OL, et al. Antinociceptive effects, metabolism and disposition of ketamine in ponies under target-controlled drug infusion. Toxicol Appl Pharmacol. 2006;216:373–86.

65. Joubert KE, Keller N, Du Plessis CJ. A retrospective case series of computer-controlled total intravenous anesthesia in dogs presented for neurosurgery. J S Afr Vet Assoc. 2004;75:85–9.

66. Musk GC, Flaherty D. Target-controlled infusion of propofol combined with variable rate infusion of remifentanil for anesthesia of a dog with patent ductus arteriosus. Vet Anaesth Analg. 2007;34:359–64.

67. Hatschbach E, Silva Fdo C, Beier SL, et al. Comparative study between target-controlled-infusion and continuous-infusion anesthesia in dogs treated with methotrimeprazine and treated with propofol and remifentanil. Acta Cir Bras. 2008;23:65–72.

68. Ribeiro LM, Ferreira DA, Bras S, et al. Correlation between clinical signs of depth of anesthesia and cerebral state index responses in dogs with different target-controlled infusions of propofol. Vet Anaesth Analg. 2012;39:21–8.

69. Beier SL, de Araujo Aguiar AJ, Vianna PT, et al. Effect of remifentanil on requirements for propofol administered by use of a target-controlled infusion system for maintaining anesthesia in dogs. Am J Vet Res. 2009;70:703–9.

70. Mannarino R, Luna SP, Monteiro ER, et al. Minimum infusion rate and hemodynamic effects of propofol, propofol-lidocaine and propofol-lidocaine-ketamine in dogs. Vet Anaesth Analg. 2012;39:160–73.

71. Reed RA, Seddighi MR, Odoi A, et al. Effect of ketamine on the minimum infusion rate of propofol needed to prevent motor movement in dogs. Am J Vet Res. 2015;76:1022–30.

72. Bettschart-Wolfensberger R, Bowen MI, Freeman SL, et al. Cardiopulmonary effects of prolonged anesthesia via propofol-medetomidine infusion in ponies. Am J Vet Res. 2001;62:1428–35.

73. Bettschart-Wolfensberger R, Freeman SL, Jaggin-Schmucker N, et al. Infusion of a combination of propofol and medetomidine for long-term anesthesia in ponies. Am J Vet Res. 2001;62:500–7.

74. Oku K, Ohta M, Yamanaka T, et al. The minimum infusion rate (MIR) of propofol for total intravenous anesthesia after premedication with xylazine in horses. J Vet Med Sci. 2005;67:569–75.

75. Yamashita K, Akashi N, Katayama Y, et al. Evaluation of bispectral index (BIS) as an indicator of central nervous system depression in horses anesthetized with propofol. J Vet Med Sci. 2009;71:1465–71.

76. Li R, Zhang WS, Liu J, et al. Minimum infusion rates and recovery times from different durations of continuous infusion of fospropofol, a prodrug of propofol, in rabbits: a comparison with propofol emulsion. Vet Anaesth Analg. 2012;39:373–84.

77. Ewing KK, Mohammed HO, Scarlett JM, et al. Reduction of isoflurane anesthetic requirement by medetomidine and its restoration by atipamezole in dogs. Am J Vet Res. 1993;54:294–9.

78. Kohrs R, Durieux ME. Ketamine: teaching an old drug new tricks. Anesth Analg. 1998;87:1186–93.

79. Rubio-Martinez LM, Hendrickson DA, Stetter M, et al. Laparoscopic vasectomy in African elephants (Loxodonta africana). Vet Surg. 2014;43:507–14.

80. Glen JB, Hunter SC. Pharmacology of an emulsion formulation of ICI 35 868. Br J Anaesth. 1984;56:617–26.

81. Kanto JH. Propofol, the newest induction agent of anesthesia. Int J Clin Pharmacol Ther Toxicol. 1988;26:41–57.

82. McCulloch MJ, Lees NW. Assessment and modification of pain on induction with propofol (Diprivan). Anesthesia. 1985;40:1117–20.

83. Mirakhur RK. Induction characteristics of propofol in children: comparison with thiopentone. Anesthesia. 1988;43:593–8.

84. Smith JA, Gaynor JS, Bednarski RM, et al. Adverse effects of administration of propofol with various preanesthetic regimens in dogs. J Am Vet Med Assoc. 1993;202:1111–5.

85. Weaver BM, Raptopoulos D. Induction of anesthesia in dogs and cats with propofol. Vet Rec. 1990;126:617–20.

86. Taylor PM, Chengelis CP, Miller WR, et al. Evaluation of propofol containing 2% benzyl alcohol preservative in cats. J Feline Med Surg. 2012;14:516–26.

87. McIntosh MP, Rajewski RA. Comparative canine pharmacokinetics-pharmacodynamics of fospropofol disodium injection, propofol emulsion, and cyclodextrin-enabled propofol solution following bolus parenteral administration. J Pharm Sci. 2012;101:3547–52.

88. Dawidowicz AL, Fornal E, Mardarowicz M, et al. The role of human lungs in the biotransformation of propofol. Anesthesiology. 2000;93:992–7.

89. Simons PJ, Cockshott ID, Douglas EJ, et al. Species differences in blood profiles, metabolism and excretion of 14C-propofol after intravenous dosing to rat, dog and rabbit. Xenobiotica. 1991;21:1243–56.

90. Veroli P, O'Kelly B, Bertrand F, et al. Extrahepatic metabolism of propofol in man during the anhepatic phase of orthotopic liver transplantation. Br J Anaesth. 1992;68:183–6.

91. Al-Jahdari WS, Yamamoto K, Hiraoka H, et al. Prediction of total propofol clearance based on enzyme activities in microsomes from human kidney and liver. Eur J Clin Pharmacol. 2006;62:527–33.

92. Chen YZ, Zhu SM, He HL, et al. Do the lungs contribute to propofol elimination in patients during orthotopic liver transplantation without veno-venous bypass? Hepatobiliary Pancreat Dis Int. 2006;5:511–4.

93. He YL, Ueyama H, Tashiro C, et al. Pulmonary disposition of propofol in surgical patients. Anesthesiology. 2000;93:986–91.

94. Hiraoka H, Yamamoto K, Miyoshi S, et al. Kidneys contribute to the extrahepatic clearance of propofol in humans, but not lungs and brain. Br J Clin Pharmacol. 2005;60:176–82.

95. Takizawa D, Hiraoka H, Goto F, et al. Human kidneys play an important role in the elimination of propofol. Anesthesiology. 2005;102:327–30.

96. Artru AA, Shapira Y, Bowdle TA. Electroencephalogram, cerebral metabolic, and vascular responses to propofol anesthesia in dogs. J Neurosurg Anesthesiol. 1992;4:99–109.

97. Pinaud M, Lelausque JN, Chetanneau A, et al. Effects of propofol on cerebral hemodynamics and metabolism in patients with brain trauma. Anesthesiology. 1990;73:404–9.

98. Strebel S, Lam AM, Matta B, et al. Dynamic and static cerebral autoregulation during isoflurane, desflurane, and propofol anesthesia. Anesthesiology. 1995;83:66–76.

99. Caines D, Sinclair M, Valverde A, et al. Comparison of isoflurane and propofol for maintenance of anesthesia in dogs with intracranial disease undergoing magnetic resonance imaging. Vet Anaesth Analg. 2014;41:468–79.

100. Kahveci FS, Kahveci N, Alkan T, et al. Propofol versus isoflurane anesthesia under hypothermic conditions: effects on intracranial pressure and local cerebral blood flow after diffuse traumatic brain injury in the rat. Surg Neurol. 2001;56:206–14.

101. Petersen KD, Landsfeldt U, Cold GE, et al. Intracranial pressure and cerebral hemodynamic in patients with cerebral tumors: a randomized prospective study of patients subjected to craniotomy in propofol-fentanyl, isoflurane-fentanyl, or sevoflurane-fentanyl anesthesia. Anesthesiology. 2003;98:329–36.

102. Raisis AL, Leece EA, Platt SR, et al. Evaluation of an anesthetic technique used in dogs undergoing craniectomy for tumour resection. Vet Anaesth Analg. 2007;34:171–80.

103. Van Hemelrijck J, Van Aken H, Merckx L, et al. Anesthesia for craniotomy: total intravenous anesthesia with propofol and alfentanil compared to anesthesia with thiopental sodium, isoflurane, fentanyl, and nitrous oxide. J Clin Anesth. 1991;3:131–6.

104. Ilkiw JE, Pascoe PJ, Haskins SC, et al. Cardiovascular and respiratory effects of propofol administration in hypovolemic dogs. Am J Vet Res. 1992;53:2323–7.

105. Muir III WW, Gadawski JE. Respiratory depression and apnea induced by propofol in dogs. Am J Vet Res. 1998;59:157–61.

106. Blouin RT, Seifert HA, Babenco HD, et al. Propofol depresses the hypoxic ventilatory response during conscious sedation and isohypercapnia. Anesthesiology. 1993;79:1177–82.

107. Taylor MB, Grounds RM, Mulrooney PD, et al. Ventilatory effects of propofol during induction of anesthesia. Comparison with thiopentone. Anesthesia. 1986;41:816–20.

108. Quandt JE, Robinson EP, Rivers WJ, et al. Cardiorespiratory and anesthetic effects of propofol and thiopental in dogs. Am J Vet Res. 1998;59:1137–43.

109. Watkins SB, Hall LW, Clarke KW. Propofol as an intravenous anesthetic agent in dogs. Vet Rec. 1987;120:326–9.

110. Cullen LK, Reynoldson JA. Xylazine or medetomidine premedication before propofol anesthesia. Vet Rec. 1993;132:378–83.

111. Davies C. Excitatory phenomena following the use of propofol in dogs. 2001. p. 48–51.

112. Smedile LE, Duke T, Taylor SM. Excitatory movements in a dog following propofol anesthesia. J Am Anim Hosp Assoc. 1996;32:365–8.

113. Bennett RA, Schumacher J, Hedjazi-Haring K, et al. Cardiopulmonary and anesthetic effects of propofol administered intraosseously to green iguanas. J Am Vet Med Assoc. 1998;212:93–8.

114. Duke T, Egger CM, Ferguson JG, et al. Cardiopulmonary effects of propofol infusion in llamas. Am J Vet Res. 1997;58:153–6.

115. Machin KL, Caulkett NA. Cardiopulmonary effects of propofol and a medetomidine-midazolam-ketamine combination in mallard ducks. Am J Vet Res. 1998;59:598–602.

116. Mama KR, Steffey EP, Pascoe PJ. Evaluation of propofol as a general anesthetic for horses. Vet Surg. 1995;24:188–94.

117. Schumacher J, Citino SB, Hernandez K, et al. Cardiopulmonary and anesthetic effects of propofol in wild turkeys. Am J Vet Res. 1997;58:1014–7.

118. Beier SL, Mattoso CR, Aguiar AJ, et al. Hemodynamic effects of target-controlled infusion of propofol alone or in combination with a constant-rate infusion of remifentanil in dogs. Can J Vet Res. 2015;79:309–15.

119. Kennedy MJ, Smith LJ. A comparison of cardiopulmonary function, recovery quality, and total dosages required for induction and total intravenous anesthesia with propofol versus a propofol-ketamine combination in healthy Beagle dogs. Vet Anaesth Analg. 2015;42:350–9.

120. Gimenes AM, de Araujo Aguiar AJ, Perri SH, et al. Effect of intravenous propofol and remifentanil on heart rate, blood pressure and nociceptive response in acepromazine premedicated dogs. Vet Anaesth Analg. 2011;38:54–62.

121. Martinez-Taboada F, Leece EA. Comparison of propofol with ketofol, a propofol-ketamine admixture, for induction of anesthesia in healthy dogs. Vet Anaesth Analg. 2014;41:575–82.

122. Wong DH, Jenkins LC. An experimental study of the mechanism of action of ketamine on the central nervous system. Can Anaesth Soc J. 1974;21:57–67.

123. Cattai A, Rabozzi R, Natale V, et al. The incidence of spontaneous movements (myoclonus) in dogs undergoing total intravenous anesthesia with propofol. Vet Anaesth Analg. 2015;42:93–8.

124. Hall LW, Chambers JP. A clinical-trial of propofol infusion anesthesia in dogs. J Small Anim Pract. 1987;28:623–37.

125. Robertson SA, Johnston S, Beemsterboer J. Cardiopulmonary, anesthetic, and postanesthetic effects of intravenous infusions of propofol in greyhounds and non-greyhounds. Am J Vet Res. 1992;53:1027–32.

126. Michou JN, Leece EA, Brearley JC. Comparison of pain on injection during induction of anesthesia with alfaxalone and two formulations of propofol in dogs. Vet Anaesth Analg. 2012;39:275–81.

127. Minghella E, Benmansour P, Iff I, et al. Pain after injection of a new formulation of propofol in six dogs. Vet Rec. 2010;167:866–7.

128. Mendes GM, Selmi AL. Use of a combination of propofol and fentanyl, alfentanil, or sufentanil for total intravenous anesthesia in cats. J Am Vet Med Assoc. 2003;223:1608–13.

129. Padilha ST, Steagall PV, Monteiro BP, et al. A clinical comparison of remifentanil or alfentanil in propofol-anesthetized cats undergoing ovariohysterectomy. J Feline Med Surg. 2011;13:738–43.

130. Ferreira TH, Aguiar AJ, Valverde A, et al. Effect of remifentanil hydrochloride administered via constant rate infusion on the minimum alveolar concentration of isoflurane in cats. Am J Vet Res. 2009;70:581–8.

131. Pascoe PJ, Ilkiw JE, Fisher LD. Cardiovascular effects of equipotent isoflurane and alfentanil/isoflurane minimum alveolar concentration multiple in cats. Am J Vet Res. 1997;58:1267–73.

132. Liehmann L, Mosing M, Auer U. A comparison of cardiorespiratory variables during isoflurane-fentanyl and propofol-fentanyl anesthesia for surgery in injured cats. Vet Anaesth Analg. 2006;33:158–68.

133. Pascoe PJ, Ilkiw JE, Frischmeyer KJ. The effect of the duration of propofol administration on recovery from anesthesia in cats. Vet Anaesth Analg. 2006;33:2–7.

134. Favetta P, Degoute CS, Perdrix JP, et al. Propofol metabolites in man following propofol induction and maintenance. Br J Anaesth. 2002;88:653–8.

135. Court MH, Greenblatt DJ. Molecular genetic basis for deficient acetaminophen glucuronidation by cats: UGT1A6 is a pseudogene, and evidence for reduced diversity of expressed hepatic UGT1A isoforms. Pharmacogenetics. 2000;10:355–69.

136. Court MH, Duan SX, Hesse LM, et al. Cytochrome P-450 2B6 is responsible for interindividual variability of propofol hydroxylation by human liver microsomes. Anesthesiology. 2001;94:110–9.

137. Hay Kraus BL, Greenblatt DJ, Venkatakrishnan K, et al. Evidence for propofol hydroxylation by cytochrome P4502B11 in canine liver microsomes: breed and gender differences. Xenobiotica. 2000;30:575–88.

138. Oda Y, Hamaoka N, Hiroi T, et al. Involvement of human liver cytochrome P4502B6 in the metabolism of propofol. Br J Clin Pharmacol. 2001;51:281–5.

139. Rutten AA, Falke HE, Catsburg JF, et al. Interlaboratory comparison of total cytochrome P-450 and protein determinations in rat liver microsomes. Reinvestigation of assay conditions. Arch Toxicol. 1987;61:27–33.

140. Correia D. Studies on propofol in sheep and rats. In: Veterinary sciences. Glasgow: University of Glasgow; 1994. p. 91–103.

141. Plummer GF. Improved method for the determination of propofol in blood by high-performance liquid chromatography with fluorescence detection. J Chromatogr. 1987;421:171–6.

142. Bley CR, Roos M, Price J, et al. Clinical assessment of repeated propofol-associated anesthesia in cats. J Am Vet Med Assoc. 2007;231:1347–53.

143. Oku K, Ohta M, Katoh T, et al. Cardiovascular effects of continuous propofol infusion in horses. J Vet Med Sci. 2006;68:773–8.

144. Umar MA, Yamashita K, Kushiro T, et al. Evaluation of cardiovascular effects of total intravenous anesthesia with propofol or a combination of ketamine-medetomidine-propofol in horses. Am J Vet Res. 2007;68:121–7.

145. Yamashita K, Muir WW. Intravenous anesthetic and analgesic adjuncts to inhalation anesthesia. In: Equine anesthesia monitoring and emergency therapy. 2nd edn. Philadelphia: Elsevier – Health Sciences Division; 2009. p. 260–276.

146. Mama KR, Pascoe PJ, Steffey EP, et al. Comparison of two techniques for total intravenous anesthesia in horses. Am J Vet Res. 1998;59:1292–8.

147. Brosnan RJ, Steffey EP, Escobar A, et al. Anesthetic induction with guaifenesin and propofol in adult horses. Am J Vet Res. 2011;72:1569–75.

148. Oku K, Kakizaki M, Ono K, et al. Clinical evaluation of total intravenous anesthesia using a combination of propofol and medetomidine following anesthesia induction with medetomidine, guaifenesin and propofol for castration in Thoroughbred horses. J Vet Med Sci. 2011;73:1639–43.

149. Bettschart-Wolfensberger R, Bowen IM, Freeman SL, et al. Medetomidine-ketamine anesthesia induction followed by medetomidine-propofol in ponies: infusion rates and cardiopulmonary side effects. Equine Vet J. 2003;35:308–13.

150. de Vries A, Taylor PM, Troughton G, et al. Real time monitoring of propofol blood concentration in ponies anesthetised with propofol and ketamine. J Vet Pharmacol Ther. 2013;36:258–66.

151. Umar MA, Fukui S, Kawase K, et al. Cardiovascular effects of total intravenous anesthesia using ketamine-medetomidine-propofol (KMP-TIVA) in horses undergoing surgery. J Vet Med Sci. 2015;77:281–8.

152. Malavasi LM. Swine. In: Grimm KA, Lamont LA, Tranquilli W, et al. editors. Veterinary anesthesia and analgesia the fifth edition of Lumb and Jones. 5th edn. Oxford: Wiley. p. 928–40.

153. Schoffmann G, Winter P, Palme R, et al. Haemodynamic changes and stress responses of piglets to surgery during total intravenous anesthesia with propofol and fentanyl. Lab Anim. 2009;43:243–8.

154. Molinaro Coelho CM, Duque Moreno JC, Goulart Dda S, et al. Evaluation of cardiorespiratory and biochemical effects of ketamine-propofol and guaifenesin-ketamine-xylazine anesthesia in donkeys (Equus asinus). Vet Anaesth Analg. 2014;41:602–12.

155. Child KJ, Currie JP, Dis B, et al. The pharmacological properties in animals of CT1341—a new steroid anesthetic agent. Br J Anaesth. 1971;43:2–13.

156. Dodman NH. Complications of saffan anesthesia in cats. Vet Rec. 1980;107:481–3.

157. Gyermek L, Soyka LF. Steroid anesthetics. Anesthesiology. 1975;42:331–44.

158. Hall LW, Clarke KW. General pharmacology of intravenous anaestthetic agents. In: Veterinary anesthesia. 9th edn. London: Saunders Ltd.; 1991. p. 80–97.

159. Prys-Roberts C, Sear J. Steroid anesthesia. Br J Anaesth. 1980;52:363–5.

160. Goodchild CS, Serrao JM, Kolosov A, et al. Alphaxalone reformulated: a water-soluble intravenous anesthetic preparation in sulfobutyl-ether-beta-cyclodextrin. Anesth Analg. 2015;120:1025–31.

161. Monagle J, Siu L, Worrell J, et al. A phase 1c trial comparing the efficacy and safety of a new aqueous formulation of alphaxalone with propofol. Anesth Analg. 2015;121:914–24.

162. Strachan FA, Mansel JC, Clutton RE. A comparison of microbial growth in alfaxalone, propofol and thiopental. J Small Anim Pract. 2008;49:186–90.

163. Zoran DL, Riedesel DH, Dyer DC. Pharmacokinetics of propofol in mixed-breed dogs and greyhounds. Am J Vet Res. 1993;54:755–60.

164. Warne LN, Beths T, Fogal S, et al. The use of alfaxalone and remifentanil total intravenous anesthesia in a dog undergoing a craniectomy for tumor resection. Can Vet J. 2014;55:1083–8.

165. Baldy-Moulinier M, Besset-Lehmann J. Study of the effects of Alfatesin on cerebral blood flow in cats. Ann Anesthesiol Fr. 1975;16:417–22.

166. Bendtsen A, Kruse A, Madsen JB, et al. Use of a continuous infusion of althesin in neuroanesthesia. Changes in cerebral blood flow, cerebral metabolism, the EEG and plasma alphaxalone concentration. Br J Anaesth. 1985;57:369–74.

167. Rasmussen NJ, Rosendal T, Overgaard J. Althesin in neurosurgical patients: effects on cerebral hemodynamics and metabolism. Acta Anaesthesiol Scand. 1978;22:257–69.

168. Sari A, Maekawa T, Tohjo M, et al. Effects of Althesin on cerebral blood flow and oxygen consumption in man. Br J Anaesth. 1976;48:545–50.

169. Muir W, Lerche P, Wiese A, et al. Cardiorespiratory and anesthetic effects of clinical and supraclinical doses of alfaxalone in dogs. Vet Anaesth Analg. 2008;35:451–62.

170. Muir W, Lerche P, Wiese A, et al. The cardiorespiratory and anesthetic effects of clinical and supraclinical doses of alfaxalone in cats. Vet Anaesth Analg. 2009;36:42–54.

171. Taboada FM, Murison PJ. Induction of anesthesia with alfaxalone or propofol before isoflurane maintenance in cats. Vet Rec. 2010;167:85–9.

172. Herbert GL, Bowlt KL, Ford-Fennah V, et al. Alfaxalone for total intravenous anesthesia in dogs undergoing ovariohysterectomy: a comparison of premedication with acepromazine or dexmedetomidine. Vet Anaesth Analg. 2013;40:124–33.

173. Kuusela E, Raekallio M, Anttila M, et al. Clinical effects and pharmacokinetics of medetomidine and its enantiomers in dogs. J Vet Pharmacol Ther. 2000;23:15–20.

174. Kuusela E, Raekallio M, Vaisanen M, et al. Comparison of medetomidine and dexmedetomidine as premedicants in dogs undergoing propofol-isoflurane anesthesia. Am J Vet Res. 2001;62:1073–80.

175. O'Hagan B, Pasloske K, McKinnon C, et al. Clinical evaluation of alfaxalone as an anesthetic induction agent in dogs less than 12 weeks of age. Aust Vet J. 2012;90:346–50.

176. O'Hagan BJ, Pasloske K, McKinnon C, et al. Clinical evaluation of alfaxalone as an anesthetic induction agent in cats less than 12 weeks of age. Aust Vet J. 2012;90:395–401.

177. Metcalfe S, Hulands-Nave A, Bell M, et al. Multicentre, randomised clinical trial evaluating the efficacy and safety of alfaxalone administered to bitches for induction of anesthesia prior to caesarean section. Aust Vet J. 2014;92:333–8.

178. Conde Ruiz C, Del Carro AP, Rosset E, et al. Alfaxalone for total intravenous anesthesia in bitches undergoing elective caesarean section and its effects on puppies: a randomized clinical trial. Vet Anaesth Analg. 2016;43:282–90.

179. Jimenez CP, Mathis A, Mora SS, et al. Evaluation of the quality of the recovery after administration of propofol or alfaxalone for induction of anesthesia in dogs anesthetised for magnetic resonance imaging. Vet Anaesth Analg. 2012;39:151–9.

180. Ndawana PS, Dzikiti BT, Zeiler G, et al. Determination of the minimum infusion rate (MIR) of alfaxalone required to prevent purposeful movement of the extremities in response to a standardised noxious stimulus in goats. Vet Anaesth Analg. 2015;42:65–71.

181. Dzikiti TB, Ndawana PS, Zeiler G, et al. Determination of the minimum infusion rate of alfaxalone during its co-administration with midazolam in goats. Vet Rec Open. 2015;2, e000065.

182. Bosing B, Tunsmeyer J, Mischke R, et al. Clinical usability and practicability of Alfaxalone for short-term anesthesia in the cat after premedication with Buprenorphine. Tierarztl Prax Ausg K Klientiere Heimtiere. 2012;40:17–25.

183. Haskins SC, Peiffer Jr RL, Stowe CM. A clinical comparison of CT1341, ketamine, and xylazine in cats. Am J Vet Res. 1975;36:1537–43.

184. Warne LN, Beths T, Holm M, et al. Comparison of perioperative analgesic efficacy between methadone and butorphanol in cats. J Am Vet Med Assoc. 2013;243:844–50.

185. Kloppel H, Leece EA. Comparison of ketamine and alfaxalone for induction and maintenance of anesthesia in ponies undergoing castration. Vet Anaesth Analg. 2011;38:37–43.

186. Leece EA, Girard NM, Maddern K. Alfaxalone in cyclodextrin for induction and maintenance of anesthesia in ponies undergoing field castration. Vet Anaesth Analg. 2009;36:480–4.

187. Dzikiti BT, Ndawana PS, Zeiler G, et al. Determination of the minimum infusion rate of alfaxalone during its co-administration with fentanyl at three different doses by constant rate infusion intravenously in goats. Vet Anaesth Analg. 2016;43:316–25.

188. Casoni D, Amen EM, Brecheisen M, et al. A combination of alfaxalone and medetomidine followed by an alfaxalone continuous rate infusion in cynomolgus monkeys (Macaca fascicularis) undergoing pharmacoMRS. Vet Anaesth Analg. 2015;42:552–4.

189. Dugdale AH. Injectable anesthetic agents. In: Veterinary anesthesia principles to practice. 1st edn. Oxford: Wiley-Blackwell; 2010. p. 45–54.

190. Reich DL, Silvay G. Ketamine: an update on the first twenty-five years of clinical experience. Can J Anaesth. 1989;36:186–97.

191. White PF, Ham J, Way WL, et al. Pharmacology of ketamine isomers in surgical patients. Anesthesiology. 1980;52:231–9.

192. White PF, Way WL, Trevor AJ. Ketamine – its pharmacology and therapeutic uses. In: Anesthesiology. 1982. p. 119–36.

193. Hirota K, Lambert DG. Ketamine: its mechanism(s) of action and unusual clinical uses. Br J Anaesth. 1996;77:441–4.

194. Baraka A, Harrison T, Kachachi T. Catecholamine levels after ketamine anesthesia in man. Anesth Analg. 1973;52:198–200.

195. Visser E, Schug SA. The role of ketamine in pain management. Biomed Pharmacother. 2006;60:341–8.

196. Bednarski RM. Dogs and cats. In: Grimm KA, Lamont LA, Tranquilli W, et al., editors. Veterinary anesthesia and analgesia the fifth edition of Lumb and Jones. 5th ed. Oxford: Wiley; 2015. p. 819–26.

197. Gutierrez-Blanco E, Victoria-Mora JM, Ibancovichi-Camarillo JA, et al. Evaluation of the isoflurane-sparing effects of fentanyl, lidocaine, ketamine, dexmedetomidine, or the combination lidocaine-ketamine-dexmedetomidine during ovariohysterectomy in dogs. Vet Anaesth Analg. 2013;40:599–609.

198. Gutierrez-Blanco E, Victoria-Mora JM, Ibancovichi-Camarillo JA, et al. Postoperative analgesic effects of either a constant rate infusion of fentanyl, lidocaine, ketamine, dexmedetomidine, or the combination lidocaine-ketamine-dexmedetomidine after ovariohysterectomy in dogs. Vet Anaesth Analg. 2015;42:309–18.

199. Wagner AE, Walton JA, Hellyer PW, et al. Use of low doses of ketamine administered by constant rate infusion as an adjunct for postoperative analgesia in dogs. J Am Vet Med Assoc. 2002;221:72–5.

200. Haskins SC, Farver TB, Patz JD. Ketamine in dogs. Am J Vet Res. 1985;46:1855–60.
201. Benson GJ, Thurmon JC, Tranquilli WJ, et al. Cardiopulmonary effects of an intravenous infusion of guaifenesin, ketamine, and xylazine in dogs. Am J Vet Res. 1985;46:1896–8.
202. Hellebrekers LJ, Sap R. Medetomidine as a premedicant for ketamine, propofol or fentanyl anesthesia in dogs. Vet Rec. 1997;140:545–8.
203. Hellebrekers LJ, van Herpen H, Hird JF, et al. Clinical efficacy and safety of propofol or ketamine anesthesia in dogs premedicated with medetomidine. Vet Rec. 1998;142:631–4.
204. Seliskar A, Nemec A, Roskar T, et al. Total intravenous anesthesia with propofol or propofol/ketamine in spontaneously breathing dogs premedicated with medetomidine. Vet Rec. 2007;160:85–91.
205. Silva Fdo C, Hatschbach E, Lima AF, et al. Continuous infusion in adult females dogs submitted to ovariohysterectomy with midazolam-xylazine and/or medetomidine pre-treated with methotrimeprazine and buprenorphine. Acta Cir Bras. 2007;22:272–8.
206. Shorrab AA, Atallah MM. Total intravenous anesthesia with ketamine-midazolam versus halothane-nitrous oxide-oxygen anesthesia for prolonged abdominal surgery. Eur J Anaesthesiol. 2003;20:925–31.
207. Brown MJ, McCarthy TJ, Bennett BT. Long term anesthesia using a continuous infusion of guaifenesin, ketamine and xylazine in cats. Lab Anim Sci. 1991;41:46–50.
208. Frizelle HP, Duranteau J, Samii K. A comparison of propofol with a propofol-ketamine combination for sedation during spinal anesthesia. Anesth Analg. 1997;84:1318–22.
209. Mortero RF, Clark LD, Tolan MM, et al. The effects of small-dose ketamine on propofol sedation: respiration, postoperative mood, perception, cognition, and pain. Anesth Analg. 2001;92:1465–9.
210. Ilkiw JE, Pascoe PJ. Cardiovascular effects of propofol alone and in combination with ketamine for total intravenous anesthesia in cats. Am J Vet Res. 2003;64:913–7.
211. Muir WW. Intravenous anesthetic drugs. In: Muir WW, Hubbell JAE, editors. Equine anesthesia monitoring and emergency therapy. 2nd ed. Philadelphia: Elsevier – Health Sciences Division; 2009. p. 243–59.
212. Staffieri F, Driessen B. Field anesthesia in the equine. Clin Tech Equine Pract. 2007;6:111–9.
213. McMurphy RM, Young LE, Marlin DJ, et al. Comparison of the cardiopulmonary effects of anesthesia maintained by continuous infusion of romifidine, guaifenesin, and ketamine with anesthesia maintained by inhalation of halothane in horses. Am J Vet Res. 2002;63:1655–61.
214. Taylor PM, Luna SP, Sear JW, et al. Total intravenous anesthesia in ponies using detomidine, ketamine and guaiphenesin: pharmacokinetics, cardiopulmonary and endocrine effects. Res Vet Sci. 1995;59:17–23.
215. Hall LW, Clarke KW, Trim CM. Intravenous anesthesia. In: Veterinary anesthesia. 10th edn. London: Saunders Ltd.; 2001. p. 33–52.
216. Hubbell JA, Aarnes TK, Lerche P, et al. Evaluation of a midazolam-ketamine-xylazine infusion for total intravenous anesthesia in horses. Am J Vet Res. 2012;73:470–5.
217. Mama KR, Wagner AE, Steffey EP, et al. Evaluation of xylazine and ketamine for total intravenous anesthesia in horses. Am J Vet Res. 2005;66:1002–7.
218. Yamashita K, Wijayathilaka TP, Kushiro T, et al. Anesthetic and cardiopulmonary effects of total intravenous anesthesia using a midazolam, ketamine and medetomidine drug combination in horses. J Vet Med Sci. 2007;69:7–13.
219. Casoni D, Spadavecchia C, Adami C. S-ketamine versus racemic ketamine in dogs: their relative potency as induction agents. Vet Anaesth Analg. 2015;42:250–9.

220. Riebold TW. Ruminants. In: Grimm KA, Lamont LA, tranquilli W, et al. editors. Veterinary anesthesia and analgesia the fifth edition of Lumb and Jones. 5th edn. Oxford: Wiley, p. 912–27.
221. Henrikson H, Jensen-Waern M, Nyman G. Anaesthetics for general anesthesia in growing pigs. Acta Vet Scand. 1995;36:401–11.
222. Thurmon JC, Tranquilli WJ, Benson GJ. Cardiopulmonary responses of swine to intravenous infusion of guaifenesin, ketamine, and xylazine. Am J Vet Res. 1986;47:2138–40.
223. Absalom AR, Sutcliffe N, Kenny GN. Closed-loop control of anesthesia using bispectral index: performance assessment in patients undergoing major orthopedic surgery under combined general and regional anesthesia. Anesthesiology. 2002;96:67–73.
224. Liu N, Chazot T, Trillat B, et al. Feasibility of closed-loop titration of propofol guided by the Bispectral Index for general anesthesia induction: a prospective randomized study. Eur J Anaesthesiol. 2006;23:465–9.
225. Morley A, Derrick J, Mainland P, et al. Closed loop control of anesthesia: an assessment of the bispectral index as the target of control. Anesthesia. 2000;55:953–9.
226. Struys MM, De Smet T, Greenwald S, et al. Performance evaluation of two published closed-loop control systems using bispectral index monitoring: a simulation study. Anesthesiology. 2004;100:640–7.
227. Carrasco-Jimenez MS, Martin Cancho MF, Lima JR, et al. Relationships between a proprietary index, bispectral index, and hemodynamic variables as a means for evaluating depth of anesthesia in dogs anesthetized with sevoflurane. Am J Vet Res. 2004;65:1128–35.
228. de Mattos-Junior E, Ito KC, Conti-Patara A, et al. Bispectral monitoring in dogs subjected to ovariohysterectomy and anesthetized with halothane, isoflurane or sevoflurane. Vet Anaesth Analg. 2011;38:475–83.
229. Greene SA, Benson GJ, Tranquilli WJ, et al. Relationship of canine bispectral index to multiples of sevoflurane minimal alveolar concentration, using patch or subdermal electrodes. Comp Med. 2002;52:424–8.
230. Greene SA, Benson GJ, Tranquilli WJ, et al. Effect of isoflurane, atracurium, fentanyl, and noxious stimulation on bispectral index in pigs. Comp Med. 2004;54:397–403.
231. Haga HA, Dolvik NI. Evaluation of the bispectral index as an indicator of degree of central nervous system depression in isoflurane-anesthetized horses. Am J Vet Res. 2002;63:438–42.
232. Lamont LA, Greene SA, Grimm KA, et al. Relationship of bispectral index to minimum alveolar concentration multiples of sevoflurane in cats. Am J Vet Res. 2004;65:93–8.
233. March PA, Muir 3rd WW. Use of the bispectral index as a monitor of anesthetic depth in cats anesthetized with isoflurane. Am J Vet Res. 2003;64:1534–41.
234. Martin-Cancho MF, Carrasco-Jimenez MS, Lima JR, et al. Assessment of the relationship of bispectral index values, hemodynamic changes, and recovery times associated with sevoflurane or propofol anesthesia in pigs. Am J Vet Res. 2004;65:409–16.
235. Williams DC, Brosnan RJ, Fletcher DJ, et al. Qualitative and quantitative characteristics of the electroencephalogram in normal horses during administration of inhaled anesthesia. J Vet Intern Med. 2016;30:289–303.
236. Sneyd JR. Recent advances in intravenous anesthesia. Br J Anaesth. 2004;93:725–36.
237. Sneyd JR, Rigby-Jones AE. New drugs and technologies, intravenous anesthesia is on the move (again). Br J Anaesth. 2010;105:246–54.
238. Lauder GR. Total intravenous anesthesia will supercede inhalational anesthesia in pediatric anesthetic practice. Paediatr Anaesth. 2015;25:52–64.

Part VI

Outcome, Education, Safety, and the Future

Advantages, Disadvantages, and Risks of TIVA/TCI

32

Ken B. Johnson

Introduction

With the introduction of sodium thiopental in 1934, intravenous anesthesia was born. Although not widely used in the mid-twentieth century, intravenous anesthesia gained more popularity as newer intravenous agents with more favorable pharmacokinetic properties were made available for clinical use. The most significant improvement was the development of "soft" drugs that were both fast and predictable with minimal risk of toxicity. Fast in the sense that onset and dissipation of effect were within minutes. One such soft drug, propofol, was first introduced in 1973. Following clinical trials with cremophor and lipid based formulations, propofol became a component of total intravenous anesthesia (TIVA) that began to gain traction as a viable anesthetic in 1984. Since then, TIVA's presence in the perioperative and procedural environments has continued to expand. In 1996, target controlled infusions were introduced and have since become commonplace worldwide as a more sophisticated approach to administering TIVA. The aim of this chapter is to review many of the clinical advantages and disadvantages of TIVA and TCI in comparison with other anesthetic techniques. A list of selected advantages and disadvantages is presented in Table 32.1.

Advantages of TIVA/TCI

Postoperative Nausea and Vomiting

Perhaps the most notable advantage of TIVA/TCI is the potential to decrease postoperative nausea and vomiting (PONV). PONV can be one of the most common and vexing problems facing patients in the post anesthesia care unit (PACU). Up to 30 % of patients experience vomiting, 50 % of patients experience nausea, and 80 % of patients at high risk will have PONV [1, 2]. For patients with a history of severe PONV or for those who meet criteria for a high risk of PONV [3], anesthesia care providers often prescribe TIVA rather than other techniques as part of their multimodal approach to minimizing PONV. Several studies support this approach.

In 2007, Apfel et al. conducted a randomized controlled trial of factorial design to explore six interactions among various antiemetic interventions in over 5000 patients, widely cited as the IMPACT study [4]. One of the interactions was a comparison between propofol versus inhalation agents. They found a reduced risk of PONV with induction and maintenance of anesthesia with propofol. To put this finding into clinical perspective, other single interactions that were also of similar benefit were the use of ondansetron, dexamethasone, or droperidol. These observations are consistent with numerous clinical trials comparing a propofol-based anesthetic with potent inhaled agents [5, 6].

In a recent set of consensus guidelines for the management of PONV prepared by the Society of Ambulatory Anesthesia, a multimodal approach is recommended for the prevention of PONV [7] based on an assessment of risk using available risk assessment scores [1, 8]. Prophylaxis in medium risk patients includes 5HT-3 antagonism (ondansetron) in combination with steroid administration (dexamethasone) or TIVA. Prophylaxis in high-risk patients includes ondansetron and dexamethasone administration in combination with TIVA. Of note, the consensus guidelines also state that TIVA consists of propofol for induction and maintenance in the absence of nitrous oxide.

Although propofol's antiemetic properties are well established, it is important to recognize that TIVA is rarely just propofol. As type A γ-aminobutyric acid (GABA$_A$) receptor agonist, propofol is primarily a sedative.

K.B. Johnson, MS, MD(✉)
Anesthesiology, University of Utah, 30 N 1900 E, Suite 3C444, Salt Lake City, UT 84132, USA
e-mail: ken.b.johnson@hsc.utah.edu

© Springer International Publishing AG 2017
A.R. Absalom, K.P. Mason (eds.), *Total Intravenous Anesthesia and Target Controlled Infusions*,
DOI 10.1007/978-3-319-47609-4_32

Table 32.1 Advantages and disadvantages and risks of TIVA/TCI

Advantages
• Reduced postoperative nausea and vomiting
• Useful in procedures that require evoked potential monitoring
• Quality of recovery from anesthesia
• Independent of an anesthesia machine
• Target controlled infusions administer intravenous drugs using target effect site concentrations, an approach this is similar to how anesthesiologists administered potent inhaled agents with a vaporizer
Disadvantages and risks
• Small increased risk of awareness, especially with neuromuscular blockade
• Hemodynamic instability with propofol, especially in the setting of severe blood loss
• Risk of hyperalgesia increased with high dose opioid techniques often used with TIVA
• Requires more equipment to deliver anesthetic (syringe infusion pumps, drug administration lines with anti-reflux and anti-syphon valves)
• Infusion rates are not automatically recorded on an electronic medical record
• Syringe pumps require frequent re-loads during long surgical procedures
• No ability to monitor drug concentrations in real time
• Dependent on continuity of functioning intravenous line
• Pain on injection with propofol
• May require processed EEG monitoring, especially with neuromuscular blockade
• Pharmacokinetic models used to drive TCI infusion pumps may inaccurately predict target concentrations in selected patients (i.e., obese patients)
• More difficult to titrate in patients with opioid or benzodiazepine tolerance
• Cost

By comparison to potent inhaled agents, propofol provides minimal analgesia. Thus TIVA often consists of a combination of propofol with an opioid or other analgesic such as ketamine. This minimizes the risk of PONV, but does not reduce the risk as if only propofol were used. Common opioids include fentanyl or one of it congeners, most notably remifentanil. One of the six interactions explored in the IMPACT study was a comparison of the incidence of PONV between remifentanil and fentanyl. The authors reported no difference in the risk of PONV [4].

The mechanism of action behind the antiemetic properties of propofol is not well defined. Potential mechanisms based in animal model work include propofol's interaction with the serotonergic or dopaminergic systems [9]. Specifically, propofol has been found to be a noncompetitive 5-hydroxytryptamine type 3 (5-HT3) receptor antagonist [10]. In addition, propofol may antagonize dopaminergic (D2) receptors in the chemoreceptor trigger zone and this may explain dystonic movements when propofol is administered in large bolus doses [11].

Neuro-Monitoring

Anesthesiologists caring for patients that require spine surgery are frequently asked to provide an anesthetic that allows continuous monitoring of motor and somatosensory evoked potentials (MEPs and SSEPs). TIVA without neuromuscular blockade is a frequent anesthetic choice in this setting for several reasons. First, propofol has less of an effect on SSEPs compared to volatile anesthetics. In fact, SSEPs remain adequate even in the presence of propofol dosed to achieve burst suppression [12]. Second, MEPs, but not SSEPs, are blunted or blocked by neuromuscular blockade and their use is discouraged in procedures that require MEP monitoring. Although they may be used at the start of a procedure for patient positioning, they are dosed such that their effect dissipates once surgery is underway. Neuromuscular blockade may be beneficial when monitoring only SSEPs as they reduce artifact from muscle movement.

A high dose opioid technique is used to minimize use of neuromuscular blockade to maintain patient akinesia. Fentanyl or one of its congeners is frequently used to achieve this effect. These are best administered as a continuous infusion as opposed to intermittent boluses to attain a more consistent analgesic profile and improved MEP monitoring conditions. Fentanyl, sufentanil, and remifentanil all can be administered as a continuous infusion to achieve and maintain profound analgesia, but have very different kinetic profiles that are especially evident once infusions are terminated at or near the end of surgery. With its rapid decline in effect, remifentanil will require a transition opioid for procedures associated with substantial postoperative pain. Hydromorphone, morphine, or fentanyl can be used to prolong opioid effect during emergence. By comparison, fentanyl and sufentanil have a slower dissipation in effect; fentanyl more so than sufentanil. A set of simulations are presented below that provides a visual expression of how the pharmacokinetic and pharmacodynamic behavior of these fentanyl congeners varies when used as part of a near equipotent TIVA.

TIVA may also have an advantage in patients with preexisting neurologic dysfunction [13]. Evoked potentials can be difficult to detect in this patient group. Investigators have used other sedatives in addition to or in place of GABA receptor agonists that include dexmedetomidine (alpha 2 agonist) and ketamine (NMDA antagonist). Clinical experience has suggested that replacing high dose opioid in this patient group may improve monitoring SSEP signals [14–16] especially in cases associated with high or low blood pressure.

Experience with dexmedetomidine in this setting has been limited to case reports and small cohort studies. Some authors suggest that in patients with persistent hypertension despite adequate opioid administration, dexmedetomidine may be useful. In a pediatric patient cohort with ages 12–17 years old, clinical researchers reported that in the presence of a propofol (100 mcg/kg/min) and remifentanil (0.2 mcg/kg/min), dexmedetomidine can suppress MEP amplitudes at higher doses (0.5 mcg/kg/h), but has no effect on SSEP amplitude or latency. They observed a substantial decrease in the bispectral index scale (BIS) values with the addition of dexmedetomidine (a drop in BIS from 58 to 31) and a 25–50 % decrease in MEP amplitude. MEP amplitudes were restored to baseline by titrating the propofol infusion to the baseline BIS value (a mean decrease from 106 to 78 mcg/kg/min) while maintaining the dexmedetomidine infusion [17]. Clinical investigators have reported similar findings in using TIVA in combination with dexmedetomidine in adults. In a study that delivered dexmedetomidine via TCI, authors report clinically relevant changes in MEPs with target plasma concentrations 0.6–0.8 ng/mL. Target concentrations of 0.4 or lower ng/mL did not reduce MEP amplitudes.

By way of summary, dexmedetomidine does not appear to adversely influence SSEPs using common dosing regimens, but does decrease MEP amplitudes. Dexmedetomidine administration should be adjusted in close consultation with the neuro-monitoring specialists to individualize dosing that allows for proper evoked potential monitoring.

With regard to ketamine, dosing recommendations in this setting vary. Some propose intermittent ketamine boluses (10 mg every hour) or low dose ketamine infusions (0.05–0.1 mg/kg/h) as an adjunct to minimize the dose of other anesthetic drugs. This may be especially useful in the setting of unwanted intraoperative hypotension with TIVA. Other authors recommend replacing propofol with ketamine at doses of 0.4–0.6 mg/kg/h [18]. The kinetic profile of ketamine is somewhat unique in comparison with other short acting sedatives. If administered by bolus, it has a slow decline in effect. Thus changes in evoked potentials (as a decrease in evoked potential amplitude) can be misinterpreted as potential nerve injury when they are simply due to changes in ketamine effect site concentrations.

Quality of Recovery from Anesthesia

In a randomized clinical trial, patient's perception of their quality of recovery was compared following a propofol-remifentanil TIVA to a desflurane anesthetic [5]. Female patients undergoing thyroid surgery were randomly allocated to one of the two anesthetic techniques and completed a Quality of Recovery-40 questionnaire (QoR-40) before and after surgery (postoperative days 1 and 2). The QoR-40 has five dimensions: emotional status, physical comfort, psychological support, physical independence, and pain. Investigators found that the total QoR-40 score on postoperative day 1 was significantly higher in the TIVA than the desflurane group. Breaking that finding down by the 5 dimensions, physical comfort, psychological support, and physical independence were significantly higher with TIVA compared to desflurane. Scores on postoperative day 2 were not significantly different. However, a breakdown by dimension revealed that physical comfort and physical independence remained significantly different. The authors concluded that quality of recovery for female thyroid surgery patients was better with TIVA compared to a desflurane-based anesthetic.

A second advantage of TIVA in the quality of recovery using intravenous agents is in the realm of managing agitated delirium in patients requiring prolonged intubation in an intensive care unit setting. In a randomized control trial, investigators explored outcomes related to mechanical ventilation with the addition of dexmedetomidine to standard sedation techniques for intubated patients. Standard sedation techniques in this study were sedation with primarily propofol with the addition of opioid and antipsychotic medications such as haloperidol. Their primary outcome was the number of ventilator free hours over a seven-day period [19]. They found that with an initial dose of 0.5 mcg/kg/h and then titrated to predetermined sedation goals, dexmedetomidine increased the number of ventilator free hours (a median difference of 17 h). Secondary outcomes of interest included time to extubation and time to resolution of delirium. They found a decrease in the time to extubation (median difference of 20 h) and a decrease in the time to resolution of delirium (median difference of 16 h). The authors concluded that their findings support the use of dexmedetomidine in patients with agitated delirium on mechanical ventilation in an intensive care unit.

Disadvantages and Risks

Awareness Under General Anesthesia

In comparison with combined techniques with potent inhaled agents, it is difficult to accurately measure the amount of drug administered using TIVA/TCI. End tidal concentrations of potent inhaled agents allow anesthetists to confirm that their patient is receiving an anesthetic and monitor changes in expired drug levels in response to changes in dose (i.e., vaporizer settings). Without the end tidal concentrations to confirm anesthetic delivery, anesthetists are left to their clinical judgment to determine the adequacy of anesthetic delivery. The major concern is that a patient receiving TIVA/TCI may have undetected awareness, especially in the presence of neuromuscular blockade.

Several studies have explored this issue with varied results. A prospective analysis published in 2008, recorded the incidence of awareness in 4001 patients undergoing general anesthesia for a variety of surgical procedures from 1995 through 2001 in a single hospital [20]. 1239 patients received TIVA and of those, 14 experienced awareness (1.1 %). The authors point out that induction and maintenance technique were not standardized and may have contributed to the incidence of awareness. To put this incidence into perspective, the authors reported an overall incidence of 0.6 % in patients presenting for elective surgery regardless of anesthetic technique. The incidence increased to 0.8 % in high-risk patients. High-risk patients were defined as patients requiring emergency surgery, patients with significant intraoperative hypotension, and patients undergoing a C-section. Awareness was more common in younger patients and anesthetics delivered at night and less common in patients pre-medicated with benzodiazepines.

In 2014, the "5th National Audit Project (NAP5) on accidental awareness during general anaesthesia" reported an incidence of 1:19,000 or 147 patients in the United Kingdom and Irish public hospitals over a one-year period for 2.8 million general anesthetics [21–23]. This analysis provided a breakout by anesthetics (Fig. 32.1). TIVA consisted of 8 % of the maintenance anesthetics, yet contributed 18 % of the patients that experienced awareness under general anesthesia (28 patients). The authors point out, that in comparison with other techniques, TIVA had a disproportionately high number of patients with awareness compared to patients anesthetized with other techniques.

Further breakdown of this group revealed that in 21 of these patients, TIVA was used for induction and maintenance and in seven of these patients, TIVA was combined with potent inhaled agents [24]. It is interesting to note that 24 of these patients experiencing awareness with TIVA were in the operating room. The main cause was felt to be "failure to deliver the intended dose of propofol." The remaining four were outside the operating room. The cause was felt primarily to be the use of neuromuscular blockade with inadequate delivery of propofol. In these cases, a manual infusion rate that was too low. All 28 of these cases of awareness were felt to be avoidable.

There are several potential explanations for the high incidence of awareness with TIVA. First, anesthesia care providers may have had an inadequate understanding of manual infusion rates or target concentrations for TCI necessary to maintain unresponsiveness. Prior studies with healthy volunteers have established that the propofol effect site concentration necessary for 50 % of volunteers to experience loss of responsiveness is near 2.2 mcg/mL using the modified observer's assessment of alertness and sedation scale [25] of less than 2 [26–28]. Propofol is known for its high degree of variability and that it requires careful titration to achieve the desired clinical effects while avoiding unwanted hemodynamic compromise especially in debilitated and elderly patients. As such, appropriate TCI dosing ranges may span effect site concentrations from 1.5 to 6 mcg/mL [29].

Second, impaired propofol and or opioid delivery may serve as a source of awareness. Vigilant monitoring of the intravenous catheter is warranted to ensure continuous administration of an anesthetic. Guiding principles for TIVA/TCI include (1) easy observation of the intravenous insertion site, (2) avoidance of pressurized or pump driven carrier infusions as they may delay detection of an infiltrated intravenous catheter, and (3) connection of drug infusion tubing to the most proximal port of the carrier infusion line to minimize infusion tubing dead space.

Third, use of neuromuscular blockade may serve as a source of awareness. Two guiding principles in management include: (1) proper monitoring of neuromuscular blockade should be utilized and (2) processed electroencephalographic monitoring may be useful when administering intermediate neuromuscular blockade.

The discrepancy in the incidence of awareness between the two studies presented above may be a function of how awareness is detected and reported. In an editorial accompanying the NAP5 analysis, Absalom and Green suggest that there are several important nuances to measuring awareness under general anesthesia [30] to include the definition of "consciousness" and the methodology used to document a case of awareness. With the single institution work presented by Errando et al., investigators used a rigorous survey system to identify and confirm awareness under anesthesia events. All patients were interviewed in the PACU. If patients reported an awareness event or details of the interview suggested a possible awareness event, follow-up interviews on postoperative day 7 and 30 were performed. By contrast, investigators in the much larger NAP5 work relied on patient self-reporting to identify

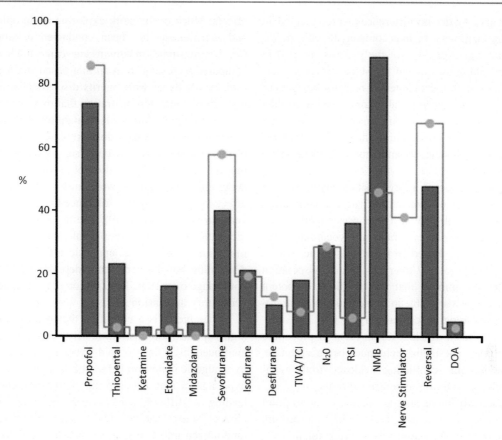

Fig. 32.1 Representation of some components of anesthesia practice in certain/probable and possible accidental awareness during general anesthesia reports (*bars*) compared with distribution of reports of awareness under anesthesia (*dots* and *lines*), reported by the NAP5 study [22]. Propofol in first bar refers to its use as an induction agent, as distinct from a later bar (TIVA) where its use is referred to for maintenance. *TIVA* total i.v. anesthesia, *TCI* target controlled infusion,

N2O nitrous oxide, *RSI* rapid sequence induction, *NMB* neuromuscular block, *DOA* specific depth of anesthesia monitor. (Reproduced from Pandit JJ, Andrade J, Bogod DG, Hitchman JM, Jonker WR, Lucas N, et al. 5th National Audit Project (NAP5) on accidental awareness during general anaesthesia: summary of main findings and risk factors. British Journal of Anaesthesia. 2014;113(4):54959 with permission from Oxford University Press)

awareness under anesthesia. This approach assumes that patients that have awareness recall the event and report it. Patients that recall awareness but did not report it are not included in the analysis. Furthermore, patients may have had awareness but are unable to recall it without prompting and also not included in the analysis. In summary, the methods and tools used to detect awareness are likely to influence the reporting of awareness. As can be appreciated, the more rigorous the monitoring technique, the more difficult it is to assess large groups of patients as was done in the NAP5 study.

Hemodynamic Consequences of Propofol

A major concern is the potential adverse effect propofol may have in patients with known or suspected myocardial disease. In patients undergoing coronary artery bypass grafting, some evidence, although not conclusive suggests the use of

volatile anesthetics can provide myocardial preconditioning. Meta-analyses of 32 randomized controlled trials suggest that this type of preconditioning can reduce troponin release and preserve myocardium [31] but were inconclusive regarding mortality. Follow-up work comparing TIVA with sevoflurane during coronary artery bypass graft procedures reported similar findings for on-pump but not off pump procedures [32]. A similar finding was observed in patients presenting for noncardiac surgery [33] and high-risk cardiac surgery [34].

In a randomized multicenter clinical trial, investigators explored the hypothesis that sevoflurane has a lower incidence of myocardial ischemia than a propofol-based anesthetic in 385 patients undergoing major noncardiac surgery [35]. Primary endpoints were myocardial ischemia as detected by electrocardiogram or elevated troponin levels over 48 h. No differences were detected between groups. Secondary endpoints were the incidence of delirium and incidence of adverse cardiovascular events for 12 months following surgery. Again, no differences were detected in these secondary endpoints. In an accompanying editorial, it was pointed out that over 70 % of the patients enrolled in this study were taking aspirin and beta-blockers. Sixty percent were taking statins and angiotensin receptor blockers or angiotensin converting enzyme inhibitors. The editorialist points out that the negative finding may represent better preoperative myocardial conditioning than a lack of difference between inhalation agents and propofol-based TIVA for this patient group.

Landoni et al. conducted a large meta-analysis of over 6000 patients undergoing noncardiac surgery comparing volatile anesthetics with TIVA. There was no difference between anesthetic techniques in rates of myocardial ischemia and infarction [36]. Based on these results, the American College of Cardiology/American Heart Association 2014 guidelines recommend that use of TIVA or potent inhaled anesthetics is reasonable in stable patients at cardiovascular risk undergoing noncardiac surgery [37]. This recommendation was rated as Class IIa, in favor of procedure (in this case, either anesthetic technique) being effective, however there is some conflicting evidence from meta-analysis or multiple randomized controlled trials.

It is widely known among anesthesiologists that propofol has hemodynamic consequences beyond the myocardium and should be used with caution when caring for patients with compromised intravascular volume. It can be especially dangerous in the setting of acute severe hemorrhagic shock. Animal models exploring the pharmacokinetics and pharmacodynamics of propofol in the presence of severe blood loss (i.e., half the blood volume) suggest that reducing up to 25 % of a normal propofol dose will lead to a near equivalent effect [38]. Of note, remifentanil, by contrast is well tolerated under similar conditions of hemorrhagic hypovolemia [39].

In summary, patients with known or suspected cardiovascular disease or decreased intravascular volume may require reduced doses of TIVA/TCI, the use of vasopressors, and heightened vigilance when monitoring cardiovascular function.

Opioid-Induced Hyperalgesia

TIVA/TCI techniques often use high dose opioids. Remifentanil, with its rapid decline in effect once an infusion is terminated is especially attractive for high dose administration with minimal residual effect. Thus it can be used to provide analgesia for very stimulating procedures with little regard to time required to emerge from anesthesia once an anesthetic is turned off. Although convenient for the anesthesia practitioner, authors have called into question the use of high dose opioids with concerns of acute opioid tolerance, hyperalgesia, and potential long-term adverse effects. Much of the work exploring acute opioid tolerance and hyperalgesia has been conducted in animal models. Confirming studies in humans are scarce and less convincing compared to results from animal based studies. That being said, this body of work merits discussion in the setting of high dose opioid administration that may occur with TIVA.

Acute opioid tolerance is thought to be of concern within hours of exposure to high dose opioids. Typical management of this phenomenon may be to simply increase opioid dosing, or the use of a small dose of ketamine to overcome the acute tolerance. Animal work in this area has explored the effects of acute morphine tolerance to a painful stimulus and ventilatory depression [40]. The most interesting finding is the appearance of differential tolerance. With a continuous morphine infusion, the analgesic effect lasted 8 h before dissipating but the ventilatory depression, by contrast, did not change over 10 h. Thus, although the analgesia was lost, ventilatory depression persisted.

Hyperalgesia is a condition that results from persistent high opioid administration. By contrast to tolerance, continued high dose opioid exposure may exacerbate the hyperalgesic condition [41]. Although not well understood, hyperalgesia may develop during the perioperative period leading to difficult pain control following surgery. In a clinical study, patients undergoing a thoracotomy were randomized into two groups: one that received a low dose remifentanil and use of an epidural throughout the procedure and another that received high dose remifentanil with use of the epidural only at the end of the procedure [42]. The authors measured the wound area with hyperalgesia and found that high dose opioid not only increased the hyperalgesic area, but also increased the risk of chronic pain at 3, 6, ad 9 months after surgery. Similar work on patients undergoing colorectal surgery provides similar results [43]. Patients were randomized to receive high or low dose remifentanil infusions in combination with sevoflurane. High dose remifentanil on average was 0.3 mcg/kg/min. They found that patients in the high dose group consumed almost twice as much morphine in the first 24 h following surgery than patients in the low dose group.

Other studies have not been so convincing. In one study, patients undergoing gynecologic surgery randomized into two groups: sevoflurane only and sevoflurane in combination with remifentanil demonstrated no difference in 24-h postoperative opioid requirements [44]. One caveat to this work was that in both groups, patients received 50 % nitrous oxide, a known N-methyl-D-aspartate (NMDA)-type glutamate receptor antagonist. A meta-analysis exploring the question of perioperative opioid administration and postoperative opioid requirements found that when combining all studies using remifentanil, doses greater than 0.3 mcg/kg/min required more postoperative opioids [45]. This was not observed for sufentanil and fentanyl, although data sets were more limited for these two opioids. One theory describing the development of hyperalgesia is the increase in pronociceptive activity by release of peptides and activation of the NMDA receptor [46]. To that end, work by Echevarría et al. found that nitrous oxide reduces postoperative opioid-induced hyperalgesia after remifentanil-propofol anesthesia in humans [47].

In summary, there is evidence to suggest that high dose opioid may lead to hyperalgesia within the perioperative period. It is probably more likely with remifentanil where high concentrations are more easily maintained throughout an anesthetic compared to other opioids. NMDA antagonists such as ketamine, nitrous oxide, or methadone along with other commonly used analgesic adjuncts may be useful to reduce opioid exposure and minimize this adverse effect.

Neurotoxicity

Exposure to anesthetics may result in an increase in expression of substances that harm neural tissue to include neuroapoptosis (cell death) and/or faulty synaptogenesis [48, 49] most likely via epigenetic mechanisms that result in synaptic and cognitive dysfunction [50]. Elderly and very young patients may be especially susceptible to neurologic injury from these proteins. Although they may appear to emerge from anesthesia neurologically intact, there can be a persistent subtle decline in cognitive abilities that reduce the quality of life.

An ideal anesthetic would be one that not only provides anesthesia but offers some degree of neuroprotection as well. In animal models of neuroapoptosis, isoflurane has been found to be more destructive than sevoflurane and desflurane [51–53]. These histologic findings have been translated to behavioral deficits in models of elderly rodents [54, 55]. One hope was that a propofol-based TIVA that avoids potent inhaled agents would be less neurotoxic or possibly provide some degree of neuroprotection. Animal work in non-human neonatal primates, however, suggests that propofol can have similar neurotoxic consequences [56]. As with isoflurane, a 5-h exposure to propofol can result in apoptotic degeneration of oligodendrocytes, especially those who are in the early phases of myelination.

Simulations

A set of simulations is presented below that illustrate two key points discussed in this chapter: The probability of responsiveness and the probability of delayed emergence and persistent ventilatory depression for various TIVA techniques. Simulations of drug effect site concentrations and selected drug effects (analgesia, ventilatory depression, and loss of responsiveness) are presented in Figs. 32.2, 32.3, and 32.4. In these simulations, propofol is combined with remifentanil, fentanyl, or sufentanil for a 4-h infusion to an

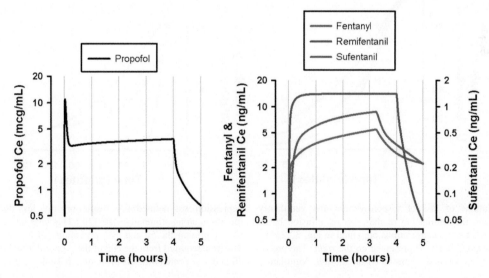

Fig. 32.2 Simulations of predicted effect site concentrations (Ce) for three different TIVA propofol-opioid techniques for a 4-h TIVA. Propofol effect site concentrations over time are presented on the *left*. The three propofol-opioid techniques consisted of fentanyl, sufentanil, and remifentanil. Opioid effect site concentrations are presented on the *right*. Opioid infusions were dosed to achieve a near equivalent high probability of analgesic effect, and the fentanyl and sufentanil were terminated 45 min before the end of the procedure to minimize the influence of excessive opioid on time to emergence from anesthesia.

Predictions of drug Ce levels and drug effects were based on published pharmacokinetic and models [58–62]. Simulations assume 30-year-old 183 cm tall 100 kg male that is otherwise healthy and does not chronically consume opioids or benzodiazepines. Induction consisted of propofol 2 mg/kg and fentanyl 150 mcg. Maintenance of anesthesia consisted of propofol 100 mcg/kg/min and an opioid infusion (remifentanil 0.2 mcg/kg/min, sufentanil 0.7 mcg/kg/h, or fentanyl 6 mcg/kg/h)

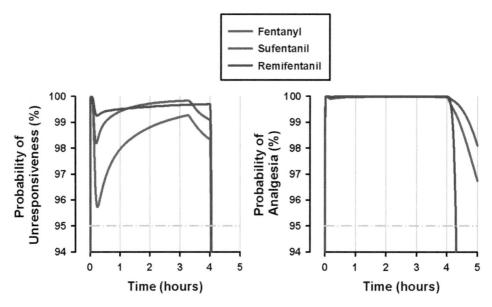

Fig. 32.3 Simulations of loss of responsiveness and analgesia over time based on the predicted effect site concentrations presented in Fig. 32.2. Loss of responsiveness was defined as a loss of response to verbal and painful stimuli (Observer's Assessment of Alertness and Sedation scale less than 2, [25]). Analgesia was defined as a loss of response to painful pressure on the anterior tibia [26]. The probability of unresponsiveness is presented on the *left*. The probability of analgesia is present on the *right*. The vertical axis presents the probabilities ranging from 94 to 100 %. The *gray horizontal dot-dash line* represents the 95 % probability of loss of responsiveness

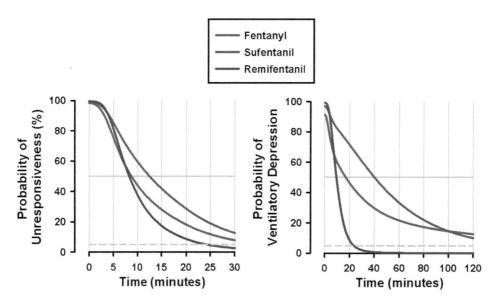

Fig. 32.4 Simulations of loss of responsiveness and ventilatory depression following the termination of the propofol infusion based on the predicted effect site concentrations presented in Fig. 32.2. The probability of unresponsiveness is presented on the *right*. The probability of ventilatory depression is presented on the *left*. Ventilatory depression was defined as a respiratory rate less than 4 breaths per minute in an un-stimulated state [28]. The *horizontal solid* and *dashed lines* represent the 50 and 5 % probability of loss of responsiveness. The time required from the end of the propofol infusion to reaching the 50 and 5 % probabilities is presented in Table 32.2

otherwise healthy male. Induction consisted of propofol 2 mg/kg and fentanyl 150 mcg. Maintenance consisted of a propofol infusion set at 100 mcg/kg/min and an opioid infusion. The opioid infusion rates were selected based on their ability to produce a near equivalent opioid effect, namely a greater than 95 % probability of analgesia and are listed in the figure legend.

Figure 32.2 presents the predicted effect site concentrations that will result from these TIVA dosing regimens. Using the predicted concentrations from Fig. 32.2, pharmacodynamic interaction models were used to create Fig. 32.3. This figure presents selected predicted effects of propofol combined with fentanyl, remifentanil, or sufentanil. The most important findings are that the

Table 32.2 Predicted times to emergence for selected TIVA techniques

Time to emergence following termination of the propofol infusion[a]	
Remifentanil	8 min
Fentanyl[b]	9 min
Sufentanil[b]	12 min
Predicted times to a 50 % probability of ventilatory depression following termination of the propofol infusion	
Remifentanil	9 min
Fentanyl[b]	17 min
Sufentanil[b]	40 min

See Fig. 32.2 legend for definitions of loss of responsiveness and ventilatory depression

[a]Emergence is defined as the time of a 50 % probability of responsiveness

[b]Infusions were terminated 45 min prior to the termination of the propofol infusion

probabilities of unresponsiveness and analgesia remain high throughout the 4 h anesthetic (well above 95 % for both effects). This is primarily a function of the interactions between propofol and high dose opioids. Specifically, the opioid effect is substantially enhanced by propofol, providing profound analgesia. By contrast, the sedation effect from propofol is somewhat enhanced by the opioid. These simulations corroborate the assumption that if administered properly, TIVA or TCI will render a patient unresponsive and analgesic. An important clinical nuance with these simulations is that in patients with known or suspected opioid or benzodiazepine tolerance from chronic use may require higher propofol and opioid doses to achieve the desired level of sedation and analgesia.

Figure 32.4 and Table 32.2 present the probability of unresponsiveness and ventilatory depression over time once the propofol infusion is terminated. Sufentanil and fentanyl infusions were turned off 45 min before the anticipated end of the anesthetic (i.e., when the propofol was turned off). This was done to minimize the impact of opioid effect on emergence from anesthesia. As dosed, emergence from each of these TIVA techniques is similar for each of the three opioids (8–12 min). By contrast, the probability of ventilatory depression remains high for a longer period after the propofol is turned off. The sufentanil and fentanyl infusions, although terminated early, contributed to a longer predicted period of ventilatory depression compared to remifentanil (Table 32.2).

Summary

TIVA/TCI has a long track record of safe and effective use [57]. The advantages of the technique make it the preferred anesthetic technique for patients with a history of or a high risk for postoperative nausea and vomiting, provide utility in procedures that require evoked potential monitoring, and improve quality of recovery. Although widely thought to be worrisome in patients with known or suspected cardiovascular disease undergoing noncardiac surgery, 2015 ACC/AHA guidelines point out that there is class IIa evidence that TIVA is as suitable in this patient group as a potent inhaled agent. Disadvantages and risks of this technique include the slightly increased risk of awareness, unwanted hypotension associated with propofol delivery, especially in patients with depleted intravascular volumes and/or compromised cardiac function, and a risk of hyperalgesia with TIVA techniques that use high dose opioids. Overall, TIVA/TCI has enjoyed widespread use and is becoming more common among anesthesia practitioners because of its ease of titration, enhanced utility over other techniques in selected clinical settings, and quality of recovery.

References

1. Koivuranta M, Laara E, Snare L, Alahuhta S. A survey of postoperative nausea and vomiting. Anaesthesia. 1997;52(5):443–9.
2. Sinclair DR, Chung F, Mezei G. Can postoperative nausea and vomiting be predicted? Anesthesiology. 1999;91(1):109–18.
3. Gan TJ, Diemunsch P, Habib AS, Kovac A, Kranke P, Meyer TA, et al. Consensus guidelines for the management of postoperative nausea and vomiting. Anesth Analg. 2014;118(1):85–113. doi:10.1213/ANE.0000000000000002.
4. Apfel CC, Korttila K, Abdalla M, Kerger H, Turan A, Vedder I, et al. A factorial trial of six interventions for the prevention of postoperative nausea and vomiting. N Engl J Med. 2004;350 (24):2441–51. doi:10.1056/NEJMoa032196. PMID: 15190136, PMCID: PMC1307533.
5. Lee WK, Kim MS, Kang SW, Kim S, Lee JR. Type of anaesthesia and patient quality of recovery: a randomized trial comparing propofol-remifentanil total i.v. anaesthesia with desflurane anaesthesia. Br J Anaesth. 2015;114(4):663–8. doi:10.1093/bja/aeu405.
6. Wu ZF, Jian GS, Lee MS, Lin C, Chen YF, Chen YW, et al. An analysis of anesthesia-controlled operating room time after propofol-based total intravenous anesthesia compared with desflurane anesthesia in ophthalmic surgery: a retrospective study. Anesth Analg. 2014;119(6):1393–406. doi:10.1213/ANE.0000000000000435.
7. Gan TJ, Meyer TA, Apfel CC, Chung F, Davis PJ, Habib AS, et al. Society for Ambulatory Anesthesia guidelines for the management of postoperative nausea and vomiting. Anesth Analg. 2007;105 (6):1615–28; table of contents. doi:10.1213/01.ane.0000295230.55439.f4.
8. Apfel CC, Laara E, Koivuranta M, Greim CA, Roewer N. A simplified risk score for predicting postoperative nausea and vomiting: conclusions from cross-validations between two centers. Anesthesiology. 1999;91(3):693–700.
9. Vasileiou I, Xanthos T, Koudouna E, Perrea D, Klonaris C, Katsargyris A, et al. Propofol: a review of its non-anaesthetic effects. Eur J Pharmacol. 2009;605(1–3):1–8. doi:10.1016/j.ejphar.2009.01.007.
10. Barann M, Dilger JP, Bonisch H, Gothert M, Dybek A, Urban BW. Inhibition of 5-HT3 receptors by propofol: equilibrium and kinetic measurements. Neuropharmacology. 2000;39(6):1064–74.
11. Borgeat A, Dessibourg C, Popovic V, Meier D, Blanchard M, Schwander D. Propofol and spontaneous movements: an EEG study. Anesthesiology. 1991;74(1):24–7.

12. Liu EH, Wong HK, Chia CP, Lim HJ, Chen ZY, Lee TL. Effects of isoflurane and propofol on cortical somatosensory evoked potentials during comparable depth of anaesthesia as guided by bispectral index. Br J Anaesth. 2005;94(2):194–7.

13. Hermanns H, Lipfert P, Meier S, Jetzek-Zader M, Krauspe R, Stevens MF. Cortical somatosensory-evoked potentials during spine surgery in patients with neuromuscular and idiopathic scoliosis under propofol-remifentanil anaesthesia. Br J Anaesth. 2007;98 (3):362–5. doi:10.1093/bja/ael365.

14. Agarwal R, Roitman KJ, Stokes M. Improvement of intraoperative somatosensory evoked potentials by ketamine. Paediatr Anaesth. 1998;8(3):263–6.

15. Erb TO, Ryhult SE, Duitmann E, Hasler C, Luetschg J, Frei FJ. Improvement of motor-evoked potentials by ketamine and spatial facilitation during spinal surgery in a young child. Anesth Analg. 2005;100(6):1634–6. doi:10.1213/01.ANE.0000149896. 52608.08.

16. Ubags LH, Kalkman CJ, Been HD, Porsius M, Drummond JC. The use of ketamine or etomidate to supplement sufentanil/N2O anesthesia does not disrupt monitoring of myogenic transcranial motor evoked responses. J Neurosurg Anesthesiol. 1997;9(3):228–33.

17. Tobias JD, Goble TJ, Bates G, Anderson JT, Hoernschemeyer DG. Effects of dexmedetomidine on intraoperative motor and somatosensory evoked potential monitoring during spinal surgery in adolescents. Paediatr Anaesth. 2008;18(11):1082–8. doi:10. 1111/j.1460-9592.2008.02733.x.

18. Penney R. Use of dexmedetomidine and ketamine infusions during scoliosis repair surgery with somatosensory and motor-evoked potential monitoring: a case report. AANA J. 2010;78 (6):446–50.

19. Reade MC, Eastwood GM, Bellomo R, Bailey M, Bersten A, Cheung B, et al. Effect of dexmedetomidine added to standard care on ventilator-free time in patients with agitated delirium: a randomized clinical trial. JAMA. 2016. doi:10.1001/jama.2016. 2707.

20. Errando CL, Sigl JC, Robles M, Calabuig E, Garcia J, Arocas F, et al. Awareness with recall during general anaesthesia: a prospective observational evaluation of 4001 patients. Br J Anaesth. 2008;101(2):178–85. doi:10.1093/bja/aen144.

21. Cook TM, Andrade J, Bogod DG, Hitchman JM, Jonker WR, Lucas N, et al. 5th National Audit Project (NAP5) on accidental awareness during general anaesthesia: patient experiences, human factors, sedation, consent, and medicolegal issues. Br J Anaesth. 2014;113(4):560–74. doi:10.1093/bja/aeu314.

22. Pandit JJ, Cook TM, Jonker WR, O'Sullivan E, 5th National Audit Project (NAP5) of the Royal College of Anaesthetists and the Association of Anaesthetists of Great Britain and Ireland. A national survey of anaesthetists (NAP5 Baseline) to estimate an annual incidence of accidentalawareness during general anaesthesia in the UK. Anaesthesia. 2013;68(4):343–53. doi:10.1111/anae. 12190.

23. Pandit JJ, Andrade J, Bogod DG, Hitchman JM, Jonker WR, Lucas N, et al. 5th National Audit Project (NAP5) on accidental awareness during general anaesthesia: summary of main findings and risk factors. Br J Anaesth. 2014;113(4):549–59. doi:10.1093/ bja/aeu313.

24. Pandit JJ, Cook TM, Jonker WR, O'Sullivan E; 5th National Audit Project (NAP5) of the Royal College of Anaesthetists and the Association of Anaesthetists of Great Britain and Ireland. Anaesthesia. 2013 Apr;68(4):343-53. doi: 10.1111/anae.12190.

25. Chernick DA, Gillings D, Laine H, Hendler J, Silver JM, Davidson AB. Validity and reliability of the Observer's Assessment of Alertness/Sedation Scale: study with intravenous midazolam. J Clin Psychopharmacol. 1990;10(4):244–51.

26. Johnson KB, Syroid ND, Gupta DK, Manyam SC, Egan TD, Huntington J, et al. An evaluation of remifentanil propofol response

surfaces for loss of responsiveness, loss of response to surrogates of painful stimuli and laryngoscopy in patients undergoing elective surgery. Anesth Analg. 2008;106(2):471–9; table of contents. doi:10.1213/ane.0b013e3181606c62. PMID: 18227302; PMCID: PMC3050649.

27. Kern SE, Xie G, White JL, Egan TD. A response surface analysis of propofol-remifentanil pharmacodynamic interaction in volunteers. Anesthesiology. 2004;100(6):1373–81.

28. LaPierre CD, Johnson KB, Randall BR, White JL, Egan TD. An exploration of remifentanil-propofol combinations that lead to a loss of response to esophageal instrumentation, a loss of responsiveness, and/or onset of intolerable ventilatory depression. Anesth Analg. 2011;113(3):490–9. doi:10.1213/ANE.0b013e318210fc45.

29. Reves JG, Glass PSA, Lubarsky DA, MvEvoy MD, Martinez-Ruiz R. In: Miller R, editor. Intravenous anesthetics. Philadelphia: Churchill Livingston; 2007.

30. Absalom AR, Green D. NAP5: the tip of the iceberg, or all we need to know? Br J Anaesth. 2014;113(4):527–30. doi:10.1093/bja/ aeu349.

31. Yu CH, Beattie WS. The effects of volatile anesthetics on cardiac ischemic complications and mortality in CABG: a meta-analysis. Can J Anaesth. 2006;53:906–18.

32. Yao YT, Li LH. Sevoflurane versus propofol for myocardial protection in patients undergoing coronary artery bypass grafting surgery: a meta-analysis of randomized controlled trials. Chin Med Sci J. 2009;24:133–41.

33. Bignami E, Landoni G, Gerli C, Testa V, Mizzi A, Fano G, et al. Sevoflurane vs. propofol in patients with coronary disease undergoing mitral surgery: a randomised study. Acta Anaesthesiol Scand. 2012;56(4):482–90. doi:10.1111/j.1399-6576.2011.02570. x.

34. Landoni G, Guarracino F, Cariello C, Franco A, Baldassarri R, Borghi G, et al. Volatile compared with total intravenous anaesthesia in patients undergoing high-risk cardiac surgery: a randomized multicentre study. Br J Anaesth. 2014;113(6):955–63. doi:10.1093/ bja/aeu290.

35. Buse GAL, Schumacher P, Seeberger E, Studer W, Schuman RM, Fassl J, et al. Randomized comparison of sevoflurane versus propofol to reduce perioperative myocardial ischemia in patients undergoing noncardiac surgery. Circulation. 2012;126:2696–704.

36. Landoni G, Fochi O, Bignami E, Calabro MG, D'Arpa MC, Moizo E, et al. Cardiac protection by volatile anesthetics in non-cardiac surgery? A meta-analysis of randomized controlled studies on clinically relevant endpoints. HSR Proc Intensive Care Cardiovasc Anesth. 2009;1(4):34–43. PMID: 23439516, PMCID: PMC3484562.

37. Fleisher LA, Fleischmann KE, Auerbach AD, Barnason SA, Beckman JA, Bozkurt B, et al. 2014 ACC/AHA guideline on perioperative cardiovascular evaluation and management of patients undergoing noncardiac surgery: executive summary: a report of the American College of Cardiology/American Heart Association Task Force on practice guidelines. Developed in collaboration with the American College of Surgeons, American Society of Anesthesiologists, American Society of Echocardiography, American Society of Nuclear Cardiology, Heart Rhythm Society, Society for Cardiovascular Angiography and Interventions, Society of Cardiovascular Anesthesiologists, and Society of Vascular Medicine Endorsed by the Society of Hospital Medicine. J Nucl Cardiol. 2015;22 (1):162–215. doi:10.1007/s12350-014-0025-z.

38. Johnson KB, Egan TD, Kern SE, McJames SW, Cluff ML, Pace NL. Influence of hemorrhagic shock followed by crystalloid resuscitation on propofol: a pharmacokinetic and pharmacodynamic analysis. Anesthesiology. 2004;101(3):647–59.

39. Johnson KB, Kern SE, Hamber EA, McJames SW, Kohnstamm KM, Egan TD. Influence of hemorrhagic shock on remifentanil: a

pharmacokinetic and pharmacodynamic analysis. Anesthesiology. 2001;94(2):322–32.

40. Kayan S, Woods LA, Mitchell CL. Morphine-induced hyperalgesia in rats tested on the hot plate. J Pharmacol Exp Ther. 1971;177 (3):509–13.

41. Hayhurst CJ, Durieux ME. Differential opioid tolerance and opioid-induced hyperalgesia: a clinical reality. Anesthesiology. 2016;124 (2):483–8. doi:10.1097/ALN.0000000000000963.

42. Salengros JC, Huybrechts I, Ducart A, Faraoni D, Marsala C, Barvais L, et al. Different anesthetic techniques associated with different incidences of chronic post-thoracotomy pain: low-dose remifentanil plus presurgical epidural analgesia is preferable to high-dose remifentanil with postsurgical epidural analgesia. J Cardiothorac Vasc Anesth. 2010;24:608–16.

43. Guignard B, Bossard AE, Coste C, Sessler DI, Lebrault C, Alfonsi P, et al. Acute opioid tolerance: intraoperative remifentanil increases postoperative pain and morphine requirement. Anesthesiology. 2000;93:409–17.

44. Cortinez LI, Brandes V, Munoz HR, Guerrero ME, Mur M. No clinical evidence of acute opioid tolerance after remifentanil-based anaesthesia. Br J Anaesth. 2001;87(6):866–9.

45. Fletcher D, Martinez V. Opioid-induced hyperalgesia in patients after surgery: a systematic review and a meta-analysis. Br J Anaesth. 2014;112:991–1004.

46. Célèrier E, Rivat C, Jun Y, Laulin JP, Larcher A, Reynier P, et al. Long-lasting hyperalgesia induced by fentanyl in rats: preventive effect of ketamine. Anesthesiology. 2000;92:465–72.

47. Echevarria G, Elgueta F, Fierro C, Bugedo D, Faba G, Iniguez-Cuadra R, et al. Nitrous oxide (N(2)O) reduces postoperative opioid-induced hyperalgesia after remifentanil-propofol anaesthesia in humans. Br J Anaesth. 2011;107(6):959–65. doi:10.1093/bja/aer323.

48. Creeley CE, Olney JW. The young: neuroapoptosis induced by anesthetics and what to do about it. Anesth Analg. 2010;110 (2):442–8. doi:10.1213/ANE.0b013e3181c6b9ca.

49. Engelhard K, Werner C, Eberspacher E, Bachl M, Blobner M, Hildt E, et al. The effect of the alpha 2-agonist dexmedetomidine and the N-methyl-D-aspartate antagonist S(+)-ketamine on the expression of apoptosis-regulating proteins after incomplete cerebral ischemia and reperfusion in rats. Anesth Anal. 2003;96 (2):524–31; table of contents.

50. Wu J, Bie B, Naguib M. Epigenetic manipulation of brain-derived neurotrophic factor improves memory deficiency induced by neonatal anesthesia in rats. Anesthesiology. 2016;124(3):624–40. doi:10.1097/ALN.0000000000000981.

51. Liang G, Ward C, Peng J, Zhao Y, Huang B, Wei H. Isoflurane causes greater neurodegeneration than an equivalent exposure of sevoflurane in the developing brain of neonatal mice. Anesthesiology. 2010;112(6):1325–34. doi:10.1097/ALN.0b013e3181d94da5. PMID: 20460994, PMCID: PMC2877765.

52. Wei H, Liang G, Yang H, Wang Q, Hawkins B, Madesh M, et al. The common inhalational anesthetic isoflurane induces apoptosis via activation of inositol 1,4,5-trisphosphate receptors. Anesthesiology. 2008;108(2):251–60. doi:10.1097/01.anes.0000299435. 59242.0e.

53. Yang H, Liang G, Hawkins BJ, Madesh M, Pierwola A, Wei H. Inhalational anesthetics induce cell damage by disruption of intracellular calcium homeostasis with different potencies. Anesthesiology. 2008;109(2):243–50. doi:10.1097/ALN. 0b013e31817f5c47. PMID: 18648233, PMCID: PMC2598762.

54. Culley DJ, Baxter MG, Crosby CA, Yukhananov R, Crosby G. Impaired acquisition of spatial memory 2 weeks after isoflurane and isoflurane-nitrous oxide anesthesia in aged rats. Anesth Analg. 2004;99(5):1393–7; table of contents. doi:10.1213/01.ANE. 0000135408.14319.CC.

55. Culley DJ, Baxter MG, Yukhananov R, Crosby G. Long-term impairment of acquisition of a spatial memory task following isoflurane-nitrous oxide anesthesia in rats. Anesthesiology. 2004;100(2):309–14.

56. Creeley C, Dikranian K, Dissen G, Martin L, Olney J, Brambrink A. Propofol-induced apoptosis of neurones and oligodendrocytes in fetal and neonatal rhesus macaque brain. Br J Anaesth. 2013;110 Suppl 1:i29–38. doi:10.1093/bja/aet173. PMID: 23722059, PMCID: PMC3667347.

57. Schnider TW, Minto CF, Struys MM, Absalom AR. The safety of target-controlled infusions. Anesth Analg. 2015. doi:10.1213/ANE. 0000000000001005.

58. Gepts E, Shafer SL, Camu F, Stanski DR, Woestenborghs R, Van Peer A, et al. Linearity of pharmacokinetics and model estimation of sufentanil. Anesthesiology. 1995;83(6):1194–204.

59. Minto CF, Schnider TW, Egan TD, Youngs E, Lemmens HJ, Gambus PL, et al. Influence of age and gender on the pharmacokinetics and pharmacodynamics of remifentanil. I. Model development. Anesthesiology. 1997;86(1):10–23.

60. Minto CF, Schnider TW, Shafer SL. Pharmacokinetics and pharmacodynamics of remifentanil. II. Model application. Anesthesiology. 1997;86(1):24–33.

61. Schnider TW, Minto CF, Gambus PL, Andresen C, Goodale DB, Shafer SL, et al. The influence of method of administration and covariates on the pharmacokinetics of propofol in adult volunteers. Anesthesiology. 1998;88(5):1170–82.

62. Schnider TW, Minto CF, Shafer SL, Gambus PL, Andresen C, Goodale DB, et al. The influence of age on propofol pharmacodynamics. Anesthesiology. 1999;90(6):1502–16.

Economics of TIVA

33

Jane Montgomery and Mary Stocker

Introduction

Whilst we all want to give the best quality clinical care to each individual patient, in the modern healthcare environment we cannot ignore the cost implication of what we are doing. In this chapter we will look at how the use of TIVA may impact on the cost efficiency of a patient's surgical treatment, not just in terms of direct costs but also in terms of the whole patient pathway which in turn has impacts on healthcare institutions and society as a whole.

Drug budgets and the costs of individual drugs are easily quantifiable and are an attractive area for managers to attempt to make cost savings as these direct costs are easily monitored and reported in both the short and long term. Some anaesthetic departments have used guidelines to restrict the use of more expensive drugs to try to contain costs and many studies have looked at the relative costs of anaesthetics drugs and disposables with varying out comes as to the comparative costs between TIVA and volatile anaesthesia. The costs of different drugs vary from country to country and indeed vary between different institutions, and with volatile anaesthesia will vary with the flow rates used. Overall TIVA is probably the more expensive option especially if the cost of disposables and wastage is taken into account, however looking solely at direct cost does not give the whole picture as it gives no measure of outcome and further economic analysis is needed.

There are four main types of economic analysis that can be applied to healthcare and anaesthesia, the first being analysis of direct costs as mentioned above and could be classed as a cost minimisation analysis. The second form of analysis would be a cost effectiveness analysis looking at numbers of patients treated and free from symptoms such as post-operative nausea and vomiting, thirdly cost benefit analysis could be applied looking money saved in the wider economy such as benefits of shorter hospital stays and earlier return to work, and finally cost-utility could be used looking at how anaesthesia impacts on quality adjusted life years.

Cost Minimisation Analysis

Looking further at cost minimisation although in most reports the costs of TIVA is higher, when the use of TIVA is seen as part of a package of care overall drug cost may not be increased by increasing use of TIVA. This hypothesis has been analysed within the day surgery community in our own unit in Torbay [1] and also by Rowe in his day surgery unit in Norwich [2]. In our own unit we recognised that we were increasing the use of TIVA over time and wanted to ascertain whether this was associated with an increase in anaesthetic drug costs over the same period. The results are shown in Table 33.1. Over the 4-year period studied, theatre activity in terms of caseload increased by 23 % and the number of cases where TIVA techniques were used increased by 25 % over the same period. The duration of the cases also increased due to more complex procedures being introduced into the day surgery unit. Despite these increases in case numbers and duration the drug cost increase was only 18 %. When analysed in terms of drug costs per hour of anaesthetic time we actually showed a slight reduction rather than increase over the time period studied despite increasing TIVA use. This led us to the conclusion that increasing the use of TIVA does not negatively impact on drug costs within our unit.

Rowe analysed the costs of providing anaesthesia using a variety of different techniques in his own day surgery unit in Norfolk and Norwich [2]. His first analysis looked simply at the cost of maintaining anaesthesia in a 70 kg individual

J. Montgomery, MBBS, FRCA, FFICM (✉) • M. Stocker, MA, MBChB, FRCA
Department of Anaesthetics, South Devon Healthcare NHS Foundation Trust, Lawes Bridge, Torquay, Devon TQ2 7AA, UK
e-mail: jane.montgomery@nhs.net; mary.stocker@nhs.net

© Springer International Publishing AG 2017
A.R. Absalom, K.P. Mason (eds.), *Total Intravenous Anesthesia and Target Controlled Infusions*,
DOI 10.1007/978-3-319-47609-4_33

Table 33.1 Analysis of drug costs with increasing TIVA usage in Torbay Day Surgery Unit

	1996/1997	1997/1998	1998/1999	1999/2000
GA case numbers	4492	4933	4916	4843
Number of TIVA cases	2587	3063	3022	3232
TIVA (%)	58	62	61	67
Mean time/case (h)	0.47	0.47	0.48	0.52
Cost/h of GA	£31.52	£34.57	£35.02	£33.50

Table 33.2 Comparative costs of different anaesthetic techniques in a Day Surgery Unit in 1994

	Fresh gas flow	Cost/h
Isoflurane	6	£14.32
Desflurane	6	£13.40
Sevoflurane	6	£28.98
Isoflurane	2	£4.77
Desflurane	2	£4.47
Sevoflurane	2	£9.66
	Infusion rate	Cost/h
Propofol	10 mg/kg/h	£13.58
	6 mg/kg/h	£8.15

using either volatile anaesthesia or propofol infusions. Whilst Rowe analysed a variety of volatile agents we have limited the data reproduced here to those commonly in practice today. He considered maintenance with both high or low fresh gas flows for volatile anaesthesia and high and low infusion rates for TIVA. Using high fresh gas flow or high TIVA infusion rates as might be appropriate for induction of anaesthesia or for short procedures before steady state is achieved, he demonstrated that the hourly cost of TIVA infusions is slightly greater than that of isoflurane or desflurane however 50 % cheaper than using sevoflurane. When low flow rates of volatile agents were considered and compared with a lower maintenance infusion rate for propofol. P, propofol anaesthesia was found to be double the cost of using isoflurane or desflurane but still cheaper than with sevoflurane (Table 33.2). It is of note that when considering day surgery anaesthesia sevoflurane is the volatile agent most commonly used for comparison purposes due to its improved side effect profile compared with the other agents combined with smooth induction and emergence and relatively quick recovery.

In a further audit Rowe analysed the cost of a common procedure (laparoscopic sterilisation) undertaken by five different anaesthetists using different anaesthetic techniques (Table 33.3). Those anaesthetists using TIVA had shorter total procedure times which may reflect a variety of factors including speed of surgeon, theatre team or anaesthetic efficiency. The mean anaesthetic cost did not vary greatly between techniques and was shown to equate to approximately 4 % of the total procedure cost when staffing and disposable costs were taken into account. Interestingly those

patients receiving the cheapest anaesthetic incurred the highest total procedure costs! Whilst the costs of all the drugs shown have changed since the time of analysis the comparisons are still we believe noteworthy.

Of particular note is that the most significant change in drugs cost since both the work of Rowe and that of ourselves back in the 1990s is that propofol came off patent which removed the requirement to use the very expensive diprifusor chipped syringes if using the Target Controlled model of delivery.

This is shown very clearly by the step change in propofol costs within the Torbay Day Surgery Unit in July 2007 (Fig. 33.1). Switching to an alternative source of propofol saved £4000/month, whilst new pumps were required their cost of £25,000 was paid for in 6 months by the propofol savings incurred. Rowe republished his data in 2006 [3] considering the use of generic propofol as shown in Table 33.4, he now demonstrates that propofol infusions for maintenance of anaesthesia are more cost effective than either sevoflurane or desflurane.

Choice of drug for induction and maintenance of anaesthesia will also have an impact on the disposables and other equipment used during the conduct of anaesthesia and this needs to be taken into account even in the most simple cost minimisation study of different anaesthetic techniques. Use of volatile anaesthesia requires certain expensive items of equipment to be available. The most obvious of these is an anaesthetic machine with the ability to deliver the anaesthetic vapours to the patient, whilst it would be unusual for most hospitals in the UK not to have anaesthetic machines readily available, this may not be the case for more financial restricted parts or the world. Even within our own hospitals it is not possible to provide an anaesthetic machine in every environment where anaesthesia may be undertaken and the simple drug delivery system of a syringe driver for TIVA administration may be preferable, desirable or the only option available. Choice of volatile anaesthesia also dictates the requirement for a more formal airway, the majority of cases undertaken using volatile anaesthesia employ either an endo-tracheal tube or laryngeal mask. Whilst short cases may be undertaken using a face mask this still requires a formal circuit and filter and commits the anaesthetist to holding the facemask for the duration of anaesthesia. With TIVA the interdependence of airway and

Table 33.3 Comparative drug costs for five different anaesthetic techniques for laparoscopic sterilisation

Anaesthetic technique	Mean time/case	Mean anaesthetic cost	Total procedure cost (drugs and disposables)	Anaesthetic costs as of total costs
Enflurane/ETT/IPPV	13 min	£13.64	£327.11	4.17 %
Enflurane/ETT/IPPV	12 min	£15.30	£323.21	4.73 %
Enflurane/SV/LMA	16.5 min	£12.43	£333.44	3.73 %
Propofol TIVA/SV/LMA	10.29 min	£13.88	£325.67	4.26 %
Propofol TIVA/SV/LMA	10.29 min	£14.90	£313.40	4.75 %

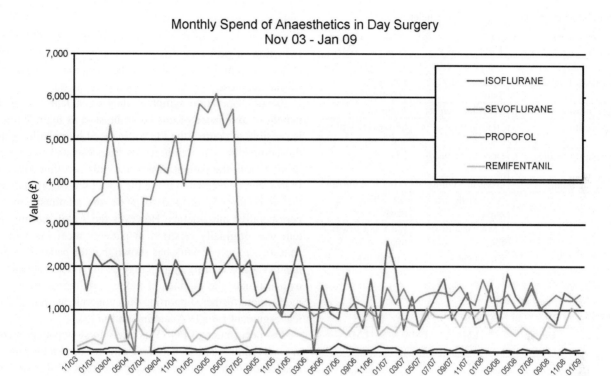

Fig. 33.1 Monthly cost of anaesthetic drugs in Torbay Hospital Day Surgery Unit

Table 33.4 Comparative costs of different anaesthetic techniques in a Day Surgery Unit in 2006

	Fresh gas flow	Cost/h
Isoflurane	6	£3.01
Desflurane	6	£17.60
Sevoflurane	6	£28.98
Isoflurane	1	£0.50
Desflurane	1	£2.53
Sevoflurane	1	£4.83
	Infusion rate	Cost/h
Propofol	14 mg/kg/h	£4.91
	6 mg/kg/h	£2.11

anaesthesia delivery is not present, hence the anaesthetist is free to select whichever airway technique is appropriate for that patient. In many cases this may simply be the use of a variable performance (Hudson type) facemask with spontaneous ventilation. This technique eliminates the cost of anaesthetic circuit/filter/face mask/laryngeal mask/endotracheal tube, etc. As this technique of airway management is commonly used in our day surgery unit we have analysed the costs of providing anaesthesia by a variety of techniques and included the costs not only of the drugs but of the associated delivery and airway management equipment required for that technique [4].

For the purpose of the study a single common procedure was selected, check cystoscopy (this of course may proceed to cystodiathermy or trans-urethral resection of bladder tumour). The costs analysed are shown in Tables 33.5 and 33.6. Table 33.5 shows the items considered to be "core" to all anaesthetic techniques, Table 33.6 shows those additional items allocated to each technique employed. Results (Table 33.7) showed that for this short procedure the most cost effective technique was TIVA

Table 33.5 Equipment items common to all cases

Core disposable costs
ECG electrodes (3)
Skin cleaning wipe
Intravenous cannula
Cannula dressing
Hudson mask

Table 33.6 Equipment specific to each technique

Additional costs for TIVA + Hudson mask	Additional costs for TIVA + LMA	Additional costs for volatile + LMA
1 % propofol 50 ml	1 % propofol 50 ml	1 % Propofol, 20 ml
Alfentanil, 1 mg/2 ml	Alfentanil, 1 mg/2 ml	Fentanyl 100 mcg/2 ml
TIVA infusion set	TIVA infusion set	Isoflurane/min
50 ml syringe	50 ml syringe	Syringes (20 ml and 2 ml)
Drawing-up needle	Drawing-up needle	Drawing-up needle ×2
Oxygen, 6 l/min	Oxygen, 6 l/min	Oxygen, 6 l/m7in
	Anaesthetic face mask	Anaesthetic face mask
	LMA and airway filter	LMA and airway filter
	Circuit costs	Circuit costs

Table 33.7 Total cost of anaesthesia delivery

	Hudson mask + TIVA	LMA + TIVA	LMA + isoflurane	LMA + sevoflurane
n	65	26	46	0
Cost/min (1 syringe)	£0.42	£0.60	£0.46	£0.55
Cost/min (2 syringes)	£0.55	£0.71		
Average cost/min	£0.43	£0.64	£0.46	£0.55
Average cost/case	£9.03	£13.44	£9.66	£11.50

with a variable performance facemask, however this cost advantage was reduced if a second syringe of propofol was required at which point the costs equalled that of a sevoflurane/laryngeal mask technique. The use of a laryngeal mask airway increased the likelihood of requiring a second syringe of propofol due to the higher boluses required at induction to enable rapid positioning of the airway and transfer to the operating theatre. When comparing LMA techniques the overall cost of the TIVA technique is £1.94 or 9 pence/min more expensive than that of Sevoflurane.

Cost Effectiveness Analysis

If we are only going to choose the drugs used on the basis of cost and use this as our primary method of economic analysis, then we have to assume that the outcomes from using one drug or another are the same. This is not the case and is why we need to consider more than a simple cost minimisation approach. If we are to undertake a cost effective analysis we need to consider the various clinical outcome measures which may vary between anaesthetic techniques.

One of the consistently reported benefits of TIVA is a reduction in post-operative nausea and vomiting (PONV) [5, 6]. We know that PONV is the symptom that patients dislike the most, with up to 72 % of patients stating that this is the post-operative symptom they most fear [7] so the benefit of avoidance of this could be seen as high. While it is possible to control the PONV induced by volatile agents this comes at a cost both in direct drug costs and an increase in the risk to the patient of adverse drug reactions. Risk of PONV can be estimated using the Apfel scoring system and this is commonly utilised to target the administration of perioperative antiemetics. However the Apfel scoring system was originally reported in patients receiving volatile anaesthesia, recent work has shown that for patients receiving TIVA this scoring system may be invalid and appears to over estimate the number of patients requiring antiemetic medication, further supporting the economic as well as clinical argument for TIVA administration [8].

The occurrence of PONV is likely to slow patient recovery and require increased nursing time to care for the patient; in addition if the planned pathway of care is for day surgery, then PONV may result in unplanned overnight stay. Quoted rates for unplanned overnight stays range from 1.8 to 7 % and PONV may account for up to 50 % of these. With an unplanned overnight stay the additional cost of an overnight bed, which is currently though to be over £250, will more than over ride any cost saving accrued by the use of agents more likely to cause PONV. Rafferty demonstrated a significant reduction in both nausea and vomiting rates and additionally unplanned admissions following assisted conception therapy with TIVA compared with volatile anaesthesia (5 % vs 21 %, $p < 0.05$) [9].

Another common post-operative symptom is pain. This may lead to prolonged hospital stay, higher rates of unplanned admission after day surgery and increased requirements for nursing care. Published work shows that patients receiving TIVA experienced reduced levels of post-operative pain than those anaesthetised with either isoflurane or sevoflurane [10, 11].

One further area where cost minimisation comparisons will give false reassurance is in the incidence of more minor morbidity following surgery, for example if a technique is chosen that avoids the requirement for instrumentation of the airway then patients are less likely to experience a sore throat or risk dental damage than when a laryngeal mask or endo-tracheal tube is required.

Moving away from the physical symptoms further cost effectiveness analysis has been studied by Epple et al. [12] who looked at patient satisfaction following either TIVA or a volatile based anaesthetic and showed that satisfaction was higher in the TIVA group than in the volatile group (93.2 % vs 65.6 %) and the cost of each satisfied patient was lower in the TIVA group by almost 100 euros.

Cost Benefit Analysis

The choice of anaesthetic agent may directly impact on theatre efficiency as some studies have shown that turn around times may be shorter for short spontaneously breathing cases where TIVA is used as opposed to volatile agents. However this will only result in economic benefit if the accrued time allows for another case to be added to the list.

Just looking at cost minimisation and cost effectiveness of anaesthetic agents loses sight of the fact that the anaesthetic costs are tiny when compared with the costs of theatre time, surgical equipment and disposables, the cost of immediate post anaesthetic care where one to one nursing is required and the hospital episode as a whole. The cost of maintaining and staffing a theatre is over £15 per minute so any analysis of the economics of anaesthetic agent must take into account theatre efficiency and time in post anaesthetic care units.

It has been estimated that the cost of anaesthetic drugs contribute less than 4 % of the total cost of a day surgery procedure [2] and that this varies very little whether the technique chosen is TIVA or a volatile based anaesthetic technique [13]. Furthermore when considering the cost of anaesthesia in more major inpatient abdominal surgery, the cost reduces to a mere 1 % of the total cost of the procedure [14]. Analysed a different way even the techniques considered more expensive in terms of drug costs equate to the equivalent of only 36 s of theatre time when compared with the cost of staffing and running our operating theatres (currently £12/min for day surgery theatres and £15/min for inpatients). This is shown using data from our own unit analysed over a 10-month period from April 2008–January 2009 (Table 33.8). The dramatic tumbling of the cost of propofol is reflected by the over 50 % reduction in cost/case from £15.40 in 2000 to £7.20 in 2009.

This further reinforces the need to consider the bigger picture when discussing financial implications of different anaesthetic techniques and to recognise that if we can improve theatre efficiency by a mere 30 s per case we could entirely negate the anaesthetic drug costs. Many would argue that the choice of TIVA enables faster turn around of cases and as

Table 33.8 Average monthly drug costs and cost per case within a day sugery unit

	Average monthly cost (£)
Isoflurane	31.1
Sevoflurane	1212
Propofol	1245
Remifentanil	601
Other drugs	560
Total	3649
GA cases	504
Cost/case	7.2
	(£15.4 in 2000!)

such could result in considerable costs savings by shaving time off a theatre list. If by helping to improve theatre efficiency, anaesthetic techniques using TIVA enable such significant time savings as to enable an additional theatre case to occur within an allocated theatre session then the additional income accrued will make any anaesthetic drug costs insignificant in the overall economical analysis of the session. In our own unit we have demonstrated that by using more efficient processes within our day surgery unit compared with those in our inpatient theatres we can operate on an additional patient when carrying out a list of hernia repairs if these patients are operated upon in the day surgery unit [15]. Whilst this increased efficiency cannot be attributed to the use of TIVA alone in the day surgery unit it demonstrates that if attention is paid to all aspects of the theatre pathway to improve efficiency huge benefits in terms of increased productivity and hence income and reductions in cost per case can be achieved, use of TIVA in expert hands can contribute significantly to these efficiency improvements.

A further part of the patient pathway where choice of anaesthetic may have an impact is recovery from anaesthesia and therefore on the efficiency of the post anaesthetic care unit. Delays in discharge from the post anaesthetic care unit may result in delays between subsequent patients on a theatre list due to anaesthetic personnel being required to remain in the unit with their patient. This will impact on theatre efficiency, it therefore makes economic sense to use anaesthetic agents where recovery is rapid and which have a low incidence of side effects such as PONV. Shortening the time required for one to one nursing may even enable larger units to reduce overall staffing numbers and thus accrue significant budgetary savings.

A further cost benefit to be considered is whether different anaesthetic techniques influence longer term outcomes and timing of return to work. There are small amounts of conflicting evidence regarding this. Whilst Carvalho et al. showed no difference in functional recovery the first week after laparoscopic sterilisation between patients groups receiving TIVA or volatile anaesthesia [16], Sung demonstrated an earlier return to work following breast biopsy in patients anaesthetised using TIVA compared with those receiving a volatile technique [17].

Conclusion

In conclusion, whilst in some circles there is a perception that TIVA techniques are more expensive than alternative methods of anaesthesia, our cost minimisation analysis has demonstrated that this is not always the case, particularly when the entire patient episode is considered rather than drug costs alone. TIVA certainly can be argued to provide a more cost effective anaesthetic by minimising the morbidity commonly associated with volatile techniques. Additionally there may be wider cost benefits in using TIVA to society as a whole by enabling faster recovery and return to work. We would advocate that if a TIVA technique is considered the most clinically appropriate for the patient and the hospital environment involved then financial considerations should not restrict its use.

References

1. Stocker ME, Houghton K. Anaesthetic drug costs in a district general hospital day surgery unit. Ambul Surg. 2001;9:87–9.
2. Rowe WL. Economics and anaesthesia. Anaesthesia. 1998;53:782–8.
3. Rowe WL. Practical pharmacoeconomics with TIVA. Abstract presented at EuroSIVA Meeting 2006.
4. Blandford C, Brown ZE, Montgomery JE, Stocker ME. A comparison of the anaesthetic costs of day case surgery: propofol total intravenous anaesthesia and volatile anaesthesia. J One Day Surg. 2013;23:25–8.
5. Sneyd JR, Carr A, Byrom WD, Bilski AJ. A meta-analysis of nausea and vomiting following maintenance of anaesthesia with propofol or inhalational agents. Eur J Anaesthesiol. 1998;15:433–45.
6. Vari A, Gazzanelli S, Cavallaro G, et al. Post-operative nausea and vomiting after thyroid surgery: a prospective randomised study comparing totally intravenous versus inhalational anesthetics. Am Surg. 2010;76:325–8.
7. Orkin FK. What do patients want? Preferences for immediate recovery. Anaesth Analg. 1992;74(S):225.
8. Field V, Barnett G, Montgomery J, Stocker M. Post operative nausea and vomiting following total intravenous anaesthesia – is the Apfel score valid? J One Day Surg. 2015.
9. Rafferty S, Sherry E. Total intravenous anaesthesia with propofol and alfentanil protects against nausea and vomiting. Can J Anaesth. 1992;39:37–40.
10. Cheng SS, Yeh J, Flood P. Anesthesia matters: patients anesthetized with propofol have less postoperative pain than those anesthetized with isoflurane. Anesth Analg. 2008;106:264–9.
11. Tan TMF, Bhinder RM, Carey MMDF, Briggs LMDF. Day surgery patients anesthetized with propofol have less postoperative pain than those anesthetized with sevoflurane. Anesth Analg. 2010;111:83–5.
12. Epple J, Kubitz J, Schmidt H, et al. Comparative analysis of costs of total intravenous anaesthesia with propofol and remifentanil vs. balanced anaesthesia with isoflurane and fentanyl. Eur J Anaesthesiol. 2001;18(1):20–2812.
13. Rowe WL. The cost of anaesthesia; which drugs should we use in the future? R Coll Anaesth Newsl. 1999;44:8–9.
14. Churnside RJ, Glendenning GA, Thwaites RMA, Watts NWR. Resource use in operative surgery. Br J Med Econ. 1996;10:83–98.
15. Dione T, McCarthy R, Stocker ME. The financial argument for day surgery; illustrated using inguinal hernia repairs. J One Day Surg. 2008:18S.
16. Carvalho B, Benton JI, Vickery PJ, et al. Long term functional recovery following day case laparoscopic sterilisation. Inhalational versus TIVA maintenance. Ambul Surg. 2002;10:45–51.
17. Sung YF, Reiss N, Tillette T. The differential cost of anaesthesia and recovery with propofol-nitrous oxide anaesthesia versus thiopental sodium-isoflurane-nitrous oxide anaesthesia. J Clin Anesth. 1991;3:391–4.

Teaching TCI with Human Patient Simulators

Wolfgang Heinrichs

Introduction

Target-controlled infusion (TCI) technology is available in most countries worldwide for clinical use during sedation and anesthesia. Pharmacokinetic models are used in this infusion mode to calculate the infusion rates necessary to reach and maintain the desired drug concentration. The calculated infusion rates during TCI are consistent with the manually controlled infusion rates. Nevertheless there may be unique safety concerns when using this technology under various clinical conditions.

A recent report of Schnider et al. [1] analyzed the available data on safety and complications occurring during TCI. Although TCI is reported to be more complex than traditional modes of drug administration, there was no evidence that the TCI mode of drug delivery introduces unique safety issues aside from selecting the wrong pharmacokinetic model. The authors state that this risk is analogous to that of selecting the wrong drug with the current, "manual" infusion pumps.

A review of the recent literature shows that selecting the appropriate model and use of the correct patient data with respect to height, weight, and LBM (lean body mass) is critical to the safe use of TCI [2–4].

Finally, for every anesthesiologist, his/her first use of TCI is a new adventure. Although he or she may be experienced in administering TIVA (total intravenous anesthesia), there are new approaches and multiple steps involved in the use of these pumps. Once these are learned, TCI can indeed be a safe and effective method.

How to learn TCI? Traditionally there are classes offered which explain the theory of TCI and pharmacological models using a traditional class room setting. This is how it first started when TCI became available in Germany. The first day was filled with theoretical lectures. On the second day participants were taken to the OR (operating room) and TCI was administered to patients and demonstrated by experienced anesthetists. Participants were allowed to work on the TCI pumps under supervision of an experienced instructor. Shortly thereafter the simulation software TIVA Trainer™ was added to the course settings. With this simulation software, participants were able to conduct virtual TCIs. The disadvantage of this method of learning was that TIVA Trainer did not show any physiological data of the patient. Overcoming this limitation, a simulation program was developed in 2005. It was developed at the AQAI simulation center in Mainz, Germany. Today this program has been adopted by several organizations.

Initially, Medical Education Technologies (formerly METI but now CAE Healthcare) simulators were used. METI simulators have realistic physiological models and are able to calculate pharmacokinetic parameters using three-compartment models. To follow the physiologic effect of the anesthesia, the BIS (Bispectral Index by Aspect Medical, now part of Medtronic, Dublin, Ireland) was applied. Special interface software (HIDEP) was able to interface with METI in order to communicate data to and from the METI HPS (HPS = human patient simulator) software. Serial communication links of various TCI pumps read the data out of the pumps and entered this data into the METI pharmacological model. Aspect Medical Systems developed a simulator to generate certain EEG (electroencephalogram) traces in order to demonstrate that BIS could interface with simulation and TCI.

The first demonstration of a full simulation of TIVA/TCI took place at a TIVA conference in Venice, Italy in 2007. Figure 34.1 shows the setup that was used in Venice. There were two simulators running in parallel: one was equipped to perform conventional TIVA and the second was used with TCI (Base Primea™ by Fresenius). Two teams performed anesthesia in parallel and the audience could compare the

W. Heinrichs, MD, PhD (✉)
AQAI Simulation Center Mainz, Wernher-von-Braun-Str 9,
D-55129 Mainz, Germany
e-mail: wh@aqai.de

© Springer International Publishing AG 2017
A.R. Absalom, K.P. Mason (eds.), *Total Intravenous Anesthesia and Target Controlled Infusions*,
DOI 10.1007/978-3-319-47609-4_34

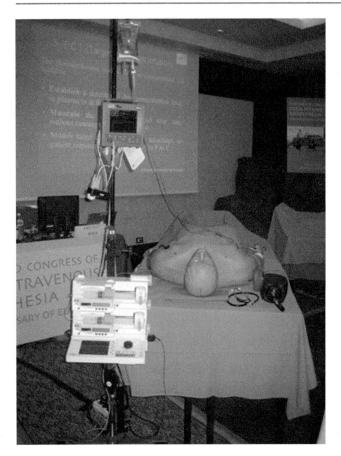

Fig. 34.1 The first demonstration of TCI and BIS simulation in Venice, Italy in 2007

and reports about a curriculum that has been developed during the past few years.

Methodological Setup of Training Environment

SIS—Simulation Interface Software is a flexible simulation software program. For details please see Fig. 34.2. The SIS software combines several modules which are used in the simulations. The most important module is the core physiological and pharmacological model which is designed like a grid, where rows are inputs, column outputs, and the cells do the calculations needed for combining inputs to calculate outputs. The system is highly flexible and can serve an almost unlimited number of situations and tasks. Attached to this, several drivers are used to communicate inputs and outputs to external devices. Input drivers include communication to iv-pumps, to maneuvers performed on the mannequin or interventions done by the participants. Output drivers include the full control of the mannequin, the EEG which is represented as BIS values and other displays such as the output of special monitors. Special monitors may show the estimated plasma- or effect-site concentration of the drugs, interactions between Propofol and Opiates and more.

Communication between the various external devices is performed by means of these devices. In most cases RS232 connections or TCP/IP network communication is used. In the simulated operating room, the setup is "life like." The participating anesthesiologists can work on the mannequin as a simulated patient, apply anesthetic drugs using TCI pumps, observe the cardiovascular reactions on the patient monitor, and follow depth of anesthesia on the BIS monitor. Normal and abnormal operations can be simulated to allow the participant in these programs to gain experience in TIVA/TCI from the level of beginners to the level of experts.

The pharmacokinetic models are open three-compartment models. If certain models are used in the TCI pumps (like Marsh for Propofol), the corresponding pharmacological model will use the constants and distribution volumes as originally published. By this the plasma or effect-site concentration can be calculated to be the same as those calculated by the commercial pumps. Input of height, weight, age, and gender supports those models that calculate the model parameters (volumes and/or rate constants) as functions of one or more of these co-variates (like Schnider model for Propofol). Many data for these drugs and models are to be found in TIVA Trainer™—simulation software for intravenous anesthesia edited by the European society for intravenous anesthesia (Euro-SIVA).

During the simulations, the data flows from the TCI pumps into the pharmacological model. This model calculates the estimated plasma and effect-site concentration

performance of both teams and follow the vital signs on two big screens. The learning objectives of this session were focused on the safe application of TCI compared to routine TIVA. In the ensuing years, this system was used by different simulation centers throughout the world.

Unfortunately METI eventually created a new software platform called Muse™ and decided not to support the HIDEP interface any longer. This decision terminated the application of METI for TCI simulation.

From 2010 AQAI started a new collaboration with Laerdal. Laerdal introduced a new family of full-scale simulators called the SimMan3G™. A physiological and pharmacological model for the use with the SimMan 3G family was developed with software which was called SIS (simulation interface software), still in use today with all Laerdal simulators that run the LLEAP™ (Laerdal learning application) platform. Thus SIS can be used with a variety of simulators of patients ranging from the baby to the adult and also the pregnant adult. For all these simulators the SIS TIVA TCI model can be applied (although TCI is not recommended in babies).

This chapter will describe the principle design of the hardware and software setup, how to simulate TCI today

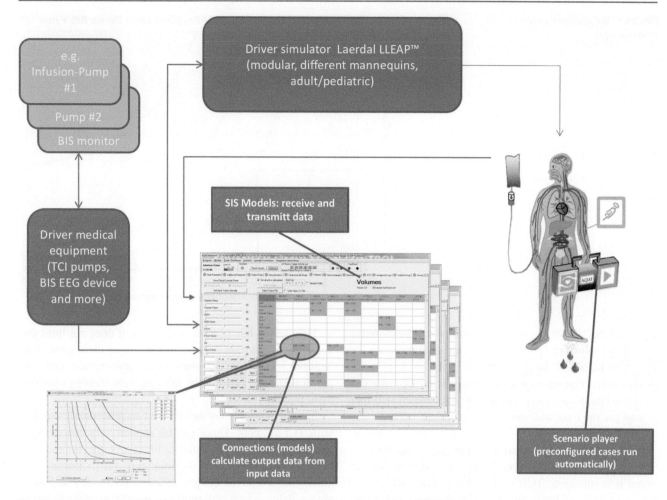

Fig. 34.2 Schematic drawing of the simulator and software setup used for TCI training. Details see text

Table 34.1 Relationship between clinical observations, propofol administration, and BIS values

Clinical situation	Dose propofol (mg/kg)	TCI effect concentration (µg/ml)	BIS
Awake/normal memory	0	<0.5	100–85
Sedation	0.5–1.0	0.5–2.5	85–65
Adequate anesthesia	1.0–2.0	2.5–5.0	65–40
Deep anesthesia	2.5–3.5	5.0–8.0	40–20
Full EEG depression	>4.0	>8.0	20–0

This table is used for procedural sedation cases using propofol alone

in parallel to the pumps. The effect-site concentrations are then used to model the clinical effects of the drugs used. For example, Propofol commonly has a heart rate and blood pressure lowering effect. With some typical nonlinear functions, the concentration of Propofol is used to modulate heart rate and blood pressure.

A special model was necessary to show the effects of Propofol on the depth of anesthesia. There is some data in the literature [5–9] and some assumptions are applied to fit data to the simulation sessions. Table 34.1 shows some relations between Propofol target concentration and depth of anesthesia.

The principles of EEG-based BIS monitoring have been selected to represent depth of sedation and anesthesia. The data flow in the model is as follows:

- IV-Pump sends drug amount administered every 10 s
- Pharmacological model calculates plasma- and effect-target concentration
- Effects of drugs are modeled to cardiovascular parameters directly
- Lookup function similar to the table given above derives BIS value
- BIS value is used to represent depth of anesthesia

Fig. 34.3 Interaction diagram
used (see text)

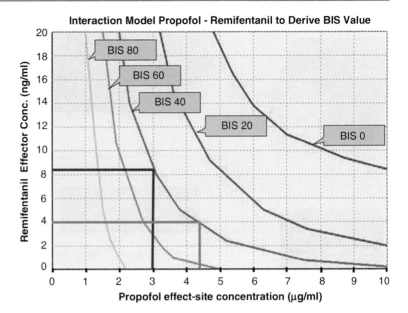

— BIS below 80: Eyes of the simulator will be closed
— BIS below 60: Depression of respiration present
— BIS below 40: Deep anesthesia, apnea
• BIS value is also used to generate a typical EEG trace that is used as input to any real BIS monitor which will then analyze the trace and show the appropriate value

With this setup, it is possible for the participants to work with Propofol in any TIVA mode (repeated boluses, conventional iv-application, TCI) as in a real patient and see and feel the results of the drugs on the mannequin and on the physiological monitoring parameters.

What about the typical combination of Propofol together with Opiates such as Remifentanil? Remifentanil on its own does not show major effects on BIS (Fig. 34.3). In combination with Propofol it is a well-known clinical effect that anesthesia is influenced by the combination of both. The work of Milne and Vuyk [8, 10] illustrated a synergistic relationship between the two with regard to the clinical effect (i.e., loss of consciousness). The following diagram shows the resulting model that is used. Propofol and Remifentanil effect-site concentration are entered into a 2-dimensional matrix to find a corresponding BIS value. In the example shown a Propofol effect concentration of 3 μg/ml with a Remifentanil concentration of approximately around 8 ng/ml will result in a BIS value of 40. The same will be true for a combination of Propofol 4.4 μg/ml and Remifentanil 4 ng/ml. Thus the lines in the model represent lines of equal BIS values. Values between the lines are derived by linear interpolation.

Similar models are used for other opioids (e.g., Alfentanil [11]). If additional sedatives (e.g., Midazolam or inhalational anesthetics) are used, the model will calculate additive effects of sedation and analgesia separately and then use an interaction model similar to the one given in the example.

This design has several advantages: it does not limit the application to certain drugs or models. Even the combination between TIVA and inhalational anesthetics can be performed, thus creating the most realistic training environment possible.

Special interest may be directed to procedural sedation with TCI systems. These can be applied very successfully and they also provide information about the interactions between Propofol and Remifentanil [12]. Borrat and colleagues looked at the gag reflex in endoscopy and were able to define levels of Remifentanil and Propofol needed to avoid this reflex during gastroscopy [13].

Basic Curriculum

The basic curriculum runs over 1 day of 8 h. Participants of the classes are mainly anesthesiologists or senior anesthesia nurses and a maximum of eight to ten participants are accepted. Pre-course material checks are performed to ensure that all participants are using TIVA in their daily practice. Most of them use TIVA pumps regularly with Propofol and Remifentanil. Some still use pumps in ml/h mode or apply repeated boluses of the drugs at least if they take care of short term procedures.

The theoretical learning goals refer to the general understanding of pharmacokinetic models, mainly open three-compartment models and how such models are applied to iv-pumps facilitating TCI. These learning goals are achieved by 2 h of lectures [14].

Basic theory lectures are followed by 6 h of practical work with the simulator-setup in the OR. At first a TCI controlled anesthesia using Propofol (Marsh model) and Remifentanil (Minto model) with two TCI pumps is demonstrated to the participants. The simulated patient is a healthy ASA I (American society of Anesthesiologists health status I) patient of 35 years undergoing some laparoscopic surgery. Muscle relaxation is achieved with Rocuronium by single bolus injection. During this demonstration there is a special focus on the handling of the TCI pumps and the technique of bolus followed by stepwise decreasing maintenance infusion rates that is unique to the TCI mode. Adaption of the level of anesthesia and how this is handled by the algorithms in the pumps supplements this session. Finally recovery is performed and the concentrations of the two drugs is observed when the simulated patient wakes up. As has been described in the previous section before, the pharmacology and the control of the mannequin simulator is handled by the SIS software automatically. The instructor works on the TCI pumps with no interaction by a simulator technician.

During the next hours the participants are divided into two groups of four to five each and they perform various TCI anesthesias of 15–45 min in length. Video recording of the scenarios is standard and debriefing sessions immediately after each anesthesia follow. In all cases the simulated drug concentrations as well as the resulting BIS values of the model together with the vital parameters and a view of the scene are recorded. These values can be used during the debriefing session, to optimize the strategy taken or to evaluate the quality of the anesthesia. This intensifies the knowledge and provides practical hints. Below are some examples of a variety of simulation scenarios, didactic goals, and debriefing objectives:

Case 1: Maria Engster; 32 years, 168 cm, 61 kg, ASA health status II; known allergy to various substances not relevant for anesthetic drugs or materials; scheduled for minor gynecological surgery (planned duration of surgery 5–10 min).

Task 1: Perform TCI with Propofol using Marsh Plasma TCI. Add 0.5 mg Alfentanil as single bolus. Use either no muscle relaxant, or a short acting muscle relaxant. Ventilate the lungs with LMA or face mask.

Learning goals 1: The participants should do everything on their own: prepare syringes and iv lines, prepare and pre-program the TCI pump. Decide with which Target concentration they want to start. Note that during the first anesthesia, just one pump is used to help participants understand the usage and the controls. Use the recovery time calculation to determine when the patient will probably return to consciousness. During this first try, no problems or complications are present.

Case 2: Alan Smith; 45 years, 175 cm, 73 kg, ASA health status I; No concomitant diseases; scheduled for minimal invasive (laparoscopic) cholecystectomy (planned duration of surgery 25–35 min).

Task 2: Perform TCI with Propofol using Marsh Plasma TCI plus Remifentanil using Minto Plasma TCI. Use muscle relaxants appropriately and intubate the trachea of the patient.

Learning goals 2: The participants will now use two TCI systems in parallel. This task is moderated by suggesting a constant Remifentanil TCI target concentration of 6–8 ng/ml, thus optimizing analgesia support first. Participants are then asked to titrate the Propofol target to clinical needs as judged by observation and vital parameters. Some changes in lung compliance due to the CO_2 peritoneum and the positioning (flat vs. anti-Trendelenburg) at typical phases of the procedure can be added. Clear statements 10 and 5 min before the end of the procedure are given and it is desired that the patient regains consciousness as soon as possible after that point.

Case 3: Clara Dryer; 31 years, 192 cm 81 kg, ASA health status I. Very similar to case 1.

Task 2: Perform TCI with Propofol using Marsh effect TCI.

Learning goals 3: Observe the difference in dosing compared to case 1 (the recorded data of case 1 will be available during the debriefing).

Case 4: Paul Iben; 53 years, 184 cm 91 kg; ASA health status II. Hypertension WHO grade I (World health organization); Very similar to case 2.

Task 4: Perform anesthesia using Marsh TCI in effect-site mode for Propofol and Minto in effect-site mode TCI for Remifentanil. In this case the Remifentanil target is no longer influenced by the course instructor but left to the discretion of the participants. Again data from case 2 can be used during the debriefing and compared to the actual course.

Learning goals 4: with case 4 participants are able to administer routine TCI safely for healthy patients. They can describe differences between plasma and effect TCI.

Case 5: Sven Moro; 74 years, 172 cm, 81 kg; ASA health status III. Hypertension WHO grade II. He had a myocardial infarction 4 months ago. Today he is scheduled for total hip replacement surgery (planned duration of surgery 45–60 min).

Task 5: Perform anesthesia using Marsh effect-site TCI for Propofol and Minto effect-site TCI for Remifentanil. Titrate the induction and determine precisely the LOC (loss of consciousness) concentration. Use these values for the recovery and determine the ROC (return of consciousness) values.

Learning goals 5: Participants have already learned during cases 3 and 4 that effect-site concentration TCI results in initially higher plasma concentrations, thus more side effects visible from the drugs. By titrating the increase of the target concentrations in steps of 1 (Propofol µg/ml; Remifentanil ng/ml) this disadvantage will be minimized. The LOC target can also be identified precisely using this technique and used to predict the moment of, and drug concentrations at, awakening (ROC target) more precisely.

Case 6: Martin Smith; 62 years, 156 cm, 69 kg; ASA health status II. Scheduled for colonoscopy. Propofol sedation desired. Expected duration 25 min (Polypectomy).

Task 6: Perform sedation using Propofol TCI.

Learning goals 6: Sedation with Propofol is standard care during endoscopy. In most cases sedation is performed by repeated boluses of Propofol. A common method comprises a preload with 0.5–1 mg/kg Propofol followed by boluses of 0.25 mg/kg at 3 min intervals. The number and the size of boluses may be varied by the sedation nurse/physician. If the duration of the procedure increases, there are several risks associated with this kind of application: either the sedation level reached is too low or the drug cumulates. TCI is well suited to overcome these disadvantages and may be superior especially in longer lasting sedations. Participants learn how to manage sedation using TCI and observe the time course of the drug administration. A second group of participants may be asked to perform the same task in the classical way. The data of both groups can be compared during the debriefing session.

Case 7: Frank Bauer; 72 years, 188 cm, 84 kg; ASA health status III. Various cardiopulmonary concomitant diseases. Scheduled for sigmoid colon resection due to cancer. Expected duration 3 h. (Participants are put in the middle of the surgery and should continue to supervise the anesthesia).

Task 7: Analyze the status and depth of the anesthesia. Continue while the surgeon starts a more painful operation period also associated with more blood loss.

Learning goals 7: During this last case, a typical error is introduced which may occur during the course of anesthesia: the Propofol syringe is replaced, during which time the pump is powered off. The participants have the task to solve this clinical problem which normally cannot be solved by re-starting the pump in TCI mode. One solution is to change the pump mode into TIVA and to continue optimally with the last infusion rate of the TCI mode before it was switched off. Alternatively, the user can use dose rates from his clinical experience. One learning goal of this scenario is also to observe TCI

pumps not only according to the target set but also to the drug usage that results from the individual target.

Advanced Curriculum

Participants to this class are regularly accepted, if they have attended the basic curriculum. If not they have to prove that they have sufficient knowledge about the basics of TCI and that they are already using TCI in their daily practice. Again this curriculum runs for 1 day of 8 h.

The lecture part of the day is very short and focuses mainly on the theory of interactions between various drugs used for TIVA. During the practical part participants have to perform two identical anesthesias: one with moderate dose Remifentanil (Target of 4 ng/ml) and titrate Propofol to achieve a BIS value between 40 and 50. The second one with high dose Remifentanil (Target 8 ng/ml) and again with the goal of titrating Propofol to BIS 40–50. Participants look at various stages of the anesthesia: side effects of induction, side effects during maintenance, dosage (target) of Propofol and recovery times.

A second lecture shows the most important facts about the idea of having different models for the same drug. To show the effects participants will conduct Propofol anesthesia in the same patient twice: Marsh Model vs. Schnider model. The task is to compare the drug usage of both models during induction and maintenance. From the simulator they learn that using Marsh may result in faster induction, but also in more pronounced side effects compared to that associated with the Schnider model. During maintenance the models behave similarly, so differences are no longer relevant.

More practical cases focus on high risk and elderly patients, patients with extreme low or high body weight and finally pediatric applications using appropriate models for children.

Case 1: Roger Simon; 76 years, 181 cm, 94 kg; ASA health status IV due to multiple cardiac diseases, hypertension, and recent myocardial infarction. Scheduled for urgent abdominal surgery.

Task 1: Perform induction in a way that cardiovascular reactions are minimized. This case may be repeated several times and different approaches may be used. What kind of maintenance level will be optimal for this patient?

Learning goals 1: This is a typical case where the Marsh model is no longer appropriate, if used in the conventional way. It may well be used with lower initial target concentrations of Propofol, thus titrating the induction slowly. An alternative is the use of the Schnider model which gives better results during induction and has some kind of "intrinsic" titration effect. As this case can be repeated using different approaches the participants will be able to derive the optimal strategy for this kind of patients.

Case 2: Mary Moulder; 39 years, 168 cm, 189 kg; ASA health status III. Scheduled for bariatric surgery.

Task 2: Perform manually controlled TIVA in this obese patient and compare it to the use of TCI models. Use Marsh or Schnider for Propofol. Observe maximum weight settings in the models.

Learning goals 2: As TCI models currently do not support extreme body weight or other extreme clinical conditions [15–18], participants have to judge the body weight they want to set for these patients. This task may be critical from a legal point of view, because the TCI system is used out of its defined boundaries. Participants have to decide, if they want to go for this kind of "Off label use" or not and use TIVA conventionally instead. Still the problem remains: a certain body weight has to be used in TIVA mode as well. In the simulation setting it can be experienced with the other models without the danger of harming a patient.

Case 3: Susan Dangler; 15 years, 172 cm, 48 kg; ASA health status III. Scheduled for a minor gynecological intervention.

Task 3: Select TCI model and perform anesthesia. The case will be performed twice: without and with access to BIS readings.

Learning goals 3: First time without having the possibility to take a look at the resulting BIS readings. Participants have to be aware that most models overestimate the effect in these patients. Consequently the danger of awareness is considerable. In the second run, participants shall be able to compare their settings from the first run with those obtained when the BIS model gives some ideas about the minimal depth of anesthesia. The simulation model itself is adapted to this special situation by a factor called "patient sensitivity."

Case 4: Maria Merrydom; 96 years, 164 cm, 59 kg; ASA health status IV due to various age dependent cardiovascular and respiratory diseases. Scheduled for repair of fractured proximal femur.

Task 4: Perform TCI using the Schnider model. Observe any cardiovascular side effects. Observe that even fairly low

TCI target concentrations may generate BIS values below 40 (that should of course be avoided).

Learning goals 4: Participants should be able to work with extreme age and adapt the settings appropriately. The Schnider model may be the better choice compared to Marsh; even special considerations may be applicable [19].

Case 5: Frederique Chapman; 8 years, 121 cm 34 kg; ASA health status I. Scheduled for hernia repair.

Task 5: Use an appropriate pediatric model. Observe the desired level of anesthesia mainly from clinical parameters. BIS is not available.

Learning goals 5: this case finally presents a child of 8 years which may be treated with TCI if an appropriate pediatric model (e.g., Paedfusor™) is selected. The case will be presented without BIS monitor, because EEG analysis in children may be less defined than in adults [20]. Nevertheless participants learn how to apply TCI to children.

Results and Experience from Classes Given

These TCI seminars have been performed regular in Germany and some other countries (such as Turkey, Bulgaria, and Italy) during the past years. The cases have been adapted according to the feedback of the participants. In general, this author has found that the feedback from the participants has been extremely positive. Participants especially like the combination of theoretical lectures explaining the basics with the practical tasks on the simulator.

In a study with 55 participants from various classes a questionnaire containing 10 multiple choice questions was used. Participants formed teams consisting of senior anesthesiologists, residents in training, and anesthesia nurses (Fig. 34.4).

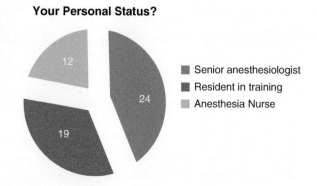

Your Personal Status?

■ Senior anesthesiologist
■ Resident in training
■ Anesthesia Nurse

Fig. 34.4 Personal status of 55 participants

The overall assessment of the basic and advanced curriculum is given in Fig. 34.5.

The results from 55 participants are shown in Fig. 34.6. The ratings range from excellent to fair. Not all participants are able to accept a mannequin being a real simulated patient.

What Is Needed to Set up Such a Program?

What is necessary to set up training like this in a center that wants to participate in this program and/or modify the cases to special interests?

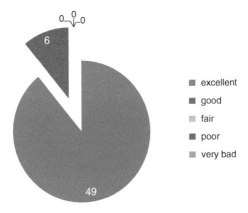

Fig. 34.5 Results of a questionnaire with 55 participants. Overall assessment is rated excellent or good. There are no negative judgements

Fig. 34.6 Relevance of cases for daily practice. These cases refer to cases 1–4 of the advance curriculum (detailed description see above). The pediatric cases were not presented to these participants

To make this training very realistic, the setup should contain a full-scale mannequin placed in an OR-like environment with the typical instruments and monitors found in an OR, respectively, in the anesthetist's working place. The mannequin simulator can be an adult or a child, male or female. There are several companies on the market which provide different simulator models. At a first sight all these simulators seem to be usable for this kind of classes. The individual differences result from the software provided by the manufacturer. This will be discussed below.

A minimum of two TIVA/TCI pumps are needed. These pumps should support the open model approach—that means the user should be able to select between the most important models and different drugs on these devices. Table 34.2 lists the most popular models that can be found on commercial TIVA/TCI pumps. It is important to have these models available in two different modes: plasma target and effect target. The differences between the models may be significant, especially during induction and it is the goal of the advanced training that participants learn the special features of these models. In principle all types of TCI pumps currently available on the market can be used.

In addition to pharmacokinetic and pharmacodynamic models, software is needed to implement a user interface, accept patient characteristics, use these to calculate model parameters, and then to run an infusion algorithm that calculates the required infusion rates (in TCI mode) or calculates blood and effect-site concentrations (manual TIVA mode) and the resulting clinical effects. Ideally the software should work like the model in the iv-pump, which makes it complicated. To this author's best knowledge,

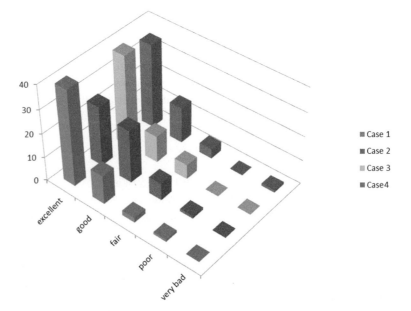

Table 34.2 Selection of models which should be supported by TCI iv-pumps

Drug	Description	Ref.
Alfentanil	Population multi study analysis	[11, 18]
Fentanyl	Fixed set	[21]
Ketamine	Racemic	[22]
Morphine	Gender differences in keo	[23]
Propofol	Diprifusor	[24]
Propofol	Population volunteers Pk/Pd	[19]
Propofol	Multicenter NONMEM analysis	[25]
Propofol	Paedfusor	[26]
Propofol	Fresenius (short keo)	[26]
Remifentanil	Population analysis	[27]
Sufentanil	Fixed set	[28]

today there are no simulators on the market which support these special needs.

Additional software is needed to control the devices together. Actually the data flow starts in the TCI pumps and continues to the mannequin resulting in certain reactions of the mannequin (like closed eyes, respiratory depression, cardiovascular reactions, etc.) provided on the mannequin itself and on the patient monitor. Once set to deliver a dedicated target, TCI pumps start by application of boluses and continue with variable running speed. This means that the amount of drugs administered to the (virtual) patient varies continuously over time. In consequence it seems to be impossible to follow these variable injection speeds manually by keying the current speed into the software of the simulator. This has to be automated and here the limitations of all currently available simulators show a big problem: even in the CAE models that support some kind of pharmacological model, it is not possible to connect TCI pumps directly. Therefore the decision about the model of simulator is exclusively determined by its ability to externally connect and communicate to the software of the mannequin.

Putting these requirements together, this author believes that Laerdal Company provides the best software interface to the mannequin software. Laerdal has recently released a new software family called LLEAP (Laerdal Learning Application) which is unique to a whole family of different simulator mannequins. It is based on the SimMan 3G software platform. That means that this program can be established on the more simple mannequins as well as on the high end types, on adult and children mannequins. The disadvantage of Laerdal is the fact that LLEAP does not provide detailed pharmacological reactions. This is why the SIS (Simulation Interface Software) was developed. With this tool all connections can be controlled by an external computer, the models run also in the external computer and the mannequin is controlled from there.

In conclusion, the simulation model can be used to simulate TIVA and TCI under realistic conditions. Thus for the beginner in TCI as well the advanced user of TCI, a setup has been created where personal experience can be gained without harming any patient. This approach is not only useful to increase the number of those who are confident in applying TCI but also helps anesthetists to be more safe in the application of TCI.

Conflict of Interest Wolfgang Heinrichs is CEO and senior developer of AQAI GmbH, Simulation Center, Mainz, Germany. AQAI has developed the models, the SIS interface software and the curriculum presented in this article. AQAI functions as supplier of these products. Wolfgang Heinrichs is also a consultant to Laerdal, Norway.

References

1. Schnider TW, Minto CF, Struys MM, Absalom AR. The safety of target-controlled infusions. Anesth Analg. 2016;122:79–85. PMID: 26516801.
2. Absalom AR, Mani V, De Smet T, Struys MM. Pharmacokinetic models for propofol-defining and illuminating the devil in the detail. Br J Anaesth. 2009;103(1):26–37. doi:10.1093/bja/aep143. PMID: 19520702, Epub 2009 Jun 10.
3. Chan SM, Lee MS, Lu CH, Cherng CH, Huang YS, Yeh CC, Kuo CY, Wu ZF. Confounding factors to predict the awakening effect-site concentration of propofol in target-controlled infusion based on propofol and fentanyl anesthesia. PLoS One. 2015;10(5):e0124343. doi:10.1371/journal.pone.0124343.eCollection2015. PMCID: PMC4418734; PMID: 25938415.
4. Rocha C, Mendonça T, Silva ME. Individualizing propofol dosage: a multivariate linear model approach. J Clin Monit Comput. 2014;28(6):525–36. doi:10.1007/s10877-013-9510-1. PMID: 24072471, Epub 2013 Sep 27.
5. Dahaba AA, Zhong T, Lu HS, Bornemann H, Liebmann M, Wilfinger G, Reibnegger G, Metzler H. Geographic differences in the target-controlled infusion estimated concentration of propofol: bispectral index response curves. Can J Anaesth. 2011;58(4):364–70. doi:10.1007/s12630-011-9453-2.Epub2011Jan25. PMID: 21264558.
6. Irwin MG, Hui TW, Milne SE, Kenny GN. Propofol effective concentration 50 and its relationship to bispectral index. Anaesthesia. 2002;57(3):242–8. PMID: 11879213.
7. Liu SH, Wei W, Ding GN, Ke JD, Hong FX, Tian M. Relationship between depth of anesthesia and effect-site concentration of propofol during induction with the target-controlled infusion technique in elderly patients. Chin Med J (Engl). 2009;122(8):935–40. PMID: 19493418.
8. Milne SE, Troy A, Irwin MG, Kenny GN. Relationship between bispectral index, auditory evoked potential index and effect-site EC50 for propofol at two clinical end-points. Br J Anaesth. 2003;90(2):127–31. PMID: 12538366.
9. Puri GD, Mathew PJ, Sethu Madhavan J, Hegde HV, Fiehn A. -Bi-spectral index, entropy and predicted plasma propofol concentrations with target controlled infusions in Indian patients. J Clin Monit Comput. 2011;25(5):309–14. doi:10.1007/s10877-011-9309-x. PMID: 21964767, Epub 2011 Oct 1.
10. Vuyk J, Mertens MJ, Olofsen E, Burm AG, Bovill JG. Propofol anesthesia and rational opioid selection. Determination of optimal EC50-EC95 propofol–opioid concentrations that assure adequate anesthesia and a rapid return of consciousness. Anesthesiology. 1997;87:1549–62.
11. Sigmond N, Baechtold M, Schumacher PM, Hartwich V, Schnider TW, Luginbühl M. Pharmacokinetic parameter sets of alfentanil

revisited: optimal parameters for use in target controlled infusion and anaesthesia display systems. Br J Anaesth. 2013;111(2):197–208. doi:10.1093/bja/aet049. PMID: 23512864, Epub 2013 Mar 19.

12. Barakat AR, Sutcliffe N, Schwab M. Effect site concentration during propofol TCI sedation: a comparison of sedation score with two pharmacokinetic models. Anaesthesia. 2007;62(7):661–6. PMID: 17567340.

13. Borrat X, Valencia JF, Magrans R, Gimenez-Mila M, Mellado R, Sendino O, Perez M, Nunez M, Jospin M, Jensen EW, Troconiz I, Gambus PL. Sedation-analgesia with propofol and remifentanil: concentrations required to avoid gag reflex in upper gastrointestinal endoscopy. Anesth Analg. 2015;121(1):90–6.

14. Struys MM, De Smet T, Depoorter B, Versichelen LF, Mortier EP, Dumortier FJ, Shafer SL, Rolly G. Comparison of plasma compartment versus two methods for effect compartment-controlled target-controlled infusion for propofol. Anesthesiology. 2000;92 (2):399–406. PMID: 10691226.

15. Bienert A, Wiczling P, Grześkowiak E, Cywiński JB, Kusza K. Potential pitfalls of propofol target controlled infusion delivery related to its pharmacokinetics and pharmacodynamics. Pharmacol Rep. 2012;64(4):782–95. PMID: 23087131.

16. Coetzee JF. Allometric or lean body mass scaling of propofol pharmacokinetics: towards simplifying parameter sets for target-controlled infusions. Clin Pharmacokinet. 2012;51(3):137–45. doi:10.2165/11596980-000000000-00000. PMID: 22316280.

17. La Colla L, Albertin A, La Colla G, Porta A, Aldegheri G, Di Candia D, Gigli F. Predictive performance of the 'Minto' remifentanil pharmacokinetic parameter set in morbidly obese patients ensuing from a new method for calculating lean body mass. Clin Pharmacokinet. 2010;49(2):131–9. doi:10.2165/11317690-000000000-00000.

18. Pérus O, Marsot A, Ramain E, Dahman M, Paci A, Raucoules-Aimé M, Simon N. Performance of alfentanil target-controlled infusion in normal and morbidly obese female patients. Br J Anaesth. 2012;109(4):551–60. doi:10.1093/bja/aes211. PMID: 22732112, Epub 2012 Jun 24.

19. Vuyk J, Schnider T, Engbers F. Population pharmacokinetics of propofol for target-controlled infusion (TCI) in the elderly. Anesthesiology. 2000;93(6):1557–60. PMID: 11149465.

20. Rigouzzo A, Girault L, Louvet N, Servin F, De-Smet T, Piat V, Seeman R, Murat I, Constant I. The relationship between bispectral index and propofol during target-controlled infusion anesthesia: a comparative study between children and young adults. Anesth Analg. 2008;106(4):1109–16, table of contents. doi:10.1213/ane.0b013e318164f388. PMID: 18349180.

21. Shafer SL, Varvel JR, Aziz N, Scott JC. Pharmacokinetics of fentanyl administered by computer-controlled infusion pump. Anesthesiology. 1990;73(6):1091–102.

22. Ihmsen H, Geisslinger G, Schüttler J. Stereoselective pharmacokinetics of ketamine: R(−)-ketamine inhibits the elimination of S(+)-ketamine. Clin Pharmacol Ther. 2001;70(5):431–8.

23. Sarton E, Romberg R, Dahan A. Gender differences in morphine pharmacokinetics and dynamics. Adv Exp Med Biol. 2003;523:71–80. Review.

24. Marsh B, White M, Morton N, Kenny GN. Pharmacokinetic model driven infusion of propofol in children. Br J Anaesth. 1991;67 (1):41–8. PMID: 1859758.

25. Schüttler J, Ihmsen H. Population pharmacokinetics of propofol: a multicenter study. Anesthesiology. 2000;92(3):727–38.

26. Absalom A, Kenny G. 'Paedfusor' pharmacokinetic data set. Br J Anaesth. 2005;95(1):110. No abstract available. PMID: 15941735.

27. Minto CF, Schnider TW, Egan TD, Youngs E, Lemmens HJ, Gambus PL, Billard V, Hoke JF, Moore KH, Hermann DJ, Muir KT, Mandema JW, Shafer SL. Influence of age and gender on the pharmacokinetics and pharmacodynamics of remifentanil. I. Model development. Anesthesiology. 1997;86(1):10–23. PMID: 9009935.

28. Gepts E, Shafer SL, Camu F, Stanski DR, Woestenborghs R, Van Peer A, Heykants JJ. Linearity of pharmacokinetics and model estimation of sufentanil. Anesthesiology. 1995;83(6):1194–204. PMID: 8533912.

Closed-Loop or Automated Titration of Intravenous Anesthesia: Background, Science, and Clinical Impact

Ngai Liu

Introduction

In 1950 the history of closed-loop intravenous anesthesia began in America. Mayo et al. reported the first clinical study of the use of a closed-loop controller on 50 patients allowing the automated titration of thiopental or ether guided by the electroencephalogram (EEG) activity [1]. EEG activity was already reported as a surrogate measure of anesthetic drug effect, allowing the quantification of depth of anesthesia on seven levels and EEG was used as output for automated anesthetic titration [2]. Thereafter it took several decades before new clinical studies with automated controllers were performed. The major milestone of closed-loop anesthesia occurred just around 2000, with the introduction of brain monitoring in clinical setting such as the Bispectral (BIS) index monitor (Covidien, Dublin, Ireland) associated with new short acting intravenous drugs with a short half-life (propofol or remifentanil) and new simple and powerful computers. To date several thousand patients worldwide have been anesthetized using different automated controllers. Despite an increasing number of clinical studies demonstrating the benefits of automated controllers, the administration of anesthetic agents during general anesthesia remains manual in routine care. However, two devices are commercially available; one was marketed for sedation during colonoscopy (Sedasys®, Jonhson and Jonhson, NJ, USA) and has been developed for non-anesthesiologists [3], the second device was developed for anesthesiologists (Concert-CL®, Veryark Technology, Guangxi, China) allowing the automated titration of propofol and rocuronium [4]. But in 2016, the company of the Sedasys® has stopped to selling the device.

N. Liu, MD, PhD (✉)
Department of Anesthesiology, Hôpital Foch,
40 Rue Worth, 92151 Suresnes, France

Outcomes Research Consortium, Cleveland, OH, USA
e-mail: n.liu@hopital-foch.org

Advantages of an Automated Anesthesia Controller

The benefit of an automated controller is to obtain precise control of the variables with continuous analysis and frequent changes in anesthetic drug concentrations. Thus, the drug infusion is titrated to the specific needs of each patient, taking into account inter- or intra-individual dynamic variability, specificity of the surgery thus avoiding drug accumulation [5]. In particular, automated continuous titration of the hypnotic drug guided by EEG activity improves anesthesia stability, and avoids over- or under-dosing episodes. Recently a multicenter trial highlighted the high variability in the performance of anesthesiologists manually titrating propofol administration while the performance of an automated controller was constant and predictable [6]. For a practitioner the titration is very active initially, thereafter the number of adjustments decreases over time, being related to the decrease of anesthesiologists' vigilance and the duration of the procedure [7]. Automated controllers are not subject to fatigue, thus maintaining the same efficiency and vigilance throughout a surgical procedure [8] and freeing the physician for the maintenance of cardiopulmonary homeostasis. The incorporation of an automated controller in a decision support system not only helps relieve the practitioner of repetitive tasks, but also provides perfectly reproducible action. Feedback control has the potential to improve similar improvements in the quality and safety of anesthesia as in the field of aeronautics by the standardization of the procedure [9].

Definitions of a Closed-Loop System

A closed-loop controller is defined as a system wherein a controller monitors one or more system variables and adjusts one or more interventions to maintain a setpoint. Closed-loop systems are ubiquitous in biology, for example

Fig. 35.1 Generic closed-loop
scheme

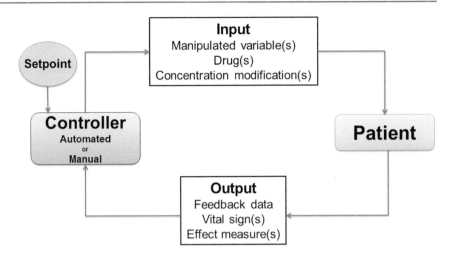

homeostasis which is present in every living organism is typically a feedback or closed-loop control. In anesthesia, the anesthesiologist himself constitutes a closed-loop controller (Fig. 35.1): the patient output is monitored in the form of vital signs and these parameters are used to titrate interventions by the practitioner [10] or an automated controller. Finally, all our therapeutic actions are by definition a closed-loop system wherein a human controller closes the loop [9]. The consequences of a human controller are that monitoring or actions are intermittent and irregular. Finally, the translation of closed-loop in medical terminology is titration and titration can be manual or automated.

The most ubiquitous controller is the Proportional-Integral-Derivative (PID) controller [11]. This controller calculates the difference between the measured output and the setpoint to adjust input value. The algorithm takes into account the present (proportional), past (integral), and future (derivative) error to adjust the correction. The artificial neural network controller is an adaptive control algorithm with a dynamic learning strategy [12]. The adaptive model-based controller [13] approximates or simulates the target system and predicts the observed response. The relationship between the propofol effect site concentration and the BIS value is determined during the induction phase and is used to construct patient-specific pharmacokinetic (PK) and pharmacodynamic (PD) models. This approach was abandoned later in favor of a Bayesian approach that optimizes the model [14]. The rule-based controller uses a set of instructions to perform its actions. A fuzzy logic controller is a system wherein the logical values true or false are not necessarily accurate but may be affected to some degree of truth. Fuzzy logic allows the imprecise information that humans use in decision-making to be formalized. This system requires testing because of the possible arbitrariness within sets. All these algorithms can be combined with each other (cascade structure) to create a specific controller to modify drug infusion rates or drug concentrations using a target-control-infusion (TCI) system.

The evaluation of the controller's performances by simulation or "in silico" studies is the first step before clinical evaluation. But, the relationship between performance obtained during simulation studies and anesthetized surgical patients is weak. Simulation studies can only determine whether the controller follows the instructions encoded in the software program [15]. It cannot always prove that the actions are logical or appropriate in anesthetized patients, many actions and results are context and time-dependent. For example in a surgical patient, a 20 mg bolus of propofol alone has virtually no effect before induction of anesthesia. After induction and during the maintenance phase, the same bolus can a significant decline in the BIS value, whereas during surgical noxious stimulation the same bolus may be inadequate so the BIS value increase despite it. Finally, controller performance can only be assessed by clinical studies because the transfer function remains unknown. In Table 35.1 we list the definitions of the most important terms used in control engineering.

Automated Intravenous Anesthesia with a Single Controller in Adult Patients

This chapter will discuss different clinical studies of a single automated controller. In particular, it will highlight randomized controlled trials but also describe observational studies.

Randomized Controlled Studies of BIS-Propofol Controllers During General Anesthesia

Since the first clinical observational study of automated titration of anesthesia using the EEG as output [1], various signals such as the median frequency of the EEG power spectrum [16] and auditory evoked potentials [17] have been used to guided automated titration of methohexital

Table 35.1 Definitions of engineering control terminology

Input	The variable entered into a function that modifies the output. In medical closed-loop systems, the inputs are the interventions of the controller (drug administration, for example)
Output	The end result of the input. In medical closed-loop systems, the outputs are the monitored patient parameters (heart rate and blood pressure, for example)
Open loop	A system wherein the measured output has no impact on the inputs
Closed-loop	A system wherein the measured output is used by a controller to determine a new input to the system. The controller which closes the loop could be manual or automated
Setpoint	Set point preset value that the control system is supposed to target
Error	The difference between the setpoint and the measured output value
PID	Proportional-integral-derivative controller. The three terms account for the present, past, and future error
Model-based	A model that approximates or simulates the target system
Rule-based	A set of defined rules organize and execute specific actions according to output changes
Artificial neural networks	An adaptive control algorithm with a dynamic learning strategy
Fuzzy logic	Systems wherein the logical values true or false are not exact and degrees of truth are permitted

[16], propofol [13, 17], or alfentanil [18]. The first randomized study reported for the use of the BIS monitor as output of automated anesthesia was performed in Hong-Kong with the collaboration of a team from New Zealand [19]. In this randomized control trial, 30 female ASA I-II patients were enrolled. In the automated group, anesthesia induction was performed manually using a mixture of propofol and alfentanil followed by a bolus of vecuronium. After tracheal intubation, the anesthesia was maintained by automated infusion of a propofol/alfentanil mixture with a setpoint of 50 for the BIS. The performance of this PID controller was similar to the manual administration of the mixture to maintain the BIS at the setpoint. No clinical advantage was found and light anesthesia episodes were more common in the closed-loop group probably related to the fact that the propofol/alfentanil ratio was fixed. This was, however, the first randomized study which demonstrated the clinical feasibility of automated intravenous titration of anesthesia guided by the BIS.

Different studies have reported the feasibility of automated propofol administration guided by the BIS during maintenance, but not induction of general anesthesia [19–21]. The induction phase is considered as a busy period during general anesthesia because the clinician needs to simultaneously control the airway, monitor and maintain hemodynamic and titrate anesthesia. A PID controller which controlled the calculated effect site concentration with the model of Schnider [22] was evaluated in a randomized control study of 40 patients specifically during the induction phase [23]. The control group received manual titration of propofol using a TCI with the model of Marsh [24]. In both groups the target BIS was 50 and a continuous infusion of remifentanil was administered. Automated induction titration of general anesthesia decreased the BIS overshoot (i.e., propofol overdosing), and reduced the mean duration of induction, whereas hemodynamic stability and

propofol consumptions were similar between the two groups. This study, which also included patients ASA III status and those taking cardiovascular medications, was the first reported of automated induction guided by the BIS. The same PID controller was used for the automated titration during induction and maintenance of general anesthesia [25]. This randomized controlled trial was performed in three centers, 83 patients were included in the automated group and remifentanil TCI was adjusted manually in both groups. The goal of the automated controller was to reach a BIS target of 50 and to maintain it in the range 40–60 which was considered to represent adequate anesthesia. During induction, the automated controller decreased propofol consumption but induction duration was longer. The mean duration of automated propofol titration was 134 min, the percentage of time of adequate anesthesia was higher with the decrease of deep anesthesia (BIS value <40) or light anesthesia (BIS > 60) during maintenance of general anesthesia. The incidences of unwanted somatic events or hemodynamic instability were similar and the time from discontinuation of propofol to tracheal extubation was shorter in the automated group. In contrast to previous studies [19–21], automated titration of propofol was performed during induction and maintenance of general anesthesia and patients undergoing major surgery, those with ASA III or worse and the elderly were not excluded. There are several physicians and anesthesia nurses who have used the controller in different centers, which demonstrates the applicability and reproducibility of the method.

Another PID controller was developed and evaluated in a study performed in India [26]. This randomized controlled study included 20 patients ASA I-II patients per group; in both groups, patients received an initial bolus of fentanyl followed by a continuous infusion. The automated controller administered less propofol and caused less overshoot of the BIS during induction. During maintenance, the automated controller decreased propofol consumption, outperformed manual titration for maintaining the BIS in the range 40–60, and facilitated earlier tracheal extubation was shorter. The same system has been used successfully in various clinical situations [26–31]. Indeed, all these studies were evaluated in the same center with the same investigators. To demonstrate the applicability and the reproducibility of the system, the authors performed a new controlled study involving multiple investigators in different centers [6]. In this randomized controlled trial the authors describe the comparison between automated and manual propofol administration guided by the BIS. This trial was performed on 242 patients undergoing elective surgery in six centers. The single closed-loop controller allowed the automated titration of propofol during induction and maintenance of GA. The automated controller outperformed a manual control to maintain the BIS around the setpoint of 50 and to maintain the heart rate and mean arterial pressure within 25 % of the baseline. The authors succeeded in delivering propofol automatically during induction and maintenance in realistic conditions.

A rule-based adaptive controller has been developed to steer propofol guided by the BIS [32]. In a controlled trial 20 ASA I-III patients, aged 54 ± 20 years, undergoing minor and major surgeries were included in the automated group. In both groups fentanyl or rocuronium boluses and propofol for induction were administered manually. The setpoint for the controller was 45 for the BIS which was deeper than in some previous studies [19, 23, 25, 26]. Propofol consumption was similar between manual and automated administration of propofol. The automated system was better able to maintain a target of BIS 45 than manual administration. Tracheal extubation was possible sooner in the automated group. Electromyogram activity measured by the monitor was integrated into the algorithm allowing the detection of artifacts.

The current trend is to evaluate automated systems in multicenter trials is to perform multicenter trial including a significant number of patients to improve the applicability and reproducibility of the results and decrease the risk of fragility of the results.

Observational Studies of BIS-Propofol Controllers During General Anesthesia

Observational clinical studies are necessary initially to assess the stability of the controller in realistic conditions such as in the operating room and to determine the proof of concept.

A study performed on female patients evaluated an adaptive model-based controller [20]. In this study a control group was available but the propofol was administered by a continuous infusion according to clinical criteria without the use of a brain monitor and therefore the control group was not considered as useful [33]. The initial patient-specific pharmacodynamic parameters were calculated during induction with a heuristic controller which had previously been used for automated sedation [34]. Propofol target concentration was increased by 0.5 µg/ml every 50 s. Once the BIS target had achieved, the system was switched to automatic feedback control, using the model parameter calculated during induction. During feedback control, the controller minimized the difference between the measured BIS and desired effect site concentration. All subsequent adjustments in propofol administration were based on the sigmoid "Hill" curve estimation. A total of 10 ASA I-II patients per group undergoing open hysterectomy were included, a continuous remifentanil infusion was administered before intubation (0.50 µg/kg/min) and during the maintenance (0.25 µg/kg/min). A bolus of rocuronium was used to facilitate tracheal intubation in both groups. During a mean duration of 113 min in the automated control group, the BIS values were better controlled using the automated controller and this method was reported to be clinically acceptable. However, the induction curve probably cannot always be obtained and this controller cannot be used in already anesthetized patients. The adaptive model-based-controller was finally improved by Bayesian optimization which overcomes the previous limitation [35]. Using a simulation protocol, all parameters of model-based adaptive controller were adjusted using specific weight calculated by the Bayesian variances. These variances determine how the model-based parameters can deviate from the population model. This algorithm was tested clinically for the automated sedation of propofol [14].

A PID controller previously tested for automated sedation of patients also receiving lumbar epidural analgesia [36] was evaluated in 20 patients undergoing body surface surgery [21]. The initial controller has a cascade structure including a PID controller which modifies target of plasma propofol concentration. In this second study the controller was modified to target the calculated effect site concentration to reduce the problem of oscillation related to the delay in equilibration between the plasma and effect site compartment. Manual induction was performed using a TCI system of propofol and remifentanil to target loss of consciousness and to tolerate the insertion of the laryngeal mask airway. The remifentanil concentration was fixed at 4 ng/ml during the maintenance phase of anesthesia. The median duration of automated administration of propofol was >27 min, the median BIS setpoint for the controller was 50 and this setpoint varied between 29 and 79. Anesthesia conditions were satisfactory for all patients except one patient who moved after the remifentanil was switched off by error. This study highlighted that targeting the effect site concentration by the controller was associated with fewer BIS oscillations.

In contrast to a PID controller, a neural network controller takes into account the nonlinearity, time variance or hysteresis, asymmetric control, delay of peak effect and uncertainty of the biological systems [12]. A comparison between a PID controller and a neural network controller using as a reinforcement learning algorithm was performed in silico [12]. In this simulated study reinforcement learning had the potential to maintain the BIS more accurately than a PID controller. Unfortunately, the relationship between controller performances during an in silico study and performance in an anesthetized patient is unknown. A neural network adaptive controller for propofol guided by the BIS has been developed and evaluated clinically [37]. This controller was tested in seven patients and was able to effectively administer propofol for induction and maintenance anesthesia during non-cardiac surgery. However, the authors reported BIS oscillation related to electromyographic noise in the BIS signal.

An adaptive proportional integral BIS control algorithm for propofol administration was developed and tested in 14 patients (30–60 years) [38]. The algorithm takes into account the present error between the setpoint and the desired BIS value and the past error. Anesthesia was induced by manual administration of propofol, remifentanil, and rocuronium. The authors reported that BIS oscillation during subsequent automatic control was probably related to the hysteresis between the infusion rate and the peak of the clinical effect. The addition of dead time or dead-time compensation after each propofol modification attenuated the BIS.

A disadvantage of these different single BIS-propofol controllers is that they only control the hypnotic component of anesthesia and the analgesic component, whereas the level of noxious stimulation varies continuously throughout surgery. During an intense noxious stimulus a single feedback propofol controller would respond by increasing the propofol to maintain the BIS at the setpoint, whereas the more appropriate action is to increase the analgesic component. Thus, tests of single propofol controller performance are in reality strongly influenced by the quality and the adequacy of analgesia policy.

Automated Intravenous Analgesia During General Anesthesia

The automated titration of opioid administration is the main challenge currently in the development of closed-loop loop anesthesia systems. At present, there is no specific parameter to directly measure analgesia in an anesthetized patient. Opioids are known to suppress the hemodynamic responses to noxious stimulation but even high opioid concentrations cannot guarantee complete control of hemodynamic responses to surgical stimulation. In clinical practice, opioid administration is titrated to hemodynamic changes after noxious stimulation which reveals the depth of antinociception.

Hemodynamic changes have been used for automated administration of alfentanil [39]. In an observational study including 11 patients, an alfentanil infusion was automatically titrated with a setpoint of mean arterial blood pressure of 70 mmHg obtained by an invasive measurement method. The controller calculated the plasma alfentanil concentration and made adjustments on the basis of a model-based predictive control algorithm. Isoflurane was titrated manually during the maintenance of anesthesia guided by the BIS. This study demonstrated the feasibility of the controller in healthy patients, during minor surgeries and with invasive mean arterial blood pressure.

By using noninvasive mean arterial blood pressure and heart rate, the Analgoscore, a score of nociception was developed allowing the automated titration of remifentanil [40]. The algorithm calculated a score related to the difference between the measured hemodynamic data and the setpoints, according to which the infusion rate of remifentanil was modified. Depending on the type of surgery and the patient's co-morbidities the clinician defined target values for mean arterial pressure and heart rate. Automated titration of remifentanil was performed in 16 patients and compared to 11 patients for whom the infusion rate of remifentanil was modified manually depending on the score given by the controller. The automated controller outperformed skilled manual titration to maintain the hemodynamic score in the desired range. This observational study reported the feasibility of this controller during minor surgeries in a limited number of healthy patients.

There are certain limitations to the use of hemodynamic changes as output for a control system. Heart rate, mean arterial pressure, and heart variability changes are not specific to analgesia needs and so are not optimal for analgesia titration. Hemodynamic status and responses can be modified by chronic hypertension, various treatments, blood loss, fluid administration, heart failure, arrhythmia, manipulation of great vessels, and a variety of drugs (inhalational and intravenous anesthetics, vasopressors, β blockers, vasodilators, etc.). An alternative to hemodynamic criteria for control of opioid administration is titration according to changes in electrocortical activity after noxious stimuli [41].

The median EEG frequency was used in 11 patients to steer alfentanil administration [18] and more recently the BIS has been used as output for a controller to steer a fixed mixture of propofol and alfentanil [19]. This latter randomized controlled trial reported no clinical advantage between automated and manual control. Use of an isoboller controller has also been described in which propofol and fentanyl administration was based on the mild-latency auditory evoked potential and a fuzzy logic algorithm that combined heart rate and mean arterial pressure, but it was tested on only one dog [42]. Currently, one of the most frequently published methods for the automated titration of remifentanil is the use of the BIS as output combined with the automated titration of propofol [43, 44]. The description of these studies will be further developed in the next section.

Multiple Automated Intravenous Controllers in Anesthesia

General anesthesia is a dynamic balance between hypnosis, analgesia, and muscle relaxation. Currently, several prototypes for the automated titration of propofol are available. The clinical relevance of automated administration of neuromuscular blocking agents is limited since the introduction of Sugammadex a specific antidote of rocuronium [45]. However, a study has reported the feasibility of combining automated titration of propofol and mivacurium [46]. In this observational study including 20 patients, the propofol was titrated automatically using a fuzzy logic-PID controller during the maintenance of general anesthesia. The control variable was the BIS, with a setpoint of 40 which was lower than in many previous studies [19–21, 25–28, 32, 35, 36]. The automated administration of mivacurium was started after tracheal intubation and neuromuscular blockade was guided by single twitch stimulation of the ulnar nerve. The setpoint for the neuromuscular controller was a train-of-four ratio of less than 10 %. Analgesia was maintained by a continuous infusion of remifentanil (0.25 µg/kg/min). No manual intervention was necessary during automated administration and operating conditions were satisfactory for all patients. The same propofol controller was combined with automated titration of a remifentanil TCI [47]. The fuzzy logic controller has a cascade structure for the automated titration of the target concentration of a remifentanil TCI. Heart rate variability, heart rate, and noninvasive blood pressure were used as output for the controller. Two fuzzy systems were implemented: one system can decrease the infusion rate during bradycardia or hypotensive episodes, the second system adjusts remifentanil administration according to tachycardia, mean arterial pressure, and heart rate variation. This controller was tested in ten patients during orthopedic surgery, was able to maintain satisfactory intraoperative conditions, and remifentanil was administered with adequate precision [47].

Recently, a randomized controlled trial reported the use of a commercial device allowing the automated titration of propofol and rocuronium during maintenance of general anesthesia [4]. In the automated group, 89 ASA I-II patients were included in three centers. The controller collected and calculated a mean BIS value during 3 min. An algorithm

then used, the calculated BIS values to control the target plasma propofol concentration using the PK model of Marsh [24]. The plasma remifentanil concentration was calculated using the PK model of Minto [41] and was titrated manually in both groups. For feedback control of rocuronium, the ulnar nerve at the wrist was stimulated every 20 s to obtain the train-of-four ratio. This study demonstrated that this new closed-loop infusion system could automatically regulate propofol and rocuronium. The automated controller achieved adequate anesthesia more accurately than manual control but no clinical advantage was found.

A controller integrating the three components of general anesthesia was evaluated and validated clinically [48]. The controller included a rule-based adaptive algorithm for the automated titration of propofol with a setpoint of 45 for the BIS value [32]. A pain score or Analgoscore® was calculated according to heart rate and mean arterial pressure and an expert-based rules algorithm allowing the automated titration of remifentanil administration [40]. The train-of-four ratio was measured every 15 min at the adductor pollicis muscle and rocuronium boluses were administered by the controller to maintain the train-of-four ratio of 0.25. A total of 186 patients were randomized and 93 ASA I-III patients were included in the automated group. This study demonstrated the feasibility of simultaneous control of hypnosis, analgesia, and muscle relaxation. The automated controller was better able to maintain the BIS around the setpoint and to maintain a target pain score and extubation time was faster than in the manual control group.

Hemodynamic changes during surgery are not always specific to analgesia and for the calculation of the pain score, the investigators need to determine the correct setpoint of heart rate and mean arterial pressure and modify the setpoint during the procedure [40]. The lack of specificity or setpoint for hemodynamic criteria during surgical procedure has given rise to other criteria. Noxious stimulus may cause cortical electrical activation with an increase of BIS values [49, 50], which indirectly reflect the level of antinociception [51]. In a randomized study including four centers, the BIS was used as output for the automated administration of propofol [25] but also for the second controller which was implemented for the automated titration of remifentanil [43]. The principle of this controller was based on the assumption that rapid BIS increase during a surgical procedure is likely to be secondary to noxious stimulation and is related to inadequate antinociception. A total of 196 patients were included in this trial and in 83 patients a PID controller with a setpoint of 50 was evaluated. The controller automatically administered both propofol and remifentanil during induction and maintenance of general anesthesia. In the automatic group, adequate anesthesia (BIS in the range 40–60) was present for a greater proportion of time, the incidence and duration period of excessively deep anesthesia and burst suppression ratio was decreased and the time to tracheal extubation was shorter than in the manual control group. However, remifentanil consumption was greater with the automated controller.

Several other clinical studies have confirmed that analyses of EEG activity can be a reasonable surrogate measure of depth of antinociception. One study involved 1494 ASA I-III patients in whom the dual controller was used [44]. In this study the initial dual PID controller [43] was also modified allowing a decrease of remifentanil administration by 20 %. The decrease of remifentanil administration by the automated controller was confirmed by another prospective study including more than 600 ASA I-III patients [52]. That these studies [43, 44, 52] were multi-centers and with many investigators supported the applicability of the controller in hands other than that of the inventors.

Previously a dual PID controller [43] used the M-Entropy analysis (GE Healthcare, Helsinki, Finland) of the EEG as output for the automated co-administration of propofol and remifentanil [7]. This randomized study reported that State Entropy can steer the automated administration of propofol, and that the difference between Response and State Entropy was a surrogate measure of depth of antinociception that can be used to steer the automated administration of remifentanil. Thirty patients were assigned to the automated group, for whom the automated controller was able to provide induction and maintenance of general anesthesia, with adequate anesthesia for a greater percentage of time, where adequate anesthesia is defined by a State Entropy value in the range 40–60. Propofol and remifentanil consumption and the incidence of hemodynamic or somatic events were similar between the two groups.

Controlled clinical studies for multiple controllers have now been performed [4, 43, 48] and the automated co-administration of propofol and remifentanil appears to be the most clinically relevant approach [43, 48]. Further evaluations are needed to determine whether hemodynamic changes or cortical electrical activation can be the most robust parameter for the automated titration of analgesia.

Automated Intravenous Sedation

Application for Surgery

The first study of automated sedation guided by the BIS was reported in Belgium [19]. It was an observational study including ten patients undergoing orthopedic surgery under spinal anesthesia. Initially, propofol administration was titrated manually to target an Observer Assessment of Alertness and Sedation scale rating 1. After that the current BIS value was used as setpoint for the automated controller. During automated sedation no episode of apnea or

hypoxemia with SpO_2 below 90 was observed. Some patients exhibited movements but no case of awareness was reported. Automated sedation was performed using a model-based adaptive controller, for a mean duration of 29 min with a maintenance dose of propofol 5.2 ± 2.7 mg/kg/h.

A PID controller initially developed for use with an auditory evoked potential monitor [17] was modified by the use of the BIS monitor instead as output allowing the feedback control of plasmatic propofol concentration [36]. The controller was evaluated in ten patients undergoing hip and knee surgery under combined epidural analgesia and sedation during a mean duration of 72 min. A lumbar epidural catheter was initiate with bupivacaine before the start of sedation. The plasma target propofol concentration was manually titrated to allow the insertion of the laryngeal mask airway and the patient breathed spontaneously. This observational study reported that the performance of the controller for different BIS setpoints (mean setpoint value was 48) was adequate and that it was able to provide clinically adequate sedation in nine patients. However, one patient moved 10 min before the end of the procedure after a noxious stimulus and in three patients BIS oscillations were observed. BIS oscillations were related to the time taken for equilibration between the calculated plasma concentration and the effect measured by the BIS. To take into account of this hysteresis between plasmatic and effect site concentration the controller was modified to steer the effect site concentration instead of the plasma concentration [21].

A model-based adaptive controller [20] was modified by Bayesian optimization [35] allowing the automated titration of propofol during induction and maintenance of sedation. This Bayesian-based controller was evaluated in 20 female patients undergoing ovarian puncture for infertility [14]. The controller continuously modified the parameters of a specific sigmoid model for the effect of propofol, and used the model to select appropriate target concentration to minimize the difference between measured BIS and the setpoint. Before the start of automated intravenous propofol administration, boluses of midazolam and alfentanil were administered. The BIS setpoint was 50 and patients maintained spontaneous ventilation during 17 min. Ability of the automated controller to maintain the BIS in the range 40–60 and to maintain cardiopulmonary stability was similar to manual control.

A new controller was developed for automated sedation of patients under spinal anesthesia [53]. This randomized controlled trial included 75 ASA I-III patients undergoing elective orthopedic lower limb surgery. An initial bolus of propofol was injected by the controller at a rate of 250 µg/kg over a period of 2 min. Afterward, an infusion rate of 50 µg/kg/min was given for 3 min and the automated maintenance sedation was started. The BIS setpoint was 65 for the automated titration of propofol and the controller included a Decision Support System which decreased automatically propofol infusion by 50 % when low respiratory rate (<8 per min) or peripheral oxygen saturation (<92 %) was detected for more than 2 min. In the automatic group, "Excellent" (BIS value 65 ± 10 %) or "Good" sedation (BIS value 65 ± 20 %) was present for a greater proportion of time.

Application for Colonoscopy

The effectiveness of a PID controller developed for sedation during surgery [36] was evaluated for sedation during colonoscopy. In an observational study automated titration of propofol for sedation was performed during maintenance in 16 adult patients ASA I-III undergoing colonoscopy. The propofol was titrated manually using a TCI system until an Observer Assessment of Alertness/Sedation rating of 3 was reached (Response only if name called loudly or repeatedly). At this point automatic control was started with the current BIS value as the setpoint for the controller [54]. The median [range] duration of automated propofol administration was 19 [7–50] min, the median setpoint for the BIS value was 80 [75–85]. The controller maintained the BIS values within 10 % of setpoint during 80 % of the maintenance duration. No episodes of apnea, hypoxemia, excessively deep sedation, or airway obstruction requiring airway support were observed. Four patients reported recall without dissatisfaction and all the endoscopists were satisfied. This study demonstrated that a PID controller combined with TCI system and the BIS allowed the automated titration of propofol during colonoscopy.

Another EEG monitor, the NeuroSense™ has been used in pediatric and adolescent patients for the automated induction and the maintenance of propofol sedation [55].

Probably the most interesting system has been the development and Food and Drug Administration approval of a commercial device: the Sedasys® (Johnson & Johnson, Los Angeles, California, USA). Sedasys® received premarket approval in 2013. This device designed for non-anesthesiologist use, to facilitate the intravenous administration of 1 % propofol [56] for intravenous sedation of adult ASA physical status I or II patients undergoing colonoscopy and esophagogastroduodenoscopy. The device continually monitors and records patient's vital signs, including oxygen saturation, respiratory rate, heart rate, noninvasive blood pressure, end-tidal carbon dioxide and patient responsiveness. The controller can automatically increase oxygen delivery when oxygen desaturation is detected, and can decrease or stop propofol administration when the controller detects signs of oversedation (oxygen desaturation, low respiratory rate/apnea or unresponsiveness to auditory prompts). However, while the user (healthcare provider) can set the system to provide additional propofol, the system itself

cannot initiate an increase in infusion rate or any additional dosing of propofol at any time. An initial evaluation of this device was performed in 48 patients in America and Belgium and the study demonstrated the proof of the concept [57]. In a randomized controlled multicenter study including 1000 patients the controller was compared to a control group [3]. After a bolus of fentanyl, the propofol was administered continuously until minimal to moderate sedation was achieved, and then the controller was started. The Sedasys® decreases the occurrence of desaturation as compared to manually administered sedation with midazolam and meperidine or fentanyl for moderate sedation for routine colonoscopy and is associated with faster recovery from sedation [3]. The Sedasys® enabled effective and safe propofol administration by non-anesthesia professionals. Those using this device are required to first undergo full training to manage the potential adverse cardiopulmonary events related to propofol. Also, an anesthesiologist must always be immediately available for clinical assistance. However, Johnson & Johnson has stopped selling the device in March 2016 related to unexpectedly slow sales and company-wide-cost-cutting (there were no safety concerns).

Application for Intensive Care Units

Sedation is an integral part of patient therapy in the intensive care unit (ICU). Mechanically ventilated patients require sedation to improve comfort, to prevent metabolic imbalance, psychological stress or post-traumatic disorders, to decrease pain in the postoperative period or during nursing procedure [58, 59]. Inadequate sedation is related to specific morbidities such as nosocomial pneumonia and withdrawal syndrome, and it also prolongs mechanical ventilation and ICU length of stay [60–62]. The amount of sedation required by instable ICU patients is related to the underlying illness and co-morbidities. It changes over time and there is a high variability of PD response to the drugs. ICU physicians and nurses have many specific responsibilities and the time allocated to sedation titration is still limited and as opposed to the operating room, there is not a dedicated anesthesiologist for administration of sedative agents. Thus, closed-loop or automated sedation has the potential to improve patient care by continuously adjusting the dosage of sedative agents to the minimum required for efficacy, thereby potentially avoiding side effects associated with overdosage. Moreover, appropriate sedation also prevents drug accumulation which facilitates neurological assessment.

In ICU patients EEG activity provides an evaluation of sedation depth. The EEG analysis given by the BIS has also been used to guide sedation in critical care patients [63, 64]. The BIS has been empirically demonstrated to correlate with behavioral measures of sedation

[65]. However, there is some controversial literature about BIS in ICU patients, related to a poor agreement between BIS index and subjective sedation scales [66, 67]. In fact BIS measures deep sedation levels (BIS < 60) more accurately than the Ramsay scale which attributes a value of 5 or 6 [68]. A BIS target between 40 and 60 thus seems to be a surrogate measurement of deep sedation in the ICU [69] and is commonly targeted. This setpoint has the further advantage of decreasing the impact of muscular activity on BIS [70] and improves agreement between BIS values and sedation scales [71–73].

The feasibility of automated ICU sedation guided by EEG activity was reported in 1999 [74]. A quantitative measure of EEG activity (median frequency of the EEG power spectrum) was used for the automated titration of propofol in 21 ICU ventilated patients. The use of a BIS monitor as output of an automated controller for postoperative sedation was reported in patients admitted to a surgical ICU after cardiac surgery [31]. In this randomized controlled study, the controller targeted a BIS value of 70 and demonstrated the feasibility of a closed-loop propofol controller guided by BIS for sedation maintenance following cardiac surgery. The authors reported a high rate of modifications per hour (above 30 per hour) required to maintain the BIS in the range but no sparing effect of propofol was found. The controller has also been validated in a pediatric cardiac surgery patient [30].

The benefit of implementing a neural network controller in an automated sedation system was suggested but never reported in ICU patients [37]. In a randomized controlled trial, our controller for the automated titration of propofol and remifentanil [43] was compared with manual control of deep sedation in ICU patients [75]. Propofol and remifentanil were guided either manually or by a computer to maintain the BIS value in the range 40–60 considered as deep sedation in the ICU. Patients were severely ill in both groups as described by the usual critical illness scores and the controller significantly outperformed manual control. The closed-loop system maintained BIS in the range 40–60 or adequate sedation for 77 % [59–82] of the total duration in compared to 36 % [22–56] in the manual group. The median duration of automated sedation was 18 h [8–24]. No adverse events were recorded during the study. Propofol consumption was 0.8 mg/kg/h, this was reduced by twofold in the automated group and automated sedation decreased the sedation drug costs. The propofol consumption was lower than that reported for sedation in cardiac surgery [31] while the setpoint was higher for the controller (BIS = 70) probably related to synergic effect with remifentanil and lower than reported during maintenance of general anesthesia [26, 43].

Reduction in propofol administration may protect patients from the risk of propofol infusion syndrome as previously described in children and more specifically in the ICU. Propofol infusion syndrome was reported in patients receiving more than 5 mg/kg/h for a prolonged period. We note a safe administration of propofol as the total regimen ranged between 0.8 and 2.6 mg/kg/h [31, 75, 76]. The use of an automated controller may decrease the duration of excessive sedation (BIS < 40) and this may improve hemodynamic stability and other adverse affects due to hypnotic overdosing. This study [75] has also reported a significant decrease of vasopressor use in the automated sedation group probably because of better hemodynamic stability or because the decrease of the workload gave the staff more time to optimize the volume status of the patients. The decrease in workload was clearly demonstrated in this study. The number of infusion rate change is notably and significantly different between closed-loop and manual control with 39 ± 29 changes per hour versus 2 ± 1, respectively, for propofol and 40 ± 9 changes for remifentanil versus 1 ± 1, respectively ($p < 0.001$). These results confirm that the continuous titration of sedation is a very difficult goal for physicians and nurses. In contrast, an automatic system reduces workload and can free time for direct patient care [77]. This study also demonstrated that the administration of anesthetic agents by ICU's nurses with a limited knowledge of propofol and remifentanil might be associated with adverse effects, whereas continuous feedback of drug effects by the controller avoids drug side effects and finally improves patient safety.

Automated sedation for ICU patients is a new concept. Clinical studies have reported the feasibility and accuracy for the automated titration of propofol and remifentanil guided by EEG activity. At present, studies have demonstrated that at least intermediate variables are improved by automated sedation. The challenge is to confirm such benefit and assess its impact on patient outcome with randomized multicenter studies.

Automated Intravenous Anesthesia in Specific Circumstances

Application for Pediatric Patients

Studies of the use of automated control of anesthesia in the pediatric population are still limited, although two randomized controlled trials in this population have now been published [30, 78]. Automated and continuous titration of intravenous anesthesia is particularly suitable in pediatric patients. Indeed the majority of published pediatric PK models have a limited predictability [79] related to the wide inter-patient variability observed in children [80]. The first successful use of an automated controller in the pediatric population was performed on a 9-year-old child (ASA

IV) requiring an emergency lung reduction in 2007 [81]. Automated titration of propofol and remifentanil was performed during induction and maintenance of general anesthesia. The duration of maintenance was 115 min and the BIS was in the range 40–60 during 77 % of the procedure despite the use of the adult PK model of Schnider for the propofol administration [22] and the adult model of Minto for the remifentanil administration [41].

The first controlled study in children involved 20 pediatric patients undergoing cardiac surgery with cardiopulmonary bypass [30]. This study compared a controller allowing the automated titration of propofol during induction and maintenance of general anesthesia with manual titration of propofol. The controller, developed initially for the adult population [27], was modified to take into account the pharmacokinetic differences of pediatric patients. In particular the distribution volume and the clearance of propofol in the model were increased as well as dosage and the maximum allowed propofol infusion rate. The mean age was 11 ± 5 years in the closed-loop group. Fentanyl was titrated manually. The automated controller decreased propofol consumption during induction and the off-cardiopulmonary bypass period and avoided overshoot of BIS during induction. Moreover in the closed-loop group the hemodynamic stability was improved with decreased phenylephrine use in the pre-cardiopulmonary bypass period.

An observational study reported automated titration of propofol guided by the NeuroSense® (NeuroWave System., Inc, Cleveland Heights, OH) in 108 pediatric patients with a median age of 12 (6–17) years undergoing gastrointestinal endoscopy [55]. A remifentanil bolus was administered followed by a continuous infusion, whereas propofol administration was automatically administered during induction and maintenance of sedation. The NeuroSense® index was in the adequate range (within 10 units of the targets) during 89 % of the time. In 85 % of the patients, no manual propofol adjustments were necessary and spontaneous breathing was maintained without manual intervention. However, as for adult patients, the control of analgesia is a strong requisite for adequate controller performance in anesthesia.

A dual controller was evaluated in pediatric and adolescent patients for the automated titration of propofol and remifentanil during induction and maintenance of general anesthesia [78]. In 23 patients with a median age of 12 [10–14] years the dual controller outperformed the ability of manual control to maintain the BIS in the range 40–60. The controller also decreased the period of deep anesthesia. Although remifentanil consumption was higher in the closed-loop group, no increase in pain scores or morphine requirements was observed in the postoperative period. In this study the controller was similar to the controller evaluated in the adult population [43], using the adult

pharmacokinetic models of Schnider [22] and Minto [41], and only the upper limits of target were increased for both drugs. Finally these different studies demonstrated the feasibility and the accuracy of automated titration of propofol [30, 55, 78] or remifentanil [78] in children older than 6 years guided by EEG activity. By a continuous titration of drug administration according to the effect measured by the EEG activity, the controller compensates for the errors when using adult pharmacokinetic models in children.

Application for Cardiac Surgery

A PID controller previously validated during orthopedic, urologic, or general surgery [26] was tested in adult patients undergoing open heart surgery with cardiopulmonary bypass [27]. In this randomized controlled trial, the single automated controller BIS-propofol was tested in 19 adult ASA I-III patients during induction and maintenance of general anesthesia and fentanyl was administered manually in both groups. The overshoot of BIS and the decline in mean arterial pressure during induction were lower with the automated controller. This was related to the decrease of propofol dose to achieve induction. During maintenance the automated controller decreased propofol consumption. The automated controller outperformed manual titration to maintain the BIS in the range of adequate anesthesia despite the use of cardiopulmonary bypass which alters propofol PK. More interestingly, this study reported a better hemodynamic stability in the automated group associated with a decrease in phenylephrine requirements. The automated controller was described as a valuable tool which improved hemodynamic stability. The same controller was also evaluated in pediatric patients [30].

Application for Obese Patients

In morbidly obese patients, the titration of intravenous anesthesia is a challenge because of difference in PK/PD parameters compared with lean patients [82]. Whether to dose the drugs based on the total body weight or the ideal body weight with or without "fictitious height" is hotly debated [83]. Moreover, the use of the PK models validated in lean patients can generate propofol overdosing during maintenance of general anesthesia in obese patients [84]. An alternative strategy is to titrate directly to a measure of depth of anesthesia or by the use of BIS-guided automatic drug administration. An automated controller is based on individual patient responses, the amounts of propofol and remifentanil given being based on individual requirement. The titration does not rely on an accurate underlying PK model or weight adjustment methods.

A dual-loop controller developed for lean patients [43] was evaluated in 30 obese patients in a prospective cohort comparison to lean patients [5]. The same controller with the PK models of Schnider [22] for propofol and Minto [41] for the remifentanil (with use of the total body weight as model input parameters in both groups) was used in both groups. The controller performance was similarly able to maintain the BIS in the range 40–60 in lean and obese patients. No propofol overdosing was reported in the obese group despite the use of the Schnider model. Using the actual true body weight, remifentanil requirement determined by the automated controller was halved. This difference disappears when the requirements were calculated using the ideal body weight.

The controller performances and anesthetic consumptions in obese patients with the dual-loop controller [5] were confirmed in another study including 117 morbidly obese patients undergoing laparoscopic sleeve gastrectomy [85]. This study reported that the incidence of postoperative nausea and vomiting (PONV) in obese patients with moderate-to-high risk of PONV was similar with or without the prophylactic combination of dexamethasone and ondansetron. Without prophylactic treatment of PONV and volatile anesthesia including obese patients with low risk factor of PONV, the incidence of PONV was 79 % [86] while the overall incidence of PONV was 50 % after automated intravenous anesthesia [85]. Automated intravenous anesthesia is a strategy to reduce PONV in obese patients.

These studies in obese patients [5, 85] demonstrated that the continuous titration by an automated controller was feasible, reliable, and safe despite the absence of a specific model or weight adjustment methods.

Application for Pheochromocytoma

Continuous titration of propofol is particularly suitable during resection of adrenal pheochromocytoma. Indeed during tumor handling, the propofol clearance increases because of the increase of liver blood flow following the sudden release of catecholamines. Conversely, after the tumor removal the propofol clearance decreases because of a decline in plasmatic catecholamines. An observational study reported the use of a BIS-propofol controller [26] in 13 patients undergoing adrenalectomy for pheochromocytoma by means of a laparoscopic procedure [28]. The automated controller was used during induction and maintenance of general anesthesia combined with thoracic epidural and intravenous fentanyl analgesia. The BIS was maintained in the range 40–60 during 87 % ±9 of the time, and moreover the investigators reported an excellent control of hemodynamic variables. All patients except one were extubated in the operating room. This study highlights the clinical interest of automated titration in this major and complex procedure.

Application for Lung Transplantation

In an observational study, a single BIS-propofol controller [25] was used in 20 patients undergoing single or bilateral lung transplantation which is a major emergency procedure [87]. The controller was used during induction and maintenance of general anesthesia. In this group of ASA IV patients, cardiopulmonary bypass was used in 5 patients; 14 patients received thoracic epidural analgesia. The percentage of time with adequate anesthesia (BIS in the range 40–60) was 84 % ±16 despite the occurrence of intraoperative events such as cardiac arrests in two patients and major bleeding (>1.5 L) in four patients. Moreover, ten patients were extubated at the end of procedure which demonstrated the absence of propofol overdosing. This study highlighted the clinical interest of automated hypnosis during prolonged procedure with major cardiopulmonary instability and in particular reported the behavior of the controller during cardiac arrest.

Application for Rigid Bronchoscopy

Most previous studies reported the use of an automated controller for a mean duration of more than 1 h [19–21, 26, 43, 44, 46, 48, 52, 88]. The use of a closed-loop controller has been rarely reported for short durations of anesthetic maintenance. Rigid bronchoscopic procedures usually require anesthesia for 30–60 min. This procedure represents a challenge for the clinician. It involves the management of patients with central airway obstruction and often major co-morbidities, the introduction and the mobilization of a rigid bronchoscope and the use of jet ventilation. In a randomized study a dual automated controller for the titration of propofol and remifentanil was evaluated in 33 ASA I-IV patients [89]. The automated controller maintained BIS in adequate range similarly to skilled manual titration and decreased the amount of propofol for induction. This study demonstrated the feasibility of automated titration for short procedures.

Application for Gigantism

The first use of the dual PID controller was reported in a patient suffering from gigantism undergoing elective hypophysectomy [90]. Automated titration of propofol and remifentanil guided by the BIS was performed during induction and maintenance of general anesthesia in a patient measuring 248 cm and weighting 125 kg. The patient was obviously not comparable to the usual population and by the use of direct measures of the effect on the cortical electrical activity, propofol and remifentanil administrations were continuously adjusted to avoid over or under-dosing.

Challenges at High Altitude

A controller allowing the automated titration of propofol guided by the BIS [26] was evaluated at high altitude [29]. In this observational study including 20 patients, fentanyl was administered manually, vecuronium bromide was given to facilitate tracheal intubation and the lungs were ventilated using 66 % of nitrous oxide in oxygen. The controller maintained the BIS value in the desired range similarly to a previous study at low altitude [26]. The performance of the controller in this observational study was in agreement with a recent randomized study including a manual group [6]. This controlled study reported the difficulty to maintain the BIS in the desired range for the manual group and the high variability of needs in patients at high altitude.

Automated Controller as Unbiased Methodology for Anesthetic Requirements

The use of an automated controller for propofol administration represents an unbiased assessment of how much propofol is required to produce similar hypnosis when an opioid or adjunct is combined with the propofol. A controller allowing the automated titration of propofol guided by auditory evoked potential was evaluated with different concentration of remifentanil [91]. Sixty patients were allocated into three groups receiving a calculated concentration of 2, 4, and 8 ng/ml of remifentanil. This robust methodology demonstrated a dose-dependent decrease in propofol requirement with increasing remifentanil concentration.

A controller allowing the automated titration of propofol during induction [23, 25, 43] was used to compare different propofol formulations [92]. In this multicenter double-blind randomized trial 217 patients were allocated into six groups. Three different formulations of 1 % propofol (Diprivan®, Propoven®,or Lipuro®) were compared with either saline solution or lidocaine 1 % added to the propofol solution. This study demonstrated by this reproducible methodology that the plain propofol formulations were not equipotent, as Propoven® required 22 % more propofol than Diprivan® or Lipuro®.

A dual PID controller guided by the BIS [43] was used to determine the sparing effect of dexmedetomidine on propofol and remifentanil consumptions. In this double-blind randomized study including 28 patients per group, one group received dexmedetomidine before induction and throughout the procedure and the second group a saline solution [93]. In both groups automated titration of propofol and remifentanil was performed during induction and maintenance of GA. Dexmedetomidine administration decreased both propofol and remifentanil requirements during induction, reduced propofol administration during maintenance of general anesthesia without an increase of hemodynamic adverse events and was associated with better postoperative analgesia.

The same dual PID controller [43] was used to determine the sparing effect of nitrous oxide on propofol and remifentanil requirements during a surgical procedure [52]. In this European (France, Belgium and Germany) randomized multicenter (10 centers) double-blind trial, 300 patients per group were randomized to receive either 40 % of oxygen in air, or a 40 and 60 % nitrous mix. Automated titration was performed in both groups during maintenance of general anesthesia to provide a similar depth of anesthesia measured by the BIS in the range 40–60. Nitrous oxide slightly reduced propofol requirement in the overall population. In fact nitrous oxide had no sparing effect in men and decreased propofol and remifentanil requirement in women was statistically significant but not clinically relevant.

The use of the automated controller is a new approach for anesthetic consumption. This methodology is robust and reproducible since investigator bias for the titration is eliminated.

Automated Titration and Outcomes

Currently, over 4100 surgical patients have been anesthetized with different automated controllers for the titration of propofol, mainly by a PID controller (82 % of the cases) and our French team has published studies involving 70 % of these patients. Since 2006 some controllers have been used to allow induction of anesthesia (Tables 35.2 and 35.3) [5, 7, 23, 25–30, 35, 37, 43, 44, 48, 52, 55, 78, 85, 89, 92, 93], others were used for patients with ASA III status and IV [7, 25, 27, 28, 32, 43, 44, 54, 85, 87, 94, 95]. The trend to assess automated controllers is to perform randomized controlled trials (Table 35.2) and to combine automated hypnosis and analgesia which now represent two thirds of the cases. However randomized controlled multicenter studies with automated induction and maintenance including patients with co-morbidities are still limited and only two controllers have been tested with this methodology [25, 43].

Automated controllers have been used for a range of different circumstances and patient population from pediatric patients [55, 78, 81], to an adult suffering from gigantism

Table 35.2 Randomized controlled trials of automated intravenous anesthesia or sedation with manual group

Study	Algorithm Output	Surgery	ASA > III	Ind	Duration	Analgesia	Multi	n
Morley et al. [19]	PID BIS	Gyn, Gen	No	M	87 [35–164] min	Mixture Propofol/alfentanil	No	30
Liu et al. [23]	PID BIS	Gen, Gyn, Uro, Orth, Tho	Yes	Auto	NA	Remifentanil TCI Variable	No	20
Liu et al. [25]	PID BIS	Gen, Gyn, Uro, Orth, Thor	Yes	Auto	136 ± 86 min	Remifentanil TCI	Yes	83
Puri et al. [26]	PID BIS	Uro, Gen, Orth	No	Auto	97 [41–298] min	Fentanyl fixed	No	20
De Smet et al. [14]	Bayesian BIS	Gyn Sedation	No	Auto	17 ± 3	Alfentanil	No	20
Agarwal et al. [27]	PID	Card	Yes	Auto	357 ± 103 min	Fentanyl	No	19
Hemmerling et al. [32]	Rule-based BIS	Gen, Thor, Uro, Orth	No	M	143 ± 57 min	Fentanyl bolus	No	20
Solanki et al. [31]	PID BIS	Sedation Card ICU	Yes	No	246 ± 152 min	Morphine	No	20
Liu et al. [43]	Dual-PID BIS	Gen, Gyn, Uro, Orth, Thor	Yes	Auto	140 ± 78 min	Auto remifentanil	Yes	83
Liu et al. [7]	Dual-PID M-Entropy	Gen, Gyn, Uro	Yes	Auto	208 [151–311] min	Auto remifentanil	No	30
Hemmerling et al. [48]	Rule-based BIS	Gen, Orth, Tho, Uro	Yes	Auto	191 [172–211] min	Auto remifentanil Auto rocuronium	No	93
Le Guen et al. [75]	Dual-PID BIS	Sedation in ICU	Yes	NA	18 [8–24] Hr	Auto remifentanil	No	15
Liu et al. [89]	Dual-PID	Rigid bronchoscopy	Yes	Auto	32 [24–51] min	Auto remifentanil	No	33
Dussaussoy et al. [96]	Dual-PID	Tho, Vasc	Yes	Auto	120 ± 50 min	Auto remifentanil	No	18
Orliaguet et al. [78]	Dual PID BIS	Gen, Orth, ENT	No	Auto	152 [114–292] min	Auto remifentanil	No	23
Liu et al. [4]	Fuzzy + PID BIS	ENT, Tho, Gen, Gyn, Uro	No	M	199 ± 96 min	Remifentanil TCI Auto rocuronium	Yes	86
Puri et al. [6]	PID BIS	Gen, Orth, ENT	No	Auto	80 [56–106] min	Fentanyl fixed Nitrous oxide	Yes	121
Zaouter et al. [53]	Rule-based BIS	Sedation Orth	Yes	Auto	119 ± 38 min	Spinal analgesia	No	75

PID proportional-integral-derivative, *Fuzzy* Fuzzy logic, *Gen* general, *Gyn* gynecologic, *Uro* urologic, *Tho* thoracic, *Orth* orthopedic, *ENT* ear nose & throat, *Card* cardiac, *Vac* vascular, *ICU* intensive care unit, *ASA > III* ASA score > III, *Ind* induction of general anesthesia, *Duration* duration of maintenance or sedation, *Auto* automated, *M* manual, *Multi* multicenter trial, *n* number of patients

[90], to pheochromocytoma surgery [28], application at high altitude [6, 29], use during lung transplantation [87], for the morbidly obese patients [5, 85] and for cardiac surgery with cardiopulmonary bypass in adult [27] and pediatric patients [30]. In adult patients automated titration results decreased in propofol doses during induction [23, 25, 26] and maintenance of general anesthesia [26]. Automated induction can also be faster than manual induction [23] and automated control of depth of anesthesia is associated with shorter time to tracheal extubation [25, 26, 32]. In adult patients scheduled for elective cardiac surgery the automated titration of propofol improves hemodynamic stability and reduces propofol and vasopressor consumption [27]. In pediatric patients scheduled for cardiac surgery, the automated titration of propofol decreases the use of phenylephrine and the amount of propofol for induction and during the off-cardiopulmonary bypass period [30]. Moreover, during major vascular or thoracic surgeries the use of an automated controller decreases the workload in particular during the induction period and improves hemodynamic stability during maintenance [96]. The use of automated intravenous sedation in ICU for severely ill patients improves the quality of sedation, reduced propofol consumption by twofold, and improved hemodynamic stability [75].

These studies highlight the clinical interest of automated control of intravenous anesthesia or sedation in patients presenting with co-morbidities or during major surgeries and show that cortical electrical activity represents a surrogate measure of hypnosis and analgesia depth. Currently all studies demonstrate that the use of automated control is potentially beneficial for the patient and that intermediate variables are improved by automated control.

Table 35.3 Observational studies of intravenous anesthesia or sedation

Study	Algorithm Output	Surgery Specificity	ASA > III	Ind	Duration Min	Analgesia	Multi	n
Mortier et al. [34]	Model-based BIS	Orth	No	M	28.8 ± 13.3	Spinal	No	10
Leslie et al. [54]	PID BIS	Sedation Colonoscopy	Yes	M	19 [7–50]	None	No	16
Struys et al. [20]	Model-based BIS	Gyn	No	M	111 ± 35	Remifentanil fixed	No	10
Absalom et al. [36]	PID BIS	Orth	No	M	72 [40–80]	Epidural	No	10
Absalom et al. [21]	PID BIS	Plast	No	M	27.5 [12–86]	Remifentanil fixed	No	20
Liu et al. [87]	PID BIS	Lung transplantation	Yes	Auto	343 ± 108	Remifentanil ± Epidural	No	20
Haddad et al. [37]	Neural BIS	No cardiac surgery	No	Auto	NA	Sufentanil or fentanyl	No	7
Pambianco et al. [57]	Rules Vital signs	Sedation Colonoscopy	No	M	12 [6–20]	Fentanyl bolus	Yes	48
Puri et al. [29]	PID BIS	Gen, orth High altitude	No	Auto	88 ± 22	Fentanyl Nitrous oxide	No	15
Hegde et al. [28]	PID BIS	Gen Pheochrom	Yes	Auto	75 [49–255]	Fentanyl and epidural	No	13
Mendez et al. [38]	PID BIS	NA	No	M	NA	Remifentanil	No	15
Pambianco et al. [3]	Rules Vital signs	Sedation Colonoscopy	No	M	13 ± 6	Fentanyl bolus	Yes	489
Besch et al. [44]	PID BIS	Gen, Gyn, Uro, Orth, Tho, Card, ENT	Yes	Auto	140 ± 78	Auto remifentanil	Yes	1494
Janda et al. [46]	Fuzzy PID BIS	Gen, Orth	No	M	129 ± 69	Remifentanil fixed Auto rocuronium	No	20
Janda et al. [47]	Fuzzy PID BIS	Orth	No	M	114 ± 27	Auto remifentanil	No	10
West et al. [55]	PID NeuroSense	Pediatric sedation Colonoscopy	No	Auto	14 to 49	Remifentanil continuous	No	108
Le Guen et al. [92]	PID BIS	Induction Propofol formulations	Yes	Auto	NA	Different propofol No analgesia	Yes	217
Liu et al. [52]	PID BIS	Gen, Gyn, Uro, Orth, ENT	Yes	Auto	128 [83–187]	Auto remifentanil Nitrous oxide	Yes	601
Le Guen et al. [93]	PID BIS	Gen, Gyn, Uro	No	Auto	170 [108–221]	Auto remifentanil Dexmedetomidine	No	56
Liu et al. [5]	PID BIS	Gen Obese/lean	Yes	Auto	147 [98–211]	Auto remifentanil	Yes	59

PID proportional-integral-derivative, *Fuzzy* Fuzzy logic, *Neural* neural network, *Gen* general, *Gyn* gynecologic, *Uro* urologic, *Tho* thoracic, *Orth* orthopedic, *ENT* ear nose & throat, *Card* cardiac, *Vac* vascular, *ICU* intensive care unit, *ASA > III* ASA score > III, *Ind* induction of general anesthesia, *Duration* duration of maintenance or sedation, *Auto* automated, *M* manual, *Multi* multicenter trial, *n* number of patients

Conclusion

Published studies have reported the clinical relevance and the technical performance of automated titration IV anesthetic agents. Automated administration of intravenous agents outperforms skilled manual control of the repetitive task of intravenous titration. This approach for anesthesia titration is feasible, in patients with co-morbidities, without fatigue, with high precision and can minimize errors. The trend is to combine automated titration of hypnosis and analgesia. Currently, one device is commercially available which demonstrates that automated titration in anesthesia is a reality. A truly collaborative effort between academic researchers and manufacturers is necessary to transform, develop, and evolve these research tools into commercial products (a photograph of the system we have developed is shown in Fig. 35.2). The possibility of having different

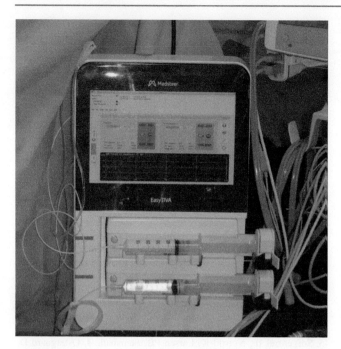

Fig. 35.2 A prototype of pumps developed by MedSteer allowing the automated titration of propofol and remifentanil

options for automated controllers provides the clinician with the opportunity to decide what type of controller best suits the environment, patients and type of surgery. The aim of of automated controllers is not in any way to replace the anesthesia provider but instead is an anesthesia adjunct to increase safety by reducing cardiopulmonary variability, thereby removing multistep processes which could be distract the anesthesiologist from other equal or more critical tasks.

The next challenge will be to determine whether the introduction of automated controllers in a clinical setting can decrease the cost, morbidity, or mortality associated with anesthesia and sedation.

Conflicts of Interest Dr Liu is the inventor and co-owner of a patent for the gain constant and control algorithm for a closed-loop anesthesia management system. Dr Liu is cofounder of MedSteer, a biomedical company which promotes research and development in Closed-loop anesthesia tools.

References

1. Mayo CW, Bickford RG, Faulconer Jr A. Electroencephalographically controlled anesthesia in abdominal surgery. J Am Med Assoc. 1950;144(13):1081–3.
2. Bickford R. Automatic electroencephalographic control of general anesthesia. Electroencephalogr Clin Neurophysiol. 1950;2:3–6.
3. Pambianco DJ, Vargo JJ, Pruitt RE, Hardi R, Martin JF. Computer-assisted personalized sedation for upper endoscopy and colonoscopy: a comparative, multicenter randomized study. Gastrointest Endosc. 2011;73(4):765–72. doi:10.1016/j.gie.2010.10.031.
4. Liu Y, Li M, Yang D, Zhang X, Wu A, Yao S, et al. Closed-loop control better than open-loop control of profofol TCI guided by BIS: a randomized, controlled, multicenter clinical trial to evaluate the CONCERT-CL closed-loop system. PLoS One. 2015;10(4), e0123862. doi:10.1371/journal.pone.0123862.
5. Liu N, Lory C, Assenzo V, Cocard V, Chazot T, Le Guen M, et al. Feasibility of closed-loop co-administration of propofol and remifentanil guided by the bispectral index in obese patients: a prospective cohort comparisondagger. Br J Anaesth. 2015;114(4):605–14. doi:10.1093/bja/aeu401.
6. Puri GD, Mathew PJ, Biswas I, Dutta A, Sood J, Gombar S, et al. A multicenter evaluation of a closed-loop anesthesia delivery system: a randomized controlled trial. Anesth Analg. 2016;122(1):106–14. doi:10.1213/ANE.0000000000000769.
7. Liu N, Le Guen M, Benabbes-Lambert F, Chazot T, Trillat B, Sessler DI, et al. Feasibility of closed-loop titration of propofol and remifentanil guided by the spectral M-Entropy monitor. Anesthesiology. 2012;116(2):286–95. doi:10.1097/ALN.0b013e318242ad4f.
8. Linkens DA, Hacisalihzade SS. Computer control systems and pharmacological drug administration: a survey. J Med Eng Technol. 1990;14(2):41–54.
9. Rinehart J, Liu N, Alexander B, Cannesson M. Review article: closed-loop systems in anesthesia: is there a potential for closed-loop fluid management and hemodynamic optimization? Anesth Analg. 2012;114(1):130–43. doi:10.1213/ANE.0b013e318230e9e0.
10. Absalom AR, De Keyser R, Struys MM. Closed loop anesthesia: are we getting close to finding the holy grail? Anesth Analg. 2011;112(3):516–8. doi:10.1213/ANE.0b013e318203f5ad.
11. Dumont GA, Ansermino JM. Closed-loop control of anesthesia: a primer for anesthesiologists. Anesth Analg. 2013;117(5):1130–8. doi:10.1213/ANE.0b013e3182973687.
12. Moore BL, Doufas AG, Pyeatt LD. Reinforcement learning: a novel method for optimal control of propofol-induced hypnosis. Anesth Analg. 2011;112(2):360–7. doi:10.1213/ANE.0b013e31820334a7.
13. Schwilden H, Stoeckel H, Schuttler J. Closed-loop feedback control of propofol anaesthesia by quantitative EEG analysis in humans. Br J Anaesth. 1989;62(3):290–6.
14. De Smet T, Struys MM, Neckebroek MM, Van den Hauwe K, Bonte S, Mortier EP. The accuracy and clinical feasibility of a new bayesian-based closed-loop control system for propofol administration using the bispectral index as a controlled variable. Anesth Analg. 2008;107(4):1200–10.
15. Liu N, Rinehart J. Closed-loop propofol administration: routine care or a research tool? What impact in the future? Anesth Analg. 2016;122(1):4–6. doi:10.1213/ANE.0000000000000665.
16. Schwilden H, Schuttler J, Stoeckel H. Closed-loop feedback control of methohexital anesthesia by quantitative EEG analysis in humans. Anesthesiology. 1987;67(3):341–7.
17. Kenny GN, Mantzaridis H. Closed-loop control of propofol anaesthesia. Br J Anaesth. 1999;83(2):223–8.
18. Schwilden H, Stoeckel H. Closed-loop feedback controlled administration of alfentanil during alfentanil-nitrous oxide anaesthesia. Br J Anaesth. 1993;70(4):389–93.
19. Morley A, Derrick J, Mainland P, Lee BB, Short TG. Closed loop control of anaesthesia: an assessment of the bispectral index as the target of control. Anaesthesia. 2000;55(10):953–9.
20. Struys MM, De Smet T, Versichelen LF, Van De Velde S, Van den Broecke R, Mortier EP. Comparison of closed-loop controlled administration of propofol using bispectral Index as the controlled variable versus "standard practice" controlled administration. Anesthesiology. 2001;95(1):6–17.
21. Absalom AR, Kenny GN. Closed-loop control of propofol anaesthesia using bispectral index: performance assessment in patients receiving computer-controlled propofol and manually controlled

remifentanil infusions for minor surgery. Br J Anaesth. 2003;90 (6):737–41.

22. Schnider TW, Minto CF, Shafer SL, Gambus PL, Andresen C, Goodale DB, et al. The influence of age on propofol pharmacodynamics. Anesthesiology. 1999;90(6):1502–16.

23. Liu N, Chazot T, Trillat B, Pirracchio R, Law-Koune JD, Barvais L, et al. Feasibility of closed-loop titration of propofol guided by the bispectral index for general anaesthesia induction: a prospective randomized study. Eur J Anaesthesiol. 2006;23(6):465–9.

24. Marsh B, White M, Morton N, Kenny GN. Pharmacokinetic model driven infusion of propofol in children. Br J Anaesth. 1991;67 (1):41–8.

25. Liu N, Chazot T, Genty A, Landais A, Restoux A, McGee K, et al. Titration of propofol for anesthetic induction and maintenance guided by the bispectral index: closed-loop versus manual control: a prospective, randomized, multicenter study. Anesthesiology. 2006;104(4):686–95.

26. Puri GD, Kumar B, Aveek J. Closed-loop anaesthesia delivery system (CLADS) using bispectral index: a performance assessment study. Anaesth Intensive Care. 2007;35(3):357–62.

27. Agarwal J, Puri GD, Mathew PJ. Comparison of closed loop vs. manual administration of propofol using the bispectral index in cardiac surgery. Acta Anaesthesiol Scand. 2009;53(3):390–7.

28. Hegde HV, Puri GD, Kumar B, Behera A. Bi-spectral index guided closed-loop anaesthesia delivery system (CLADS) in pheochromocytoma. J Clin Monit Comput. 2009;23(4):189–96.

29. Puri GD, Jayant A, Tsering M, Dorje M, Tashi M. Closed loop anaesthesia at high altitude (3505 m above sea level): performance characteristics of an indigenously developed closed loop anaesthesia delivery system. Indian J Anaesth. 2012;56(3):238–42. doi:10. 4103/0019-5049.98765IJA-56-238.

30. Biswas I, Mathew PJ, Singh RS, Puri GD. Evaluation of closed-loop anesthesia delivery for propofol anesthesia in pediatric cardiac surgery. Paediatr Anaesth. 2013. doi:10.1111/pan.12265.

31. Solanki A, Puri GD, Mathew PJ. Bispectral index-controlled postoperative sedation in cardiac surgery patients: a comparative trial between closed loop and manual administration of propofol. Eur J Anaesthesiol. 2010;27(8):708–13. doi:10.1097/EJA. 0b013e328335b2d4.

32. Hemmerling TM, Charabati S, Zaouter C, Minardi C, Mathieu PA. A randomized controlled trial demonstrates that a novel closed-loop propofol system performs better hypnosis control than manual administration. Can J Anaesth. 2010;57(8):725–35. doi:10. 1007/s12630-010-9335-z.

33. Glass PS, Rampil IJ. Automated anesthesia: fact or fantasy? Anesthesiology. 2001;95(1):1–2.

34. Mortier E, Struys M, De Smet T, Versichelen L, Rolly G. Closed-loop controlled administration of propofol using bispectral analysis. Anaesthesia. 1998;53(8):749–54.

35. De Smet T, Struys MM, Greenwald S, Mortier EP, Shafer SL. Estimation of optimal modeling weights for a Bayesian-based closed-loop system for propofol administration using the bispectral index as a controlled variable: a simulation study. Anesth Analg. 2007;105(6):1629–38, table of contents. doi:10.1213/01.ane. 0000287269.06170.0f.

36. Absalom AR, Sutcliffe N, Kenny GN. Closed-loop control of anesthesia using bispectral index: performance assessment in patients undergoing major orthopedic surgery under combined general and regional anesthesia. Anesthesiology. 2002;96(1):67–73.

37. Haddad WM, Bailey JM, Hayakawa T, Hovakimyan N. Neural network adaptive output feedback control for intensive care unit sedation and intraoperative anesthesia. IEEE Trans Neural Netw. 2007;18(4):1049–66.

38. Mendez JA, Torres S, Reboso JA, Reboso H. Adaptive computer control of anesthesia in humans. Comput Methods Biomech Biomed Engin. 2009;1.

39. Luginbuhl M, Bieniok C, Leibundgut D, Wymann R, Gentilini A, Schnider TW. Closed-loop control of mean arterial blood pressure during surgery with alfentanil: clinical evaluation of a novel model-based predictive controller. Anesthesiology. 2006;105(3):462–70.

40. Hemmerling TM, Charabati S, Salhab E, Bracco D, Mathieu PA. The Analgoscore: a novel score to monitor intraoperative nociception and its use for closed-loop application of remifentanil. J Comput. 2009;4(4):311–8.

41. Minto CF, Schnider TW, Egan TD, Youngs E, Lemmens HJ, Gambus PL, et al. Influence of age and gender on the pharmacokinetics and pharmacodynamics of remifentanil. I. Model development. Anesthesiology. 1997;86(1):10–23.

42. Zhang XS, Roy RJ, Huang JW. Closed-loop system for total intravenous anesthesia by simultaneous administering two anesthetic drugs. IEEE Eng Med Biol Soc. 1998;6:3052–5.

43. Liu N, Chazot T, Hamada S, Landais A, Boichut N, Dussaussoy C, et al. Closed-loop coadministration of propofol and remifentanil guided by bispectral index: a randomized multicenter study. Anesth Analg. 2011;112(3):546–57. doi:10.1213/ANE.0b013e318 205680b.

44. Besch G, Liu N, Samain E, Pericard C, Boichut N, Mercier M, et al. Occurrence of and risk factors for electroencephalogram burst suppression during propofol-remifentanil anaesthesia. Br J Anaesth. 2011;107(5):749–56. doi:10.1093/bja/aer235.

45. Sorgenfrei IF, Norrild K, Larsen PB, Stensballe J, Ostergaard D, Prins ME, et al. Reversal of rocuronium-induced neuromuscular block by the selective relaxant binding agent sugammadex: a dose-finding and safety study. Anesthesiology. 2006;104(4):667–74.

46. Janda M, Simanski O, Bajorat J, Pohl B, Noeldge-Schomburg GF, Hofmockel R. Clinical evaluation of a simultaneous closed-loop anaesthesia control system for depth of anaesthesia and neuromuscular blockade. Anaesthesia. 2011;66(12):1112–20. doi:10.1111/j. 1365-2044.2011.06875.x.

47. Janda M, Schubert A, Bajorat J, Hofmockel R, Noldge-Schomburg GF, Lampe BP, et al. Design and implementation of a control system reflecting the level of analgesia during general anesthesia. Biomed Tech (Berl). 2013;58(1):1–11. doi:10.1515/bmt-2012-0090/j/bmte.2013.58.issue-1/bmt-2012-0090/bmt-2012-0090.xml.

48. Hemmerling TM, Arbeid E, Wehbe M, Cyr S, Taddei R, Zaouter C. Evaluation of a novel closed-loop total intravenous anaesthesia drug delivery system: a randomized controlled trial. Br J Anaesth. 2013;110(6):1031–9. doi:10.1093/bja/aet001aet001.

49. Iselin-Chaves IA, Flaishon R, Sebel PS, Howell S, Gan TJ, Sigl J, et al. The effect of the interaction of propofol and alfentanil on recall, loss of consciousness, and the bispectral index. Anesth Analg. 1998;87(4):949–55.

50. Guignard B, Menigaux C, Dupont X, Fletcher D, Chauvin M. The effect of remifentanil on the bispectral index change and hemodynamic responses after orotracheal intubation. Anesth Analg. 2000;90(1):161–7.

51. Hagihira S. Changes in the electroencephalogram during anaesthesia and their physiological basisdagger. Br J Anaesth. 2015;115 Suppl 1:i27–31. doi:10.1093/bja/aev212.

52. Liu N, Le Guen M, Boichut N, Genty A, Herail T, Schmartz D, et al. Nitrous oxide does not produce a clinically important sparing effect during closed-loop delivered propofol-remifentanil anaesthesia guided by the bispectral index: a randomized multicentre study. Br J Anaesth. 2014;112(5):842–51. doi:10. 1093/bja/aet479.

53. Zaouter C, Taddei R, Wehbe M, Arbeid E, Cyr S, Giunta F, et al. A novel system for automated propofol sedation: hybrid sedation system (HSS). J Clin Monit Comput. 2016. doi:10.1007/s10877-016-9858-0.

54. Leslie K, Absalom A, Kenny GN. Closed loop control of sedation for colonoscopy using the bispectral index. Anaesthesia. 2002;57 (7):693–7.

55. West N, Dumont GA, van Heusden K, Petersen CL, Khosravi S, Soltesz K, et al. Robust closed-loop control of induction and maintenance of propofol anesthesia in children. Paediatr Anaesth. 2013;23(8):712–9. doi:10.1111/pan.12183.

56. Goudra BG, Singh PM, Gouda G, Borle A, Gouda D, Dravida A, et al. Safety of non-anesthesia provider-administered propofol (NAAP) sedation in advanced gastrointestinal endoscopic procedures: comparative meta-analysis of pooled results. Dig Dis Sci. 2015. doi:10.1007/s10620-015-3608-x.

57. Pambianco DJ, Whitten CJ, Moerman A, Struys MM, Martin JF. An assessment of computer-assisted personalized sedation: a sedation delivery system to administer propofol for gastrointestinal endoscopy. Gastrointest Endosc. 2008;68(3):542–7. doi:10.1016/j.gie.2008.02.011.

58. Jacobi J, Fraser GL, Coursin DB, Riker RR, Fontaine D, Wittbrodt ET, et al. Clinical practice guidelines for the sustained use of sedatives and analgesics in the critically ill adult. Crit Care Med. 2002;30(1):119–41.

59. Kress JP, Pohlman AS, O'Connor MF, Hall JB. Daily interruption of sedative infusions in critically ill patients undergoing mechanical ventilation. N Engl J Med. 2000;342(20):1471–7. doi:10.1056/NEJM200005183422002.

60. Soliman HM, Melot C, Vincent JL. Sedative and analgesic practice in the intensive care unit: the results of a European survey. Br J Anaesth. 2001;87(2):186–92.

61. Kollef MH, Levy NT, Ahrens TS, Schaiff R, Prentice D, Sherman G. The use of continuous i.v. sedation is associated with prolongation of mechanical ventilation. Chest. 1998;114 (2):541–8.

62. Cammarano WB, Pittet JF, Weitz S, Schlobohm RM, Marks JD. Acute withdrawal syndrome related to the administration of analgesic and sedative medications in adult intensive care unit patients. Crit Care Med. 1998;26(4):676–84.

63. Karamchandani K, Rewari V, Trikha A, Batra RK. Bispectral index correlates well with Richmond agitation sedation scale in mechanically ventilated critically ill patients. J Anesth. 2010;24(3):394–8. doi:10.1007/s00540-010-0915-4.

64. Trouiller P, Fangio P, Paugam-Burtz C, Appere-de-Vecchi C, Merckx P, Louvet N, et al. Frequency and clinical impact of preserved bispectral index activity during deep sedation in mechanically ventilated ICU patients. Intensive Care Med. 2009;35 (12):2096–104. doi:10.1007/s00134-009-1636-8.

65. LeBlanc JM, Dasta JF, Kane-Gill SL. Role of the bispectral index in sedation monitoring in the ICU. Ann Pharmacother. 2006;40 (3):490–500. doi:10.1345/aph.1E491.

66. Frenzel D, Greim CA, Sommer C, Bauerle K, Roewer N. Is the bispectral index appropriate for monitoring the sedation level of mechanically ventilated surgical ICU patients? Intensive Care Med. 2002;28(2):178–83. doi:10.1007/s00134-001-1183-4.

67. Olson DM, Thoyre SM, Peterson ED, Graffagnino C. A randomized evaluation of bispectral index-augmented sedation assessment in neurological patients. Neurocrit Care. 2009;11 (1):20–7. doi:10.1007/s12028-008-9184-6.

68. Tonner PH, Weiler N, Paris A, Scholz J. Sedation and analgesia in the intensive care unit. Curr Opin Anaesthesiol. 2003;16 (2):113–21.

69. Consales G, Chelazzi C, Rinaldi S, De Gaudio AR. Bispectral Index compared to Ramsay score for sedation monitoring in intensive care units. Minerva Anestesiol. 2006;72(5):329–36.

70. Liu N, Chazot T, Huybrechts I, Law-Koune JD, Barvais L, Fischler M. The influence of a muscle relaxant bolus on bispectral and datex-ohmeda entropy values during propofol-remifentanil induced loss of consciousness. Anesth Analg. 2005;101(6):1713–8. doi:10.1213/01.ANE.0000184038.49429.8F.

71. Sackey PV. Frontal EEG, for intensive care unit sedation: treating numbers or patients? Crit Care. 2008;12(5):186. doi:10.1186/cc7029.

72. Tonner PH, Wei C, Bein B, Weiler N, Paris A, Scholz J. Comparison of two bispectral index algorithms in monitoring sedation in postoperative intensive care patients. Crit Care Med. 2005;33(3):580–4.

73. Nasraway Jr SA, Jacobi J, Murray MJ, Lumb PD. Task Force of the American College of Critical Care Medicine of the Society of Critical Care M, the American Society of Health-System Pharmacists ACoCP. Sedation, analgesia, and neuromuscular blockade of the critically ill adult: revised clinical practice guidelines for 2002. Crit Care Med. 2002;30(1):117–8.

74. Albrecht S, Ihmsen H, Suchodolski K, Frenkel C, Schuttler J. Analgo-sedation in intensive care: a quantitative, EEG-based trial with propofol 1% and 2%. Anaesthesist. 1999;48(11):794–801. doi:10.1007/s001010050787.

75. Le Guen M, Liu N, Bourgeois E, Chazot T, Sessler DI, Rouby J, et al. Automated sedation outperforms manual administration of propofol and remifentanil in critically ill patients with deep sedation: a prospective randomized phase II trial. Intensive Care Med. 2013;39:454–62.

76. Albrecht S, Frenkel C, Ihmsen H, Schuttler J. A rational approach to the control of sedation in intensive care unit patients based on closed-loop control. Eur J Anaesthesiol. 1999;16(10):678–87.

77. Vasile B, Rasulo F, Candiani A, Latronico N. The pathophysiology of propofol infusion syndrome: a simple name for a complex syndrome. Intensive Care Med. 2003;29(9):1417–25. doi:10.1007/s00134-003-1905-x.

78. Orliaguet GA, Lambert FB, Chazot T, Glasman P, Fischler M, Liu N. Feasibility of closed-loop titration of propofol and remifentanil guided by the bispectral monitor in pediatric and adolescent patients: a prospective randomized study. Anesthesiology. 2014. doi:10.1097/ALN.0000000000000577.

79. Rigouzzo A, Servin F, Constant I. Pharmacokinetic-pharmacodynamic modeling of propofol in children. Anesthesiology. 2010;113(2):343–52. doi:10.1097/ALN.0b013e3181e4f4ca.

80. van Heusden K, Ansermino JM, Soltesz K, Khosravi S, West N, Dumont GA. Quantification of the variability in response to propofol administration in children. IEEE Trans Biomed Eng. 2013;60(9):2521–9. doi:10.1109/TBME.2013.2259592.

81. Liu N, Bourgeois E, Chazot T, Murat I, Fischler M. Closed-loop administration of propofol and remifentanil guided by the bispectral index in patient requiring an emergency lung volume reduction. Paediatr Anaesth. 2007;17(9):909–10. doi:10.1111/j.1460-9592.2007.02303.x.

82. Hanley MJ, Abernethy DR, Greenblatt DJ. Effect of obesity on the pharmacokinetics of drugs in humans. Clin Pharmacokinet. 2010;49(2):71–87. doi:10.2165/11318100-000000000-00000.

83. La Colla L, Albertin A, La Colla G, Ceriani V, Lodi T, Porta A, et al. No adjustment vs. adjustment formula as input weight for propofol target-controlled infusion in morbidly obese patients. Eur J Anaesthesiol. 2009;26(5):362–9. doi:10.1097/EJA.0b013e328326f7d0.

84. Absalom AR, Mani V, De Smet T, Struys MM. Pharmacokinetic models for propofol--defining and illuminating the devil in the detail. Br J Anaesth. 2009;103(1):26–37. doi:10.1093/bja/aep143.

85. Bataille A, Letourneulx JF, Charmeau A, Lemedioni P, Leger P, Chazot T, et al. Impact of prophylactic combination of dexamethasone-ondansetron on postoperative nausea and vomiting in obese adult patients undergoing laparoscopic sleeve gastrectomy during closed-loop propofol-remifentanil anaesthesia: a randomised double-blind placebo study. Eur J Anaesthesiol. 2016. doi:10.1097/EJA.0000000000000427.

86. Mendes MN, Monteiro Rde S, Martins FA. Prophylaxis of postoperative nausea and vomiting in morbidly obese patients undergoing laparoscopic gastroplasties: a comparative study among three methods. Rev Bras Anestesiol. 2009;59(5):570–6.

87. Liu N, Chazot T, Trillat B, Michel-Cherqui M, Marandon JY, Law-Koune JD, et al. Closed-loop control of consciousness during lung transplantation: an observational study. J Cardiothorac Vasc Anesth. 2008;22(4):611–5.

88. Reboso JA, Mendez JA, Reboso HJ, Leon AM. Design and implementation of a closed-loop control system for infusion of propofol guided by bispectral index (BIS). Acta Anaesthesiol Scand. 2012;56(8):1032–41. doi:10.1111/j.1399-6576.2012.02738.x.

89. Liu N, Pruszkowski O, Leroy JE, Chazot T, Trillat B, Colchen A, et al. Automatic administration of propofol and remifentanil guided by the bispectral index during rigid bronchoscopic procedures: a randomized trial. Can J Anaesth. 2013;60(9):881–7. doi:10.1007/s12630-013-9986-7.

90. Declerck A, Liu N, Gaillard S, Chazot T, Laloe PA, Fischler M, et al. Closed-loop titration of propofol and remifentanil guided by bispectral index in a patient with extreme gigantism. J Clin Anesth. 2009;21(7):542–4. doi:10.1016/j.jclinane.2009.02.008.

91. Milne SE, Kenny GN, Schraag S. Propofol sparing effect of remifentanil using closed-loop anaesthesia. Br J Anaesth. 2003;90(5):623–9.

92. Le Guen M, Grassin-Delyle S, Cornet C, Genty A, Chazot T, Dardelle D, et al. Comparison of the potency of different propofol formulations: a randomized, double-blind trial using closed-loop administration. Anesthesiology. 2014;120(2):355–64. doi:10.1097/01.anes.0000435741.97234.04.

93. Le Guen M, Liu N, Tounou F, Auge M, Tuil O, Chazot T, et al. Dexmedetomidine reduces propofol and remifentanil requirements during bispectral index-guided closed-loop anesthesia: a double-blind, placebo-controlled trial. Anesth Analg. 2014;118(5):946–55. doi:10.1213/ANE.0000000000000185.

94. Locher S, Stadler KS, Boehlen T, Bouillon T, Leibundgut D, Schumacher PM, et al. A new closed-loop control system for isoflurane using bispectral index outperforms manual control. Anesthesiology. 2004;101(3):591–602.

95. Madhavan JS, Puri GD, Mathew PJ. Closed-loop isoflurane administration with bispectral index in open heart surgery: randomized controlled trial with manual control. Acta Anaesthesiol Taiwan. 2011;49(4):130–5. doi:10.1016/j.aat.2011.11.007.

96. Dussaussoy C, Peres M, Jaoul V, Liu N, Chazot T, Picquet J, et al. Automated titration of propofol and remifentanil decreases the anesthesiologist's workload during vascular or thoracic surgery: a randomized prospective study. J Clin Monit Comput. 2013. doi:10.1007/s10877-013-9453-6.

Health Care Technology, the Human–Machine Interface, and Patient Safety During Intravenous Anesthesia

Craig S. Webster

Introduction

Modern healthcare clearly benefits the vast majority of patients. In fact, the ever increasing complexity and sophistication of healthcare technology means that more powerful and effective treatments are continually becoming available for a wider array of ailments [1]. Tempering these benefits is the realization that for a variety of reasons treatment does not always proceed as planned and too many patients are injured and killed as a result of their care [2–6]. Much of this treatment-related harm is exacerbated by emergency conditions and numerous environmental factors that set up a situation of an accident waiting to happen, and the human and financial costs of such harm are large. The extent of treatment-related harm has been famously estimated in the USA at 44,000–98,000 preventable deaths per year [2]. However, other estimates based on more recent data have put the death toll higher still, and the financial cost of such harm is in the tens of billions of dollars a year when the cost of the loss of quality of life is taken into account in cases of non-fatal injury [7, 8]. Errors and failures in the administration of drugs to patients are known to be a leading cause of treatment-related harm [2, 3, 9], and this is of particular concern during anesthesia due to the potency of the agents used, the multiple drug administrations made per anesthetic, and the large number of anesthetics provided globally [2, 3, 10]. Drug administration during anesthesia makes substantial use of intravenous injection and infusion systems, but unlike in other hospital settings, this often occurs without technological safety checks, such as electronic physician order entry systems. The number of surgical procedures being conducted around the world is also on the increase due to a larger proportion of the world's population now suffering from the diseases of an industrialized society, including ischemic heart disease, cerebrovascular disease, and cancer, thus exposing a greater number of patients to the attendant risks of treatment [10, 11]. It has recently been estimated that 234 million surgical operations are undertaken each year around the world, with Americans being disproportionately represented in this total at 50 million surgical operations a year, or an average of seven operations in each person's lifetime [1, 10]. The wider use of more sophisticated and powerful healthcare therapies also creates new and more dangerous ways in which therapies can fail when things go wrong, suggesting that safety strategies in healthcare have not kept pace with many advances in technology [1, 12]. The specialty of anesthesia has a long established reputation for being a leader in patient safety, and the introduction of new healthcare technologies presents new opportunities to extend and consolidate such safety initiatives [13, 14]. However, despite technological advances in a number of areas, many aspects of intravenous anesthesia have changed little in decades and remain unnecessarily error prone. In the following I consider the extent and nature of drug administration error during intravenous anesthesia, and a number of approaches to safety improvement that have shown evidence of efficacy, including drawing on a program of safety research pursued by our own group.

Estimating the Extent of Drug Administration Error During Anesthesia

Phenomena with a low incidence, such as those occurring at a rate of less than 1 %, pose a number of methodological problems in accurately estimating their rate. This is particularly the case when such phenomena lead only infrequently to harm, since harmful events are more likely to be reported

C.S. Webster, BSc, MSc, PhD (✉)
Centre for Medical and Health Sciences Education, University of Auckland, Private Bag 92-019, Auckland 1142, New Zealand

Department of Anaesthesiology, University of Auckland, Auckland, New Zealand
e-mail: c.webster@auckland.ac.nz

© Springer International Publishing AG 2017
A.R. Absalom, K.P. Mason (eds.), *Total Intravenous Anesthesia and Target Controlled Infusions*,
DOI 10.1007/978-3-319-47609-4_36

than non-harmful ones. Such estimations cannot be done causally, but are the important first step in safety improvement, since they allow the detection of improvements in rates over time due to a safety intervention. Clinical impressions are a poor substitute for a formal estimate of the rate of rare phenomena [15]. For example, a drug error which harms a patient will not be seen often or at all by any particular clinician. Thus a clinician who has never harmed a patient in this way may therefore suffer from optimist bias and underestimate the true rate of drug error—perhaps also believing this is because their practice is safer than average [16]. If the clinician has been unfortunate enough to have had perhaps two or three bad experiences with drug errors, they are likely to overestimate the rate of drug error. The true rate of the phenomenon will lie somewhere between these two extreme impressions, but to quantify its incidence accurately large data sets must be collected. Statistical methods exist to estimate how large a denominator, or sample size, needs to be to gain a reasonable estimate of any particular low incidence phenomenon, but even reasonable estimates often require data collection from thousands of patients, which can prohibit such studies [17, 18]. In addition, difficulties in obtaining sufficient statistical power also mean that, even when relatively large studies are undertaken, it is often difficult to determine significant differences between important subgroups of interest (see Box 36.1).

Box 36.1: Methodological Difficulties in Studying Rare, Dangerous Phenomena

Perforation of the heart or blood vessels is a dangerous, rare, but persistent complication of the use of central venous catheters (CVCs). Published estimates of the rate of perforation vary widely from 1 in 100 to 1 in 10,000 patients [19–31]. In one prospective audit of 1000 consecutive patients who received a CVC, two perforations were seen, each caused by a different kind of catheter at a different site—one of the right atrium by a triple-lumen CVC and one of the pulmonary artery by a pulmonary artery catheter (PAC) [32]. This allowed the estimation of the overall incidence of perforation at 0.2 % (95 % confidence interval [CI] 0.02–0.7 %). Owing to the relatively large sample size and prospective data collection, this estimate of the incidence of perforation is likely to be more accurate, and has a narrower confidence interval, than many previously published estimates. However, the confidence interval is still relatively wide, and even larger numbers of patients would need to be studied in order to reduce it. Assuming the point estimate of 0.2 % is correct for the rate of perforation, 10,000

Box 36.1 (continued)
patients would need to be studied to achieve a 95 % CI of 0.1–0.3 %. At our hospital, data collection alone for such a study would take many years.

Another consequence of this requirement for large numbers is that a 1000-patient study was not able to quantify the risk of perforation in different subgroups of CVCs even though evidence suggests that differences do exist. PACs are thought to perforate by mechanisms different from those of other CVCs and may carry a higher risk of perforation [33–36]. However, the rate of perforation by a PAC in this 1000-patient study (1 in 223 patients who received one, or 0.4 %, 95 % CI 0.01–2.5 %) could not be statistically distinguished from the rate of perforation by other study CVCs (1 in 1000 patients, or 0.1 %, 95 % CI 0.003–0.6 %—Fisher's exact test, $p > 0.3$) [32]. Given that rare phenomena lead to small numerators there is always a risk that no cases of the event under study will be seen, even during a relatively large study. In this case a useful rule-of-thumb to estimate the upper 95 % CI for a zero numerator is given by $3/n$, where this approximation is most accurate for total $n > 30$ [18]. For example, if no cases of vascular perforation were seen in 1000 patients, the upper 95 % confidence interval could be approximated at 3/1000 or 0.3 %.

Many of the studies of drug administration error in anesthesia have been based on surveys, interviews, or incident reporting, but which have not allowed the capture of the denominator of the number of patient cases associated with the errors identified [9, 37–45]. While these studies can be useful in identifying problem areas for immediate safety improvement, and do suggest that dose and substitution error are prominent types of drug administration error, they do not allow any estimate of the baseline rate of error. Longitudinal methods of safety improvement do require an accurate base rate and denominator. However, even when denominator data are available and large-scale studies are conducted, a number of methodological considerations are important in establishing an accurate estimate. Retrospective studies tend to underestimate the true rate of drug administration error. For example, the two large-scale *retrospective* incident monitoring studies of 113,074 and 64,285 cases of anesthesia found rates of drug administration error of 0.01 % and 0.08 % per case, respectively [46, 47]. These rates are a magnitude lower than many other, *prospective* incident monitoring studies that have estimated the rate of drug error in anesthesia at between 0.11 % and 0.16 % of cases

[48–51]. However, even these prospective rates are likely to be underestimates because they are based on incident data that were collected as part of a wider incident monitoring scheme, rather than during a study dedicated to estimating the rate of drug error in anesthesia. In 2001 our study group published an estimate of drug administration error in anesthesia based on prospective incident data, which included a denominator and was conducted solely for the purpose of studying drug administration error [52]. We called our method *facilitated incident monitoring* because we supplied incident forms in all locations where anesthesia took place in our hospital, allowing the anonymous return of a form for every anesthetic conducted, the vast majority of which indicated that no incident had occurred. Also, a dedicated staff member would follow up on anesthetic records that were filed without an accompanying incident form. These strengths address many of the previous methodological weaknesses of incident reporting [53]. In particular, anonymous reporting means that the identity of those making the reports is not legally discoverable, and further protections for reporters may be possible if the incident study is registered as a quality assurance activity [54]. Thus, in a study of 10,806 anesthetics, we estimated that a drug administration error occurred once for every 133 anesthetic cases conducted (or 0.75 %), and this estimate remains the highest of its kind in the world. The great majority of the reported errors (83 %) were made by the intravenous (IV) route—either by bolus injection (63 %) or by infusion administration (20 %)—underscoring the importance of the intravenous route in terms of its contribution to patient harm during anesthesia. Two patients received a drug by the wrong route—both given IV instead of epidurally. Incorrect dose error and substitution error (where another drug is given instead of the one intended) were the two most common types of drug administration error, making up 59 % of errors overall. However, perhaps the most concerning findings were that within substitution errors, 11 of 16 (69 %) involving an intravenous bolus and 3 of 4 (75 %) involving an infusion, occurred *between* different pharmacological classes of drug, with obvious potential for patient harm.

Consequences of Errors

No death or permanent injury to a patient was attributed to a drug error during this study. However, one patient suffered awareness. Other published estimates suggest that about 1 % of drug errors cause injury to patients [8, 55]. This is consistent with the finding that one of the 81 errors in this study caused important harm (awareness). In New Zealand, many anesthesiologists administer approximately 1000 anesthetics a year [56]. Given one drug administration error per 133 anesthetics, an individual anesthesiologist can be expected to make approximately seven drug administration errors a year. Over a 30-year career, this amounts to over 200 drug administration errors. If 1 % of these errors lead to significant injury, *every* anesthesiologist might therefore expect to injure an average of two patients in his or her career.

A series of studies have subsequently been conducted using similar facilitated incident reporting methods, and all studies of this type that I know of are shown in Table 36.1 [52, 57–60]. Some of the similarities in these studies are worth noting. Three of the five studies show a very similar rate of drug administration error (0.61–0.75 %), despite having been conducted in three different countries. Four of the five studies indicate that incorrect dose and substitution error are the two most common forms of error, and the fifth study indicates that these are among the top three most common. One study indicates that in the 29 cases where a drug administration error resulted in an unintended drug effect, 14 (48 %) of these events occurred through error in administration by infusion pump [57]. Finally the top three contributing factors associated with reported errors in all five studies also appear similar, including distraction, inattention, production pressure, and failure to check (Table 36.1). Only one study indicated inadequate knowledge as its third most common contributing factor, suggesting that drug errors do not generally occur because of a lack of training or expertise (hence "further training" for those who make such errors is unlikely to be effective in preventing them). Although the reported contributing factors in Table 36.1 could be interpreted as indicating human failures in the genesis of errors (and often in health care this is the typical interpretation), I would suggest that in fact they indicate a work environment that relies too heavily on sheer human effort to maintain appropriate levels of safety. A better designed working environment would take into account the strengths and weaknesses of human nature and better support work activities, including the maintenance of safety, such that workload and production pressure is better managed, and patient safety does not solely rely on the clinician being super human and never succumbing to distraction or inattention. For example, one study in Table 36.1 indicates that 37 % of drug administration errors were due to the misidentification of the drug ampoule [58]. Why is it that drug ampoules, among other equipment in the clinical work environment, are so poorly designed? This is a question we will return to later in the chapter. These studies reinforce the fact that despite the many technological advances of modern anesthesia, certain aspects of drug administration have changed little in decades, and that drug administration error during anesthesia remains a persistent and concerning problem.

Table 36.1 Estimates of drug administration error in anesthesia using dedicated, prospective incident reporting[a]

Year of report	Country of study	Response rate	Number of anesthetics studied	Number of drug errors reported	Error rate per anesthetic (%)	Top three error types (%)	Top three contributing factors (if reported)
2001	New Zealand [52]	72 %	10,806	81	1/133 (0.75 %)	1. Incorrect dose (32 %) 2. Substitution (27 %) 3. Omission (18 %)	1. Failure to check 2. Distraction 3. Inattention
2003	United States [57]	90 %	6709	41	1/163 (0.61 %)	1. Incorrect dose (43 %) 2. Substitution (17 %) 3. Insertion (drug not intended) (9 %)	–
2009	South Africa [58]	53 %	30,412	66	1/450 (0.22 %)	1. Substitution (60 %) 2. Incorrect dose (23 %) 3. Repetition/incorrect route (13 %)	–
2012	United States [60]	83 %	10,574	35	1/302 (0.33 %)	1. Incorrect dose (37 %) 2. Substitution (25 %) 3. Omission (19 %)	1. Distraction 2. Production pressure 3. Misread label
2013	China [59]	68 %	24,380	179	1/137 (0.73 %)	1. Omission (27 %) 2. Incorrect dose (23 %) 3. Substitution (20 %)	1. Haste 2. Inattention 3. Inadequate knowledge

[a]Some studies reported an overall rate combining errors and near-misses, however for the purpose of comparison all rates reported here have been calculated in the same way as total errors per total number of anesthetics in the study period

Lessons from Other Industries

Systematic approaches to the prevention of injury and accidents have a long history in the industrial setting. Some of the first studies of industrial accidents were conducted in the USA in the 1920s by Herbert Heinrich, who went on to become an industrial safety pioneer. In his capacity as an inspector for the Travelers Insurance Company, Heinrich studied accidents across many industries, and in 1931 published the first edition of his book entitled "Industrial Accident Prevention – A Scientific Approach," which became a landmark text in the field [61]. In this book Heinrich describes the relationship between near misses, minor accidents, and major accidents with his 300-29-1 ratio—which states that for every major injury there will be, on average, 29 minor injuries and 300 no-injury accidents or near misses. Collecting information about near misses allows problem areas to be identified and even remedied before harm occurs. By the fourth edition of his book, published in 1959, Heinrich was able to claim that "industrial accident prevention has come of age" and that "safety begins with safe tools, safe machines, safe processes and safe environment" [61]. Both early and modern work in safety and human factors suggest that a more fruitful and abundant source of evidence for understanding the potential for harm lies in the study of near misses, in addition to accidents. Although the ratio of near misses to cases of harm is likely to be different for different work environments, the collection and analysis of near misses goes a long way to solving the problem of the requirement

for very large numbers in studies considering only errors. For example, it has been estimated that incidents occur 3300 times more often in healthcare than do actual errors such as those in Table 36.1 [62].

Incident reporting is widely used in anesthesia as a safety improvement approach, and specialized web-based tools are now available for reporting incidents in various areas of practice [63, 64]. However, even taking into account the methodological pitfalls discussed above, incident reporting has its detractors—reporting rates can be low, leading to less useful or representative data, and contextual factors relevant to understanding the reported events may be lacking [65–67]. There are many ways to collect data on particular healthcare systems, each with its own advantages and disadvantages, and many inherited from other industries and disciplines—some proactive and theory driven, others reactive and using existing data sources [68–72]. The use of continuous observation to identify incidents of interest yields higher rates of events than the self-reporting of incidents, but is an expensive method of data collection that is typically not sustainable in the long term. A middle road of data collection involves clinical surveillance, which comprises the collection of data by appropriately trained staff at regular intervals from activities at key points in care delivery [73]. Clinical surveillance has the advantage of collecting data on the dual aspects of both compliance with the steps involved in delivering safe care, and in patient outcome—although issues of statistical power needed to detect improvements still apply. However, there is no single perfect measure of safety, and so a combination of measures often works best [74]. Other sources of data with which to determine safety and quality include data from electronic medical records, chart review, administrative data, and morbidity and mortality data—and I will touch of some of these later in the chapter [70].

The Double-Human Interface

Perhaps the most significant difference between the industrial setting and anesthesia lies in what might be called the double-human interface, and describes the nature of the interaction of humans and technology. The study of human factors and ergonomics typically focuses on the interface between a human operator and the technology being operated. In Fig. 36.1 this traditional human/technology interface is shown by the double-ended arrow labeled x, indicating the interaction between the anesthesiologist (A) and the technology of drug administration and monitoring. However, during an anesthetic there is importantly, another human functionally connected to the traditional human/technology system, that is the patient (y in Fig. 36.1). The patient is on the receiving end of the technology of anesthesia, forming a bio-technological system—this fact has a number of important consequences in terms of the behavior of the system and the anesthesiologist's ability to maintain the stability of the system (Fig. 36.1).

The first consequence of the nature of the bio-technological system relates to complexity. A complex system may be defined as one where the behavior of the system is difficult or impossible to predict accurately from a knowledge of the system's constituent parts [75]. A human body contains many physiological subsystems that are robustly

homeostatic under normal conditions. However, an anesthetized patient has had the control of a number of normally self-regulating subsystems suspended, altered or taken over by the technology of the anesthetic. For example, during general anesthesia, the ventilator ventilates the patient's lungs when the muscles around the lungs are paralyzed by anesthetic drugs—loss of such homeostasis creates a biological source of potentially unpredictable system behavior.[1] Furthermore, even our best machines tend to be less reliable and require greater oversight than the physiological subsystems of our bodies, thus creating a technological source of potentially unpredictable system behavior. The bio-technological system of the anesthetized patient is therefore a complex and potentially unpredictable system capable of departing from the desired path of operation and transitioning to an unanticipated state (System 2 in Fig. 36.2). In addition, the patient will typically be undergoing surgery or treatment for a pathology—both the treatment and the pathology have the potential to destabilize the patient's condition. Even the task of determining which state or step such a bio-technological system is in at any given time can be difficult. This difficulty can be seen clearly during clinical diagnosis of a patient during a crisis, when it is known only that the patient is in trouble, but when the cause of the problem remains unknown [12]. The nature and behavior of the overall system comprising the double-human interface is therefore substantially more complex and unpredictable than that typically considered in human/technology interfaces in an industrial setting [75, 76]. Despite this, health care has a relatively under-developed culture of safety compared with other safety-critical industries [77, 78].

The Culture of Denial and Effort

A large part of the difficulty in improving the safety of healthcare is due to a culture that typically places the entire burden of responsibility for patient care on the individual clinician's heroic shoulders. Traditionally efforts aimed at reducing error in medicine have tended to involve exhortation to be more careful at worst, or the creation of new safety procedures and protocols at best [79, 80]. Both these approaches to safety focus on the individual rather than the wider system or work environment in which the individual is expected to operate, and so are consistent with what has been called the person-centered approach to safety. The person-centered approach holds that all error is due to forgetfulness, inattention, poor motivation, carelessness, negligence, and recklessness [81]—paying more attention

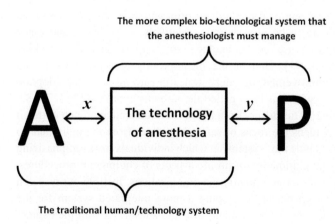

The more complex bio-technological system that the anesthesiologist must manage

The traditional human/technology system

Fig. 36.1 A conceptual diagram of the double-human interface of anesthesia, showing the more complex construct of the anesthesiologist (A) interacting with the technology of anesthesia which in turn interacts with the second human in the system, the patient (P), forming a bio-technological system. The extent of the traditional human/technology system, as typically studied by the disciplines of ergonomics and human factors, is indicated by the *lower bracket*

---

[1] Note that such alteration of self-regulating systems extends to the level of pharmacology and physiological receptors.

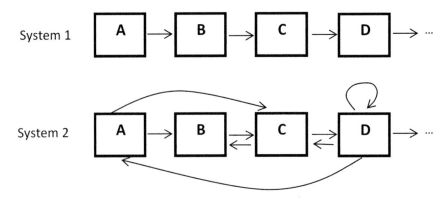

Fig. 36.2 Linear and complex systems. System 1 has linear interaction between subsystems or operational states—operation of the system moves through a set of fixed steps through to completion (a post-office-like system). System 2 has complex, non-linear causal interaction between subsystems—it is much less clear which path will be taken to achieve completion, or even how many steps will be involved or exactly how long the process might take (a system like an anesthetized patient)

or following lengthy safety protocols is therefore expected to stop error. I have called such a culture in health care the culture of denial and effort because, under such a culture, it is often denied that safety devices are needed—because the presence of the doctor is seen as the ultimate safety device—and it is presumed that appropriate levels of safety can be maintained simply through sheer effort on the part of the clinician. The culture of denial and effort is therefore the antithesis of the culture of safety in the aviation industry, has stifled the development of safety systems in health care, and persists despite the inherent complexity of health care [6, 82].

Poor Labeling

A long-standing safety concern in anesthesia involves the labeling of drug ampoules and syringes. The influence of the culture of denial and effort can be seen in this context in the view that safety will actually be improved by work environments that are deliberately made more error prone, thus forcing clinicians to be at their *most* vigilant. An early example of this view appeared in a published comment by a then editor of the journal *Anaesthesia* in 1981, and stated, "there are very sound arguments for recommending that all ampoules should be identical in appearance... Such a practice would compel users to read the inscription" [83]. The source of such "sound arguments" is not mentioned, but it could certainly not have been the evidence available in the fields of psychology, industrial accident prevention or human factors, which, even in 1981, directly contradicted such an idea [2, 3, 84–86]. In a 1996 editorial in *Anaesthesia*, we see another example of this safety counter-culture: "if we are giving an injection we must continually retrain ourselves to read the words. We should ensure that we do not read what we expect, but inspect what we read" [87]. More recently, in the *British Medical Journal* in 2002, we are informed that

"Doctors must read drug labels, not whinge about them" [88]. The message underlying these examples is that doctors are a special breed, able to overcome normal human fallibility by sheer effort alone. However, despite the decades long promulgation of this view, drug administration errors continue unabated [6, 89, 90]. Without question, the vast majority of doctors are conscientious professionals doing their absolute best. However, an insistence on being the only backstop for patient safety, in combination with the reality that human error is statistically inevitable, actually guarantees that iatrogenic harm will continue—hence, sheer effort is not enough.

Systematic Approaches to Improve Patient Safety During Anesthesia

Conventional methods of drug administration in anesthesia tend to be idiosyncratic, relatively error prone, and make little use of technology to support manual checking [75, 91]. One of the most promising approaches to the improvement of safety in health care involves the adoption of what has been called the systems approach [2, 3, 76, 82, 92]. This differs from the person-centered approach in that it widens the focus of safety initiatives from the individual to include the "system" in which individuals work, emphasizing the elimination of unsafe aspects of equipment, procedures, work environments, and organizations. In 1996 our research group began developing a more integrated system for the delivery of intravenous drugs in anesthesia with the express aim of reducing error and facilitating safe practice [93]. The new system's design is based on lessons from empirical incident reporting [52], the psychological mechanisms underlying human error [84] and the principles of safe-system design developed in other safety-critical industries such as nuclear power generation and aviation [85, 94–97].

Design Principles

The specific features of the new system are summarized in Table 36.2, these comprise physical components and operational rules [91]. The new system was designed to be modular, in the sense that any module can be used in isolation or in combination with others, many at little or no cost, without leaving the anesthesiologist worse off than when using conventional methods alone. Physical aspects of the new system include customized drug trays designed to encourage a better organized workspace and the maintenance of aseptic technique. These trays allow a zone for the storage of drugs that are intended to be given later in the case (a prompt zone), a zone for syringes currently in use, and a zone for ampoules of drug that have already been given—thus creating a tray that acts as a physical record of the anesthetic at-a-glance as it progresses. The tray's "in use" area is raised, hence allowing storage of syringes while avoiding contact of their tips with contaminated surfaces. The new system also includes pre-filled syringes for the most commonly used drugs, thus saving time and removing substantial opportunity for error during their preparation. All drug labels incorporate color-coding by pharmacological class of drug, consistent with the international and Joint Commission color code standards for anesthetic labels—and identical color-coding is used on computer screen displays and drug trolley compartments [91, 98, 99]. A special label for the administration of drugs by infusion pump was developed which represents weight and dose as a nomogram, thereby removing the need for the completion of error prone dose calculations [100]. A barcode reader allows an auditory cross-check of each drug prior to its administration, by playing a voice recording of the drug name upon scanning of the barcode on the syringe label. We chose such a voice cue in order that it would stand out against other common tone alarms in the operating room, and because an anesthesiologist could listen to the voice announcement in order to complete the drug identity cross-check while engaged in other tasks, without the need to glance at a computer screen [91, 101]. Completing the cross-check also adds the drug administration event to an automated computerized anesthetic record. The software of the new system also generates a visual and auditory warning within 15 min of the beginning of the anesthetic if an antibiotic has not been administered.

Evidence of Safety Gains

The new system was assessed for suitability for use in the clinical setting by having anesthesiologists use it in a high-fidelity human-patient simulator [103]. We then continued collecting facilitated incident reports at two hospitals during which time we introduced the new system at one. In 74,478 anesthetics we found a significant overall reduction in drug administration errors with the new system compared with conventional methods—specifically, 58 errors in an estimated 183,852 drug administrations (or 0.032 %) with the new system versus 268 errors in 550,105 drug administrations with conventional methods (or 0.049 %)—a relative reduction in drug error of 35 % ($p = 0.002$) [104]. Omission errors and dose errors were significantly reduced with the use of the new system. We also found evidence in our results for the value of drug class-specific color-coding. There were five substitution errors between differently colored drug classes with the new system versus 47 with conventional methods (with the same denominators as above, $p = 0.01$). No major adverse outcomes from these errors were reported with the new system while 11 were

Table 36.2 Features of a new multimodal system designed to improve safety during anesthesia[a]

Physical aspects
1. Customized drug trays designed to promote a well-organized anesthetic workspace and aseptic technique
2. Pre-filled syringes for the most commonly used anesthetic drugs
3. Large legible drug labels, color-coded according to the international color standard for anesthetic labels
4. A barcode reader linked to a computer to provide automatic auditory and visual verification of the selected drug immediately before each administration and to record its administration
5. An on-screen visual and auditory warning if an antibiotic has not been administered within 15 min of the start of anesthesia
6. Purpose designed drug trolley drawers including color-coding consistent with the international standard for anesthetic drug labels
7. Drug infusion labels which represent weight and dose as a nomogram obviating the need for dose calculations
8. Automatic compilation of an anesthetic record, on screen in real time and available as a paper print-out
Operational rules
1. Ampoules appropriately laid out at the start of the case
2. All empty ampoules and syringes retained for reconciliation
3. All syringes should be labeled
4. Computerized voice cross-check audible throughout each anesthetic
5. Drug label scanned before each drug administration

[a]Adapted from Merry et al. [102]

reported with conventional methods ($p = 0.055$). These 11 adverse outcomes included two cases of awareness (one when a neuromuscular blocking drug was given before induction, and one when the propofol infusion was inadvertently switched off), four cases of prolonged patient stay in the post-anesthetic care unit (three due to an overdose of neuromuscular blocking drug, and one due to a substitution error with neostigmine), and one case of anaphylactoid reaction when the patient was given an antibiotic for which they had a known allergy.

A further observational study conducted in 1075 cases confirmed lower rates of error with the use of the new system, but also found evidence of the value of the auditory cross-check [102]. Rates of errors in drug administration and recording were lower when anesthesiologists consistently scanned the drug barcode before administering each drug and kept the voice prompt active, than when they did not—a mean of 6 errors per 100 drug administrations versus 9.7, respectively ($p = 0.004$). These results provide substantial evidence for the effectiveness of a systematic approach to the reduction of drug administration error in anesthesia by supporting the actions of anesthesiologists through appropriate automation, better prompts and checking, than is possible with manual methods alone.

Consistent Color-Coding

To my knowledge, the above result showing fewer interclass drug substitution errors with the use of drug class-specific color-coding represents the first evidence of the safety benefits of the international and Joint Commission color code standard for anesthetic drugs [98, 99, 104]. This is particularly pleasing given the potentially dangerous consequences of some of the interclass substitution errors that have appeared in incident reports—e.g., giving neostigmine instead of rocuronium, nitroglycerine instead of ephedrine, and suxamethonium instead of fentanyl. Although color coding to reduce errors in health care has been in use for a number of decades, for example in blood bank services [105], there has been considerable debate up until quite recently about its appropriateness and how it should be implemented in anesthesia [106–108]. Some commentators were concerned that color coding would distract from the important task of reading the label, while others were concerned that there were simply not enough different colors or combinations of color to meaningfully differentiate all drugs used in anesthesia [109]. Although the international color code standard has now been adopted in most Western countries for *user-applied labels* in anesthesia, drug manufacturers continue to make little use of color code standards in their design of drug ampoule labels and packing [106, 108]. Labels for drug containers are typically designed to promote brand names and product lines, often with the information critical to the clinician in the smallest print on the label [110, 111].

Over 10 years ago I pointed out that ampoule labeling standards are such that the labels on ampoules themselves could carry color-coding consistent with the international user-applied labeling standard [108]. This would have significant ergonomic benefits for anyone drawing up a drug from a color-coded ampoule into a syringe with an identically color-coded label, and there is no reason why such consistency of color-coding cannot exist. Recommendations have emerged in recent years that all drug administration lines should also be labeled and color-coded, and standards have been developed for this [112]. More robust barriers than color-coding are also available to prevent the administration of drugs by the wrong route. For example, different connectors for intrathecal drug administration lines have been proposed which physically prevent cross connection with intravenous connectors, thus avoiding the devastating drug error of the injection of the chemotherapeutic drug vincristine into the spine—an error, which until recently has occurred approximately once a year in Britain alone [82, 113]. The value of physically different connectors is not restricted to the administration of chemotherapeutic agents, but could also prevent the administration of drugs by cross connected intravenous and epidural lines, something we know happens more often in the operating room than errors involving intrathecal administration [52].

The Codonics Label System

Recently a number of reports have appeared on another labeling system for anesthesia that uses labels containing barcodes and drug class-specific color-coding consistent with the international and Joint Commission color standards [99, 114, 115]. This system prints each syringe label when an ampoule of drug is scanned and drawn up. The labeled syringe can then be scanned when it is administered and the system provides an auditory cross-check by playing a voice recording of the drug name. Two of these reports offer evaluative data concerned primarily with compliance with the operating principles of the label system. The third is an observation study of 277 procedures that allows an estimation of the rate of adverse drug events and potential for patient harm, but without reporting evidence of the effectiveness of the new label system in preventing such events [115]. The paper concludes that future work should address the root causes of error in order to reduce the incidence of adverse events. Although these reports do not offer data on the ability of the Codonics label system to reduce drug administration error, given the use of drug class-specific color-coded labels and an auditory cross-check of drug identity, this system could be expected to show similar safety benefits as reported above for these specific aspects.

The Triumph of Software

The more software a device contains, the more complex the functions it is capable of performing, but also the more likely it is that the user will find it difficult to operate. This is the primary reason why it is more difficult to use a personal computer than a microwave oven—the former contains much more software than the latter. Some commentators have suggested that a solution to the problem of overly complex software is to have a specialized computer, or the so-called information appliance, for each task or application, with a simple and intuitive interface, rather than using a single general-purpose computer to run many different kinds of software (the current personal-computer approach) [116, 117]. Computers are now inexpensive enough that information appliances are viable, and perhaps the first commercial examples of information appliances were early mobile phones. However, as the functionality of mobile phones rapidly increased to include many "smart" features such as e-mail access, apps, games, pictures and video, they quickly became more like general-purpose computers rather than information appliances. "Up-grading" to software with more features is so ingrained in our sense of staying up to date and so integral to the commercial viability of so many high technology industries that it would seem Luddite to many even to question the need to do so. However, many common software applications are now so bloated with features that they run slower than previous versions even on the fastest available computer processors [118]. This is despite the fact that most users make use of only a small fraction of the features of most software products.

In the electronics industry a rule of thumb known as Moore's Law states that the number of transistors on a new computer chip will double every 18–24 months, and this exponential regularity is now used as a benchmark with which manufacturers judge their own competitiveness in the market [119]. A number of high technology manufacturers also use an analogue of Moore's Law to describe the increasing number of lines of software code in their goods. For commercial aircraft manufacturers to remain competitive, for example, new aircraft should be lighter, have more features and be more expensive than previous models. To achieve this there is no better-suited addition to the design of a new aircraft than software—which weighs nothing, but adds perceived value because of the new features it brings and the fact that software is an expensive commodity to produce [120, 121].

Software code generally costs between $25 and $100 per line. However, with safety critical systems, such as aircraft, nuclear power plants and weapons systems, the price per line can be many times higher because of the exhaustive, formal validation processes intended to rid the software of errors or "bugs" [122]. Formal validation is a combinatorial problem—the effort and expense required increases very rapidly with the increasing number of lines of software code [123]. The software for NASA's space shuttle flight control system cost approximately $1000 per line because of formal validation, and is some of the safest software in existence. Yet, it is estimated that even this software contains about 50 bugs [120]. By comparison, most commercial software is not considered to be safety-critical and contains millions of lines of code—a number that is impossible to formally validate (at least with current methods). For example, Microsoft Office 2013 contains 45 million lines of code [124]. Even if it were possible to formally validate this amount of software it would still contain in the order of 20,000 bugs at the end of the process. In reality, it is certain that Microsoft Office 2013 contains many times this number of bugs because of the inability to formally validate a program of this size.

The versatility of software is its greatest advantage—software systems tend to have more features, are more easily re-configured and upgraded, and are cheaper and faster to produce than mechanical systems. However, it is also the inherent lack of physical constraints on the ways in which software can go wrong that make it so difficult to generate completely safe and error-free software. This complexity of software makes any system that contains it more functionally opaque—that is, users and experts alike have difficulty in understanding what is going on inside the system if it begins to perform in an unexpected way. Even software experts will often simply reboot or re-install software when the system begins to behave inexplicably, because no one fully understands what has actually gone wrong or how to fix it. A single error in software code can be enough to cause a catastrophic software failure or a "crash," and so software can be the unavoidable weakest link that brings down an entire system [120, 125]. For example, it was recently discovered that the software for Boeing's new $200 million Dreamliner passenger aircraft contains a software bug which could cause all onboard power generators to go into fail-safe mode after 248 days of continual operation—potentially leading to catastrophic loss of control of the aircraft if such an event took place during flight [126, 127]. The solution proposed by Boeing is to reboot the aircraft every 3 months.

Software in Hospitals

The promise of software makes its introduction into hospitals and health care inevitable, but given the known risks and difficulties such introduction needs to proceed with caution. The problems of software in health care are often compounded by the fact that computerized solutions are typically produced by committees of technology experts with inadequate consultation with the intended users. This approach may work if the product is completely new and so doesn't conflict with the way users already do things, or if users are relatively unskilled and so can be trained on how to use the new software. However, in the case of the introduction of software systems into hospitals, neither of these points is true: the intended users are highly skilled clinicians who have established and very specific ways of doing things, usually for very good reason. Health care is a highly complex work environment, both in terms of the skill levels of practitioners and in the greatly varying needs of patients [75]. Patients are not car bodies and clinicians are not assembly line workers—yet it is from such an industrial model that much of the technological skill that creates many software systems typically comes. It is also an industrial model that is often attractive to hospital management who usually introduce computerized systems specifically with the intention of increasing efficiency and decreasing costs. However, computerized systems in health care often fail because they are not able to accommodate the complexities inherent in health care [128]. Issues of the controllability and reliability of software in health care are certain to become more important in the near future, not only with the introduction of hospital-wide patient information systems and electronic health records, but with an increase in the number of software-controlled medical devices, including high technology applications such as clinical diagnoses by artificial neural networks and the use of virtual reality and robotics in surgery [129–132].

Software in Anesthesia

The operating room is one of the most high technology work environments in any hospital and so the encroachment of software into anesthesia can only be expected to increase. Recently, fully computerized, "state of the art" anesthetic machines have been introduced into some hospitals. These machines have had much of the mechanical control layer replaced by sophisticated software, including electronically represented rotameters. In some hospitals, after a number of power cuts and "software malfunctions" with these new computerized anesthetic machines, it has become common practice to insure that there is an Ambubag or similar manual ventilation equipment within easy reach on the back of the machine [133]. Unreliable software can significantly increase the unpredictability of the bio-technological system under the anesthesiologist's control (Fig. 36.1).

Syringe pumps and Target Controlled Infusion (TCI) systems in anesthesia are another essential piece of anesthetic technology that contains a substantial amount of software. Modern infusion pumps contain around 100,000 lines of computer code, and this is likely to increase with the introduction of more sophisticated closed-loop drug infusion systems [134, 135]. While the dosing algorithms, which these computerized pumps contain, deliver safe anesthesia in a vast number of operating rooms every day throughout the world, the use of such pumps is not without adverse event [136–138]. Approximately 11,000 adverse event reports are made to the United States Food and Drug Administration (FDA) every year concerning infusion pumps, including events that result in patient injury and death (Table 36.3 contains a summary of reported problem events) [139]. It is worth noting that relatively few reported problems in Table 36.3 are related to physical or software failure of the pump—that is, the pump was behaving as it was designed to do. But rather the great majority of reported problems are concerned with user confusion over some aspect of the complexity of the device—e.g., "nuisance" or unintelligible alarms, confusing screen displays and programming options, or incomplete understanding of the pump's default settings. Like with other forms of drug administration error in anesthesia, trying harder is unlikely to eliminate these problems. The events in Table 36.3 suggest that modern pump interfaces are just too complex and that substantially more effort needs to go into designing displays and programming sequences that are more intuitive. This should involve some standardization of screen displays and drug libraries across brands and models [128, 140]. A further difficulty with infusion pumps was identified in a systematic review of the user-interfaces of these devices—a problem the authors called the "virtuality" of the systems [139]. This is related to a general property of software in that there are few constraints on the ways that software can fail—many impossible or meaningless modes can be entered into without the system preventing such an occurrence. This is unlike a physical system that prevents a great number of meaningless and dangerous states simply because the system's components can be arranged in only a finite number of configurations (Fig. 36.3). For example, confusion over the units of grams versus milligrams when programming infusion pumps has resulted in 1000× overdose being delivered [141]. The solution to this problem lies in appropriately designed forcing functions that simplify and constrain sequences of user interaction to avoid meaningless or dangerous configurations. This requires the designers of the pumps to have a deeper understanding of the way the pumps are in fact used, so that such forcing functions are helpful and not a hindrance. Drug infusion pumps are ideally suited to being information appliances.

Table 36.3 Examples of problems with various types of infusion pump as reported to the FDA[a]

Software problems

- An error message states that the pump is inoperable in the absence of any identifiable problem
- The infusion pump interprets a single keystroke as multiple keystrokes (a problem called "key bounce") leading to errors such as the administration of 100 mL/h instead of 10 mL/h

Alarm errors

- The infusion pump fails to generate an audible alarm for a critical problem (e.g., clamped or occluded tubing, or air bubbles in line)
- The infusion pump generates an occlusion alarm in the absence of an occlusion

Inadequate user interface design

- The design of the screen display confuses the user, or the pump does not respond as it should (i.e., with a warning) when inappropriate data is entered
- The screen display doesn't clearly indicate which units of measurement are expected (e.g., lbs or kg)
- Pump labels or components become damaged under routine use or during "normal" cleaning making user labeling unreadable
- User instructions or cues for mechanical setup are not clear enough—for example, resulting in clamped tubing
- Inadequately designed alarm functions and settings causing users to miss problems or respond too late—for example, an alarm indicating a low battery may not display in time for the user to prevent pump shut-off of a critical infusion during patient transport
- The infusion display and buttons are poorly positioned leading to user errors and delays in therapy—for example, the "start button" may be located next to the "power" key, resulting in the user turning the pump off instead of starting the infusion, leading to all settings being lost, and requiring programming to start again
- Warnings or "nuisance alarms" occur so often, or are sufficiently unintelligible that users ignore them
- Warning messages are ambiguous, or have double meanings, such that it is unclear what pressing "confirm" will actually initiate
- User manuals are confusing, inadequate, outdated, or unavailable
- Aspects of the pump's default settings are not adequately communicated to the user

Broken components

- The infusion pump may have been dropped or damaged during use, resulting in over- or under-infusion being delivered when the pump continues to be used without being repaired
- Water enters the plastic case of the infusion pump and cause malfunction
- Improperly aligned tubing causes stress on the pump case when closed, leading to cracks

Electrical faults

- A design fault causes batteries to overheat and fail prematurely
- The battery is not replaced during the recommended lifetime leading to failure
- The user receives an electrical shock when plugging or unplugging the pump from the power outlet
- Sparks, burning smell or flames are noticed during pump operation

[a]Summarized from incident reports on the website of the US Food and Drug Administration—http://www.fda.gov

The Alarm Problem

Although much is often made of attempts to adopt the aviation safety culture in health care, the "cockpit" of anesthesia is very different to the cockpit of an aircraft. The most striking difference is in the lack of integration of the technologies and devices used in the operating room. Typically medical devices are made by various different manufacturers and few integrate or co-ordinate with each other in any kind of meaningful way. One of the most obvious failures of integration can be seen in the alarm problem [128, 142]. Anesthetic machines, drug infusion pumps, and other devices in the operating room deliver tone alarms for any deviation from the pre-programmed operating parameters, including many problems which are apparently absent, unknown, or unimportant to the anesthesiologist (Table 36.3). In his book *The Digital Doctor*, Dr Robert Wachter discusses the design of alarms in modern aircraft cockpits with Captain Chesley "Sully" Sullenberger,

famed pilot of the "Miracle on the Hudson" airline ditching in 2009 [128]. Sully explains "false positives are one of the worst things you can do to any warning system"—carefully avoiding them is the only way to avoid alarm fatigue when operators quickly begin ignoring alarms or switching them off [143]. Avoiding false positives in aviation is achieved by agreement between engineers and pilots about exactly what needs to be alerted to the pilot from all aircraft systems and what does not. In modern aircraft, agreed alarms are then integrated into a strict hierarchy, with many being reported only as "cautions" or "advisories" which appear in color-coded text on a screen and without any auditory alert—these are not time-critical events and can be dealt with when the pilot is free to do so. The system then provides a checklist on the screen for each event advising the pilot of standard or preferred options for resolving the problem. Only conditions posing a threat to the flight path reach the top alarm level—for example, an impending stall leads to red lights, a red text message, a voice warning, and the shaking of the steering

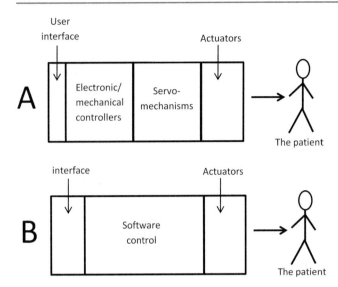

Fig. 36.3 Schematic representation of mechanical control (**A**) versus software control (**B**) in a healthcare device (e.g., an anesthetic machine or drug infusion pump). Software subsumes all calculation and control functions, removing the need for many electronic and mechanical parts, while simultaneously offering more complex functions and programming options accessed through nested menus in the user interface (hence in (**B**) software replaces many electronic and mechanical parts shown in (**A**) and a more extensive user interface is indicated). Disadvantages of software control stem from the greater complexity of such devices, including greater propensity for user confusion, and a larger number of ways in which such devices can fail (see text)

column—doing nothing in this condition would lead to the aircraft falling out of the sky. Even an event as apparently serious as an engine failure in a multi-engine aircraft will not result in a top level alarm, but only a caution, due to the fact that this does not require immediate pilot intervention [128]. By contrast in the anesthetic "cockpit," the lack of integration of alarms means that alarms on multiple individual devices trigger without any prioritization, filtering or co-ordination—often resulting in a cacophony of beeps and tones, where trivial alarms can drown out important ones because they all look and sound similar.

Environments That Audit Themselves

Many devices in modern operating rooms, including infusion pumps, continuously collect information on the way they are used, and this information can already be built into a picture of clinical activities [128, 141, 144]. New approaches have been suggested to extend and supplement this automated data collection by placing Radiofrequency Identification (RFID) sensors and transmitters in various locations around the operating room in order to track the movements and activities of staff [145]. RFID sensors can also be attached to the patient, and in combination with

wirelessly networked devices could lead to what has been called a pervasive computing system or "network of things" in the operating room—essentially a high technology environment capable of continually monitoring and auditing itself (Fig. 36.4) [146, 147]. There is no shortage of possible uses for such self-audit data. For example, if such a pervasive computing system was able to connect and regulate all devices in the operating room, it could impose a hierarchical control over alerts and alarms, in order to rationalize and prioritize them in a similar way to an aircraft cockpit, thus solving the current alarm problem. Real time analysis of the data flowing from the network of devices in combination with historical datasets could better identify subtle, and sometimes not-so-subtle, signs of patient risk and these could be prioritized and fed to a display in the anesthesiologist's work area (with or without an auditory alert). For example, a 10× overdose of a drug running on an infusion pump could be spotted by such a system if it were capable of reading the dose being delivered and also knew the patient's weight or other physiological parameters. Similar intelligent processing of patient information is also envisaged by Wachter in other hospital areas such as the hospital ward [128].

New Risks and Dangers

We must be cautious, however, in trying to solve technological problems with yet more technology. This is not to say that the increase in technology in health care should stop—this seems both undesirable and impossible [148]. What we need is more good technology and not more bad—and technology that takes into account the complexities of the double-human interface, and the subtle and variable needs of patients. We must also carefully anticipate new risks and dangers, and appreciate that almost all technology can be a double-edged sword. For example, RFID technology is potentially very useful in the operating room and other hospital locations, but existing RFID tags can cause radiofrequency interference capable of "crashing" existing drug infusion pumps—and perhaps what is of more concern is that switching the pump off and on again may not clear the problem [149, 150]. There is also evidence that use of RFID technology can cause clinically significant interference in the operation of implantable pacemakers [151]. Wireless connectivity for infusion pumps is considered an essential safety feature by some commentators because it allows the software in the pumps to be automatically updated in real time by the manufacturer through the hospital's WiFi network [141]. However, this feature may also place certain WiFi enabled pumps at risk of computer hacker attacks, where it may be possible to remotely send instructions to the pump to administer a lethal dose of a drug to the patient [152].

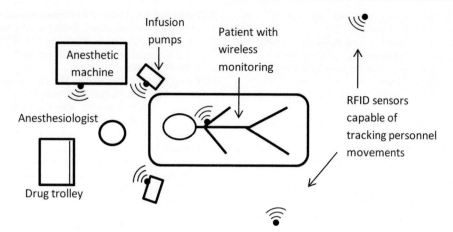

Fig. 36.4 A bird's eye view of an example of an operating room capable of auditing itself. Radiofrequency identification (RFID) devices used for patient monitoring and placed in strategic locations around the room could supplement devices with wireless network capability, such as infusion pumps and anesthetic monitors, to form a network of things. Such a network could have access to patient data and would be capable of monitoring personnel movements, recording operating room usage patterns, and identifying potentially dangerous anomalies such as an infusion pump delivering a dose of drug outside the expected range for a particular patient's weight. If such a network were also capable of coordinating devices, it could manage alerts and alarms in a way similar to the cockpit of an aircraft, thereby avoiding alarm fatigue (see text)

Conclusion

The specialty of anesthesia has a long established and well-earned reputation for being a leader in patient safety. Yet despite recent technological advances, many aspects of intravenous anesthesia have changed little in decades and remain unnecessarily error prone. The complexity of modern anesthesia is such that the traditional person-centered approach to safety is inadequate, and more sophisticated approaches to safety need to be adopted more widely. The application of human factors principles to the delivery of anesthesia has demonstrated evidence of safety gains in reduced rates of drug administration error through better workspace organization, cueing, checking, and color-coding. However, better integration of technology in the operating room could bring substantial additional safety benefits, and this appears to be an area where further lessons from the aviation industry can be applied—for example, in the management of patient alarms. Humans and machines have very different capacities. Machines are good at doing monotonous tasks such as making records, tracking events, and checking information. Humans are bad at the monotonous, but good at planning and dealing with the unpredictable. A safer way to achieve a division of the task of delivering an anesthetic between the anesthesiologist and theater systems should consider the capacities of each and divide the task accordingly. Anesthesiologists should not be expected to behave like machines or like super humans, and the design of the technology of anesthesia should take this into account and better support anesthesiologists in their work.

Acknowledgements CSW was involved in the development and assessment of the anesthesia safety system mentioned in references [91, 102, 104] in this chapter and owns a small number of shares in the company which now offers it commercially. Work for this chapter was completed without funding.

References

1. Gawande A. The Checklist Manifesto – how to get things right. New York: Metropolitan Books; 2009.
2. Institute of Medicine. To err is human – building a safer health system. Washington: National Academy Press; 2000.
3. Department of Health. An organisation with a memory – report of an expert group on learning from adverse events in the NHS. London: Stationery Office; 2000.
4. Bates DW. Frequency, consequences and prevention of adverse drug events. J Qual Clin Pract. 1999;19:13–7.
5. Merry AF, McCall Smith A. Errors, medicine and the law. Cambridge: Cambridge University Press; 2001.
6. Webster CS. The iatrogenic-harm cost equation and new technology. Anaesthesia. 2005;60:843–6.
7. Andel C, Davidow SL, Hollander M, Moreno DA. The economics of health care quality and medical errors. J Health Care Finance. 2012;39:39–50.
8. James JT. A new, evidence-based estimate of patient harms associated with hospital care. J Patient Saf. 2013;9:122–8.
9. Wheeler SJ, Wheeler DW. Medication errors in anaesthesia and critical care. Anaesthesia. 2005;60:257–73.
10. Weiser TG, Regenbogen SE, Thompson KD, Haynes AB, Lipsitz SR, Berry WR, et al. An estimation of the global volume of surgery: a modelling strategy based on available data. Lancet. 2008;372:139–44.
11. Gawande AA, Thomas EJ, Zinner MJ, Brennan TA. The incidence and nature of surgical adverse events in Colorado and Utah in 1992. Surgery. 1999;126:66–75.
12. Webster CS. The nuclear power industry as an alternative analogy for safety in anaesthesia and a novel approach for the conceptualisation of safety goals. Anaesthesia. 2005;60:1115–22.

13. Bagshaw RJ. Systems theory and the anaesthetist. Acta Anaesthesiol Scand. 1980;24:379–92.

14. Cooper JB, Gaba D. No myth – anesthesia is a model for addressing patient safety. Anesthesiology. 2002;97:1335–7.

15. Altman DG, Bland JM. Absence of evidence is not evidence of absence. Br Med J. 1995;311:485.

16. Webster CS, Grieve DJ. Attitudes to error and patient safety. Prometheus. 2005;23:253–63.

17. Bach LA, Sharpe K. Sample size for clinical and biological research. Aust N Z J Med. 1989;19:64–8.

18. Hanley JA, Lippmann-Hand A. If nothing goes wrong is everything all right? Interpreting zero numerators. JAMA. 1983;249:1743–5.

19. Rutherford JS, Merry AF, Occleshaw CJ. Depth of central venous catheterization: an audit of practice in a cardiac surgical unit. Anaesth Intensive Care. 1994;22:267–71.

20. Sitzmann JV. The technique of managing central venous lines. J Crit Illness. 1986;1:50–5.

21. Pellegrini RV, Marcelli G, Di Marco RF, Bekoe S, Grant K, Marrangoni AG. Swan-Ganz catheter induced pulmonary hemorrhage. J Cardiovasc Surg (Torino). 1987;28:646–9.

22. Karnauchow PN. Cardiac tamponade from central venous catheterization. Can Med Assoc J. 1986;135:1145–7.

23. Ellis LM, Vogel SB, Copeland EM. Central venous catheter vascular erosions – diagnosis and clinical course. Ann Surg. 1989;209:475–8.

24. Merry AF, Webster CS, Van Cotthem IC, Holland RL, Beca JS, Middleton NG. A prospective randomized clinical assessment of a new pigtail central venous catheter in comparison with standard alternatives. Anaesth Intensive Care. 1999;27:639–45.

25. Mukau L, Talamini MA, Sitzmann JV. Risk factors for central venous catheter-related vascular erosions. J Parenter Enteral Nutr. 1991;15:513–6.

26. Fraser RS. Catheter-induced pulmonary artery perforation: pathologic and pathogenic features. Hum Pathol. 1987;18:1246–51.

27. Shah KB, Rao TLK, Laughlin S, El-Etr AA. A review of pulmonary artery catheterization in 6,245 patients. Anesthesiology. 1984;61:271–5.

28. Sirivella S, Gielchinsky I, Parsonnet V. Management of catheter-induced pulmonary artery perforation: a rare complication in cardiovascular operations. Ann Thorac Surg. 2001;72:2056–9.

29. Sekkal S, Cornu E, Christidès C, Laskar M, Serhal C, Ghossein Y, et al. Swan-Ganz catheter induced pulmonary artery perforation during cardiac surgery concerning two cases. J Cardiovasc Surg. 1996;37:313–7.

30. Choh JH, Khazei AH, Ihm HJ, Thatcher WC, Batty PR. Catheter induced pulmonary arterial perforation during open heart surgery. J Cardiovasc Surg. 1994;35:61–4.

31. Malbezin S, Gauss T, Smith I, Bruneau B, Mangalsuren N, Diallo T, et al. A review of 5434 percutaneous pediatric central venous catheters inserted by anesthesiologists. Paediatr Anaesth. 2013;23:974–9.

32. Webster CS, Merry AF, Emmens DJ, Van Cotthem IC, Holland RL, Middleton NG. A prospective clinical audit of central venous catheter use and complications in 1000 consecutive patients. Anaesth Intensive Care. 2003;31:80–6.

33. Cohen JA, Blackshear RH, Gravenstein N, Woeste J. Increased pulmonary artery perforating potential of pulmonary artery catheters during hypothermia. J Cardiothorac Vasc Anesth. 1991;5:234–6.

34. Chernow B. Pulmonary artery flotation catheters: a statement by the American college of chest physicians and the American Thoracic Society [editorial]. Chest. 1997;111:261–2.

35. Barash PG, Nardi D, Hammond G, Walker-Smith G, Capuano D, Laks H, et al. Catheter-induced pulmonary artery perforation: mechanisms, management, and modifications. J Thorac Cardiovasc Surg. 1981;82:5–12.

36. Polderman KH, Girbes ARJ. Central venous catheter use – part 1: mechanical complications. Intensive Care Med. 2002;28:1–17.

37. Cooper JB, Newbower RS, Long CD, McPeek B. Preventable anesthesia mishaps – a study of human factors. Anesthesiology. 1978;49:399–406.

38. Utting JE, Gray TC, Shelley FC. Human misadventure in anaesthesia. Can Anaesth Soc J. 1979;26:472–8.

39. Cooper JB, Newbower RS, Kitz RJ. An analysis of major errors and equipment failures in anesthesia management – considerations for prevention and detection. Anesthesiology. 1984;60:34–42.

40. Chopra V, Bovill JG, Spierdijk J, Koornneef F. Reported significant observations during anaesthesia – a prospective analysis over an 18-month period. Br J Anaesth. 1992;68:13–7.

41. Currie M, Mackay P, Morgan C, Runciman WB, Russell WJ, Sellen A, et al. The "wrong drug" problem in anaesthesia – an analysis of 2000 incident reports. Anaesth Intensive Care. 1993;21:596–601.

42. Short TG, O'Regan A, Jayasuriya JP, Rowbottom M, Buckley TA, Oh TE. Improvements in anaesthetic care resulting from a critical incident reporting programme. Anaesthesia. 1996;51:615–21.

43. Sinclair M, Simmons S, Cyna A. Incidents in obstetric anaesthesia and analgesia – an analysis of 5000 AIMS reports. Anaesth Intensive Care. 1999;27:275–81.

44. Orser BA, Chen RJB, Yee DA. Medication errors in anesthetic practice: a survey of 687 practitioners. Can J Anaesth. 2001;48:139–46.

45. Abeysekera A, Bergman IJ, Kluger MT, Short TG. Drug error in anaesthetic practice – a review of 896 reports from the Australian Incident Monitoring Study database. Anaesthesia. 2005;60:220–7.

46. Sakaguchi Y, Tokuda K, Yamaguchi K, Irita K. Incidence of anesthesia-related medication errors over a 15-year period in a university hospital. Fukuoka Igaku Zasshi. 2008;99:58–66.

47. Chopra V, Bovill JG, Spierdijk J. Accidents, near accidents and complications during anaesthesia. Anaesthesia. 1990;45:3–6.

48. Craig J, Wilson ME. A survey of anaesthetic misadventures. Anaesthesia. 1981;36:933–6.

49. Kumar V, Barcellos WA, Mehta MP, Carter JG. An analysis of critical incidents in a teaching department for quality assurance – a survey of mishaps during anaesthesia. Anaesthesia. 1988;43:879–83.

50. Short TG, O'Regan A, Lew J, Oh TE. Critical incident reporting in an anaesthetic department quality assurance programme. Anaesthesia. 1993;48:3–7.

51. Fasting S, Gisvold SE. Adverse drug errors in anesthesia, and the impact of coloured syringe labels. Can J Anesth. 2000;47:1060–7.

52. Webster CS, Merry AF, Larsson L, McGrath KA, Weller J. The frequency and nature of drug administration error during anaesthesia. Anaesth Intensive Care. 2001;29:494–500.

53. Morag I, Gopher D, Spillinger A, Auerbach-Shpak Y, Laufer N, Lavy Y, et al. Human factors-focused reporting system for improving care quality and safety in hospital wards. Hum Factors. 2012;54:195–213.

54. Runciman B, Merry A, McCall Smith A. Improving patients' safety by gathering information – anonymous reporting has an important role. Br Med J. 2001;323:298.

55. Bates DW. Medication errors – how common are they and what can be done to prevent them. Drug Saf. 1996;15:303–10.

56. Merry AF, Peck DJ. Anaesthetists, errors in drug administration and the law. N Z Med J. 1995;108:185–7.

57. Bowdle A, Kruger C, Grieve R, Emmens D, Merry A. Anesthesia drug administration error in a university hospital. Anesthesiology. 2003;99:A1358.

58. Llewellyn RL, Gordon PC, Wheatcroft D, Lines D, Reed A, Butt AD, et al. Drug administration error – a prospective survey from

three South African teaching hospitals. Anaesth Intensive Care. 2009;37:93–8.

59. Zhang Y, Dong YJ, Webster CS, Ding XD, Liu XY, Chen WM, et al. The frequency and nature of drug administration error during anaesthesia in a Chinese hospital. Acta Anaesthesiol Scand. 2013;57:158–64.

60. Cooper L, DiGiovanni N, Schultz L, Taylor AM, Nossaman B. Influences observed on incidence and reporting of medication errors in anesthesia. Can J Anaesth. 2012;59:562–70.

61. Heinrich HW. Industrial accident prevention – a scientific approach. 4th ed. New York: McGraw-Hill; 1959.

62. Barach P, Small SD. Reporting and preventing medical mishaps – lessons from non-medical near miss reporting systems. Br Med J. 2000;320:759–63.

63. Mason KP, Green SM, Piacevoli Q, International Sedation Task Force. Adverse event reporting tool to standardize the reporting and tracking of adverse events during procedural sedation: a consenses document from the World SIVA International Sedation Task Force. Br J Anaesth. 2012;108:13–20.

64. WebAIRS. Anaesthetic Incident Reporting System, Australasian and New Zealand College of Anaesthetists (ANZCA). Demonstration page: http://www.anztadc.net/Demo/IncidentTabbed.aspx. Accessed 18 Feb 2016.

65. Shojania KG. The frustrating case of incident-reporting systems. Qual Saf Health Care. 2008;17:400–2.

66. Kringos DS, Sunol R, Wagner C, Mannion R, Michel P, Klazinga NS, et al. The influence of context on the effectiveness of hospital quality improvement strategies: a review of systematic reviews. BMC Health Serv Res. 2015;15:277. doi:10.1186/s12913-015-0906-0.

67. Sittig DF, Singh H. A new sociotechnical model for studying health information technology in complex adaptive healthcare systems. Qual Saf Health Care. 2010;19:i68–74.

68. Boyd M. A method for prioritizing interventions following root cause analysis (RCA) – lessons from philosophy. J Eval Clin Pract. 2015;21:461–9.

69. Jeffs L, Berta W, Lingard L, Baker GR. Learning from near misses: from quick fixes to closing off the Swiss-cheese holes. BMJ Qual Saf. 2012;21:287–94.

70. Thomas EJ, Petersen LA. Measuring errors and adverse events in health care. J Gen Intern Med. 2003;18:61–7.

71. Reason J. Understanding adverse events: human factors. Qual Health Care. 1995;4:80–9.

72. Keers RN, Williams SD, Cooke J, Walsh T, Ashcroft DM. Impact of interventions designed to reduce medication administration errors in hospitals: a systematic review. Drug Saf. 2014;37:317–32.

73. Thomas EJ. The future of measuring patient safety: prospective clinical surveillance. BMJ Qual Saf. 2015;24:244–5.

74. Vincent C, Burnett S, Carthey J. Safety measurement and monitoring in healthcare: a framework to guide clinical teams and healthcare organisations in maintaining safety. BMJ Qual Saf. 2014;23:670–7.

75. Webster CS, Anderson BJ, Stabile MJ, Merry AF. Improving the safety of pediatric sedation – human error, technology and clinical microsystems. In: Mason KP, editor. Pediatric sedation outside of the operating room: a multispecialty international collaboration. New York: Springer Science; 2015. p. 587–612.

76. Webster CS. Why anaesthetising a patient is more prone to failure than flying a plane. Anaesthesia. 2002;57:819–20.

77. Weaver SJ, Lubomksi LH, Wilson RF, Pfoh ER, Martinez KA, Dy SM. Promoting a culture of safety as a patient safety strategy: a systematic review. Ann Intern Med. 2013;158:369–74.

78. Pronovost P, Vohr E. Safe patients, smart hospitals. London: Hudson Street Press; 2010.

79. Webster CS. Human psychology applies to doctors too. Anaesthesia. 2000;55:929–30.

80. Anderson DJ, Webster CS. A systems approach to the reduction of medication error on the hospital ward. J Adv Nurs. 2001;35:34–41.

81. Reason J. Human error – models and management. Br Med J. 2000;320:768–70.

82. Webster CS. Doctors must implement new safety systems, not whinge about them. Anaesthesia. 2002;57:1231–2.

83. Nott MR. The labelling of ampoules. Anaesthesia. 1981;36:223–4.

84. Reason J. Human error. New York: Cambridge University Press; 1990.

85. Sagan SD. The limits of safety – organizations, accidents, and nuclear weapons. Princeton: Princeton University Press; 1993.

86. Reason J. The contribution of latent human failures to the breakdown of complex systems. Philos Trans R Soc Lond B. 1990;327:475–84.

87. Nunn DS, Baird WLM. Ampoule labelling [editorial]. Anaesthesia. 1996;51:1–2.

88. Wildsmith JAW. Doctors must read drug labels, not whinge about them. Br Med J. 2002;324:170.

89. Norman DA. The psychology of everyday things. New York: Basic Books; 1998.

90. Rasmussen J, Pejtersen AM, Goodstein LP. Cognitive systems engineering. New York: Wiley; 1994.

91. Merry AF, Webster CS, Mathew DJ. A new, safety-oriented, integrated drug administration and automated anesthesia record system. Anesth Analg. 2001;93:385–90.

92. Spath PL. Error reduction in health care – a systems approach to improving patient care. San Francisco: Jossey-Bass; 2000.

93. Merry AF, Webster CS. Anaesthetists and drug administration error—towards an irreducible minimum. In: Keneally J, Jones M, editors. Australasian anaesthesia. Melbourne: Australian and New Zealand College of Anaesthetists; 1996. p. 53–61.

94. Perrow C. Normal accidents – living with high risk technologies. New York: Basic Books; 1984.

95. Chiles JR. Inviting disaster – lessons from the edge of technology. New York: Harper Collins Publishers; 2001.

96. Takano K, Reason J. Psychological biases affecting human cognitive performance in dynamic operational environments. J Nucl Sci Tech. 1999;36:1041–51.

97. Pronovost PJ, Hudson DW. Improving healthcare quality through organisational peer-to-peer assessment: lessons from the nuclear power industry. BMJ Qual Saf. 2012;21:872–5.

98. Anonymous. Anaesthetic and respiratory equipment – user-applied labels for syringes containing drugs used during anaesthesia – colours, design and performance (ISO 26825:2008): International Organization for Standardization, 2008. Available from: http://www.iso.org. Accessed 18 Feb 2016.

99. Jelacic S, Bowdle A, Nair BG, Kusulos D, Bower L, Togashi K. A system for anesthesia drug administration using barcode technology: the Codonics Safe Label System and Smart Anesthesia Manager. Anesth Analg. 2015;121:410–21.

100. Merry AF, Webster CS, Connell H. A new infusion syringe label system designed to reduce task complexity during drug preparation. Anaesthesia. 2007;62:486–91.

101. Li B, Parmentier FBR, Zhang M. Behavioral distraction by auditory deviance is mediated by the sound's informational value. Exp Psychol. 2013;60:260–8.

102. Merry AF, Webster CS, Hannam J, Mitchell SJ, Edwards K, Jardim A, et al. Multimodal system designed to reduce errors in recording and administration of drugs in anaesthesia: a prospective randomised clinical evaluation. BMJ. 2011;343:d5543. doi:10.1136/bmj.d5543.

103. Merry AF, Webster CS, Weller J, Henderson S, Robinson B. Evaluation in an anaesthetic simulator of a prototype of a new drug administration system designed to reduce error. Anaesthesia. 2002;57:256–63.

104. Webster CS, Larsson L, Frampton CM, Weller J, McKenzie A, Cumin D, et al. Clinical assessment of a new anaesthetic drug administration system: a prospective, controlled, longitudinal incident monitoring study. Anaesthesia. 2010;65:490–9.

105. Hunter DT, Sumsion EG. A color code system in blood banking. Transfusion. 1967;7:451–2.

106. Webster CS. Manufacturers' obligations to colour-code prefilled syringes correctly. Anaesthesia. 2013;68:783–4.

107. Merry AF, Webster CS. Labelling and drug administration error. Anaesthesia. 1996;51:987–8.

108. Webster CS, Mathew DJ, Merry AF. Effective labelling is difficult, but safety really does matter. Anaesthesia. 2002;57:201–2.

109. Smellie GD, Lees NW, Smith EM. Drug recognition by nurses and anaesthetists. Anaesthesia. 1982;37:206–8.

110. Webster CS, Anderson DJ. A practical guide to the implementation of an effective incident reporting scheme to reduce medication error on the hospital ward. Int J Nurs Pract. 2002;8:176–83.

111. James RH, Rabey PG. Illegibility of drug ampoule labels. Br Med J. 1993;307:658–9.

112. Merry AF, Shipp DH, Lowinger JS. The contribution of labelling to safe medication administration in anaesthetic practice. Best Pract Res Clin Anaesthesiol. 2011;25:145–59.

113. Lanigan CJ. Safer epidural and spinal connectors. Anaesthesia. 2002;57:567–71.

114. Ang SBL, Hing WC, Tun SY, Park T. Experience with the use of the Codonics Safe Label System to improve labelling compliance of anaesthesia drugs. Anaesth Intensive Care. 2014;42:500–6.

115. Nanji KC, Patel A, Shaikh S, Seger DL, Bates DW. Evaluation of perioperative medication errors and adverse drug events. Anesthesiology. 2016;124:25–34.

116. Norman DA. The invisible computer. Cambridge: MIT Press; 1999.

117. Bergman E. Information appliances and beyond. San Francisco: Morgan Kaufmann; 2000.

118. Negroponte N. Hack out the useless extras – bloated software is swamping hard-won advances in computing power. N Sci. 2004;182:26.

119. Moore's Law. https://en.wikipedia.org/wiki/Moore%27s_law. Accessed 18 Feb 2016.

120. Wiener LR. Digital woes – why we should not depend on software. New York: Addison-Wesley; 1993.

121. Campbell-Kelly M, Aspray-Kelly W. Computer – a history of the information machine. New York: Basic Books; 1996.

122. Leveson NG. Safeware – system safety and computers. New York: Addison-Wesley; 1995.

123. Patton R. Software testing. Indianapolis: Sams Publishing; 2000.

124. Information is Beautiful. http://www.informationisbeautiful.net/visualizations/million-lines-of-code/. Accessed 18 Feb 2016.

125. Neumann PG. Computer related risks. New York: Addison-Wesley; 1995.

126. Gibbs S. US aviation authority: Boeing 787 bug could cause 'loss of control', 2015. *The Guardian.* http://www.theguardian.com/business/2015/may/01/us-aviation-authority-boeing-787-dreamliner-bug-could-cause-loss-of-control. Accessed 18 Feb 2016.

127. Goodin D. Boeing 787 Dreamliners contain a potentially catastrophic software bug, 2015. *ARS Technica.* http://arstechnica.com/information-technology/2015/05/boeing-787-dreamliners-contain-a-potentially-catastrophic-software-bug/. Accessed 18 Feb 2016.

128. Wachter RM. The digital doctor: hope, hype, and harm at the dawn of medicine's computer age. USA: McGraw-Hill; 2015.

129. Baxt WG. Application of artificial neural networks to clinical medicine. Lancet. 1995;346:1135–8.

130. McCloy R, Stone R. Virtual reality in surgery. Br Med J. 2001;323:912–5.

131. Buckingham RA, Buckingham RO. Robots in operating theatres. Br Med J. 1995;311:1479–82.

132. Catchpole K, Perkins C, Bresee C, Solnik MJ, Sherman B, Fritch J, et al. Safety, efficiency and learning curves in robotic surgery: a human factors analysis. Surg Endosc. 2015. doi:10.1007/s00464-015-4671-2.

133. Langford R. All in the name of progress. Anaesthesia. 2002;57:313.

134. United States Food and Drug Administration. http://www.fda.gov/MedicalDevices/ProductsandMedicalProcedures/GeneralHospitalDevicesandSupplies/InfusionPumps/ucm202511.htm. Accessed 18 Feb 2016.

135. Liu N, Rinehart J. Closed-loop propofol administration: routine care or a research tool? What impact in the future? Anesth Analg. 2016;122:4–6.

136. Absalom AR, Glen JI, Zwart GJ, Schnider TW, Struys MM. Target-controlled infusion: a mature technology. Anesth Analg. 2016;122:70–8.

137. Schnider TW, Minto CF, Struys MM, Absalom AR. The safety of target-controlled infusions. Anesth Analg. 2016;122:79–85.

138. Ohashi K, Dalleur O, Dykes PC, Bates DW. Benefits and risks of using smart pumps to reduce medication error rates – a systematic review. Drug Saf. 2014;37:1011–20.

139. Schraagen JM, Verhoeven F. Methods for studying medical devices technology and practitioner cognitition – the case of user-interface issues with infusion pumps. J Biomed Inform. 2013;46:181–95.

140. Manrique-Rodriguez S, Sanchez-Galindo A, Fernandez-Llamazares CM, Lopez-Herce J, Garcia-Lopez I, Carrillo-Alvarez A, et al. Developing a drug library for smart pumps in a pediatric intensive care unit. Artif Intell Med. 2012;54:155–61.

141. Mansfield J, Jarrett S. Using smart pumps to understand and evaluate clinician practice patterns to ensure patient safety. Hosp Pharm. 2013;48:942–50.

142. Woods DD. The alarm problem and directed attention in dynamic fault management. Ergonomics. 1995;38:2371–93.

143. Rayo MF, Moffatt-Bruce SD. Alarm system management: evidence-based guidance encouraging direct measurement of informativeness to improve alarm response. BMJ Qual Saf. 2015;24:282–6.

144. Catlin AC, Malloy WX, Arthur KJ, Gaston C, Young J, Fernando S, et al. Comparative analytics of infusion pump data across multiple hospital systems. Am J Health Syst Pharm. 2015;72:317–24.

145. Houliston BR, Parry DT, Merry AF. TADAA: Towards automated detection of anaesthetic activity. Methods Inf Med. 2011;5:464–71.

146. Agarwal S, Joshi A, Finin T, Yesha Y, Ganous T. A pervasive computing system for the operating room of the future. Mobile Netw Appl. 2007;12:215–28.

147. Reicher J, Reicher D, Reicher M. Use of radio frequency identification (RFID) tags in bedside monitoring of endotracheal tube position. J Clin Monit Comput. 2007;21:155–8.

148. Webster CS. Resistance is futile – the future and post-humanity. Prometheus. 2006;24:341–8.

149. Houliston B, Parry D, Webster CS, Merry AF. Interference with the operation of medical devices resulting from the use of radio frequency identification technology. N Z Med J. 2009;122:9–16.

150. van der Togt R, van Lieshout EJ, Hensbroek R, Beinat E, Binnekade JM, Bakker PJM. Electromagnetic interference from

radio frequency identification inducing potentially hazardous incidents in critical care medical equipment. JAMA. 2008;299:2884–90.

151. Seidman SJ, Brockman R, Lewis BM, Guag J, Shein MJ, Clement WJ, et al. In vitro tests reveal sample radiofrequency identification readers inducing clinically significant electromagnetic interference to implantable pacemakers and implantable cardioverter-defibrillators. Heart Rhythm. 2010;7:99–107.

152. Armstrong D. Hospital drug pump can be hacked through network, *FDA Warns*. http://www.bloomberg.com/news/articles/2015-07-31/hospital-drug-pump-can-be-hacked-on-wireless-network-fda-warns. Accessed 18 Feb 2016.

Can IV Sedatives Affect Outcome?

37

Christopher G. Hughes, Christina J. Hayhurst, and Pratik P. Pandharipande

Properties of IV Analgesics and Sedatives

Analgesics

Intravenous opioid analgesics are the mainstay of pain therapy for patients undergoing procedures or requiring hospitalization for acute illness. Opioids, however, have a number of adverse effects. Respiratory depression is commonly seen and often worsened by administration of additional sedative agents. Opioid administration can lead to hypotension from decreased sympathetic tone or vasodilation from histamine release. Other common side effects include decreased gastrointestinal motility, pruritus, flushing, urinary retention, and delirium. The most commonly used intravenous opioid agents include morphine, hydromorphone, fentanyl, sufentanil, and remifentanil. See Table 37.1 for important characteristics of common opioids.

Morphine and hydromorphone are most often utilized as intermittent injections. Morphine is often given in doses of 2–5 mg IV every 5–15 min until the pain is controlled, followed by similar doses on a scheduled basis every 2–4 h. Morphine is characterized by hepatic metabolism and renal excretion with intermediate volume of distribution. Its effects can be prolonged in patients with renal or hepatic impairment or obesity [1]. It has an active metabolite (morphine-6-glucuronide) that can cause analgesia and sedation and also has a second metabolite (morphine-3-glucoronide) that may result in seizures, and both metabolites can accumulate in patients with renal failure. Hydromorphone is a more potent congener of morphine with similar pharmacokinetic and pharmacodynamic profiles [2]. Its lack of

histamine release and decreased incidence of central nervous system side effects make it a useful alternative to morphine, with typical dosing ranges of 0.2–1 mg IV every 10–15 min until pain is controlled followed by similar doses every 2–4 h. Unlike morphine, hydromorphone does not have clinically active metabolites; thus, it is has an improved safety profile in patients with end-organ disease.

Fentanyl is a synthetic opioid with a rapid onset (5–15 min) and a short duration of action (30–60 min). It is frequently used as intermittent injections in the operating rooms, for procedural sedation, and in the intensive care unit due to its rapid onset and potency. It is also commonly used as a continuous infusion secondary to its short half-life and ease of titration. In general, intermittent doses of 25–100 µg of fentanyl are given every 5–10 min until the pain is controlled, followed by infusion rates of 25–250 µg/h if required. It has a large volume of distribution secondary to its lipophilicity, while its clearance correlates most closely with pharmacokinetic mass (similar to lean body mass); therefore, significant drug accumulation and a prolonged context sensitive half-life can occur with prolonged infusions [3]. However, because it causes less histamine release than morphine and does not undergo renal elimination, it is the preferred opioid analgesic in hemodynamically unstable patients or those with renal insufficiency. Sufentanil is an extremely potent derivative of fentanyl with a smaller volume of distribution and shorter context sensitive half-life than fentanyl, despite its high lipophilicity due to increased protein binding [4]. Furthermore, its pharmacokinetics are linear with weight, and dosing does not need to be adjusted for lean body mass [5]. These qualities are beneficial for infusion (0.3–1.5 µg/kg/h) in the operating room for analgesia or as part of a total intravenous anesthetic. Remifentanil, also a derivative of fentanyl, is unique as an opioid secondary to its metabolism by non-specific blood and tissue esterases. It is utilized primarily as an infusion (0.05–2 µg/kg/min) and has an elimination half-life of less than 10 min regardless of infusion duration.

C.G. Hughes, MD • C.J. Hayhurst, MD • P.P. Pandharipande, MD, MSCI (✉)
Department of Anesthesiology, Division of Anesthesiology Critical Care Medicine, Vanderbilt University School of Medicine, 1211 21st Ave. South, 526 MAB, Nashville, TN 37212, USA
e-mail: christopher.hughes@vanderbilt.edu; christina.hayhurst@vanderbilt.edu; Pratik.pandharipande@vanderbilt.edu

© Springer International Publishing AG 2017
A.R. Absalom, K.P. Mason (eds.), *Total Intravenous Anesthesia and Target Controlled Infusions*,
DOI 10.1007/978-3-319-47609-4_37

Dosing regimens for the infusion should be based on ideal body weight or lean body mass [6], and hypotension and bradycardia are the most common side effects seen with remifentanil administration. Importantly and secondary to its ultra-short half-life, supplemental analgesic medication is required at the conclusion of a remifentanil infusion. Higher cost and reports of withdrawal [7] and hyperalgesia [8] have limited the widespread utilization of remifentanil for analgesia.

Sedatives

Intravenous sedative medications most commonly administered for patients undergoing procedures or requiring sedation in the intensive care unit include propofol, dexmedetomidine, and benzodiazepines. See Table 37.1 for important characteristics of commonly used sedatives.

Propofol is a diisopropylphenol anesthetic and a γ-aminobutyric acid (GABA) agonist. Its rapid onset (1–2 min) and short duration of action (2–8 min) are advantageous, and it is typically given as a bolus injection of 40–100 mg IV followed by an infusion of 25–75 μg/kg/min. Its volume of distribution is large with a short distribution half-life. Emergence from propofol sedation when used as bolus or low dose infusion is related to redistribution from the brain and blood to peripheral tissues and not metabolic clearance, which can be advantageous in patients with renal or hepatic dysfunction. Emergence from longer infusion durations is related to metabolic clearance once saturation of peripheral tissues occurs [9]. Side effects from propofol administration include significant respiratory depression and hypotension. Propofol does not directly act on the vasculature [10] but inhibits sympathetic activity and decreases heart rate responses to blood pressure changes [11]. It increased pulse pressure variation in a dose-dependent

Table 37.1 Characteristics of commonly used IV analgesic and sedative medications

Agent	Mechanism	Metabolism	Duration of action	Advantages	Disadvantages
Morphine	μ-opioid receptor agonist	Glucuronidation Renal elimination	2–4 h	Familiarity Low cost	Histamine release Active metabolites Seizure risk
Hydromorphone	μ-opioid receptor agonist	Glucuronidation Renal elimination	2–4 h	No histamine release Increased potency	Higher cost than morphine Longer onset than fentanyl
Fentanyl	μ-opioid receptor agonist	CYP 3A4	30–60 min	Rapid onset No renal elimination Hemodynamic stability High potency	Large V_D Long context sensitive $T_{1/2}$
Sufentanil	μ-opioid receptor agonist	CYP 3A4	30–60 min	Rapid onset Smaller V_D and shorter context sensitive $T_{1/2}$ than fentanyl	Very high potency Uncommon outside the OR
Remifentanil	μ-opioid receptor agonist	Nonspecific esterases	<10 min	Rapid onset Very short context sensitive $T_{1/2}$	High cost Hyperalgesia Withdrawal Bradycardia
Propofol	GABA agonist	Glucuronidation Renal elimination	<10 min	Rapid onset Rapid redistribution Fast offset	Respiratory depression Oversedation PRIS No analgesia
Dexmedetomidine	α_2 receptor agonist	CYP2A6 Glucuronidation	2–4 h	No respiratory depression Analgesia No renal elimination Fast offset	Slow onset Infusion and not bolus dosing Bradycardia
Midazolam	GABA agonist	CYP3A4 Glucuronidation Renal elimination	30–80 min	Minimal respiratory depression Hemodynamic stability	Slow offset Active metabolites Deliriogenic No analgesia
Ketamine	N-methyl-D-aspartate antagonist	CYP3A4	5–45 min	No respiratory depression Strong analgesia	Sympathetic activation Deliriogenic Salivation Active metabolite

Abbreviations: *CYP* cytochrome P450, *GABA* γ-aminobutyric acid, *OR* operating room, *PRIS* propofol infusion syndrome, $T_{1/2}$ half-life, V_D volume of distribution fashion and increased heart rate without affecting vascular resistance or contractility in an animal model of septic shock [12]. Propofol can increase pro-inflammatory cytokine production [13], exacerbate reactive oxygen species production and apoptosis [14], and impair bacterial clearance [15]. Hypertriglyceridemia may also result from propofol administration either due to the intralipid carrier or altered hepatic lipid metabolism which can be seen with the propofol infusion syndrome (PRIS) [1]. PRIS is associated with high doses of propofol (>75 µg/kg/min or >5 mg/kg/h), pediatric sedation, critical illness with concomitant steroid and vasopressor administration, and prolonged infusions (>48 h) and is characterized by impaired tissue metabolism, severe lactic acidosis, and rhabdomyolysis [1]. High mortality rates are associated with PRIS, and supportive management and discontinuation of propofol are the mainstays of therapy. When high dosage or prolonged infusions are being used, it is recommended to regularly monitor serum pH, lactate, creatinine kinase, triglyceride levels, and the electrocardiogram (Brugada-type changes) [16].

Dexmedetomidine is an alpha-2 receptor agonist that acts on presynaptic neurons in the locus ceruleus and spinal cord. It causes sedation and analgesia without significant respiratory depression. Infusion rates of 0.2–1.5 µg/kg/h are required for sedation. Initiation of sedation frequently requires dosage in the higher end of this range to achieve therapeutic target and subsequent decrease in dosing as tolerated. Alternatively, a bolus of 1 µg/kg over 10–20 min may be utilized but with likely higher incidence of hemodynamic effects. Studies have shown safety with doses up to 2 µg/kg/h, although with increased incidence of bradycardia (most common side effect) and hypotension [17]. Hypertension can also result from stimulation of post-junctional alpha-2 receptors located on arterial and venous smooth muscle; this is more likely to be seen with bolus dosing and has led numerous providers to routinely avoid bolus dosing in the ICU. Dexmedetomidine may attenuate blood pressure and heart rate responses to temporarily reduce blood flow [18] but did not affect pulse pressure variation in an animal model of septic shock [12]. It possesses anti-inflammatory properties [19–21] and may improve bacterial clearance [22]. Dexmedetomidine is metabolized by the liver; thus, patients with severe liver disease require lower dosing, but there is no need for dose adjustment in patients with renal dysfunction [23].

Intravenous benzodiazepines used for sedation include midazolam, lorazepam, and diazepam. They are agonists to the GABA receptor and are metabolized in the liver to active metabolites (lorazepam being the exception with no active metabolite). These metabolites can lead to prolongation of their sedative effects, especially in patients with renal failure. The use of lorazepam is limited by the fact it is dissolved in propylene glycol which can accumulate to produce metabolic acidosis and renal dysfunction [24]. They have a dose-dependent respiratory depressant effect and cause a modest reduction in arterial blood pressure and an increase in heart rate from decreased systemic vascular resistance [25]. These effects may be exaggerated by concomitant administration of opioids. Benzodiazepines impair inflammatory signaling and blunt bacterial clearance [26, 27]. Benzodiazepines may increase mortality in bacterial infection [28, 29] or increase susceptibility to secondary infections [30]. Benzodiazepines, in particular midazolam, are frequently used for procedural sedation outside of operating rooms due to their hemodynamic stability and less respiratory depression than propofol. Routine use in the intensive care unit for sedation, however, is no longer indicated due to their association with worse patient outcomes which will be detailed later in this chapter [31].

Ketamine is an adjunct sedative agent used for analgesia and procedural sedation. It is an N-methyl-D-aspartate antagonist that produces a dissociative state and has significant analgesic properties. Ketamine does not cause the respiratory depression seen with other intravenous sedative medications and is thus most commonly utilized for sedation for painful procedures (e.g., burn debridement, fracture realignment) or for opioid reduction in patients with acute pain. It has direct myocardial depressant properties but causes sympathetic system activation potentially leading to tachycardia, hypertension, myocardial ischemia, and raised intracranial pressure [32, 33].

IV Sedation in the Operating Room

Propofol and other intravenous agents (e.g., remifentanil or sufentanil) are often used as continuous infusions in the operating room to perform general anesthesia (total intravenous anesthetic or TIVA) or to provide sedation after regional or neuraxial blockade. One common indication of TIVA is for spinal surgery that requires motor evoked potential monitoring, thus prohibiting standard administration of inhaled anesthetics. Use of these intravenous agents for sedation in the operating room has been studied with regard to various patient outcomes. See Table 37.2.

Recovery After General Anesthesia

Several studies have examined the effects of TIVA versus inhaled anesthetics with regard to recovery from general anesthesia. One study compared TIVA vs. sevoflurane or desflurane anesthesia using the Trieger Dot Test and the Digit Symbol Substitution Test to assess cognitive function [34]. Cognitive function with TIVA was higher at 60 min but

Table 37.2 Key clinical outcomes associated with IV analgesic and sedative medications

Setting	Associated outcomes
Operating room	• TIVA with propofol and lighter depth of sedation may lead to faster recovery and less postoperative delirium • Propofol TIVA reduces postoperative nausea and vomiting • Propofol and opioid TIVA may reduce postoperative pain levels
Procedural sedation	• Benzodiazepines and propofol are responsible for most oversedation, with highest incidence when multiple medications are co-administered • Benzodiazepines and dexmedetomidine are preferred agents for radiological testing due to less respiratory compromise than propofol • General anesthesia is preferred for cerebral aneurysm coiling, with inhaled anesthetics potentially leading to more rapid recovery than TIVA • Moderate sedation is associated with improved mortality and functional outcomes compared to general anesthesia in acute ischemic stroke requiring intra-arterial endovascular intervention • Propofol infusion with bolus for defibrillator placement may decrease procedural duration and complications • Propofol administered by trained personnel or computer-assisted devices is associated with faster recovery times and higher satisfaction in patients undergoing endoscopy
ICU sedation	• Fentanyl and remifentanil have displayed equal efficacy for achieving sedation with no difference in extubation times • Analgosedation regimens likely reduce time on mechanical ventilation • Propofol and dexmedetomidine increase time at target sedation and reduce time on mechanical ventilation • Dexmedetomidine use is associated with less delirium and improved arousability and communication • Dexmedetomidine use after cardiac surgery has been associated with reduced complications and mortality • Incidence of clinically significant bradycardia and hypotension are similar between propofol and dexmedetomidine • Propofol and dexmedetomidine are associated with per patient cost reduction despite higher drug costs

TIVA total intravenous anesthetic

no significant differences were found at 90 min, suggesting patients receiving TIVA recovered their cognitive function faster than those receiving inhaled anesthetics. A study of patients undergoing office-based ambulatory surgery randomized patients to propofol induction and TIVA, propofol induction and sevoflurane/nitrous oxide maintenance, or sevoflurane induction with sevoflurane/nitrous oxide maintenance [35]. This study found no significant differences to early recovery signs such as eye opening amongst the three groups. The study did find, however, that the propofol TIVA group had a significantly shorter time to tolerating fluids, recovery room stay, and time to discharge and that the sevoflurane only group had longer time to "home ready" [35]. A large study of 1158 patients randomized people to either propofol induction and maintenance, propofol induction and isoflurane/N$_2$O or sevoflurane/N$_2$O maintenance, or inhalational sevoflurane induction and maintenance [36]. They found no difference in rate of recovery. Another large study of over 2000 patients randomized to TIVA or isoflurane/nitrous oxide found that the cost of TIVA was three times that of an inhalational technique, which was not recouped despite shorter post-anesthesia care unit (PACU) stays in the TIVA group [37]. In overweight patients undergoing minor peripheral surgery, propofol TIVA was associated with impaired early postoperative lung function and lower oxygen saturation though the differences were not likely clinically significant [38]. One study examined the effects of TIVA vs. inhalational anesthesia on patient's "well being" after surgery [39]. Patients undergoing minor gynecologic or orthopedic procedures were randomized to either a propofol

infusion or sevoflurane. Adjective Mood Scale (AMS) and the State-Trait-Anxiety Inventory (STAI) were measured at baseline, at 90 min after anesthesia, and 24 h after anesthesia. This study found a significantly lower AMS and STAI at 90 min after TIVA, which indicated improved well-being and less anxiety as compared with inhalation anesthesia [39]. TIVA has been compared to desflurane in cardiac surgery patients [40]. This study found no difference in delirium on postoperative day 1 between groups, a higher incidence of cognitive dysfunction on postoperative days 3–7 in the propofol group, and no difference in cognitive dysfunction at 3 months. Intravenous sedation has also been used to provide a comfortable experience for patients undergoing surgery with a regional or neuraxial anesthesia. While IV sedation is not needed for anesthesia, it is used for anxiolysis and occasionally amnesia, which improves patient comfort [41]. Depth of this sedation, however, may affect brain function after surgery. A study of elderly patients undergoing hip fracture repair under spinal anesthesia randomized the patients to either deep sedation (Bispectral Index of 50) or light sedation (Bispectral Index of 80). The light sedation group had 50 % less postoperative delirium than the deep sedation group [42]. Monitoring depth of anesthesia with processed electroencephalography (and presumably avoiding oversedation) also reduced the incidence and duration of postoperative delirium but found no difference in long-term cognitive impairment [43]. Thus while TIVA and lighter depth of sedation likely leads to faster recovery from anesthesia and less postoperative delirium, the effects of TIVA on cost and long-term cognitive function are less clear.

Postoperative Nausea

Approximately one third of patients that undergo surgery will have postoperative nausea and vomiting (PONV) [44]. In one study, vomiting was rated by patients as being more undesirable than pain or gagging on the endotracheal tube after surgery [45]. Several studies have looked at the relationship between PONV and TIVA vs. inhalational anesthesia. TIVA vs. isoflurane/nitrous oxide anesthesia was found to significantly decrease PONV early in their recovery period [37]. In the previously mentioned study of patients undergoing minor gynecologic or orthopedic procedures, the occurrence of both nausea and vomiting was significantly lower 90 min and 24 h after anesthesia in the TIVA group compared to inhalation anesthesia [39]. In a study of over 4000 people undergoing general anesthesia, antiemetics such as ondansetron, dexamethasone, and droperidol were shown to reduce PONV by about 26 %, while TIVA with propofol reduced PONV by 19 % [44]. In a meta-analysis of over 6000 patients, the number needed to treat to reduce PONV by using propofol TIVA vs. other anesthetics was only 5 [46]. Additionally, when added to a PONV prophylaxis regimen, TIVA with propofol, ketamine, and dexmedetomidine was able to further reduce PONV by 17.3 % compared to inhalational anesthesia with opioids with the same PONV prophylaxis regimen [47]. PONV is a common problem and one of the most undesirable complications of anesthesia, and propofol as part of a TIVA has been shown to reliably reduce PONV, even when compared with inhalational anesthesia with an antiemetic prophylaxis regimen.

Postoperative Pain

There have been few studies in humans looking at differences in pain after TIVA or inhalational anesthesia. Patients undergoing minor gynecologic or orthopedic procedures had comparable postoperative pain intensity with propofol or sevoflurane [39]. In a small study of patients undergoing uterine surgery that were randomized to propofol and fentanyl vs. isoflurane and fentanyl, patients who were anesthetized with propofol had less postoperative pain at 24 h and used less morphine within 24 h [48]. The authors postulated that the effect was related to a possible immediate hyperalgesia caused by volatile anesthetics upon emergence or the synergistic activity of propofol and opioids on nociceptive neuronal transmission. A trial of middle ear surgery patients randomized to TIVA vs. volatile anesthetics noted worse pain scores in patients who received inhalational anesthesia [49]. A larger randomized controlled trial compared TIVA with propofol and remifentanil to sevoflurane (both groups had epidural analgesia with ropivacaine and sufentanil) and their effects on chronic post-thoracotomy pain syndrome [50]. At both 3 and 6 months, those patients who had undergone TIVA had less post-thoracotomy pain than those who were anesthetized with sevoflurane. Again, the authors suggest the outcome might be related to depression of nociceptive neuronal transmission by acting on GABA receptors. They also suggest propofol could have some anti-oxidizing effects or act upon the NMDA receptor, thus preventing remifentanil-induced hyperalgesia. Overall, data supports reduced pain levels after propofol and opioid TIVA anesthetics, although the mechanism is not fully elucidated and the clinical significance of these findings is unclear in a wide range of patient populations.

IV Sedatives for Procedural Sedation

With advances in medical technology, limited operating room space, and increasing numbers of outpatient procedures, medically complex patients are increasingly undergoing diagnostic and therapeutic procedures outside the operating rooms [51]. The requirements of the procedure and the health of the patient will determine which intravenous analgesic and sedative medications are most appropriate, but several underlying considerations are also present for the clinician providing sedation for these nonoperating-room cases. See Table 37.2. Importantly, procedural sedation is not defined by specific medications or doses but rather by levels of consciousness achieved. The rapid onset and narrow therapeutic window of many agents mandate proper provider education, availability of emergency equipment, and close hemodynamic monitoring. Minimal sedation is the first step on the continuum of depth of sedation, followed by moderate sedation, deep sedation, and general anesthesia.

Procedural sedation can progress to general anesthesia at any point, and clinicians administering procedural sedation are required to possess the skills necessary to rescue unstable patients according to the Joint Commission on Accreditation of Hospital Organizations [52]. Upon review of the American Society for Anesthesiologists Closed Claims database, the greatest number of claims (33 %) for nonoperating-room cases was from inadequate oxygenation or ventilation secondary to the effects of administered drugs, and the proportion of death was significantly increased in these cases (54 % versus 24 %) when compared to operating room claims [51]. This illustrates the need for clinicians to have education and experience in airway management and cardiopulmonary resuscitation in order to perform safe sedation. Benzodiazepines and propofol utilized as single agents were responsible for oversedation in 9 % of patients; however, the addition of another drug to propofol increased the incidence of oversedation to 50 % [52]. Respiratory compromise from propofol was less than that from using the combination of benzodiazepines and opioids. Increased age (>70 years), American Society of Anesthesiologists physical status III or higher, and obesity were associated with negative events, which correlates with their increased risk from intravenous sedative agents [52].

Radiology

Sedation is often required for patients undergoing radiographic imaging to prevent movement during examination and to relieve anxiety and symptoms of claustrophobia. The efficiency of the procedure depends on the interval of drug administration to the patient being ready to scan and the time required for emergence after the procedure. Propofol has the advantage of a fast onset and short recovery profile, but relatively high doses (approximately 100 mcg/kg/min) are required to prevent involuntary movement, increasing the incidence of respiratory depression [53]. The inaccessibility of patients in the scanner can create problems with patient visualization and airway management in patients receiving propofol [54]. Benzodiazepines can produce moderate sedation without significant respiratory depression but have been found to have a high percentage of prolonged sedation, unsteadiness, and hyperactivity, thus decreasing their efficacy for radiological testing [53]. Due to its lack of respiratory depression, dexmedetomidine should be considered in patients at high risk for airway obstruction and respiratory failure, especially in locations with obstacles to airway management.

For interventional radiology and neuroradiology procedures, the primary sedation goals for these cases are to alleviate patient anxiety and discomfort while providing appropriate patient cooperation or immobility. These procedures additionally require rapid awakening to obtain neurological exams. General anesthesia is preferred for cerebral aneurysm coiling secondary to the requirement for an immobile patient and control of respiratory and hemodynamic profiles [55]. Sevoflurane inhaled anesthetic maintenance led to a more rapid recovery when compared to propofol infusion in one interventional neuroradiology study of patients requiring general anesthesia for embolization procedures [56]. When neurological testing is required during the procedure, dexmedetomidine may be advantageous as patients are often arousable and cooperative when stimulated. In patients with acute ischemic stroke requiring intra-arterial endovascular interventions, patients receiving general anesthesia appear to have worse outcomes than patients receiving moderate sedation, including over two times higher odds of death, respiratory complications, and poor functional outcome [57, 58]. Stroke severity at the onset of treatment may confound the comparison between general anesthesia and moderate sedation in these studies, as patients with worse neurological deficits from their ischemic strokes typically require intubation for airway protection.

Cardiac Procedures

For cardiac procedures, the severity of the underlying medical condition and the urgency of the procedure often determine the optimal plan for procedural sedation. In patients undergoing cardiac catheterization or short electrophysiology studies, midazolam and fentanyl are most commonly utilized due to their lack of significant hemodynamic alterations and the requirement for moderate levels of sedation. Hemodynamic or respiratory instability may necessitate intubation and general anesthesia. For insertion of implantable defibrillators, most cases can be performed under local anesthesia or moderate sedation with deepening of sedation during the defibrillator check. This technique likely decreases procedure duration and complications compared to general anesthesia [59, 60]. Because of its rapid onset and offset, low dose propofol infusions with boluses during defibrillation work well for this procedure. Longer duration electrophysiology studies often require general anesthesia for patient comfort over the several-hour time span as well as for cessation of ventilation. Transesophageal echocardiography requires deep sedation for patient tolerance but is a brief procedure, making propofol the preferred sedative agent.

Endoscopy

Benzodiazepines and opioids are used for the majority of endoscopies but often produce deeper levels of sedation than planned (68 % of patients inadvertently progressed to deep sedation when sedated with midazolam and meperidine) [61]. In addition to potential respiratory compromise during the procedure, this leads to prolonged recovery times. Due to its rapid onset and offset, propofol utilization is increasing for endoscopy cases, but its narrow therapeutic index requires it to be administered by trained personnel. The quality of sedation was higher and recovery time shorter in patients sedated with propofol versus midazolam and meperidine [62]. Two large studies reported the safety of nurse-administered propofol infusions but did not elucidate the total number of patients with hypoxemia, thus likely grossly underestimating the number of respiratory events [63, 64]. A review of procedural sedation with benzodiazepines and opioids, however, found similar incidence of respiratory events to that reported with propofol [52]. In one study examining remifentanil versus propofol infusion for colonoscopy, respiratory function and pain scores were superior in the remifentanil group, but patients receiving propofol had increased amnesia and lower nausea and vomiting [65]. Moderate/deep sedation with remifentanil and propofol versus TIVA with midazolam, fentanyl, and propofol was compared for colonoscopy [66]. The sedation group experienced higher pain scores but was discharged approximately 15 min faster than the TIVA group. The sedation group also had less change in hemodynamics and less respiratory depression. Deep sedation with propofol for colonoscopy was more recently found to increase the risk of aspiration pneumonia compared to moderate sedation in a large population-based analysis of patients undergoing colonoscopy without polypectomy [67]. Newer techniques that include patient controlled sedation and analgesia with propofol and fentanyl have been shown to be effective and safe for upper GI endoscopy [68, 69]. Furthermore, computer-assisted devices that integrate propofol delivery with patient monitoring enable personalized sedation and the safe administration of propofol by endoscopist/nurse teams in patients requiring minimal to moderate sedation for upper endoscopy and colonoscopy. Compared to moderate sedation with benzodiazepines and opioids, the SEDASYS system had less oxygen desaturation, higher patient and clinician satisfaction, and faster recovery times [70].

IV Sedation in the Intensive Care Unit

Pain and agitation can contribute to increased catecholamine activity, increased oxygen demand and consumption, and hypermetabolism. Furthermore, agitation may place patients and clinicians at risk of injury. Intravenous analgesic and sedative medications are therefore administered to provide patient comfort and ensure patient safety. See Table 37.2. Unpredictable pharmacokinetics and pharmacodynamics in critically ill patients with impaired organ function, fluctuating volume status, hemodynamic instability, and potential drug interactions complicate sedative administration in this setting. Administration of intravenous sedative agents is associated with longer time on mechanical ventilation and in the ICU, increased radiological evaluation for altered mental status, and higher rates of delirium [71, 72]. Clinicians can improve patients outcomes by incorporating analgesia and sedation protocols, targeting light sedation levels, performing daily interruption of sedation and spontaneous breathing trials, assessing and preventing delirium, and performing early mobilization [73–79]. Furthermore, patient care strategies should focus on providing adequate analgesia and incorporating propofol or dexmedetomidine to reach light sedation targets, thus reducing benzodiazepine exposure [30, 80, 81]. The Society for Critical Care Medicine's clinical practice guidelines outline sedation methods to optimize patient care and safety while minimizing negative outcomes associated with sedative agents [31].

Analgesia

The selection of an opioid for systemic analgesia depends on the pharmacology of the specific opioid, the likely required duration, and the amount of discomfort. Few comparative trials between opioid regimens have been performed in the intensive care unit. Remifentanil provided better outcomes than morphine with regard to time at sedation target, use of supplemental sedation, and duration of mechanical ventilation in one randomized double blind study [82]. Meanwhile, remifentanil and fentanyl have displayed equal efficacy in achieving time at target sedation with no difference in extubation times [83]. Patients receiving fentanyl required more frequent administration of additional sedatives but experienced less pain after extubation compared to those receiving remifentanil [83]. Data are inconsistent on the role of opioids on delirium outcomes. Patients who received higher morphine equivalents per day were less likely to develop delirium than patients who received less analgesic medications in a study of elderly hip fracture patients [84]. Trauma and burn critically ill patients may benefit from morphine and methadone with regard to delirium [85, 86]. However, meperidine and morphine have been associated with increasing the risk of delirium [87, 88]. Thus, analgesia with opioids in patients with acute pain may be protective of acute brain dysfunction while excessive administration to achieve sedation may be detrimental. This may be especially true in the perioperative setting, where poor pain control has been associated with increased rates of postoperative delirium [89, 90].

Analgosedation

The use of analgesic-based sedative regimens to perform light sedation protocols is increasing. In a randomized controlled study comparing analgesia only (remifentanil with rescue propofol) versus analgesia and sedation (titrated propofol or benzodiazepine infusion with as needed opioid), the analgesia only group had decreased length of stay in the intensive care unit, more days alive without mechanical ventilation, and improved sedation scores [91]. Other multicenter trials comparing analgesia-based regimens versus sedative regimens have also demonstrated that analgosedation regimens can shorten the duration of mechanical ventilation [92, 93]. Recently, a single center randomized controlled trial compared a morphine-based analgesia protocol versus propofol sedation and similarly

Fig. 37.1 Days in the ICU with analgosedation vs. traditional (Reproduced from Strom T, Martinussen T, Toft P. A protocol of no sedation for critically ill patients receiving mechanical ventilation: a randomised trial. *Lancet.* 2010;375(9713):475–480 [80] with permission from Elsevier)

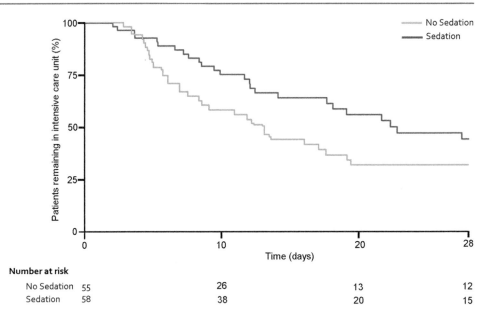

Number at risk

No Sedation	55	26	13	12
Sedation	58	38	20	15

found shorter times on mechanical ventilation and in the ICU in the morphine analgesia group (Fig. 37.1) [80].

Sedatives

When compared to benzodiazepines, propofol has been shown to increase time at sedation target, decrease time spent on mechanical ventilation, and decrease costs despite higher drug costs [94–96]. Dexmedetomidine has been compared to benzodiazepines in multiple randomized controlled trials. Compared to lorazepam and midazolam, patients sedated with dexmedetomidine had lower probability of developing delirium [30, 81]. Dexmedetomidine patients also had decreased duration of mechanical ventilation, less tachycardia and hypertension, and less bacterial superinfection [30]. Subgroup analysis showed increased survival in septic patients with dexmedetomidine use compared to lorazepam [29].

A study comparing dexmedetomidine and propofol sedation in post-surgical patients showed similar time at sedation target, but patients sedated with dexmedetomidine required less supplemental analgesia [97]. When compared to propofol in post-cardiac surgical patients, patients sedated with dexmedetomidine had decreased use of beta blockers and epinephrine [98]. The Dexmedetomidine Compared to Morphine (DEXCOM) study demonstrated a reduction in hypotension and norepinephrine requirement in patients sedated with dexmedetomidine compared to morphine after cardiac surgery [99]. In a large retrospective cohort study of patients who underwent cardiac surgery, dexmedetomidine administration in the perioperative period was associated with reduced in-hospital, 30-day, and 1-year mortality along with reduced risk of overall complications

[100]. Major adverse cardiocerebral events (stroke, coma, perioperative myocardial infarction, heart block, or cardiac arrest) were not statistically different between groups [100]. This study was limited by significant clinical and procedural differences between groups (e.g., greater incidence of previous myocardial infarct, congestive heart failure, and low ejection fraction in those receiving dexmedetomidine). More recently, a randomized controlled trial of dexmedetomidine vs. propofol for ICU sedation after cardiac surgery demonstrated a 50 % decrease in the incidence of delirium and a 1-day reduction in delirium duration with dexmedetomidine sedation [101]. This leads to a reduction in ICU time and cost related to delirium.

Two large multicenter randomized controlled trials recently compared dexmedetomidine to midazolam and propofol for light to moderate sedation in patients requiring mechanical ventilation for greater than 24 h [102]. Time at sedation target was equivalent between dexmedetomidine and the control groups though patients in the dexmedetomidine group had overall lighter levels of sedation. Patients in the dexmedetomidine group required rescue drug more often than propofol group, and discontinuation due to lack of efficacy was more common in patients sedated with dexmedetomidine than those sedated with midazolam or propofol. Arousability, communication, and patient cooperation were all significantly improved with dexmedetomidine sedation. Dexmedetomidine reduced duration of mechanical ventilation compared to midazolam, and time to extubation was faster with dexmedetomidine than either midazolam or propofol. Overall, length of intensive care unit and hospital stay and mortality were similar between groups.

Two recent studies have examined the role of dexmedetomidine in treating hyperactive delirium. The first randomized patients on mechanical ventilation who

Fig. 37.2 Dexmedetomidine vs. placebo for hyperactive delirium during mechanical ventilation (Reproduced from Reade MC, Eastwood GM, Bellomo R, et al. Effect of Dexmedetomidine Added to Standard Care on Ventilator-Free Time in Patients With Agitated Delirium: A Randomized Clinical Trial. *JAMA*. 2016 [103] with permission from the American Medical Association)

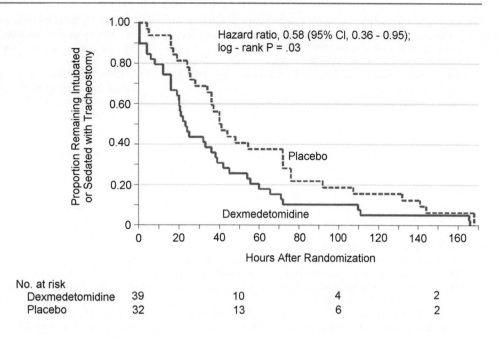

could not be extubated due to hyperactive delirium to either dexmedetomidine or placebo in addition to their ongoing standard sedative regimen (most commonly propofol) [103]. Patients randomized to dexmedetomidine had faster resolution of delirium, required less antipsychotic medications, were extubated earlier, and had an increase in ventilator-free days (Fig. 37.2). The second study examined non-intubated ICU patients with hyperactive delirium [104]. Patients were first administered intravenous boluses of haloperidol for symptom control. Those with improved agitation after haloperidol received a haloperidol infusion, and those whose agitation did not improve received dexmedetomidine in addition to a haloperidol infusion. Patients receiving dexmedetomidine were less likely to fail the regimen, had more time with satisfactory sedation, had less oversedation and noninvasive positive pressure ventilation requirement, had on average a 3-day shorter ICU stay, and had significantly lower total costs despite higher drug costs.

The most common clinical concerns with dexmedetomidine are bradycardia and cost. Bradycardia was a common side effect in several studies, but there were no significant differences between the comparator groups with regard to bradycardia necessitating treatment (atropine, glycopyrrolate, or pacing) [30, 81, 102]. Furthermore, neither the incidence of bradycardia nor that of hypotension was significantly different between dexmedetomidine and propofol [102]. With regard to cost, several studies have showed a significant per patient cost reduction with dexmedetomidine use despite higher drug costs [94, 101, 104, 105]. Future studies comparing outcomes, including cost, between propofol and dexmedetomidine are necessary to further delineate their potential advantages and disadvantages in different ICU patient populations.

Conclusions

Intravenous medications for analgesia and sedation are commonly administered in clinical practice for general anesthesia, procedural sedation, and in the care of the critically ill. Their pharmacokinetic, pharmacodynamic, and side effect profiles must be taken into consideration by clinicians to balance the benefits and risks of these medications. Clinical outcome data are available to guide clinicians in the administration of these agents in different healthcare settings in order to maximize patient care.

Acknowledgments Dr. Hughes is supported by American Geriatrics Society Jahnigen Career Development Award, and National Institutes of Health HL111111 and R03AG045085 (Bethesda, Maryland, USA). Dr. Pandharipande is supported by the National Institutes of Health AG035117 and HL111111 (Bethesda, Maryland, USA).

Conflict of Interest
Christopher G. Hughes and Christina J. Hayhurst declare that they have no conflict of interest and Pratik P. Pandharipande receives research grant from Hospira Inc.

References

1. Diedrich DA, Brown DR. Analytic reviews: propofol infusion syndrome in the ICU. J Intensive Care Med. 2011;26(2):59–72.
2. Horn E, Nesbit SA. Pharmacology and pharmacokinetics of sedatives and analgesics. Gastrointest Endosc Clin N Am. 2004;14(2):247–68.
3. Shibutani K, Inchiosa Jr MA, Sawada K, Bairamian M. Pharmacokinetic mass of fentanyl for postoperative analgesia in lean and obese patients. Br J Anaesth. 2005;95(3):377–83.

4. Hughes MA, Glass PS, Jacobs JR. Context-sensitive half-time in multicompartment pharmacokinetic models for intravenous anesthetic drugs. Anesthesiology. 1992;76(3):334–41.

5. Gepts E, Shafer SL, Camu F, et al. Linearity of pharmacokinetics and model estimation of sufentanil. Anesthesiology. 1995;83(6):1194–204.

6. Egan TD, Huizinga B, Gupta SK, et al. Remifentanil pharmacokinetics in obese versus lean patients. Anesthesiology. 1998;89(3):562–73.

7. Delvaux B, Ryckwaert Y, Van Boven M, De Kock M, Capdevila X. Remifentanil in the intensive care unit: tolerance and acute withdrawal syndrome after prolonged sedation. Anesthesiology. 2005;102(6):1281–2.

8. Fletcher D, Martinez V. Opioid-induced hyperalgesia in patients after surgery: a systematic review and a meta-analysis. Br J Anaesth. 2014;112(6):991–1004.

9. Barr J. Propofol: a new drug for sedation in the intensive care unit. Int Anesthesiol Clin. 1995;33(1):131–54.

10. Robinson BJ, Ebert TJ, O'Brien TJ, Colinco MD, Muzi M. Mechanisms whereby propofol mediates peripheral vasodilation in humans. Sympathoinhibition or direct vascular relaxation? Anesthesiology. 1997;86(1):64–72.

11. Sato M, Tanaka M, Umehara S, Nishikawa T. Baroreflex control of heart rate during and after propofol infusion in humans. Br J Anaesth. 2005;94(5):577–81.

12. Yu T, Li Q, Liu L, et al. Different effects of propofol and dexmedetomidine on preload dependency in endotoxemic shock with norepinephrine infusion. J Surg Res. 2015;198:185–91.

13. Helmy SA, Al-Attiyah RJ. The immunomodulatory effects of prolonged intravenous infusion of propofol versus midazolam in critically ill surgical patients. Anaesthesia. 2001;56(1):4–8.

14. Wang X, Cheng Y, Liu X, Yang J, Munoz D, Zhang C. Unexpected pro-injury effect of propofol on vascular smooth muscle cells with increased oxidative stress. Crit Care Med. 2011;39(4):738–45.

15. Kelbel I, Koch T, Weber A, Schiefer HG, van Ackern K, Neuhof H. Alterations of bacterial clearance induced by propofol. Acta Anaesthesiol Scand. 1999;43(1):71–6.

16. Fudickar A, Bein B. Propofol infusion syndrome: update of clinical manifestation and pathophysiology. Minerva Anestesiol. 2009;75(5):339–44.

17. Tan JA, Ho KM. Use of dexmedetomidine as a sedative and analgesic agent in critically ill adult patients: a meta-analysis. Intensive Care Med. 2010;36:926–39.

18. Kato J, Ogawa Y, Kojima W, Aoki K, Ogawa S, Iwasaki K. Cardiovascular reflex responses to temporal reduction in arterial pressure during dexmedetomidine infusion: a double-blind, randomized, and placebo-controlled study. Br J Anaesth. 2009;103(4):561–5.

19. Memis D, Hekimoglu S, Vatan I, Yandim T, Yuksel M, Sut N. Effects of midazolam and dexmedetomidine on inflammatory responses and gastric intramucosal pH to sepsis, in critically ill patients. Br J Anaesth. 2007;98(4):550–2.

20. Venn RM, Bryant A, Hall GM, Grounds RM. Effects of dexmedetomidine on adrenocortical function, and the cardiovascular, endocrine and inflammatory responses in post-operative patients needing sedation in the intensive care unit. Br J Anaesth. 2001;86(5):650–6.

21. Qiao H, Sanders RD, Ma D, Wu X, Maze M. Sedation improves early outcome in severely septic Sprague Dawley rats. Crit Care. 2009;13(4):R136.

22. Nishina K, Akamatsu H, Mikawa K, et al. The effects of clonidine and dexmedetomidine on human neutrophil functions. Anesth Analg. 1999;88(2):452–8.

23. Maze M, Scarfini C, Cavaliere F. New agents for sedation in the intensive care unit. Crit Care Clin. 2001;17(4):881–97.

24. Yahwak JA, Riker RR, Fraser GL, Subak-Sharpe S. Determination of a lorazepam dose threshold for using the osmol gap to monitor for propylene glycol toxicity. Pharmacotherapy. 2008;28(8):984–91.

25. Olkkola KT, Ahonen J. Midazolam and other benzodiazepines. Handb Exp Pharmacol. 2008;182:335–60.

26. Kim SN, Son SC, Lee SM, et al. Midazolam inhibits proinflammatory mediators in the lipopolysaccharide-activated macrophage. Anesthesiology. 2006;105(1):105–10.

27. Finnerty M, Marczynski TJ, Amirault HJ, Urbancic M, Andersen BR. Benzodiazepines inhibit neutrophil chemotaxis and superoxide production in a stimulus dependent manner; PK-11195 antagonizes these effects. Immunopharmacology. 1991;22(3):185–93.

28. Laschi A, Descotes J, Tachon P, Evreux JC. Adverse influence of diazepam upon resistance to Klebsiella pneumoniae infection in mice. Toxicol Lett. 1983;16(3–4):281–4.

29. Pandharipande PP, Sanders RD, Girard TD, et al. Effect of dexmedetomidine versus lorazepam on outcome in patients with sepsis: an a priori-designed analysis of the MENDS randomized controlled trial. Crit Care. 2010;14(2):R38.

30. Riker RR, Shehabi Y, Bokesch PM, et al. Dexmedetomidine vs midazolam for sedation of critically ill patients: a randomized trial. JAMA. 2009;301(5):489–99.

31. Barr J, Fraser GL, Puntillo K, et al. Clinical practice guidelines for the management of pain, agitation, and delirium in adult patients in the intensive care unit. Crit Care Med. 2013;41(1):263–306.

32. Hirota K, Lambert DG. Ketamine: new uses for an old drug? Br J Anaesth. 2011;107(2):123–6.

33. Laskowski K, Stirling A, McKay WP, Lim HJ. A systematic review of intravenous ketamine for postoperative analgesia. Can J Anaesth. 2011;58:911–23.

34. Larsen B, Seitz A, Larsen R. Recovery of cognitive function after remifentanil-propofol anesthesia: a comparison with desflurane and sevoflurane anesthesia. Anesth Analg. 2000;90(1):168–74.

35. Tang J, Chen L, White PF, et al. Recovery profile, costs, and patient satisfaction with propofol and sevoflurane for fast-track office-based anesthesia. Anesthesiology. 1999;91(1):253–61.

36. Moore JK, Elliott RA, Payne K, et al. The effect of anaesthetic agents on induction, recovery and patient preferences in adult day case surgery: a 7-day follow-up randomized controlled trial. Eur J Anaesthesiol. 2008;25(11):876–83.

37. Visser K, Hassink EA, Bonsel GJ, Moen J, Kalkman CJ. Randomized controlled trial of total intravenous anesthesia with propofol versus inhalation anesthesia with isoflurane-nitrous oxide: postoperative nausea with vomiting and economic analysis. Anesthesiology. 2001;95(3):616–26.

38. Zoremba M, Dette F, Hunecke T, Eberhart L, Braunecker S, Wulf H. A comparison of desflurane versus propofol: the effects on early postoperative lung function in overweight patients. Anesth Analg. 2011;113(1):63–9.

39. Hofer CK, Zollinger A, Buchi S, et al. Patient well-being after general anaesthesia: a prospective, randomized, controlled multicentre trial comparing intravenous and inhalation anaesthesia. Br J Anaesth. 2003;91(5):631–7.

40. Royse CF, Andrews DT, Newman SN, et al. The influence of propofol or desflurane on postoperative cognitive dysfunction in patients undergoing coronary artery bypass surgery. Anaesthesia. 2011;66(6):455–64.

41. Hohener D, Blumenthal S, Borgeat A. Sedation and regional anaesthesia in the adult patient. Br J Anaesth. 2008;100(1):8–16.

42. Sieber FE, Zakriya KJ, Gottschalk A, et al. Sedation depth during spinal anesthesia and the development of postoperative delirium in elderly patients undergoing hip fracture repair. Mayo Clin Proc. 2010;85(1):18–26.

43. Radtke FM, Franck M, Lendner J, Kruger S, Wernecke KD, Spies CD. Monitoring depth of anaesthesia in a randomized trial

decreases the rate of postoperative delirium but not postoperative cognitive dysfunction. Br J Anaesth. 2013;110 Suppl 1:i98–105.

44. Apfel CC, Korttila K, Abdalla M, et al. A factorial trial of six interventions for the prevention of postoperative nausea and vomiting. N Engl J Med. 2004;350(24):2441–51.

45. Macario A, Weinger M, Carney S, Kim A. Which clinical anesthesia outcomes are important to avoid? The perspective of patients. Anesth Analg. 1999;89(3):652–8.

46. Tramer M, Moore A, McQuay H. Propofol anaesthesia and postoperative nausea and vomiting: quantitative systematic review of randomized controlled studies. Br J Anaesth. 1997;78(3):247–55.

47. Ziemann-Gimmel P, Goldfarb AA, Koppman J, Marema RT. - Opioid-free total intravenous anaesthesia reduces postoperative nausea and vomiting in bariatric surgery beyond triple prophylaxis. Br J Anaesth. 2014;112(5):906–11.

48. Cheng SS, Yeh J, Flood P. Anesthesia matters: patients anesthetized with propofol have less postoperative pain than those anesthetized with isoflurane. Anesth Analg. 2008;106(1):264–69, table of contents.

49. Mukherjee K, Seavell C, Rawlings E, Weiss A. A comparison of total intravenous with balanced anaesthesia for middle ear surgery: effects on postoperative nausea and vomiting, pain, and conditions of surgery. Anaesthesia. 2003;58(2):176–80.

50. Song JG, Shin JW, Lee EH, et al. Incidence of post-thoracotomy pain: a comparison between total intravenous anaesthesia and inhalation anaesthesia. Eur J Cardiothorac Surg. 2012;41(5):1078–82.

51. Robbertze R, Posner KL, Domino KB. Closed claims review of anesthesia for procedures outside the operating room. Curr Opin Anaesthesiol. 2006;19(4):436–42.

52. Pino RM. The nature of anesthesia and procedural sedation outside of the operating room. Curr Opin Anaesthesiol. 2007;20(4):347–51.

53. Melloni C. Anesthesia and sedation outside the operating room: how to prevent risk and maintain good quality. Curr Opin Anaesthesiol. 2007;20(6):513–9.

54. Gooden CK, Dilos B. Anesthesia for magnetic resonance imaging. Int Anesthesiol Clin. 2003;41(2):29–37.

55. Varma MK, Price K, Jayakrishnan V, Manickam B, Kessell G. Anaesthetic considerations for interventional neuroradiology. Br J Anaesth. 2007;99(1):75–85.

56. Castagnini HE, van Eijs F, Salevsky FC, Nathanson MH. Sevoflurane for interventional neuroradiology procedures is associated with more rapid early recovery than propofol. Can J Anaesth. 2004;51(5):486–91.

57. Brinjikji W, Murad MH, Rabinstein AA, Cloft HJ, Lanzino G, Kallmes DF. Conscious sedation versus general anesthesia during endovascular acute ischemic stroke treatment: a systematic review and meta-analysis. AJNR Am J Neuroradiol. 2015;36(3):525–9.

58. van den Berg LA, Koelman DL, Berkhemer OA, et al. Type of anesthesia and differences in clinical outcome after intra-arterial treatment for ischemic stroke. Stroke. 2015;46(5):1257–62.

59. Fox DJ, Davidson NC, Royle M, et al. Safety and acceptability of implantation of internal cardioverter-defibrillators under local anesthetic and conscious sedation. Pacing Clin Electrophysiol. 2007;30(8):992–7.

60. Manolis AS, Maounis T, Vassilikos V, Chiladakis J, Cokkinos DV. Electrophysiologist-implanted transvenous cardioverter defibrillators using local versus general anesthesia. Pacing Clin Electrophysiol. 2000;23(1):96–105.

61. Patel S, Vargo JJ, Khandwala F, et al. Deep sedation occurs frequently during elective endoscopy with meperidine and midazolam. Am J Gastroenterol. 2005;100(12):2689–95.

62. Sipe BW, Rex DK, Latinovich D, et al. Propofol versus midazolam/meperidine for outpatient colonoscopy: administration by nurses supervised by endoscopists. Gastrointest Endosc. 2002;55(7):815–25.

63. Rex DK, Heuss LT, Walker JA, Qi R. Trained registered nurses/endoscopy teams can administer propofol safely for endoscopy. Gastroenterology. 2005;129(5):1384–91.

64. Walker JA, McIntyre RD, Schleinitz PF, et al. Nurse-administered propofol sedation without anesthesia specialists in 9152 endoscopic cases in an ambulatory surgery center. Am J Gastroenterol. 2003;98(8):1744–50.

65. Akcaboy ZN, Akcaboy EY, Albayrak D, Altinoren B, Dikmen B, Gogus N. Can remifentanil be a better choice than propofol for colonoscopy during monitored anesthesia care? Acta Anaesthesiol Scand. 2006;50(6):736–41.

66. Rudner R, Jalowiecki P, Kawecki P, Gonciarz M, Mularczyk A, Petelenz M. Conscious analgesia/sedation with remifentanil and propofol versus total intravenous anesthesia with fentanyl, midazolam, and propofol for outpatient colonoscopy. Gastrointest Endosc. 2003;57(6):657–63.

67. Cooper GS, Kou TD, Rex DK. Complications following colonoscopy with anesthesia assistance: a population-based analysis. JAMA Intern Med. 2013;173(7):551–6.

68. Agostoni M, Fanti L, Arcidiacono PG, et al. Midazolam and pethidine versus propofol and fentanyl patient controlled sedation/analgesia for upper gastrointestinal tract ultrasound endoscopy: a prospective randomized controlled trial. Dig Liver Dis. 2007;39(11):1024–9.

69. Fanti L, Gemma M, Agostoni M, et al. Target controlled infusion for non-anaesthesiologist propofol sedation during gastrointestinal endoscopy: the first double blind randomized controlled trial. Dig Liver Dis. 2015;47(7):566–71.

70. Pambianco DJ, Vargo JJ, Pruitt RE, Hardi R, Martin JF. - Computer-assisted personalized sedation for upper endoscopy and colonoscopy: a comparative, multicenter randomized study. Gastrointest Endosc. 2011;73(4):765–72.

71. Kollef MH, Levy NT, Ahrens TS, Schaiff R, Prentice D, Sherman G. The use of continuous i.v. sedation is associated with prolongation of mechanical ventilation. Chest. 1998;114(2):541–8.

72. Pandharipande P, Shintani A, Peterson J, et al. Lorazepam is an independent risk factor for transitioning to delirium in intensive care unit patients. Anesthesiology. 2006;104(1):21–6.

73. Payen JF, Bosson JL, Chanques G, Mantz J, Labarere J. Pain assessment is associated with decreased duration of mechanical ventilation in the intensive care unit: a post Hoc analysis of the DOLOREA study. Anesthesiology. 2009;111(6):1308–16.

74. Treggiari MM, Romand JA, Yanez ND, et al. Randomized trial of light versus deep sedation on mental health after critical illness. Crit Care Med. 2009;37(9):2527–34.

75. Kress JP, Pohlman AS, O'Connor MF, Hall JB. Daily interruption of sedative infusions in critically ill patients undergoing mechanical ventilation. N Engl J Med. 2000;342(20):1471–7.

76. Girard TD, Kress JP, Fuchs BD, et al. Efficacy and safety of a paired sedation and ventilator weaning protocol for mechanically ventilated patients in intensive care (Awakening and Breathing Controlled trial): a randomised controlled trial. Lancet. 2008;371(9607):126–34.

77. Schweickert WD, Pohlman MC, Pohlman AS, et al. Early physical and occupational therapy in mechanically ventilated, critically ill patients: a randomised controlled trial. Lancet. 2009;373(9678):1874–82.

78. Balas MC, Vasilevskis EE, Olsen KM, et al. Effectiveness and safety of the awakening and breathing coordination, delirium monitoring/management, and early exercise/mobility bundle. Crit Care Med. 2014;42:1024–36.

79. Shehabi Y, Bellomo R, Reade MC, et al. Early intensive care sedation predicts long-term mortality in ventilated critically ill patients. Am J Respir Crit Care Med. 2012;186(8):724–31.

80. Strom T, Martinussen T, Toft P. A protocol of no sedation for critically ill patients receiving mechanical ventilation: a randomised trial. Lancet. 2010;375(9713):475–80.

81. Pandharipande PP, Pun BT, Herr DL, et al. Effect of sedation with dexmedetomidine vs lorazepam on acute brain dysfunction in mechanically ventilated patients: the MENDS randomized controlled trial. JAMA. 2007;298(22):2644–53.

82. Dahaba AA, Grabner T, Rehak PH, List WF, Metzler H. Remifentanil versus morphine analgesia and sedation for mechanically ventilated critically ill patients: a randomized double blind study. Anesthesiology. 2004;101(3):640–6.

83. Muellejans B, Lopez A, Cross MH, Bonome C, Morrison L, Kirkham AJ. Remifentanil versus fentanyl for analgesia based sedation to provide patient comfort in the intensive care unit: a randomized, double-blind controlled trial [ISRCTN43755713]. Crit Care. 2004;8(1):R1–11.

84. Morrison RS, Magaziner J, Gilbert M, et al. Relationship between pain and opioid analgesics on the development of delirium following hip fracture. J Gerontol A Biol Sci Med Sci. 2003;58(1):76–81.

85. Agarwal V, O'Neill PJ, Cotton BA, et al. Prevalence and risk factors for development of delirium in burn intensive care unit patients. J Burn Care Res. 2010;31(5):706–15.

86. Pandharipande P, Cotton BA, Shintani A, et al. Prevalence and risk factors for development of delirium in surgical and trauma intensive care unit patients. J Trauma. 2008;65(1):34–41.

87. Dubois MJ, Bergeron N, Dumont M, Dial S, Skrobik Y. Delirium in an intensive care unit: a study of risk factors. Intensive Care Med. 2001;27(8):1297–304.

88. Marcantonio ER, Juarez G, Goldman L, et al. The relationship of postoperative delirium with psychoactive medications. JAMA. 1994;272(19):1518–22.

89. Lynch EP, Lazor MA, Gellis JE, Orav J, Goldman L, Marcantonio ER. The impact of postoperative pain on the development of postoperative delirium. Anesth Analg. 1998;86(4):781–5.

90. Vaurio LE, Sands LP, Wang Y, Mullen EA, Leung JM. Postoperative delirium: the importance of pain and pain management. Anesth Analg. 2006;102(4):1267–73.

91. Rozendaal FW, Spronk PE, Snellen FF, et al. Remifentanil-propofol analgo-sedation shortens duration of ventilation and length of ICU stay compared to a conventional regimen: a centre randomised, cross-over, open-label study in the Netherlands. Intensive Care Med. 2009;35(2):291–8.

92. Breen D, Karabinis A, Malbrain M, et al. Decreased duration of mechanical ventilation when comparing analgesia-based sedation using remifentanil with standard hypnotic-based sedation for up to 10 days in intensive care unit patients: a randomised trial [ISRCTN47583497]. Crit Care. 2005;9(3):R200–10.

93. Karabinis A, Mandragos K, Stergiopoulos S, et al. Safety and efficacy of analgesia-based sedation with remifentanil versus standard hypnotic-based regimens in intensive care unit patients with brain injuries: a randomised, controlled trial [ISRCTN50308308]. Crit Care. 2004;8(4):R268–80.

94. Bioc JJ, Magee C, Cucchi J, et al. Cost effectiveness of a benzodiazepine vs a nonbenzodiazepine-based sedation regimen for mechanically ventilated, critically ill adults. J Crit Care. 2014;29 (5):753–7.

95. Barrientos-Vega R, Mar Sanchez-Soria M, Morales-Garcia C, Robas-Gomez A, Cuena-Boy R, Ayensa-Rincon A. Prolonged sedation of critically ill patients with midazolam or propofol: impact on weaning and costs. Crit Care Med. 1997;25(1):33–40.

96. Carson SS, Kress JP, Rodgers JE, et al. A randomized trial of intermittent lorazepam versus propofol with daily interruption in mechanically ventilated patients. Crit Care Med. 2006;34 (5):1326–32.

97. Venn RM, Grounds RM. Comparison between dexmedetomidine and propofol for sedation in the intensive care unit: patient and clinician perceptions. Br J Anaesth. 2001;87(5):684–90.

98. Herr DL, Sum-Ping ST, England M. ICU sedation after coronary artery bypass graft surgery: dexmedetomidine-based versus propofol-based sedation regimens. J Cardiothorac Vasc Anesth. 2003;17(5):576–84.

99. Shehabi Y, Grant P, Wolfenden H, et al. Prevalence of delirium with dexmedetomidine compared with morphine based therapy after cardiac surgery: a randomized controlled trial (DEXmedetomidine COmpared to Morphine-DEXCOM Study). Anesthesiology. 2009;111(5):1075–84.

100. Ji F, Li Z, Nguyen H, et al. Perioperative dexmedetomidine improves outcomes of cardiac surgery. Circulation. 2013;127(15):1576–84.

101. Djaiani G, Silverton N, Fedorko L, et al. Dexmedetomidine versus propofol sedation reduces delirium after cardiac surgery: a randomized controlled trial. Anesthesiology. 2016;124(2):362–8.

102. Jakob SM, Ruokonen E, Grounds RM, et al. Dexmedetomidine vs midazolam or propofol for sedation during prolonged mechanical ventilation: two randomized controlled trials. JAMA. 2012;307 (11):1151–60.

103. Reade MC, Eastwood GM, Bellomo R, et al. Effect of dexmedetomidine added to standard care on ventilator-free time in patients with agitated delirium: a randomized clinical trial. JAMA. 2016;315:1460–8.

104. Carrasco G, Baeza N, Cabre L, et al. Dexmedetomidine for the treatment of hyperactive delirium refractory to haloperidol in nonintubated ICU patients: a nonrandomized controlled trial. Crit Care Med. 2016;44:1295–306.

105. Dasta JF, Kane-Gill SL, Pencina M, et al. A cost-minimization analysis of dexmedetomidine compared with midazolam for long-term sedation in the intensive care unit. Crit Care Med. 2010;38 (2):497–503.

The Benefit and Future of Pharmacogenetics

Janko Samardzic, Dubravka Svob Strac, and John N. van den Anker

Introduction

In recent years pharmacogenetics has received major attention in many areas of medicine, giving the potential basis of precision medicine in the near future. Determination of genetic factors of prognostic value for a target drug choice and dosing regimen will improve the safe and effective use of medicines in patients of all ages. Individual differences in pharmacological responses might lead to serious clinical problems such as difficulties in reaching optimal efficacy, appearance of drug interactions, and adverse drug reactions (ADRs). Based upon the current knowledge, it is clear that an early adjustment of a therapy regimen using genetic characteristics of a patient can help prevent some of these side effects [1]. Thus, the application of pharmacogenetics might have a great potential in helping providers to reduce and prevent ADRs and to improve therapeutic drug efficacy [2].

The therapeutic response of an individual patient to a certain drug is influenced by numerous factors such as pharmacokinetics, age, gender, ethnicity, as well as multiple drug therapy [3]. Even when taking all of these factors into account, it is still hard to assess the probability of appearance of ADRs as well as the efficacy of a certain drug in different individuals. The differences in response of a patient to pharmacotherapy could, at least in part, be explained by genetically determined differences in drug metabolism and distribution, or by variability in target proteins responsible for the drug's mechanism of action [4]. The impact of genetically determined factors on the efficacy of drugs was already established in 1956, when it was shown that the hemolytic reaction to the antimalarial drug primaquine could be attributed to the hereditary deficiency of glucose-6-phosphate dehydrogenase [5]. Furthermore, it has been well established that individual variations of drug serum concentrations among patients may arise from genetically determined variations in the cytochrome P450 (CYP450) family.

The link between activity of drugs and genetic polymorphisms of transporter proteins, drug metabolizing enzymes, and drug target molecules has attracted a lot of attention during the last decades. Genetically determined variations of enzymes responsible for the metabolism of drugs, as well as proteins participating in the transport of drugs, could significantly change the pharmacokinetic (PK) properties of drugs [6]. Alterations at the level of target proteins can lead to reduced affinity of the specific drug at the site of its action, therefore having an effect on the pharmacodynamic (PD) properties of that drug [7]. Moreover, a connection between genes that are responsible for the severity of illness and efficacy of drugs has also been established, despite the fact that these genes do not have a direct influence upon the PK and PD properties of a drug.

J. Samardzic, MD, PhD
Institute of Pharmacology, Clinical Pharmacology and Toxicology, Medical Faculty, University of Belgrade, Dr Subotica 1, Belgrade, Serbia

Division of Paediatric Pharmacology and Pharmacometrics, University of Basel Children's Hospital, Spitalstrasse 33, Basel CH-4056, Switzerland

D. Svob Strac, PhD
Laboratory for Molecular Neuropharmacology, Division of Molecular Medicine, Rudjer Boskovic Institute, Bijenicka cesta 54, Zagreb, Croatia

J.N. van den Anker, MD, PhD (✉)
Division of Paediatric Pharmacology and Pharmacometrics, University of Basel Children's Hospital, Spitalstrasse 33, Basel CH-4056, Switzerland

Division of Pediatric Clinical Pharmacology, Children's National Medical Center, Washington, DC, USA

Intensive Care and Department of Pediatric Surgery, Erasmus MC Sophia Children's Hospital, Rotterdam, The Netherlands
e-mail: JVandena@childrensnational.org

© Springer International Publishing AG 2017
A.R. Absalom, K.P. Mason (eds.), *Total Intravenous Anesthesia and Target Controlled Infusions*,
DOI 10.1007/978-3-319-47609-4_38

Pharmacogenetics and Pharmacogenomics

Pharmacology is the study of how drugs work in the body and genetics is the study of how characteristics that result from the action of genes acting together are inherited and how they function in human cells. Pharmacogenetics itself represents the study of genetic variations that are responsible for variable responses to drugs among patients [8]. According to the FDA-approved definitions, pharmacogenetics is the study of variations in DNA sequence as related to drug response. This term is commonly used synonymously with pharmacogenomics. However, pharmacogenetics generally refers to the variations of a single gene or few genes influencing the response to drugs, whereas pharmacogenomics focuses on genome-wide alterations in drug response, i.e. the whole spectrum of genes that will determine drug efficacy and safety by their mutual interaction [9]. Moreover, epigenetic factors can also cause profound alterations of drug action. The majority of current research that examines the link between genes and patient responses to a drug therapy are essentially pharmacogenetic studies. Considering the fact that there are a large number of proteins needed for eliciting a drug response, an increasing number of researchers start to refer to a pharmacogenomics approach in order to clarify this complex connection between genetic variations and patient responses to a drug. Finally, the ultimate goal of pharmacogenetics/pharmacogenomics is the same—optimizing therapy and reducing the incidence of ADRs and toxic effects. The results of genetic research will eventually enable clinicians to use genetic tests in order to anticipate patient's response to a therapy and to select appropriate drugs based on the patient's DNA profile, as well as to develop new strategies for treating and preventing diseases by adjusting the drug therapy to the patient's genotype [10].

Types of Genetic Variability

The term pharmacogenomics is used to describe how inherited variations in genes modulating drug actions are related to inter-individual variability in drug response. Such variability in drug action may be pharmacokinetic (PK) or pharmacodynamic (PD). PK variability refers to variability in a drug's absorption, distribution, metabolism, and excretion that mediates its efficacy and toxicity. The molecules involved in these processes include drug metabolizing enzymes and drug transport molecules that mediate drug uptake into and efflux from intracellular sites. Pharmacodynamic variability refers to variable drug effects despite equivalent drug delivery to molecular sites of action. This may reflect variability in the function of the molecular target of the drug or in the pathophysiological context in which the drug interacts with its target molecule [11] (Fig. 38.1).

Pharmacokinetic Variability due to Genetic Polymorphisms

Polymorphisms of enzymes responsible for the metabolism of drugs represent the first studied examples of genetic variations that cause changes in the effect and/or toxicity of drugs. The majority of enzymes belonging to phase I metabolism are enzymes of the CYP superfamily, while glutathione-S-transferase, N-acetyltransferase and thiopurine-S-methyltransferase are examples of enzymes involved in phase II metabolism of drugs, showing genetic polymorphisms [12]. Although over 50 CYP isoforms have been characterized, only five of them appear to be responsible for most of all P450 activity. CYP3A4/5 is the most abundant (36 %), followed by CYP2D6 (19 %), CYP2C8/9 (16 %), CYP1A1/2 (11 %), and CYP2C19 (8 %). The remaining CYP-mediated metabolism is carried out primarily by CYP2A6, CYP2B6, and CYP2E1 [13] (Fig. 38.2).

The activities of CYP enzymes are genetically determined, and for some isoforms, the existence of a genetic polymorphism has been demonstrated. Functional genetic polymorphism has been established for CYP1A2, CYP2A6, CYP2C9, CYP2C19, CYP2D6, CYP3A4/5 [14, 15]. A polymorphism represents the occurrence of two or more alleles at one locus in the same population with a frequency of more than 1 % [16]. In the presence of a genetic polymorphism, individuals within a given population are divided into at least two phenotypes, poor metabolizers and extensive metabolizers, according to their abilities to metabolize a specific probe drug. Poor or slow metabolizers have deficient metabolizing ability and generally will have higher parent drug concentrations and are more likely to exert side effects or toxicity when the parent compound is metabolized exclusively by the polymorphic enzyme. On the other hand, extensive metabolizers may show subtherapeutic levels at usual doses or need higher doses to obtain a therapeutic response. Besides the P450 genes, other phase I enzymes are polymorphic, such as alcohol dehydrogenases, acetaldehyde dehydrogenase and dihydropyrimidine dehydrogenase, relevant for the clearance of ethanol and some anticancer drugs [17].

There are several enzyme families that conjugate drugs or their oxidative metabolites. N-acetyltransferase (NAT) was the first drug metabolizing enzyme for which a genetic polymorphism was discovered. Slow acetylators show a greater therapeutic response than fast acetylators to several drugs but may be more susceptible to side-effects [18]. Furthermore, there are 15 human uridine diphosphate glucuronosyltransferases (UGTs), broadly classified into the UGT1 and UGT2 families [19, 20]. The clinical implications of polymorphisms of these drug metabolizing enzymes may be therapeutic failure and drug toxicity.

Fig. 38.1 Pharmacogenetics: PK-PD interface

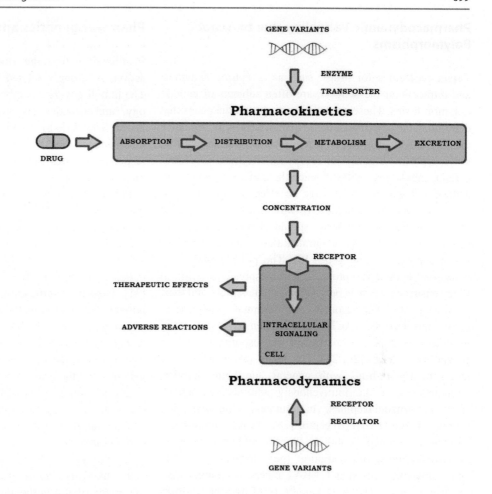

However, the clinical relevance depends on the therapeutic ratio of the drug [21].

Different transmembrane proteins facilitate transport of drugs through the gastrointestinal tract, passage through the blood–brain barrier, and excretion through bile and urine. Genetic variations can affect drug distribution, as well its concentration on its site of action. There are also genetic variations in transporters genes, and current studies indicate that membrane transporters influence drug absorption in different body compartments as well as the speed of absorption [10]. The best studied protein showing polymorphism due to genetic variations is P-glycoprotein also called multi-drug resistant P-glycoprotein. It represents an ATP-dependent efflux pump and can be found in many cells, such as proximal tubular cells, intestinal enterocytes, and endothelial cells of the blood–brain barrier [22–24]. At the blood–brain barrier, P-glycoprotein may influence the uptake of drugs into the brain: reduced P-glycoprotein activity could lead to abnormally increased accumulation in the brain and undesired side effects of a drug, while high P-glycoprotein levels may limit the uptake of sufficient amounts of the desired drug into the brain [25].

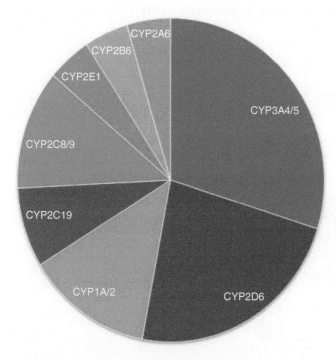

Fig. 38.2 Cytochrome P450 (CYPs) family

Pharmacodynamic Variability due to Genetic Polymorphisms

Target molecules for drugs, such as receptors, enzymes, and intracellular messengers, are often subjects of genetic polymorphisms. These genes interacting with the genes that determine the pharmacokinetic parameters will influence the final effect of a drug. Current research has shown that polymorphism of genes for receptors, enzymes, and intracellular messengers will influence the patient's response to a drug and will therefore have an effect on efficacy and safety of the applied therapy. However, it should be noted that the appearance of ADRs should also be attributed to genetic polymorphisms of intracellular signal protein and ion transporter coding genes [6]. The polymorphisms in genes that encode receptors cause widespread variation in drug sensitivity, such as beta-adrenergic receptors and their sensitivity to beta-agonists in asthma, angiotensin converting enzyme (ACE) and its sensitivity to ACE inhibitors, or 5-HT receptors and the response to certain psychotropic drugs [26, 27]. The major candidate for the target of most drugs with general anesthetic activity, including all of the intravenously administered agents such as benzodiazepines, barbiturates, etomidate and propofol is the GABA$_A$ receptor [28]. As receptor subunit composition influences both the function and pharmacology of GABA$_A$ receptors, variation (polymorphisms) in the genes encoding different GABA$_A$ receptor subunits may underlie pharmacodynamic variability of anesthetic drugs (Fig. 38.3).

Pharmacogenetics and Intravenous Anesthesia

Pharmacogenetics, the study of genetic effects on drug action, is strongly related to the field of anesthesia [29]. The first discoveries combining anesthesiology, pharmacology, and genetics appeared in 1959, when a German researcher, Friedrich Vögel, defined the concept of pharmacogenetics, as a science of genetically conditioned responses to drugs. Shortly after, Simpson and Kalow [30] in their studies on a muscle relaxing drug—succinylcholine, discovered the polymorphism of hydrolysis associated with plasma pseudocholinesterase which fails to guarantee appropriate metabolism of this agent. As a consequence, an appropriate dose of succinylcholine can lead to undesirable side effects due to excessively decreased biotransformation in patients suffering from cholinesterase enzymopathy [31]. Further identification of metabolic pathways made it possible to determine the specific genes that encode the enzymes involved in drug metabolism. These discoveries were accompanied by the development of nucleic acid analysis methods that resulted in the sequencing of the human genome, and the characterization of over 3.1 million human single nucleotide polymorphisms [32]. Mapping the genome enabled a lot of research that accelerated the discovery of genetic variations influencing pathogenesis and therapy of certain diseases.

Besides pseudocholinesterase deficiency, another genetically linked disorder in the field of anesthesiology, seen as a major contributor to the advancement of pharmacogenetics, is malignant hyperthermia (MH) [33]. MH is a rare

Fig. 38.3 The binding sites of anesthetic drugs on GABA$_A$ receptor

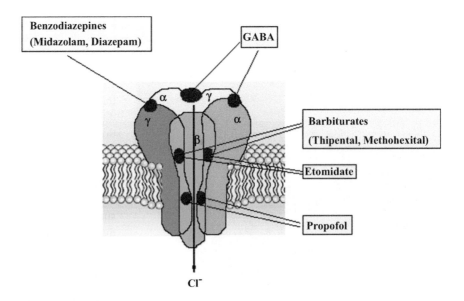

Table 38.1 Pharmacogenetically relevant CYP/UGT enzymes involved in the metabolism of intravenous anesthetics

CYP/UGT Enzymes	Intravenous anesthetics	References
CYP2A6	Ketamine, dexmedetomidine	[110, 119, 121–123]
CYP3A4/5	Ketamine, midazolam, diazepam	[65–71, 110]
CYP2B6	Propofol, ketamine	[38, 43, 107, 108]
CYP2C9	Propofol, diazepam, etomidate	[27, 38, 41, 88]
CYP2C19	Ketamine, diazepam, barbiturates	[27, 72, 73, 110]
UGT1A9	Propofol	[27, 43]
UGT2B4, 2B7, 2B15	Lorazepam	[75–77]

autosomal dominant genetic disease of skeletal muscle calcium metabolism that is triggered by application of halogenated inhalation agents and/or succinylcholine in susceptible individuals. MH susceptibility was initially linked to the ryanodine receptor gene locus on chromosome 19q, but it is becoming increasingly clear that it results from a complex interaction between multiple genes and environmental factors. There are almost 50 mutations that have been found to be associated with MH [34]. Because of polygenic determinism and variable penetrance, direct DNA testing in the general population for MH susceptibility is currently not recommended. However, the caffeine halothane contracture test may be useful for identification of people with MH susceptibility. Although the test is very specific, only about 25 % of the people at risk for MH are detected because of the multiple areas of MH mutations [35].

In total intravenous anesthesia, special attention is focused on the individual metabolic variability that is increasingly reported in the literature (Table 38.1). It has been shown that the metabolism of the applied substances depends on genetic polymorphisms of enzymes involved in the biotransformation of the intravenous anesthetics, or mediating its action such as receptor proteins [36–38]. Furthermore, an understanding of the CYP system and its substrates is also a key factor in the prevention of important drug–drug interactions, either as a result of enzyme induction or inhibition. It is also important to take into consideration to what extent aging and environmental factors (smoking, alcohol, diet, or other drugs) interact with genetic factors to modulate drug effects. Therefore, we summarize here the current available information related to pharmacogenetics/pharmacogenomics (PG) and its application to anesthetic agents commonly used in total intravenous anesthesia.

Propofol

Propofol (2,6-diisopropylphenol) is one of the most commonly applied agents in intravenous general anesthesia [39]. It is usually available as a 1 or 2 % emulsion which contains soya bean oil and purified egg phosphatide. It was introduced into clinical practice in the 1970s, and an important advantage is its rapid onset of deep anesthesia. The recovery from propofol is rapid and the incidence of nausea, vomiting is extremely low, particularly when it is used as the sole anesthetic agent [40]. Pain on injection occurs in a high proportion of patients when the drug is injected into small hand veins; this can be minimized by injection into larger veins or by prior administration of 1 % lidocaine. Propofol causes a proportional reduction in cerebral metabolism, cerebral blood flow and intracranial pressure, but the associated decrease in systemic blood pressure may also decrease cerebral perfusion pressure. Cortical EEG changes produced by propofol resemble those of barbiturates and its neuroprotective effect may reflect antioxidant properties. It produces dose-dependent depression of ventilation, and apnea occurs in 25–35 % of patients after induction of anesthesia. Propofol does not trigger MH and may be considered the induction drug of choice in patients who are susceptible to MH [11].

About 70 % of propofol serum concentration is metabolized into propofol glucuronide, for which UDP-glucuronosyltransferase, coded by the UDP glucuronosyltransferase 1 family, polypeptide A9 (UGT1A9) gene is responsible [41]. An alternative pathway of propofol biotransformation (approximately 29 %) is dependent on enzymes coded by CYP2C9, CYP2B6, NQO1, and SULT1A genes. So far experiments indicate a relationship between patients' response to propofol during general anesthesia and polymorphisms of these genes [38]. After the action of CYP2B6 and CYP2C9 enzymes, 4-hydroxypropofol is formed and the end-products include: 2,6-diisopropyl-1,4-benzoquinone with the NQO1 participation, 1- and 4-hydroxypropofol 1-O-β-D-glucuronide with the UGT participation and 4-hydroxypropofol sulfate as a result of the action of the SULT1A enzyme [41, 42]. However, a recent pilot study by Loryan et al. [43] showed no significant effects of CYP2B6 and UGT1A9 single nucleotide polymorphisms or age on propofol biotransformation, but there was a pronounced effect of sex as an important factor for the systemic clearance of propofol, indicating higher amounts of propofol glucuronide in women.

It is well known that the mechanism of propofol action is based on its interaction with the $GABA_A$ (gamma-aminobutyric acid type A) ionotropic receptor inhibiting the transfer of nerve impulses between neurons in the central nervous system [44]. In recent years, the complex structure and function of GABA$_A$ receptor complex and its binding sites have been elucidated [45]. GABA$_A$ receptor complex is made up of pentameric transmembrane proteins that make the associated ion channel selectively permeable to chloride anion. These are mainly localized in synapses, especially on the postsynaptic membrane [46]. Activation of GABA$_A$ receptors leads to a change in the conformational state of the associated ion channel, which results in an increased permeability for chloride ions [47]. So far, 19 subunits of GABA$_A$ receptor complex have been cloned, which are classified into several structurally related subfamilies, that comprise highly homologous isoforms (α 1–6, β 1–3, γ 1–3, δ, ε, θ, π, ρ 1–3) [48]. The dominant receptor isoform in the central nervous system consists of $\alpha1$, $\beta2$, and $\gamma2$ subunits. The activity of the receptor is regulated by the binding of GABA, but it also contains domains recognizing anesthetics. In the case of propofol, these include mainly $\beta3$ and $\beta2$ subunits but also $\beta1$ [49]. Receptor activation results in the hyperpolarization of the neuron membrane and, hence, prevents the development of an action potential. It takes place as the result of the intensification of the influence of GABA on its receptor or by way of a direct induction caused by the anesthetic agent [50]. It was proven that the activation of the receptor as a result of propofol action (3 µg/ml) was the strongest after 2 min and the hyperpolarization of the neuron membrane lasted up to 10 s [38].

Genetic mutations of GABA$_A$ receptors have been implicated in multiple disorders, as described in a recent review [51]. Genes encoding GABA$_A$ receptor subunits are situated in cluster forms on 5q34, Xq28, 4p12, and 15 chromosomes. Nineteen genes have been discovered so far including GABRB2 coding subunit $\beta2$ as well as GABRA1, GABRA3, GABRB3, GABRG1, and GABRG3 genes [52]. Data from the literature indicate that the course of general anesthesia is also affected by GABRG2 gene polymorphism. Furthermore, the four polymorphic variations (20118C/T, 20326C/T, 20502 A/T, and 358G/T) in the GABRE gene showed no statistically significant correlation with the anesthesia induction time, but the impact of this gene on propofol anesthesia cannot be excluded [53].

Barbiturates

Thiopental and methohexital are derivatives of barbituric acid, formulated as alkaline racemic mixtures of their water-soluble sodium salts. They are both potent hypnotics, although methohexital is about 3 times more potent than thiopental. Hence, a dose of 3–5 mg/kg of thiopental and 1–1.5 mg/kg of methohexital usually produces anesthesia within 30 s after i.v. injection. Recovery after a single dose is relatively rapid (5–10 min with thiopental and 2–3 min with methohexital) due to redistribution, and there is a low incidence of restlessness, nausea, and vomiting. Due to their dose-dependent CNS depression ranging from sedation to general anesthesia, barbiturates are clinically applied for rapid intravenous induction of anesthesia. However, a continuous i.v. infusion of barbiturates to maintain anesthesia is rarely used because of their long context-sensitive half-time and prolonged recovery period.

In plasma, both thiopental and methohexital are predominantly (65–85 %) bound to protein, mostly albumin. Metabolism of these barbiturates occurs mainly in the liver by oxidation, but also by N-dealkylation, desulfuration, and destruction of the barbituric acid ring structure. The resulting metabolites are inactive and excreted mainly by kidneys in the urine or, conjugated to glucuronic acid and excreted in bile. In standard induction doses first order kinetics are observed, whereas at higher doses metabolism follows zero order kinetics, which means that a constant amount of drug is being eliminated per hour, irrespective of the plasma concentration [54]. Methohexital is cleared more rapidly by the liver in comparison to thiopental, and has a shorter elimination half-time [55]. Regarding the metabolism of barbiturates, they produce time-dependent effects on the hepatic microsomal enzyme system (cytochrome P450 (CYP) enzymes). The impact of their genetic polymorphisms on barbiturate metabolism still remains to be further elucidated [56]. In addition, barbiturates interact with various CYPs, and may inhibit the biotransformation of other CYP substrates and vice versa. Chronic barbiturate treatment produces induction of the microsomal enzymes (CYPs 1A2, 2C9, 2C19, and 3A4) increasing the metabolism of drugs metabolized by these enzymes. Consequently, larger dosages of those medications are required in order to achieve therapeutic effect, and barbiturate tolerance may develop due to increased barbiturate metabolism. On the other hand, barbiturate dose requirements could be reduced by pharmacokinetic effects due to anemia, hypoproteinemia, low cardiac output or shock [55].

Barbiturates are relatively non-selective compounds that bind to an entire superfamily of ligand-gated ion channels, and act by both enhancement of inhibitory neurotransmission and inhibition of excitatory transmission [57, 58]. Barbiturates mediate their anesthetic action by acting as positive allosteric modulators, and at higher doses as agonists at the inhibitory GABA$_A$ receptor, as well as by blocking AMPA and kainate glutamate receptors. The binding of barbiturates to the distinct binding site on GABA$_A$ receptor requires the β subunit [59]. In addition, a mutation in the GABA$_A$ α subunit abolishes the action of barbiturates [60]. Genetic variation in the genes encoding various subunits of GABA$_A$ receptor may be important for the sensitivity to barbiturates [27]. For instance, a human GABA$_A$

receptore subunit, encoded by the GABRE gene on chromosome Xq28 [61], confers insensitivity to the potentiating effects of i.v. anesthetic agents on GABAergic transmission.

Via stimulation of δ-aminolevulinic acid (ALA) synthetase, the rate-limiting enzyme of heme synthesis in the liver, barbiturates, especially thiopental, can increase the production of porphyrins and should therefore not be administered to patients susceptible to development of acute porphyria. The porphyrias are a group of genetic disorders characterized by overproduction and excretion of porphyrins as a consequence of partial deficiencies in the heme biosynthesis pathway [62]. Acute Intermittent Porphyria (AIP) is caused by a deficiency in porphobilinogen PBG deaminase, and has an incidence of 1:20,000 in Europe. It is an autosomal dominant disease encoded by gene located on chromosome 11. On the other hand, in South Africa Variegate Porphyria is the most common porphyria with an incidence of around 1: 250 to 1:500 and it is due to a deficiency in protoporphyrinogen oxidase. The gene for this enzyme is found on chromosome 1. The genes, encoding for the deficient enzymes in hereditary and plumboporphyria, are both situated on chromosome 9. Barbiturates such as thiopental are contraindicated in patients with porphyria as they may precipitate an attack, manifested by severe abdominal pain, nausea, vomiting, psychiatric disorders, and neurologic abnormalities [63]. The effect of thiopental in other hereditary diseases should also be considered. As such, thiopental should be used with caution in patients with dystrophia myotonica, myasthenia gravis, and familiar periodic paralysis.

Benzodiazepines

The typical benzodiazepines (BDZs) of primary interest to anesthesiologists are midazolam, diazepam, and lorazepam. These drugs are primarily used as preoperative medication and adjuvant therapy because of their anxiolytic, amnestic, and sedative effects [11]. Midazolam is a water-soluble agent that produces minimal irritation after intramuscular or intravenous injection. Once exposed to physiologic pH it becomes more lipid-soluble. Diazepam and lorazepam are lipid-soluble and their formulations contain propylene glycol, a tissue irritant that causes venous irritation and pain on injection site. BDZs generally undergo hepatic metabolism via oxidation and glucuronide conjugation [40]. The hepatic clearance rate of midazolam is ten times greater than that of diazepam and five times greater than that of lorazepam. The primary metabolite of midazolam is 1-hydroxymethylmidazolam and it has some CNS depressant activity, and diazepam is metabolized to active metabolites, which may prolong its effects. Lorazepam is directly conjugated to glucuronide acid to form inactive metabolites. The half-life

for diazepam and lorazepam is prolonged compared to midazolam, therefore only midazolam should be used for continuous infusion [11].

BDZs decrease cerebral metabolism and cerebral blood flow analogous to propofol and barbiturates, but they do not show neuroprotective activity in humans. BDZs produce dose-dependent depression of ventilation. In contrast to all other sedative-hypnotic drugs like barbiturates, there is a specific antagonist for BDZs—flumazenil [64]. It has a high affinity for the benzodiazepine binding site of GABA$_A$ receptors and possesses minimal intrinsic activity. It acts as a competitive antagonist in the presence of benzodiazepine agonist compounds. Most BDZs are highly lipophilic and undergo extensive metabolism by CYP enzymes to increase elimination. There are wide interindividual variations in their biotransformation, resulting in pronounced differences in plasma concentrations. They are primarily metabolized by the polymorphically expressed CYP2C19 and CYP3A4/5. Other CYPs, especially CYP1A2 and CYP2C9, may also contribute to the metabolism of some BDZs [65].

Midazolam is being extensively used in premedication for operations and sedation for minor surgical procedures. The metabolites of midazolam are 1'-hydroxymidazolam and 4'-hydroxymidazolam. It has been shown that CYP3A5 converted midazolam to 1'-hydroxymidazolam more than CYP3A4 did in an in vitro experiment [66]. Kuehl et al. [67] reported that the midazolam hydroxylation activity was more than twofold higher in livers with CYP3A5*1/*3 genotype than in those with CYP3A5*3/*3. Similarly, Wong et al. [68] demonstrated that midazolam clearance after an oral or intravenous dose was about 1.5 times higher in the CYP3A5*1/*3 genotype than in the CYP3A5*3/*3 genotype in patients receiving chemotherapy. However, some research groups have shown that the pharmacokinetics of midazolam and 1'-hydroxymidazolam after an intravenous or oral dose of midazolam was independent of the number of the CYP3A5*3 allele [65, 69, 70]. Therefore, the effect of the polymorphism of CYP3A5 on the pharmacokinetics of midazolam is still inconclusive.

For diazepam, N-demethylation is catalyzed by CYP3A4 and CYP2C19, whereas the 3-hydroxylation is catalyzed mainly by CYP3A4 in liver microsomes [71]. Poor metabolizers of CYP2C19 showed significantly lower clearance (12 vs. 26 mL/min) and longer elimination half-life (88 vs. 41 h) of diazepam than extensive metabolizers after a single oral dose [72]. Furthermore, poor metabolizers had lower clearance and longer elimination half-life of desmethyldiazepam. It was reported that the area under the plasma concentration–time curve (AUC) and elimination half-life of both diazepam and desmethyldiazepam increased significantly according to the increase in mutated CYP2C19 alleles, suggesting significant effects of the gene-dose of

CYP2C19 on their metabolism [73]. These studies suggest that the CYP2C19 polymorphism affects the disposition of both diazepam and desmethyldiazepam. Nevertheless, pharmacodynamic effects were not evaluated in these studies, thus the clinical significance of the pharmacokinetic changes observed remains to be elucidated.

Lorazepam is a 3-hydroxy-1,4-benzodiazepine. Owing to the presence of the 3-hydroxy group, lorazepam exists as pairs of enantiomers: S,R-lorazepam. It is cleared predominantly by conjugation with glucuronic acid in humans [74]; however, the enantioselective glucuronidation of lorazepam needs attention. It was demonstrated that both S- and R-lorazepam were glucuronidated by UGT2B15, 2B7, and 2B4, whereas R-lorazepam was additionally metabolized by extrahepatic enzymes UGT1A7 and 1A10 [75]. A significant contribution of UGT2B15 to lorazepam glucuronidation is supported by the observation that the lorazepam clearance was 42 % lower in subjects homozygous for the UGT2B15*2 allele compared with subjects who were homozygous for wild-type UGT2B15*1 [76]. An investigation of the influence of UGT2B7 polymorphism on lorazepam disposition demonstrated that its clearance was not significantly different between subjects with the UGT2B7*1 and *2 genotypes [77]. The effect of polymorphisms of UGT2B4, 1A7, and 1A10 on the pharmacokinetics of lorazepam is still inconclusive. Since altered lorazepam clearance may impact efficacy and safety, further studies were performed to investigate potential drug–drug interactions arising from inhibition of lorazepam glucuronidation. Inhibition of lorazepam glucuronidation was characterized by known substrates and/or inhibitors of UGT2B enzymes, such as fluconazole, ketoconazole, morphine, codeine, methadone, ketamine, valproic acid, and zidovudine. However, it was suggested that of these drugs only ketoconazole had the potential to inhibit lorazepam clearance to a clinically significant extent [75].

Genetic variations in the gene encoding for the subunits of a GABA-receptor complex may be of importance for the sensitivity to many intravenous anesthetic agents, such as benzodiazepines, barbiturates, propofol, as well as susceptibility to alcohol addiction [56, 78]. Most intravenous anesthetics act selectively through a different binding site on the $GABA_A$ receptor. As previously discussed with propofol and barbiturates, $GABA_A$ receptor complex is made up of pentameric transmembrane proteins that makes the ion channel selectively permeable to chloride anion. So far, 19 subunits of $GABA_A$ receptor complex have been cloned, which are classified into several structurally related subfamilies, that comprise highly homologous isoforms (α 1–6, β 1–3, γ 1–3, δ, ε, θ, π, ρ 1–3) [48]. BDZs and other non-benzodiazepine analogs that bind to BDZ site, placed at the interface between α and a γ subunits, allosterically increase GABA-receptor affinity [79]. The result of this modulatory influence is an increased opening frequency of the ion channel in the presence of a given neurotransmitter concentration, i.e. increased efficiency of GABAergic neurotransmission. Several experimental models with genetic mutations on certain $GABA_A$ receptor complex subunits have been created. Knockout of the $GABA_A$ γ2 receptor subunit gene resulted in mice that were completely insensitive to the sedative-hypnotic actions of BDZs [80]. Although $GABA_A$ receptor activity depends on γ2 subunit presence, the selectivity by which BDZs bind to $GABA_A$ receptors mainly depends on six different α subunits (α 1–6) [81]. Therefore, diazepam selectively binds to $GABA_A$ receptors containing γ2, β, α1, α2, α3, or α5 subunit (BDZ-sensitive receptors), but they do not bind to receptors containing α4 or α6 subunits (BDZ-insensitive receptors). Consequently, polymorphisms in genes encoding BDZ-sensitive receptors may cause variation in the sensitivity to BDZs among patients. In conclusion, further studies on the effects of genetic polymorphisms on the pharmacokinetics and pharmacodynamics of BDZs are warranted. Those studies will generate data that may help in more tailored dosing of appropriate BDZs to optimize the therapeutic effects and to reduce their side-effects or toxicity.

Etomidate

Etomidate is a carboxylated imidazole derivative which has two optical isomers. However, as (R)-etomidate is tenfold more potent than the (S)-enantiomer, it is prepared as $D(+)$ stereoisomer, which has hypnotic properties. Due to its sedative and hypnotic properties and hemodynamic stability etomidate is applied for the rapid intravenous induction of general anesthesia and sedation. After application of an i.v. induction dose (0.2–0.3 mg/kg), the onset of unconsciousness occurs usually within 30 s. Awakening after a single i.v. dose is rapid, with minor residual depressant effects. Short duration of action (2–3 min) is due predominately to rapid distribution, although it is also eliminated rapidly from the body [55].

Etomidate is a potent cerebral vasoconstrictor and decreases the cerebral blood flow and intracranial pressure. Although it suppresses the cerebral metabolic rate for oxygen, the results of the studies investigating its neuroprotective properties are contradictory [82]. Myoclonic movements occur in more than 50 % of patients receiving etomidate. Etomidate has fewer cardiovascular and respiratory depressant effects in comparison to thiopental. The depressant action of etomidate on ventilation is not pronounced, although apnea may occasionally occur following rapid i.v. drug administration. Due to its minimal effects on heart rate, cardiac output, myocardial contractility, and arterial blood pressure, it is used for anesthesia in patients with a compromised cardiovascular system. It is also suitable for outpatient anesthesia [83]. However, it does not demonstrate analgesic properties and postoperative nausea and vomiting may be more common [41]. Etomidate is suitable for use as a continuous infusion, but mainly because of its endocrine side effects it is not widely used anymore. The activity of adrenal mitochondrial 11-β-hydroxylase, a cytochrome P450 enzyme necessary for the conversion of cholesterol to cortisol, is transiently inhibited by a single dose of etomidate, with consecutive adrenal suppression [84]. This effect is due to binding of a nitrogen atom in etomidate's imidazole ring to the Fe^{2+} within the heme ring of the 11-b-hydroxylase enzyme resulting in the inhibition of steroid formation. Observed suppression may be either desirable for stress-free anesthesia or undesirable if it prevents useful protective responses against stresses that accompany the perioperative period, such as synthesis of cortisol and response to adrenocorticotrophic hormone [85]. Some analogues of etomidate, such as methoxy-carbonyl-etomidate (MOC etomidate) and carboetomidate, with minimal adrenocortical suppression have been developed as novel i.v. anesthetic agents; however, further investigation is still necessary [86, 87].

Etomidate is redistributed rapidly in the body. Approximately 76 % is bound to protein, primarily to albumin. It is metabolized in the plasma and liver, mainly by esterase hydrolysis and hepatic microsomal enzymes to inactive metabolites which are excreted in the urine (78 %) and bile (22 %). Less than 3 % is excreted as unchanged drug in urine [55]. Clearance of etomidate is about five times greater than that for thiopental and the terminal elimination half-life is 2.4–5 h. The recent data from a case report showed that CYP2C9 polymorphisms could potentially affect the pharmacokinetics of etomidate [88]. CYP2C9 is one of the clinically significant drug metabolizing enzymes that demonstrates genetic variants with significant phenotype and clinical outcomes [89]. However, no consistent data are currently available about the relationship between CYP2C9 polymorphism and the etomidate metabolism. Etomidate primarily acts through enhancement of GABA-activated chloride currents, decreasing neuronal activity by producing hyperpolarization of the neuronal membrane [60]. It has been shown to markedly prolong the decay of GABAergic IPSPs in hippocampal slices [90]. The fact that the ratio of anesthetic potencies of the two etomidate enantiomers was mimicked by their potencies as GABA modulators strongly supports the involvement of $GABA_A$ receptor in etomidate action [91]. At low concentrations etomidate is a modulator at $GABA_A$ receptors [41], while at higher concentrations it can elicit currents in the absence of GABA and behaves as an allosteric agonist. Its binding site on $GABA_A$ receptor is located in the transmembrane region between the alpha and beta subunits [92]. On the other hand, cardiovascular stability of the etomidate is due to its activation of α2B adrenergic receptors [93]. Moreover, it has been demonstrated that in wild-type mice etomidate raises blood pressure, in contrast to mice lacking α2B adrenoreceptors.

The studies expressing various subunits of $GABA_A$ receptors in cell culture revealed that receptors containing β2 and β3 subunits were sensitive to etomidate, while those containing β1 subunits were insensitive [94]. Using knock-in mice, researchers identified several amino acids which determine receptor sensitivity to etomidate [95], by introducing mutations in the β2 or β3 peptide sequences that changed the asparagine at position 265 to methionine (M) or serine (S) [96]. Transgenic β3 (N265M) mice were insensitive to the immobilizing and respiratory depressant action and have a reduced sensitivity to the hypnotic action of etomidate [97]. These results indicated that β3-containing $GABA_A$ receptors are involved in the anesthetic actions of etomidate, while β2-containing receptors are involved in sedative effects [98]. In addition, transgenic mice lacking $GABA_A$ receptor α5 subunit are resistant to the amnestic, but not hypnotic effects of etomidate [99]. Hence, pharmacodynamic variability in the amnestic, hypnotic, sedative, or other effects of etomidate might be due to genetic polymorphisms located in the genes encoding various $GABA_A$ receptor subunits.

Ketamine

Ketamine is a phencyclidine derivative and an antagonist of the N-methyl-D-aspartate (NMDA) receptor. In anesthetic doses it produces a trance-like state known as dissociative anesthesia, in which patient may remain conscious, though amnesic and insensitive to pain [100]. Anesthesia usually persists for up to 15 min after a single intravenous injection, characterized by profound analgesia. In contrast to most other anesthetic drugs, ketamine may produce tachycardia and increases blood pressure and cardiac output. The cardiovascular effects of ketamine are accompanied by an increase in plasma noradrenaline concentration. Ketamine increases intracranial and intraocular pressure, and produces no muscular relaxation [40]. The main drawback of ketamine, in spite of the safety associated with a lack of overall depressant activity, is that hallucinations, and sometimes delirium and irrational behavior are common during recovery. These effects limit the usefulness of ketamine, but they might be less marked in children. Therefore, ketamine, often in conjunction with benzodiazepines, is frequently used for minor procedures in pediatrics [100].

Sub-anesthetic doses of ketamine are currently used in the treatment of patients with postoperative pain in opioid tolerant patients and complex regional pain syndrome, in emergency room treatments, and recently it has been suggested as an anti-depressant in patients with treatment-resistant bipolar depression [101–104]. However, the clinical response to sub-anesthetic doses is highly variable with approximately 33 % of the patients failing treatment [101, 105, 106]. A potential explanation for this high variability in response is inter-individual differences in ketamine metabolism due to factors such as genetic polymorphisms and metabolic drug interactions. Furthermore, genetic variations in the gene encoding for the subunits of an NMDA receptor may be of importance for the sensitivity to ketamine; however, no consistent data are currently available on NMDA receptor polymorphism and anesthetic response to ketamine.

For some clinically used drugs, including ketamine, CYP2B6 single nucleotide polymorphisms have been shown to be useful predictor of pharmacokinetics and drug response [107]. Cytochrome isoenzyme CYP2B6 belongs to the minor drug metabolizing P450s in liver. However, it is one of the most polymorphic CYP genes in humans. Expression is highly variable between individuals, owing to genetic polymorphisms, inducibility, and irreversible inhibition by many compounds [108]. The pharmacogenetic mechanisms are complex, and appear on several levels of gene expression from initial mRNA transcript to altered proteins. The most common functionally deficient allele is CYP2B6*6, which occurs at frequencies of 15–60 % in different populations [107]. It leads to lower expression in the liver due to erroneous splicing. However, the effect of the polymorphism of CYP2B6 on the pharmacokinetics of ketamine is still inconclusive. CYP2B6 is strongly inducible by several drugs including typical inducers such as rifampicin, phenytoin, and phenobarbital involving a so-called phenobarbital-responsive enhancer module at -1.7 kb of the CYP2B6 gene promoter [107]. Furthermore, ketamine itself has been shown to induce CYPs [109]. Besides CYP2B6, other CYP isoforms involved in the metabolism of ketamine are: CYP3A4, CYP3A5, CYP2A6, and CYP2C19 [110]. The impact of their genetic polymorphisms on ketamine metabolism remains to be elucidated.

Dexmedetomidine

Dexmedetomidine is a highly selective α2 adrenergic agonist with anesthetic properties, introduced in 1999 [111–113]. It is an active S-enantiomer of medetomidine, which is used in veterinary medicine [114]. This drug produces dose-dependent sedation, hypnosis, anxiolysis, amnesia, and analgesia [115, 116], and therefore is used as a premedication, as an anesthetic adjunct for general and regional anesthesia, and as a postoperative sedative and analgesic [113]. It provides a unique "conscious sedation"

state in which patients administered dexmedetomidine become alert and can respond to commands following modest stimulation such as shaking [113, 117]. Moreover, dexmedetomidine has analgesic effects (best described as opioid-sparing), without respiratory depression. In addition, increasing evidence suggests that dexmedetomidine has protective effects against ischemic and hypoxic injury, including cardioprotection, neuroprotection, and renoprotection [111].

Dexmedetomidine is water soluble and is commonly used for i.v. anesthesia initiation with a 1 μg/kg loading dose, administered over 10 min, followed by a maintenance infusion of 0.2–1.0 μg/kg/h [55]. It decreases cerebral blood flow without significant changes in intracranial pressure and cerebral metabolic rate of oxygen. After initial hypertension and reflex bradycardia, dexmedetomidine infusion usually produces moderate decreases in heart rate and systemic vascular resistance and, consequently, decreases in systemic blood pressure. Dexmedetomidine does not induce respiratory depression. The effects of dexmedetomidine on the respiratory system are a small to moderate decrease in tidal volume, and very little change in the respiratory rate. Moreover, dexmedetomidine suppresses shivering, possibly by its activity at α2b receptors in the hypothalamic thermoregulatory center of the brain [111].

Following i.v. administration, dexmedetomidine is rapidly distributed with a half-life of 6 min and a terminal elimination half-life of approximately 2 h [118]. Approximately 94 % of dexmedetomidine is protein bound, primarily to serum albumin and α1-acid glycoprotein. Dexmedetomidine shows linear or zero order kinetics, which means that a constant amount of drug is being eliminated per hour rather than first order kinetics, meaning that a constant fraction of the drug is eliminated per hour [111]. It undergoes rapid hepatic metabolism involving conjugation, N-methylation, and hydroxylation, followed by conjugation. After almost complete biotransformation by direct glucuronidation (the major pathway) as well as cytochrome P450 mediated metabolism, metabolites are excreted in urine (95 %) and feces (4 %) [55]. Dexmedetomidine is primarily metabolized by CYP2A6, which is also responsible for the metabolism of valproic acid, nicotine and coumarin, whereas CYP2A6 can be induced by dexamethasone and phenobarbital. Furthermore, several polymorphisms with significant inter-individual variations that affect drug metabolism have been reported [119]. A meta-analysis by Carter et al. [120] reported that the polymorphism CYP2A6*2 and CYP2A6*4 were associated with poor metabolism of CYP2A6 metabolized drugs. Two studies have evaluated the role of CYP2A6 polymorphisms in dexmedetomidine metabolism [121, 122]. Both studies determined that there was no significant impact of polymorphisms on dexmedetomidine metabolism, but these studies suffer from a small patient population size. Therefore, the effect of the polymorphism of CYP2A6 on the pharmacokinetics of dexmedetomidine is still inconclusive. However, this may contribute to dexmedetomidine's clinical response variability [119, 123].

Dexmedetomidine produces its selective α2-agonist effects through activation of CNS α2-receptors of the locus ceruleus and spinal cord and therefore causes sedation and analgesia, respectively [118, 124]. It is approximately eight times more specific for α2 adrenoceptors than the chemically related drug clonidine. The α2 selectivity of dexmedetomidine is observed following slow intravenous infusion of low and medium doses, while both α1 and α2 activities are observed following high doses or rapid i.v. administration of dexmedetomidine. The agonistic action of dexmedetomidine on α2a receptor subtype promotes sedation, hypnosis, analgesia, sympatholysis, neuroprotection and inhibition of insulin secretion, while agonism at the α2b receptor suppresses shivering, promotes analgesia and induces vasoconstriction in peripheral arteries. The α2c receptor subtype is associated with modulation of cognition sensory processing, mood and stimulant-induced locomotor activity, and regulation of epinephrine outflow from the adrenal medulla. On the other hand, inhibition of norepinephrine release is equally influenced by all three α2 receptor subtypes [125]. Moreover, as dexmedetomidine also incorporates an imidazoline structure, it also has an agonist effect on imidazoline receptors. It also displays a low affinity for beta-adrenergic, muscarinic, dopaminergic and serotonergic receptors [111]. Co-administration of anesthetics, sedatives, hypnotics or opioids and other drugs, such as vasodilators or negative chronotropic agents, with dexmedetomidine is likely to lead to additive pharmacodynamic effects and enhancement of their actions. Hence, a reduction in dosage with these agents is required.

The variable vasoconstrictor response to dexmedetomidine has been observed in individuals with a genetic variation in α2B-AR gene [126, 127]. A 301–303 deletion polymorphism has been identified in the coding region of the α2B-AR gene (ADRA2B), encoding for α-2B adrenergic receptor and has functional effects in vitro and in vivo. Human α2B-AR deletion (D) allele has been associated with loss of short-term agonist-promoted receptor desensitization, which may lead to increased vasoconstriction on α2 activation [128]. Moreover, a common 12 base-pair deletion in the coding region of the α2C-AR gene (ADRA2C) results in the deletion of four amino acids (del322–325) and a receptor that has markedly decreased agonist-mediated responses in vitro [129]. This common ADRA2C del322–325 variant is associated with pain perception both at baseline and after administration of dexmedetomidine.

Some studies determined that two mice strains exhibit a binary difference in their ability to stay awake following administration of dexmedetomidine during an arousal-promoting activity (maintaining their posture in a rotating tube). The C57BL/6 strain resisted dexmedetomidine-induced loss of righting reflex (LORR) only when given a sufficiently strong arousal stimulus, whereas another strain, 129X1, could be kept awake with just minimal stimulation [130]. There was a region identified on chromosome 4 that correlates with the mice being more resistant to dexmedetomidine-induced LORR which contains 26 genes bearing SNPs and 11 genes with CNVs polymorphic between the two strains [130].

Conclusion

For many years anesthesiologists have witnessed individual differences in response to anesthetics and other pharmacologic agents used during anesthesia. We know now that many of these drug-related phenomena are due to individual patient's genetic predisposition affecting drug absorption, distribution, metabolism, excretion, receptor binding, clinical effects, and toxicity. Pharmacogenetics (or pharmacogenomics) aims to understand the inherited basis for variability in drug response in terms of safety, efficacy, and pharmacokinetics, and to individualize therapy based on the patient's specific genetic profile, by matching the right drug to the right patient at the right time. Anesthesiology has contributed significantly to the development of this rapidly evolving science, recently empowered by the development and accessibility of molecular biotechnologies (DNA chips/microarrays, genetic manipulation using transgenic animals), high-throughput screening systems, and advanced bioinformatics.

The great promise of pharmacogenetics towards personalized medicine resides in promoting an individualized therapeutic approach, highly predictive for more efficient and safer drugs for a precisely predicted, homogenously genotyped, segment of patients who are responders to the therapy, rather being focused on each individual specifically. Although it plays a pivotal role in drug development, elucidation of therapeutic efficacy and constraining the risks of adverse drug reactions, the ultimate clinical applicability and cost-effectiveness of pharmacogenetic testing remains to be determined. An identification of genetic markers associated with drug response does not always equate to useful predictors of clinical outcomes. The main challenges to clinical implementation of pharmacogenetics are illustrated in Fig. 38.4.

Clinical validity refers to a test's ability to detect/predict the clinical disorder or phenotype associated with the genotype, while utility is a widely used measure of its usefulness

Fig. 38.4 The main challenges to clinical implementation of pharmacogenetics

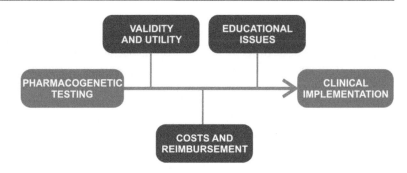

in clinical practice [131]. However, because most drug response phenotypes are multifactorial, it is not always easy to achieve the high clinical validity and utility for pharmacogenetic testing. Furthermore, the current significance of pharmacogenetics is not well accepted by some clinicians who may not understand how to manage a patient based on pharmacogenetics results. Finally, insurance coverage for pharmacogenetic testing is currently sporadic. Further pharmacoeconomic studies are therefore necessary to adequately assess the cost-effectiveness and impact of pharmacogenetic testing on the healthcare system. As large number of patients has been introduced to anesthesia, often once only, and frequently only for a short period of time, a genetic screening is not likely to represent a cost-effective method for reducing morbidity. However, once some genetic conditions are documented, family screening becomes a logical follow-up. Moreover, although it is not likely that pharmacogenetics will have a major impact on the way anesthesia is practiced today, it may help to elucidate interpatient variability in drug response, optimize therapeutic approach particularly in patients with repeated procedures under anesthesia, and influence new drug development and clinical trial designs.

Acknowledgements Janko Samardzic is supported by the Ministry of Education, Science and Technological Development of the Republic of Serbia (Grant No. 175076). Dubravka Svob Strac is supported by the Ministry of Science, Education and Sports of the Republic of Croatia (Grant No. 098-0000000-2448) and WWN/SFN Collaborative Research Program (CRNP), IBRO. John van den Anker is supported by NIH (K24DA027992, R01HD048689, U54HD071601) and the European Commission (TINN [223614], TINN2 [260908], NEUROSIS [223060]). The authors declare no conflict of interest regarding the content of this chapter.

References

1. Evans WE, McLeod HL. Pharmacogenomics – drug disposition, drug targets, and side effects. N Engl J Med. 2003;348(6):538–49.
2. Meyer UA. Pharmacogenetics – five decades of therapeutic lessons from genetic diversity. Nat Rev Genet. 2004;5(9):669–76.
3. Weinshilboum R. Inheritance and drug response. N Engl J Med. 2003;348(6):529–37.
4. Weber WW. Pharmacogenetics. New York: Oxford University Press; 1997.
5. Alving AS, Carson PE, Flanagan CL, Ickes CE. Enzymatic deficiency in primaquine-sensitive erythrocytes. Science. 1956;124 (3220):484–5.
6. Grbovic L, Radenkovic M, Djokic J, et al. New bearings in pharmacotherapeutic strategies: pharmacogenetics and gene therapy. Vojnosanit Pregl. 2007;64(10):707–13. [Serbian].
7. Johnson JA, Zineh I, Puckett BJ, et al. Beta 1-adrenergic receptor polymorphisms and antihypertensive response to metoprolol. Clin Pharmacol Ther. 2003;74(1):44–52.
8. Price Evans DA. Genetic factors in drug therapy: clinical and molecular pharmacogenetics. Cambridge: Cambridge University Press; 1993.
9. Streetman DS. Emergence and evolution of pharmacogenetics and pharmacogenomics in clinical pharmacy over the past 40 years. Ann Pharmacother. 2007;41(12):2038–41.
10. Ama T, Bounmythavong S, Blaze J, et al. Implications of pharmacogenomics for anesthesia providers. AANA J. 2010;78 (5):393–9.
11. Barash PG, Cullen BF, Stoelting RK, et al. Handbook of clinical anesthesia. 6th ed. Philadelphia: Lippincott Williams & Wilkins; 2009.
12. Wilkinson GR. Pharmacokinetics: the dynamics of drug absorption, distribution, and elimination. In: Hardman JG, Limbird LE, Gilman AG, editors. Goodman & Gilman's the pharmacological basis of therapeutics. 10th ed. New York: McGraw-Hill; 2001.
13. Kashuba D, Bertino JS. Mechanisms of drug interactions. In: Piscitelli J, Rodvold K, Masur H, editors. Drug interaction in infectious disease. Totowa: Humana Press; 2001.
14. Sata F, Sapone A, Elizondo G, et al. CYP3A4 allelic variants with amino acid substitutions in exons 7 and 12: evidence for an allelic variant with altered catalytic activity. Clin Pharmacol Ther. 2000;67(1):48–56.
15. Nelson DR. Comparison of P450s from human and fugu: 420 million years of vertebrate P450 evolution. Arch Biochem Biophys. 2003;409(1):18–24.
16. Strachan T, Read AP. Human molecular genetics. 3rd ed. - New York: Garland Science; 2004.
17. Ingelman-Sundberg M. Pharmacogenetics: an opportunity for a safer and more efficient pharmacotherapy. J Intern Med. 2001;250:186–200.
18. Hein DW, Doll MA, Fretland AJ, et al. Molecular genetics and epidemiology of the NAT1 and NAT2 acetylation polymorphisms. Cancer Epidemiol Biomarkers Prev. 2000;9:29–42.
19. De Wildt SN, Kearns GL, Leeder JS, et al. Glucuronidation in humans. Clin Pharmacokinet. 1999;36:439–52.
20. Tukey RH, Strassburg CP. Human UDP-glucuronosyltransferases: metabolism, expression, and disease. Annu Rev Pharmacol Toxicol. 2000;40:581–616.

21. Tucker GT. Clinical implications of genetic polymorphism in drug metabolism. J Pharm Pharmacol. 1994;46(1):417–24.

22. Larsen UL, Hyldahl Olesen L, Guldborg Nyvold C, et al. Human intestinal P-glycoprotein activity estimated by the model substrate digoxin. Scand J Clin Lab Invest. 2007;67(2):123–34.

23. Mrozikiewicz PM, Seremak-Mrozikiewicz A, Semczuk A, et al. The significance of C3435T point mutation of the MDR1 gene in endometrial cancer. Int J Gynecol Cancer. 2007;17(3):728–31.

24. Turgut S, Yaren A, Kursunluoglu R, Turgut G. MDR1 C3435T polymorphism in patients with breast cancer. Arch Med Res. 2007;38(5):539–44.

25. Brinkmann U. Functional polymorphism of the human multidrug resistance (MDR1) gene: correlation with P glycoprotein expression and activity in vivo. Novartis Found Symp. 2002;243:207–10.

26. Fagerlund TH, Braaten O. No pain relief from codeine ...? An introduction to pharmacogenomics. Acta Anaesthesiol Scand. 2001;45:140–9.

27. Iohom G, Fitzgerald D, Cunningham AJ. Principles of pharmaco-genetics—implications for the anaesthetist. Br J Anaesth. 2004;93 (3):440–50.

28. Olsen RW, Li GD. GABA(A) receptors as molecular targets of general anesthetics: identification of binding sites provides clues to allosteric modulation. Can J Anaesth. 2011;58(2):206–15.

29. Chidambaran V, Ngamprasertwong P, Vinks AA, Sadhasivam S. Pharmacogenetics and anesthetic drugs. Curr Clin Pharmacol. 2012;7(2):78–101.

30. Simpson NE, Kalow W. The "silent" gene for serum cholinesteraze. Am J Hum Genet. 1964;16:180–8.

31. Kalow W. Pharmacogenetics and anesthesia. Anesthesiology. 1964;25:377–87.

32. International Human Genome Sequencing Consortium, Lander ES, Linton LM, Birren B, et al. Initial sequencing and analysis of the human genome. Nature. 2001;409(6822):860–921.

33. Galley HF, Mahdy A, Lowes DA. Pharmacogenetics and anesthesiologists. Pharmacogenomics. 2005;6(8):849–56.

34. Greenbaum I, Weigl Y, Pras E. The genetic basis of malignant hyperthermia. Isr Med Assoc J. 2007;9(1):39–41.

35. Litman RS, Rosenberg H. Malignant hyperthermia: update on susceptibility testing. JAMA. 2005;293(23):2918–24.

36. Ingelman-Sundberg M. Polymorphism of cytochrome P450 and xenobiotic toxicity. Toxicology. 2002;181–182:447–52.

37. Landau R. Pharmacogenetics: implications for obstetric anesthesia. Int J Obstet Anesth. 2005;14(4):316–23.

38. Mikstacki A, Skrzypczak-Zielinska M, Tamowicz B, et al. The impact of genetic factors on response to anaesthetics. Adv Med Sci. 2013;58(1):9–14.

39. Watson KR, Shah MV. Clinical comparison of 'single agent' anaesthesia with sevoflurane versus target controlled infusion of propofol. Br J Anaesth. 2000;85(4):541–6.

40. Bennett PN, Brown MJ, Sharma P. Clinical pharmacology. 11th ed. Edinburgh: Churchill Livingstone; 2012.

41. Vanlersberghe C, Camu F. Etomidate and other non-barbiturates. Handb Exp Pharmacol. 2008;182:267–82.

42. Guitton J, Buronfosse T, Desage M, et al. Possible involvement of multiple human cytochrome P450 isoforms in the liver metabolism of propofol. Br J Anaesth. 1998;80(6):788–95.

43. Loryan I, Lindqvist M, Johansson I, et al. Influence of sex on propofol metabolism, a pilot study: implications for propofol anesthesia. Eur J Clin Pharmacol. 2012;68(4):397–406.

44. Franks NP. Molecular targets underlying general anaesthesia. Br J Pharmacol. 2006;147(1):S72–81.

45. Samardzic J, Strac DS, Obradovic M, et al. DMCM, a benzodiazepine site inverse agonist, improves active avoidance and motivation in the rat. Behav Brain Res. 2012;235(2):195–9.

46. Fritschy JM, Brunig I. Formation and plasticity of GABAergic synapses: physiological mechanisms and pathophysiological implications. Pharmacol Ther. 2003;98:299–323.

47. Olsen RW, Sieghart W. International Union of Pharmacology. LXX. Subtypes of gamma-aminobutyric acid(A) receptors: classification on the basis of subunit composition, pharmacology, and function. Update. Pharmacol Rev. 2008;60(3):243–60.

48. Samardzic J. Behavioural effects of the inverse agonists of benzodiazepine receptors. Belgrade: ZaduzbinaAndrejevic; 2015.

49. Bali M, Akabas MH. Defining the propofol binding site location on the GABAA receptor. Mol Pharmacol. 2004;65(1):68–76.

50. Krasowski MD, Koltchine VV, Rick CE, et al. Propofol and other intravenous anesthetics have sites of action on the gamma-aminobutyric acid type A receptor distinct from that for isoflurane. Mol Pharmacol. 1998;53(3):530–8.

51. Macdonald RL, Kang JQ, Gallagher MJ. Mutations in GABAA receptor subunits associated with genetic epilepsies. J Physiol. 2010;588(11):1861–9.

52. Tsang SY, Ng SK, Xu Z, Xue H. The evolution of GABAA receptor-like genes. Mol Biol Evol. 2007;24(2):599–610.

53. Iohom G, Ni Chonghaile M, O'Brien JK, et al. An investigation of potential genetic determinants of propofol requirements and recovery from anaesthesia. Eur J Anaesthesiol. 2007;24 (11):912–9.

54. Williams GW, Williams ES. Basic anesthesiology examination review. New York: Oxford University Press; 2016.

55. Miller R, Pardo M. Basics of anesthesia. 6th ed. Philadelphia: Elsevier; 2011.

56. Restrepo JG, Garcia-Martín E, Martínez C, Agúndez JA. Polymorphic drug metabolism in anaesthesia. Curr Drug Metab. 2009;10(3):236–46.

57. Sato Y, Kobayashi E, Murayama T, et al. Effect of N-methyl-D-aspartate receptor epsilon1 subunit gene disruption of the action of general anesthetic drugs in mice. Anesthesiology. 2005;102 (3):557–61.

58. Yamakura T, Bertaccini E, Trudell JR, Harris RA. Anesthetics and ion channels: molecular models and sites of action. Annu Rev Pharmacol Toxicol. 2001;41:23–51.

59. Carlson BX, Engblom AC, Kristiansen U, et al. A single glycine residue at the entrance to the first membrane-spanning domain of the gamma-aminobutyric acid type A receptor beta(2) subunit affects allosteric sensitivity to GABA and anesthetics. Mol Pharmacol. 2000;57(3):474–84.

60. Zhou C, Liu J, Chen XD. General anesthesia mediated by effects on ion channels. World J Crit Care Med. 2012;1(3):80–93.

61. Wilke K, Gaul R, Klauck SM, Poustka A. A gene in human chromosome band Xq28 (GABRE) defines a putative new subunit class of the GABAA neurotransmitter receptor. Genomics. 1997;45(1):1–10.

62. Welch E. Anaesthetic genetics and genomics. South Afr J Anaesth Analg. 2011;17(5):339–42.

63. Bush GH. Pharmacogenetics and anaesthesia. Proc R Soc Med. 1968;61(2):171–4.

64. Pericic D, Lazic J, Strac DS. Chronic treatment with flumazenil enhances binding sites for convulsants at recombinant alpha(1) beta(2)gamma(2S) GABA(A) receptors. Biomed Pharmacother. 2005;59(7):408–14.

65. Fukasawa T, Suzuki A, Otani K. Effects of genetic polymorphism of cytochrome P450 enzymes on the pharmacokinetics of benzodiazepines. J Clin Pharm Ther. 2007;32(4):333–41.

66. Wandel C, Böcker R, Böhrer H, et al. Midazolam is metabolized by at least three different cytochrome P450 enzymes. Br J Anaesth. 1994;73(5):658–61.

67. Kuehl P, Zhang J, Lin Y, et al. Sequence diversity in CYP3A promoters and characterization of the genetic basis of polymorphic CYP3A5 expression. Nat Genet. 2001;27(4):383–91.

68. Wong M, Balleine RL, Collins M, et al. CYP3A5 genotype and midazolam clearance in Australian patients receiving chemotherapy. Clin Pharmacol Ther. 2004;75(6):529–38.

69. Shih PS, Huang JD. Pharmacokinetics of midazolam and 1'-hydroxymidazolam in Chinese with different CYP3A5 genotypes. Drug Metab Dispos. 2002;30(12):1491–6.

70. Yu KS, Cho JY, Jang IJ, et al. Effect of the CYP3A5 genotype on the pharmacokinetics of intravenous midazolam during inhibited and induced metabolic states. Clin Pharmacol Ther. 2004;76(2):104–12.

71. Jung F, Richardson TH, Raucy JL, Johnson EF. Diazepam metabolism by cDNA-expressed human 2C P450s: identification of P4502C18 and P4502C19 as low K(M) diazepam N-demethylases. Drug Metab Dispos. 1997;25(2):133–9.

72. Bertilsson L, Henthorn TK, Sanz E, et al. Importance of genetic factors in the regulation of diazepam metabolism: relationship to S-mephenytoin, but not debrisoquin, hydroxylation phenotype. Clin Pharmacol Ther. 1989;45(4):348–55.

73. Qin XP, Xie HG, Wang W, et al. Effect of the gene dosage of CgammaP2C19 on diazepam metabolism in Chinese subjects. Clin Pharmacol Ther. 1999;66(6):642–6.

74. Greenblatt DJ. Clinical pharmacokinetics of oxazepam and lorazepam. Clin Pharmacokinet. 1981;6(2):89–105.

75. Uchaipichat V, Suthisisang C, Miners JO. The glucuronidation of R- and S-lorazepam: human liver microsomal kinetics, UDP-glucuronosyltransferase enzyme selectivity, and inhibition by drugs. Drug Metab Dispos. 2013;41(6):1273–84.

76. Chung JY, Cho JY, Yu KS, et al. Effect of the UGT2B15 genotype on the pharmacokinetics, pharmacodynamics, and drug interactions of intravenous lorazepam in healthy volunteers. Clin Pharmacol Ther. 2005;77(6):486–94.

77. Chung JY, Cho JY, Yu KS, et al. Pharmacokinetic and pharmacodynamic interaction of lorazepam and valproic acid in relation to UGT2B7 genetic polymorphism in healthy subjects. Clin Pharmacol Ther. 2008;83(4):595–600.

78. Iwata N, Cowley DS, Radel M, et al. Relationship between a GABAA alpha 6 Pro385Ser substitution and benzodiazepine sensitivity. Am J Psychiatry. 1999;156:1447–9.

79. Svob Strac D, Vlainic J, Jazvinsćak Jembrek M, Pericic D. Differential effects of diazepam treatment and withdrawal on recombinant GABAA receptor expression and functional coupling. Brain Res. 2008;1246:29–40.

80. Gunther U, Benson J, Benke D, et al. Benzodiazepine-insensitive mice generated by targeted disruption of the γ2 subunit of γ-aminobutyric acid type A receptors. Proc Natl Acad Sci U S A. 1995;92:7749–53.

81. Pericic D, Strac DS, Jembrek MJ, Vlainic J. Allosteric uncoupling and up-regulation of benzodiazepine and GABA recognition sites following chronic diazepam treatment of HEK 293 cells stably transfected with alpha1beta2gamma2S subunits of GABA (A) receptors. Naunyn Schmiedebergs Arch Pharmacol. 2007;375(3):177–87.

82. Bilotta F, Stazi E, Zlotnik A, et al. Neuroprotective effects of intravenous anesthetics: a new critical perspective. Curr Pharm Des. 2014;20(34):5469–75.

83. Yeung JK, Zed PJ. A review of etomidate for rapid sequence intubation in the emergency department. Can J Emerg Med. 2002;4(3):194–8.

84. Molenaar N, Bijkerk RM, Beishuizen A, et al. Steroidogenesis in the adrenal dysfunction of critical illness: impact of etomidate. Crit Care. 2012;16:R121.

85. Fragen RJ, Shanks CA, Molteni A, Avram MJ. Effects of etomidate on hormonal responses to surgical stress. Anesthesiology. 1984;61(6):652–6.

86. Khan KS, Hayes I, Buggy DJ. Pharmacology of anaesthetic agents. I: intravenous anaesthetic agents. Contin Educ Anaesth Crit Care Pain. 2013.

87. Sneyd JR, Rigby-Jones AE. New drugs and technologies, intravenous anaesthesia is on the move (again). Br J Anaesth. 2010;105 (3):246–54.

88. Ferreira T, Arede MJ, Oliveira V, et al. Etomidate induction in an adult patient carrier of a CYP 2C9 polymorphism – case report: 9AP3-7. Eur J Anaesthesiol. 2013;30:147.

89. Wang B, Wang J, Huang SQ, et al. Genetic polymorphism of the human cytochrome P450 2C9 gene and its clinical significance. Curr Drug Metab. 2009;10(7):781–834.

90. Proctor WR, Mynlieff M, Dunwiddie TV. Facilitatory action of etomidate and pentobarbital on recurrent inhibition in rat hippocampal pyramidal neurons. J Neurosci. 1986;6 (11):3161–8.

91. Tomlin SL, Jenkins A, Lieb WR, Franks NP. Stereoselective effects of etomidate optical isomers on gamma-aminobutyric acid type A receptors and animals. Anesthesiology. 1998;88 (3):708–17.

92. Li GD, Chiara DC, Sawyer GW, et al. Identification of a GABAA receptor anesthetic binding site at subunit interfaces by photolabeling with an etomidate analog. J Neurosci. 2006;26:11599–605.

93. Paris A, Philipp M, Tonner PH, et al. Activation of alpha 2B-adrenoceptors mediates the cardiovascular effects of etomidate. Anesthesiology. 2003;99:889–95.

94. Hill-Venning C, Belelli D, Peters JA, Lambert JJ. Subunit-dependent interaction of the general anaesthetic etomidate with the gamma-aminobutyric acid type A receptor. Br J Pharmacol. 1997;120(5):749–56.

95. Belelli D, Lambert JJ, Peters JA, et al. The interaction of the general anesthetic etomidate with the gamma-aminobutyric acid type A receptor is influenced by a single amino acid. Proc Natl Acad Sci U S A. 1997;94(20):11031–6.

96. Jurd R, Arras M, Lambert S, et al. General anesthetic actions in vivo strongly attenuated by a point mutation in the GABA (A) receptor beta3 subunit. FASEB J. 2003;17:250–2.

97. Zeller A, Arras M, Lazaris A, et al. Distinct molecular targets for the central respiratory and cardiac actions of the general anesthetics etomidate and propofol. FASEB J. 2005;19 (12):1677–9.

98. Reynolds DS, Rosahl TW, Cirone J, et al. Sedation and anesthesia mediated by distinct GABA(A) receptor isoforms. J Neurosci. 2003;23:8608–17.

99. Cheng VY, Martin LJ, Elliott EM, et al. Alpha5GABA-A receptors mediate the amnestic but not sedative- effects of the general anesthetic etomidate. J Neurosci. 2006;26:3713–20.

100. Dale MM, Rang H, Dale MM. Rang & Dale's pharmacology. 7th ed. Edinburgh: Churchill Livingstone; 2012.

101. Diazgranados N, Ibraham L, Brutsche NE, et al. A randomized add-on trial of an N-methyl-D-asparate antagonist in treatment-resistant bipolar depression. Arch Gen Psychiatry. 2010;67:793–801.

102. Lester L, Braude DA, Niles C, Crandall CS. Low-dose ketamine for analgesia in the ED: a retrospective case series. Am J Emerg Med. 2010;28:820–7.

103. Loftus RW, Yeager MP, Clark JA, et al. Intraoperative ketamine reduces perioperative opiate consumption in opiate-dependent patients with chronic back pain undergoing back surgery. Anesthesiology. 2010;113:639–46.

104. Sabia M, Hirsh RA, Torjman MC, et al. Advances in translational neuropathic research: example of enantioselective pharmacokinetic-pharmacodynamic modeling of ketamine-induced pain relief in complex regional pain syndrome. Curr Pain Headache Rep. 2011;15:207–14.

105. Goldberg ME, Torjman MC, Schwartzman RJ, et al. Pharmacodynamic profiles of ketamine (R)-(−)- and (S)-(+)

with 5 day inpatient infusion for the treatment of complex regional pain syndrome. Pain Phys. 2010;13:379–87.

106. Goldberg ME, Torjman MC, Schwartzman RJ, et al. Enantioselective pharmacokinetics of (R)- and (S)-ketamine after a 5-day infusion in patients with complex regional pain syndrome. Chirality. 2011;23:138–43.

107. Zanger UM, Klein K. Pharmacogenetics of cytochrome P450 2B6 (CYP2B6): advances on polymorphisms, mechanisms, and clinical relevance. Front Genet. 2013;4:24.

108. Zanger UM, Klein K, Saussele T, et al. Polymorphic CYP2B6: molecular mechanisms and emerging clinical significance. Pharmacogenomics. 2007;8(7):743–59.

109. Chen JT, Chen RM. Mechanisms of ketamine-involved regulation of cytochrome P450 gene expression. Expert Opin Drug Metab Toxicol. 2010;6:273–81.

110. Desta Z, Moaddel R, Ogburn ET, et al. Stereoselective and regiospecific hydroxylation of ketamine and norketamine. Xenobiotica. 2012;42(11):1076–87.

111. Afonso J, Reis F. Dexmedetomidine current role in anesthesia and intensive care. Rev Bras Anestesiol. 2012;62(1):118–33.

112. Correa-Sales C, Rabin BC, Maze M. A hypnotic response to dexmedetomidine, an alpha 2 agonist, is mediated in the locus coeruleus in rats. Anesthesiology. 1992;76(6):948–52.

113. Kamibayashi T, Maze M. Clinical uses of alpha2-adrenergic agonists. Anesthesiology. 2000;93:1345–9.

114. Clarke KW, Hall LW. "Xylazine" – a new sedative for horses and cattle. Vet Rec. 1969;85:512–7.

115. Khan ZP, Ferguson CN, Jones RM. Alpha2 and imidazoline recreptor agonists: their pharmacology and therapeutic role. Anaesthesia. 1999;54:146–65.

116. Maze M, Scarfini C, Cavaliere F. New agents for sedation in the intensive care unit. Crit Care Clin. 2001;7:221–6.

117. Venn RM, Grounds RM. Comparison between dexmedetomidine and propofol for sedation in the intensive care unit: patient and clinician perceptions. Br J Anaesth. 2001;87(5):684–90.

118. Naaz S, Ozair E. Dexmedetomidine in current anaesthesia practice – a review. J Clin Diagn Res. 2014;8(10):GE01–4.

119. Holliday SF, Kane-Gill SL, Empey PE, et al. Interpatient variability in dexmedetomidine response: a survey of the literature. Scientific World Journal. 2014;2014:805013.

120. Carter B, Long T, Cinciripini P. A meta-analytic review of the CYP2A6 genotype and smoking behavior. Nicotine Tob Res. 2004;6(2):221–7.

121. Choi L, Caffo BS, Kohli U, et al. A Bayesian hierarchical nonlinear mixture model in the presence of artifactual outliers in a population pharmacokinetic study. J Pharmacokinet Pharmacodyn. 2011;38(5):613–36.

122. Kohli U, Pandharipande P, Muszkat M, et al. CYP2A6 genetic variation and dexmedetomidine disposition. Eur J Clin Pharmacol. 2012;68(6):937–42.

123. Raunio H, Rautio A, Gullstén H, Pelkonen O. Polymorphisms of CYP2A6 and its practical consequences. Br J Clin Pharmacol. 2001;52(4):357–63.

124. Mizobe T, Maghsoudi K, Sitwala K, et al. Antisense technology reveals the alpha2A adrenoceptor to be the subtype mediating the hypnotic response to the highly selective agonist, dexmedetomidine, in the locus coeruleus of the rat. Invest. 1996;98(5):1076–80.

125. Panzer O, Moitra V, Sladen RN. Pharmacology of sedative-analgesic agents: dexmedetomidine, remifentanil, ketamine, volatile anesthetics, and the role of peripheral mu antagonists. Crit Care Clin. 2009;25:451–69.

126. Muszkat M, Kurnik D, Sofowora GG, et al. Desensitization of vascular response in vivo: contribution of genetic variation in the [alpha]2B-adrenergic receptor subtype. J Hypertens. 2010;28(2):278–84.

127. Talke P, Stapelfeldt C, Lobo E, et al. Alpha-2B adrenoceptor polymorphism and peripheral vasoconstriction. Pharmacogenet Genomics. 2005;15(5):357–63.

128. Talke P, Stapelfeldt C, Lobo E, et al. Effect of alpha2B-adrenoceptor polymorphism on peripheral vasoconstriction in healthy volunteers. Anesthesiology. 2005;102(3):536–42.

129. Small KM, Wagoner LE, Levin AM, et al. Synergistic polymorphisms of beta1- and alpha2C-adrenergic receptors and the risk of congestive heart failure. N Engl J Med. 2002;347 (15):1135–42.

130. Gelegen C, Gent TC, Ferretti V, et al. Staying awake--a genetic region that hinders α2 adrenergic receptor agonist-induced sleep. Eur J Neurosci. 2014;40(1):2311–9.

131. Scott SA. Personalizing medicine with clinical pharmacogenetics. Genet Med. 2011;13(12):987–95.

Lessons From Drug Interaction Displays

39

Ross Kennedy

Introduction

The Kinetics of Most Anaesthetic Drugs Are Complex

Most anaesthesia practitioners have an understanding of the general principles and theory of pharmacokinetics (PK) and pharmacodynamics (PD) and how these relate to individual drugs. They would recognize that the time course of many drugs in the plasma can be described by a tri-exponential equation with the form:

$$C_t = Ae^{-\alpha t} + Be^{-\beta t} + Ge^{-\gamma t}$$

Used on a data set [1] for propofol this becomes

$$C_t = 4.7\,e^{-0.324.t} + 0.80e^{-0.016.t} + 0.86e^{-0.0026.t}$$

However for most practitioners this equation, which describes only one of several drugs used during a typical anaesthetic, has little practical meaning.

Furthermore, as clinicians we are not really interested in plasma levels but with effects. The hysteresis (delay) between plasma levels and effect adds further complexity (and another exponential equation). A common way of dealing with the complexity of the relationship between drug dosing and effect is to develop standard recipes or sequences of drug dosing. These are empirically derived (essentially trial and error) but are frequently handed down to new trainees as ideal solutions.

Demonstrating the Relationship Between Dose and Effect

A range of tools have been developed to illustrate the relationship between drug doses and plasma and effect-site concentrations in various settings. The role of these systems, including StanPump, TIVAtrainer, Rugloop, and IVA-SIM, has been summarized [2]. To these can be added a plethora of home grown solutions. These tools have been used for research and for teaching and demonstrating drug kinetics both in real time and for "off-line" teaching. More recently various "apps" have been developed which allow users to carry kinetic simulations in their pocket making these simulations available for everyday use by the enthusiast.

For individual drugs, commercial TCI systems are an attempt to address this complexity in ways that can be used and understood by all users. The displays of TCI devices often illustrate the history and predictions of both plasma and effect-site levels, giving the user an insight into the underlying kinetics and potentially allow better matching of drug delivery to changing requirements, at different stages of a surgical procedure.

Anaesthesia Involves Multiple Drugs—and Multiple Effects

Anaesthesia is not about single drugs. Most general anaesthetics involve administration of at least two classes of drugs, typically a hypnotic and an opioid. The interactions between these groups of drugs have been well demonstrated [3, 4] and shown to be synergistic [5].

To further complicate matters, anaesthesia "depth" is not a single dimension [6]. Glass describes three endpoints [7]

1. lack of explicit recall, primarily mediated in the cortex
2. lack of response to noxious stimuli (both motor and sympathetic response), primarily mediated in the spinal cord
3. providing optimal operating condition

R. Kennedy, MB, ChB, PhD
Department of Anaesthesia, Christchurch Hospital and University of Otago: Christchurch, Private Bag 4076, Rolleston Ave, Christchurch 8140, New Zealand
e-mail: ross.kennedy@cdhb.health.nz

© Springer International Publishing AG 2017
A.R. Absalom, K.P. Mason (eds.), *Total Intravenous Anesthesia and Target Controlled Infusions*,
DOI 10.1007/978-3-319-47609-4_39

It is difficult enough to appreciate the time course of effect of one or more bolus doses of an individual drug, it is equally difficult to get a true perception of the potency of synergy. As an example a single bolus of 1.5 mcg/kg of fentanyl will reduce MAC (a measure of the amount of a volatile agent required to block the motor response to a given noxious stimulus) by around 50 % for 5 min.

Over recent years the technique of response surface modeling [8, 9] has allowed interactions between drugs to be quantified over a wide range of doses for each drug. Most of this work has been performed by two groups, one based at the University of Utah and the other based in Switzerland, Belgium and the Netherlands. These groups have used response-surface methodology to investigate a wide range of opioid–hypnotic interactions [10–16].

In 2004 Schumacher and Bouillon described the concept of an interaction display [17] while the drug kinetic display described by Syroid et al. in 2002 [18] which incorporated a graphic of individual drug effects was easily adapted to incorporate response surface models.

These two prototypes, incorporating the results of ongoing work, became the basis for the two commercial devices released in the past 10 years.

These devices, Navigator Application Suite (GE Healthcare, Helsinki, Finland) and SmartPilot View (Dräger Medical GmbH, Lübeck, Germany) have made PK/PD interaction available to the more casual user. In both systems "lack of consciousness" is defined as no response to "shake-and-shout", or an Observer's Assessment of Alertness/Sedation (OAA/S) score [19] ≤ 1.

Both devices collect information on volatile anaesthetic delivery and measured concentrations from anaesthesia machines and monitors. Many types of infusion pumps can be directly connected to allow continuous input of infusion data. This is especially useful with TCI pumps as the infusion rates can change frequently. Bolus drug doses and infusions not directly logged can be entered manually.

Although there is much that appeals about these devices, to date there is little published work to help determine the true place in routine clinical practice. Much of the rest of this chapter are personal observations based on the use of both systems, but predominantly Navigator, in a large number of anaesthetics over the past six years by an enthusiast for this technology [20] (Figs. 39.1 and 39.2) [21].

What These Devices Show Us

SmartPilot View and Navigator have much in common although the systems display the information in quite different ways. Although promoted as demonstrations of drug interactions these devices show the user a wide range of other information, some of which are discussed below.

Displaying Effect-Site Concentration: Making the Effect Site Normal

The systems start by calculating and displaying past, present, and future effect-site concentrations. Both systems have chosen to display only effect-site concentrations which is appropriate as, to some extent, the dosing and plasma levels that produce the effect are of limited interest and value.

Seeing the Time Course of Individual Drugs

We often only see binary effects of drugs such as propofol (the patient goes to sleep). It is difficult to appreciate the actual time course of effect (Fig. 39.3) [22]. Interaction displays present this information to the user every time a bolus is given (see Figs. 39.1 and 39.2) and help users develop an understanding of the relationship between dose and effect.

An Advisory System for Manual Target Control

The trend display and predictions of individual drug contraptions allow the user to make intelligent changes to drug delivery. The consequences of change are immediately obvious and the input (or dosing) can be altered until the desired profile of effect-site concentration is achieved. We developed a system to guide delivery of inhalational agents incorporating model based forward prediction using vaporizer setting, fresh gas flow, and measured end-tidal concentration [23]. Users made step changes with this system more rapidly than without the display [24].

Manual targeting allows the user to control the rate of change more easily than on many TCI systems which are set up to achieve the target as soon as possible. This can be useful when a gradual change in concentration is desirable such as using a fixed rate infusion of propofol just until the point a patient becomes unresponsive to avoid the haemodynamic consequence of larger doses. This type of display may also allow many of the advantages of TCI in areas where TCI is not currently available or licensed, such as the USA (see Fig. 39.4).

Target Control of Drugs Not Modeled in TCI Systems

Many drugs used in anaesthesia and for which kinetic and PK/PD models exist are not included in TCI systems. Fentanyl and neuromuscular blockers are examples of these. Use of real time modeling may allow better matching of drug dosing to requirement, and as with TCI may reduce total

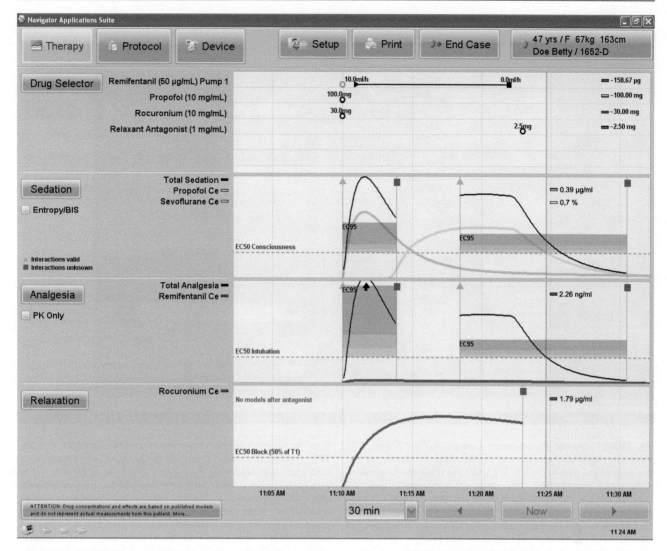

Fig. 39.1 The standard demonstration example of the Navigator (GE) screen. In this example induction was with boluses of propofol, remifentanil and rocuronium. Anaesthesia was maintained with a remifentanil infusion and sevoflurane. Delivery of both drugs stopped at around 11:22. The *top pane* shows drug dosing with totals on the right. The *second pane* is labelled "sedation" and is based on response to shake-and-shout (OAA/S $\leq$ 1) and the *third* "analgesia" (response to intubation with a positive response being gross movement or a rise in pule rate or blood pressure >20 % above baseline). The *bottom pane* relates to neuromuscular blockade. *Coloured lines* in the three drug panels are the modeled effect-site levels of individual drugs based on the drug doses, which can be entered manually or directly from up to three syringe drivers, and the patient anthropomorphic data shown in the top right of the screen. The division between the white background and yellow background is the current time, with lines to the right representing forward predictions. Current effect-site levels for the individual drugs are shown on the right of each panel. From top to bottom these are propofol, sevoflurane, remifentanil, and rocuronium. In the second (sedation/consciousness) and third (analgesia/noxious stimulus) panes the *black lines* represent the combined, or synergistic,

effect of the opioid and hypnotic on that effect. The *shaded areas* show the band in which 50 % (lower) to 95 % (upper) of subjects will *not* respond to the stimulus (shake-and-shout or intubation). The combined effects (*black lines*) are plotted on the same effect scale as individual drugs. In this example, the sevoflurane effect-site concentration is above the EC95 from around 11:16 until 11:22. At the current time (11:25) about 50 % of subjects would be unresponsive to this level of sevoflurane but given the (reducing) remifentanil levels it will be a further 1–2 min before the combined effect reaches this 50 % likelihood of response level. Although opioid levels are plotted in the "analgesia" pane, they seldom get far above the baseline as very large doses of opioids alone are needed to block the response to intubation. The check box labeled "PK only" allows display of individual opioid concentrations, but without the interaction effect. The break in the *shaded areas* and *black lines* is a zone where the algorithm is unable to calculate a combined effect because of moderate levels of both propofol and sevoflurane. Once either agent drops below a threshold that agent is ignored. Image provided by and printed with permission of GE Healthcare, Helsinki Finland

consumption. Additionally once users become aware of the large swings in drug concentration and the duration of effect of a given bolus, we start to see smaller doses used to control the duration of effect.

Several authors have quantified fentanyl levels at emergence after various procedures [25, 26]. Suggesting a target of 1–1.5 ng/ml of fentanyl at emergence is meaningless to most practitioners. A continuous effect-site display allows

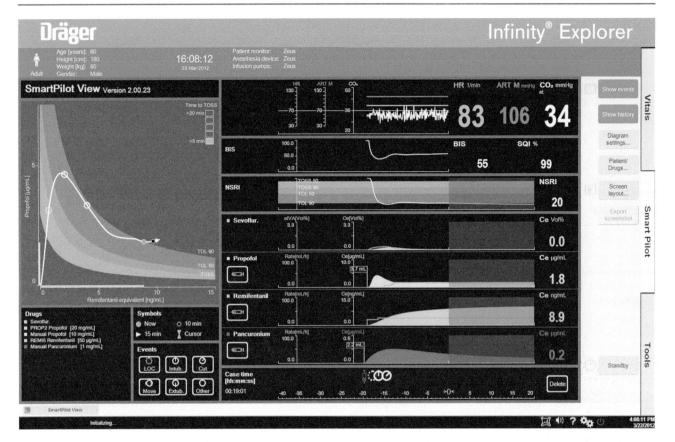

Fig. 39.2 A standard demonstration SmartPilot View Screen. The interaction between hypnotic and opioid drugs is shown on the two-dimensional plot on the left. The *white line* illustrates progression of the patient through time. The *orange dot* is the current time; the *black dot* and the *arrowhead* represent 10 and 15 min, respectively, in the future. Various events in the past are marked by the *white circles* on the 2-D surface and on the time line. The likelihood of tolerance to stimulus (TOL = tolerance of laryngoscopy, TOSS = tolerance of shake-and-shout) response (or the absence of response) is indicated by the *shaded bands*. "TOSS" = 50 % likelihood of response to shake & shout, "TOL 90" and "TOL 50" the level at which 90 % and 50 % of patients would tolerate laryngoscopy. The *coloured bands* on the axes indicate the current hypnotic (expressed as propofol or sevoflurane equivalents) and opioid (in remifentanil equivalents) effect-site levels. The boxes in the top right of the 2-D display estimate the time to 50 % response to shake-and-shout, if drug delivery stopped, in this case < 5 min. This display is equivalent to the decrement time (the time to fall from the current value to a preset concentration) displayed by many TCI systems, typically preset to a propofol concentration of 1 mcg/ml. Individual drug dosing and effect-site levels are plotted over time. Dosing is shown with *grey lines* and the coloured areas the effect-site levels. The *shaded background* represents future "predictions" while the values shown are estimates of the current levels. In addition to the monitored variables shown in the upper two panels, "NSRI" or noxious stimulus response index [21] is plotted. NSRI is a modification of the hypnotic–opioid interaction to allow for intensity of stimulus. NSRI has been shown to be a better predictor of response to noxious stimulus (the "analgesic" component of anaesthesia) than EEG based measures. (Used with permission from Dräger. Source: ©Drägerwerk AG & Co KGaA, Lubeck. All rights reserved. No portion hereof may be reproduced, saved, or stored in a data processing system, electronically or mechanically copied or otherwise recorded by any other means without our express prior written permission.)

practitioners to "target" specific levels. They also start to understand the consequences of different dosing regimes (see Fig. 39.5).

Bolus or Infusion

Both the display of the individual effect-site concentrations and the interaction displays demonstrate wide swings in drug concentrations seen with boluses (Figs. 39.6 and 39.7). Smaller boluses (Fig. 39.5) reduce this variability but at a cost of decreased duration.

Illustrating Compartmental Kinetics

For most drugs administered by fixed rate infusion, as opposed to TCI delivery, the rate required to maintain a given concentration decreases over time. In Fig. 39.7 the need to reduce the rocuronium infusion illustrates this point. This is a useful illustration of the concept of faster compartments filling first and of redistribution. It also demonstrates to users the type of changes TCI pumps need to make to achieve and maintain a set concentration.

Fig. 39.3 The effect-site propofol concentration after a single 150 mg (*red*) or 100 mg (*blue*) bolus in a 80 kg, 170 cm male aged 40 yr modeled using the Schneider parameters [22]. As a first approximation assume the patient is unconscious (no response to shake-and-shout) when the propofol concentration is >4 ng/ml. The casual user only "knows" that the patient became unrousable after about 25 s with the 150 mg bolus and 10 s later with 100mg (40 % longer!) and has no way of knowing how long the effect will last

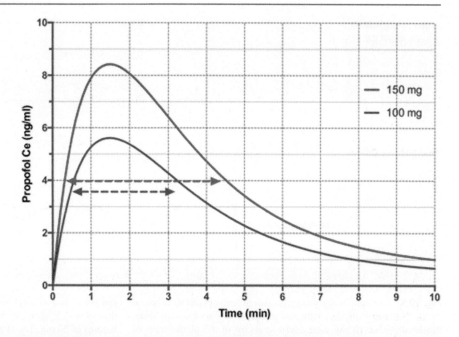

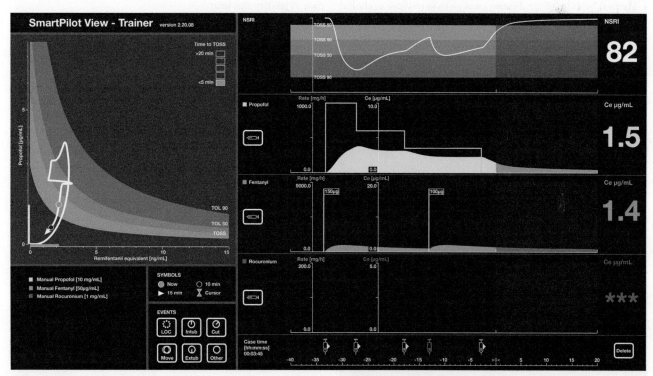

Fig. 39.4 A SmartPilot View example of a series of fixed rate propofol infusions guided by a combination of predicted effect-site levels and patient response. The initial infusion rate was 100 ml/h, reduced to 60 ml/h at 6 min and 35 ml/h at 15 min. (Used with permission from Dräger. Source: ©Drägerwerk AG & Co KGaA, Lubeck. All rights reserved. No portion hereof may be reproduced, saved, or stored in a data processing system, electronically or mechanically copied or otherwise recorded by any other means without our express prior written permission.)

Opioid Combinations

For the purposes of the interaction modeling, both systems convert all opioids into remifentanil equivalents. The user can observe the effect on the measure of total analgesia with different opioid combinations and choose the mix that is most appropriate at different stages of the procedure and for the early postoperative period. This is illustrated in Fig. 39.6.

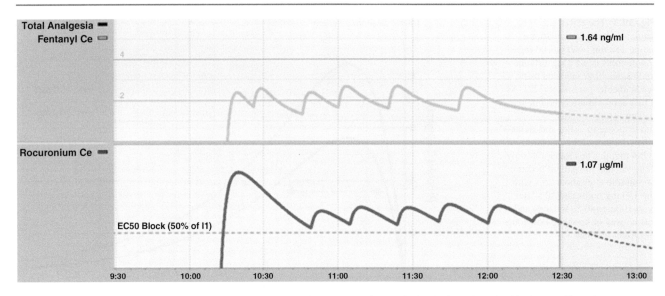

Fig. 39.5 An example of repeated boluses of fentanyl and rocuronium in the Navigator display. After an initial 40 mg rocuronium dose, further doses of 10 mg were given at return of T2 of the train of 4. The final bolus was 5 mg. Fentanyl was given in response to clinical end points and with the intention of achieving an effect-site concentration of 1–1.5 ng/ml at the completion of surgery followed by two boluses of 50 mg. The "PK only" box was checked in the "Analgesia" pane to produce this image

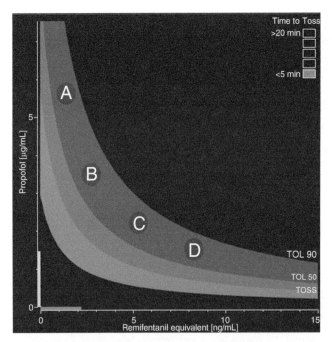

Fig. 39.6 A segment of the 2-D display from Smart-Pilot View. The oscillations illustrate the effect of repeated fentanyl boluses. (Used with permission from Dräger. Source: ©Drägerwerk AG & Co KGaA, Lubeck. All rights reserved. No portion hereof may be reproduced, saved, or stored in a data processing system, electronically or mechanically copied or otherwise recorded by any other means without our express prior written permission.)

Pump Setting Errors

In both systems the user needs to tell the device the contents of a given syringe. Even if the syringe driver is performing TCI, the interaction systems use only the rate information from the pump and recalculate effect-site levels. A difference between pump and device programming shows up as an unusual pattern and can alert the user to search for problems. An occasional error of this type is to place a syringe of propofol into a pump programmed for remifentanil before inserting the syringes.

Interaction Display

Titration to Effect

New users of these systems frequently ask "what number should I target?" As with much of anaesthesia drug delivery, initial doses and concentrations are no more than places to start with further dosing based on the response of the patient. The interaction display is one more tool to help guide this process. Thinking about responses in terms of probabilities also helps the user understand patient variability. It rapidly becomes clear to the user that the interaction is a useful end point for titration of anaesthesia with an individual patient

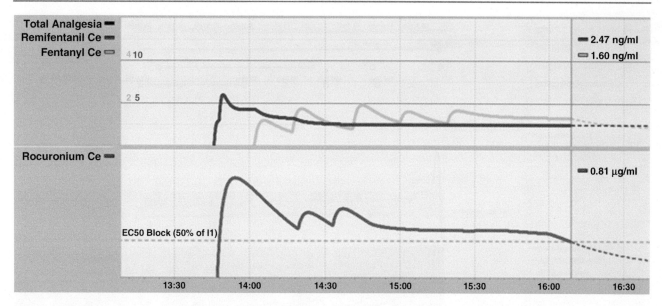

Fig. 39.7 A Navigator screenshot where after number of boluses infusions of rocuronium (*lower panel*) and fentanyl (*upper panel*) were commenced. Following initial boluses of rocuronium of 40 mg, 10 mg, and 10 mg, the rocuronium infusion commenced at 25 mg/h at 1445. This was reduced to 20 mg/h at 1530 and turned off at 1555. Three fentanyl boluses of 100 mg were followed by two of 50 mg. A fentanyl infusion of 100 mcg/h ran from 1515 until 1605. A remifentanil infusion was also used

tending to stay in a given region. This is seen in Figs. 39.7 and 39.8.

Coppens et al. considered that

> The major strength of effect-site controlled TCI lies not in predicting the resulting hypnotic effect in the individual patient but rather in its ability to maintain the pharmacological condition once a predetermined clinical effect has been reached [27].

Finding the optimal part of the response surface for a specific patient and procedure is a multi-dimensional version of this process.

Using Different Combinations of Hypnotic and Opioid

In the surface in Fig. 39.9 four areas are labeled. These zones have equivalent probabilities of response to laryngoscopy but are achieved with different combinations of hypnotic and opioid, falling approximately on the same isobol. There is a four-fold difference in the propofol and remifentanil concentrations between zone A and zone D. Although the hypnotic axis of Fig. 39.9 is labeled propofol, an equivalent pattern is seen with inhalational agents.

An empirical observation is that an individual practitioner will tend to give most anaesthetics in a particular area of the surface. Furthermore, practice in an individual institution will tend towards a particular zone, which may be different from that seen in another institution. Because isobols are nonlinear, moving between individual points can be challenging with users reluctant to make sufficient change in the hypnotic component for the change they have made in opioid. Thus if attempting to move from A - > C, the user will tend to a point above C. Because the patient is now receiving more anaesthetic, they may have a lower blood pressure and a longer time to awake than expected. Conversely in moving from C - > A the practitioner may not increase the hypnotic component of anaesthesia sufficiently.

Moving along isobols also occurs during a case. The example in Fig. 39.2 (SmartPilot View demo) starts as predominantly propofol based and shifts down and to the right as propofol decreases and remifentanil increases. This transition becomes a smooth "slide" very close to a single isobol.

Interaction displays allow the user to readily move between zones in the interaction space. This makes selecting the agents and appropriate zone for a given patient and procedure much more straightforward. This is a further example of the way in which "..these tools translate the wealth of PK/PD research (into) usable tools for everyday clinical practice" [28].

Combining Measures of Effect with Models of Effect

Various aspects of interaction displays, such as response probabilities, the SmartPilot NSRI and individual drug levels represent various models of drug effect. These can be combined with direct measures of effect to improve titration of drug delivery to effect. A straightforward

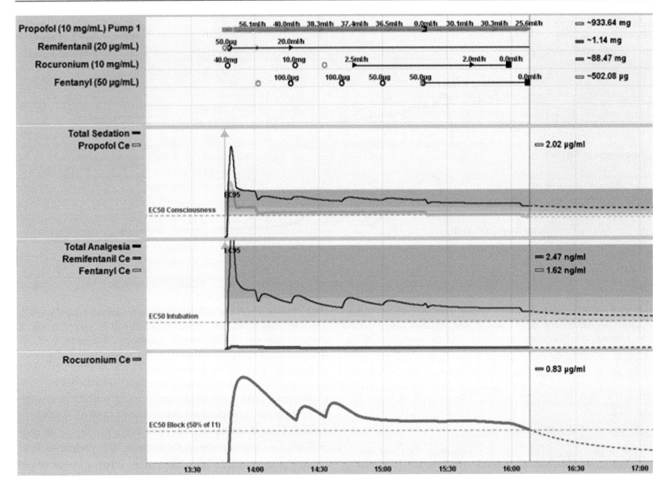

Fig. 39.8 This is the same case as Fig. 39.7, including the dosing and "sedation" panes and with the "analgesic" effect shown. Note that both "effects" remain within the same broad bands for most of the case and become less variable once the fentanyl infusion commenced at about 1520. The oscillation in "analgesic" effect at that time is exaggerated by a change in the propofol target at the same time as the propofol syringe was changed

example is using the concentration of neuromuscular blocking drugs in combination with quantitative measurement of neuromuscular blockade to guide delivery of neuromuscular blocking drugs.

Similarly the response probability to shake-and-shout (consciousness) frequently parallels EEG based measures such as BIS and spectral entropy while sympathetic activity, as measured by pulse rate and blood pressure, is the effect approximated by the response to noxious stimulus.

Both the underlying drug models and the interaction models themselves have limitations. Much work is being done to overcome model deficiencies and to make them applicable to wider populations. Although models will improve it is unlikely they will be able to perfectly account variability between patients. Automated control systems combine models and direct measures of effect [29–31] and we have advocated the use of this same approach by clinicians [32]. Interaction models are a useful part of this approach.

Interaction Displays as a Form of Monitoring

An extension of this concept is to consider interaction displays as monitors. The delivery of anaesthesia remains a clinical skill involving the integration of inputs from a range of devices. We seldom base decisions on a single device. For instance, blood pressure and pulse rate are often considered together and the pulse rate may determine the treatment path for a low blood pressure. Interaction display also makes the variability in response of individual patients explicit by presenting information in terms of population probabilities.

Consider a 70-year-old patient needing some degree of pharmacological support for their blood pressure despite receiving only 0.4MAC (age adjusted) of volatile and small amounts of opioids. This information alone would raise concern about possible awareness. The BIS is 45, which appears surprisingly low for the small amount of anaesthesia being administered. An interaction display would place this patient near the 75 % probability of not

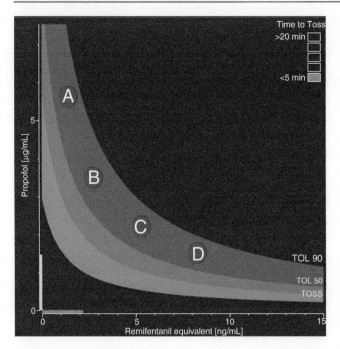

Fig. 39.9 A SmartPilot View 2-D surface with four zones with equivalent probability of response

responding to "shake-and-shout," adding support to the BIS value and making the anaesthesia provider more comfortable with the amount of anaesthesia being delivered. Conversely, an example where the patient requires large amounts of anaesthetic to control sympathetic responses and keep EEG parameters within reasonable limits are seen on occasions. Such patients may sit at the 95 % or even 99 % area on the population distribution.

Interaction Displays as Tools for Teaching, Comprehension, and Practice Change

As discussed above interaction displays reveal many details of everyday anaesthetic practice. They allow individual reflection and optimization while providing many useful talking and education points.

For example, "standard" trainee induction doses of propofol and fentanyl make patients 99.9 % likely to be unrousable but 50–60 % likely to not respond to airway manipulation. When the patient moves in response to attempt LMA insertion the standard response is more propofol, which increases the non-response probability to 80 % or so while pushing rousability off the scale. The interaction display provides a useful tool for discussing drug dosing and Gordon's assertion that an ultra-short acting opioid should be used for every airway manipulation [33].

As examples of changes in practice, Cirillo et al. [34] found users reduced end-tidal sevoflurane concentrations by

30 % when either SmartPilot View or Navigator were used and Obara et al. [35] found that at the end of surgery patients were at a lower probability of non-response with their own interaction display. Furthermore patients had lower isoflurane levels and higher propofol levels when the display was present.

When practitioners with some anaesthesia experience first meet these devices we suggest not making immediate changes to individual practice. Instead they should observe the predictions of response and relate these to drug dosing and clinical observations. Once these relationships start to be understood then incremental changes away from standard recipes can start.

Limitations

As with any device it is useful to understand the limitations of the system. Some of these are underlying issues while others are choices made in the implementation of these displays.

What Do Probabilities Mean?

The first issue is to understand what the interaction displays mean and to appreciate that the probabilities shown are the likelihood that an individual with the characteristics and drug doses entered into the system would respond or not to the given stimulus. Of 100 patients at the 75 % probability for not responding to shake-and-shout, 1 in 4 will respond. These displays say nothing about the individual patient, a patient at the 75 % probability is not 1/4 awake! The responses modeled are all or nothing events in an individual.

Predicting Vapour Concentration

Although these systems are designed to work in tandem with the anaesthesia delivery and monitoring systems from the same provider, the forward prediction of inhaled agents varies and is generally much less precise than for intravenous drugs. Although forward modeling of vapour concentration based on vaporizer and fresh gas flow setting is feasible [24], only the Drager Zeus and Perseus (if equipped with an appropriate vaporizer) do this type of modeling. In other Drager machines and all GE machines, the forward prediction of vapour concentration appears to be based on forward prediction of the trend of measured end-tidal concentrations.

The Transition Gap and Other Limitations of the Models

As illustrated in the Navigator example above, the response of patients when there are moderate concentrations of both propofol and volatile is less well defined. Schumacher et al. have studied the propofol–sevoflurane interaction [13]. Studies of combinations of propofol, volatile and opioids are ongoing which, when completed, will be able to be implemented in the commercial display systems.

This is part of the more general problem of extending the use of models beyond the population from which they were derived. All the studies underpinning interaction displays are derived from finite numbers (usually < 100) of subjects who will not be evenly spread across the range of covariates such as age, height, and weight. Furthermore these studies are performed in volunteers exposed to specific stimuli in a laboratory setting and not with sustained noxious stimulus [36].

Drug Equivalence

These systems make the reasonable assumption that all the opioids modeled (remifentanil, fentanyl, alfentanil and sufentanil) have equivalent effects when mapped to remifentanil equivalents based on mu receptor effects. This assumption is also made with inhalational agents by converting to sevoflurane equivalents, based on relative MAC values. Given that inhalational agents have significant effects on both major anaesthetic end points (the cerebral effect on recall and the spinal effect on response to stimulus), it is possible that different agents will have a different mix of these effects.

Choice of Model

Unlike many TCI systems, the interaction displays do not give the user a choice of drug model to use. Both systems use the Schneider propofol model [37] as this model was used in the studies which underpin the interaction displays.

Opioid Concentrations with Navigator

As noted in Fig. 39.1 opioid concentrations in Navigator are plotted within the "analgesia" panel. The user needs to toggle the "PK only" box to see both the "analgesic effect" and opioid concentrations.

Not All Drugs Are Modeled

In particular morphine, pethidine, and alpha-2 agonists, all of which may influence response to noxious stimulus and arousal are not included in the models. Atracurium is not included in the modeled neuromuscular blocking agents.

The Future

Much has been learned from widespread use of these devices, which represent the first generation of commercial interaction monitor. We hope that second generation devices incorporate the feedback that has been provided to the manufacturers. Ongoing work on modeling of individual drugs and further expanding the range of drug combinations investigated in response studies will improve the applicability of these devices.

In the same way that the Open-TCI initiative has combined the data from many studies of individual drugs, there may be value in combining the different datasets behind the two competing interaction displays.

And finally there is a need for further clinical studies investigating the value of these systems.

Conclusion

An important objective of anaesthesia delivery should be to match drug delivery to the individual patient needs at different stages of their procedure. Giving too much may slow recovery and potentially have other detrimental effects. Too little risks awareness and unnecessary sympathetic activity. Any tools which allow us to better optimize anaesthesia delivery are useful. These interaction displays help fill this need.

These devices may help us learn the "art" (trial, error, and experience) of anaesthesia more rapidly, and encourage us to use a wider palette of drugs. (and)... may produce a tangible improvement in outcome [20].

Acknowledgments All screenshots are simulations. Thanks to Christian Ulke of Drager Medical and Tali Gordon of GE Healthcare for producing a range of images, not all of which I used, and for organizing permission for publication of these images. Several of the Navigator simulations were performed by the author. I am especially grateful to the clinicians and researchers whose vision and work underpins the devices discussed in this chapter.

References

1. Kay NH, Sear JW, Uppington J, Cockshott ID, Douglas EJ. Disposition of propofol in patients undergoing surgery. A comparison in men and women. Br J Anaesth. 1986;58(10):1075–9.
2. Struys MM, De Smet T, Mortier EP. Simulated drug administration: an emerging tool for teaching clinical pharmacology during anesthesiology training. Clin Pharmacol Ther. 2008;84(1):170–4.
3. Vuyk J. Pharmacokinetic and pharmacodynamic interactions between opioids and propofol. J Clin Anesth. 1997;9 (6 Suppl):23S–6.

4. Kazama T, Ikeda K, Morita K. The pharmacodynamic interaction between propofol and fentanyl with respect to the suppression of somatic or hemodynamic responses to skin incision, peritoneum incision, and abdominal wall retraction. Anesthesiology. 1998;89 (4):894–906.

5. Hendrickx JF, Eger EI, Sonner JM, Shafer SL. Is synergy the rule? A review of anesthetic interactions producing hypnosis and immobility. Anesth Analg. 2008;107(2):494–506.

6. Sleigh JW. Depth of anesthesia: perhaps the patient isn't a submarine. Anesthesiology. 2011;115(6):1149–50.

7. Glass PS. Anesthetic drug interactions: an insight into general anesthesia--its mechanism and dosing strategies. Anesthesiology. 1998;88(1):5–6.

8. Minto CF, Schnider TW, Short TG, Gregg KM, Gentilini A, Shafer SL. Response surface model for anesthetic drug interactions. Anesthesiology. 2000;92(6):1603–16.

9. Short TG, Ho TY, Minto CF, Schnider TW, Shafer SL. Efficient trial design for eliciting a pharmacokinetic-pharmacodynamic model-based response surface describing the interaction between two intravenous anesthetic drugs. Anesthesiology. 2002;96 (2):400–8.

10. Bouillon TW, Bruhn J, Radulescu L, Andresen C, Shafer TJ, Cohane C, et al. Pharmacodynamic interaction between propofol and remifentanil regarding hypnosis, tolerance of laryngoscopy, bispectral index, and electroencephalographic approximate entropy. Anesthesiology. 2004;100(6):1353–72.

11. Kern SE, Xie G, White JL, Egan TD. A response surface analysis of propofol-remifentanil pharmacodynamic interaction in volunteers. Anesthesiology. 2004;100(6):1373–81.

12. Manyam SC, Gupta DK, Johnson KB, White JL, Pace NL, Westenskow DR, et al. Opioid-volatile anesthetic synergy: a response surface model with remifentanil and sevoflurane as prototypes. Anesthesiology. 2006;105(2):267–78.

13. Schumacher PM, Dossche J, Mortier EP, Luginbuehl M, Bouillon TW, Struys MM. Response surface modeling of the interaction between propofol and sevoflurane. Anesthesiology. 2009;111 (4):790–804.

14. Syroid ND, Johnson KB, Pace NL, Westenskow DR, Tyler D, Bruhschwein F, et al. Response surface model predictions of emergence and response to pain in the recovery room: an evaluation of patients emerging from an isoflurane and fentanyl anesthetic. Anesth Analg. 2010;111:380–6.

15. Ting C-K, Johnson KB, Teng W-N, Synoid ND, Lapierre C, Yu L, et al. Response surface model predictions of wake-up time during scoliosis surgery. Anesth Analg. 2014;118(3):546–53.

16. Heyse B, Proost JH, Schumacher PM, Bouillon TW, Vereecke HEM, Eleveld DJ, et al. Sevoflurane remifentanil interaction: comparison of different response surface models. Anesthesiology. 2012;116(2):311–23.

17. Struys MMRF, Sahinovic M, Lichtenbelt BJ, Vereecke HEM, Absalom AR. Optimizing intravenous drug administration by applying pharmacokinetic/pharmacodynamic concepts. Br J Anaesth. 2011;107(1):38–47.

18. Syroid ND, Agutter J, Drews FA, Westenskow DR, Albert RW, Bermudez JC, et al. Development and evaluation of a graphical anesthesia drug display. Anesthesiology. 2002;96(3):565–75.

19. Chernik DA, Gillings D, Laine H, Hendler J, Silver JM, Davidson AB, et al. Validity and reliability of the Observer's Assessment of Alertness/Sedation Scale: study with intravenous midazolam. J Clin Psychopharmacol. 1990;10(4):244–51.

20. Kennedy RR. Seeing the future of anesthesia drug dosing: moving the art of anesthesia from impressionism to realism. Anesth Analg. 2010;111(2):252–5.

21. Luginbuhl M, Schumacher PM, Vuilleumier P, Vereecke H, Heyse B, Bouillon TW, et al. Noxious stimulation response index: a novel anesthetic state index based on hypnotic-opioid interaction. Anesthesiology. 2010;112(4):872–80.

22. Schnider TW, Minto CF, Shafer SL, Gambus PL, Andresen C, Goodale DB, et al. The influence of age on propofol pharmacodynamics. Anesthesiology. 1999;90(6):1502–16.

23. Kennedy RR, French RA. The development of a system to guide volatile anaesthetic administration. Anaesth Intensive Care. 2011;39(2):182–90.

24. Kennedy RR, French RA, Gilles S. The effect of a model-based predictive display on the control of end-tidal sevoflurane concentrations during low-flow anesthesia. Anesth Analg. 2004;99(4):1159–63.

25. Iwakiri H, Nagata O, Matsukawa T, Ozaki M, Sessler DI. Effect-site concentration of propofol for recovery of consciousness is virtually independent of fentanyl effect-site concentration. Anesth Analg. 2003;98:1651–5.

26. Johnson KB, Syroid ND, Gupta DK, Manyam SC, Egan TD, Huntington J, et al. An evaluation of remifentanil propofol response surfaces for loss of responsiveness, loss of response to surrogates of painful stimuli and laryngoscopy in patients undergoing elective surgery. Anesth Analg. 2008;106(2):471–9.

27. Coppens M, Van Limmen JGM, Schnider T, Wyler B, Bonte S, Dewaele F, et al. Study of the time course of the clinical effect of propofol compared with the time course of the predicted effect-site concentration: performance of three pharmacokinetic-dynamic models. Br J Anaesth. 2010;104(4):452–8.

28. Gin T. Clinical pharmacology on display. Anesth Analg. 2010;111 (2):256–8.

29. Hemmerling TM, Arbeid E, Wehbe M, Cyr S, Taddei R, Zaouter C. Evaluation of a novel closed-loop total intravenous anaesthesia drug delivery system: a randomized controlled trial. Br J Anaesth. 2013;110(6):1031–9.

30. Dussaussoy C, Peres M, Jaoul V, Liu N, Chazot T, Picquet J, et al. Automated titration of propofol and remifentanil decreases the anesthesiologist's workload during vascular or thoracic surgery: a randomized prospective study. J Clin Monit Comput. 2014;28:35–40.

31. Dumont GA, Ansermino JM. Closed-loop control of anesthesia. Anesth Analg. 2013;117:1130–8.

32. Kennedy RR. Individualising target-controlled anaesthesia. Better models or better targets? Anaesth Intensive Care. 2010;38 (3):421–2.

33. Gordon RJ. Anesthesia dogmas and shibboleths: barriers to patient safety? Anesth Analg. 2012;114(3):694–9.

34. Cirillo V, Zito Marinosci G, De Robertis E, Iacono C, Romano GM, Desantis O, et al. Navigator® and SmartPilot® View are helpful in guiding anesthesia and reducing anesthetic drug dosing. Minerva Anestesiol. 2015;81:1163–9.

35. Obara S, Syroid ND, Johnson KB, Westenskow D, Albert R, Ogura T, Agutter J, Egan TD. A clinical pharmacology display system changes anesthesiologists' technique and is associated with high user satisfaction. Anesthesiology. 2011;A1274. http://www.asaabstracts.com/strands/asaabstracts/searchArticle.htm;jsessionid= AEC4D2F116F777A122370968590E2687?index=3&highlight= true&highlightcolor=0&bold=true&italic=false. Accessed 1 Mar 2016.

36. Short TG. Using response surfaces to expand the utility of MAC. Anesth Analg. 2010;111(2):249–51.

37. Schnider TW, Minto CF, Gambus PL, Andresen C, Goodale DB, Shafer SL, et al. The influence of method of administration and covariates on the pharmacokinetics of propofol in adult volunteers. Anesthesiology. 1998;88(5):1170–82.

Claudia Spies, Susanne Koch, Alissa Wolf, Rudolf Mörgeli, and Björn Weiss

The Role of Intravenous Agents in Delirium

Delirium and Cognitive Dysfunction

Since decades, anesthesiologists have been concerned about cognitive disturbances associated with anesthesia. The first notable publication was from 1955, when Bedfort and Leeds published a detailed analysis in the Lancet concerning 18 patients who suffered postoperative cognitive decline [1]. In their renowned conclusion, they provided recommendations for the prevention of surgery-related long-term cognitive impairment (Table 40.1).

Remarkably, after 60 years and over 12,000 published manuscripts relating to the topic, Bedfort and Leeds' recommendations remain the major preventive foundations of postoperative cognitive dysfunction.

Our knowledge about this condition has grown exponentially in the last decades, and today it is well known that perioperative stress—including anesthesia—can cause adverse cerebral effects. Although major risk factors have been identified, only recently has the staggering incidence of postoperative cognitive dysfunctions been fully recognized [2, 3]. The exact pathophysiology remains elusive, but landmark studies and theories within the last decade promise a more comprehensive understanding of how surgery and anesthesia impact cognitive function, both in the short and long terms [4]. During Bedford's time, volatile anesthetics were the only option to conduct general anesthesia, whereas today there is the additional possibility of using iv agents. This chapter is going to explain the role of postoperative delirium (POD) in the perioperative setting and focus on the role of iv agents and total intravenous anesthesia.

Spectrum of Cognitive Disorders Following Surgery

Cognitive complications that arise in the context of surgery are usually classed as direct brain insults, which have a clear causation (e.g., hypoxia, medication), or as aberrant stress responses, which tend to be multifactorial and show no clear etiology (e.g., peripheral infection) [5, 6]. These postoperative brain injuries can be subdivided in short-term and long-term cognitive disorders, whereas short term includes inadequate emergence (IE) and postoperative delirium (POD) and long term can be summarized as postoperative cognitive dysfunction (POCD) (Fig. 40.1). However, when considering the entire spectrum of these complications, the term "cognitive complication" is misleading, as the spectrum is by no means limited to cognition and may also have pronounced effects in awareness and motor skills (e.g., delirium).

Inadequate emergence describes a state of altered mental status immediately following anesthesia, which can be further classified as either hyperactive or hypoactive emergence. In literature, IE is often cited as emergence delirium, though the criteria for delirium are not always entirely fulfilled. IE is especially prevalent in the pediatric population, and aside from acute injury, its implications have not been thoroughly analyzed [7–9].

The most common type of short-term cerebral dysfunction following surgery is the *postoperative delirium* (POD) and involves a manifestation of delirium within 5–7 days following surgery. POD has a high prevalence and is the typical clinical manifestation of "acute brain failure" after anesthesia and surgery. The occurrence of delirium 8–9 days after surgery is typically due to factors such as immobilization or consecutive pneumonia and thus only indirectly linked to the anesthesia and surgical intervention. It remains

C. Spies, MD (✉) • S. Koch, MD • A. Wolf, MD • R. Mörgeli, MD
B. Weiss, MD
Department of Anesthesiology and Intensive Care Medicine, Charité—Universitätsmedizin Berlin, Campus Charité Mitte and Campus Virchow-Klinikum, Berlin, Germany
e-mail: claudia.spies@charite.de

© Springer International Publishing AG 2017
A.R. Absalom, K.P. Mason (eds.), *Total Intravenous Anesthesia and Target Controlled Infusions*,
DOI 10.1007/978-3-319-47609-4_40

Table 40.1 Bedford and Leeds recommendations vs. recent considerations

Bedford and Leeds recommendations	Recent considerations
• Careful risk-benefit analysis for surgery on elderly patients	• Frailty assessment • Consideration of the risk of postoperative cognitive dysfunction
• No routine pre- or postoperative medication	• Patient tailored pre- or postoperative medication • Avoidance of anticholinergic side effects
• Cautious choice of drugs to avoid suppression of vital centers	• Neuromonitoring-guided anesthesia to generate adequate depth of anesthesia • Goal-directed anesthesia and analgesia with TCI and neuromonitoring • Usage of adjuvants such as alpha-2 agonists to reduce stress and to provide goal-directed depth of anesthesia • Usage of adjuvants such as alpha-2 agonists and ketamine to reduce POD • Avoidance of anticholinergic side effects
• Tight fluid, electrolyte, and hemodynamic management	• Tight fluid, electrolyte, and hemodynamic management
• Proper prevention and treatment of postoperative confusion	• Proper prevention and timely pharmacological and non-pharmacological treatment of postoperative delirium

Fig. 40.1 Spectrum of cognitive dysfunction after surgery. Immediately post anesthesia, the inadequate emergence affect in particular preschool children. Mostly postoperative delirium occurs hours after surgical procedures. Postoperative delirium and its subsequent outcomes like prolonged hospital stay, higher mortality, and posttraumatic stress disorder are a risk factor for long-term impairment. Postoperative cognitive dysfunction is characterized by cognitive impairment compared to the baseline performance. Recently naturally brain aging process and postoperative cognitive dysfunction in the elderly cannot be discriminated exactly

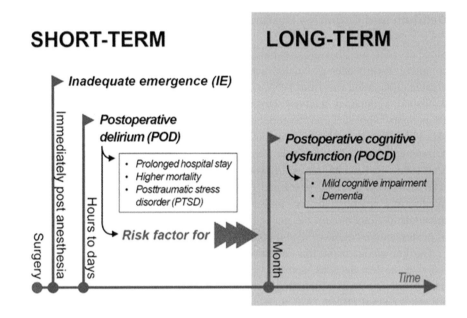

prudent to maintain preventive measures in place during this late postoperative phase.

Cognitive impairment with effects lasting weeks to months following surgery is usually referred to as *postoperative cognitive dysfunction* (POCD). Whereas delirium is a clearly defined syndrome, POCD has no formal definition and requires cognitive testing before and after the operative intervention in order to assess the extent of the cognitive impact. If clinically manifest, POCD is usually classified as either mild cognitive impairment or dementia [10, 11]. The link between delirium, i.e., not only the rate but in particular the duration of delirium, and POCD has been shown in the postoperative and the critical care setting, even long-term cognitive decline 1 year after treatment [12–14].

Although the mechanism is poorly understood and teeming with confounders, the surgical trauma, inadequate anesthesia (e.g., too deep, with painful stimuli), and insufficient stress reduction have a profound, and sometimes permanent, impact on the brain. The analysis of POCD is critical to obtain insight into the role of acute stressors in the cognitive trajectory, as well as to find new techniques to limit or prevent long-term cognitive impairment.

Defining Delirium

Delirium is the most common clinical manifestation of brain dysfunction following surgery. Delirium is not a disease, but a syndrome, in the sense that it comprises a typical reaction of the brain to disturbances. The concept of delirium as a syndrome is necessary to understand its association to other underlying medical conditions such as sepsis, intoxication, withdrawal, and other systemic illnesses.

Both the Diagnostic and Statistical Manual of Mental Disorders, Fifth Edition (DSM-5) [11], and the International Statistical Classification of Diseases and Related Health

Table 40.2 Gold standard of delirium definition

Diagnostic and Statistical Manual, 5th Edition, 95	10th revision of the International Statistical Classification of Diseases and Related Health Problems
	Delirium, not induced by alcohol and other psychoactive drugs and not superimposed on dementia
(Code 596)	(F05.0)
A–E must be fulfilled	An etiologically nonspecific organic cerebral syndrome characterized by concurrent disturbances of consciousness and attention, perception, thinking, memory, psychomotor behavior, emotion, and sleep-wake schedule. The duration is variable, and the degree of severity ranges from mild to very severe
A. Disturbance in attention (i.e., reduced ability to direct, focus, sustain, and shift attention) and awareness (reduced orientation to the environment)	A. Clouding of consciousness, i.e., reduced clarity of awareness of the environment, with reduced ability to focus, sustain, or shift attention
B. The disturbance develops over a short period of time (usually hours to a few days), represents an acute change from baseline attention and awareness, and tends to fluctuate in severity during the course of a day	B. Disturbance of cognition, manifest by both: (1) Impairment of immediate recall and recent memory, with relatively intact remote memory (2) Disorientation in time, place, or person
C. An additional disturbance in cognition (e.g., memory deficit, disorientation, language, visuospatial ability, or perception)	C. At least one of the following psychomotor disturbances: (1) Rapid, unpredictable shifts from hypoactivity to hyperactivity (2) Increased reaction time (3) Increased or decreased flow of speech (4) Enhanced startle reaction
D. The disturbances in criteria A and C are not better explained by a preexisting, established, or evolving neurocognitive disorder and do not occur in the context of a severely reduced level of arousal such as coma	D. Disturbance of sleep or the sleep-wake cycle manifests by at least one of the following: (1) Insomnia, which in severe cases may involve total sleep loss, with or without daytime drowsiness or reversal of the sleep-wake cycle (2) Nocturnal worsening of symptoms (3) Disturbing dreams and nightmares which may continue as hallucinations or illusions after awakening
E. There is evidence from the history, physical examination, or laboratory findings that the disturbance is a direct physiological consequence of another medical condition, substance intoxication or withdrawal (i.e., due to a drug of abuse or to a medication) or exposure to a toxin or is due to multiple etiologies	E. Rapid onset and fluctuations of the symptoms over the course of the day
	F. Objective evidence from history, physical and neurological examination, or laboratory tests of an underlying cerebral or systemic disease (other than psychoactive substance related) that can be presumed to be responsible for the clinical manifestations in A–D

Diagnostic and Statistical Manual, 5th Edition, 95 (DSM-5) and the 10th revision of the International Statistical Classification of Diseases and Related Health Problems (ICD-10) delirium definitions

Problems, 10th revision (ICD-10) [15], define delirium as a psychiatric syndrome (Table 40.2). Recently, a comparison of the ICD-10 and DSM-IV criteria for the diagnosis of delirium revealed that the DSM-IV definition is more comprehensive than that from ICD-10 and thus better suited to identify patients that will eventually suffer from an impaired outcome [16–19]. At the moment, there is discussion as to whether the DSM-5 criteria have a comparable diagnostic validity to the previous version. The DSM-5 defines delirium using five core criteria. The primary features are inattentiveness and reduced awareness, with an additional cognitive disturbance (e.g., memory, orientation, perception). These symptoms must not be attributable to a previously known underlying illness (e.g., dementia), but rather present acutely, and with fluctuating severity, in the context of a developing medical condition. From the clinical point of view, there is a hyperactive, a hypoactive, and a mixed

form of delirium, whereas hypoactive delirium is considered to be particularly dangerous, as it is often overlooked in clinical practice [20–23].

The level of consciousness is critical for the DSM-5 definition, as delirium cannot be diagnosed under a severely reduced level of arousal, such as a state of coma (Table 40.3). As this limitation has the potential to overlook purely hypoactive forms of delirium, the DSM-5 criteria have been often criticized by some authors as less inclusive [24, 25]. The joint statement of the American Delirium Society and the European Delirium Association (EDA) summarizes that the "conceptualization of delirium must extend beyond what can be assessed through cognitive testing (attention) and accept that altered arousal is fundamental" [26]. This comprehensive requirement is an important factor, not only as the diagnosis of delirium is often missed but also because failure to timely diagnose delirium severely

Table 40.3 The Richmond Agitation and Sedation Scale (RASS)

+4 Combative	Violent, immediate danger to staff
+3 Very agitated	Pulls or removes tube (tubes) or catheter (catheters), aggressive
+2 Agitated	Frequent non-purposeful movement, fights ventilator
+1 Restless	Anxious, apprehensive but movements not aggressive or vigorous
0	Alert and calm
−1 Drowsy	Not fully alert but has sustained awakening to voice (eye opening and contact for more than or exactly 10 s)
−2 Light sedation	Briefly awakens to voice (eye opening and contact for less than 10 s)
−3 Moderate sedation	Movement or eye opening to voice (but no eye contact)
−4 Deep sedation	No response to voice but movement or eye opening to physical stimulation
−5 Unarousable	No response to voice or physical stimulation

The RASS is used to assess sedation, respectively, level of consciousness. Sedation aims depend on the individual requirements. Usually in general anesthesia unarousability (RASS -5) is favored, while ICU patients should be alert (RASS 0/−1) to participate in their recovery

increases the risk of mortality and impaired functional outcome for the patient.

Diagnosis

The diagnosis of delirium in clinical routine was traditionally made on the basis of clinical observations, though it is now well recognized that these unstructured clinical observations are inadequate to detect such a complex disorder with a sufficient diagnostic validity [27]. Although the DSM-5 criteria are the reference standard for the diagnosis of delirium, a psychiatrist or a well-trained expert is required for the proper assessment of these criteria, and thus it is not easily applicable in clinical routine. These limitations are due to the fact that the clinical presentation of delirium is heterogeneous, and especially patients presenting with the hypoactive subtype of delirium do not necessarily behave conspicuously [23]. This form of delirium, also known as *silent delirium*, is the most common subtype in ventilated patients [22]. Even patients with a mixed form of delirium, which is the most common subtype in non-ventilated patients, might be overseen during hypoactive periods. Only the pure form of hyperactive delirium is easily recognizable, where the patients are agitated and arouse the attention of the staff. Hyperactive delirium comprises less than 5 % of all delirious patients [20, 22] (Fig. 40.2). In order to solve this predicament, several delirium screening tools have been developed.

There are several guidelines that recommend screening with a validated tool in critical care [28]. The "Clinical Practice Guideline for the Management of Pain, Agitation, and Delirium in Adult Patients in the Intensive Care Unit" shows the results of a psychometric testing of the available tools as well as their scope of application [29, 30]. The most commonly applied scores for the diagnosis of delirium are the Confusion Assessment Method for the Intensive Care Unit (CAM-ICU) [31, 32] (Fig. 40.3), the Intensive Care Delirium Screening Checklist (ICDSC) [33], and the Nursing Delirium Screening Scale (Nu-DESC) [34] (Table 40.4). Although these screening tools have been originally validated in critically ill patients [35], there are

SUBTYPES OF DELIRIUM

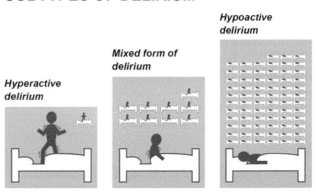

Fig. 40.2 Subtypes of delirium. Depending on the health status, the subtypes of delirium diversify. Frequently mechanically ventilated ICU patients present the hypoactive form of delirium, which is characterized by anhedonia and decreased activity. On peripheral ward the mixed form of delirium with fluctuation over the course of the day between hypo- and hyperactivity is predominant. Hyperactive delirium despite being well known is quite rare

studies assessing their validity in the recovery room, alluding that these tools may also be applicable in other settings [36–38]. These scores do not restrict the screening process to physicians but also allow for routine staff members, such as nurses and physiotherapists, to adequately identify POD with high diagnostic validity. This is an important aspect, as another key challenge for the diagnosis is that patients are regularly transferred to different units following surgery (e.g., recovery room, ward, postanesthesia care unit). These short periods of observation by constantly shifting staff impair the ability of staff to detect trends or acute changes in the state of the patient. Accounting for the time period in which POD can arise, this highlights the importance of simple and universal tools for the assessment of POD throughout the entire perioperative period, allowing for proper evaluation not only in the recovery room but also in the peripheral wards.

CAM-ICU Worksheet

Feature 1: Acute Onset or Fluctuating Course	Score	Check here if Present
Is the patient different than his/her baseline mental status? OR Has the patient had any fluctuation in mental status in the past 24 hours as evidenced by fluctuation on a sedation/level of consciousness scale (i.e.,	**Either question Yes >>**	☐
Feature 2: Inattention		
Letters Attention Test (See training manual for alternate **Pictures**) Directions: Say to the patient, "I am going to read you a series of 10 letters. Whenever you hear the letter 'A', indicate by squeezing my hand." Read letters from the following letter list in a normal tone 3 seconds apart. **S A V E A H A A R T** or **C A S A B L A N C A** or **A B A D B A D A A Y** **Errors are counted when patient fails to squeeze on the letter "A" and when the patient sqeezes on any letter other than "A."**	**Number of Errors >2 >>**	☐
Feature 3: Altered Level of Consciousness		
Present if the Actual RASS score is anything other than alert and calm (zero)	**RASS anything other than zero >>**	☐
Feature 4: Disorganized Thinking		
Yes/No Questions (See training manual for alternate set of questions) 1. Will a stone float on water? 2. Are there fish in the sea? 3. Does one pound weigh more than two pounds? 4. Can you use a hammer to pound a nail? **Errors are counted when the patient the incorrectly answer a question.** **Command** Say to patient: "Hold up this many fingers" (Hold 2 fingers in front of patient) "Now do the same thing with other hand" (Do not repeat number of fingers) *if the patient is unable to move both arms, for 2nd part of command ask patient to "Add one more finger" **An error is counted if patient is unable to complete the entire Command.**	**Combined number of errors >1 >>**	☐

Overall CAM-ICU Feature 1 plus 2 and either 3 or 4 present = CAM-ICU positive	Criteria Met >>	**CAM-ICU Positive** (Delirium Present) ☐
	Criteria Not Met >>	**CAM-ICU Negative** (No Delirium) ☐

Fig. 40.3 Confusion Assessment Method for the Intensive Care Unit (CAM-ICU). (Used with permission from Wesley Ely. Copyright© 2013, E. Wesley Ely, MD, MPH, all rights reserved)

Staff training and validation setting remain important factors regarding the proper use of these diagnostic scores. Each of these tools has different requirements in respect to staff training, and studies have revealed that these scores drastically lose diagnostic power if used inadequately [39]. It is also important to account for the setting in which the score has been validated. As these current scores cannot be simply extrapolated from the intensive care unit to the recovery room, there has been a demand for evidence-based guidelines in other settings. The "European Society of Anaesthesiology (ESA)" has established a task force to formulate guidelines on delirium management for the postanesthesia period [40]. This guideline will provide the first recommendations specifically designed for the postoperative context.

Table 40.4 Scores that have been evaluated in the recovery room and the peripheral ward

Recovery room	Peripheral ward
Nursing Delirium Screening Scale (Nu-DESC)	Nursing Delirium Screening Scale (Nu-DESC)
Confusion Assessment Method (CAM)	Confusion Assessment Method (CAM)—short form
Delirium Rating Scale (DRS-98)	Delirium Symptom Interview (DSI)
Memorial Delirium Assessment Scale (MDAS)	

While most reliable and validated scoring tools were designed for the ICU context, several have been deemed appropriate for use in the recovery room and peripheral wards. As long as all medical practitioners are trained in the standardized application of the scoring tool, the choice of test is unimportant. Consistent application and stringent treatment consequences of scoring results are essential. Assessment should be performed on all recovery room patients and should take place at least once per shift on peripheral wards

Incidence

Identifying the incidence of delirium is an extremely challenging issue. The condition is chronically underdiagnosed, and the available data is usually specific to certain patient collectives or particular surgical procedures, so that projections vary drastically.

To exemplify the dependency on patient population, one meta-analysis study assessing the incidence of delirium among elderly patients with hip fracture showed results between 16.0 and 43.9 % [41]. Among patients undergoing cardiac surgery, reported incidences are relatively constant, lying between 45 and 50 % [42–44]. While about a quarter of major abdominal surgery patients is affected [45], elderly patients undergoing major abdominal and trauma surgery show incidences of about 40 % [46]. The highest incidences of delirium have been reported among medical critically ill patients, where almost every patient suffered from delirium during their ICU stay [47, 48].

These estimates underline the importance of an adequate and consistent diagnostic assessment.

Short- and Long-Term Consequences

With few exceptions, delirium was for decades belittled as a trivial side effect of surgery and anesthesia. During the 1990s, there was a growing amount of evidence regarding the ramifications of delirium. Although most of these early landmark studies were performed in the geriatric and critical care context, and not in the perioperative setting, these studies revealed nonetheless that delirium has severe implications [49, 50] and is by no means an inconsequential issue.

Studies revealed that delirious patients have a significantly higher risk of mortality [51] and that even the "dose of delirium" has an impact on this mortality risk [52]. Pisani and co-workers revealed that every additional day in delirium leads to a significantly increased probability of death (hazard ratio 1.1 for each day) [52]. In the critical care context, delirious patients require increased periods of mechanical ventilation, as well as an increased intensive care unit and hospital stay [53]. In 2010, Witlox and co-workers published a meta-analysis showing the association between delirium and long-term outcomes [2]. They focused on elderly patients (mean age ≥ 65 years), using seven studies to estimate the relationship between mortality and delirium, and found an increased long-term mortality (mean follow-up time of the studies was 22.7 months) with a hazard ratio of 1.95 for delirious patients. Additionally, they found that patients suffering from delirium were more often institutionalized (seven studies, OR 2.41) following discharge and had a higher risk of developing dementia (two studies, OR 12.52). Recently the rate of posttraumatic stress disorder following POD was also shown to be significantly increased [54].

Studies regarding the long-term consequences of delirium in the postoperative setting also showed an impact on mortality [2, 52, 55–57]. Furthermore, it was also found that POD has a severe detrimental influence on the long-term cognitive trajectory, although the measurements used to assess cognitive performance were heterogeneous among these studies [13, 55, 58]. This shows that postoperative delirium can signal and/or trigger the development of long-term postoperative cognitive dysfunction (s.f. 1.1) and ultimately heralds all the severe individual and socioeconomic consequences of this disorder.

Special attention must be given to the evidence gathered by the "International Study of Postoperative Cognitive Dysfunction (ISPOCD)" group, which specifically sought to assess long-term cognitive dysfunctions related to surgery [3]. Among their study population of 1218 patients, the authors found a higher rate of early (25.8 %) and late cognitive dysfunction (9.9 %). Cognitive test batteries were applied 1 week and 3 months after surgery, and in a follow-up of the study (for a mean of more than 8 years), they found an association for late POCD and higher mortality (OR 1.63). Interestingly, they also found an increased probability of early departure from the labor market. The odds ratio for leaving the market was higher for patients with early POCD (OR: 2.26), which also accounted for social transfer payments [3, 59]. Although the original ISPOCD publication did not primarily account for delirium, the results nevertheless highlight that factors impairing long-term cognitive function, such as delirium, should be carefully monitored and prevented.

In summary, there is robust evidence that delirium significantly increases cognitive and noncognitive morbidity, as well as mortality, irrespective of the observed collective.

Pathophysiology of Delirium

Despite considerable research, the pathogenesis of delirium remains elusive. As there are several conditions that can lead to delirium, it is likely that no single cause, but rather numerous distinctive mechanisms, conjoins in a final pathway that induces cerebral dysfunction.

Inflammatory Pathway

There is mounting evidence that the common pathway leading to delirium is an activation of microglia cells—cerebral immune cells with the capacity to launch local reactions—with subsequent neuroinflammation [4, 60, 61].

Peripheral inflammation can have a profound influence on the brain through the dissemination of cytokines—namely, interleukin 1β, interleukin 6, and tumor necrosis factor-α (TNF-α) [61]. These proinflammatory cytokines are released by trauma, surgery, or infection, initiating a systemic response that also activates microglia in the central nervous system (Fig. 40.4). It is important to note that this communication is not limited to humoral processes, but can also occur directly via afferent neural pathways. Microglial cells are extremely sensitive to a variety of coexisting factors, so that a previous insult can prime these cells and a relatively mild subsequent insult could trigger an exponential reaction [4].

Willard et al. showed that by administering a peripheral injection of lipopolysaccharide in rats, an acute and chronic neuroinflammation could be triggered [62]. The levels of TNF-α, which has an established role in microglial activation, rose considerably in the periphery and in the brain, whereas the levels in the brain remained elevated for months thereafter [63]. The effects of a neuroinflammation through cytotoxic agents are not only acute, but can also persist due to structural damage to synapses and neuronal apoptosis. The chronic inflammation in Willard's experiment induced a time-dependent, and not dose-dependent, neuronal loss of both choline acetyltransferase (responsible for acetylcholine synthesis) and p75-immunoreactive cells (responsible for the inhibition of apoptosis).

The cholinergic anti-inflammatory pathway, as presented by Tracey et al., showed that cholinergic inhibition of this inflammatory processes is key for limiting the extent of the reaction, thus avoiding an exaggerated response with excessive inflammation [61]. The role of this cholinergic inhibition has also been well established: it has been shown that stimulation of the vagus nerve suppresses inflammatory response, that a vagotomy exacerbates cytokine release

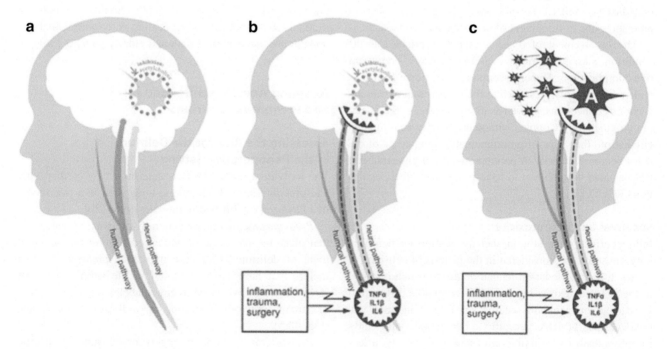

Fig. 40.4 Model of delirium genesis. While the full pathogenesis of delirium is still not clear, some onset pathways are generated. The microglial cells are inhibited by the neurotransmitter acetylcholine, which keeps them in a resting state. In case of trauma, surgery and infection proinflammatory cytokines named TNF-α, interleukin 6, and interleukin 1β are disseminated. Via humoral pathway, these cytokines overcome the blood-brain barrier and stimulate the microglial cells to activation. Proinflammatory cytokines of a lower dosage can be sensed by afferent nerves. Activated microglia cause local inflammatory effects like changes on tight junctions of astrocytes and influences of neuronal functions. This results in changes in awareness, attention, and behavior and in the worst case delirium. Long-term damage can be explained by an over-activation of pre-damaged microglial cells

[64], and that microglia itself is deactivated in the presence of the parasympathetic neurotransmitter acetylcholine [65]. This cholinergic inhibition can be hampered by a variety of factors, such as through medication (e.g., anticholinergic drugs, benzodiazepines), preexisting conditions (e.g., dementia, substance withdrawal), previous inflammation (prior structural damage, priming of microglia), or simply old age—predisposing the brain for delirium.

As postulated by van Gool, an additional insult to an already predisposed brain allows microglia—now unchecked by the cholinergic pathway—to become abnormally active, releasing cytokines that activate further microglia, thus entering a vicious cycle by triggering a sustained local inflammation with subsequent neurodegeneration, with further damage to cholinergic pathways [4]. This uncontrolled neuroinflammation, with neurochemical and synaptic disturbances, can explain the behavioral effects, as well as short- and long-term consequences of delirium and POCD. Additionally, this provides a plausible explanation as to the roles of many recognized risk factors, such as advanced age and the use of anticholinergic drugs, in the genesis of delirium.

Metabolic Factors

Metabolic disorders also appear to play a significant role in the pathophysiology of delirium. Aging, neurological maladies, as well as diabetes and hyperglycemia seem to predispose the development of cognitive dysfunction.

The involvement of diabetes is not surprising, as this condition is known to induce vascular, sensory, and cognitive complications. Hyperglycemia is also known to affect a wide range of structures, such as the blood-brain barrier and synaptic connections, as well as directly increase the release of cytokines [66]. Coupled with neurotoxicity and impaired circulation, the scope of proinflammatory properties of diabetes becomes evident. A perioperative tight glycemic control has also been shown to have protective effects against POD/POCD.

Sedatives and Neurotoxicity

Indirect effects of anesthesia, such as sedation and neurotoxicity, must also be considered in the genesis of delirium.

Much like the sedation-related delirium, which is known in the ICU context as being rapidly reversible, every hypnotic agent, or agent with sedative side effects, interacts with GABA and NMDA receptors. Interaction with those receptors leads to an inhibition of neuronal activity, affecting attention, qualitative and quantitative consciousness, as well as cognition [67]. By intermittently setting perfusion pump on and off, an acute onset and a fluctuating level of attention and/or consciousness over the day are easily produced, finally fulfilling all DSM-5 criteria for delirium. This

form of delirium is a reaction to the termination of sedation and thus also related to emergence delirium.

Preclinical experimental work raised growing concerns regarding cognitive and behavioral impairments due to anesthesia. Several experimental trials established a link between time in anesthesia and dose-dependent calcium dysregulation and neuroapoptosis in growing mice brains [68, 69]. This effect has also been shown for surgery, surgical stress, and neuroapoptosis [70]. The significance of these animal studies for humans is still unclear, and there are ongoing prospective clinical trials aiming to clarify this issue.

Depth of Anesthesia

The role of anesthesia must also be considered in the context of delirium pathophysiology. Extended periods in deep anesthesia, as expressed in a burst suppression pattern and duration in EEG monitoring, are also associated with postoperative delirium [71–74]. Burst suppression pattern represents a massive reduction of central activity and neuronal metabolic rate. Deep anesthesia may cause disturbance of neuronal homeostasis with the detrimental complication of POD. Studies published by Monk et al. show that cumulative time in burst suppression in noncardiac surgery patients significantly increased mortality within a 1-year period [75]. These results advocate that the use of EEG for the monitoring of anesthesia depth should be employed routinely, but especially when dealing with more vulnerable populations, such as the infant and elderly patients [76].

Avoiding Anesthesia-Related Risks and Preventing Delirium

Assessing the Risk for the Delirium in the Perioperative Setting

The individual risk of POD is determined by predisposing and precipitating risk factors, as suggested in a risk model that has been established in the late 1990s [50].

Predisposing factors are generally preexisting conditions that place the patient at an increased risk for the development of delirium. There are numerous predisposing risk factors that have been identified in the surgical context, including cognitive impairment, diabetes, anemia, history of stroke, previous delirium, as well as advanced age (Fig. 40.5).

Precipitating factors are triggers for delirium in a specific treatment framework, developing in the context of the medical treatment. Though these may be modifiable under certain circumstances, they are not always avoidable. Precipitating factors include, for example, the use of drugs with anticholinergic activity, burst suppression rate and duration under

PREDISPOSITIONING RISK FACTORS

- Chronic immobility
- Sensorial deficiency
- Malnutrition
- Frailty
- Atrial fibrillation
- Diabetes mellitus
- Poly-medication
- Alcohol use disorders

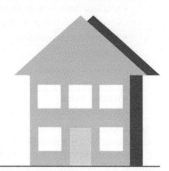

Fig. 40.5 Predispositioning risk factors for POD. Several predispositioning risk factors had been identified in association with POD. Immobility, sensorial deficiency, diabetes mellitus and malnutrition, frailty, atrial fibrillation, and poly-medication belong to these risk factors as well as alcohol and/or benzodiazepine use disorders. Early anticipation of individuals on POD risk contributes to forced special care or treatment

PRECIPITATION FACTORS

- Preoperative fluid fasting and dehydration
- Premedication with benzodiazepines
- Duration of deep anesthesia
- Altered sleep-wake cycle
- Altered sodium balance
- Intraoperative bleeding
- Anxiety
- Stress
- Pain
- Emergency surgery
- Duration of surgery
- Side of surgery

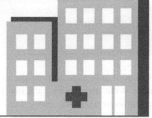

Fig. 40.6 Precipitation factors for POD. These factors are those the patient suffers during the medical treatment. If ever possible the precipitation factors should be minimized or avoided if conclusive. Reduction of precipitation factors contributes to effective POD prevention

anesthesia, a prolonged period of fluid fasting, as well as poorly managed postoperative pain (Fig. 40.6).

A special consideration must be given to advanced age, as it is—from the quantitative point—an important and frequently reported risk factor [2, 3, 17, 37, 50, 77, 78]. However, current evidence suggests that chronological age should not be viewed strictly as a risk factor, but rather as a surrogate marker for comorbidity, multimorbidity, and a loss of functional reserve [79, 80]. Undoubtedly, both comorbidity and functional impairment are more often present with advanced age, but these factors are surely not limited to elderly patients. There is a high heterogeneity among the older population, which requires the inclusion of a detailed assessment in order to properly estimate the

PREDISPOSITIONING RISK FACTORS - RELATED TO AGE: **FRAILTY**

- impaired activity of daily living
- reduced functional status
- poly-medication
- comorbidity

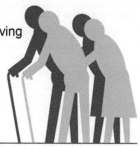

Fig. 40.7 Predispositioning risk factor age surrogates for frailty. Considering the wide range of physiological status in the elderly, many seniors are healthy and participate in all aspects of social life. On the other side some elderly suffer from comorbidities and are on poly-medication. The usual activities of daily living are impaired. Using a mobile phone or driving is too challenging for them. They cannot care for their nutrition or finances. Those elderly are frail and need more medical support. Frailty is known to be a risk factor for POD and POCD

overall risk [81]. The reduction of the "functional cognitive reserve" is the one of the most important factors to be considered in elderly patients. This means that fewer or less severe precipitating factors might suffice to induce delirium in those patients.

This increased vulnerability is not exclusively related to comorbidities like dementia (which can indeed occur at any age), but rather the loss of physiological functions. The functional status includes several domains, such as cognition, sensory functions, mobility, and malnutrition [49]. "Frailty" indicates a severely impaired functional status that is not limited to one organ system, but rather denotes a systemic condition. It seems critical to understand that not all elderly patients are frail, but only a fraction (normally between 5 and 30 % in the general population) [82]. In the in-hospital surgical setting, it is estimated that about half of the elderly patients suffer from frailty (Fig. 40.7) [78, 80].

Finally, the role of age as a predisposition condition is caused by the higher likelihood of an accumulation of age-related risk factors, linked to comorbidity and functional impairment. Therefore, a detailed functional assessment in elderly patients is of utmost importance. This includes functional tests focusing on mobility and coordination, such as the "timed up and go" test; a cognitive screening with validated tools, such as the Minimal Mental State Examination (MMSE); and a detailed medical history accounting for malnutrition, sensory and hearing loss, as well as psychiatric disorders and comorbidities (Table 40.5) [83].

In clinical routine, it would be desirable to use validated tools that predict the actual risk for the development of POD for each individual patient. There are several risk prediction

Table 40.5 Possible frailty assessment tools

Functional domain	Test examples
Cognitive impairment, dementia	• Minimal Mental State Examination (MMSE) • Clock completion test (Watson)
Mobility and risk of drop	• "Timed up and go" test
Handgrip strength as surrogate for general muscle strength	• Dynamometer
Hand-eye coordination, fine motor skills, and motor processing	• Grooved pegboard • Trail making test A & B
Activity of daily living	• Barthel Index • Instrumental Activities of Daily Living (Lawton and Brody)

Frailty comprises a geriatric symptom complex which includes several functional domains. Screening and assessment is necessary to identify frailty in the elderly. A battery of easy and short-to-perform tests for functional domains are validated and proven in frailty assessment. For example, to screen swiftly for impaired cognition, the Minimal Mental State Examination (MMSE) or the clock completion test can be used. To diagnose dementia elaborated neuropsychiatric assessment is mandatory. Frailty is accompanied with impaired mobility, muscle strength, and nutrition and increased need for help in activities of daily living

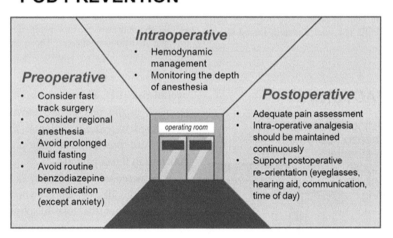

Fig. 40.8 POD prevention. To reduce harm and costs, POD prevention should be on focus in all patients and specially in those identified to be on risk of POD. In the surgical context, the actions can be discriminated in pre-, intra-, and postoperative assessments. POD prevention is multi-professional, from the nurse on ward giving care on sensorial aids and fluids to the surgeon choosing the adequate procedure to the anesthesiological management of blood pressure, analgesia, and anesthesia agents; every link in the medical chain needs to be aware of POD prevention

models that have been developed in different contexts. A recent systematic review and meta-analysis found 37 risk prediction models for POD, although the authors found only seven were either internally or externally validated [84].

While those models might indeed be more suitable for risk evaluation than an individual clinical decision [85], currently there is still no risk prediction model that adequately covers all patients. While a comprehensive risk model remains unavailable, the risk assessment should continue to be evaluated on an individual basis in the clinical setting (Fig. 40.8).

Anesthesia and Delirium

Postoperative delirium was first attributed to anesthesia rather than to the surgical procedure itself. In their article from 1955, Bedfort and Leeds attributed the risk of a patient developing delirium solely to the general anesthesia [1].

In the later phase of POD research, it became evident that it is rather the inflammatory stress induced by a surgical procedure that causes POD. Nevertheless, anesthesia and anesthesia-related factors are important aspects that can either place patients at risk or exert protective effects. The most important factors in this context are the type of anesthesia, hemodynamic management, neuromonitoring, and postoperative pain management [71, 86–88].

EEG Monitoring and Delirium

Monitoring the brain activity via electroencephalography (EEG) during administration of phenobarbital was first reported by Berger in 1931, where he described systematic changes comparable to those associated with sleep stages [89]. But even though it is clear that EEG recording is the most feasible approach for tracking brain states under general anesthesia, currently it is still not part of routine practices in anesthesiology. Instead of a thorough analysis, a single number has been derived from frontal EEG recordings, intended to represent the level of consciousness [90–92]. When compared with the non-EEG-based standard of monitoring—where depth of anesthesia is based on changes in heart rate, blood pressure, and muscle tone—his simplistic approach has been shown to be ineffective in reducing the incidence of intraoperative awareness [93]. Further, these indices are less reliable in pediatric populations, since they have been developed exclusively from cohorts of adult patients [94].

Nevertheless, the widely used EEG-based indices monitoring depth of anesthesia assume that the same index value defines the same level of consciousness for all anesthetics as well as patients of all ages. Since it is known that different anesthetics interact with different molecular targets to induce changes in neuronal circuits, it is important to develop methods for the more detailed analysis of raw EEG data. Slower EEG oscillations are generally assumed to indicate a more profound state of general anesthesia. Ketamine and nitrous oxide, however, commonly induce faster EEG oscillations and, therefore, generally produce increased EEG-derived indices [95, 96]. These elevated EEG indices are misleading in regard to the level of consciousness, frequently leading clinicians to doubt the EEG index reading. In contrast, dexmedetomidine can produce profound slowing of EEG oscillations, leading to low EEG indices, though patients can still easily be aroused [97].

Nonetheless, it is important to note that such an index-based EEG neuromonitoring has been shown to decrease the risk of developing POD in several, large randomized studies [71, 98, 99], where it was found that depth of anesthesia is one of the main risk factors contributing to the incidence of POD and POCD. In these three large randomized trials, elderly patients receiving an elective surgery were included and randomized either in a "BIS-guided" group or a "BIS-blinded" group. In the "BIS-guided" group, the anesthetist was allowed to use the BIS data to guide anesthesia, whereas in the "BIS-blinded" group, the BIS monitor was covered, and patients received routine care during anesthesia. All studies mentioned a decrease in the incidence of POD, as excessive depth of anesthesia could be avoided by processed EEG guiding. Furthermore, the frequency and duration of burst suppression during anesthesia correlated significantly with the POD incidence [71, 100]. These data provide a clear suggestion as to the potential of EEG as a monitoring tool in anesthesia.

Furthermore, BIS monitoring used in combination with TCI systems during anesthesia leads to a significant reduction of applied hypnotics and opioids [101]. These results underline the potential capability of EEG monitoring as a primary parameter to define unconscious states during anesthesia. In a similar study using TCI systems for propofol anesthesia, additional monitoring using auditory evoked potentials led to less patient movement and better sedation [102]. This data provides a clear suggestion as to the potential of neuromonitoring in anesthesia.

Neuromonitoring is not inferior to a combination of TCI with neuromonitoring. TCI systems may be particularly useful for inexperienced personnel (e.g., non-anesthetist sedation providers) or in settings where neuromonitoring is not available or not implemented. TCI algorithms can provide an automatization of dosage, thus reducing alpine blood pressures caused by bolus-wise administration of anesthetics.

The term *burst suppression* describes an electroencephalographic (EEG) pattern consisting of a continuous alternation between high-voltage slow waves and depressed electrographic activity. It is noticed in various conditions as coma, cerebral anoxia, cerebral trauma, drug intoxication, encephalopathy, hypothermia, and deep anesthesia. The presence of an ongoing oscillation in subcortical structures (hippocampal neurons) during cortical isoelectric line has been noted [103]. Importantly, it has been shown that a propofol-induced burst suppression state is associated with a state of cortical hyperexcitability and that the bursts are triggered by subliminal stimuli reaching the hyperexcitable cortex [104]. Bursts triggered by propofol anesthesia can be asynchronous across the cortex and may even occur in a limited cortical region. This happens while other areas maintain ongoing continuous activity, indicating that different cortical and subcortical circuits express different sensitivities to high doses of anesthetics [105, 106].

During anesthesia, awareness is suppressed by hypnotics, whereas arousal is mainly attenuated by analgesics. There is currently no EEG-derived single parameter which can effectively define the level of arousability. EEG activity is generally influenced by many factors during anesthesia, where the primary contributing factors are age and the choice of anesthetics and analgesics used. If EEG monitoring would be further developed to account for influencing parameters, such as age and anesthetics used, in the index calculation, it could well become an ideal tool for monitoring the level of consciousness.

Age-Related Changes

It is of interest to note that elderly patients are more likely to experience burst suppression during anesthesia [107]. Age-related changes during anesthesia with propofol and sevoflurane are related to EEG power and coherence. EEG power is defined as a function of EEG wave amplitudes and frequencies, whereas coherence can be seen as a frequency-dependent correlation or as a measure of synchrony between two signals at the same frequency (e.g., alpha-band) in

Fig. 40.9 EEG neuromonitoring during propofol anesthesia. Intraoperative frontal EEG recording with slow oscillations. *Upper screen*: raw EEG show a theta-delta activity during deep sedation with propofol. *Lower screen right*: spectrogram during propofol-induced unconsciousness with increase of power in the low-frequency alpha-band and mainly in the theta and delta band. *Lower screen left*: EEG-derived index D1 or 51

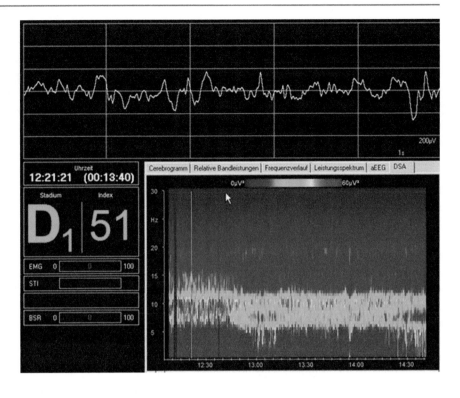

different regions of the brain. Purdon and colleagues [107] examined 155 patients, aged 18–90 years old, while receiving either propofol or sevoflurane anesthesia. For both anesthetics, they found a marked reduction in EEG signal power for all frequency bands ($a = 8\text{–}12\,\text{Hz}, b = 13\text{–}35\,\text{Hz}, q = 4\text{–}7\,\text{Hz}, d < 4\,\text{Hz}, g > 35\,\text{Hz}$) with increasing age. The effect was most pronounced in the alpha-frequency band, where they found a loss of coherence, as well as a lower peak coherent frequency in elderly patients, as compared to the younger patients. They proposed that the age-related EEG power reduction might be caused by a decline in synaptic density, changes in dendritic dynamics, or a decline in neurotransmitter synthesis within the cortex. The frontal alpha-band changes are thought to be mediated through the frontal GABA (gamma-aminobutyric acid) thalamocortical circuits [108], so that these age-related changes might reflect a functional alteration in the GABA-dependent fronto-thalamocortical circuits. In the propofol group, these occurrences were more pronounced, which can be related to the different underlying molecular mechanisms of both drugs: while propofol acts primarily as an activator on the GABA receptor, sevoflurane and other inhalative anesthetics show an additional inhibition on NMDA receptors [109].

Propofol-Related Changes

Propofol binds postsynaptically to GABA receptors, hyperpolarizing postsynaptic neurons and thus leading to inhibition [109]. EEG signatures of propofol-induced loss of consciousness show an increase in low-frequency power, a loss of coherent occipital coherent alpha-oscillation, and

the appearance of coherent frontal alpha-oscillation, which is reversed during regain of consciousness [110]. Additionally, there is a disruption of frontoparietal feedback connectivity, which also recovers during regain of consciousness (Fig. 40.9) [111].

Dexmedetomidine-Related Changes

Dexmedetomidine is an alpha-2-adrenoceptor agonist that gives rise to similarly slow oscillations and spindle-like activity during sedation [112]. In contrast to propofol, dexmedetomidine is clinically known to induce a sedation state comparable to non-rapid eye movement sleep, in which patients can easily be aroused with verbal or tactile stimuli. Both anesthetics are associated with slow/delta oscillation during induced unconsciousness, even though the amplitude power of slow wave oscillation was much larger in propofol anesthesia. Similar to sleep-induced spindles, unconsciousness induced by dexmedetomidine triggers spindles with a maximum power and coherence at 13 Hz, in contrast to propofol, where the peak frequency is at 11 Hz [97]. The authors propose that propofol enables a deeper state of unconsciousness, as seen by large-amplitude slow wave oscillation, whereas dexmedetomidine places patients into a more plane brain state of sedation.

Ketamine-Related Changes

Ketamine acts primarily via the inhibition of NMDA receptors, inducing a "dissociative anesthesia" [109]. This difference in molecular interaction can be seen in EEG analysis, where a reduction in alpha-power as well as an increase in gamma-power can be noted. But despite the molecular and neurophysiological differences to the other major classes of anesthetics, the frontoparietal feedback connectivity was gradually diminished during induction with ketamine anesthesia and was inhibited after loss of consciousness [113].

Target-controlled infusion (TCI) systems have been developed for intravenous drugs, where a set of pharmacokinetic parameters has been selected for computer simulation of an infusion scheme. The selected model is incorporated into the infusion pump, where it is used to predict the drug concentration in the plasma and at the drug target site. This allows it to calculate the needed concentration of anesthetics to reach an unconscious state. Monitoring the depth of anesthesia, or unconscious state during anesthesia, may be defined as the probability of nonresponse to stimulation [114] and, therefore, is dependent on the intensity of the stimulus, as well as the nature of response. Anesthesia may well induce unresponsiveness and amnesia, but the extent to which it causes unconsciousness remains uncertain [109].

Therefore, it may be more reliable in the future to focus on parameters that are directly related to the level of consciousness, such as the EEG, in order to monitor depth of anesthesia/unconscious state. In order to ensure more reliable results, it is important to use EEG signatures that are specific to age and to the anesthetic of choice.

To measure "arousability," which is the balance between noxious stimulation and nociceptive suppression by analgesics, it is necessary to analyze responses evoked by a strong painful stimulus. Since analgesics primarily act at a subcortical level, it seems appropriate to assess electrophysiological reflexes at the subcortical/spinal level to achieve this goal.

Target-Controlled Infusions and Delirium

Target-Controlled Infusions

In the last decades, the availability of short-acting drugs with a high degree of performance prediction, such as propofol [115], allowed for the development of novel approaches to anesthesia. Aside from total intravenous anesthesia (TIVA), these advancements allowed for the development of target-controlled infusion (TCI) systems, which employ multi-compartment pharmacokinetic models to predict anesthetic doses [116, 117], as described in Chaps. 6 and 8.

Since the first computer-based infusions were developed in the 1980s [118, 119], increasingly more accurate and reliable models have expanded the prospects of TCI, and today there are regimens available for the drug delivery of

several substances, such as sedatives, analgesics, antiarrhythmics, antibiotics, and chemotherapeutics (see Chap. 8).

Anesthesia is attained by a balanced mixture use of hypnotics and analgesics, whereas the ideal dosage is generally estimated using vegetative signs as surrogate markers, such as heart rate and blood pressure fluctuations. Monitoring the depth of anesthesia in this fashion is challenging and has several limitations, so that much skill is needed to properly recognize and interpret stress signals in a broad patient collective. While an insufficient depth of anesthesia increases the risk of awareness and subsequent complications [93, 120], excessive anesthesia, expressed as burst suppression patterns in EEG analysis, is associated with POD [72, 100]. Therefore, inadequate dosage of these substances in either side of the target range can have severe effects on patient outcome [40]. There are promising new monitoring approaches, such as the noxious stimulation response index (NSRI) [121] and surgical pleth index (SPI) [122, 123], which may be helpful devices in future anesthetic assessments.

By properly defining target doses, TCI offers an elegant solution to this predicament, with the potential to decrease complication rates and improve patient outcome. One major limitation of the most commonly used TCI algorithms is that anesthesiologists utilize algorithms that were designed for the use of one opioid (mostly remifentanil) and one hypnotic (mostly propofol). Usually, the target plasma concentrations do not allow an automatic correction for co-analgesics and co-hypnotics, so that these have to be manually adjusted. Especially for patients with a high risk for delirium, these co-substances might play an important role by blocking proinflammatory pathways, thus providing beneficial effects for patients. This can explain the protective effect of iv agents (e.g., ketamine, dexmedetomidine) *and* also their sparing effect on hypnotics with a considerable risk for burst suppression (e.g., propofol).

When using a TCI model in a patient with a significant risk for POD, the additional use of an EEG-controlled monitoring is recommended in order to avoid excessive anesthesia and to better titrate analgesia to avoid pain and overdosing of opioids by reduction of anticholinergic side effects, as well as to allow for manual adjustments of the target concentrations, if necessary.

Background Information: Pediatrics

Children have a particular high risk of experiencing inadequate emergence after surgery [7, 9]. IE can be further divided as *pediatric emergence delirium* (paedED) and *emergence agitation* (EA). EA, which occurs more frequently than paedED [40], is a behavioral disturbance seen as excessive motor activity caused by discomfort, pain, or anxiety [124].

In the case of paedED, however, all the DSM-5 criteria for delirium are entirely fulfilled. This complication usually affects preschool children following anesthesia with sevoflurane and is associated with consecutive maladaptive behavioral changes [125]. Thus, prevention is essential.

The employment of TCI in pediatrics is promising, but remains limited [126, 127]. Intravenous anesthesia has been shown to have beneficial effects on children, including a decrease in the rate of paedED, and postoperative nausea and vomiting (PONV) [126]. Reduced rates of paedED have also been shown under premedication with midazolam [128–130] or alpha-2 agonists [131–134]. Intraoperative application of propofol and ketamine and adequate perioperative pain management also provide protection [135, 136]. The development of proper TCI models for pediatric patients, however, has been hindered due to essential differences in pharmacokinetics and pharmacodynamics, as well as limitations on anesthesia monitoring in this patient collective [126, 127, 137].

TCI Substances and Delirium

Propofol

Propofol is a highly lipid-soluble substrate that readily permeates biomembranes such as the blood-brain barrier, so that the onset of anesthetic effects is equivalent to the blood circulation time. This property also allows for the rapid redistribution to the periphery, so that patients can readily recover from anesthetic states.

Propofol has been extensively studied in the context of anesthesiology and critical care. It is seen as the gold standard hypnotic for total intravenous anesthesia and is also frequently used for short-term sedation in critical care. The use is limited to short-term sedation, as prolonged use carries the risk of a severe complication known as *propofol infusion syndrome* (PRIS). The pathophysiology of this condition is not understood comprehensively, but it is mitochondria related and characterized by a massive lactate acidosis, lipidemia, and severe myolysis, leading ultimately to multi-organ dysfunction with a high mortality [138]. The risk of PRIS is increased if propofol is given in high doses or for prolonged periods of time. Therefore, the use is generally limited for both dosage and application period (≤ 4 mg/kg/h for sedation in intensive care and limited for use only up to 7 days) [139]. The risk of developing PRIS is generally higher in children [140], and, therefore, strict indications for prolonged sedation is critical.

Propofol has vasodilatative properties, which can lead to a severe decrease in blood pressure and heart rate, as well as a strong respiratory depression. When compared to sevoflurane, propofol reduces cerebral blood flow [105, 141], whereas the combination of propofol and remifentanil induces a low-flow state preserving the pressure-flow autoregulation. In contrast, sevoflurane induces a certain degree of luxury perfusion. Further, propofol reduces cerebral oxygenation compared to sevoflurane [142]. Preexisting impairment of cerebral oxygenation in elderly patients has been proven to be related with a higher risk of POD and POCD [3, 143]. These findings might have important implications to the development of POD/POCD, and it may be useful to assess the preexisting cerebral blood flow and oxygenation parameters, so as to allow anesthesiologists to select an appropriate medication in an individual basis. Although these experimental pharmacodynamic findings suggest a link between POD and propofol, there is nearly no evidence supporting this thesis. Propofol is usually seen as a reference standard substance in the ICU context, as it has the delirium risk profile of a "non-benzodiazepine" sedative, so that it is even recommended for ICU sedation.

Interestingly, although propofol binds the same receptors as benzodiazepines, causes a reduced cerebral blood flow, and lowers cerebral oxygenation, there is still no evidence showing that propofol is a risk factor for delirium.

Propofol TCI and Delirium

Pharmacokinetic and pharmacodynamic models for propofol drug delivery in adults have been available for decades [117, 144]. These propofol TCI models have been shown to correlate significantly with BIS readings [145], where the effects of age on target concentrations have been highlighted. When compared to younger patients, the elderly required less propofol to lose consciousness, in spite of higher BIS indices [146, 147]. Concerns that propofol may induce neuroapoptosis in infants are still being investigated [137]. The currently available TCI regimens for children vary considerably and lack proper validation, so that there is still a need for improved monitoring techniques before TCI may be implemented in pediatric anesthesia [126].

Although there are several studies regarding propofol TCI sedation, none showed direct evidence that it reduces the risk or incidence of postoperative delirium. In combination with remifentanil, however, it has been established that propofol TCI regimens have the potential to reduce the risk of burst suppression by reducing dosages [142, 148], which would indirectly also affect the risk for POD. This remains controversial, as there are also studies indicating that TCI may in fact increase total propofol doses, so that additional investigations are still required to determine whether TCI is indeed superior to conventional anesthesia [149].

Alpha-2 Agonists

Alpha-2 agonists (A2As) are a group of substances that bind to presynaptic alpha-2 receptors and exert its effect via the inhibition of presynaptic noradrenaline release. By understanding that A2As reduce the activity of the sympathetic tone, it is not surprising that these substances have not been introduced into the market as an iv sedative, but rather as an antihypertensive. Their first release took place more than 50 years ago. However, in the modern management of sedation, A2As are more important than ever.

Dexmedetomidine is currently available for iv use both in the US and European markets. It is a lipophilic imidazole derivative that has, compared to clonidine, a higher affinity for the alpha-2 receptor [150].

The sedative effect of A2A is delivered independently from the GABA receptor, but due to stimulation of presynaptic noradrenaline receptors, essentially in the locus coeruleus. The sedation properties of A2As are a result of reduced firing in the neurons of the locus coeruleus, which is part of the ascending reticular activating system (ARAS). Incidentally, the drugs do not directly interfere with the cortex, but rather increase the threshold for stimulation, thus promoting a condition similar to natural non-rapid eye movement (NREM) sleep. On the Richmond Agitation-Sedation Scale, the minimum achievable RASS with the exclusive use of an A2A is "−3" [150].

The side effects can be explained by the fact that alpha-2 adrenoreceptors are not exclusively located in the locus coeruleus, but can also be found throughout the body. Therefore, a decrease in blood pressure, heart rate, and orthostatic dysregulations are typical side effects, whereas these side effects tend to be mild, and the tolerance of the substances is excellent [151–153].

Clonidine, a prototype substance that is still used in Europe, differs from dexmedetomidine not only in regard to their affinity to alpha-2 receptors but also concerning their pharmacokinetic properties. Clonidine has also been shown to attenuate early proinflammatory response in cardiac patients [154].

Dexmedetomidine is very lipophilic and, therefore, quickly distributed throughout the body. Although the termination is dependent on its distribution effect in short-term use, such as during anesthesia, the elimination of dexmedetomidine is also rapid, shown to be completed within about 2 h in healthy volunteers. In contrast, clonidine has a half-life of up to 72 h.

A2As play a significant role in the concept of "early goal-directed sedation" [30], which aims at an awake and attentive patient from the very beginning of an intensive care treatment [155]. Additionally, it is also approved for procedural sedation, as it has a near complete lack of respiratory depression. Dexmedetomidine has also been studied in the context of fiber-optic intubations for anticipated difficult airways, as the patients remain well cooperative and able to tolerate tubes and stimuli [156–160]. From the intensive

care context, it has been shown that patients treated with dexmedetomidine have lower mortality rates, although further trials are necessary to confirm this finding, as thus far this could only be shown in a subgroup analysis of a randomized controlled trial [161]. The possible neuroprotective effects of dexmedetomidine have been hypothesize, as it might mitigate the inflammatory response of the brain to peripheral stimuli. Experimental in vitro trials showed dexmedetomidines' potential to attenuate lipopolysaccharide (LPS)-induced inflammatory response in activated microglia [162–164].

Finally, dexmedetomidine is also one of the selected substances that showed effectiveness in the symptom-orientated treatment of delirium. Dexmedetomidine and other A2A class substances are seen as the most promising drugs for neuroprotection and delirium prevention [165]. The reduced levels of stress caused by A2A minimize the proinflammatory response. A formal recommendation regarding the use of A2A as potential neuroprotective co-sedatives is still not available, as corroborating studies are still ongoing.

Alpha-2 Agonists TCI and Delirium

The use of A2S has been relatively well established in the TCI context, where it is usually employed in a three-compartment model [166, 167]. Dexmedetomidine TCI has been shown to have several beneficial effects, including reduced anesthetic requirement, less postoperative pain, and reduced ICU length of stay, mechanical ventilation, and occurrence of delirium [168–172]. Even in children, dexmedetomidine/propofol TCI was able to reduce the rate of intra- and postoperative complications in comparison to fentanyl [131].

The hemodynamic stability and lack of respiratory suppression provided by dexmedetomidine have also been noted, so that it can be safely used for sedation during potentially stressful procedures, such as awake fiber-optic intubations [129, 173–175]. The mild hemodynamic side effects also favor the use of dexmedetomidine in the ICU, where it can be used as an adjuvant in order to reduce dosage of other substances, such as propofol and benzodiazepines (for alcohol withdrawal) [153, 176]. Though this effect is largely beneficial, the reduced need for other substances carries the risk of accidental overdosage with consecutive complications, such as burst suppression. Therefore, the use of a dexmedetomidine TCI requires careful monitoring via EEG [177].

In conclusion, the use of dexmedetomidine TCI has the potential to reduce several risk factors for delirium. Especially its opioid- and hypnotic-sparing and stress-reducing effect makes it interesting as an adjuvant for prevention and risk reduction.

Benzodiazepines

Anesthesiologists use benzodiazepines primarily for anxiolysis and premedication. Traditionally, almost every patient received an oral bolus of a benzodiazepine approximately half an hour before scheduled surgery. A well-known side effect of benzodiazepines is the possibility of paradoxical reactions, generally occurring in children and elderly patients [178–180]. This dose-dependent phenomenon of paradox excitation is a subset of hyperactive-sedation-related delirium [67]. Additionally, there is strong evidence for an increased risk for ICU delirium if lorazepam or midazolam is used in the context of critical care [181, 182].

Aside from these complications, benzodiazepines have nevertheless a sedative, anxiolytic, anticonvulsant, and relaxing pharmacological profile, also known for mediation of analgesic effects on a spinal level [183–185]. The distinct characteristics of substances from this class are due to their individual affinity for particular GABA subtypes [183, 186, 187]. There are at least five distinctive GABA-A-alpha receptors, each with different subtypes mediating different therapeutic actions. For instance, benzodiazepines with a high affinity toward the GABA-A-alpha 1 receptor possess strong sedative properties, whereas GABA-A-alpha 2/3 agonists are more adequate for the induction of anxiolysis [184].

Many anesthesiologists favor benzodiazepines due to their broad therapeutic range. When compared to other substance classes, benzodiazepines have less prominent respiratory and cardio-depressive effects [188]. Especially due to their beneficial effects on hemodynamics, benzodiazepines are sometimes used for the induction of anesthesia in patients with severe cardiovascular comorbidities. This can be a feasible method, especially in cardiac anesthesia.

In addition to cardiac surgery, the advantageous hemodynamic stability of benzodiazepines led to an extensive use of lorazepam and midazolam for sedation in the intensive care unit [189]. Long-term sedation is particularly relevant in this context, as propofol has limitations regarding the duration of treatment and dosage. However, studies have repeatedly shown that long-term sedation with midazolam and lorazepam is independently correlated with an increased incidence for ICU delirium [181]. It is important to note that only these two substances, lorazepam and midazolam, have been extensively studied in this context, thus acting as surrogates for the entire substance class.

From the pharmacodynamic point, benzodiazepines and propofol are both GABA agonists, so it is surprising to note a significant difference in their type of action. This major difference is due to their binding affinity and the pharmacokinetics. Per example, both midazolam and the alpha-OH-hydroxymidazolam (the first metabolite, which is still active) are known to undergo the cytochrome P450-dependent breakdown, a notoriously stagnant metabolic pathway, which leads to accumulation and extensive prolongation of their half-life. A 3-day midazolam infusion can result in elevated plasma levels of these active metabolites for more than a week [190].

Although the evidence is currently inconsistent, benzodiazepines should be used reservedly. The bolus-wise use of these substances can be indicated to provide a stress-free environment, particularly for patients suffering from anxiety or stress, though their routine administration cannot be recommended.

Benzodiazepines TCI and Delirium

There is controversial data regarding the use of benzodiazepine TCI systems. Though often used in the context of premedication and sedation, benzodiazepines have a notorious deliriogenic reputation. However, studies involving midazolam TCI systems in the ICU have shown that these systems are capable of avoiding deliriogenic dosages [191] and the three-compartment models have been deemed feasible and safe for sedation in the ICU [192].

The question of whether or not benzodiazepines induce delirium due to their long half-life (sedation-related delirium) or through their potentially precipitating effect on neuroinflammation is still the object of current investigations, whereas there is evidence supporting both mechanisms. Also noteworthy is that benzodiazepines have dependence potential, which can subsequently trigger severe withdrawal delirium [193]. In this context, it is interesting to note the innovations in the field of benzodiazepines , where anxiolytic and analgesic experimental benzodiazepines with an increased affinity to certain sub-receptor types are recently under development. These could be suitable for preoperative anxiolysis, without the negative sedating side effect.

Additionally, a new substance called "remimazolam" is undergoing trials in Japan for procedural sedation as an ultrashort-acting benzodiazepine [194]. Though further trials are needed, this drug might play a significant role in the future of "total intravenous anesthesia" in instable patients.

The postoperative use of midazolam also demonstrated a sparing effect on hypnotics and opioids, though this effect was not as pronounced as that of alpha-2 agonists [195, 196].

Taking these factors under account, further research is needed to safely assess the benefits of midazolam TCI systems without inducing delirium. Currently, however, the independent association between benzodiazepines and delirium leads to the recommendation that a continuous application of benzodiazepines should be avoided in intensive care [30, 197].

Ketamine

Ketamine exists in two isomers, S(+) and the R(−), whereas the S(+) isomer has a higher affinity to N-methyl-D-aspartate (NMDA) receptor and thus exhibits a higher potency than R (−) ketamine. The effects of ketamine are unfolded by an interaction of muscarinic, opioid, and voltage-gated receptors. The "dissociative anesthesia" is caused by the antagonism of NMDA receptors. Ketamine combines hypnotic and analgesic properties, as well as altered amnestic and psychomimetic functions. These properties offer ketamine-wide and interesting applications, especially in the prehospital setting. In the perioperative context, ketamine is favored for its bronchodilation and lack of respiratory suppression.

The sympathetic nervous and cardiovascular systems are slightly stimulated by ketamine, though recent findings reveal no intraocular or intracranial pressure rise when it is used carefully and in combination with other anesthetics [198, 199].

In the field of psychiatry, there is an ongoing study examining ketamine infusion in combination with clonidine as an option for treatment-resistant depression [200]. Ketamine seems to be particularly effective in the treatment of fatigue in individuals with treatment-resistant bipolar depression [201].

Ketamine TCI and Delirium

Outside of the operating room, ketamine TCI systems are used for procedural sedation in gastrointestinal endoscopy, as well as for children undergoing MRI examinations and interventional radiology [202, 203].

In the perioperative context, ketamine is used as a potent adjuvant in general anesthesia, effective in reducing intra- and postoperative opioid requirement, as well as lowering postoperative pain scores [204]. When compared to propofol or midazolam, EEG guidance during sedation induction with ketamine can be challenging, as there is no change in the BIS index after loss of consciousness. Therefore, other monitoring methods, such as auditory evoked potentials, can be necessary [205].

As for postoperative pain treatment, the addition of ketamine to morphine/hydromorphone PCA reduced the rate of PONV, as well as reduced opioid requirements [206]. This analgesic-sparing effect of ketamine helps to avoid pro-deliriogenic opiate oversedation. A systematic review recently revealed that perioperative application of ketamine, dexmedetomidine, and antipsychotics may reduce the risk of POD [207], whereas dexamethasone remains controversial [208].

Compared to sevoflurane, children treated with ketamine anesthesia had a reduced risk of experiencing emergence delirium [136]. For the elderly patients undergoing cardiac anesthesia, a high-risk collective, single bolus of ketamine during induction of general anesthesia showed reductions in the rate of POD [209, 210].

Opioids

A sufficient analgesic treatment is imperative, as pain has severe effects on the development of complications such as delirium [50]. However, the administration of substances with sedative properties must be critically evaluated, as they have also been shown to increase the risk of delirium [211, 212].

In the perioperative and ICU settings, opioids are routinely favored for their unrivaled analgesic effect, their little cardiovascular influence, as well as their lack of liver and kidney toxicity [213]. They may also be used in combination with regional anesthesia [214] and allow for a patient-controlled administration, which can and should be implemented on patients who are sufficiently awake [215].

Opioids were originally derived from opium, though currently several synthetic and semisynthetic alternatives are available. The effects of opioids are unfolded through binding on opioid receptors in the brain stem, in the subcortex, and on the spinal level, which are physiologically the binding sites of several ligands, such as endorphins and enkephalins [213, 216]. Differences among opioids are due primarily to their relative affinity to particular receptors, but also due to their pharmacodynamic properties. While there are several types of opioid receptors, the μ and kappa receptors are the most relevant in anesthesia, as both can elicit analgesia and sedation [217].

Remifentanil is the opioid with the shortest half-life (3–4 min), and due to its degradation by plasma esterases, it provides excellent controllability while eliminating the danger of accumulation [218].

The associated side effects of opioids are related to unspecific binding of receptors. For example, while the binding of μ1 receptors induces the desired analgesia, μ2 receptors are responsible for respiratory depression and reduced gastrointestinal motility [219]. Other side effects include postoperative nausea and vomiting, thorax rigidity, and substance dependency.

Opioid TCI and Delirium

The continuous iv application of opioids is known in the perioperative context, primarily as part of a total intravenous anesthesia during surgery, as well as in the postoperative management of pain via (patient-controlled) infusion pumps.

Remifentanil is the opioid of choice for use in total intravenous anesthesia, and it has been shown to reduce the incidence of POD [220]. It was shown to be secure and feasible for rescue therapies [221] and also shows synergetic effects with hypnotics, allowing for a significant dosage reduction [148, 222]. This sparing effect was shown to be more pronounced with remifentanil than with other opioids, such as fentanyl [223], though no clear benefit over sufentanil could be seen [224]. Other substances, such as hydromorphone, also showed satisfactory results as TCI in the management of postoperative pain [225].

Aside from meperidine, which has been shown to be more prone to trigger delirium than other opioids [226], there is no evidence of a clear advantage among substances in this class in regard to deliriogenic effect [227]. A clear superiority of automated over manual systems could not be established [228]. As compared to an oral intake, however, studies have shown that the iv administration of opioids in the postoperative setting is linked to a higher incidence of POCD [87].

The inadequate pain management in anesthesiology and ICU settings may result in more delirium, either due to insufficient dosage with subsequent pain or due to excessive dosage with subsequent anticholinergic effect.

Summary

TCI systems have the potential to reduce significant risk factors for delirium, such as overdosage and alpine blood pressure. The use of adjuvants, such as ketamine and dexmedetomidine, is particularly promising in achieving dosage reduction and neuroprotection, though most of the drug delivery models currently available are restricted to only two substances (generally a hypnotic and an opioid). For now, this constraint still limits the potential of TCI to reduce delirium rates.

Finally, it is advisable to combine the use of TCI systems with neuromonitoring so as to harmonize dosage adaptation, depth of anesthesia, hemodynamic stability, and neuroprotection. If neuromonitoring is not available or not implemented, TCI can be useful. However, TCI should always be used in combination with neuromonitoring when used in patients at risk for delirium.

References

1. Bedford PD. Adverse cerebral effects of anaesthesia on old people. Lancet. 1955;269:259–63.
2. Witlox J, Eurelings LSM, de Jonghe JFM, Kalisvaart KJ, Eikelenboom P, van Gool WA. Delirium in elderly patients and the risk of postdischarge mortality, institutionalization, and dementia: a meta-analysis. JAMA. 2010;304:443–51.
3. Moller J, Cluitmans P, Rasmussen L, et al. Long-term postoperative cognitive dysfunction in the elderly: ISPOCD1 study. Lancet. 1998;351:857–61.
4. van Gool WA, van de Beek D, Eikelenboom P. Systemic infection and delirium: when cytokines and acetylcholine collide. Lancet. 2010;375:773–5.
5. Maclullich AMJ, Anand A, Davis DHJ, Jackson T, Barugh AJ, Hall RJ, Ferguson KJ, Meagher DJ, Cunningham C. New horizons in the pathogenesis, assessment and management of delirium. Age Ageing. 2013;42:667–74.
6. Maclullich AMJ, Ferguson KJ, Miller T, de Rooij SEJA, Cunningham C. Unravelling the pathophysiology of delirium: a focus on the role of aberrant stress responses. J Psychosom Res. 2008;65:229–38.
7. Radtke FM, Franck M, Hagemann L, Seeling M, Wernecke KD, Spies CD. Risk factors for inadequate emergence after anesthesia: emergence delirium and hypoactive emergence. Minerva Anestesiol. 2010;76:394–403.
8. Lepousé C, Lautner CA, Liu L, Gomis P, Leon A. Emergence delirium in adults in the post-anaesthesia care unit. Br J Anaesth. 2006;96:747–53.
9. Hudek K. Emergence delirium: a nursing perspective. AORN J. 2009;89:509–16. Quiz 517–519.
10. Silverstein JH, Deiner SG. Perioperative delirium and its relationship to dementia. Prog Neuropsychopharmacol Biol Psychiatry. 2013;43:108–15.
11. American Psychiatric Association. Diagnostic and statistical manual of mental disorders. 5th ed. Arlington, VA: American Psychiatric Association; 2013.
12. Kratz T, Diefenbacher A. Acute and long-term cognitive consequences of treatment on intensive care units. Nervenarzt. 2016;87(3):246–52. doi:10.1007/s00115-016-0078-0.
13. Wacker P, Nunes PV, Cabrita H, Forlenza OV. Post-operative delirium is associated with poor cognitive outcome and dementia. Dement Geriatr Cogn Disord. 2006;21:221–7.
14. Bryson GL, Wyand A, Wozny D, Rees L, Taljaard M, Nathan H. A prospective cohort study evaluating associations among delirium, postoperative cognitive dysfunction, and apolipoprotein E genotype following open aortic repair. Can J Anaesth. 2011;58:246–55.
15. Organization WH. The ICD-10 classification of mental and behavioural disorders: clinical descriptions and diagnostic guidelines. Geneva: World Health Organization; 1992.
16. Kazmierski J, Kowman M, Banach M, Fendler W, Okonski P, Banys A, Jaszewski R, Rysz J, Sobow T, Kloszewska I. The use of DSM-IV and ICD-10 criteria and diagnostic scales for delirium among cardiac surgery patients: results from the IPDACS study. J Neuropsychiatry Clin Neurosci. 2010;22:426–32.
17. Laurila JV, Pitkala KH, Strandberg TE, Tilvis RS. Impact of different diagnostic criteria on prognosis of delirium: a prospective study. Dement Geriatr Cogn Disord. 2004;18:240–4.
18. Cole MG, Dendukuri N, McCusker J, Han L. An empirical study of different diagnostic criteria for delirium among elderly medical inpatients. J Neuropsychiatry Clin Neurosci. 2003;15:200–7.
19. Morandi A, Davis D, Taylor JK, et al. Consensus and variations in opinions on delirium care: a survey of European delirium specialists. Int Psychogeriatr. 2013;25:2067–75.
20. Robinson TN, Raeburn CD, Tran ZV, Brenner LA, Moss M. Motor subtypes of postoperative delirium in older adults. Arch Surg. 2011;146:295–300.
21. Meagher DJ, Maclullich AMJ, Laurila JV. Defining delirium for the international classification of diseases, 11th Revision. J Psychosom Res. 2008;65:207–14.
22. Pandharipande P, Cotton BA, Shintani A, Thompson J, Costabile S, Truman Pun B, Dittus R, Ely EW. Motoric subtypes of delirium in mechanically ventilated surgical and trauma intensive care unit patients. Intensive Care Med. 2007;33:1726–31.
23. Stagno D, Gibson C, Breitbart W. The delirium subtypes: a review of prevalence, phenomenology, pathophysiology, and treatment response. Palliat Support Care. 2004;2:171–9.
24. Neufeld KJ. Delirium classification by the diagnostic and statistical manual—a moving target. Int Psychogeriatr. 2015;27:881–2.

25. Blazer DG, van Nieuwenhuizen AO. Evidence for the diagnostic criteria of delirium: an update. Curr Opin Psychiatry. 2012;25:239–43.

26. European Delirium Association, American Delirium Society. The DSM-5 criteria, level of arousal and delirium diagnosis: inclusiveness is safer. BMC Med. 2014;12:1–4.

27. Devlin JW, Marquis F, Riker RR, Robbins T, Garpestad E, Fong JJ, Didomenico D, Skrobik Y. Combined didactic and scenario-based education improves the ability of intensive care unit staff to recognize delirium at the bedside. Crit Care Lond Engl. 2008;12: R19.

28. Luetz A, Balzer F, Radtke FM, Jones C, Citerio G, Walder B, Weiss B, Wernecke K-D, Spies C. Delirium, sedation and analgesia in the intensive care unit: a multinational, two-part survey among intensivists. PLoS One. 2014;9, e110935.

29. Barr J, Fraser GL, Puntillo K, et al. Clinical practice guidelines for the management of pain, agitation, and delirium in adult patients in the intensive care unit. Crit Care Med. 2013;41:263–306.

30. DAS-Taskforce 2015, Baron R, Binder A, et al. Evidence and consensus based guideline for the management of delirium, analgesia, and sedation in intensive care medicine. Revision 2015 (DAS-Guideline 2015)—short version. Ger Med Sci. 2015; 13: Doc 19.

31. Inouye SK, van Dyck CH, Alessi CA, Balkin S, Siegal AP, Horwitz RI. Clarifying confusion: the confusion assessment method. A new method for detection of delirium. Ann Intern Med. 1990;113:941–8.

32. Ely EW, Margolin R, Francis J, May L, Truman B, Dittus R, Speroff T, Gautam S, Bernard GR, Inouye SK. Evaluation of delirium in critically ill patients: validation of the Confusion Assessment Method for the Intensive Care Unit (CAM-ICU). Crit Care Med. 2001;29:1370–9.

33. Bergeron N, Dubois MJ, Dumont M, Dial S, Skrobik Y. Intensive Care Delirium Screening Checklist: evaluation of a new screening tool. Intensive Care Med. 2001;27:859–64.

34. Gaudreau J-D, Gagnon P, Harel F, Tremblay A, Roy M-A. Fast, systematic, and continuous delirium assessment in hospitalized patients: the nursing delirium screening scale. J Pain Symptom Manage. 2005;29:368–75.

35. Gusmao-Flores D, Salluh JIF, Chalhub RÁ, Quarantini LC. The confusion assessment method for the intensive care unit (CAM-ICU) and intensive care delirium screening checklist (ICDSC) for the diagnosis of delirium: a systematic review and meta-analysis of clinical studies. Crit Care. 2012;16:R115.

36. Radtke FM, Franck M, Schust S, et al. A comparison of three scores to screen for delirium on the surgical ward. World J Surg. 2010;34:487–94.

37. Neufeld KJ, Leoutsakos J-MS, Sieber FE, Wanamaker BL, Gibson Chambers JJ, Rao V, Schretlen DJ, Needham DM. Outcomes of early delirium diagnosis after general anesthesia in the elderly. Anesth Analg. 2013;117:471–8.

38. Stukenberg S, Franck M, Spies CD, Neuner B, Myers I, Radtke FM. How to advance prediction of postoperative delirium? A secondary analysis comparing three methods for very early assessment of elderly patients after surgery and early prediction of delirium. Minerva Anestesiol. 2016.

39. van Eijk MM, van den Boogaard M, van Marum RJ, et al. Routine use of the confusion assessment method for the intensive care unit: a multicenter study. Am J Respir Crit Care Med. 2011;184:340–4.

40. European Society of Anaesthesiology. European Society of Anaesthesiology, Guideline on reduction of post-operative delirium—in press. http://www.esahq.org/. Accessed 27 Feb 2016.

41. Bruce AJ, Ritchie CW, Blizard R, Lai R, Raven P. The incidence of delirium associated with orthopedic surgery: a meta-analytic review. Int Psychogeriatr. 2007;19:197–214.

42. Rudolph JL, Jones RN, Levkoff SE, et al. Derivation and validation of a preoperative prediction rule for delirium after cardiac surgery. Circulation. 2009;119:229–36.

43. Saczynski JS, Marcantonio ER, Quach L, Fong TG, Gross A, Inouye SK, Jones RN. Cognitive trajectories after postoperative delirium. N Engl J Med. 2012;367:30–9.

44. Maldonado JR, Wysong A, van der Starre PJA, Block T, Miller C, Reitz BA. Dexmedetomidine and the reduction of postoperative delirium after cardiac surgery. Psychosomatics. 2009;50:206–17.

45. Morimoto Y, Yoshimura M, Utada K, Setoyama K, Matsumoto M, Sakabe T. Prediction of postoperative delirium after abdominal surgery in the elderly. J Anesth. 2009;23:51–6.

46. Luetz A, Heymann A, Radtke FM, et al. Different assessment tools for intensive care unit delirium: which score to use? Crit Care Med. 2010;38:409–18.

47. Girard TD, Pandharipande PP, Ely EW. Delirium in the intensive care unit. Crit Care. 2008;12 Suppl(3):S3.

48. Ely EW, Girard TD, Shintani AK, et al. Apolipoprotein E4 polymorphism as a genetic predisposition to delirium in critically ill patients. Crit Care Med. 2007;35:112–7.

49. Inouye SK, Peduzzi PN, Robison JT, Hughes JS, Horwitz RI, Concato J. Importance of functional measures in predicting mortality among older hospitalized patients. JAMA. 1998;279:1187–93.

50. Inouye SK, Charpentier PA. Precipitating factors for delirium in hospitalized elderly persons. Predictive model and interrelationship with baseline vulnerability. JAMA. 1996;275:852–7.

51. Ely EW, Shintani A, Truman B, Speroff T, Gordon SM, Harrell FE, Inouye SK, Bernard GR, Dittus RS. Delirium as a predictor of mortality in mechanically ventilated patients in the intensive care unit. JAMA. 2004;291:1753–62.

52. Pisani MA, Kong SYJ, Kasl SV, Murphy TE, Araujo KLB, Van Ness PH. Days of delirium are associated with 1-year mortality in an older intensive care unit population. Am J Respir Crit Care Med. 2009;180:1092–7.

53. Ely EW, Gautam S, Margolin R, Francis J, May L, Speroff T, Truman B, Dittus R, Bernard R, Inouye SK. The impact of delirium in the intensive care unit on hospital length of stay. Intensive Care Med. 2001;27:1892–900.

54. Drews T, Franck M, Radtke FM, Weiss B, Krampe H, Brockhaus WR, Winterer G, Spies CD. Postoperative delirium is an independent risk factor for posttraumatic stress disorder in the elderly patient: a prospective observational study. Eur J Anaesthesiol. 2015;32:147–51.

55. Kat MG, Vreeswijk R, de Jonghe JFM, van der Ploeg T, van Gool WA, Eikelenboom P, Kalisvaart KJ. Long-term cognitive outcome of delirium in elderly hip surgery patients. A prospective matched controlled study over two and a half years. Dement Geriatr Cogn Disord. 2008;26:1–8.

56. Bellelli G, Mazzola P, Morandi A, et al. Duration of postoperative delirium is an independent predictor of 6-month mortality in older adults after hip fracture. J Am Geriatr Soc. 2014;62:1335–40.

57. Krzych LJ, Wybraniec MT, Krupka-Matuszczyk I, Skrzypek M, Bolkowska A, Wilczyński M, Bochenek AA. Detailed insight into the impact of postoperative neuropsychiatric complications on mortality in a cohort of cardiac surgery subjects: a 23,000-patient-year analysis. J Cardiothorac Vasc Anesth. 2014;28:448–57.

58. Bickel H, Gradinger R, Kochs E, Förstl H. High risk of cognitive and functional decline after postoperative delirium. A three-year prospective study. Dement Geriatr Cogn Disord. 2008;26:26–31.

59. Steinmetz J, Christensen KB, Lund T, Lohse N, Rasmussen LS, ISPOCD Group. Long-term consequences of postoperative cognitive dysfunction. Anesthesiology. 2009;110:548–55.

60. Cunningham C. Systemic inflammation and delirium: important co-factors in the progression of dementia. Biochem Soc Trans. 2011;39:945–53.

61. Tracey KJ. The inflammatory reflex. Nature. 2002;420:853–9.

62. Willard LB, Hauss-Wegrzyniak B, Wenk GL. Pathological and biochemical consequences of acute and chronic neuroinflammation within the basal forebrain cholinergic system of rats. Neuroscience. 1999;88:193–200.

63. Qin L, Wu X, Block ML, Liu Y, Breese GR, Hong J-S, Knapp DJ, Crews FT. Systemic LPS causes chronic neuroinflammation and progressive neurodegeneration. Glia. 2007;55:453–62.

64. Watkins LR, Maier SF. Implications of immune-to-brain communication for sickness and pain. Proc Natl Acad Sci U S A. 1999;96:7710–3.

65. De Simone R, Ajmone-Cat MA, Carnevale D, Minghetti L. Activation of α7 nicotinic acetylcholine receptor by nicotine selectively up-regulates cyclooxygenase-2 and prostaglandin E2 in rat microglial cultures. J Neuroinflammation. 2005;2:4.

66. Gandhi GK, Ball KK, Cruz NF, Dienel GA. Hyperglycaemia and diabetes impair gap junctional communication among astrocytes. ASN Neuro. 2010;2(2), e00030. doi:10.1042/AN20090048.

67. Patel SB, Poston JT, Pohlman A, Hall JB, Kress JP. Rapidly reversible, sedation-related delirium versus persistent delirium in the intensive care unit. Am J Respir Crit Care Med. 2014;189:658–65.

68. Lu LX, Yon J-H, Carter LB, Jevtovic-Todorovic V. General anesthesia activates BDNF-dependent neuroapoptosis in the developing rat brain. Apoptosis. 2006;11:1603–15.

69. Wei H. The role of calcium dysregulation in anesthetic-mediated neurotoxicity. Anesth Analg. 2011;113:972–4.

70. Kalb A, von Haefen C, Sifringer M, Tegethoff A, Paeschke N, Kostova M, Feldheiser A, Spies CD. Acetylcholinesterase inhibitors reduce neuroinflammation and -degeneration in the cortex and hippocampus of a surgery stress rat model. PLoS One. 2013;8, e62679.

71. Radtke FM, Franck M, Lendner J, Krüger S, Wernecke KD, Spies CD. Monitoring depth of anaesthesia in a randomized trial decreases the rate of postoperative delirium but not postoperative cognitive dysfunction. Br J Anaesth. 2013;110 Suppl 1:i98–105.

72. Andresen JM, Girard TD, Pandharipande PP, Davidson MA, Ely EW, Watson PL. Burst suppression on processed electroencephalography as a predictor of postcoma delirium in mechanically ventilated ICU patients. Crit Care Med. 2014;42:2244–51.

73. Kertai MD, Pal N, Palanca BJA, Lin N, Searleman SA, Zhang L, Burnside BA, Finkel KJ, Avidan MS, B-Unaware Study Group. Association of perioperative risk factors and cumulative duration of low bispectral index with intermediate-term mortality after cardiac surgery in the B-Unaware Trial. Anesthesiology. 2010;112:1116–27.

74. Leslie K, Myles PS, Forbes A, Chan MTV. The effect of bispectral index monitoring on long-term survival in the B-aware trial. Anesth Analg. 2010;110:816–22.

75. Monk TG, Saini V, Weldon BC, Sigl JC. Anesthetic management and one-year mortality after noncardiac surgery. Anesth Analg. 2005;100:4–10.

76. American Geriatrics Society. Postoperative delirium in older adults: best practice statement from the American Geriatrics Society. J Am Coll Surg. 2015;220:136–48.

77. Nobili A, Marengoni A, Tettamanti M, et al. Association between clusters of diseases and polypharmacy in hospitalized elderly patients: results from the REPOSI study. Eur J Intern Med. 2011;22:597–602.

78. Sündermann S, Dademasch A, Praetorius J, Kempfert J, Dewey T, Falk V, Mohr F-W, Walther T. Comprehensive assessment of frailty for elderly high-risk patients undergoing cardiac surgery. Eur J Cardiothorac Surg. 2011;39:33–7.

79. Mannucci PM, Nobili A, Investigators REPOSI. Multimorbidity and polypharmacy in the elderly: lessons from REPOSI. Intern Emerg Med. 2014;9:723–34.

80. Makary MA, Segev DL, Pronovost PJ, et al. Frailty as a predictor of surgical outcomes in older patients. J Am Coll Surg. 2010;210:901–8.

81. Jankowski CJ, Trenerry MR, Cook DJ, Buenvenida SL, Stevens SR, Schroeder DR, Warner DO. Cognitive and functional predictors and sequelae of postoperative delirium in elderly patients undergoing elective joint arthroplasty. Anesth Analg. 2011;112:1186–93.

82. Santos-Eggimann B, Cuénoud P, Spagnoli J, Junod J. Prevalence of frailty in middle-aged and older community-dwelling Europeans living in 10 countries. J Gerontol A Biol Sci Med Sci. 2009;64:675–81.

83. Brimblecombe CN, Lim WK, Sunderland Y. Preoperative comprehensive geriatric assessment: outcomes in elective lower limb joint replacement surgery for complex older adults. J Am Geriatr Soc. 2014;62:1396–8.

84. van Meenen LCC, van Meenen DMP, de Rooij SE, ter Riet G. Risk prediction models for postoperative delirium: a systematic review and meta-analysis. J Am Geriatr Soc. 2014;62:2383–90.

85. Grove WM, Zald DH, Lebow BS, Snitz BE, Nelson C. Clinical versus mechanical prediction: a meta-analysis. Psychol Assess. 2000;12:19–30.

86. Ellard L, Katznelson R, Wasowicz M, Ashworth A, Carroll J, Lindsay T, Djaiani G. Type of anesthesia and postoperative delirium after vascular surgery. J Cardiothorac Vasc Anesth. 2014;28:458–61.

87. Wang Y, Sands LP, Vaurio L, Mullen EA, Leung JM. The effects of postoperative pain and its management on postoperative cognitive dysfunction. Am J Geriatr Psychiatry. 2007;15:50–9.

88. Wang N-Y, Hirao A, Sieber F. Association between intraoperative blood pressure and postoperative delirium in elderly hip fracture patients. PLoS One. 2015;10, e0123892.

89. Berger H. Über das Elektrenkephalogramm des Menschen. Arch Für Psychiatr Nervenkrankh. 1933;98:231–54.

90. Glass PS, Bloom M, Kearse L, Rosow C, Sebel P, Manberg P. Bispectral analysis measures sedation and memory effects of propofol, midazolam, isoflurane, and alfentanil in healthy volunteers. Anesthesiology. 1997;86:836–47.

91. Schultz B, Grouven U, Schultz A. Automatic classification algorithms of the EEG monitor Narcotrend for routinely recorded EEG data from general anaesthesia: a validation study. Biomed Tech (Berl). 2002;47:9–13.

92. Revuelta M, Paniagua P, Campos JM, Fernández JA, Martínez A, Jospin M, Litvan H. Validation of the index of consciousness during sevoflurane and remifentanil anaesthesia: a comparison with the bispectral index and the cerebral state index. Br J Anaesth. 2008;101:653–8.

93. Avidan MS, Jacobsohn E, Glick D, et al. Prevention of intraoperative awareness in a high-risk surgical population. N Engl J Med. 2011;365:591–600.

94. Tirel O, Wodey E, Harris R, Bansard JY, Ecoffey C, Senhadji L. Variation of bispectral index under TIVA with propofol in a paediatric population. Br J Anaesth. 2008;100:82–7.

95. Yamamura T, Fukuda M, Takeya H, Goto Y, Furukawa K. Fast oscillatory EEG activity induced by analgesic concentrations of nitrous oxide in man. Anesth Analg. 1981;60:283–8.

96. Tsuda N, Hayashi K, Hagihira S, Sawa T. Ketamine, an NMDA-antagonist, increases the oscillatory frequencies of alpha-peaks on the electroencephalographic power spectrum. Acta Anaesthesiol Scand. 2007;51:472–81.

97. Akeju O, Pavone KJ, Westover MB, et al. A comparison of propofol- and dexmedetomidine-induced electroencephalogram

dynamics using spectral and coherence analysis. Anesthesiology. 2014;121:978–89.

98. Sieber FE, Zakriya KJ, Gottschalk A, Blute M-R, Lee HB, Rosenberg PB, Mears SC. Sedation depth during spinal anesthesia and the development of postoperative delirium in elderly patients undergoing hip fracture repair. Mayo Clin Proc. 2010;85:18–26.

99. Whitlock EL, Torres BA, Lin N, Helsten DL, Nadelson MR, Mashour GA, Avidan MS. Postoperative delirium in a substudy of cardiothoracic surgical patients in the BAG-RECALL clinical trial. Anesth Analg. 2014;118:809–17.

100. Soehle M, Dittmann A, Ellerkmann RK, Baumgarten G, Putensen C, Guenther U. Intraoperative burst suppression is associated with postoperative delirium following cardiac surgery: a prospective, observational study. BMC Anesthesiol. 2015;15:61.

101. Karwacki Z, Niewiadomski S, Rzaska M, Witkowska M. The effect of bispectral index monitoring on anaesthetic requirements in target-controlled infusion for lumbar microdiscectomy. Anaesthesiol Intensive Ther. 2014;46:284–8.

102. Lin B-F, Huang Y-S, Kuo C-P, Ju D-T, Lu C-H, Cherng C-H, Wu C-T. Comparison of A-line autoregressive index and observer assessment of alertness/sedation scale for monitored anesthesia care with target-controlled infusion of propofol in patients undergoing percutaneous vertebroplasty. J Neurosurg Anesthesiol. 2011;23:6–11.

103. Kroeger D, Florea B, Amzica F. Human brain activity patterns beyond the isoelectric line of extreme deep coma. PLoS One. 2013;8, e75257.

104. Kroeger D, Amzica F. Hypersensitivity of the anesthesia-induced comatose brain. J Neurosci Off J Soc Neurosci. 2007;27:10597–607.

105. Conti A, Iacopino DG, Fodale V, Micalizzi S, Penna O, Santamaria LB. Cerebral haemodynamic changes during propofol-remifentanil or sevoflurane anaesthesia: transcranial Doppler study under bispectral index monitoring. Br J Anaesth. 2006;97:333–9.

106. Lewis LD, Ching S, Weiner VS, Peterfreund RA, Eskandar EN, Cash SS, Brown EN, Purdon PL. Local cortical dynamics of burst suppression in the anesthetized brain. Brain J Neurol. 2013;136:2727–37.

107. Purdon PL, Pavone KJ, Akeju O, Smith AC, Sampson AL, Lee J, Zhou DW, Solt K, Brown EN. The Ageing Brain: age-dependent changes in the electroencephalogram during propofol and sevoflurane general anaesthesia. Br J Anaesth. 2015;115 Suppl 1:i46–57.

108. Ching S, Cimenser A, Purdon PL, Brown EN, Kopell NJ. Thalamocortical model for a propofol-induced alpha-rhythm associated with loss of consciousness. Proc Natl Acad Sci U S A. 2010;107:22665–70.

109. Alkire MT, Gruver R, Miller J, McReynolds JR, Hahn EL, Cahill L. Neuroimaging analysis of an anesthetic gas that blocks human emotional memory. Proc Natl Acad Sci U S A. 2008;105:1722–7.

110. Purdon PL, Pierce ET, Mukamel EA, et al. Electroencephalogram signatures of loss and recovery of consciousness from propofol. Proc Natl Acad Sci U S A. 2013;110:E1142–51.

111. Ku S-W, Lee U, Noh G-J, Jun I-G, Mashour GA. Preferential inhibition of frontal-to-parietal feedback connectivity is a neurophysiologic correlate of general anesthesia in surgical patients. PLoS One. 2011;6, e25155.

112. Huupponen E, Maksimow A, Lapinlampi P, et al. Electroencephalogram spindle activity during dexmedetomidine sedation and physiological sleep. Acta Anaesthesiol Scand. 2008;52:289–94.

113. Lee U, Ku S, Noh G, Baek S, Choi B, Mashour GA. Disruption of frontal-parietal communication by ketamine, propofol, and sevoflurane. Anesthesiology. 2013;118:1264–75.

114. Shafer SL, Stanski DR. Defining depth of anesthesia. Handb Exp Pharmacol. 2008;182:409–23.

115. Kay B, Rolly G. I.C.I. 35868, a new intravenous induction agent. Acta Anaesthesiol Belg. 1977;28:303–16.

116. Schwilden H. A general method for calculating the dosage scheme in linear pharmacokinetics. Eur J Clin Pharmacol. 1981;20:379–86.

117. Schnider TW, Minto CF, Gambus PL, Andresen C, Goodale DB, Shafer SL, Youngs EJ. The influence of method of administration and covariates on the pharmacokinetics of propofol in adult volunteers. Anesthesiology. 1998;88:1170–82.

118. Schüttler J, Schwilden H, Stoekel H. Pharmacokinetics as applied to total intravenous anaesthesia. Practical implications. Anaesthesia. 1983;38(Suppl):53–6.

119. Shafer SL, Siegel LC, Cooke JE, Scott JC. Testing computer-controlled infusion pumps by simulation. Anesthesiology. 1988;68:261–6.

120. Whitlock EL, Rodebaugh TL, Hassett AL, et al. Psychological sequelae of surgery in a prospective cohort of patients from three intraoperative awareness prevention trials. Anesth Analg. 2015;120:87–95.

121. Luginbühl M, Schumacher PM, Vuilleumier P, Vereecke H, Heyse B, Bouillon TW, Struys MMRF. Noxious stimulation response index: a novel anesthetic state index based on hypnotic-opioid interaction. Anesthesiology. 2010;112:872–80.

122. Wu Y, Zhang F, Sun K, Yu L, Zhang H, Yan M. Evaluation of pleth variability index for predicting hypotension during induction of anesthesia in surgical patients. Zhonghua Yi Xue Za Zhi. 2014;94:3167–70.

123. Maughan BC, Seigel TA, Napoli AM. Pleth variability index and fluid responsiveness of hemodynamically stable patients after cardiothoracic surgery. Am J Crit Care. 2015;24:172–5.

124. Wong DDL, Bailey CR. Emergence delirium in children. Anaesthesia. 2015;70:383–7.

125. Dahmani S, Delivet H, Hilly J. Emergence delirium in children: an update. Curr Opin Anaesthesiol. 2014;27:309–15.

126. Anderson BJ, Hodkinson B. Are there still limitations for the use of target-controlled infusion in children? Curr Opin Anaesthesiol. 2010;23:356–62.

127. Anderson BJ. Pediatric models for adult target-controlled infusion pumps. Paediatr Anaesth. 2010;20:223–32.

128. Arai Y-CP, Fukunaga K, Hirota S. Comparison of a combination of midazolam and diazepam and midazolam alone as oral premedication on preanesthetic and emergence condition in children. Acta Anaesthesiol Scand. 2005;49:698–701.

129. Chen K, Shen X. Dexmedetomidine and propofol total intravenous anesthesia for airway foreign body removal. Ir J Med Sci. 2014;183:481–4.

130. Ko YP, Huang CJ, Hung YC, Su NY, Tsai PS, Chen CC, Cheng CR. Premedication with low-dose oral midazolam reduces the incidence and severity of emergence agitation in pediatric patients following sevoflurane anesthesia. Acta Anaesthesiol Sin. 2001;39:169–77.

131. Ali AR, El Ghoneimy MN. Dexmedetomidine versus fentanyl as adjuvant to propofol: comparative study in children undergoing extracorporeal shock wave lithotripsy. Eur J Anaesthesiol. 2010;27:1058–64.

132. Pasin L, Febres D, Testa V, Frati E, Borghi G, Landoni G, Zangrillo A. Dexmedetomidine vs midazolam as preanesthetic medication in children: a meta-analysis of randomized controlled trials. Paediatr Anaesth. 2015;25:468–76.

133. Dahmani S, Brasher C, Stany I, Golmard J, Skhiri A, Bruneau B, Nivoche Y, Constant I, Murat I. Premedication with clonidine is superior to benzodiazepines. A meta analysis

of published studies. Acta Anaesthesiol Scand. 2010;54:397–402.

134. Sun L, Guo R, Sun L. Dexmedetomidine for preventing sevoflurane-related emergence agitation in children: a meta-analysis of randomized controlled trials. Acta Anaesthesiol Scand. 2014;58:642–50.

135. Dahmani S, Stany I, Brasher C, Lejeune C, Bruneau B, Wood C, Nivoche Y, Constant I, Murat I. Pharmacological prevention of sevoflurane- and desflurane-related emergence agitation in children: a meta-analysis of published studies. Br J Anaesth. 2010;104:216–23.

136. Costi D, Cyna AM, Ahmed S, Stephens K, Strickland P, Ellwood J, Larsson JN, Chooi C, Burgoyne LL, Middleton P. Effects of sevoflurane versus other general anaesthesia on emergence agitation in children. Cochrane Database Syst Rev. 2014;9, CD007084.

137. Chidambaran V, Costandi A, D'Mello A. Propofol: a review of its role in pediatric anesthesia and sedation. CNS Drugs. 2015;29:543–63.

138. Vanlander AV, Okun JG, de Jaeger A, et al. Possible pathogenic mechanism of propofol infusion syndrome involves coenzyme q. Anesthesiology. 2015;122:343–52.

139. Kam PCA, Cardone D. Propofol infusion syndrome. Anaesthesia. 2007;62:690–701.

140. Bray RJ. Propofol infusion syndrome in children. Paediatr Anaesth. 1998;8:491–9.

141. Rasmussen M, Juul N, Christensen SM, Jónsdóttir KY, Gyldensted C, Vestergaard-Poulsen P, Cold GE, Østergaard L. Cerebral blood flow, blood volume, and mean transit time responses to propofol and indomethacin in peritumor and contra-lateral brain regions: perioperative perfusion-weighted magnetic resonance imaging in patients with brain tumors. Anesthesiology. 2010;112:50–6.

142. Guo J-Y, Fang J-Y, Xu S-R, Wei M, Huang W-Q. Effects of propofol versus sevoflurane on cerebral oxygenation and cognitive outcome in patients with impaired cerebral oxygenation. Ther Clin Risk Manag. 2016;12:81–5.

143. Monk TG, Weldon BC, Garvan CW, Dede DE, van der Aa MT, Heilman KM, Gravenstein JS. Predictors of cognitive dysfunction after major noncardiac surgery. Anesthesiology. 2008;108:18–30.

144. Marsh B, White M, Morton N, Kenny GN. Pharmacokinetic model driven infusion of propofol in children. Br J Anaesth. 1991;67:41–8.

145. Liu S, Wei W, Ding G, Ke J, Hong F, Tian M. Relationship between depth of anesthesia and effect-site concentration of propofol during induction with the target-controlled infusion technique in elderly patients. Chin Med J (Engl). 2009;122: 935–40.

146. Yang N, Yue Y, Pan JZ, Zuo M-Z, Shi Y, Zhou S-Z, Peng W-P, Gao J-D. Changes in the bispectral index in response to loss of consciousness and no somatic movement to nociceptive stimuli in elderly patients. Chin Med J (Engl). 2016;129:410–6.

147. Gotoda T, Okada H, Hori K, et al. Propofol sedation with a target-controlled infusion pump and bispectral index monitoring system in elderly patients during a complex upper endoscopy procedure. Gastrointest Endosc. 2015;83(4):756–64. doi:10.1016/j.gie.2015.08.034.

148. Büttner N, Schultz B, Grouven U, Schultz A. EEG-adjusted target-controlled infusion: propofol target concentration with different doses of remifentanil. Anaesthesist. 2010;59:126–34.

149. Leslie K, Clavisi O, Hargrove J. Target-controlled infusion versus manually-controlled infusion of propofol for general anaesthesia or sedation in adults. Cochrane Database Syst Rev. 2008; CD006059.

150. Maze M, Virtanen R, Daunt D, Banks SJ, Stover EP, Feldman D. Effects of dexmedetomidine, a novel imidazole sedative-

anesthetic agent, on adrenal steroidogenesis: in vivo and in vitro studies. Anesth Analg. 1991;73:204–8.

151. Klinger RY, White WD, Hale B, Habib AS, Bennett-Guerrero E. Hemodynamic impact of dexmedetomidine administration in 15,656 noncardiac surgical cases. J Clin Anesth. 2012;24:212–20.

152. Yu T, Huang Y, Guo F, Yang Y, Teboul J-L, Qiu H. The effects of propofol and dexmedetomidine infusion on fluid responsiveness in critically ill patients. J Surg Res. 2013;185:763–73.

153. Triltsch AE, Welte M, von Homeyer P, Grosse J, Genähr A, Moshirzadeh M, Sidiropoulos A, Konertz W, Kox WJ, Spies CD. Bispectral index-guided sedation with dexmedetomidine in intensive care: a prospective, randomized, double blind, placebo-controlled phase II study. Crit Care Med. 2002;30:1007–14.

154. von Dossow V, Baehr N, Moshirzadeh M, von Heymann C, Braun JP, Hein OV, Sander M, Wernecke K-D, Konertz W, Spies CD. Clonidine attenuated early proinflammatory response in T-cell subsets after cardiac surgery. Anesth Analg. 2006;103:809–14.

155. Shehabi Y, Bellomo R, Reade MC, et al. Early goal-directed sedation versus standard sedation in mechanically ventilated critically ill patients: a pilot study*. Crit Care Med. 2013;41:1983–91.

156. Bajwa SJS, Gupta S, Kaur J, Singh A, Parmar S. Reduction in the incidence of shivering with perioperative dexmedetomidine: a randomized prospective study. J Anaesthesiol Clin Pharmacol. 2012;28:86–91.

157. Soliman RN, Hassan AR, Rashwan AM, Omar AM. Prospective, randomized study to assess the role of dexmedetomidine in patients with supratentorial tumors undergoing craniotomy under general anaesthesia. Middle East J Anaesthesiol. 2011;21:325–34.

158. Ngwenyama NE, Anderson J, Hoernschemeyer DG, Tobias JD. Effects of dexmedetomidine on propofol and remifentanil infusion rates during total intravenous anesthesia for spine surgery in adolescents. Paediatr Anaesth. 2008;18:1190–5.

159. Tufanogullari B, White PF, Peixoto MP, Kianpour D, Lacour T, Griffin J, Skrivanek G, Macaluso A, Shah M, Provost DA. Dexmedetomidine infusion during laparoscopic bariatric surgery: the effect on recovery outcome variables. Anesth Analg. 2008;106:1741–8.

160. Bergese SD, Patrick Bender S, McSweeney TD, Fernandez S, Dzwonczyk R, Sage K. A comparative study of dexmedetomidine with midazolam and midazolam alone for sedation during elective awake fiberoptic intubation. J Clin Anesth. 2010;22:35–40.

161. Pandharipande PP, Sanders RD, Girard TD, McGrane S, Thompson JL, Shintani AK, Herr DL, Maze M, Ely EW, MENDS investigators. Effect of dexmedetomidine versus loraze-pam on outcome in patients with sepsis: an a priori-designed analysis of the MENDS randomized controlled trial. Crit Care. 2010;14:R38.

162. Taniguchi T, Kidani Y, Kanakura H, Takemoto Y, Yamamoto K. Effects of dexmedetomidine on mortality rate and inflammatory responses to endotoxin-induced shock in rats. Crit Care Med. 2004;32:1322–6.

163. Taniguchi T, Kurita A, Kobayashi K, Yamamoto K, Inaba H. Dose- and time-related effects of dexmedetomidine on mortality and inflammatory responses to endotoxin-induced shock in rats. J Anesth. 2008;22:221–8.

164. Peng M, Wang Y-L, Wang C-Y, Chen C. Dexmedetomidine attenuates lipopolysaccharide-induced proinflammatory response in primary microglia. J Surg Res. 2013;179:e219–25.

165. Al-Qadheeb NS, Balk EM, Fraser GL, Skrobik Y, Riker RR, Kress JP, Whitehead S, Devlin JW. Randomized ICU trials do not demonstrate an association between interventions that reduce delirium duration and short-term mortality: a systematic review and meta-analysis. Crit Care Med. 2014;42:1442–54.

166. Dyck JB, Maze M, Haack C, Azarnoff DL, Vuorilehto L, Shafer SL. Computer-controlled infusion of intravenous dexmedetomidine hydrochloride in adult human volunteers. Anesthesiology. 1993;78:821–8.

167. Hannivoort LN, Eleveld DJ, Proost JH, Reyntjens KMEM, Absalom AR, Vereecke HEM, Struys MMRF. Development of an optimized pharmacokinetic model of dexmedetomidine using target-controlled infusion in healthy volunteers. Anesthesiology. 2015;123:357–67.

168. Park HY, Kim JY, Cho SH, Lee D, Kwak HJ. The effect of low-dose dexmedetomidine on hemodynamics and anesthetic requirement during bis-spectral index-guided total intravenous anesthesia. J Clin Monit Comput. 2015;30(4):429–35. doi:10. 1007/s10877-015-9735-2.

169. Apan A, Doganci N, Ergan A, Büyükkoçak U. Bispectral index-guided intraoperative sedation with dexmedetomidine and midazolam infusion in outpatient cataract surgery. Minerva Anestesiol. 2009;75:239–44.

170. Khan ZP, Munday IT, Jones RM, Thornton C, Mant TG, Amin D. Effects of dexmedetomidine on isoflurane requirements in healthy volunteers. 1: pharmacodynamic and pharmacokinetic interactions. Br J Anaesth. 1999;83:372–80.

171. Fragen RJ, Fitzgerald PC. Effect of dexmedetomidine on the minimum alveolar concentration (MAC) of sevoflurane in adults age 55 to 70 years. J Clin Anesth. 1999;11:466–70.

172. Constantin J-M, Momon A, Mantz J, Payen J-F, De Jonghe B, Perbet S, Cayot S, Chanques G, Perreira B. Efficacy and safety of sedation with dexmedetomidine in critical care patients: a meta-analysis of randomized controlled trials. Anaesth Crit Care Pain Med. 2016;35:7–15.

173. Hayama HR, Drumheller KM, Mastromonaco M, Reist C, Cahill LF, Alkire MT. Event-related functional magnetic resonance imaging of a low dose of dexmedetomidine that impairs long-term memory. Anesthesiology. 2012;117:981–95.

174. Kunisawa T, Nagashima M, Hanada S, Suzuki A, Takahata O, Iwasaki H. Awake intubation under sedation using target-controlled infusion of dexmedetomidine: five case reports. J Anesth. 2010;24:789–92.

175. Tsai C-J, Chu K-S, Chen T-I, Lu DV, Wang H-M, Lu I-C. A comparison of the effectiveness of dexmedetomidine versus propofol target-controlled infusion for sedation during fibreoptic nasotracheal intubation. Anaesthesia. 2010;65:254–9.

176. Bielka K, Kuchyn I, Glumcher F. Addition of dexmedetomidine to benzodiazepines for patients with alcohol withdrawal syndrome in the intensive care unit: a randomized controlled study. Ann Intensive Care. 2015;5:33.

177. Wang T, Ge S, Xiong W, Zhou P, Cang J, Xue Z. Effects of different loading doses of dexmedetomidine on bispectral index under stepwise propofol target-controlled infusion. Pharmacology. 2013;91:1–6.

178. Hall RC, Zisook S. Paradoxical reactions to benzodiazepines. Br J Clin Pharmacol. 1981;11 Suppl 1:99S–104.

179. Greenblatt DJ, Harmatz JS, Shader RI. Clinical pharmacokinetics of anxiolytics and hypnotics in the elderly. Therapeutic considerations (Part II). Clin Pharmacokinet. 1991;21:262–73.

180. Massanari M, Novitsky J, Reinstein LJ. Paradoxical reactions in children associated with midazolam use during endoscopy. Clin Pediatr (Phila). 1997;36:681–4.

181. Pandharipande P, Shintani A, Peterson J, Pun BT, Wilkinson GR, Dittus RS, Bernard GR, Ely EW. Lorazepam is an independent risk factor for transitioning to delirium in intensive care unit patients. Anesthesiology. 2006;104:21–6.

182. Pandharipande P, Cotton BA, Shintani A, Thompson J, Pun BT, Morris JA, Dittus R, Ely EW. Prevalence and risk factors for development of delirium in surgical and trauma intensive care unit patients. J Trauma. 2008;65:34–41.

183. Knabl J, Witschi R, Hösl K, et al. Reversal of pathological pain through specific spinal GABAA receptor subtypes. Nature. 2008;451:330–4.

184. Ralvenius WT, Benke D, Acuña MA, Rudolph U, Zeilhofer HU. Analgesia and unwanted benzodiazepine effects in point-mutated mice expressing only one benzodiazepine-sensitive GABAA receptor subtype. Nat Commun. 2015;6:6803.

185. Nandi S, Harvey WF, Saillant J, Kazakin A, Talmo C, Bono J. Pharmacologic risk factors for post-operative delirium in total joint arthroplasty patients: a case-control study. J Arthroplasty. 2014;29:268–71.

186. Fritschy J-M. Significance of GABA$_A$ receptor heterogeneity: clues from developing neurons. Adv Pharmacol. 2015;73:13–39.

187. Rudolph U, Crestani F, Benke D, Brünig I, Benson JA, Fritschy JM, Martin JR, Bluethmann H, Möhler H. Benzodiazepine actions mediated by specific gamma-aminobutyric acid(A) receptor subtypes. Nature. 1999;401:796–800.

188. Amatya A, Marhatta MN, Shrestha GS, Shrestha A, Amatya A. A comparison of midazolam co-induction with propofol priming in propofol induced anesthesia. J Nepal Health Res Counc. 2014;12:44–8.

189. Martin J, Franck M, Fischer M, Spies C. Sedation and analgesia in German intensive care units: how is it done in reality? Results of a patient-based survey of analgesia and sedation. Intensive Care Med. 2006;32:1137–42.

190. Bauer TM, Ritz R, Haberthür C, Ha HR, Hunkeler W, Sleight AJ, Scollo-Lavizzari G, Haefeli WE. Prolonged sedation due to accumulation of conjugated metabolites of midazolam. Lancet. 1995;346:145–7.

191. Somma J, Donner A, Zomorodi K, Sladen R, Ramsay J, Geller E, Shafer SL. Population pharmacodynamics of midazolam administered by target controlled infusion in SICU patients after CABG surgery. Anesthesiology. 1998;89:1430–43.

192. Zomorodi K, Donner A, Somma J, Barr J, Sladen R, Ramsay J, Geller E, Shafer SL. Population pharmacokinetics of midazolam administered by target controlled infusion for sedation following coronary artery bypass grafting. Anesthesiology. 1998;89:1418–29.

193. Lonergan E, Luxenberg J, Areosa Sastre A, Wyller TB. Benzodiazepines for delirium. Cochrane Database Syst Rev. 2009; CD006379.

194. Wiltshire HR, Kilpatrick GJ, Tilbrook GS, Borkett KM. A placebo- and midazolam-controlled phase I single ascending-dose study evaluating the safety, pharmacokinetics, and pharmacodynamics of remimazolam (CNS 7056): part II. Population pharmacokinetic and pharmacodynamic modeling and simulation. Anesth Analg. 2012;115:284–96.

195. Frank T, Thieme V, Radow L. Premedication in maxillofacial surgery under total intravenous anesthesia. Effects of clonidine compared to midazolam on the perioperative course. Anästhesiol Intensivmed Notfallmedizin Schmerzther. 2000;35:428–34.

196. Grottke O, Müller J, Dietrich PJ, Krause TH, Wappler F. Comparison of premedication with clonidine and midazolam combined with TCI for orthopaedic shoulder surgery. Anästhesiol Intensivmed Notfallmedizin Schmerzther. 2003;38:772–80.

197. Zaal IJ, Devlin JW, Hazelbag M, Klein Klouwenberg PMC, van der Kooi AW, Ong DSY, Cremer OL, Groenwold RH, Slooter AJC. Benzodiazepine-associated delirium in critically ill adults. Intensive Care Med. 2015;41:2130–7.

198. Altiparmak B, Akça B, Yilbaş AA, Çelebi N. All about ketamine premedication for children undergoing ophthalmic surgery. Int J Clin Exp Med. 2015;8:21525–32.

199. Cohen L, Athaide V, Wickham ME, Doyle-Waters MM, Rose NGW, Hohl CM. The effect of ketamine on intracranial and cerebral perfusion pressure and health outcomes: a systematic review. Ann Emerg Med. 2015;65:43–51.e2.

200. Lenze EJ, Farber NB, Kharasch E, Schweiger J, Yingling M, Olney J, Newcomer JW. Ninety-six hour ketamine infusion with co-administered clonidine for treatment-resistant depression: a pilot randomised controlled trial. World J Biol Psychiatry. 2016;17(3):230–8.

201. Saligan LN, Luckenbaugh DA, Slonena EE, Machado-Vieira R, Zarate CA. An assessment of the anti-fatigue effects of ketamine from a double-blind, placebo-controlled, crossover study in bipolar disorder. J Affect Disord. 2016;194:115–9.

202. Garnier M, Bonnet F. Management of anesthetic emergencies and complications outside the operating room. Curr Opin Anaesthesiol. 2014;27:437–41.

203. Mahmoud M, Mason KP. A forecast of relevant pediatric sedation trends. Curr Opin Anaesthesiol. 2016;29 Suppl 1:S56–67.

204. Kator S, Correll DJ, Ou JY, Levinson R, Noronha GN, Adams CD. Assessment of low-dose i.v. ketamine infusions for adjunctive analgesia. Am J Health Syst Pharm. 2016;73:S22–9.

205. Matsushita S, Oda S, Otaki K, Nakane M, Kawamae K. Change in auditory evoked potential index and bispectral index during induction of anesthesia with anesthetic drugs. J Clin Monit Comput. 2015;29:621–6.

206. Wang L, Johnston B, Kaushal A, Cheng D, Zhu F, Martin J. Ketamine added to morphine or hydromorphone patient-controlled analgesia for acute postoperative pain in adults: a systematic review and meta-analysis of randomized trials. Can J Anaesth. 2016;63:311–25.

207. Orena EF, King AB, Hughes CG. The role of anesthesia in the prevention of postoperative delirium: a systematic review. Minerva Anestesiol. 2016;82(6):669–83.

208. Ottens TH, Dieleman JM, Sauër AM, Peelen LM, Nierich AP, de Groot WJ, Nathoe HM, Buijsrogge MP, Kalkman CJ, van Dijk D, Dexamethasone for Cardiac Surgery (DECS) Study Group. Effects of dexamethasone on cognitive decline after cardiac surgery: a randomized clinical trial. Anesthesiology. 2014;121 (3):492–500.

209. Rascón-Martínez DM, Fresán-Orellana A, Ocharán-Hernández ME, Genis-Zarate JH, Castellanos-Olivares A. The effects of ketamine on cognitive function in elderly patients undergoing ophthalmic surgery: a pilot study. Anesth Analg. 2016;122 (4):969–75. doi:10.1213/ANE.0000000000001153.

210. Hudetz JA, Patterson KM, Iqbal Z, Gandhi SD, Byrne AJ, Hudetz AG, Warltier DC, Pagel PS. Ketamine attenuates delirium after cardiac surgery with cardiopulmonary bypass. J Cardiothorac Vasc Anesth. 2009;23:651–7.

211. Pisani MA, Murphy TE, Araujo KLB, Slattum P, Van Ness PH, Inouye SK. Benzodiazepine and opioid use and the duration of ICU delirium in an older population. Crit Care Med. 2009;37:177–83.

212. Leung JM, Sands LP, Lim E, Tsai TL, Kinjo S. Does preoperative risk for delirium moderate the effects of postoperative pain and opiate use on postoperative delirium? Am J Geriatr Psychiatry. 2013;21:946–56.

213. Freye E. Opioids in medicine: a comprehensive review on the mode of action and the use of analgesics in different clinical pain states. Dordrecht: Springer; 2008.

214. Pöpping DM, Elia N, Marret E, Remy C, Tramèr MR. Protective effects of epidural analgesia on pulmonary complications after abdominal and thoracic surgery: a meta-analysis. Arch Surg. 2008;143:990–9. Discussion 1000.

215. Hudcova J, McNicol E, Quah C, Lau J, Carr DB. Patient controlled opioid analgesia versus conventional opioid analgesia for postoperative pain. Cochrane Database Syst Rev. 2006; CD003348.

216. Janecka A, Fichna J, Janecki T. Opioid receptors and their ligands. Curr Top Med Chem. 2004;4:1–17.

217. Dhawan BN, Cesselin F, Raghubir R, Reisine T, Bradley PB, Portoghese PS, Hamon M. International Union of Pharmacology. XII. Classification of opioid receptors. Pharmacol Rev. 1996;48:567–92.

218. Michelsen LG, Hug CC. The pharmacokinetics of remifentanil. J Clin Anesth. 1996;8:679–82.

219. Chen W, Chung H-H, Cheng J-T. Opiate-induced constipation related to activation of small intestine opioid μ2-receptors. World J Gastroenterol. 2012;18:1391–6.

220. Radtke FM, Franck M, Lorenz M, Luetz A, Heymann A, Wernecke K-D, Spies CD. Remifentanil reduces the incidence of post-operative delirium. J Int Med Res. 2010;38:1225–32.

221. Motamed C, Weil G, Deschamps F, Billard V. Remifentanil target-controlled infusion: a safe rescue protocol for unexpected severe postoperative pain. J Opioid Manag. 2014;10:284–8.

222. Yang L, Wei B, Zhang L, Bi S, Lu W, Guo X. Pharmacodynamic interaction between propofol and remifentanil on the tolerance response to electrical tetanus stimuli. Beijing Da Xue Xue Bao. 2010;42:547–53.

223. Del Gaudio A, Ciritella P, Perrotta F, Puopolo M, Lauta E, Mastronardi P, De Vivo P. Remifentanil vs fentanyl with a target controlled propofol infusion in patients undergoing craniotomy for supratentorial lesions. Minerva Anestesiol. 2006;72: 309–19.

224. De Baerdemaeker LEC, Jacobs S, Pattyn P, Mortier EP, Struys MMRF. Influence of intraoperative opioid on postoperative pain and pulmonary function after laparoscopic gastric banding: remifentanil TCI vs sufentanil TCI in morbid obesity. Br J Anaesth. 2007;99:404–11.

225. Jeleazcov C, Ihmsen H, Saari TI, Rohde D, Mell J, Fröhlich K, Krajinovic L, Fechner J, Schwilden H, Schüttler J. Patient-controlled analgesia with target-controlled infusion of hydromorphone in postoperative pain therapy. Anesthesiology. 2016;124:56–68.

226. Eisendrath SJ, Goldman B, Douglas J, Dimatteo L, Van Dyke C. Meperidine-induced delirium. Am J Psychiatry. 1987;144:1062–5.

227. Fong HK, Sands LP, Leung JM. The role of postoperative analgesia in delirium and cognitive decline in elderly patients: a systematic review. Anesth Analg. 2006;102:1255–66.

228. Liu N, Pruszkowski O, Leroy JE, Chazot T, Trillat B, Colchen A, Gonin F, Fischler M. Automatic administration of propofol and remifentanil guided by the bispectral index during rigid bronchoscopic procedures: a randomized trial. Can J Anaesth. 2013;60:881–7.

Perioperative Cardioprotective Strategies in Noncardiac Surgery

41

Stefan De Hert

Introduction

Worldwide, noncardiac surgery has been reported to be associated with an average overall complication rate of about 11 % and a mortality rate of 1.5 % [1]. Despite benefits associated with the introduction of safety procedures and improved surgical techniques, major perioperative complications continue to occur. Of these, perioperative cardiac events account for one third of perioperative deaths [2] and are associated with increased hospital stay [3] and long-term mortality rates [4]. As a consequence, there is a major interest in an efficient preoperative risk stratification that uses available clinical information to stratify the risk of perioperative cardiac complications in order to tailor potential protective strategies. Unfortunately, the currently available preoperative risk prediction models have limitations and do not allow for an accurate individual patient risk stratification [5, 6].

Measurements of sensitive biomarkers have been shown to be of additional help in identifying the patient at risk for adverse postoperative outcome [7, 8], and preliminary data suggest that intensification of therapy in those patients improves outcome [9].

Taking into account the major implications of perioperative cardiac events and the fact that occurrence of these events can be modulated, maximal efforts should be directed toward the prevention and treatment of perioperative myocardial ischemia.

Pathophysiology of Perioperative Myocardial Ischemia

In nonoperative myocardial infarctions, 64–100 % of patients present with coronary artery plaque fissuring, and in 65–95 % an acute luminal thrombus is present [10, 11]. The pathophysiology underlying perioperative myocardial infarction (PMI) seems to be more complex. Some studies on the coronary pathology underlying fatal PMIs revealed important coronary artery disease without obvious plaque fissuring and presence of intraluminal thrombosis in only a limited proportion of patients [12, 13]. These findings suggest that fatal PMIs may primarily be the result of a myocardial oxygen supply–demand imbalance in the setting of fixed coronary artery stenoses. Angiographic data, on the other hand, observed that the majority of nonfatal PMIs occurred in the presence of coronary arteries without high-grade stenoses [14], suggesting that plaque fissuring and acute coronary artery thrombosis are involved as the causal mechanism.

As a consequence, it seems that two distinct mechanisms may lead to PMI: the acute coronary syndrome and the prolonged myocardial oxygen supply–demand imbalance in the presence of stable coronary artery disease [15–18] (Fig. 41.1). These two types have been designated type 1 and type 2 myocardial infarction by the universal definition of myocardial infarction [19].

Acute Coronary Syndrome (Type 1 Myocardial Infarction)

This will occur when an unstable plaque undergoes spontaneous rupture, fissuring, or erosion. The consequence is an acute coronary thrombosis with myocardial ischemia and finally infarction. Central in the process of plaque instability is the intraplaque inflammation, but external factors occurring in the perioperative period may trigger the event. These factors include tachycardia and hypertension, the

S. De Hert, MD, PhD (✉)
Department of Anesthesiology, Ghent University Hospital, Ghent University, De Pintelaan 185, 9000 Ghent, Belgium
e-mail: stefan.dehert@ugent.be

© Springer International Publishing AG 2017
A.R. Absalom, K.P. Mason (eds.), *Total Intravenous Anesthesia and Target Controlled Infusions*,
DOI 10.1007/978-3-319-47609-4_41

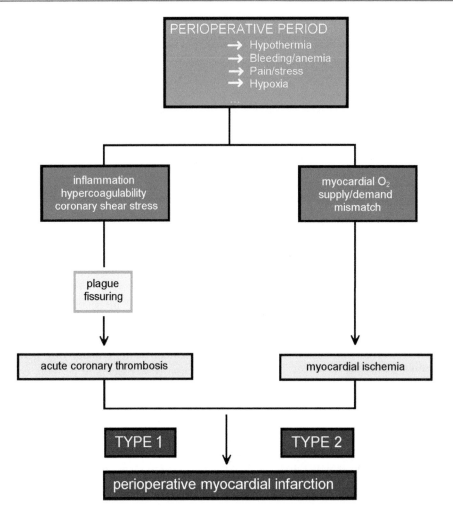

Fig. 41.1 Schematic representation of the events leading to type 1 and type 2 perioperative myocardial infarction. The acute coronary syndrome (type 1 myocardial infarction) will occur when an unstable plaque undergoes spontaneous rupture or fissuring. The consequence is an acute coronary thrombosis with myocardial ischemia and finally infarction. Central in the process of plaque instability is the intraplaque inflammation, but external factors occurring in the perioperative period may trigger the event. These factors include tachycardia and hypertension, the release of stress hormones, and the increase in procoagulant factors. Myocardial oxygen supply–demand imbalance (type 2 myocardial infarction) will occur whenever myocardial oxygen demand exceeds oxygen supply. Tachycardia is the most common cause of such an imbalance. Perioperative hypotension (hypovolemia or systemic vasodilation) or hypertension (elevated stress hormones, vasoconstriction), anemia, hypoxemia, and hypercarbia may also trigger or aggravate myocardial ischemia and aggravate pre-existing diastolic and systolic dysfunction

release of stress hormones, and the increase in procoagulant factors [20–23].

Myocardial Oxygen Supply–Demand Imbalance (Type 2 Myocardial Infarction)

Tachycardia is the most common cause of an imbalance in the myocardial oxygen supply–demand ratio [24, 25]. Perioperative hypotension (hypovolemia or systemic vasodilation) or hypertension (elevated stress hormones, vasoconstriction), anemia, hypoxemia, and hypercarbia may also trigger or aggravate myocardial ischemia and aggravate pre-existing diastolic and systolic dysfunction [17].

Timing of Perioperative Myocardial Ischemic Events

Perioperative myocardial ischemia predominantly occurs in the postoperative period [26]. Postoperative ischemia and infarction often start shortly after the end of surgery, at a moment when sympathetic discharge and procoagulant activity increase [24, 27]. Le Manach et al. distinguished two types of PMI according to time of appearance and rate of increase in troponin I [28]. Early PMI occurs in the early postoperative period (<24 h) and is not preceded by subinfarction myocardial damage, whereas delayed PMI occurs later (>24 h) and is preceded by a period of myocardial damage in which biomarkers are increased.

They postulated that the mechanism underlying the early PMI pattern is that of the vulnerable plaque, whereas the biomarker release pattern of delayed PMI is more consistent with a prolonged myocardial oxygen demand–supply imbalance. In addition to these two patterns, some patients showed a prolonged period of subinfarction troponin I release, indicative for prolonged subclinical myocardial damage but without the development of PMI [28, 29].

Combining all available data on perioperative ischemia and infarction in patients undergoing noncardiac surgery, the following time sequence has been proposed [15]. First, ischemia starts in most patients (~67 %) immediately after the end of surgery and during emergence from anesthesia. Such ischemia is most often silent and can only be detected by continuous electrocardiographic monitoring. In most instances ischemia is preceded by an increase in heart rate. Because the ischemic ST changes usually revert back to baseline in almost all cases (even in patients who later develop increased levels of biomarkers), this episode may be easily missed in the absence of continuous monitoring. Patients with a prolonged period of myocardial ischemia may subsequently develop an increase in biomarkers, signifying myocardial damage. An increased value for cardiac troponin is defined as a measurement exceeding the 99th percentile of a normal reference population [19].

Only about 50 % of PMI patients will show symptoms of myocardial infarction, while the other 50 % of PMIs are silent and will remain unnoticed in the absence of electrocardiographic ST segment or biomarker analysis. The increase in troponin starts mostly within 8–24 h after the end of surgery [15]. When the increase in troponin occurs shortly after the prolonged period of ST segment depression, without sudden conversion to ST segment elevation, stress-induced ischemia and not plaque rupture is the most likely cause of PMI. The peak incidence of mortality in these patients is in the first 1–3 postoperative days. In patients in whom plaque rupture or coronary thrombosis is the cause of fatal PMI (~50 %), the timing of death is evenly distributed in the postoperative period, with no special correlation to the end of surgery [15].

Pathophysiology of Ischemia–Reperfusion Injury

Prolonged and unresolved interruption of blood supply to the myocardium without reperfusion ultimately causes myocyte cell death. Early restoration of blood flow to the ischemic myocardium is therefore necessary to prevent myocardial cell death to occur. However, reperfusion itself may lead to additional tissue injury beyond that generated by the ischemic event (Fig. 41.2). This phenomenon is called reperfusion injury, and it may manifest as arrhythmias, reversible contractile dysfunction (myocardial stunning), endothelial dysfunction, and ultimately irreversible reperfusion injury with myocardial cell death. This lethal reperfusion injury may result from two mechanisms which are necrosis and apoptosis.

The pathogenesis of reperfusion injury still is not fully elucidated, but several mechanisms have been shown to be involved [30, 31]. The major consistent metabolic abnormality that has been observed in the stunned myocardium is a reduction of the adenosine triphosphate concentration in the cells [32]. Because this resolves with a time course that is roughly parallel to that of the functional recovery [33], emphasis was initially placed on a potential role of high energy phosphates stores in the development of myocardial stunning. However, several lines of evidence have made it quite clear that adenosine triphosphate depletion has no major pathogenetic role in the development of reperfusion injury [34–36].

More recently the focus has turned to a potential role of reactive oxygen species and the disruption of the normal intracellular calcium homeostasis as major mechanisms involved in the pathogenesis of reperfusion injury. The oxygen paradox hypothesis is based on the observation that oxygen—while it is essential for tissue survival—may also be harmful during reperfusion of the ischemic myocardium [30, 31]. Indeed, upon reperfusion, molecular oxygen undergoes a sequential reduction with formation of reactive oxygen species, which interact with cell membrane lipids and essential proteins. This results in myocardial cell damage, initially with depressed myocardial function but ultimately leading to irreversible tissue damage. Although the role of reactive oxygen species in the pathogenesis of myocardial stunning has been established, the mechanisms by which oxygen-derived free radicals produce contractile dysfunction at the cellular level are still not fully understood. Since calcium is the major ion involved in the force generation by the myocardium, it seems likely that a change in extracellular calcium influx, intracellular calcium release, or reuptake by the sarcoplasmic reticulum or an alteration in myofilament sensitivity to calcium is also involved in the pathogenesis of depressed function with myocardial stunning [37].

In the last years, numerous reports provided solid evidence on the key role of the mitochondrial permeability transition pore (MPTP) in myocardial injury caused by ischemia and reperfusion. Following an acute episode of sustained myocardial ischemia, the opening of the MPTP in the first few minutes of reperfusion has been shown to mediate cell death. Opening of the MPTP renders the inner mitochondrial membrane nonselectively permeable resulting in a collapse of the mitochondrial membrane potential, thereby uncoupling oxidative phosphorylation, leading to adenosine triphosphate depletion and cell death. Another important effect of MPTP opening is mitochondrial matrix

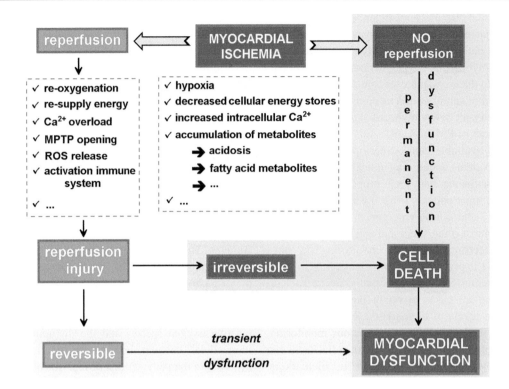

Fig. 41.2 Schematic representation of the different factors contributing to myocardial dysfunction and/or damage with ischemia–reperfusion injury. During ischemia, the hypoxic conditions result in a decrease and depletion of the energy stores and an accumulation of metabolites resulting in tissue acidosis. If no reperfusion occurs, the myocardial cell will ultimately die resulting in permanent myocardial dysfunction. Even if reperfusion is restored, there will be a period of transient myocardial dysfunction as a consequence of the ischemia–reperfusion injury. Upon reperfusion, the tissue reoxygenation triggers a burst of reactive oxygen species release and mitochondrial permeability transition pore (MPTP) opening (see Fig. 41.3), leading to disturbance of the electrochemical gradients over the mitochondrial membrane and swelling of the mitochondrial intermembrane space

swelling and rupture of the outer mitochondrial membrane resulting in the deposition of proapoptotic factors into the cytosol, thereby initiating cell death [38–42] (Fig. 41.3).

Perioperative Cardioprotective Strategies

It is obvious that prevention of ischemic events is the primary prerequisite of a cardioprotective strategy. This is basically obtained by keeping the myocardial oxygen demand–supply ratio in balance. Whenever myocardial ischemia occurs, treatment should not only be directed toward a prompt restoration of blood flow to the ischemic area but should also include measures to prevent or minimize the extent of reperfusion injury.

Modulation of the Myocardial Oxygen Demand–Supply Ratio

Modulation of the myocardial oxygen demand–supply ratio will primarily aim at optimizing oxygen supply to the myocardium while keeping myocardial oxygen demand

to a minimum. The latter will be obtained by avoiding hemodynamic instability and prevent tachycardia and hyper- or hypotension.

Most anesthetic techniques reduce sympathetic tone, which leads to a vasodilation with the potential development of a deceased blood pressure. Therefore, anesthesiological management must ensure proper maintenance of organ flow and perfusion pressure [43]. There is no universal target blood pressure value to define intraoperative arterial hypotension, but percentage decreases >20 % of mean arterial pressure, or mean arterial pressure values <60 mmHg for cumulative durations of >30 min are associated with an increased risk of postoperative complications such as myocardial infarction, stroke, and death [44–46].

Spinal or epidural anesthesia also induces sympathetic blockade. The benefit of neuraxial anesthesia versus general anesthesia is highly debated in the literature with proponents of a beneficial effect of neuraxial techniques and opponents who claim a lack of effect on criteria such as mortality or severe morbidity such as myocardial and pulmonary complications. Given the ongoing debate, the ESC/ESA guidelines gave a grade IIb recommendation, meaning that neuraxial anesthesia and analgesia may be considered for the

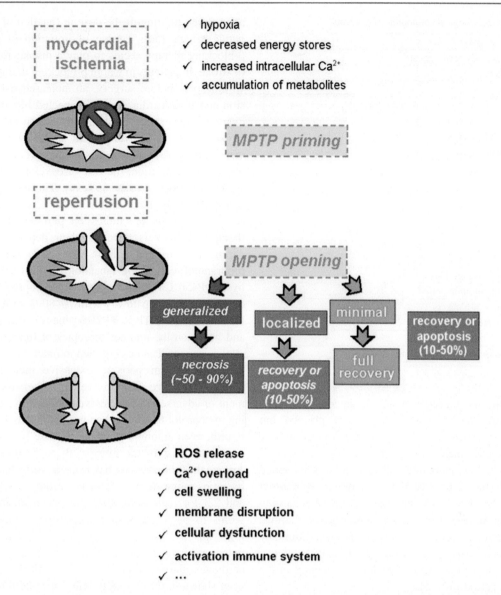

- ✓ hypoxia
- ✓ decreased energy stores
- ✓ increased intracellular Ca²⁺
- ✓ accumulation of metabolites

✓ ROS release
✓ Ca²⁺ overload
✓ cell swelling
✓ membrane disruption
✓ cellular dysfunction
✓ activation immune system
✓ ...

Fig. 41.3 *Schematic* representation of the presumed role of the mitochondrial permeability transition pore (MPTP) in the pathogenesis of ischemia–reperfusion injury. In normal conditions the MPTP is in a closed state. Also during the period of ischemia, the MPTP remains closed keeping mitochondrial integrity intact at this level. Upon reperfusion, the tissue reoxygenation triggers a burst of reactive oxygen species release, and the MPTP opens, leading to disturbance of the electrochemical gradients over the mitochondrial membrane and swelling of the mitochondrial intermembrane space. As a consequence, the supramolecular complex, containing the proton pump, ATP synthase, adenine nucleotide transporter, and mitochondrial creatine kinase, will disrupt, and normal mitochondrial function is lost. If the MPTP opening is minimal, full functional recovery of the cell may occur. When MPTP opening occurs in 10–50 % of the mitochondria, either recovery or apoptosis may occur depending on the extent of damage. However, if MPTP opening occurs in more than 50 %, necrosis of cell will occur leading to irreversible damage of the myocardium

management of patients with cardiovascular risk factors or diseases, provided no contraindications are present for the application of these techniques [43].

Several pharmacological strategies have been proposed to help stabilizing the perioperative hemodynamic conditions, in order to preserve the myocardial oxygen supply–demand ratio (Table 41.1).

β-Blockers

Despite the lack of unequivocal evidence [47], international guidelines [48, 49] have put an important emphasis on the place of β-blockers in the prevention of perioperative cardiac complications. The generally accepted protective effect of perioperative β-blockade was seriously questioned by the results of the POISE study [50]. Perioperative treatment

Table 41.1 Pharmacological cardioprotective agents

✓	Anesthetic agents
✓	Hemodynamically active agents
→	β-Blockers
→	Nitrates
→	Angiotensin-converting enzyme inhibitors
→	Angiotensin receptor blockers
→	Calcium channel blockers
→	α_2-Receptor agonists
✓	Others
→	Statins
→	Aspirin

Table 41.2 Causes of heterogeneity with regard to protective effects of perioperative β-blocking therapy

✓	Low-bias versus high-bias-risk trials
✓	Length of the titration period
✓	Metabolism of β-blockers
✓	β_1 to β_2 receptor selectivity
✓	Perioperative anemia
✓	Patient risk factors and type of surgery

with metoprolol did indeed decrease the incidence of perioperative myocardial infarction compared to placebo, but this was at the expense of an increased mortality mainly related to a higher incidence of stroke in the metoprolol-treated patients. This increased incidence of stroke seemed to be related to the occurrence of intraoperative hypotension and bradycardia. Moreover, the concerns raised regarding the reliability of the Dutch Echocardiographic Cardiac Risk Evaluation Applying Stress Echocardiography (DECREASE) studies [51] further prompted skepticism regarding the appropriateness of β-blocking therapy in the perioperative period [52–55].

Clearly, the issue of perioperative β-blocking therapy is more complex than initially assumed [56]. Reasons for the heterogeneity of results among different studies on perioperative β-blocking therapy include influences of bias, length of the titration period, metabolism of the different β-blocking compounds, ratio of β_1 to β_2 selectivity, and others (Table 41.2). First, conclusions with regard to the beneficial effects of perioperative β-blocking therapy seem to have been skewed by a number of trials with a high risk of bias. Indeed, the results of the low-bias-risk studies clearly show that the beneficial effect on perioperative myocardial infarction rate is associated with an increased mortality and an increased rate of perioperative stroke, an observation which is blunted by the inclusion of high-bias-risk studies [47]. Second, the risk of adverse events with perioperative β-blocking therapy seems to be related to the length of the titration period. In the POISE study, the β-blocking therapy was initiated just before surgery at a fixed dose without

appropriate titrating of the dose in function of the hemodynamic effects [50]. Timing of initiation of perioperative β-blocking therapy seems to play a pivotal role in the risk of stroke. In patients in whom β-blocking therapy is initiated within hours before surgery, an increased risk of hypotension and bradycardia is to be expected because of insufficient careful titration of the drugs with an increased risk of stroke as result. Conversely, in studies where β-blockers were started at least a week before surgery, allowing for more careful titration, the risk of developing perioperative stroke was not increased [57–59]. Thirdly, metabolism of β-blockers may be a factor to take into account when analyzing results of studies on perioperative β-blocking therapy. β-Blockers differ in their dependency on cytochrome P450 for metabolism. Many β-blockers (metoprolol, propranolol, carvedilol, labetalol, timolol) are metabolized by the P450 CYP2D6 isoenzyme. Metoprolol is the most dependent on this pathway with 70–80 % of its metabolism by CYP2D6 [60]. The CYP2D6 gene is highly polymorphic, and based on the number of copies of functional CYP2D6 alleles, patients can be classified in function of the degree of metabolism from poor to extensive metabolizers. Poor metabolizers have an up to fivefold higher risk for development of adverse effects (bradycardia and hypotension) during metoprolol treatment than normal metabolizers [61–63]. Fourth, even among β-blockers that are β_1 cardioselective, variations exist in the ratio of β_1 to β_2 receptor affinity. Among the β-blockers used perioperatively, the β_1 to β_2 affinity ratios range from 13.5 for bisoprolol to 4.7 for atenolol and 2.3 for metoprolol [64]. Incidence of adverse events seems to be lower with perioperative β-blockers with a high β_1 to β_2 ratio [56, 65–67]. Finally, genetic polymorphisms at the level of β-receptors may determine cardiovascular outcome [68, 69] though they have not yet been shown to differentially affect specific β-blockers [56]. More important is the interaction of perioperative β-blocking therapy with the occurrence of intraoperative anemia. The beneficial effect of perioperative β-blocking therapy may revert to a deleterious effect on perioperative mortality in the presence of acute anemia with intraoperative bleeding [70, 71]. Finally, the protective effects of perioperative β-blockade seem to depend on the risk profile of the patient and the type of surgery involved. β-Blocking therapy was associated with lower mortality only in nonvascular surgery, and protection seemed more pronounced in the presence of a higher revised cardiac risk index score [72]. Similarly, among patients with ischemic heart disease undergoing noncardiac surgery, perioperative protective effects were only observed in patients with heart failure or recent myocardial infarction [73].

Currently, the guidelines give a class Ib recommendation to continue β-blocking therapy perioperatively in those patients who already receive this medication.

There is indeed evidence of an increased mortality when preoperative β-blocking therapy is withdrawn [74–76]. In patients without clinical risk factors or undergoing low risk surgery, initiation of β-blocking therapy is not recommended [43]. Things are less obvious for intermediate risk patients. If the decision is made to initiate β-blocking therapy, the drug should be slowly uptitrated starting at a low dose in order to achieve a resting heart rate between 60 and 70 beats per minute. β_1-Selective blockers without intrinsic sympathomimetic activity are favored, and evidence indicates that atenolol and bisoprolol are superior to metoprolol [65, 66]. Because of the need of slow uptitration to appropriate heart rate and blood pressure targets, initiation of treatment should be at least 1 week up to 30 days before surgery.

Other Vasoactive Drugs

Although *nitrates* are well known to reverse myocardial ischemia, the effect of perioperative intravenous nitroglycerine on perioperative ischemia is debated, and no effect has been demonstrated on the incidence of myocardial infarction or cardiac death. In addition, perioperative administration of the drug may impair the hemodynamic stability of the patient because of hypotension and tachycardia [43].

Perioperative use of *angiotensin-converting enzyme inhibitors* and *angiotensin receptor blockers* carries a risk of severe hypotension under anesthesia. Hypotension is less common when the drugs are discontinued the day before surgery, the reason why some consider withdrawal 24 h before surgery [43].

The beneficial effects of *calcium channel blockers* on the myocardial oxygen balance make them theoretically suitable for perioperative risk reduction strategies. However, the relevance of the available evidence is limited by the small size of the trials, the lack of risk stratification, and the absence of systematic reporting of adverse effects and complications. A meta-analysis of 11 randomized trials (1007 patients) showed a reduction in episodes of myocardial ischemia and supraventricular tachycardia, but decrease in mortality and myocardial infarction only reached statistical significance when both endpoints were combined [77]. Another study in elective aortic aneurysm surgery showed that dihydropyridine use was independently associated with an increased incidence of perioperative mortality [78]. Therefore, it is recommended to avoid the use of short-acting dihydropyridines, in particular, nifedipine [43].

α_2-*Receptor agonists* reduce postganglionic noradrenaline output and may therefore be helpful in preventing perioperative hemodynamic instability. Perioperative administration of mivazerol did not reduce the incidence of death or myocardial infarction in the entire study population but seemed to have a protective effect in the subgroup of vascular surgery patients [79]. In a small study in 190 patients, perioperative administration of clonidine was shown to be associated with a reduction of perioperative cardiac morbidity and postoperative death in patients at risk for coronary artery disease undergoing noncardiac surgery [80]. However, more recently, the results of the POISE-2 trial clearly indicated that clonidine did not reduce the incidence of perioperative myocardial infarction or death but instead was associated with an increased incidence of important hypotension and nonfatal cardiac arrest [81]. Although some early data suggest that dexmedetomidine may be helpful in hemodynamic management of vascular surgery patients [82], to date, no firm evidence has demonstrated a perioperative cardioprotective action of the drug. A systematic review and meta-analysis of 20 studies including a total of 840 patients found no statistically significant evidence for improved cardiac outcomes but an increased evidence for perioperative hypotension and bradycardia [83]. Therefore, it was suggested that at this moment insufficient data are available to recommend the use of α_2-receptor agonists in perioperative cardioprotective strategies [43].

Apart from pharmacological strategies aiming at a stabilization of the patient's perioperative hemodynamic status, prevention of perioperative cardiac complications also includes avoiding the occurrence of thromboembolic events. Several drugs are available that—at least theoretically—may be of help in stabilizing the coronary plaques and/or prevent the occurrence of thromboembolic events.

3-Hydroxy-3-methylglutaryl coenzyme A reductase inhibitors or *statins* are widely prescribed in patients with or at risk for ischemic heart disease. They also induce coronary plaque stabilization through pleiotropic effects, thereby preventing perioperative plaque fissuring or rupture and subsequent myocardial infarction. Several studies have shown a beneficial effect of perioperative statin therapy on mortality and cardiovascular complications [84–89]. Even more, statin withdrawal more than 4 days is associated with a threefold increased risk of postoperative myocardial ischemia [90]. According to the current guidelines, patients with peripheral artery disease should receive statins. In patients not previously treated, statins should be initiated preferably at least 2 weeks before the procedure for maximal plaque-stabilizing effects and continued for at least 1 month after surgery. In patients undergoing nonvascular surgery, there is no evidence to support preoperative statin treatment if there is no other indication [43].

Aspirin is an antiplatelet drug prescribed to patients with established cardiovascular disease (secondary prevention) or with certain cardiovascular disease risk factors (primary prevention) to reduce major adverse thrombotic events such as myocardial infarction and stroke. Whereas the use of aspirin for secondary prevention of thrombotic events is based on high-quality evidence [91–95], the evidence supporting the use of aspirin for primary prevention is less robust [96, 97]. Data to guide the use of aspirin during the perioperative period are limited, and as a consequence, controversy exists on this issue [98, 99]. A large meta-analysis, including 41 studies in 49,590 patients, which compared periprocedural withdrawal versus bleeding risks of aspirin, observed that the risk of bleeding complications with aspirin was increased by 1.5, but that this did not result in a higher severity of bleeding complications. In subjects at risk of proven ischemic heart disease, aspirin nonadherence/withdrawal was associated with a threefold higher risk of major adverse cardiac events [100]. The POISE-2 trial, including 10,010 patients, found no difference in the composite endpoint of death or nonfatal myocardial infarction between placebo- and aspirin-treated patients. However, major bleeding occurred more often in the aspirin group [101]. On the basis of these results, it was concluded that the risk of continuing perioperative aspirin may not outweigh the risk of cessation [101]. These conclusions, however, have been challenged [102, 103], and the current guidelines recommend that the use of low-dose aspirin in patients undergoing noncardiac surgery should be based on an individual decision that depends on the perioperative bleeding risk weighed against the risk of thrombotic complications [43].

Modulation of Ischemia–Reperfusion Injury

During the past decades it has become increasingly obvious that important cellular damage may occur upon reperfusion after a period of myocardial ischemia. Interestingly, the extent of ischemia–reperfusion injury can be modulated by an intrinsic defense mechanism which is *conditioning* of the organ (Fig. 41.4). In 1986, Murry et al. observed that in an in vivo dog model, four 5 min occlusions of the circumflex coronary artery, each separated by 5 min of reperfusion, followed by a sustained 40 min occlusion were associated with a 25 % lower infarct size of that seen in a control group that received a single 40 min occlusion [104]. This phenomenon has been termed *ischemic preconditioning*. This study initiated extensive research—both experimentally and clinically—with regard to underlying mechanisms and potential clinical relevance.

It was only in 2003 that Zhao et al. introduced the concept of *ischemic postconditioning*. In an open chest dog model, three cycles of 30 s reocclusion were applied at the start of reperfusion after a 60 min occlusion of the left anterior descending artery [105]. Compared to a control group without reocclusion, a similar reduction in infarct size was observed as with an ischemic preconditioning protocol. This protective mechanism has since then been widely studied in order to determine both the pathways involved and its potential clinical applications.

This concept of endogenous cardioprotection was further refined by the intriguing observation that similar degrees of cardioprotection could be achieved by applying brief episodes of nonlethal ischemia and reperfusion to an organ or tissue remote from the heart. Skeletal muscle has been investigated as the most appropriate remote site for generation of such cardioprotection. In experimental studies, the application of an ischemic stimulus to skeletal muscle both before (*remote ischemic preconditioning*) and immediately after (*remote ischemic postconditioning*) myocardial ischemia has been shown to induce cardioprotective effects [106, 107]. More than direct ischemic conditioning, the concept of remote ischemic conditioning may constitute an attractive protective strategy to reduce the extent of ischemia–reperfusion injury [108], though the conclusions of these studies might be influenced by methodological issues [109].

The alternative of ischemic conditioning is to mimic its effects by the use of pharmacological agents that modulate one or more of the different steps involved in ischemic pre- and postconditioning [110–114]. Over the years different pharmacological compounds have been tested that may either inhibit or activate different steps in the pathways involved in ischemic conditioning, such as adenosine receptor agonists, K_{ATP} channel openers, activators of protein kinases including protein kinase C, p38 mitogen-activated protein kinases and tyrosine kinases, free radical scavengers, and others. However, none of these compounds has entered clinical practice up to now, either because of the occurrence of substantial side effects or because of the lack of measurable clinical benefit. Interestingly, there is now some recent evidence suggesting that direct modulation of the mitochondrial permeability transition pore by inhibition of its opening with cyclosporine A is capable of substantially reducing myocardial infarction size [115–117].

In the laboratory setting, it has been extensively shown that volatile anesthetics have both pre- and postconditioning effects and are capable of substantially reducing the deleterious effects of myocardial ischemia–reperfusion injury. Numerous experimental papers have been published further characterizing this phenomenon of anesthetic cardioprotection and its underlying mechanisms. It became evident that ischemic and anesthetic pre- and postconditioning share many common pathways [110, 111, 113, 114, 118, 119].

In the setting of coronary artery bypass surgery, it has been shown that the use of a volatile anesthetic regimen is associated with a lower extent of myocardial damage, a lower incidence of myocardial infarction, and a lower in-hospital and long-term mortality [120–131]. These cardioprotective effects have—until now—not been confirmed in noncardiac surgery. One small study in vascular surgery patients observed a lower incidence of major cardiac events in patients anesthetized with a volatile anesthetic agent compared with an intravenous anesthetic agent [132],

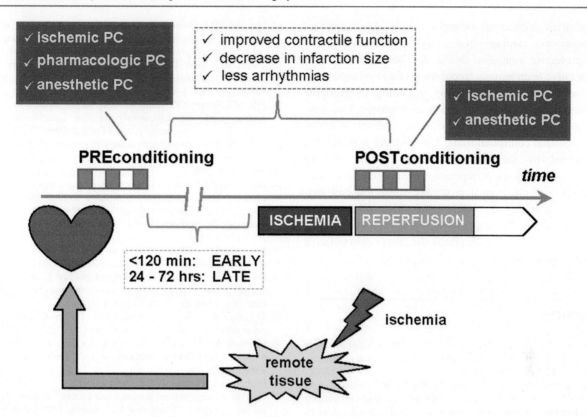

Fig. 41.4 Schematic representation of the principle of organ protection by the "conditioning" mechanism. Both preconditioning (PC) and postconditioning (PoC) are intrinsic defense mechanisms that help to attenuate the extent of ischemia–reperfusion injury. At the level of the heart, this will manifest as better preservation of contractile function, a decreased myocardial infarction size, and less occurrence of arrhythmias after the ischemic event. The phenomenon was first described as ischemic preconditioning after the observation that a number of short bursts of ischemia alternated with short periods of reperfusion resulted in protection against the consequences of a prolonged period of myocardial ischemia. Several protocols with varying time of repetitive ischemia and reperfusion have been proposed. Essential for the preconditioning is the washout period, i.e., the period between the last ischemic preconditioning trigger and the insult of prolonged myocardial ischemia. Depending on the length of the time interval between preconditioning and the actual ischemic insult, a distinction is made between "early" (<120 min) and "late" (24–72 h) preconditioning. Postconditioning involves the same principle, but now the ischemic trigger is applied after the event of myocardial ischemia. Since the concept of ischemic conditioning involves an additional

ischemic burden to an already jeopardized, intensive research has been performed to possibilities of pharmacological modulation of the mechanistic pathways involved in the phenomenon of preconditioning. Several compounds have been tested such as adenosine receptor agonists, K_{ATP} channel openers, protein kinase C agonists, etc. However, all the compounds tested showed important side effects prohibiting their use for "pharmacological" preconditioning in clinical practice. Only cyclosporine A (an inhibitor of MPTP opening) is capable of providing pharmacological protection against the extent of myocardial ischemia–reperfusion injury. Interestingly, volatile anesthetic agents have also been shown to confer direct (independent of the modulation of the myocardial oxygen balance) cardioprotective effects via a pre- and a postconditioning pathway. Especially in coronary surgery patients, application of this strategy seems to protect the heart with less myocardial damage and better functional recovery after ischemia. A similar cardioprotective effect can be obtained by an ischemic trigger in a tissue distant from the heart. This strategy is termed "remote ischemic preconditioning." Typically, this ischemic trigger is applied on the skeletal muscle either of the upper or lower limb

but other studies in noncardiac surgery observed no difference in outcome [133–136]. However, the conclusions of these studies have been challenged for several pertinent methodological issues [136–139] among others because of the fact that the overall incidence of perioperative events was too low to address the relationship between choice of anesthetic agent and patient outcome [140].

The evidence about direct (independent from modulation of the myocardial O₂ balance) cardioprotective effects of intravenous anesthetic agents is less straightforward. Some experimental studies have suggested such effects for

propofol [141–143] and dexmedetomidine [144, 145], but evidence for a translation in clinically relevant cardioprotection is limited, both for propofol [146–148] and dexmedetomidine [149, 150].

Conclusion

During the last decades, perioperative cardioprotective strategies have undergone substantial changes, thanks to our better understanding of the pathophysiology of perioperative myocardial ischemic events. Assessment of perioperative cardiac risk and identification of cardioprotective strategies should best be developed by a perioperative team approach consisting of a close collaboration and shared decision-making according to available evidence-based guidelines. However, evidence for these guidelines frequently lacks the basis and strength of multiple randomized controlled trials. This problem was recently underscored by the dramatic change in the role of β-blocking therapy as perioperative cardioprotective strategy. Also with other cardioprotective strategies, new evidence is challenging the validity of recommendations that have been made for many years. Therefore continuing research is needed to further clarify the proper perioperative care of surgical patients.

References

1. Haynes AB, Weiser TG, Berry WR, et al. A surgical safety checklist to reduce morbidity and mortality in a global population. N Engl J Med. 2009;360:491–9.
2. Devereaux PJ, Yang H, Yusuf S, POISE Study Group, et al. Effects of extended-release metoprolol succinate in patients undergoing non-cardiac surgery (POISE trial). Lancet. 2008;371:1839–47.
3. Fleishmann KE, Goldman L, Young B, et al. Association between cardiac and noncardiac complications in patients undergoing non-cardiac surgery: outcomes and effects on length of stay. Am J Med. 2003;115:515–20.
4. Landesberg G, Shatz V, Akopnik I, et al. Association of cardiac troponin, CK-MB, and postoperative myocardial ischemia with long-term survival after major vascular surgery. J Am Coll Cardiol. 2003;42:1547–54.
5. Gordon HS, Johnson ML, Wray NP, et al. Mortality after noncardiac surgery: prediction from administrative versus clinical data. Med Care. 2005;43:159–67.
6. Ford MK, Beattie WS, Wijeysundera DN. Systematic review: prediction of perioperative cardiac complications and mortality by the revised cardiac risk index. Ann Intern Med. 2010;152:26–35.
7. Vascular Events In Noncardiac Surgery Patients Cohort Evaluation (VISION) Study Investigators. Association between postoperative troponin levels and 30-day mortality among patients undergoing noncardiac surgery. Lancet. 2012;307:2295–304.
8. Rodseth RN, Biccard BM, Chu R, et al. Postoperative B-type natriuretic peptide for prediction of major cardiac events in patients undergoing noncardiac surgery. Systematic review and individual patient meta-analysis. Anesthesiology. 2013;119:270–83.
9. Foucrier A, Rodseth R, Aissaoui M, et al. The long-term impact of early cardiovascular therapy intensification for postoperative troponin elevation after major vascular surgery. Anesth Analg. 2014;119:1053–63.
10. Davies MJ, Woolf N, Robertson WB. Pathology of acute myocardial infarction with particular reference to occlusive coronary thrombi. Br Heart J. 1976;38:659–64.
11. Falk E. Plaque rupture with severe pre-existing stenosis precipitating coronary thrombosis. Characteristics of coronary atherosclerotic plaques underlying fatal occlusive thrombi. Br Heart J. 1983;50:127–34.
12. Dawood MM, Gutpa DK, Southern J, et al. Pathology of fatal perioperative myocardial infarction: implications regarding pathophysiology and prevention. Int J Cardiol. 1996;57:37–44.
13. Cohen MC, Aretz TH. Histological analysis of coronary artery lesions in fatal postoperative myocardial infarction. Cardiovasc Pathol. 1999;8:133–9.
14. Ellis SG, Hertzer NR, Young JR, et al. Angiographic correlates of cardiac death and myocardial infarction complicating major nonthoracic vascular surgery. Am J Cardiol. 1996;77:1126–8.
15. Landesberg G. The pathophysiology of perioperative myocardial infarction: facts and perspectives. J Cardiothor Vasc Anesth. 2003;17:90–100.
16. Devereaux PJ, Goldman L, Cock DJ, et al. Perioperative cardiac events in patients undergoing noncardiac surgery: a review of the magnitude of the problem, the pathophysiology of the events and methods to estimate and communicate risk. CMAJ. 2005;173:627–34.
17. Landesberg G, Beattie S, Mosseri M, et al. Perioperative myocardial infarction. Circulation. 2009;119:2936–44.
18. De Hert S, Moerman A, De Baerdemaeker L. Postoperative complications in cardiac patients undergoing non-cardiac surgery. Curr Opin Crit Care. 2016;22(4):357–64.
19. Thygesen K, Alpert JS, White HD. Universal definition of myocardial infarction. J Am Coll Cardiol. 2007;22:2173–95.
20. Chernow B, Alexander HR, Smallridge RC, et al. Hormonal responses to graded surgical stress. Arch Intern Med. 1987;147:1273–8.
21. Gibbs NM, Crawford GP, Michalopoulos N. Postoperative changes in coagulant and anticoagulant factors following abdominal aortic surgery. J Cardiothor Vasc Anesth. 1992;6:680–5.
22. Sametz W, Metzler H, Gries M, et al. Perioperative catecholamine changes in cardiac risk patients. Eur J Clin Invest. 1999;29:582–7.
23. Fukumoto Y, Hiro T, Fujii T, et al. Localized elevation of shear stress is related to coronary plaque rupture. J Am Coll Cardiol. 2008;51:645–50.
24. Landesberg G, Mosseri M, Zahger D, et al. Myocardial infarction following vascular surgery: the role of prolonged, stress-induced, ST-depression-type ischemia. J Am Coll Cardiol. 2001;37:1839–45.
25. Feringa HH, Bax JJ, Boersma E, et al. High-dose beta-blockers and tight heart rate control reduce myocardial ischemia and troponin T release in vascular surgery patients. Circulation. 2006;114 (Suppl):I-344–9.
26. Mangano DT, Wong MG, London MJ, et al. Perioperative myocardial ischemia in patients undergoing noncardiac surgery. II. Incidence and severity during the 1th week after surgery. The study of perioperative ischemia (SPI) research group. J Am Coll Cardiol. 1991;17:851–7.
27. Badner NH, Knill RL, Brown JE, et al. Myocardial infarction after noncardiac surgery. Anesthesiology. 1998;88:572–8.
28. Le Manach Y, Perel A, Coriat P, et al. Early and delayed myocardial infarction after abdominal aortic surgery. Anesthesiology. 2005;102:885–91.
29. Longhitano S, Coriat P, Agro F. Postoperative myocardial infarction: pathophysiology, new diagnostic criteria, prevention. Minerva Anestesiol. 2006;72:965–83.
30. Park JL, Lucchesi BR. Mechanisms of myocardial reperfusion injury. Ann Thorac Surg. 1999;68:1905–12.
31. De Hert S. Myocardial protection from ischemia and reperfusion injury. In: Mebazaa A, Gheorghiade M, Zannad FM, Parillo JE, editors. Acute heart failure. London: Springer; 2008.
32. Kloner RA, Deboer LWV, Darsee JR, et al. Prolonged abnormalities of myocardium salvages by reperfusion. Am J Physiol. 1981;241:H591–9.
33. Ellis SG, Henschke CI, Sandor T, et al. Time course of functional and biochemical recovery of myocardium salvaged by reperfusion. J Am Coll Cardiol. 1983;1:1047–55.

34. Przyklenk K, Kloner RA. Superoxide dismutase plus catalase improve contractile function in the canine model of "stunned" myocardium. Circ Res. 1986;58:148–56.

35. Ambrosio G, Jacobus WE, Mitchell MC, et al. Effects of ATP precursors on ATP and free ADP content and functional recovery of postischemic hearts. Am J Physiol. 1989;256:H560–6.

36. Kusuoka H, Marban E. Cellular mechanisms of myocardial stunning. Annu Rev Physiol. 1992;54:243–56.

37. Gross GJ, Kersten JR, Warltier DC. Mechanisms of postischemic contractile dysfunction. Ann Thorac Surg. 1999;68:1898–904.

38. Hausenloy DJ, Yellon DM. The mitochondrial permeability transition pore: its fundamental role in mediating cell death during ischaemia and reperfusion. J Mol Cell Cardiol. 2003;35:339–41.

39. Honda HM, Korge P, Weiss JN. Mitochondria and ischemia/reperfusion injury. Ann N Y Acad Sci. 2005;1047:248–58.

40. Ong S-B, Samangouei P, Kalkhoran SB, et al. The mitochondrial permeability transition pore and its role in myocardial ischemia reperfusion injury. J Mol Cell Cardiol. 2015;78:23–34.

41. Halestrap AP, Richardson AP. The mitochondrial permeability transition: a current perspective on its identity and role in ischemia/reperfusion injury. J Mol Cell Cardiol. 2015;78:129–41.

42. Heusch G. Molecular basis of cardioprotection. Signal transduction in ischemic pre-, post-, and remote conditioning. Circ Res. 2015;116:674–99.

43. Kristensen SD, Knuuti J, Saraste A, et al. ESC/ESA guidelines on non-cardiac surgery: cardiovascular assessment and management. Eur J Anaesthesiol. 2014;31:517–73.

44. Bijker JB, Persoons S, Peelen LM, et al. Intraoperative hypotension and perioperative ischemic stroke after general surgery: a nested case-control study. Anesthesiology. 2012;116:658–64.

45. Sessler DI, Sigl JC, Kelley SD, et al. Hospital stay and mortality are increased in patients having a "triple low" of low blood pressure, low bispectral index, and low minimum alveolar concentration of volatile anesthesia. Anesthesiology. 2012;116:1195–203.

46. Walsh M, Devereaux PJ, Garg AX, et al. Relationship between intraoperative mean arterial pressure and clinical outcomes after noncardiac surgery: toward an empirical definition of hypotension. Anesthesiology. 2013;119:507–15.

47. Bangalore S, Wetterslev J, Pranesh S, et al. Perioperative β-blockers in patients having noncardiac surgery: a meta-analysis. Lancet. 2008;372:1962–76.

48. Fleisher LA, Beckman JA, Brown KA, et al. AAC/AHA 2007 guidelines on perioperative cardiovascular evaluation and care for noncardiac surgery: a report of the American College of Cardiology/American Heart Association task force on practice guidelines. Circulation. 2007;116:e418–500.

49. Poldermans D, Bax JJ, Boersma E, et al. Guidelines for pre-operative cardiac risk assessment and perioperative cardiac management in non-cardiac surgery. Eur Heart J. 2009;30:2769–812.

50. Devereaux PJ, Yang H, Yusuf S, et al. Effects of extended-release metoprolol succinate in patients undergoing non-cardiac surgery (POISE trial): a randomised controlled trial. Lancet. 2008;371:1839–47.

51. Bouri S, Shun-Shin MJ, Cole GD, et al. Meta-analysis of secure randomized controlled trials of β-blockade to prevent perioperative death in non-cardiac surgery. Heart. 2014;100:456–64.

52. Nowbar AN, Cole GD, Shun-Shin MJ, et al. International RCT-based guidelines for use of preoperative stress testing and perioperative beta-blockers and statins in non-cardiac surgery. Int J Cardiol. 2014;172:138–43.

53. Cole GD, Francis DP. Perioperative β-blockade: guidelines do not reflect the problems with the evidence from the DECREASE trials. BMJ. 2014;349:g5210.

54. Cole GD, Francis DP. The challenge of delivering reliable science and guidelines: opportunities for all to participate. Eur Heart J. 2014;35:2433–40.

55. Lüscher TF, Gersh B, Landmesser U, et al. Is the panic about beta-blockers in perioperative care justified? Eur Heart J. 2014;35:2442–4.

56. Badgett RG, Lawrence VA, Cohn SL. Variations in pharmacology of β-blockers may contribute to heterogeneous results in trials of perioperative blockade. Anesthesiology. 2010;113:585–92.

57. Poldermans D, Schouten O, van Lier F, et al. Perioperative strokes and β-blockade. Anesthesiology. 2009;111:910–5.

58. Flu W-J, van Kuijk P-J, Chonchol M, et al. Timing of pre-operative beta-blocker treatment in vascular surgery patients. Influence on post-operative outcome. J Am Coll Cardiol. 2010;56:1922–9.

59. Ellenberger C, Tait G, Beattie S. Chronic β-blockade is associated with a better outcome after elective noncardiac surgery than acute β-blockade. Anesthesiology. 2011;114:817–23.

60. Shin J, Johnson JA. Pharmacogenetics of beta-blockers. Pharmacotherapy. 2007;27:874–87.

61. Wuttke H, Rau T, Heide R, et al. Increased frequency of cytochrome P450 2D6 poor metabolizers among patients with metoprolol-associated adverse effects. Clin Pharmacol Ther. 2002;72:429–37.

62. Fux R, Mörike K, Pröhmer AM, et al. Impact of CYP2D6 genotype on adverse effects during treatment with metoprolol: a prospective clinical study. Clin Pharmacol Ther. 2005;78:378–87.

63. Rau T, Wuttke H, Michels LM, et al. Impact of CYP2D6 genotype on the clinical effects of metoprolol: a prospective longitudinal study. Clin Pharmacol Ther. 2009;85:269–72.

64. Baker JG. The selectivity of beta-adrenoceptor antagonists at the human beta1, beta2, and beta3 adrenoceptors. Br J Pharmacol. 2005;144:317–22.

65. Wallace AW, Au S, Cason BA. Perioperative β-blockade: atenolol is associated with reduced mortality when compared to metoprolol. Anesthesiology. 2011;114:824–36.

66. Ashes C, Judelman S, Wijeysundera DN, et al. Selective β_1-antagonism with bisoprolol is associated with fewer postoperative strokes than atenolol or metoprolol. A single-center cohort study of 44,092 consecutive patients. Anesthesiology. 2013;119:777–87.

67. Mashour GA, Sharifpour M, Freundlich RE, et al. Perioperative metoprolol and risk of stroke after noncardiac surgery. Anesthesiology. 2013;119:1340–6.

68. Lanfear DE, Spertus JA, McLeod HL. Beta2-adrenergic receptor genotype predicts survival: implications and future directions. J Cardiovasc Nurs. 2006;21:474–7.

69. Zaugg M, Bestmann L, Wacker J, et al. Adrenergic receptor genotype but not perioperative bisoprolol therapy may determine cardiovascular outcome in at-risk patients undergoing surgery with spinal Block: the Swiss beta blocker in spinal anesthesia (BBSA) study: a double-blinded, placebo-controlled, multicenter trial with 1-year follow-up. Anesthesiology. 2007;107:33–44.

70. Beattie WS, Wijeysundera DN, Karkouti K, et al. Acute surgical anemia influences the cardioprotective effects of β-blockade. Anesthesiology. 2010;112:25–33.

71. Le Manach Y, Collins GS, Ibanez C, et al. Impact of perioperative bleeding on the protective effect of β-blockers during infrarenal aortic reconstruction. Anesthesiology. 2012;117:1203–11.

72. London MJ, Hur K, Schwartz GG, et al. Association of perioperative beta-blockade with mortality and cardiovascular morbidity following major noncardiac surgery. JAMA. 2013;309:1704–13.

73. Andersson C, Mérie C, Jorgensen M, et al. Association of β-blocker therapy with risks of adverse cardiovascular events and deaths in patients with ischemic heart disease undergoing noncardiac surgery: a Danish nationwide cohort study. JAMA Intern Med. 2014;174:336–44.

74. Shammash JB, Trost JC, Gold JM, et al. Perioperative beta-blocker therapy and mortality after major noncardiac surgery. Am Heart J. 2001;141:148–53.

75. Wallace AW, Au S, Cason BA. Association of the pattern of use of perioperative beta-blockade and postoperative mortality. Anesthesiology. 2010;113:794–805.

76. Kwon S, Thompson R, Florence M, et al. β-blocker continuation after noncardiac surgery: a report from the surgical care and outcomes assessment program. Arch Surg. 2012;147:467–73.

77. Wijeysundera DN, Beattie WS. Calcium channel blockers for reducing cardiac morbidity after noncardiac surgery: a meta-analysis. Anesth Analg. 2003;97:634–41.

78. Kertai MD, Westerhout CM, Varga KS, et al. Dihydropyridine calcium-channel blockers and perioperative mortality in aortic aneurysm surgery. Br J Anaesth. 2008;101:458–65.

79. Oliver MF, Goldman L, Julian DG, et al. Effect of mivazerol on perioperative cardiac complications during non-cardiac surgery in patients with coronary heart disease: the European Mivazerol Trial (EMIT). Anesthesiology. 1999;91:951–61.

80. Wallace AW, Galindez D, Salahieh A, et al. Effect of clonidine on cardiovascular morbidity and mortality after noncardiac surgery. Anesthesiology. 2004;101:284–93.

81. Devereaux PJ, Sessler DI, Leslie K, et al. Clonidine in patients undergoing noncardiac surgery. N Engl J Med. 2014;370:1504–13.

82. Talke P, Li J, Jain U, et al. Effects of perioperative dexmedetomidine infusion in patients undergoing vascular surgery. The Study of Perioperative Ischemia Research Group. Anesthesiology. 1995;82:620–33.

83. Biccard BM, Goga S, de Beurs J. Dexmedetomidine and cardiac protection for non-cardiac surgery: a meta-analysis of randomised controlled trials. Anaesthesia. 2008;63:4–14.

84. Lindenauer PK, Pekow P, Wang K, et al. Lipid-lowering therapy and in-hospital mortality following major noncardiac surgery. JAMA. 2004;291:2092–9.

85. Durazzo AE, Machado FS, Ikeoka DT, et al. Reduction in cardiovascular events after vascular surgery with atorvastatin: a randomized trial. J Vasc Surg. 2004;39:967–75.

86. Hindler K, Shaw AD, Samuels J, et al. Improved postoperative outcomes associated with preoperative statin therapy. Anesthesiology. 2006;105:1260–72.

87. Desai H, Aronow WS, Ahn C, et al. Incidence of perioperative myocardial infarction and of 2-year mortality in 577 elderly patients undergoing noncardiac vascular surgery treated with and without statins. Arch Gerontol Geriatr. 2010;51:149–51.

88. Winchester DE, Wen X, Xie L, et al. Evidence of preprocedural statin therapy: a meta-analysis of randomized trials. J Am Coll Cardiol. 2010;56:1099–109.

89. Chopra V, Wesorick DH, Sussman JB, et al. Effect of perioperative statins on death, myocardial infarction, atrial fibrillation, and length of stay: a systematic review and meta-analysis. Arch Surg. 2012;147:181–9.

90. Le Manach Y, Godet G, Coriat P, et al. The impact of postoperative discontinuation or continuation of chronic statin therapy on cardiac outcome after major vascular surgery. Anesth Analg. 2007;104:1326–33.

91. Antithrombotic Trialists Collaboration. Collaborative meta-analysis of randomized trials of antiplatelet therapy for prevention of death, myocardial infarction, and stroke in high risk patients. BMJ. 2002;324:71–86.

92. Smith Jr SC, Benjamin EJ, Bonow RO, et al. AHA/ACCF secondary prevention and risk reduction therapy for patients with coronary and other atherosclerotic vascular disease: 2011 update: a guideline from the American Heart Association and American College of Cardiology Foundation. Circulation. 2011;124:2458–73.

93. Vandvik PO, Lincoff AM, Gore JM, et al. Primary and secondary prevention of cardiovascular disease: antithrombotic therapy and prevention of thrombosis, 9th ed: American College of Chest Physicians Evidence-Based Clinical Practice Guidelines. Chest. 2012;141:e637S–68.

94. Berger JS. Aspirin, clopidogrel and ticagrelor in acute coronary syndromes. Am J Cardiol. 2013;112:737–45.

95. Tai WA, Albers GW. Secondary prevention of atherothrombotic or cryptogenic stroke. Circulation. 2014;129:527–31.

96. Pignone M, Alberts MJ, Colwell JA, et al. Aspirin for primary prevention of cardiovascular events in people with diabetes: a position statement of the American Diabetes Association, a scientific statement of the American Heart Association, and an expert consensus document of the American College of Cardiology Foundation. Circulation. 2010;121:2694–701.

97. Pignone M. Aspirin for primary prevention: a challenging decision. J Am Heart Assoc. 2014;3:1–3.

98. Oscarsson A, Gupta A, Fredrikson M, et al. To continue or discontinue aspirin in the perioperative period: a randomized, controlled trial. Br J Anaesth. 2010;104:305–12.

99. Mantz J, Samama CM, Tubach F, et al. Impact of preoperative maintenance or interruption of aspirin on thrombotic and bleeding events after elective non-cardiac surgery: the multicentre, randomized, blinded, placebo-controlled, STRATAGEM trial. Br J Anaesth. 2011;107:899–910.

100. Burger W, Chemnitius JM, Kneissl GD, et al. Low-dose aspirin for secondary cardiovascular prevention—cardiovascular risks after its perioperative withdrawal versus bleeding risks with its continuation—review and meta-analysis. J Int Med. 2005;257:399–414.

101. Devereaux PJ, Mrkobrada M, Sessler DI, et al. Aspirin in patients undergoing noncardiac surgery. N Engl J Med. 2014;370:1494–503.

102. Gerstein NS, Charlton GA. Questions linger over POISE-2 and perioperative aspirin management. Evid Based Med. 2014;19:224–5.

103. Gerstein NS, Carey MC, Cigarroa JE, et al. Perioperative aspirin management after POISE-2: some answers, but questions remain. Anesth Analg. 2015;120:570–5.

104. Murry CE, Jennings RB, Reimer KA. Preconditioning with ischemia: a delay of lethal cell injury in ischemic myocardium. Circulation. 1986;74:1124–36.

105. Zhao Z-Q, Corvera JS, Halkos ME, et al. Inhibition of myocardial injury by ischemic postconditioning during reperfusion: comparison with ischemic preconditioning. Am J Physiol Heart Circ Physiol. 2003;285:H579–88.

106. Birnbaum Y, Hale SL, Kloner RA. Ischemic preconditioning at a distance: reduction of myocardial infarct size by partial reduction of blood supply combined with rapid stimulation of the gastrocnemius muscle in the rabbit. Circulation. 1997;96:1641–6.

107. Andreka G, Vertesaljai M, Szantho G, et al. Remote ischaemic postconditioning protects the heart during acute myocardial infarction in pigs. Heart. 2007;93:749–52.

108. Twine CP, Ferguson S, Boyle JR. Benefits of remote ischaemic preconditioning in vascular surgery. Eur J Vasc Endovasc Surg. 2014;48:215–9.

109. De Hert S, De Baerdemaeker L. Benefits of remote ischaemic preconditioning are related to methodological issues. Eur J Vasc Endovasc Surg. 2014;48:712–3.

110. Zaugg M, Lucchinetti E, Uecker M, et al. Anaesthetics and cardiac preconditioning. Part I. Signalling and cytoprotective mechanisms. Br J Anaesth. 2003;91:551–65.

111. De Hert SG, Turani F, Mathur S, et al. Cardioprotection with volatile anesthetics: mechanisms and clinical implications. Anesth Analg. 2005;100:1584–93.

112. Hausenloy DJ, Yellon DM. Preconditioning and postconditioning: underlying mechanisms and clinical application. Atherosclerosis. 2009;204:334–41.

113. Fräßdorf J, De Hert S, Schlack W. Anaesthesia and myocardial ischaemia/reperfusion injury. Br J Anaesth. 2009;103:89–98.

114. De Hert S, Moerman A. Myocardial injury and protection related to cardiopulmonary bypass. Best Pract Res Clin Anaesthesiol. 2015;29:137–49.

115. Piot C, Croisille P, Staat P, et al. Effect of cyclosporine on reperfusion injury in acute myocardial infarction. N Engl J Med. 2008;359:473–81.

116. Mewton N, Croisille P, Gahide G, et al. Effect of cyclosporine on left ventricular remodeling after reperfused myocardial infarction. J Am Coll Cardiol. 2010;55:1200–5.

117. Hausenloy DJ, Kunst G, Boston-Griffiths E, et al. The effect of cyclosporine-A on perioperative myocardial injury in adult patients undergoing coronary artery bypass graft surgery: a randomized controlled clinical trial. Heart. 2014;100:544–9.

118. Bienengraeber MW, Weihrauch D, Kersten JR, et al. Cardioprotection by volatile anesthetics. Vasc Pharmacol. 2005;42:243–52.

119. Pagel PS. Postconditioning by volatile anesthetics: salvaging ischemic myocardium at reperfusion by activation of prosurvival signaling. J Cardiothorac Vasc Anesth. 2008;22:753–65.

120. De Hert SG, ten Broecke PW, Mertens E, et al. Sevoflurane but not propofol preserves myocardial function in coronary surgery patients. Anesthesiology. 2002;97:42–9.

121. Julier K, da Silva R, Garcia C, et al. Preconditioning by sevoflurane decreases biochemical markers for myocardial and renal dysfunction in coronary artery bypass graft surgery: a double-blinded, placebo-controlled, multicenter study. Anesthesiology. 2003;98:1315–27.

122. De Hert SG, Van der Linden PJ, Cromheecke S, Meeus R, ten Broecke PW, De Blier IG, Stockman BA, Rodrigus IE. Choice of primary anesthetic regimen can influence intensive care unit length of stay after coronary surgery with cardiopulmonary bypass. Anesthesiology. 2004;101:9–20.

123. De Hert SG, Van der Linden PJ, Cromheecke S, et al. Cardioprotective properties of sevoflurane in patients undergoing coronary surgery with cardiopulmonary bypass are related to the modalities of its administration. Anesthesiology. 2004;101:299–310.

124. Bein B, Renner J, Caliebe D, et al. Sevoflurane but not propofol preserves myocardial function during minimally invasive direct coronary artery bypass surgery. Anesth Analg. 2005;100:610–6.

125. Garcia C, Julier K, Bestmann L, et al. Preconditioning with sevoflurane decreases PECAM-1 expression and improves one-year cardiovascular outcome in coronary artery bypass graft surgery. Br J Anaesth. 2005;94:159–65.

126. Landoni G, Biondi-Zoccai GG, Zangrilla A, et al. Desflurane and sevoflurane in cardiac surgery: a meta-analysis of randomized clinical trials. J Cardiothorac Vasc Anesth. 2007;21:502–11.

127. De Hert S, Vlasselaers D, Barbé R, et al. A comparison of volatile and non volatile agents for cardioprotection during on-pump coronary surgery. Anaesthesia. 2009;64:953–60.

128. De Hert SG. Is anaesthetic cardioprotection clinically relevant? Another futile search for a magic bullet? Eur J Anaesthesiol. 2011;28:616–7.

129. Bein B. Clinical application of the cardioprotective effects of volatile anaesthetics-PRO: get an extra benefit from a proven anaesthetic free of charge. Eur J Anaesthesiol. 2011;28:620–2.

130. Van Rompaey N, Barvais L. Clinical application of the cardioprotective effects of volatile anaesthetics—CON: TIVA or not TIVA to anaesthetise a cardiac patient? Eur J Anaesthesiol. 2011;28:623–7.

131. Landoni G, Greco T, Biondi-Zoccai G, et al. Anaesthetic drugs and survival: a Bayesian network meta-analysis of randomized trials in cardiac surgery. Br J Anaesth. 2013;111:886–96.

132. Van der Linden PJ, Dierick A, Wilmin S, et al. A randomized controlled trial comparing an intraoperative goal-directed strategy with routine clinical practice in patients undergoing peripheral artery surgery. Eur J Anaesthesiol. 2010;27:788–93.

133. Zangrillo A, Testa V, Aldrovandi V, et al. Volatile agents for cardiac protection in noncardiac surgery: a randomized controlled study. J Cardiothor Vasc Anesth. 2011;126:2696–704.

134. Lurati Buse GA, Schumacher P, Seeberger E, et al. Randomized comparison of sevoflurane versus propofol to reduce perioperative myocardial ischemia in patients undergoing noncardiac surgery. Circulation. 2012;126:2696–704.

135. Lindholm EE, Aune E, Norén CB, et al. The anesthesia in abdominal aortic surgery (ABSENT) study. A prospective, randomized, controlled trial comparing troponin T release with fentanyl-sevoflurane and propofol-remifentanil anesthesia in major vascular surgery. Anesthesiology. 2013;119:802–12.

136. De Hert S, Moerman A. Sevoflurane. F1000Res. 2015;4(F1000 Faculty Rev):626.

137. Zaugg M, Lucchinetti E. Letter by Zaugg and Lucchinetti regarding the article: randomized comparison of sevoflurane versus propofol to reduce perioperative myocardial ischemia in patients undergoing noncardiac surgery. Circulation. 2013;127, e875.

138. Zaugg M, Lucchinetti E. Sevoflurane- compared with propofol-based anesthesia reduces the need for inotropic support in patients undergoing abdominal aortic aneurysm repair: evidence of cardioprotection by volatile anesthetics in noncardiac surgery. Anesthesiology. 2014;120:1289–90.

139. Xue FS, Cui XL, Cheng Y, Wang SY. Comparing cardioprotective effects of anesthesia methods in patients undergoing elective abdominal aortic surgery. Anesthesiology. 2014;120:1291–2.

140. De Hert SG. Cardioprotection by volatile anesthetics: what about noncardiac surgery? J Cardiothor Vasc Anesth. 2011;25:899–901.

141. Kokita N, Hara A, Abiko Y, et al. Propofol improves functional and metabolic recovery in ischemic reperfused isolated rat hearts. Anesth Analg. 1998;86:252–8.

142. Mathur S, Farhangkgoee P, Karmazyn M. Cardioprotective effects of propofol and sevoflurane in ischemic and reperfused rat hearts: role of K(ATP) channels and interaction with the sodium-hydrogen exchange inhibitor HOE642 (cariporide). Anesthesiology. 1999;91:1349–60.

143. Lemoine S, Zhu L, Gress S, et al. Mitochondrial involvement in propofol-induced cardioprotection: an in vitro study in human myocardium. Exp Biol Med. 2016;241:527–38.

144. Guler L, Bozkirli F, Berdirli N, et al. Comparison of the effects of dexmedetomidine versus ketamine in cardiac ischemia-reperfusion injury in rats: preliminary study. Adv Clin Exp Med. 2014;23:683–9.

145. Riquelme JA, Westermeier F, Hall AR, et al. Dexmedetomidine protects the heart against ischemia-reperfusion injury by an endothelial eNOS/NO dependent mechanism. Pharmacol Res. 2016;103:318–27.

146. Ansley DM, Sun J, Visser WA, et al. High dose propofol enhances red cell antioxidant capacity during CPB in humans. Can J Anaesth. 1999;46:641–8.

147. Xia Z, Huang Z, Ansley DM. Large-dose propofol during cardiopulmonary bypass decreases biochemical markers of myocardial injury in coronary surgery patients: a comparison with isoflurane. Anesth Analg. 2006;103:527–32.

148. Ansley DM, Raedschelders K, Choi PT, et al. Propofol cardioprotection for on-pump aortocoronary bypass surgery in patients with type 2 diabetes mellitus (PRO-TECT II): a phase 2 randomized-controlled trial. Can J Anaesth. 2016;63:442–53.

149. Xu L, Hu Z, Shen J, et al. Does dexmedetomidine have a cardiac protective effect during non-cardiac surgery? A randomized controlled trial. Clin Exp Pharmacol Physiol. 2014;41:879–83.

150. Chen S, Hua F, Lu J, et al. Effect of dexmedetomidine on myocardial ischemia-reperfusion injury. Int J Clin Exp Med. 2015;8:21166–72.

Philippe Richebe and Cyrip Rivat

Introduction

For decades opioids have been used to treat chronic pain as well as perioperative pain. More recently the phenomenon of opioid-induced hyperalgesia (OIH) was introduced in the literature: the demonstration of diffuse hyperalgesia after chronic exposure to morphine (or other opioids), OIH, was linked to evidence of central sensitization detected by changes in heat tolerance thresholds and temporal summation tests [1–4]. To date, preexisting OIH, in the perioperative period, has not been well reported in the anesthesia literature. However, experimental studies suggest that sensitivity to pain is greater in those animals who have been exposed to opioids perioperatively as compared to those who were unexposed animals [5–7].

Our challenge is to differentiate chronic OIH and tolerance induced by chronic opiate exposure from the acute OIH induced by high doses of opioids used in the perioperative setting.

In this chapter, we will differentiate the OIH originating from chronic opiate exposure from the OIH of acute exposure to high dose of opioids.

This chapter will focus only on OIH that occurs preoperatively in these "naive" patients who have not received opioids prior to surgery but who were subsequently exposed to high doses of opioids intra- and postoperatively. The aim will be to propose recommendations on the use of perioperative opioids in order to prevent the development of OIH and its consequences in opioid-naive patients.

Definitions of Pain Sensitization, Allodynia, and Hyperalgesia

Acute intraoperative and postoperative pain is known to induce peripheral and central pain sensitization, similar to that seen in chronic pain conditions. The clinical symptoms encountered are called allodynia and hyperalgesia.

Allodynia is defined by the International Association for the Study of Pain (IASP) as "pain due to a stimulus that does not normally provoke pain." For example, as a perioperative consequence, it might be defined as a non-painful mechanical stimulation that becomes painful after tissue injury.

Hyperalgesia is referred to as a slightly painful mechanical stimulation which becomes much more painful or "hyper"-painful after tissue injury. Indirect markers of pain hypersensitivity include pain scores at rest and/or on movement and overall opioid consumption (opioid titration, patient controlled analgesia, or rescue analgesia).

It is important to differentiate peripheral from central sensitization in the clinical setting. In the context of postoperative pain, peripheral sensitization is correlated with hypersensitivity generated at the peripheral nerve level and can be evaluated by exerting mechanical stimulations next to the wound, 1–2 cm apart. This is called "primary hyperalgesia." Central sensitization occurs at the central nervous system level (spinal and supraspinal level) and is evaluated distal to the wound, beyond the immediate area of inflammation. The area of hyperalgesia is then measured, and an index can be calculated [8, 9]. More complex tools have also been reported in order to evaluate this central sensitization (RIII reflex, etc. [10–12]). Some authors developed experimental models in human volunteers in order to evaluate the therapeutic impact of "anti-hyperalgesic" drugs [12].

P. Richebe, MD, PhD (✉) • C. Rivat, MD, PhD
Maisonneuve Rosemont Hospital, CIUSSS de l'Est-de-l'ile-de-Montreal, 5414, Boulevard de l'Assomption, Montreal, QC H1t2M4, Canada

Department of Anesthesiology, University of Montreal, Montreal, QC, Canada
e-mail: philipperichebe@live.com

© Springer International Publishing AG 2017
A.R. Absalom, K.P. Mason (eds.), *Total Intravenous Anesthesia and Target Controlled Infusions*,
DOI 10.1007/978-3-319-47609-4_42

For clinician anesthesiologists, it is important to have a basic knowledge of pain sensitization processes, because the development of postoperative hypersensitivity to pain has been reported as a risk factor to develop persistent postsurgical pain (PPSP) [13, 14].

In the clinical perioperative setting, this chapter will illustrate that most of the clinical trials reported on indirect evaluation of hyperalgesia by assessing pain scores and morphine equivalent consumption for 24 or 48 h after surgery. There are only a few studies which evaluate the area of postoperative hyperalgesia in humans, although there is extensive [15] data from animal studies, which will be reviewed in this chapter.

Opioid-Induced Hyperalgesia in Experimental Studies

Surgery acts as an intense and repeated peripheral painful stimulus that induces central sensitization by changing the release of neurotransmitters in the spinal synaptic cleft and modifying the activity of pre- and postsynaptic receptors such as α-amino-3-hydroxy-5-methyl-4-isoxazolepropionic acid (AMPA) receptors and N-methyl-D-aspartate (NMDA) receptors.

As a consequence of this sustained stimulation from the periphery, changes in gene transcription in sensory neurons (in the dorsal root ganglia, DRG, and spinal cord) augment the release of excitatory neurotransmitters and decrease inhibitory ones, enhancing neuronal excitability for days. This neuronal plasticity continues over time and leads to changes in neuronal function and structure, thereby creating PPSP [4, 16–18].

More recently, numerous authors have reported that glial cells (microglia and astrocytes), activated by inflammatory responses to the surgical insult, play an important role in the induction and the maintenance of the central sensitization that leads to PPSP. This process is initiated by inflammation which activates macrophages. These macrophages activate microglial cells in DRGs and astrocytes in the central nervous system (CNS). Activated microglial cells induce an increase in pro-inflammatory cytokines such as IL-1β, IL-6 (IL for interleukins), TNFα (tumor necrosis factor), and brain-derived neurotrophic factor (BDNF). These cytokines contribute to the development of the neuronal central hyperexcitability that exists in neuropathic pain and PPSP [17, 19, 20].

Interestingly, anesthesia might also be responsible for some part of the activation of NMDA receptors and/or glial cells. More precisely, higher doses of opioid have been reported to increase the level of central sensitization at the spinal and supraspinal level. In animal and human volunteer studies, this opioid-induced hyperalgesia (OIH) was shown with all types of opioids (e.g., fentanyl, remifentanil, etc.) [7, 21–24], regardless of the route of administration (subcutaneous, intravenous, intrathecal) [24–26]. Implication of NMDA receptors in the development of OIH was reported early [27], and more recently, the ability of intraoperative opioids to activate glial cells was demonstrated [19]. OIH is dose dependent and time exposure dependent [26].

Usually opioids act on specific receptors and activate specific intracellular G-proteins. This leads to a hyperpolarization of the neuron, an inhibition of excitatory neurotransmitter release (glutamate, Substance P), and a reduction of the sensatory neuron at the spinal and supraspinal level. OIH might result from the conjunction of several mechanisms:

1. Desensitization and internalization of opioid receptors after phosphorylation of these receptors by a protein kinase C (PKC).
2. Activation of adenylcyclase: the Gs protein activated by the opioid induces an overproduction of AMPc which stimulates the release of the pronociceptive neurotransmitter: glutamate.
3. Activation of NMDA receptors [24]: phosphorylation of these receptors by PKC, activation of NO synthase (increase of NO and decrease of μ-opioid receptors' function).
4. Release of anti-opioid peptides: production of pronociceptive peptides such as cholecystokinin (CCK), FF neuropeptide (NPFF), orphanin, etc.
5. Increase activity of the descending pathways with predominant activity of ON-cells in the RVM (Fig. 42.1, from [42]).

Shen and Crain were the first to report that ultralow doses of morphine produced hyperalgesia via cellular changes at the dorsal root ganglia level [28–30]. Strong evidences indicate that opioid receptor can be interconverted rapidly between inhibitory Gi/o coupled and excitatory (Gs coupled) mode, following physiological alterations in the concentration of cAMP/PKA-dependent glycolipid GM1 ganglioside in neuronal sensory cell membranes [28–30].

At the supraspinal level, different mechanisms in the periaqueductal gray (PAG) have been reported to explain the excitatory effects of morphine. NMDA receptors and MOR have been shown to coexist in the PAG within single neurons [31]. In brain slices, the excitatory action of NMDA on PAG neurons is potentiated by a MOR (μ opioid receptor) agonist at low nanomolar concentration [32]. A molecular interaction has been shown to take place in the PAG, between NMDA and opioid receptors to mediate morphine-induced acute nociception [33]. Ultralow dose morphine has been shown to increase pERK1 contents in the PAG [34]. This data suggests that the NMDA receptors in the PAG play a critical role in the mediation of excitatory effects of

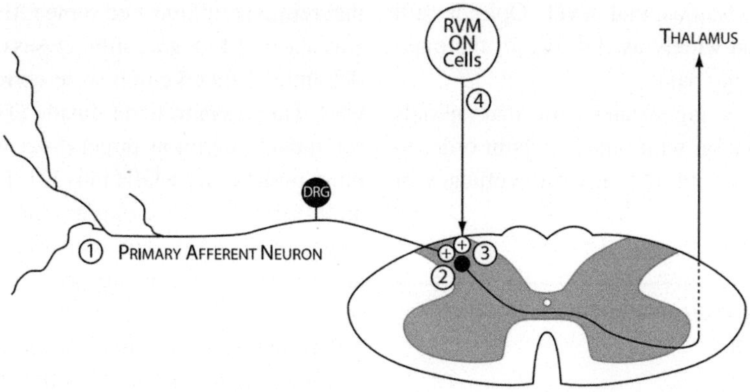

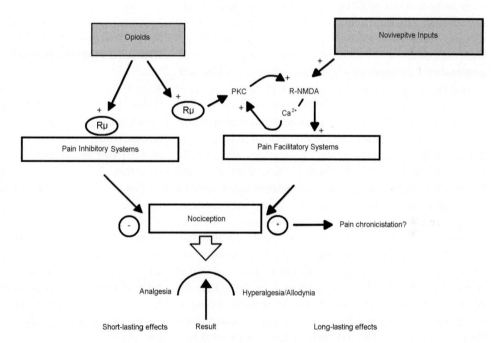

Fig. 42.1 Possible molecular mechanisms for opioid-induced hyperalgesia. Some mechanisms that have been studied include (*1*) sensitization of primary afferent neurons, (*2*) enhanced production and release of excitatory neurotransmitters and diminished reuptake of neurotransmitters, (*3*) sensitization of second order neurons to excitatory neurotransmitters, and (*4*) neuroplastic changes in the rostral ventromedial medulla that may increase descending facilitation via "on-cells" leading to upregulation of spinal dynorphin and enhanced primary afferent neurotransmitter release and pain (Reproduced from [42] with permission from Wolters Kluwer Health, Inc.)

Fig. 42.2 Schematic view of how analgesic opioids may activate not only pain inhibitory systems (analgesia) but also pain facilitatory systems (hyperalgesia/allodynia) via activation of the NMDA receptors. The analgesic effect of a first opioid administration would result from the activation of these two opposing systems. R-NMDA, NMDA receptor; Rμ, mu-opioid receptor; PKC, protein kinase C-γ (Reproduced from [40] with permission from Wolters Kluwer Health, Inc.)

morphine, thereby supporting the beneficial effects of systematically administrated NMDA receptor antagonists such as ketamine in blocking opioid-induced pain hypersensitivity [7, 24, 35–38]. Recently, neuroinflammatory responses in the PAG indicate that vlPAG glia regulate morphine tolerance development via TLR4 signaling [39]. Since TLR4 activation has been implicated in hyperalgesia, these findings may represent novel cellular mechanisms by which morphine may produce pain hypersensitivity after injection in the PAG.

In conclusion, several animal studies have reported that opioids activate pain facilitatory systems originating from PAG and the RVM [40–43] to produce pain hypersensitivity (Fig. 42.2, from [40]).

As proposed by Célèrier et al., the net effects of morphine after systemic administration may be a result of the balance between the activation of pain inhibitory systems and the concomitant activation of pain excitatory systems [35].

Systemic administration of opioids may produce centrally mediated analgesia via the involvement of the hypothalamus, subdivision of the PAG, for instance, but would also activate the medium septum, some subdivision of the PAG leading to decreased opioids analgesia.

Research still remains to be done in an order to better understand the effects (analgesic and hyperalgesic) of opioids at the spinal and supraspinal level. Opioids still remain the most potent and widely used drugs for the management of acute and chronic pain.

Nevertheless, it is becoming clearer now that opioids should be used in combination with other drugs in order to limit their excitatory effects and to enhance the efficacy of the pain relief.

The Clinical Perioperative Reality of Opioid-Induced Hyperalgesia

For the last 15 years, clinical trials have reported on postoperative hypersensitivity to surgical pain, called OIH and on acute opioid tolerance (AOT). Most reported higher pain scores, higher opioid consumption, and higher postoperative acute hyperalgesia for 2 or 3 days postoperatively after receiving higher intraoperative doses of opioids [15, 44–48].

A meta-analysis of 2014 identified 27 randomized controlled trials (RCTs) from a variety of surgeries (cesarean section, gynecology, CABGs, colorectal surgery, etc.) and compared different regimens of intrathecal and intravenous administered intraoperative opioids (fentanyl, remifentanil, sufentanil) with groups that received a placebo or a lower dose. Of 27 studies, at least 7 had poor methodology and were eliminated from analysis. The aim of this meta-analysis was to determine whether higher doses of an intraoperative opioid might affect postoperative pain scores, acute opioid tolerance and opioid/analgesics consumption, and hyperalgesia [15]. This review and meta-analysis selected 18 studies that looked at OIH following intraoperative remifentanil administration. Six RCTs evaluated OIH after Fentanyl use, three of which received intrathecal fentanyl. Three RCTs received IV sufentanil. Hyperalgesia after surgery was not evaluated directly (area of hypersensitivity) in a majority of the studies. Nevertheless, in those that did assess this parameter, higher doses of intraoperative opioids increased the risk of developing OIH. Higher intraoperative doses were associated with slightly higher pain scores at rest, despite equivalent morphine consumption at 24 h. Conclusions on fentanyl and sufentanil were unable to be drawn because the limited studies and varied techniques. The review concluded that an association between high doses of IV remifentanil and increased postoperative pain, morphine consumption, and hyperalgesia might exist. Remifentanil might not be the only narcotic to be implicated in postoperative OIH, as it was well demonstrated with other narcotics in preclinical experimental studies [7, 24, 49]. More clinical studies are needed to conclude whether fentanyl and sufentanil can induce OIH.

In 2014, another systematic review evaluated OIH and AOT after intraoperative use of remifentanil [50]. It cited studies done in human volunteers [51, 52] that demonstrated

that remifentanil induced some OIH and AOT when the dose was above 0.1 mcg/kg/min. Doses of remifentanil infusion at 0.3 and 0.4 mcg/kg/min were correlated with postoperative OIH. Target-controlled infusion (TCI) of remifentanil, when set above 3 ng/ml as target dose, was also shown to induce more postoperative OIH [44, 53]. The authors calculated that an infusion of 0.2 mcg/kg/min might be equivalent to a TCI target of 4 ng/ml. The conclusion of their review is that anesthesiologists should be cautioned not to exceed 0.1 mcg/kg/min of remifentanil. Although this may seem highly precautious, based on the published RCTs on OIH, a dose above the threshold of 0.2 mcg/kg/min [8] may likely contribute postoperative OIH and AOT.

Finally, only two studies reported on the influence of high intraoperative doses on the risk of developing PPSP [45, 54]. More studies are required in order to determine whether acute OIH might participate to the development of PPSP.

Any Strategy to Prevent Perioperative Opioid-Induced Hyperalgesia?

Kim et al. concluded in a systematic review [50] that remifentanil induced AOT and OIH could be reduced with "coadministered anesthetic drugs, such as propofol and nitrous oxide, or by using TCI." The pharmacologic basis of OIH can be attributed to modulation via the NMDA receptors.

The key receptors involved in the activation of central pain sensitization processes are the glutamate receptors, such as NMDA receptors. NMDA receptors are activated when high intensity of painful stimulation occurs intra- and postoperatively. High doses of opioids given during and after surgery have also been shown to activate NMDA receptors and, as a consequence, to induce higher level of central pain sensitization and postoperative hyperalgesia, thereby increasing the risk of developing chronic pain.

NMDA receptors modulation and/or blockade might be an interesting perioperative strategy to reduce central pain sensitization and to improve pain management intra- and postoperatively. Future studies examining this strategy are needed.

NMDA Modulators as Adjuvants of Postoperative Pain Management

Ketamine

Ketamine is a NMDA receptor antagonist. It blocks this receptor channel by acting on a specific subunit of the receptor. Plasma concentration of ketamine at 30 ng/ml seems to be sufficient to achieve a minimal analgesic effect [55] and to obtain a decrease in pain and opioid consumption after surgery [56, 57].

Administered during and after surgery, ketamine has been shown to reduce hyperalgesia when tested around the surgical wound [8, 58, 59].

Several recent meta-analyses demonstrated that the beneficial effect of ketamine on postoperative pain and opioid consumption endured beyond the elimination half-life of the drug [60–64]. These findings suggest that the pharmacologic effect of ketamine is outlasting by its ability to block pain sensitization after surgery. As a consequence, ketamine demonstrate long-lasting effects on the development of long-term pain sensitization. The most recent meta-analysis indicates that a large majority of clinical trials favor the use of perioperative ketamine for perioperative acute pain management [64].

There is considerable variability of the ketamine regimens published to obtain an anti-hyperalgesic effect and to reduce acute postoperative pain and opiates. These findings have been demonstrated in rat models [24] (Fig. 42.3, from [24]).

Some tables published by various authors [65] present regimens that appear to be practical and relevant [64]. Intra- and postoperative low doses of IV ketamine can reduce the development of chronic pain at 6 or 12 months after laparotomies [9, 66]. Finally, the epidural administration of ketamine reported to effectively block pain sensitization [67, 68]. However, has been this is not a recommended mode of usage, due to the possible neurotoxic effect of the various solutions used in different countries. There are reports on the use of S-ketamine. Regular ketamine is a racemic mixture of $S(+)$ ketamine and $R(-)$ ketamine. $S(+)$ ketamine alone is now available in some countries. Its NMDA receptor affinity is four times greater than that of $R(-)$ ketamine, and the analgesic effect is said to be 2–3 times greater than the racemic presentation of the drug. More clinical studies are needed to understand the role that $S(+)$ ketamine will play in perioperative pain management.

Ketamine has psychomimetic and hallucinogenic side effects when used in anesthetic doses. However, some studies note these side effects when only small sub-anesthetic doses were used [69, 70]. To minimize these side effects, it is recommended not to exceed intra- and postoperatively the recommended sub-anesthetic ketamine doses.

The combinations of ketamine with opioid in PCA appear inferior to a continuous infusion of ketamine alone, delivered separately from opioid PCA. Therefore, the administration of ketamine and opioid in the same solution cannot be recommended [71, 72].

The future challenge will be to choose the patient population that will maximally benefit from perioperative ketamine utilization. Meta-analyses locate reports in favor of

ketamine as a means to improve postoperative pain management [64]. Unfortunately, these meta-analyses do not identify preoperative risk factors, nor do they differentiate high from low-risk patients with the respect to pain development and persistence. It nevertheless seems likely that a patient with a high preoperative risk for pain sensitization (e.g., a patient with chronic pain condition and chronic opioid tolerance) would benefit more from ketamine administration than would a low-risk patient. One recent study [73] demonstrated ketamine's beneficial effects on postoperative pain management in high-risk patients with chronic pain and chronic opioid exposure.

As a patient is only once in his life "naïve" in terms of pain sensitization, i.e., before he undergoes his first "major surgery," this author suggests that NMDA blockade or modulation should be given to everybody perioperatively. Future studies are needed to determine, whether ketamine should only be used for specific, high-risk populations or for all patients.

Other NMDA Antagonists and Perioperative Pain Management

Memantine (NMDA receptor antagonist), amantadine (antiviral drug originally used to treat flu symptoms, antiparkinsonian drug, weak NMDA receptor antagonist effects), and methadone (μ-receptor opioid agonist and NMDA receptor antagonist) also antagonize NMDA receptors. Because of the limited literature addressing the utilization of these drugs, no recommendation for clinical practice can be made to date in the perioperative setting. Dextromethorphan has also been proposed as an adjuvant for postoperative pain management because of its anti-NMDA properties [74]. This drug has been abandoned and removed from the market in some European countries. Recommendation for clinical use cannot be made at this time because of limited supporting literature.

Magnesium

Magnesium is the physiological blocker of the inactive NMDA receptor. A recent study demonstrated that IV magnesium does not cross the blood–brain barrier [75].

Most animal studies which administered magnesium to block NMDA receptors report outstanding results [76–79]. Evidence from RCTs is conflicting, with some supporting the use of IV magnesium to improve postoperative pain [80–82] and others failing to support its use [83–85]. This lack of effect of IV magnesium might be attributed to its failure to cross the blood–brain barrier. Nevertheless, a recent meta-analysis reported that perioperative administration of IV magnesium could reduce both the overall 24 h morphine consumption by 24.4 % and the postoperative pain intensity (4.2 at rest, 9.2 on movement on a scale of 100) [86]. In most studies, magnesium is administered as an

Fig. 42.3 Effects of ketamine on the fentanyl enhancement of mechanical hyperalgesia (**a**), tactile allodynia (**b**), and weightbearing changes (**c**) induced by hind paw plantar incision. A hind paw plantar incision was realized on rats during halothane anesthesia on D_0. One fentanyl (100 g/kg) or saline injection was performed four consecutive times every 15 min, resulting in a total dose of 400 g/kg subcutaneously administered (n 12). Surgery was performed just after the second fentanyl injection. Three ketamine (3×10 mg/kg; n 12) or saline boluses (n 12) were subcutaneously administered. The first one was performed 30 min before surgery, and the following injections were performed every 5 h. The three pain parameters were evaluated before surgery on D_2, D_1, and D_0; 2, 4, 6, and 10 h after the surgery on D_0; and subsequently once daily for 8 days. At the end of the experiment (D_8), all rats were injected with naloxone (1 mg/kg subcutaneous), and the three pain parameters were measured 5 min later. (*Inset*) Algesic index showing the variations of mechanical hyperalgesia, tactile allodynia, and weight bearing on the days after the incision. Pain parameters values and algesic index are expressed as mean SD. # Dunnett test, $P < 0.05$ compared with the D_0 basal value. *Dunnett test, $P < 0.05$ for comparison between groups. $ Mann–Whitney test for comparison algesic indexes, $P < 0.05$. Filled circles saline–fentanyl-treated rats; open diamond ketamine–fentanyl-treated rats (Reproduced from [24] with permission from Wolters Kluwer Health, Inc.)

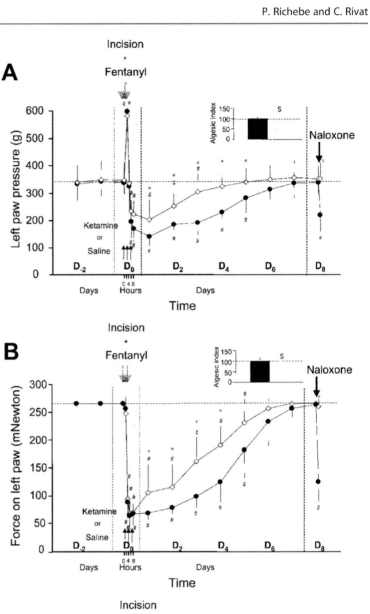

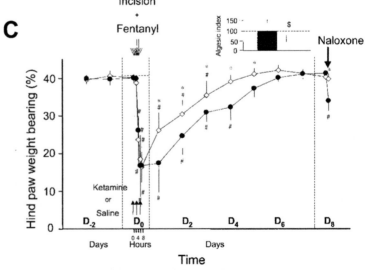

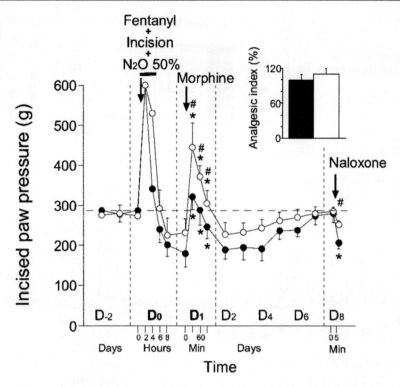

Fig. 42.4 Effect of premixed 50/50 % N_2O–O_2 treatment on fentanyl–incision-induced hyperalgesia and acute morphine tolerance at D_1. The fentanyl or saline injections were performed on D_0 (total dose: 4×100 g/kg or same saline volume). The first injection was done 15 min before incision and then every 15 min. Nitrous oxide or air was administered to rats from 15 min before the first fentanyl injection and for 4 h. Morphine (3 mg/kg subcutaneously) was injected on D_1. Nociceptive threshold was assessed on D_2, D_1, and D_0; every 30 min after the first fentanyl injection and to 8 h on D_0; every 30 min after morphine injection on D_1 for 1 h 30 min; and subsequently once daily

for 8 days. On D_8, all rats were injected with naloxone (1 mg/kg subcutaneously), and the nociceptive threshold was evaluated 5 min later. Nociceptive threshold is expressed as mean and SD. *Dunnett test, $P < 0.05$ compared with the D_1 basal value. # Dunnett test, $P < 0.05$ for comparison between groups. Open circles N_2O–O_2–incision–fentanyl-treated rats ($n = 10$); filled circles air–incision–fentanyl-treated rats ($n = 10$). Analgesic indexes: *black square* air–incision–fentanyl-treated rats; white square N_2O–O_2–incision–fentanyl-treated rats (Reproduced from [23] with permission from Wolters Kluwer Health, Inc.)

IV bolus of 30–50 mg/kg at the time of anesthesia induction and continued intra- and postoperatively with an average of 500 mg/h for 24 h [86].

When administered intrathecally or epidurally in humans, magnesium might have beneficial effect in perioperative pain management, but more studies are needed to support this specific route of administration [87–91].

Nitrous Oxide

Nitrous oxide (N_2O) has been used in anesthesia for more than 150 years. It has sedative, analgesic, and anxiolytic properties. It is an NMDA receptor antagonist [92, 93]. Animal studies reported promising anti-hyperalgesic effect and an improvement of opioid tolerance in the animals that only receive N_2O intraoperatively (Fig. 42.4, from [23]).

In humans, there is still no study as of as yet that has been designed to look at the impact of its intraoperative administration on postoperative pain, hyperalgesia, and opioid consumption. Future studies should address this question in clinical practice.

Regional Anesthesia

One recent experimental study evaluated the effect of sciatic nerve blocks on postoperative acute hyperalgesia and development of persistent central pain sensitization (a surrogate for chronic pain) following surgery (Fig. 42.5, from [94]).

In this study, animals underwent hind paw surgery under sciatic nerve block using "single shot" or "multiple shots" of bupivacaine. The latter was used to simulate a continuous local anesthetic infusion. The sciatic nerve blocks were all placed before surgery. Surgery was performed under isoflurane anesthesia without opioids. The "continuous" (multiple shots) sciatic nerve block reduced postoperative hyperalgesia and decreased the risk of central pain sensitization. This study also demonstrated that intraoperative fentanyl, when administrated during general anesthesia, eliminated the decrease in central sensitization, even in the presence of the sciatic nerve block [94]. These findings suggest that opioids enhance central pain sensitization, reducing the preventative effect of nerve blocks on the development of chronic pain. Thus, peripheral nerve blocks

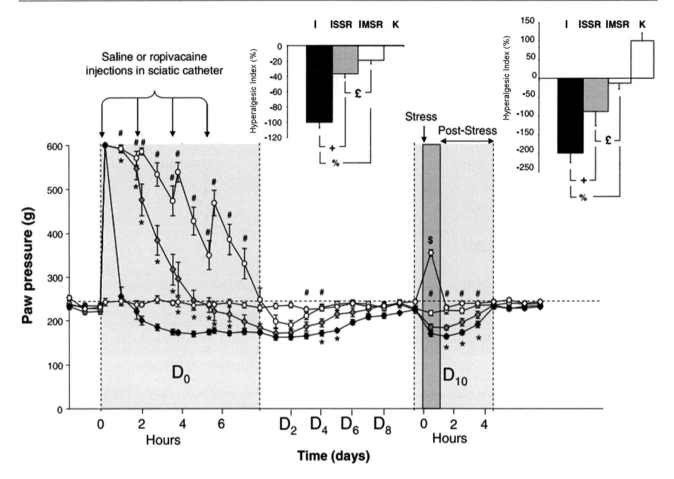

Fig. 42.5 Effects of regional anesthesia on D_0: (**a**) on the development of acute hyperalgesia for hours and days after the incisional pain model in rats and (**b**) on the variations of the nociceptive threshold (NT) after stress exposure on D_{10}. The NT of animals was measured on the incised left-hind paw (or sham), and values are given in grams. Ropivacaine (0.2 mL, 0.5 %) (or saline) was injected in the sciatic nerve catheter 5 min before surgery and then every 2 h. No animal received SC fentanyl around the surgery on D_0; they were all treated with SC saline instead of fentanyl (four injections SC 15 min apart around surgery). White diamonds: saline in sciatic nerve catheter, no plantar surgery, and SC saline (control animals, group K1). Black diamonds: saline in sciatic nerve catheter, plantar surgery, and SC saline (group I). *Gray diamonds*: single-shot ropivacaine (SSR), plantar surgery, and SC saline (group ISSR). *White circles*: multiple-shot ropivacaine (MSR, one injection every 2 h, four injections total), plantar surgery, and SC saline (group IMSR). "*" indicates Newman–Keuls test, P G 0.05 for comparison between I and ISSR. "#" indicates Newman–Keuls test, P G 0.05 for comparison between ISSR and IMSR. Mann–Whitney U test was used for comparison of area above the curve for postoperative hyperalgesia, from D_1 to D_{10}, and for comparison of area above the curve for NT after stress on D_{10}: "%," "+," and "U" represent P G 0.05 for I versus IMSR, I versus ISSR, and ISSR versus IMSR, respectively (Reproduced from [94] with permission from Wolters Kluwer Health, Inc.)

may reduce chronic pain following surgery: (1) by decreasing pain sensitization induced by the surgery itself and (2) by decreasing intraoperative use and opioid-induced hyperalgesia.

Neuraxial analgesia (epidural) used pre- and postsurgery led not only to better pain relief right after thoracic surgery but also to a smaller incidence of chronic pain 6 months after the surgical insult, as compared to a control group that received high doses of opioids intraoperatively [45]. These findings reinforce the theory that higher doses of intraoperative opioids increase the likelihood of developing OIH [8, 9, 54] and PPSP [54]. Neuraxial analgesia plays a major role in protecting against PPSP development [9, 45, 95–97].

Conclusion

As reported by experimental data of the last 20 years and confirmed by the two most recent meta-analyses or systematic reviews, OIH and AOT are real phenomena that anesthesiologists should consider when making a personalized plan for their patient's anesthesia. Whether remifentanil induces more OIH than fentanyl or sufentanil is unclear as there is a bias from more publications on remifentanil. Animal studies tend to show that all opioids, when given at higher doses, will induce OIH and AOT.

The number one strategy for the anesthesiologist should be to reduce opioids doses (for remifentanil, the author suggests below 0.15 mcg/kg/min) by combining strategies to block NMDA receptors (ketamine, N_2O, magnesium, etc.) and utilize regional anesthesia whenever possible.

References

1. Chu LF, Clark DJ, Angst MS. Opioid tolerance and hyperalgesia in chronic pain patients after one month of oral morphine therapy: a preliminary prospective study. J Pain. 2006;7(1):43–8.
2. Compton P, Charuvastra VC, Ling W. Pain intolerance in opioid-maintained former opiate addicts: effect of long-acting maintenance agent. Drug Alcohol Depend. 2001;63(2):139–46.
3. Chen L, et al. Altered quantitative sensory testing outcome in subjects with opioid therapy. Pain. 2009;143(1–2):65–70.
4. Woolf CJ. Central sensitization: implications for the diagnosis and treatment of pain. Pain. 2011;152(3 Suppl):S2–15.
5. Laboureyras E, et al. Long-term pain vulnerability after surgery in rats: prevention by nefopam, an analgesic with antihyperalgesic properties. Anesth Analg. 2009;109(2):623–31.
6. Celerier E, et al. Long-lasting hyperalgesia induced by fentanyl in rats: preventive effect of ketamine. Anesthesiology. 2000;92(2):465–72.
7. Rivat C, et al. Fentanyl enhancement of carrageenan-induced long-lasting hyperalgesia in rats: prevention by the N-methyl-D-aspartate receptor antagonist ketamine. Anesthesiology. 2002;96(2):381–91.
8. Joly V, et al. Remifentanil-induced postoperative hyperalgesia and its prevention with small-dose ketamine. Anesthesiology. 2005;103(1):147–55.
9. Lavand'homme P, De Kock M, Waterloos H. Intraoperative epidural analgesia combined with ketamine provides effective preventive analgesia in patients undergoing major digestive surgery. Anesthesiology. 2005;103(4):813–20.
10. Dirks J, et al. Mechanisms of postoperative pain: clinical indications for a contribution of central neuronal sensitization. Anesthesiology. 2002;97(6):1591–6.
11. Skljarevski V, Ramadan NM. The nociceptive flexion reflex in humans—review article. Pain. 2002;96(1–2):3–8.
12. Koppert W, et al. A new model of electrically evoked pain and hyperalgesia in human skin: the effects of intravenous alfentanil, S(+)-ketamine, and lidocaine. Anesthesiology. 2001;95(2):395–402.
13. Eisenach JC. Preventing chronic pain after surgery: who, how, and when? Reg Anesth Pain Med. 2006;31(1):1–3.
14. Kehlet H, Jensen TS, Woolf CJ. Persistent postsurgical pain: risk factors and prevention. Lancet. 2006;367(9522):1618–25.
15. Fletcher D, Martinez V. Opioid-induced hyperalgesia in patients after surgery: a systematic review and a meta-analysis. Br J Anaesth. 2014;112(6):991–1004.
16. Ji RR, et al. Central sensitization and LTP: do pain and memory share similar mechanisms? Trends Neurosci. 2003;26(12):696–705.
17. Wen YR, et al. Microglia: a promising target for treating neuropathic and postoperative pain, and morphine tolerance. J Formos Med Assoc. 2011;110(8):487–94.
18. Latremoliere A, Woolf CJ. Central sensitization: a generator of pain hypersensitivity by central neural plasticity. J Pain. 2009;10(9):895–926.
19. Romero A, et al. Glial cell activation in the spinal cord and dorsal root ganglia induced by surgery in mice. Eur J Pharmacol. 2013;702(1–3):126–34.
20. Ji RR, Berta T, Nedergaard M. Glia and pain: is chronic pain a gliopathy? Pain. 2013;154 Suppl 1:S10–28.
21. Cabanero D, et al. The pro-nociceptive effects of remifentanil or surgical injury in mice are associated with a decrease in delta-opioid receptor mRNA levels: prevention of the nociceptive response by on-site delivery of enkephalins. Pain. 2009;141(1–2):88–96.
22. Cabanero D, et al. Pronociceptive effects of remifentanil in a mouse model of postsurgical pain: effect of a second surgery. Anesthesiology. 2009;111(6):1334–45.
23. Richebe P, et al. Nitrous oxide revisited: evidence for potent antihyperalgesic properties. Anesthesiology. 2005;103(4):845–54.
24. Richebe P, et al. Ketamine improves the management of exaggerated postoperative pain observed in perioperative fentanyl-treated rats. Anesthesiology. 2005;102(2):421–8.
25. Van Elstraete AC, et al. A single dose of intrathecal morphine in rats induces long-lasting hyperalgesia: the protective effect of prior administration of ketamine. Anesth Analg. 2005;101(6):1750–6.
26. Ishida R, et al. Intravenous infusion of remifentanil induces transient withdrawal hyperalgesia depending on administration duration in rats. Anesth Analg. 2012;114(1):224–9.
27. Celerier E, et al. Opioid-induced hyperalgesia in a murine model of postoperative pain: role of nitric oxide generated from the inducible nitric oxide synthase. Anesthesiology. 2006;104(3):546–55.
28. Crain SM, Shen KF. Modulation of opioid analgesia, tolerance and dependence by Gs-coupled, GM1 ganglioside-regulated opioid receptor functions. Trends Pharmacol Sci. 1998;19(9):358–65.
29. Crain SM, Shen KF. Antagonists of excitatory opioid receptor functions enhance morphine's analgesic potency and attenuate opioid tolerance/dependence liability. Pain. 2000;84(2–3):121–31.
30. Crain SM, Shen KF. Neuraminidase inhibitor, oseltamivir blocks GM1 ganglioside-regulated excitatory opioid receptor-mediated hyperalgesia, enhances opioid analgesia and attenuates tolerance in mice. Brain Res. 2004;995(2):260–6.
31. Rodriguez-Munoz M, et al. The mu-opioid receptor and the NMDA receptor associate in PAG neurons: implications in pain control. Neuropsychopharmacology. 2012;37(2):338–49.
32. Kow LM, et al. Potentiation of the excitatory action of NMDA in ventrolateral periaqueductal gray by the mu-opioid receptor agonist. DAMGO Brain Res. 2002;935(1–2):87–102.
33. Galeotti N, et al. Signaling pathway of morphine induced acute thermal hyperalgesia in mice. Pain. 2006;123(3):294–305.
34. Sanna MD, Ghelardini C, Galeotti N. Regionally selective activation of ERK and JNK in morphine paradoxical hyperalgesia: a step toward improving opioid pain therapy. Neuropharmacology. 2014;86:67–77.
35. Celerier E, et al. Evidence for opiate-activated NMDA processes masking opiate analgesia in rats. Brain Res. 1999;847(1):18–25.
36. Li X, Angst MS, Clark JD. A murine model of opioid-induced hyperalgesia. Brain Res Mol Brain Res. 2001;86(1–2):56–62.
37. Wala EP, Holtman Jr JR. Buprenorphine-induced hyperalgesia in the rat. Eur J Pharmacol. 2011;651(1–3):89–95.
38. Ahmadi S, et al. N-methyl-D-aspartate receptors involved in morphine-induced hyperalgesia in sensitized mice. Eur J Pharmacol. 2014;737:85–90.
39. Eidson LN, Murphy AZ. Blockade of Toll-like receptor 4 attenuates morphine tolerance and facilitates the pain relieving properties of morphine. J Neurosci. 2013;33(40):15952–63.
40. Simonnet G, Rivat C. Opioid-induced hyperalgesia: abnormal or normal pain? Neuroreport. 2003;14(1):1–7.
41. Ossipov MH, et al. Underlying mechanisms of pronociceptive consequences of prolonged morphine exposure. Biopolymers. 2005;80(2–3):319–24.
42. Chu LF, Angst MS, Clark D. Opioid-induced hyperalgesia in humans: molecular mechanisms and clinical considerations. Clin J Pain. 2008;24(6):479–96.

43. Bannister K. Opioid-induced hyperalgesia: where are we now? Curr Opin Support Palliat Care. 2015;9(2):116–21.
44. Richebe P, et al. Target-controlled dosing of remifentanil during cardiac surgery reduces postoperative hyperalgesia. J Cardiothorac Vasc Anesth. 2011;25(6):917–25.
45. Salengros JC, et al. Different anesthetic techniques associated with different incidences of chronic post-thoracotomy pain: low-dose remifentanil plus presurgical epidural analgesia is preferable to high-dose remifentanil with postsurgical epidural analgesia. J Cardiothorac Vasc Anesth. 2010;24(4):608–16.
46. Angst MS, Clark JD. Opioid-induced hyperalgesia: a qualitative systematic review. Anesthesiology. 2006;104(3):570–87.
47. Chia YY, et al. Intraoperative high dose fentanyl induces postoperative fentanyl tolerance. Can J Anaesth. 1999;46(9):872–7.
48. Guignard B, et al. Acute opioid tolerance: intraoperative remifentanil increases postoperative pain and morphine requirement. Anesthesiology. 2000;93(2):409–17.
49. Laulin JP, Maurette P, Corcuff JB, Rivat C, Chauvin M, Simonnet G. The role of ketamine in preventing fentanyl-induced hyperalgesia and subsequent acute morphine tolerance. Anesth Analg. 2002;94(5):1263–9.
50. Kim SH, et al. Intraoperative use of remifentanil and opioid induced hyperalgesia/acute opioid tolerance: systematic review. Front Pharmacol. 2014;5:108.
51. Koppert W, et al. Differential modulation of remifentanil-induced analgesia and postinfusion hyperalgesia by S-ketamine and clonidine in humans. Anesthesiology. 2003;99(1):152–9.
52. Angst MS, et al. Short-term infusion of the mu-opioid agonist remifentanil in humans causes hyperalgesia during withdrawal. Pain. 2003;106(1–2):49–57.
53. Shin SW, et al. Maintenance anaesthetics during remifentanil-based anaesthesia might affect postoperative pain control after breast cancer surgery. Br J Anaesth. 2010;105(5):661–7.
54. van Gulik L, et al. Remifentanil during cardiac surgery is associated with chronic thoracic pain 1 yr after sternotomy. Br J Anaesth. 2012;109(4):616–22.
55. Suzuki M, et al. Determining the plasma concentration of ketamine that enhances epidural bupivacaine-and-morphine-induced analgesia. Anesth Analg. 2005;101(3):777–84.
56. Clements JA, Nimmo WS. Pharmacokinetics and analgesic effect of ketamine in man. Br J Anaesth. 1981;53(1):27–30.
57. Owen H, et al. Analgesia from morphine and ketamine. A comparison of infusions of morphine and ketamine for postoperative analgesia. Anaesthesia. 1987;42(10):1051–6.
58. Stubhaug A, et al. Mapping of punctuate hyperalgesia around a surgical incision demonstrates that ketamine is a powerful suppressor of central sensitization to pain following surgery. Acta Anaesthesiol Scand. 1997;41(9):1124–32.
59. Ozyalcin NS, et al. Effect of pre-emptive ketamine on sensory changes and postoperative pain after thoracotomy: comparison of epidural and intramuscular routes. Br J Anaesth. 2004;93(3):356–61.
60. Schmid RL, Sandler AN, Katz J. Use and efficacy of low-dose ketamine in the management of acute postoperative pain: a review of current techniques and outcomes. Pain. 1999;82(2):111–25.
61. Bell RF, et al. Peri-operative ketamine for acute post-operative pain: a quantitative and qualitative systematic review (Cochrane review). Acta Anaesthesiol Scand. 2005;49(10):1405–28.
62. Elia N, Tramer MR. Ketamine and postoperative pain—a quantitative systematic review of randomised trials. Pain. 2005;113 (1–2):61–70.
63. Himmelseher S, Durieux ME. Ketamine for perioperative pain management. Anesthesiology. 2005;102(1):211–20.
64. Laskowski K, et al. A systematic review of intravenous ketamine for postoperative analgesia. Can J Anaesth. 2011;58 (10):911–23.
65. Chauvin M, et al. How can we use antihyperalgesic drugs? Ann Fr Anesth Reanim. 2009;28(1):e13–25.
66. De Kock M, Lavand'homme P, Waterloos H. 'Balanced analgesia' in the perioperative period: is there a place for ketamine? Pain. 2001;92(3):373–80.
67. Kawana Y, et al. Epidural ketamine for postoperative pain relief after gynecologic operations: a double-blind study and comparison with epidural morphine. Anesth Analg. 1987;66(8):735–8.
68. Islas JA, Astorga J, Laredo M. Epidural ketamine for control of postoperative pain. Anesth Analg. 1985;64(12):1161–2.
69. Bowdle TA, et al. Psychedelic effects of ketamine in healthy volunteers: relationship to steady-state plasma concentrations. Anesthesiology. 1998;88(1):82–8.
70. Webb AR, et al. The addition of a small-dose ketamine infusion to tramadol for postoperative analgesia: a double-blinded, placebo-controlled, randomized trial after abdominal surgery. Anesth Analg. 2007;104(4):912–7.
71. Mion G, Tourtier JP, Rousseau JM. Ketamine in PCA: what is the effective dose? Eur J Anaesthesiol. 2008;25(12):1040–1.
72. Carstensen M, Moller AM. Adding ketamine to morphine for intravenous patient-controlled analgesia for acute postoperative pain: a qualitative review of randomized trials. Br J Anaesth. 2010;104 (4):401–6.
73. Loftus RW, et al. Intraoperative ketamine reduces perioperative opiate consumption in opiate-dependent patients with chronic back pain undergoing back surgery. Anesthesiology. 2010;113 (3):639–46.
74. Duedahl TH, et al. A qualitative systematic review of peri-operative dextromethorphan in post-operative pain. Acta Anaesthesiol Scand. 2006;50(1):1–13.
75. Mercieri M, et al. Changes in cerebrospinal fluid magnesium levels in patients undergoing spinal anaesthesia for hip arthroplasty: does intravenous infusion of magnesium sulphate make any difference? A prospective, randomized, controlled study. Br J Anaesth. 2012;109(2):208–15.
76. Begon S, et al. Magnesium increases morphine analgesic effect in different experimental models of pain. Anesthesiology. 2002;96 (3):627–32.
77. Begon S, et al. Assessment of the relationship between hyperalgesia and peripheral inflammation in magnesium-deficient rats. Life Sci. 2002;70(9):1053–63.
78. Begon S, et al. Role of spinal NMDA receptors, protein kinase C and nitric oxide synthase in the hyperalgesia induced by magnesium deficiency in rats. Br J Pharmacol. 2001;134(6):1227–36.
79. Begon S, et al. Magnesium and MK-801 have a similar effect in two experimental models of neuropathic pain. Brain Res. 2000;887 (2):436–9.
80. Tauzin-Fin P, et al. Intravenous magnesium sulphate decreases postoperative tramadol requirement after radical prostatectomy. Eur J Anaesthesiol. 2006;23(12):1055–9.
81. Steinlechner B, et al. Magnesium moderately decreases remifentanil dosage required for pain management after cardiac surgery. Br J Anaesth. 2006;96(4):444–9.
82. Mikkelsen S, et al. Effect of intravenous magnesium on pain and secondary hyperalgesia associated with the heat/capsaicin sensitization model in healthy volunteers. Br J Anaesth. 2001;86 (6):871–3.
83. Tramer MR, Glynn CJ. An evaluation of a single dose of magnesium to supplement analgesia after ambulatory surgery: randomized controlled trial. Anesth Analg. 2007;104(6):1374–9.
84. Lysakowski C, Dumont L, Czarnetzki C, Tramèr MR. Magnesium as an adjuvant to postoperative analgesia: a systematic review of randomized trials. Anesth Analg. 2007;104(6):1532–9.
85. Wilder-Smith CH, Knopfli R, Wilder-Smith OH. Perioperative magnesium infusion and postoperative pain. Acta Anaesthesiol Scand. 1997;41(8):1023–7.

86. Albrecht E, et al. Peri-operative intravenous administration of magnesium sulphate and postoperative pain: a meta-analysis. Anaesthesia. 2013;68(1):79–90.

87. Sun J, et al. A comparison of epidural magnesium and/or morphine with bupivacaine for postoperative analgesia after cesarean section. Int J Obstet Anesth. 2012;21(4):310–6.

88. Yousef AA, Amr YM. The effect of adding magnesium sulphate to epidural bupivacaine and fentanyl in elective caesarean section using combined spinal-epidural anaesthesia: a prospective double blind randomised study. Int J Obstet Anesth. 2010;19(4):401–4.

89. Bilir A, et al. Epidural magnesium reduces postoperative analgesic requirement. Br J Anaesth. 2007;98(4):519–23.

90. Arcioni R, et al. Combined intrathecal and epidural magnesium sulfate supplementation of spinal anesthesia to reduce postoperative analgesic requirements: a prospective, randomized, double-blind, controlled trial in patients undergoing major orthopedic surgery. Acta Anaesthesiol Scand. 2007;51(4):482–9.

91. Albrecht E, et al. The analgesic efficacy and safety of neuraxial magnesium sulphate: a quantitative review. Anaesthesia. 2013;68 (2):190–202.

92. Jevtovic-Todorovic V, et al. Nitrous oxide (laughing gas) is an NMDA antagonist, neuroprotectant and neurotoxin. Nat Med. 1998;4(4):460–3.

93. Ranft A, et al. Nitrous oxide (N2O) pre- and postsynaptically attenuates NMDA receptor-mediated neurotransmission in the amygdala. Neuropharmacology. 2007;52(3):716–23.

94. Meleine M, et al. Sciatic nerve block fails in preventing the development of late stress-induced hyperalgesia when high-dose fentanyl is administered perioperatively in rats. Reg Anesth Pain Med. 2012;37(4):448–54.

95. Senturk M, Ozcan PE, Talu GK, Kiyan E, Camci E, Ozyalçin S, Dilege S, Pembeci K. The effects of three different analgesia techniques on long-term postthoracotomy pain. Anesth Analg. 2002;94(1):11–5.

96. Ju H, et al. Comparison of epidural analgesia and intercostal nerve cryoanalgesia for post-thoracotomy pain control. Eur J Pain. 2008;12(3):378–84.

97. Lu YL, Wang XD, Lai RC. Correlation of acute pain treatment to occurrence of chronic pain in tumor patients after thoracotomy. Ai Zheng. 2008;27(2):206–9.

Memory, Awareness and Intravenous Anesthetics

43

Michael Wang

Introduction

It is clear that there are increased risks of accidental awareness under general anaesthesia when a total intravenous anaesthetic or even target-controlled infusion technique is being used [1, 2] especially in the presence of neuromuscular blockade. Typically, the problems include compromise of infusion patency due to tube kinking, infiltration at the cannula site, underdosing or even frank human error such as failure to turn on the pump, connect the pump or drug administration lines or incorrect pump programming. In contrast to volatile inhaled anaesthetic techniques, where end-tidal agent concentration monitoring is available, for TIVA, there are no indicators of adequate dose or alarms which alert the anaesthetist to a problem. It is therefore imperative that the anaesthetist regularly checks the infusion line and ensures that it is visible. The cannula site should also be checked frequently to ensure patency of infusion. The pump itself also needs to be checked throughout that it is actually delivering the infusion and the correct programme parameters have been selected. In addition it is a National Institute for Health and Care Excellence (NICE UK) recommendation that some additional technique for monitoring depth of anaesthesia is employed, especially when neuromuscular blockade is included [3]. In most cases this will be a processed EEG monitor such as the bispectral index (Medtronic, Minneapolis, USA). The Royal College of Anaesthetists' National Audit Project 5 (Accidental Awareness during General Anaesthesia) expert panel also recommends the use of the isolated forearm technique, despite the general reluctance on the part of the profession to use this [2]. However, the IFT remains the only direct and reliable indication of mental state and consciousness during

a general anaesthetic when a muscle relaxant is administered. It is relatively simple to implement, making use of equipment that can be found in all operating theatres and anaesthetic rooms, and is inexpensive. Nevertheless, there are many myths about the IFT which give rise to a lack of enthusiasm for the technique [4]. These include the fallacies that it cannot be used for more than 20 min, it does not correlate with post-operative patient interview, and it cannot be used when both arms are needed for surgical or anaesthetic purposes. Another important obstacle for many is concern about losing face in front of surgical colleagues: shouldn't the competent anaesthetist know that their patient is unconscious without having to interrogate the patient on the table? A simple way to overcome this concern is to use a recurrent pre-recorded message supplied through headphones using a digital recorder, thus making verbal commands inconspicuous. Nevertheless, it is always important to observe the tourniqued limb throughout to identify movement. NAP5 has also emphasised the importance of the use of a nerve stimulator to monitor paralysis.

One of the key findings from the UK and Ireland National Audit Project was the predominance of neuromuscular blockade in cases of accidental awareness: 96 % of awareness reports were associated with the use of a muscle relaxant, in contrast with the national activity survey [5] result of only 48 % of all general anaesthetics in the UK. In the sample of awareness patients who had received a total intravenous anaesthetic (TIVA), 87 % had been administered a muscle relaxant. This finding reinforces the NICE (UK) advice that if TIVA is used with neuromuscular blockade, some additional monitor such as processed EEG or the isolated forearm technique should be employed. This finding is also consistent with my own clinical practice in which the experience of awake paralysis is commonly the most psychologically traumatic aspect of anaesthetic awareness for the patient: perhaps counterintuitively, it is not generally the pain experienced during accidental awareness that causes so much of the psychological problem. Even today, despite

M. Wang, BSc, MSc, PhD (✉)
Clinical Psychology Unit, University of Leicester, Centre for Medicine, Lancaster Road, Leicester LE1 7HA, UK
e-mail: mw125@le.ac.uk

© Springer International Publishing AG 2017
A.R. Absalom, K.P. Mason (eds.), *Total Intravenous Anesthesia and Target Controlled Infusions*,
DOI 10.1007/978-3-319-47609-4_43

lurid and sensational media reporting concerning anaesthetic awareness, most patients are unaware of the routine use of muscle relaxants and their effects. When the patient accidentally becomes conscious and notices she is unable to move, she may have catastrophic ideas about what has happened: she may believe the surgeon has accidently cut her spinal cord or that there has been some unusual interaction between the anaesthetic drugs, rendering her paralysed *for the rest of her life*. Often patients think they are suffocating despite being mechanically ventilated along with pulse oximeter monitoring indicating adequate oxygenation. The subsequent return of movement and voluntary breathing does not ameliorate the intraoperative trauma—the psychological damage has been done, and typically the patient will be left with flashbacks and nightmares which may continue for months if not years. Emergence awareness may be accompanied by the sensation of suffocation and impending death. Another insight revealed by the British and Irish National Audit Project data is that some patients actually believe they have died on the operating table during their awareness experience. Most patients, even undergoing a relatively trivial procedure but under general anaesthesia, will have the thought "I might die" at some point prior to their operation [6]. They lose consciousness following induction and, on awakening, find that they are in darkness (eyelids taped shut), unable to move, but can hear the voices of theatre staff. They conclude they have died on the operating table, and the state they are now experiencing will be permanent, for eternity. These experiences along with catastrophic ideation produce severe psychological trauma which can be very difficult to resolve.

There were a number of awareness reports in the National Audit Project dataset from medical or healthcare professionals who had undergone general anaesthesia: invariably these patients suffered minimal post-operative psychological difficulty, because they understood what was happening to them, knew it was temporary and reversible and were protected from erroneous speculation concerning their intraoperative condition [7].

Detailed analysis of individual awareness cases from the National Audit Project dataset involving TIVA demonstrates increased risk when general anaesthesia is induced outwith the operating room (e.g. in the radiology department) or during transfer (e.g. between OR and ICU). Typically in these cases patients were paralysed and an inappropriately low dose of anaesthetic transfused, giving rise to awareness.

In 35 % of AAGA cases, an uncommon TIVA technique was employed with unorthodox drugs or using repeat bolus rather than continuous infusion, or partial TIVA mixed with volatile anaesthesia. In 13 % of cases, a change in anaesthetic technique occurred part way through the operation. In another 13 %, the TIVA dose was reduced due to concern about hypotension. In 13 % of cases, there was failure of the cannula or the line, usually undetected by the anaesthetist until after awareness had occurred [2].

Incidence of Awareness During Total Intravenous Anaesthesia or Target-Controlled Infusion

Sandin and Nordström [8] described five cases of awareness identified from around 2500 successive TIVA anaesthetics. In the majority of these (1727), patients were asked on two occasions during the first 2 days post-operatively if they had "slept well". No formal Brice protocol was used. This gives an incidence of 0.2 %, but this should be treated with caution as it is likely to be an underestimate due to the methodology. Sandin and Nordstrom describe each of their awareness cases in some detail and conclude that two cases resulted from inability to deliver the target dose of anaesthetics, while the patient's need for anaesthetics was greater than anticipated in three. They felt that all five cases had been avoidable and were a function of inexperience of the anaesthetist.

Miller et al. [9] discontinued their study prematurely when 6 out of 90 arthroscopy patients (6.7 %) receiving propofol TIVA were found to have been conscious with recall in their comparison of different doses of midazolam and a placebo group. Four of these were in the placebo group ($n = 21$, incidence of 19.1 %).

Nordstrom et al. [10] exclusively studied anaesthetic awareness in a sample of 1000 TIVA cases. They used a Brice interview protocol at emergence and then again 1–2 days later. In 500 of their cases, a third interview took place at seven to eight days post-anaesthetic. They found an overall rate of 0.2 %; however, one of the two AAGA cases did not describe explicit recall until the eighth day, raising the possibility that one or more cases might have been found in the 500 in whom the 1-week follow-up was omitted.

Errando et al. [11] found that propofol TIVA was a significant risk factor for accidental awareness in their sample of 4001 general anaesthetics (incidence of 1.1 % compared with 0.59 % for volatile anaesthesia). They had interviewed their patients immediately after surgery, at 7 and 30 days post-operatively in an uncontrolled observational study.

The incidence of accidental awareness with TIVA in China is reported as high as 1 %; a recent Chinese study using the BIS found an incidence of 0.36 % [12]. A Japanese questionnaire survey found 21/24 reported awareness cases involved TIVA with only three inhalational awareness cases [13].

These studies of TIVA awareness incidence (Table 43.1) are small in number, and the results are variable. Study design and methodology are of variable quality, making

Table 43.1 Incidence of awareness during TIVA

Authors	N	Incidence (%)
Sandin and Nordström [8]	1727	0.2
Miller et al. [9]	90	6.7
Nordstrom et al. [10]	1000	0.2
Errando et al. [11]	4001	1.1
Zhang et al. [12]	5228	0.36

the drawing of reliable conclusions problematic. Nevertheless, overall, there are indications that TIVA is associated with a moderately raised risk of accidental awareness.

Case Examples from the British and Irish National Audit Project TIVA Reports

NAP5 provided a unique opportunity to evaluate many cases of accidental awareness in some detail and specifically in the context of TIVA. The following is a selection of cases which provide important clues as to the psychological mechanisms underlying the patient's subsequent psychological difficulties—or otherwise. An absence of sequelae is often as instructive as in those where profound trauma is reported.

Case 1

The TIVA dose was reduced to manage intraoperative hypotension in a critically ill patient. A depth of anaesthesia monitor (not employed) may have helped in this complex case with neuromuscular blockade. Fortunately, the patient understood the nature of the paralysis and therefore suffered no psychological sequelae.

The patient stated: "I woke up and had a lot of pain, wanted to ask for pain killers, but couldn't speak nor move; I couldn't move a hand. I heard voices talking about drugs, saw bright light through my [closed] eyelids, I was vaguely clear that it was during the operation, and that you are supposed to be paralysed when you have an anaesthetic". So this patient was not very distressed and protected psychologically because she understood the role, effect and reversibility of muscle relaxants. On close questioning, she was not aware at all of the tracheal tube, nor of being ventilated.

Case 2

The TIVA dose was reduced to manage hypotension. The TIVA technique used was described as TCI but in fact was not: the target was expressed in "ml/hr". The patient was obese, receiving numerous chronic pain drugs and therefore at risk of accidental awareness; nevertheless, there was no depth of anaesthesia monitoring.

The patient reported coming out of anaesthesia which resulted in a major complication. The patient reported a brief episode of severe pain and a sense of something going on around her. She did not report any memory of voices or specific intraoperative events.

The patient suffered flashbacks and post-traumatic stress disorder as a result of her awareness experience.

Case 3

The patient underwent a wisdom teeth extraction procedure. There appears to have been incomplete or ineffective reversal towards the end of the anaesthetic, and the patient continued to experience paralysis on emergence. No nerve stimulator was used to monitor neuromuscular blockade. There was poor preoperative communication with the patient and failure to shape patient expectations. The consultant anaesthetist left the operating theatre before the end of the procedure, and the TIVA was discontinued too soon, allowing the patient to experience awake paralysis.

The patient was left with the impression she had become conscious during her operation and that she had been "held down" by surgical staff. This was probably her attribution of the paralysis.

No post-operative psychological sequelae were reported.

Case 4

In this case, the muscle relaxant was given late so reversal and extubation were delayed.

The patient stated: "I felt very frightened, I couldn't breathe, I felt I was going to die".

Immediately on waking up from the anaesthetic, the patient spontaneously remarked "I knew I was in trouble and I wanted to tell you, but I couldn't move".

The following day, the patient, on being questioned specifically by the anaesthetist, was unable to recall any details of the event and apparently was dismissive of the event saying "It must have been just me".

No post-operative psychological sequelae were reported.

Case 5

Remifentanil and propofol TIVA was used but programmed wrongly for each. Tiredness of the anaesthetist could have been a factor in the error.

The patient remembered waking up and feeling unable to move or communicate, but thought "I'll come round soon", so she didn't feel overly distressed.

No post-operative psychological sequelae were reported.

These cases illustrate a number of key points:

1. The importance of the experience of conscious paralysis as the principal cause of post-operative psychological trauma
2. The role of misattribution and misunderstanding of neuromuscular blockade during this experience of conscious paralysis in mediating acute psychological trauma, which can be obviated if the patient already has an accurate understanding of the use and effects of muscle relaxants
3. The importance of human error giving rise to TIVA underdosing or infusion failure which goes undetected because of the presence of paralysis, preventing body movement to indicate the patient's predicament

Management of Accidental Awareness

The National Audit Project reporting prevalence (1:15,000; [2]) is completely at odds with that indicated by prospective Brice interview studies (1:600; [14]), which underscores the fact that the vast majority of those who have intraoperative memories are unmotivated or reluctant to complain or inform anaesthetic or surgical staff of what they have experienced [15]. When a patient does report that they have unexpected intraoperative memories, they may be experiencing acute distress in the recovery area or on the receiving ward. Typically it is the nursing staff who are first made aware that there has been a problem. The anaesthetist responsible for the awareness incident may well also be traumatised themselves by the report from the nurses and understandably will feel reluctant to see the patient (they too require care and support). However, it is advisable for both medicolegal and psychological welfare reasons for the anaesthetist to meet with the patient as soon as possible. It is also advisable that they take another member of staff as a witness. The anaesthetist should take a compassionate and empathic approach, making it clear that they wish to hear and understand what the patient has experienced. They should avoid being defensive, and seek to establish the facts of what has happened and accept that the patient experience is very real, irrespective of any misunderstandings on the patient's part. The anaesthetist should avoid jumping to conclusions about what has happened at this early stage. They should feel able to apologise without admitting liability, given that this is the official stance of the medical defence union in these circumstances. Sometimes there has been some confusion on the patient's part when, for example, perioperative experiences have been mistaken as intraoperative. Such misunderstanding must be handled gently and with great care, seeking to explain what has happened sensitively. If the patient's account clearly indicates an episode of AAGA has occurred, the anaesthetist

may wish to consult the anaesthetic record, the theatre equipment and colleagues, in order to investigate what may have gone wrong, before making any definitive comment to the patient. However, it is important that at the earliest opportunity, some explanation is provided to the patient. Sometimes no explanation will be immediately apparent, in which case it is necessary to communicate this. It is crucial that the anaesthetist makes it clear to the patient at all times that they believe the patient's account, that they regret this has happened and that they are as anxious as the patient to understand what has gone wrong (see Fig. 43.1).

The patient should be followed up during the following two weeks via outpatient appointment or telephone interview. It is common for traumatised patients to experience nightmares and flashbacks of intraoperative events during this period; however, in many the frequency and intensity of these phenomena will decline, and they may not need any specific intervention. It is always helpful to provide contact details of a psychologist or psychiatrist who is experienced in the treatment of PTSD, whether or not this option is called upon. If there is no improvement in PTSD symptoms over the first two weeks, referral is recommended [7, 16].

Psychologists or psychiatrists receiving such a referral should offer exposure-based cognitive behavioural therapy (CBT) or eye movement desensitisation and reprocessing (EMDR, as recommended by NICE [17]). The key common feature of these techniques is the repeated and deliberate evocation of the most traumatic aspect of the experience to encourage habituation, emotional processing and resolution of the conditioned fear response, along with the development of more rational and adaptive cognitive understandings and thoughts about the experience.

Death Fear

Some of the NAP5 awareness patients reported that during their experience of conscious paralysis, they actually believed they had died on the operating theatre table: that what they were experiencing (immobility, darkness but still being able to hear) was actually what death is like and that they would be in this condition for the rest of eternity. This relates to a very primitive and basic fear of death that commonly arises in children aged 7–11 when they first become aware of their own mortality [18, 19]. Typically children at this age do not conceptualise the cessation of consciousness but imagine permanent oblivion in which consciousness is preserved in the absence of perception, sensation or agency: a kind of eternal darkness of the soul, of which they are understandably terrified. It is possible that this primitive death fear lies within many of us, despite the later development of more adult conceptualisations and accommodation with our own mortality. Moreover, anaesthetic drugs may tend to depress frontal brain

Fig. 43.1 NAP5 psychological support pathway

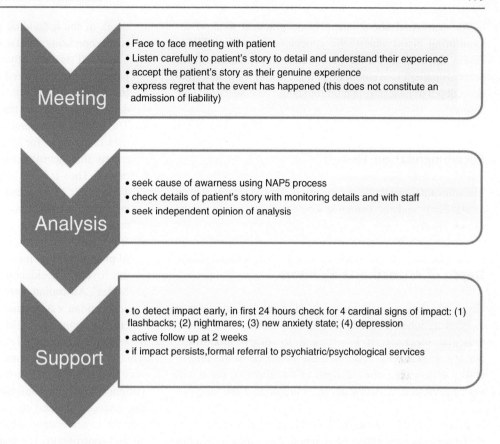

Meeting
- Face to face meeting with patient
- Listen carefully to patient's story to detail and understand their experience
- accept the patient's story as their genuine experience
- express regret that the event has happened (this does not constitute an admission of liability)

Analysis
- seek cause of awarness using NAP5 process
- check details of patient's story with monitoring details and with staff
- seek independent opinion of analysis

Support
- to detect impact early, in first 24 hours check for 4 cardinal signs of impact: (1) flashbacks; (2) nightmares; (3) new anxiety state; (4) depression
- active follow up at 2 weeks
- if impact persists, formal referral to psychiatric/psychological services

structures first (including rational adult cognition) and in a partially anaesthetised state, older, more primitive structures of the midbrain particularly concerned with emotional processing may be left intact. This partially anaesthetised state may allow primitive childhood memory and emotional processing to re-emerge. This state may therefore provide fertile ground for the emergence of an underlying fearful conception of death, reinforced by darkness, and an inability to move, which gives rise to profound psychological trauma, even though this state proves to be temporary and reversible. This may account for the severity of psychological and emotional impact of accidental awareness and its devastating effects on post-operative quality of life in some patients.

National Audit Project TIVA Recommendations

NAP5 made four key recommendations which will be reviewed here.

Recommendation 18.1

All anaesthetists should be trained in the maintenance of anaesthesia with intravenous infusions.

TIVA and TCI are not presently compulsory components of the anaesthetic curriculum in the UK: NAP5 advises that

this should change, since most anaesthetists at some point in their practice will find themselves expected to use one or the other. There are a number of common errors with TIVA administration, and proper training should reduce these risks.

Recommendation 18.2

When using total intravenous anaesthesia, wherever practical, anaesthetists should ensure that the cannula used for drug delivery is visible and patent at all times.

The most common cause of TIVA accidental awareness is human error, particularly in relation to incorrect connection, line patency and programming errors. Visual checking of the line and infusion flow should provide early warning of a problem.

Recommendation 18.3

Depth of anaesthesia monitoring should be considered in circumstances where patients undergoing TIVA may be at higher risk of accidental awareness. These include use of neuromuscular blockade, at conversion of volatile anaesthesia to TIVA and during use of TIVA for transfer of patients.

As mentioned above, there is no practical method for monitoring blood anaesthetic concentration during TIVA. Given the added risk of neuromuscular blockade which prevents patient movement as an indicator of light anaesthesia, a depth of anaesthesia monitor should be considered (see below).

Recommendation 18.4

The relevant anaesthetic organisations should establish a set of standards and recommendations for best practice in the use of TIVA.

Depth of Anaesthesia Monitors

Given the key recommendation of depth of anaesthesia monitoring when TIVA is used in conjunction with neuromuscular blockade, it is pertinent to review monitoring options. Please note that given the evidence of the unreliability of so-called clinical signs of wakefulness, these will not be reviewed here as a serious monitoring method.

1. Processed EEG Monitors (BIS, Narcotrend, Entropy)
   These monitors collect EEG signals from the forehead or scalp and process them to produce a number between 0 and 100. Typically the processing involves transforming raw EEG into a power spectrum, and then a probability algorithm is used to determine the numerical indicator of depth of anaesthesia. The manufacturers of the BIS state that the target range for surgical anaesthesia is 40–60. Most of the validation studies have been conducted using the BIS, and it is assumed (e.g. by NICE) that other processed EEG monitors share the same validity characteristics. This assumption may be risible.
   There are some key points that should be borne in mind when considering the characteristics of processed EEG monitors and their output:
   a. The studies compare, standardise and validate the processed EEG against post-operative amnesia, not intraoperative consciousness. This is an important issue since the two are not the same—it is perfectly possible (and even common) to have an intraoperatively conscious patient who subsequently has no explicit recall of such experience/events. Thus, a BIS reading of 40 may mean the patient has no memory, but may not guarantee intraoperative unconsciousness.
   b. The processed EEG output number represents a statistical average probability of the likelihood of anaesthesia, not a reliable indication of the actual anaesthetic depth of the individual patient. Thus each numerical score represents the statistical mean of a normal distribution. It is perfectly possible that the individual patient being monitored lies on the tail of the distribution and is therefore significantly more lightly or deeply anaesthetised than the number suggests.
   c. The frontalis electromyogram signal is included in the beta component for determining the BIS index. This means that neuromuscular blockade affects the BIS output. Thus it is no surprise that there are reports of a BIS index of 40 in conscious but paralysed volunteer anaesthetists who have received muscle relaxant but no anaesthetic [20, 21].
   d. It remains controversial as to whether the routine use of processed EEG monitoring makes any difference to the overall accidental awareness incidence, with Myles' Australian group arguing strongly in favour and Avidan's American group arguing equally vociferously against [22, 23].

2. The Isolated Forearm Technique (IFT) (Fig. 43.2)
   This is a remarkably simple, inexpensive and obvious way to identify consciousness in an otherwise paralysed patient where neuromuscular blockade is being used during intended general anaesthesia. It is so obvious, it is difficult to understand why it has evoked so much hostility and controversy. Using an available limb (and it could be a leg if necessary), a sphygmomanometer cuff is used as a pneumatic tourniquet. It should be applied to the forearm (or below the knee in the case of a leg) and inflated to around 200 mmHg or at least 10 mmHg above the patient's systolic blood pressure. A protective pad of cotton wool should also be placed between the tourniquet and the skin. The tourniquet is applied and the forelimb isolated just before muscle relaxant injection, thus preserving the potential for movement in the

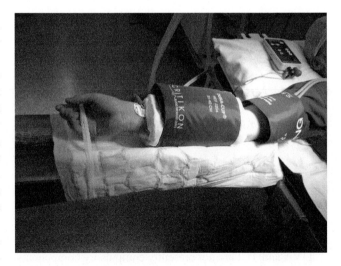

Fig. 43.2 The isolated forearm technique

forelimb and hand/foot. It is also important to use a nerve stimulator to allow for periodic monitoring of the presence of motor function of the isolated limb: stimulator electrodes should be placed immediately distal to the tourniquet on the ventral surface of the forelimb, with the ground electrode located near to the antecubital fossa [or knee]. A digital audio recorder and headphones are then used to present the instruction "[patient's first name], if you can hear my voice, open and close the fingers of your right/left hand [or move the big toe on your right/left foot]". Typically the message is presented once every minute during the GA. The tourniquet should not be applied for more than 20 min continuously, since after this time typically a functional ischaemia and nerve block occurs, rendering the limb effectively immobile. However, the tourniquet can be released after this period, the blood supply to the limb refreshed for a few minutes, and if further paralysis is required, the tourniquet can be reinflated and more muscle relaxant administered. Providing a non-depolarising modern muscle relaxant is employed, the limb will continue to be potentially mobile, despite the period of blood flow cessation. This cycle can be repeated for surgeries lasting several hours. I will not discuss the numerous myths and misunderstandings regarding the IFT here, but the interested reader is directed to the detailed article by Russell [4]. In summary, the IFT is a perfectly practical, inexpensive and reliable method for monitoring depth of anaesthesia which could be used for routine anaesthesia with neuromuscular blockade, particularly where risk of accidental awareness is previously identified. For those with direct experience of the technique, it remains the gold standard for depth of anaesthesia monitoring against which all other monitors, including processed EEG should be validated. NAP5 recommends that it should be included in the curriculum for all trainee anaesthetists as an option to be considered for depth of anaesthesia monitoring.

Summary

- TIVA with neuromuscular blockade represents a significant risk for accidental awareness.
- The cause of TIVA accidental awareness is underdosing as a result of impaired infusion patency or programming error. This can be obviated by regular visual inspection of the TIVA line and cannula and the use of a depth of anaesthesia monitor such as the IFT or a processed EEG monitor, although there is significant doubt concerning the reliability of the latter.
- It is the experience of awake paralysis that is the main cause of psychological trauma. It is vital that whenever neuromuscular blockade is employed, a nerve stimulator is used, particularly prior to emergence.
- If a case of awake paralysis occurs, the NAP5 care pathway should be implemented.
- Awake paralysis may produce severe PTSD, in some cases because the patient has thought they died, or were dying, during their awareness experience.

References

1. Pandit JJ, Andrade J, Bogod DG, Hitchman JM, Jonker WR, Lucas N, Mackay JH, Nimmo AF, O'Connor K, O'Sullivan EP, Paul RG, Palmer JH, Plaat F, Radcliffe JJ, Sury MR, Torevell HE, Wang M, Cook TM. 5th National Audit Project (NAP5) on accidental awareness during general anaesthesia: protocol, methods, and analysis of data. Br J Anaesth. 2014;113:540–8.
2. Pandit JJ, Andrade J, Bogod DG, Hitchman JM, Jonker WR, Lucas N, Mackay JH, Nimmo AF, O'Connor K, O'Sullivan EP, Paul RG, Palmer JH, Plaat F, Radcliffe JJ, Sury MR, Torevell HE, Wang M, Hainsworth J, Cook TM. 5th National Audit Project (NAP5) on accidental awareness during general anaesthesia: summary of main findings and risk factors. Br J Anaesth. 2014;113:549–59.
3. National Institute for Health and Care Excellence (NICE), Diagnostics guidance [DG6]: Depth of anaesthesia monitors—Bispectral Index (BIS), E-Entropy and Narcotrend-Compact M. 2012. https://www.nice.org.uk/guidance/DG6.
4. Russell IF. Fourteen fallacies about the isolated forearm technique, and its place in modern anaesthesia (Editorial). Anaesthesia. 2013;68:677–88.
5. Sury MR, Palmer JH, Cook TM, Pandit JJ. The state of UK anaesthesia: a survey of National Health Service activity in 2013. Br J Anaesth. 2014;113:575–84.
6. Ramsay MAE. A survey of pre-operative fear. Anaesthesia. 1972;27:396–402.
7. Cook TM, Andrade J, Bogod DG, Hitchman JM, Jonker WR, Lucas N, Mackay JH, Nimmo AF, O'Connor K, O'Sullivan EP, Paul RG, Palmer JH, Plaat F, Radcliffe JJ, Sury MR, Torevell HE, Wang M, Hainsworth J, Pandit JJ. 5th National Audit Project (NAP5) on accidental awareness during general anaesthesia: patient experiences, human factors, sedation, consent, and medicolegal issues. Br J Anaesth. 2014;113:560–74.
8. Sandin R, Nordström O. Awareness during total i.v. anaesthesia. Br J Anaesth. 1993;71:782–7.
9. Miller DR, Blew PG, Martineau RJ, Hull KA. Midazolam and awareness with recall during total intravenous anaesthesia. Can J Anaesth. 1996;43(9):946–53.
10. Nordstrom O, Engstrom AM, Persson S, Sandin R. Incidence of awareness in total i.v. anaesthesia based on propofol, alfentanil and neuromuscular blockade. Acta Anaesthesiol Scand. 1997;41 (8):978–84.
11. Errando CL, Sigl JC, Robles M, Calabuig E, Garcıa J, Arocas F, Higueras R, del Rosario E, Lopez D, Peiro CM, Soriano JL, Chaves S, Gil F, Garcıa-Aguado R. Awareness with recall during general anaesthesia: a prospective observational evaluation of 4001 patients. Br J Anaesth. 2008;101(2):178–85.
12. Zhang C, Xu L, Ma YQ, Sun YX, Li YH, Zhang L, Feng CS, Luo B, Zhao ZL, Guo JR, Jin YJ, Wu G, Yuan W, Yuan ZG, Yue Y.

Bispectral index monitoring prevent awareness during total intravenous anesthesia: a prospective, randomized, double-blinded, multicenter controlled trial. Chin Med J (Engl). 2011;124(22):3664–9.

13. Morimoto Y, Nogami Y, Harada K, Tsubokawa T, Masui K. Awareness during anesthesia: the results of a questionnaire survey in Japan. J Anesth. 2011;2011(25):72–7.

14. Sebel PS, Bowdle TA, Ghoneim MM, Rampil IJ, Padilla RE, Gan TJ, Domino KB. The incidence of awareness during anesthesia: a multicenter united states study. Anesth Analg. 2004;99:833–9.

15. Absalom AR, Green D. NAP5: the tip of the iceberg, or all we need to know? Br J Anaesth. 2014;113(4):527–30.

16. Wang M. The psychological consequences of explicit and implicit memories of events during surgery. In: Ghoneim M, editor. Awareness during anesthesia. Woburn, MA: Butterworth-Heinemann; 2001.

17. National Institute for Health and Care Excellence (NICE): Posttraumatic stress disorder: management NICE guidelines [CG26]. 2005. https://www.nice.org.uk/guidance/cg26.

18. Gullone E. The development of normal fear: a century of research. Clin Psychol Rev. 2000;20(4):429–51.

19. Slaughter V, Griffiths M. Death understanding and fear of death in young children. Clin Child Psychol Psychiatry. 2007;12(4):525–35.

20. Messner M, Beese U, Romstock J, Dinkel M, Tschaikowsky K. The bispectral index declines during neuromuscular block in fully awake persons. Anesth Analg. 2003;97:488–91.

21. Schuller PJ, Newell S, Strickland PA, Barry JJ. Response of bispectral index to neuromuscular block in awake volunteers. Br J Anaesth. 2015;115 Suppl 1:i95–103.

22. Avidan MS, Zhang L, Burnside BA, Finkel KJ, Searleman AC, Selvidge JA, Saager L, Turner MS, Rao S, Bottros M, Hantler C, Jacobsohn E, Evers AS. Anesthesia awareness and the bispectral index. N Engl J Med. 2008;358:1097–108.

23. Myles PS. Prevention of awareness during anaesthesia. Best Pract Res Clin Anaesthesiol. 2007;21(3):345–55.

Awareness and Dreaming During TIVA

Kate Leslie

Introduction

Total intravenous anaesthesia (TIVA) became popular after the introduction of propofol in 1986. In this chapter we will not distinguish between TIVA administered by simple manual infusions and TIVA administered using target-controlled infusion (TCI) technology. Soon after the introduction of propofol, reports of awareness and dreaming during TIVA began to appear [1–4]. Awareness is the postoperative recall of events occurring during intended general anaesthesia and is a subjective phenomenon that is defined by either spontaneous or elicited patient report [5]. The modified Brice questionnaire is the most commonly used questionnaire to measure the incidence of awareness [6]. The incidence of awareness during modern general anaesthesia (0.1–0.2 %) was established in three large cohort studies published in the period 2000–2004 [7–9]. The reported incidence of awareness during TIVA varies between 0 and 1.1 %—potentially a higher incidence than during volatile anaesthesia. Patients who have been aware recall touch, pain, thoughts and emotions that occurred during the awareness event [10]. The consequences of awareness include early and late psychological symptoms and post-traumatic stress disorder (PTSD) [11]. Therefore measures should be taken to prevent unintended awareness during general anaesthesia. Avoidance of awareness during TIVA is dependent upon the acquisition and maintenance of key knowledge, skills and behaviours. This includes thorough preoperative assessment of the patient, careful preparation and administration of TIVA, vigilance for signs of inadequate anaesthesia and prompt action to deepen anaesthesia if appropriate. Some guideline writers have recommended the use of processed electroencephalographic (EEG) monitoring to prevent awareness in all patients having general anaesthesia with TIVA [12].

Anaesthetic dreaming is defined as any experience, other than awareness, that a patient is able to recall postoperatively, which he or she thinks was a dream and which occurred between induction of anaesthesia and the first moment of consciousness after anaesthesia [13, 14]. The timing of the interview for dreaming is important because anaesthesia-related dreams, like the dreams of sleep, are quickly forgotten. Dreaming is reported by 25–60 % of patients during emergence from general anaesthesia with TIVA [15–22], but only 1.3–2.7 % of patients 1 day later [23–25]. Dreaming is also reported by 19–40 % of patients during emergence from sedation with TIVA [26–28]. TIVA does not increase the incidence of dreaming [19]. Most dreams reported during anaesthesia are short and the content relates to everyday life: family, friends, work and leisure activities [16, 18, 19, 21, 29–31]. They lack the hallucinatory quality and emotional intensity of the dreams of rapid eye movement sleep. As dreaming during anaesthesia is usually pleasant but quickly forgotten, there is no need to prevent dreaming. If the patient suffers adverse consequences from dreaming, then appropriate counselling should be provided.

Awareness

Definition

Awareness is the postoperative recall of events occurring during intended general anaesthesia. This phenomenon is also called 'awareness with recall' [32], 'awareness with explicit recall' [25], 'explicit recall' [33] and 'accidental awareness during general anaesthesia' [34, 35]. Several related phenomena are also described. One is intraoperative wakefulness where patients may move in response to command, but not have any postoperative recall [5]. Another is unconscious (or 'implicit') learning during anaesthesia

K. Leslie, MD, FRANZCA (✉)
Department of Anaesthesia and Pain Management, Royal Melbourne Hospital, Grattan St, Parkville, VIC 3050, Australia
e-mail: kate.leslie@mh.org.au

© Springer International Publishing AG 2017
A.R. Absalom, K.P. Mason (eds.), *Total Intravenous Anesthesia and Target Controlled Infusions*,
DOI 10.1007/978-3-319-47609-4_44

where patients may retain information that affects subsequent behaviour or performance on testing [5].

An important distinction exists between postoperative recall of events occurring during intended general anaesthesia and postoperative recall of events occurring during sedation that is not intended to guarantee unconsciousness. The latter is not defined as 'awareness' as general anaesthesia was not intended. Nevertheless it is frequently confused with awareness by patients and carers and is important in this context because TIVA is commonly used to provide sedation for diagnostic and interventional procedures.

Awareness may be subclassified in a variety of ways by adjudicators other than the patient. For example, awareness reports are frequently classified using terms like 'definite', 'probable', 'possible' or 'unlikely' and different combinations of these types of awareness comprise the primary outcome variable for the study [25, 36, 37]. Alternatively awareness may be classified in terms of its clinical characteristics. For example, Mashour et al. [38] developed a classification system for awareness that included the following categories, with 'D' added to indicate emotional distress:

- Class 0: No awareness
- Class 1: Isolated auditory perceptions
- Class 2: Tactile perceptions (e.g. surgical manipulation or endotracheal tube)
- Class 3: Pain
- Class 4: Paralysis (e.g. feeling one cannot move, speak or breathe)
- Class 5: Paralysis and pain

The definition and classification of awareness does not differ between patients who are maintained with TIVA or with volatile anaesthetics.

Measurement

Awareness is a subjective phenomenon that is defined by either spontaneous or elicited patient report. The measurement instrument used affects the incidence of awareness recorded [39], although there is no evidence that the performance of any measurement tool differs between patients maintained with TIVA or with volatile anaesthetics.

The Brice Questionnaire
The modified Brice questionnaire is the most commonly used questionnaire to measure the incidence of awareness. The original questionnaire was developed in patients administered inhaled anaesthetics [6], but has since been used extensively in patients receiving TIVA. The original questionnaire included the following questions:

- What was the last thing you remembered happening before you went to sleep?
- What is the first thing you remember happening on awakening?
- Did you dream or have any other experiences whilst you were asleep?
- What was the worst thing about your operation?
- What was the next worst thing?

Subsequently the questionnaire was modified to include a direct question about awareness [40]. This form of the questionnaire has been used in recent studies that have investigated the incidence of awareness during TIVA [24, 30, 41]:

- What was the last thing you remember before you went to sleep for your operation?
- What was the first thing you remember after your operation?
- Can you remember anything in between these two periods?
- Did you dream during your operation?
- What was the worst thing about your operation?

The Brice questionnaire is usually administered on a number of occasions postoperatively (e.g. in the PACU, a few hours or days after the surgery and after 30 days). A report of awareness on any or all of these occasions is usually classified as awareness [25, 36, 37]. Because the Brice questionnaire provides contextual clues, especially if the patient was prepared by a research informed consent process, it may lead to false attribution of memories [42]. This has not been proven although it is a frequently expressed concern.

Other Questionnaires
Some research and quality assurance methods systematically offer all patients the opportunity to mention awareness without specifically asking about it. For example, Pollard et al. [43] examined clinical quality improvement data for 87,361 patients treated in a regional medical system. As part of routine care, patients were asked questions about dreaming and difficulty with anaesthesia but were not asked a direct question about awareness. Similarly Mashour et al. [44] examined electronic medical records of 44,006 patients at their academic medical centre for reports of awareness. These patients were asked about their experience of anaesthesia but were not asked a direct question about awareness. Mashour et al. [39] subsequently demonstrated an increased incidence of awareness detected by the modified Brice questionnaire over the quality assurance approach in the same patients. However few, if any, patients received TIVA in these studies [39, 43, 44].

Spontaneous Reports

Finally various measurement methods rely on spontaneous reports by patients or ad hoc questioning by anaesthetists. For example, the 5th National Audit Project (NAP5) study counted awareness events that were voluntarily reported to healthcare providers or were elicited by them during routine patient care (Box 44.1). Many of these patients were administered TIVA. The incidence of awareness has also been measured via surveys of anaesthetists [35, 45–48], where they are asked to recall awareness cases in a certain time period or over their whole career. Finally the American Society of Anesthesiologists (ASA) has established an anaesthesia awareness registry at which patients may self-report awareness experiences.

Box 44.1: The 5th National Audit Project (NAP5): Accidental Awareness During General Anaesthesia
NAP5 was a collaboration between the Royal College of Anaesthetists and the Association of Anaesthetists of Great Britain and Ireland which was conducted in three steps.

STEP 1: Surveys of anaesthetists were conducted in the United Kingdom and Ireland that retrospectively recorded the numbers of awareness cases reported during 2011. The numbers of patients receiving anaesthesia in the same time period were estimated from NAP4 (UK) and an anaesthesia activity survey (Ireland). Using this method, the incidences of awareness in the United Kingdom and Ireland were 1:15,414 and 1:23,366 respectively.

STEP 2: Reports of awareness were collected prospectively between June 2012 and May 2013. Events occurring before this period that were reported for the first time during this period were also admissible. Reports were classified by likelihood, contributory factors and preventability.

STEP 3: Anaesthesia activity surveys were conducted in the United Kingdom and Ireland to determine the numbers of general anaesthetics given at participating centres during the study period. Based on these data, the incidences of awareness in the United Kingdom and Ireland were 1:19,600 and 1: 31,200, respectively.

The protocol and results of NAP5 were co-published in the *British Journal of Anaesthesia and Anaesthesia* with accompanying editorials.

Incidence

Intended General Anaesthesia

The benchmark incidence of awareness during modern general anaesthesia was established in three large cohort studies published in the period 2000–2004 [7–9]. The incidence of awareness in these studies was 0.1–0.2 %. The majority of the included patients received volatile anaesthetics and few were monitored with a processed EEG monitor. A single question about awareness was used in two studies [7, 8] and the third used the modified Brice questionnaire [9]. More recently three large randomised controlled trials of bispectral index (BIS)-guided versus end-tidal anaesthetic agent-guided anaesthesia reported similar incidences of awareness (0.1–0.2 %) [36, 49, 50]. Some of these patients were selected because they were at higher than usual risk of awareness. All completed the modified Brice questionnaire.

Awareness was reported during TIVA shortly after the introduction of propofol in 1986 [2–4]. The reported incidence of awareness during TIVA varies between 0 and 1.1 %. Enlund and Hassan [51] studied 5216 patients presenting for short-stay surgical procedures. All of the patients received TIVA for maintenance of anaesthesia, but only 7 % received muscle relaxants and none were monitored with a processed EEG monitor. There were no recorded awareness events. In contrast Errando et al. [32] and Xu et al. [52] reported incidences of awareness of 1.1 and 1.0 %, respectively, in patients receiving TIVA. In these studies most patients received muscle relaxants (97 and 100 %) and none were monitored with a processed EEG monitor. The incidence of awareness was significantly lower in the patients in these studies who received volatile anaesthetics (0.59 and 0.2 %). These studies all used the modified Brice questionnaire.

The influence of TIVA on the incidence of awareness was also investigated in NAP5 [34]. The anaesthesia activity study identified a low rate (8 %) of TIVA in the United Kingdom and Ireland [53]. However the use of TIVA appeared to be overrepresented among the patients with reported awareness in the prospective study (18 %). The NAP5 study has several major weaknesses with respect to estimating the incidence of awareness overall and in TIVA patients [54, 55]. Firstly, the numerator included reports from previous years as well as reports from the data collection year. Secondly, the denominator (annual number of anaesthetics) was estimated from an anaesthesia activity survey over a 2-day period. And finally, the investigators relied on spontaneous reports of awareness and reports elicited by ad hoc questioning by anaesthetists, with the potential for follow-up bias with respect to patients receiving

Table 44.1 Incidence of awareness during TIVA

Author (year)	n	Patients	Relaxants (%)	TIVA (%)	Awareness (%)
Sandin and Nordstrom [41]	1727	Undifferentiated	100	100	0.3
Nordstrom et al. [24]	1000	Undifferentiated	100	100	0.2
Sandin et al. [8]	11,785	Undifferentiated	66	2.8	0 (V: 0.17)
Sebel et al. [9]	19,575	Undifferentiated	Not reported	Not reported	4 cases (V: 21 cases)
Ekman et al. [33]	4945	Undifferentiated	96	5.2	0 (V: 0.04)
Myles et al. [37]	2463	High risk of awareness	100	35[a]	0.36 (V: 0.64)
Enlund and Hassan [51]	5216	Short stay	7	100	0
Errando et al. [32]	4001	Undifferentiated	97	37	1.1 (V: 0.59)
Ye et al. [56]	1800	Undifferentiated	?	79	?
Xu et al. [52]	11,101	Undifferentiated	100	22	1.0 (V: 0.2)
Zhang et al. [25]	5228	Undifferentiated	93	100	0.36
Pandit et al. [34]	2,452,700[b]	Undifferentiated	49	0.7	0.01 (V: 0.004)

TIVA total intravenous anaesthesia, *TCI* target-controlled anaesthesia, *GA* general anaesthesia, *BIS* bispectral index

[a]35 % of B-Aware Trial patients were administered propofol TIVA without any inhaled anaesthetics. 2398 patients had at least one postoperative interview. Three of the 13 confirmed awareness patients received propofol TIVA without any inhaled anaesthetics (unpublished data)

[b]The denominator in the NAP5 study was derived from an anaesthesia activity survey. The awareness reports of the 1-year study period included first reports of cases occurring before the study period

volatile-based anaesthesia versus TIVA. These factors mean that the estimates of awareness from NAP5 are unreliable.

These observational studies suffer from the risk of several biases. In these studies, patients at a different risk of awareness from the overall study population might be administered TIVA rather than volatile anaesthetics. In addition, patients at higher risk of awareness might be monitored with a processed EEG monitor. A randomised controlled trial of TIVA versus volatile-based general anaesthesia would be required to overcome these issues, but such a study has not been done. In order to be feasible, such a study would need to recruit patients at higher than average risk of awareness presenting for surgery under relaxant general anaesthesia (in order to increase the event rate). Given the potential impact of processed EEG monitoring on the incidence of awareness, especially during TIVA [25], this monitoring would most likely be mandated for all patients in the study, unless the study was conducted in a region where this monitoring was not available or routinely used (Table 44.1).

Intended Sedation

TIVA is frequently used to provide sedation for diagnostic and interventional procedures. The sedative effects of propofol and other intravenous drugs occur on a continuum from mild drowsiness to deep unconsciousness with the threshold for amnesia occurring at a lighter depth of sedation than loss of response to command [57]. Consequently, light sedation can be associated with amnesia for perioperative events [58], but very deep sedation is required if the risk of recall is to be reduced to very low levels. This depth of sedation is usually commensurate with general anaesthesia.

Self-reporting of procedural recall occurs at the same rate following sedation and general anaesthesia. For example, in a retrospective medical record review conducted at an

academic medical centre, the documented incidence of awareness following general anaesthesia was 0.02 % and following other forms of anaesthesia was 0.03 % (relative risk 0.74 [95 % CI 0.28, 2.0]) [44]. These low incidences are likely due to the self-reporting methodology.

When systemic direct questioning about recall is applied, the reported incidence of recall is higher but still varies widely. Studies involving light to moderate sedation reported recall incidences of 14–50 % [59], whereas studies investigating deep sedation reported recall incidences of 3–4 % [26, 28]. Adjuvant drugs varied between these studies and none were randomised trials. Recently Allen et al. [60] randomised adult patients presenting for elective outpatient colonoscopy to light (BIS 70–80) or deep (BIS <60) propofol and fentanyl-based sedation. The incidence of recall was 12 % in the light group and 1 % in the deep group (risk difference for recall 0.11 [90 % CI 0.06, 0.17]). Data such as these support the notion that patients should be advised about the risk of recall during the consent process prior to sedation.

Risk Factors

Conceptually the risk of awareness increases when there is an imbalance between anaesthetic requirement and anaesthetic delivery. Patients with normal anaesthetic requirement are at risk of awareness when anaesthetic delivery is insufficient. Patients with high anaesthetic requirement are at risk of awareness at anaesthetic doses or concentrations that are sufficient for most people. Patients with low anaesthetic requirement are at risk of awareness when very low anaesthetic doses or concentrations are delivered (Table 44.2).

Table 44.2 Causes of awareness during TIVA

Requirement	Delivery	Causes
Normal	Low	Equipment malfunction Anaesthetist errors • Knowledge (e.g. inappropriate target concentrations) • Skills (e.g. inadequate iv access) • Behaviours (e.g. lack of vigilance)
High	Normal	*In addition to equipment malfunction and anaesthetist errors* Genetic predisposition Acquired drug tolerance
Low	Very low	*In addition to equipment malfunction and anaesthetist errors* Caesarean section Cardiovascular instability

Identifying risk factors for awareness is difficult in individual cohort studies and randomised controlled trials because awareness is such a rare event. To overcome this impediment, Ghoneim et al. [61] undertook a review of 271 case reports of awareness published in the English-language, peer-reviewed literature between 1950 and 2005. Aware patients were compared with two control populations totalling 19,504 patients. Apart from a possible association between younger age and female sex, and the reporting of awareness, there were no patient characteristics associated with awareness except for a past history of awareness. Cardiac and obstetric surgeries were overrepresented relative to the control population. More than 25 % of the cases received no potent hypnotic agent during surgery, but no comment was made about volatile anaesthesia versus TIVA.

Incident monitoring studies and case reports highlight the specific issues arising during TIVA that put patients at risk of awareness. These include inadequate intravenous access, failure of the intravenous delivery system, failure of the infusion device, inappropriate programming of the infusion device, errors in drug preparation and lack of real-time anaesthetic concentration monitoring for propofol [62, 63].

Clinical Features

The Patient Experience

Patients who have been aware recall touch, pain, body position and body movement (or inability to move), sound and sometimes light during intended general anaesthesia. Patients also recall thoughts and emotions that occurred during the awareness event [10]. When recounting the event, the patient may experience a range of emotions from calm acceptance to extreme distress. There is no evidence that the patient experience of awareness varies between patients maintained with TIVA or volatile anaesthetic

agents. A case of awareness during TIVA that illustrates all these features is summarised in Box 44.2.

> **Box 44.2: Awareness During Propofol TCI: A Case Report**
>
> A medical practitioner reported her experience of awareness during laparoscopic cholecystectomy under relaxant general anaesthesia with propofol TCI. Following placement of the intravenous cannula, the patient felt the sting of propofol administration but did not lose consciousness. As the muscle relaxant took effect, she became apnoeic and unable to move. She recalled endotracheal intubation, skin preparation and surgery and believed that she was conscious for up to 30 min. During this time, she felt panic, terror and despair as well as experiencing excruciating pain. She awoke extremely distressed and has significant and on-going psychological sequelae.
>
> The anaesthetist noted tachycardia, hypertension and sweating after induction of anaesthesia and bigeminy after endotracheal intubation, and he checked the patient's pupillary signs several times during the awareness episode. After some time, a fault with the Graseby 3500 infusion pump was identified. The display on the pump indicated that the targeted dose had been administered, but the syringe driver had not moved after initial 5 mL bolus was delivered. Subsequently testing revealed a defect in the pump mechanism and the local distributor of the device recommended repair of all pumps at risk of this failure.

Clinical Observations During an Awareness Event

Anaesthetists and other personnel in the operating room may notice sweating, lacrimation and pupillary dilation and movement, including swallowing, coughing and straining, if the patient is not paralysed. The routine monitored variables that may change include the respiratory rate, tidal volume, end-tidal partial pressure of carbon dioxide, heart rate and arterial blood pressure. The anaesthetist may notice a problem with anaesthetic delivery, such as a non-functioning intravenous cannula, propofol leakage or an infusion pump that is not infusing sufficient propofol for some reason. However, none of these clinical features is a reliable predictor of postoperative recall in patients having TIVA [5].

The EEG and Awareness

The raw EEG can be displayed by most anaesthesia EEG monitoring systems and may change in recognisable ways before or during an episode of inadequate anaesthesia [64]. Slow, repetitive delta waves are the cardinal feature of deep anaesthesia. Together with sleep spindles, which are bursts of 12–14 Hz oscillatory brain activity, they provide significant reassurance that the patient is adequately anaesthetised. The presence of a flat EEG, either intermittently (burst suppression) or continuously (isoelectricity), provides additional confirmation of adequate or even excessively deep anaesthesia. During an awareness episode, the anaesthetist may notice an increase in the frequency and a decrease in the amplitude of the raw EEG trace, along with loss of sleep spindles. In the unparalysed patient, electromyographic (EMG) interference and movement artefacts may appear. From the perspective of a clinical anaesthetist using an anaesthesia EEG monitor, changes in the raw EEG are indistinguishable during TIVA and volatile anaesthesia [19].

Processed EEG index values are designed to increase with decreasing anaesthetic effect-site concentration and increasing noxious stimulation, thus alerting the anaesthetist to the possibility of inadequate anaesthesia [57]. They are also designed to be agent independent: this was tested during the development phase on patients receiving TIVA and volatile anaesthetics [57]. Index values typically range from 100 (awake) to 0 (isoelectric) with values less than 60 considered to represent an extremely low probability of consciousness.

Reports of index values above the recommended range during episodes of awareness have been published. For example, a B-Aware Trial patient, who was randomised to BIS-guided anaesthesia and was anaesthetised with TIVA, had BIS values of 79–82 during the awareness episode (he recalled a piece of 'cold metal' being placed in his mouth at the start of his rigid bronchoscopy) [37]. Similarly Ekman et al. [33] reported two patients who recalled endotracheal intubation under TIVA anaesthesia where BIS values were >60, and Zhang et al. [25] reported four cases of awareness during various phases of TIVA where BIS values were >60 (one for up to 106 min).

Reports of index values within the recommended range during episodes of awareness have also been published. For example, a patient in the study of Zhang et al. [25], who was randomised to the routine care group, recalled that she 'felt hurt as a needle puncturing her navel' (sic). This patient recorded BIS values below 60 throughout the operation (although values were recorded in the 55–60 range at the relevant time).

As TIVA is commonly implemented in combination with muscle relaxants, the effect of these drugs on processed EEG indices is important. The frequency spectrum of EMG substantially overlaps with the upper end of the EEG frequency range. Artefact from EMG has the potential to obscure the underlying raw EEG and make it difficult to interpret. EMG can also be interpreted by processed EEG algorithms as evidence of high-frequency EEG activity suggesting wakefulness [65]. The administration of a muscle relaxant has been associated with a decrease in the BIS in patients under TIVA [66] and in unanaesthetised volunteers [67, 68].

Consequences

Consequences for the Patient

The early studies establishing that some patients suffer adverse sequelae after awareness recruited patients anaesthetised before the TIVA era [69, 70]. However the adverse consequences of awareness during TIVA were reported soon after the introduction of propofol in 1986 [71]. These consequences range from short-term psychological, emotional and sleep problems to long-term PTSD.

PTSD is a serious psychiatric condition that may follow a variety of severe traumatic events and is characterised by re-experiencing, avoidance and physiological hyperarousal. The condition was first formally diagnosed in awareness patients by Osterman et al. [69]. The reported incidence of PTSD of awareness varies widely (0–78 %) [11, 30, 70–77], but the incidence of PTSD in patients receiving TIVA and volatile anaesthetics has not been directly investigated.

The B-Aware Trial included a large number of patients who received TIVA (43 %) [37]. A long-term follow-up study of the B-Aware Trial revealed that 5 of the 7 confirmed awareness patients (71 %) and 3 of the 25 controls (12 %) fulfilled the criteria for PTSD at the time of the interview (adjusted odds ratio 13.3 [95 % CI 1.4–650]; $P < 0.02$) [76]. One of the control patients and two of the confirmed awareness patients received TIVA during the index surgery. The median onset time of symptoms was 14 days (range 7–243 days) after surgery and the median duration of symptoms was 4.7 years (range 4.4–5.6 years).

Recall of events during sedation that is not intended to guarantee unconsciousness may also result in adverse psychological consequences. Kent et al. [78] analysed self-reports of awareness to the ASA anaesthesia awareness registry and found that patients often mistakenly reported events that had occurred during sedation or regional anaesthesia. They reported that 78 % of sedation/regional anaesthesia patients and 94 % of general anaesthesia patients experienced distress and approximately 40 % of patients in each group had persistent psychological sequelae.

Consequences for the Anaesthetist

An awareness event can be very distressing for the anaesthetist and other staff looking after the patient. In particular the anaesthetist may be disappointed by his or her failure to correctly implement TIVA or failure to recognise and treat inadequate anaesthesia in a timely manner. Awareness figures among the most common patient claim for compensation [63, 79]. There is no evidence that claims for compensation vary between patients maintained with TIVA or volatile anaesthetics.

Prevention and Treatment

Training and Continuing Education

Avoidance of awareness during TIVA is dependent upon the acquisition and maintenance of key knowledge, skills and behaviours. An understanding of the pharmacology of intravenous hypnotic and analgesic drugs and the basics of cerebral electrophysiology is required. Trainee must practice the technical aspects of implementing TIVA and learn to avoid and detect technical errors. They must learn to assess patients preoperatively with a view to eliciting any past history of awareness and to include discussions about awareness in consent conversations. Finally trainees must learn behaviours, such as vigilance, conscientiousness and decisiveness in complex uncertain situations, and develop good communication skills.

Preoperative Preparation

Preoperatively it is important to identify patients at particular risk of awareness, such as patients with a past history of awareness, patients with altered drug tolerance due to prior exposure to hypnotic and/or analgesic drugs and patients in whom cardiovascular instability during anaesthesia can be anticipated. Aranake et al. [80] recently demonstrated that a past history of awareness was associated with an increased risk of awareness (relative risk 5.0 [95 % CI 1.2, 19.9]) in patients administered volatile anaesthetics. This raises the prospect that awareness may have a genetic aetiology in some cases.

As part of the consent process, anaesthetists should consider whether the risk of awareness is material to the patient and therefore should be mentioned. An ASA practice advisory published in 2006 revealed that ASA members and consultants were equivocal about advising low-risk patients about awareness but in favour of advising high-risk patients [81]. However, given that patients receiving TIVA are thought to be at higher than average risk [25], it may be indicated to advise all these patients about awareness. Finally as patients frequently seem to misunderstand the risk of awareness during sedation and may be adversely affected by recall of intra-procedure events, a detailed discussion of these issues with sedation patients is warranted.

Careful preparation of equipment for TIVA is essential in the prevention of awareness. The anaesthetist must check that the lines are primed and free of blockages from clamps, three-way taps and the like. The TIVA device should be carefully programmed with accurate information about the patient. This is particularly true when TCI technology is used, when it is prudent to recheck the device or ask a colleague to check it in order to avoid using the wrong infusion algorithm (e.g. a remifentanil model to infuse propofol) and/or the wrong data. It is also prudent to have a spare syringe of propofol prepared and to have ready access to further drug supplies for longer cases. The NAP5 investigators proposed a checklist for awareness to be undertaken by the team at the start of each case [82]. This did not meet with universal agreement [55].

General Intraoperative Management

The key to intraoperative monitoring is to take into account all the information about the patient when making decisions about anaesthetic depth: clinical signs such as sweating, lacrimation, pupillary dilation and movement, as well as monitored variables such as respiratory rate, tidal volume, heart rate and blood pressure and raw or processed EEG information if available [81]. The experienced anaesthetist also is vigilant to changes in surgical stimulation or surgical complications as they arise. In this way the anaesthetist can balance anaesthetic delivery with TIVA to individual requirements of the patient and the surgery.

Muscle relaxants are an important adjunct to anaesthesia but should only be used when necessary to improve patient safety and facilitate surgery. In particular the anaesthetist should check the depth of anaesthesia before administering muscle relaxants either initially or during the case. This is particularly important during induction or if the patient is moving.

In many respects the use of TCI should help to reduce the incidence of awareness because the infusion device takes care of the transition between induction and maintenance, particularly during prolonged intubation attempts. However there has been no research to support this assertion. If inadequate anaesthesia is suspected, the anaesthetist should act promptly as there is some evidence that memory traces take seconds or minutes to be laid down.

Only one trial of a drug to prevent awareness has been undertaken. Wang et al. [83] investigated the use of penehyclidine hydrochloride, a centrally acting anticholinergic drug, to prevent awareness in Chinese women having breast cancer surgery under TIVA. The incidence of awareness with penehyclidine hydrochloride (0/456 patients, 0 %) was significantly lower than with placebo (5/452, 1.1 %), $P = 0.030$. However the incidence of awareness in the placebo group was high for this group of relatively low-risk patients.

Intraoperative EEG Monitoring

As mentioned above, the raw EEG can be displayed by most anaesthesia EEG monitoring systems and may change in recognisable ways before or during an episode of inadequate anaesthesia [64]. However the raw EEG has not been investigated as a tool for preventing awareness in patients anaesthetised with TIVA.

The BIS is the only processed EEG index that has been investigated for the prevention of awareness during TIVA. Punjasawadwong et al. [84] conducted a systematic review of clinical trials comparing BIS-guided anaesthesia with standard practice. In the four studies using clinical signs as standard practice, BIS significantly reduced the risk of intraoperative awareness (7761 participants, odds ratio 0.24, 95 % CI 0.12, 0.48). This effect was not demonstrated in the four studies using end-tidal anaesthetic gas monitoring as standard practice (26,530 participants, odds ratio 1.13, 95 % CI 0.56, 2.26).

Two of the studies comparing BIS with clinical signs included patients maintained with TIVA [25, 37]. In the B-Aware Trial, 35 % of patients were administered propofol TIVA without any inhaled anaesthetics. There were three confirmed awareness cases. There were two reports of awareness in the BIS-guided group and 11 reports in the routine care group ($P = 0.022$). BIS-guided anaesthesia reduced the risk of awareness by 82 % (95 % CI 17–98 %). Three confirmed awareness patients received propofol TIVA without any inhaled anaesthetic (0.36 %) versus ten confirmed awareness patients who received inhaled anaesthetics with or without TIVA (0.64 %). One hundred percent of patients in the study of Zhang et al. were administered TIVA. In 5228 patients there were four cases of confirmed awareness (0.14 %) in the BIS-guided group and 15 (0.65 %) in the control group (odds ratio 0.21, 95 % CI 0.07, 0.63, $P = 0.002$,).

Opinion is divided about the need for BIS monitoring to prevent awareness during anaesthesia. In 2006 the practice advisory issued by the ASA did not support the routine use of EEG-based monitoring to monitor the depth of anaesthesia or prevent awareness, instead recommended that the decision to use EEG-based monitoring be made on a case-by-case basis [81]. In contrast the Australian and New Zealand College of Anaesthetists made the recommendation that 'When clinically indicated, equipment to monitor the anaesthetic effect on the brain should be available for use on patients at high risk of awareness during general anaesthesia' [85]. These organisations did not distinguish between patients maintained with TIVA or volatile anaesthetics. The National Institute on Care and Excellence in the United Kingdom recommended EEG-based monitors as an option 'during any type of general anaesthesia in patients considered at higher risk of adverse outcome' and 'in all patients receiving total intravenous anaesthesia' [12]. The use of EEG-based monitors during TIVA was recommended because it was deemed to be cost-effective (by reducing anaesthetic delivery) and because real-time monitoring of anaesthetic concentration is not possible in TIVA patients.

Australian anaesthetists were surveyed in 2014 about their use of depth of anaesthesia monitoring [86]. Twenty-nine percent (95 % CI 24 %, 34 %) of respondents thought that such monitoring was indicated in all cases under relaxant general anaesthesia, but 74 % (95 % CI 69 %, 79 %) thought that it should be mandatory during TIVA TCI.

Postoperative Management

The postoperative management of awareness is the same regardless of the agent used to maintain general anaesthesia. Institutions should develop protocols for the management of awareness patients and make sure that all clinicians caring for the patient are aware of them. Patients may be reluctant to report their experience of awareness to their anaesthetist [87] and anaesthetists are reluctant to ask their patients direct questions about awareness [48, 81]. However it is vital to foster open and safe two-way communication between patients and their anaesthetists on this subject. Systematic feedback from patients about their experience with anaesthesia is increasingly sought. This gives patients an opportunity to report their awareness experience. Anaesthetists should also consider specifically questioning patients about awareness (using the modified Brice questionnaire) if the patient was at high risk preoperatively or if any concerning signs were evident during or after anaesthesia. In either case the patient should be allowed to relate their experience in their own words first of all and should be offered acknowledgement of their distress, and an apology if this is appropriate. Patients who have confirmed awareness, and any other patients who are concerned about their experiences, should be followed up by the anaesthetist and referred for counselling [10, 11, 78].

As part of risk management and continuous improvement, cases of awareness should be reported through departmental and institutional channels to the appropriate groups. It is vital to 'close the loop' by informing the reporting anaesthetist (and if appropriate the patient) about the changes to policy and procedure that have ensued. This particularly important in the case of TIVA where reporting may lead to recall and repair of TIVA equipment [88].

Significance

Awareness during TIVA is a significant problem. In patients at high risk of awareness or with high anxiety about the potential for awareness, propofol TIVA should be implemented with the utmost care. Because of the ability to monitor end-tidal concentrations, it may be preferable to maintain anaesthesia with volatile anaesthetics in these patients if there is no contraindication.

Dreaming

Definition

Dreaming is defined as 'any type of cognitive activity occurring during sleep' [89]. Anaesthetic-related dreaming is defined as any experience, other than awareness, that a patient is able to recall postoperatively, which he or she thinks was a dream and which occurred between induction of anaesthesia and the first moment of consciousness after anaesthesia [13, 14]. Observers report that the patient appears to be unconscious or asleep during the period when the dream is postulated to have been experienced. Dreaming differs from hallucinations in that patients who report hallucinations believe that they were awake and believe that the experience actually happened. These patients also appear awake to observers. The definition of dreaming does not differ between patients in whom anaesthesia was maintained with TIVA or volatile anaesthetics.

Measurement

Like awareness dreaming is a subjective phenomenon, relying on the report of the patient. The incidence of dreaming is commonly measured using the modified Brice questionnaire [9, 37]. The narrative report of the dream is a recorded verbatim without synthesis by the observer and is later adjudicated by an independent panel.

The timing of measurement affects the incidence of dreaming although there is no evidence that the timing of measurement differently affects the incidence of dreaming reported after TIVA or volatile anaesthesia. The timing of questioning is important because anaesthesia-related dreams, like the dreams of sleep, are quickly forgotten. Patients should be questioned as soon as they are conscious and orientated after emergence from anaesthesia. Sometimes patients report different dreams at a second interview: these dreams likely occurred after the first dream and during the recovery period [29].

The characteristics of the dream can be measured by a number of scales that have been appropriated from sleep and dreaming science. These classify the dream according to criteria such as emotional content, memorability, visual vividness, amount of sound, emotional intensity, meaningfulness, amount of movement and strangeness [90].

Incidence

The reported incidence of dreaming during TIVA varies very widely. Dreaming is reported by 25–60 % of patients during emergence from general anaesthesia with TIVA [15–22], but only 1.3–2.7 % of patients 1 day later [23–25]. Dreaming is also reported by 19–40 % of patients during emergence from sedation with TIVA [26–28] (Table 44.3).

Risk Factors

Early case reports raised the possibility that dreaming is more commonly experienced by patients having TIVA than volatile anaesthesia [98]. Large studies in which the agent used for maintenance of anaesthesia was not controlled also suggested an increased incidence of dreaming with TIVA [37]. For example, in a study of patients at high risk of awareness, dreaming was reported by 4.2 % of patients 2–4 h postoperatively and TIVA was associated with higher odds of awareness than volatile anaesthesia (odds ratio 2.40 [95 % CI 1.34, 4.30]; $P = 0.0003$) [29]. Similarly in a study of healthy patients presenting for elective noncardiac surgery [18], TIVA patients had higher odds of dreaming than patients receiving volatile anaesthesia (odds ratio 3.42 [95 % CI 1.40, 8.37]; $P = 0.007$).

However observational studies may be misleading because patients at high risk of dreaming may be preferentially anaesthetised with TIVA. Randomised controlled trials therefore are required. Small studies, which randomised patients to TIVA or longer-acting volatile agents and which did not standardise anaesthetic depth during surgery, reported conflicting results [15–17, 20, 23]. Luginbühl et al. [23] compared TIVA with desflurane (a volatile anaesthetic with a more rapid offset of action) and standardised the depth of anaesthesia using BIS monitoring, but reported no difference in the incidence of awareness. However, these patients were interviewed on the first postoperative day. Subsequently a study was initiated where 300 healthy patients were randomised to TIVA or desflurane, depth of anaesthesia was standardised using BIS and interviews were conducted on emergence from anaesthesia [19]. The incidence of dreaming in this study was 27 % in the TIVA group and 28 % in the desflurane group.

Dreaming is reported more commonly by younger patients [9, 18, 29, 30], healthier patients [18, 29, 30], women [29–31], those with high home dream recall [18, 19] and those who emerge rapidly from anaesthesia [18, 19]. Ketamine-based anaesthesia is also associated with a high incidence of dreaming [99]. There is no evidence for an interaction between these factors and TIVA.

Much has been written about the influence of anaesthetic depth on the incidence of dreaming and whether dreaming signifies near-miss awareness. This has been supported by dreaming reports that include events or conversations occurring anaesthesia. For example, Leslie et al. [18] reported that

'a female patient remembered dreaming about "driving on a road. The road just swallowed her up. The doctor said she was okay but the car was wrecked. She couldn't move—she was trying to tell the driver to stop but he couldn't hear her...." This patient moved and developed tachycardia during abdominal closure, coinciding with less than 1 min of BIS values near 60. At this time, the anesthesiologist administered propofol and told the patient, "Everything is okay." Although the patient believed that she had been dreaming, an awareness report was completed, and all three adjudicators believed that awareness was "possible"'.

Several studies have evaluated the association between anaesthetic depth and dreaming; however none have

Table 44.3 Incidence of dreaming during TIVA

Author (year)	n	Patients	Interview	TIVA	Dreaming
De Grood et al. [1]	30	ENT	Within 3 h	50 %	TIVA: 6.7 % Volatile: 0 %
Millar and Jewkes [91]	130	Day case	2 h	50 %	TIVA: 6.2 % Volatile: 6.2 %
Galletly and Short [92]	50	Upper GI	Not stated	100 %	All: 6 %
Ensink et al. [93]	150	All comers	PACU	33 %	All: 18 %
Marsch et al. [20]	60	ENT	Emergence, PACU	50 %	TIVA: 43 %, 10 % Volatile: 10 %, 3 %
Oddby-Muhrbeck and Jakobsson [94]	60	Laparoscopy	Not stated	50 %	TIVA: 10 % Volatile: 3.3 %
Oxorn et al. [95]	56	Uterine D&C	1, 24 h	50 %	TIVA: 21 %, 17 % Volatile: 15 %, 18 %
Kasmacher et al. [17]	230	Minor surgery	PACU	50 %	TIVA: 60 % Volatile: 21 %
Oxorn et al. [21]	60	Uterine D&C	Emergence, PACU, day 1	100 %	25 %, 12 %, 12 %
Brandner et al. [15]	112	Varicose veins	Emergence	33 %	TIVA: 56 % Volatile: 26 %
Nordstrom et al. [24]	1000	All comers	24 h	100 %	All: 2.7 %
Munte et al. [96]	60	Lumbar discectomy	6–8 h	100 %	All: 3.3 %
Hellwagner et al. [16]	50	Breast	Emergence	50 %	TIVA: 40 % Volatile: 24 %
Luginbühl and Schnider[23]	160	Gynaecology	Day 1	50 %	TIVA: 1.3 % Volatile: 5 %
Leslie et al. [18]	300	Noncardiac	Emergence	12 %	TIVA: 36 % Volatile: 20 %
Aceto [97]	58	Lap chole	24 h	100 %	All: 10.3 %
Toscano et al. [22]	97	Gynaecology	PACU, 6 h	100 %	All: 23.7 %, 24.7 %
Stait et al. [28]	200	Sedation	PACU	100 %	All: 25.5 %
Leslie et al. [19]	300	Noncardiac	Emergence	50 %	TIVA: 27 % Volatile: 28 %
Eer et al. [26]	200	Sedation	PACU	100 %	All: 19 %
Kim et al. [27]	215	Sedation	Emergence, 30 min	50 %	Propofol: 39.8 % Midazolam: 12.1 %
Zhang et al. [25]	5228	All comers	Day 1, 4	100 %	All: 3.1 %

ENT ear nose and throat surgery, *TIVA* total intravenous anaesthesia, *TCI* target-controlled infusion, *GI* gastrointestinal, *PACU* post-anaesthesia care unit, *D&C* dilatation and curettage

provided evidence of an interaction between anaesthetic depth and the use of TIVA. In patients having caesarean section, for example, provoked lower oesophageal contractility above 13 mmHg (a sign of light anaesthesia) predicted dreaming [100]. In contrast other studies reported no association between anaesthetic depth and dreaming. In the B-Aware Trial, there was no difference in maintenance BIS values in dreamers and non-dreamers who were randomised to the intervention group [101]. This issue was resolved by a 300-patient cohort study in which BIS values were measured intraoperatively and patients were interviewed immediately postoperatively for evidence of awareness and dreaming [19]. Dreaming was reported by 22 % of patients, but there was no difference in median BIS values between dreamers and non-dreamers (37 [18, 19, 22–55, 57–60] vs. 38 [18, 19, 22–55, 57–60]; $P = 0.68$) nor the duration of BIS >60 (0 [0–7] vs. 0 [0–31] min; $P = 0.38$).

Most dreams were similar to the dreams of sleep and none were suggestive of awareness.

Clinical Features

Most dreams reported during anaesthesia are short and easily forgotten. The content is about everyday life: family, friends, work and leisure activities [16, 18, 19, 21, 29–31]. Anaesthetic dreams do not usually contain the hallucinatory, delusional or highly emotional elements of the dreams of sleep. Occasionally dreams contain information that could only have been acquired during intraoperative wakefulness. They are really awareness episodes that have been interpreted as dreams [29, 102]. When scales are used to measure the form of anaesthetic dreams, they are consistently reported as having low strangeness and memorability,

Table 44.4 Dreams reported after anaesthesia

Author (year)	Dream report
Harris et al. [13]	'One dreamed that he was at a fairground and someone was throwing darts at his stomach though there was no association with pain'
Hellwagner et al. [16]	'Meadow in summer, walking with her dog'
Myles et al. [37]	'I dreamt that I was having a conversation with my anaesthetist about the research trial. The dream was interrupted by the anaesthetist's voice trying to wake me up'
Leslie et al. [18]	'Catching a few fish on a river in the city … the water was really rough'
Stait et al. [28]	I was at a farm doing work. The investigator was in it, just checking on me
Eer et al. [26]	Dreamt I was at the office working on a laptop

although reports of emotional content, visual vividness and movement vary [18, 27] (Table 44.4).

There are no routinely monitored variables that can detect anaesthetic dreaming as it is happening. BIS values during anaesthesia do not vary between patients who do and do not report dreaming postoperatively [18]. This has been interpreted as signifying that dreaming occurs during emergence from anaesthesia [18]. Careful analysis of the raw EEG has revealed some differences between dreaming and non-dreaming patients. Leslie et al. extensively analysed the raw EEG of patients reporting and not reporting dreaming [19]. The most significant differences between dreamers and non-dreamers were observed just before the postoperative interview, when the EEG of dreamers revealed more high-frequency (30 Hz) spectral power and fewer lower-frequency (10.68 Hz) spindles than non-dreamers. These are signs of cortical activation, which also occur during rapid eye movement sleep. However there was no interaction between the agent used to maintain anaesthesia (propofol or desflurane) and the EEG correlates of dreaming.

Consequences

Dreaming during anaesthesia is usually without any consequences, either positive or negative, as dreams are usually forgotten. If the patient interprets the dream as awareness, or is otherwise emotionally traumatised by the dream, then he or she may develop postoperative psychological or emotional sequelae or even PTSD [10, 78]. In one study, dreaming was associated with lower satisfaction with care; however these patients were at high risk of awareness and also other complications [29].

Prevention and Treatment

As anaesthetic dreams are usually pleasant and ephemeral, little attention has been given to preventing them. BIS monitoring was associated with a lower incidence of dreaming in the B-Aware Trial, but these patients were at high risk of awareness, so the generalisability of this finding is not clear. Toscano et al. [22] randomised patients having TIVA to scopolamine or atropine and interviewed them on emergence about dreaming. None of the scopolamine patients and 47 % of the atropine patients reported dreaming. This finding was consistent with studies in non-surgical settings where centrally acting anticholinergic agents were associated with suppression of dreaming [22]. Patients who report dreaming only require treatment if they are distressed by their experience, and this treatment would be similar to the treatment provided for aware patients.

Significance

Dreams are a fascinating but insignificant part of anaesthesia as far as the patient is concerned. The only real interest for anaesthetists is separating dreams from inaccurately interpreted awareness and in elucidating the underlying causes of unconsciousness, dreaming and anaesthetic action.

References

1. De Grood P, Mitsukuri S, Van Egmond J, Rutten J, Crul J. Comparison of etomidate and propofol for anaesthesia in microlaryngeal surgery. Anaesthesia. 1987;42:366–72.
2. Kelly JS, Roy RC. Intraoperative awareness with propofol-oxygen total intravenous anesthesia for microlaryngeal surgery. Anesthesiology. 1992;77:207–9.
3. Rupreht J. Awareness with amnesia during total intravenous anaesthesia with propofol [letter]. Anaesthesia. 1989;44:1005.
4. Schafer HG, Marsch SC. Awareness in total intravenous anesthesia. Anaesthesist. 1990;39:617–8.
5. Ghoneim M. Awareness during anesthesia. Anesthesiology. 2000;92:597–602.
6. Brice D, Hetherington R, Utting J. A simple study of awareness and dreaming during anaesthesia. Br J Anaesth. 1970;42:535–42.
7. Myles P, Williams D, Hendrata M, Anderson H, Weeks A. Patient satisfaction after anaesthesia and surgery: results of a prospective survey of patients. Br J Anaesth. 2000;84:6–10.
8. Sandin R, Enlund G, Samuelsson P, Lennmarken C. Awareness during anaesthesia: a prospective case study. Lancet. 2000;355:707–11.

9. Sebel P, Bowdle T, Ghoneim M, Rampil I, Padilla R, Gan T, Domino K. The incidence of awareness during anesthesia: a multicenter United States study. Anesth Analg. 2004;99:833–9.

10. Kent CD, Posner KL, Mashour GA, Mincer SL, Bruchas RR, Harvey AE, Domino KB. Patient perspectives on intraoperative awareness with explicit recall: report from a North American anaesthesia awareness registry. Br J Anaesth. 2015;115 Suppl 1: i114–21.

11. Samuelsson P, Brudin L, Sandin R. Late psychological symptoms after awareness among consecutively included surgical patients. Anesthesiology. 2007;106:26–32.

12. National Institute of Care and Excellence. NICE diagnostics guidance 6: depth of anaesthesia monitors—Bispectral Index (BIS), E-Entropy and Narcotrend-Compact M. London: National Institute of Care and Excellence; 2012.

13. Harris T, Brice D, Hetherington R, Utting J. Dreaming associated with anaesthesia: the influence of morphine premedication and two volatile adjuvants. Br J Anaesth. 1971;43:172–8.

14. Leslie K, Skrzypek H. Dreaming during anaesthesia in adult patients. Best Pract Res Clin Anaesthesiol. 2007;21:403–14.

15. Brandner B, Blagrove M, McCallum G, Bromley L. Dreams, images and emotions associated with propofol anaesthesia. Anaesthesia. 1997;52:750–5.

16. Hellwagner K, Holzer A, Gustorff B, Schroegendorfer K, Greher M, Weindlmayr-Goettel M, Saletu B, Lackner F. Recollection of dreams after short general anaesthesia: influence on patient anxiety and satisfaction. Eur J Anaesthesiol. 2003;20:282–8.

17. Kasmacher H, Petermeyer M, Decker C. Incidence and quality of dreaming during anaesthesia with propofol compared with enflurane. Anaesthetist. 1996;45:146–53.

18. Leslie K, Skrzypek H, Paech M, Kurowski I, Whybrow T. Dreaming during anesthesia and anesthetic depth in elective surgery patients: a prospective cohort study. Anesthesiology. 2007;106:33–42.

19. Leslie K, Sleigh J, Paech M, Voss L, Lim CW, Sleigh C. Dreaming and electroencephalographic changes during anesthesia maintained with propofol or desflurane. Anesthesiology. 2009;111:547–55.

20. Marsch S, Schaefer H, Tschan C, Meier B. Dreaming and anaesthesia: total iv anaesthesia with propofol vs balanced volatile anaesthesia with enflurane. Eur Journal Anaesthesiol. 1992;9:331–3.

21. Oxorn D, Ferris L, Harrington E, Orser B. The effects of midazolam on propofol-induced anesthesia: propofol dose requirements, mood profiles, and perioperative dreams. Anesth Analg. 1997;85:553–9.

22. Toscano A, Pancaro C, Peduto V. Scopolamine prevents dreams during general anesthesia. Anesthesiology. 2007;106:952–5.

23. Luginbühl M, Schnider T. Detection of awareness with the bispectral index: two case reports. Anesthesiology. 2002;96:241–3.

24. Nordstrom O, Engstrom A, Persson S, Sandin R. Incidence of awareness in total i.v. anaesthesia based on propofol, alfentanil and neuromuscular blockade. Acta Anaesthesiol Scand. 1997;41:978–84.

25. Zhang C, Xu L, Ma YQ, Sun YX, Li YH, Zhang L, Feng CS, Luo B, Zhao ZL, Guo JR, Jin YJ, Wu G, Yuan W, Yuan ZG, Yue Y. Bispectral index monitoring prevent awareness during total intravenous anesthesia: a prospective, randomized, double-blinded, multi-center controlled trial. Chin Med J. 2011;124:3664–9.

26. Eer AS, Padmanabhan U, Leslie K. Propofol dose and incidence of dreaming during sedation. Eur J Anaesthesiol. 2009;26:833–6.

27. Kim DK, Joo Y, Sung TY, Kim SY, Shin HY. Dreaming in sedation during spinal anesthesia: a comparison of propofol and midazolam infusion. Anesth Analg. 2011;112:1076–81.

28. Stait M, Leslie K, Bailey R. Dreaming and recall during sedation for colonoscopy. Anaesth Intensive Care. 2008;36:685–90.

29. Leslie K, Myles P, Forbes A, Chan M, Swallow S, Short T. Dreaming during anaesthesia in patients at high risk of awareness. Anaesthesia. 2005;60:239–44.

30. Ranta S, Laurila R, Saario J, Ali-Melkkila T, Hynynen M. Awareness with recall during general anesthesia: incidence and risk factors. Anesth Analg. 1998;86:1084–9.

31. Wilson S, Vaughan R, Stephen C. Awareness, dreams, and hallucinations associated with general anesthesia. Anesth Analg. 1975;54:609–17.

32. Errando C, Sigl J, Robles M, Calabuig E, Garcia J, Arocas F, Higueras R, del Rosario E, Lopez D, Peiro C, Soriano J, Chaves S, Gil F, Garcia-Aguado R. Awareness with recall during general anaesthesia: a prospective observational evaluation of 4001 patients. Br J Anaesth. 2008;101:178–85.

33. Ekman A, Lindholm M, Lennmarken C, Sandin R. Reduction in the incidence of awareness using BIS monitoring. Acta Anaesthesiol Scand. 2004;48:20–6.

34. Pandit JJ, Andrade J, Bogod DG, Hitchman JM, Jonker WR, Lucas N, Mackay JH, Nimmo AF, O'Connor K, O'Sullivan EP, Paul RG, Palmer JH, Plaat F, Radcliffe JJ, Sury MR, Torevell HE, Wang M, Hainsworth J, Cook TM. 5th National Audit Project (NAP5) on accidental awareness during general anaesthesia: summary of main findings and risk factors. Br J Anaesth. 2014;113:549–59.

35. Pandit JJ, Cook TM, Jonker WR, O'Sullivan E. A national survey of anaesthetists (NAP5 baseline) to estimate an annual incidence of accidental awareness during general anaesthesia in the UK. Br J Anaesth. 2013;110:501–9.

36. Avidan M, Zhang L, Burnside B, Finkel K, Searleman A, Selvidge J, Saager L, Turner M, Rao S, Bottros M, Hantler C, Jacobsohn E, Evers A. Anesthesia awareness and the bispectral index. N Engl J Med. 2008;358:1097–108.

37. Myles P, Leslie K, McNeil J, Forbes A, Chan M, Group B-AT. A randomised controlled trial of BIS monitoring to prevent awareness during anaesthesia: the B-Aware Trial. Lancet. 2004;363:1757–63.

38. Mashour G, Esaki R, Tremper K, Glick D, O'Connor M, Avidan M. A novel classification instrument for intraoperative awareness events. Anesth Analg. 2010;110:813–5.

39. Mashour GA, Kent C, Picton P, Ramachandran S, Tremper K, Turner C, Shanks A, Avidan M. Assessment of intraoperative awareness with explicit recall: a comparison of 2 methods. Anesth Analg. 2013;116:889–91.

40. Liu W, Thorp T, Graham S, Aitkenhead A. Incidence of awareness with recall during general anaesthesia. Anaesthesia. 1991;46:435–7.

41. Sandin R, Nordstrom O. Awareness during total iv anaesthesia. Br J Anaesth. 1993;71:782–7.

42. Pryor KO, Hemmings Jr HC. NAP5: intraoperative awareness detected, and undetected. Br J Anaesth. 2014;113:530–3.

43. Pollard R, Coyle J, Gilbert R, Beck J. Intraoperative awareness in a regional medical system. A review of 3 years' data. Anesthesiology. 2007;106:269–74.

44. Mashour G, Wang L, Turner C, Vandervest J, Shanks A, Tremper K. A retrospective study of intraoperative awareness with methodological implications. Anesth Analg. 2009;108:521–6.

45. Jonker WR, Hanumanthiah D, O'Sullivan EP, Cook TM, Pandit JJ. A national survey (NAP5-Ireland baseline) to estimate an annual incidence of accidental awareness during general anaesthesia in Ireland. Anaesthesia. 2014;69:969–76.

46. Lau K, Matta B, Menon DK, Absalom AR. Attitudes of anaesthetists to awareness and depth of anaesthesia monitoring in the UK. Eur J Anaesthesiol. 2006;23:921–30.

47. Morimoto Y, Nogami Y, Harada K, Tsubokawa T, Masui K. Awareness during anesthesia: the results of a questionnaire survey in Japan. J Anesth. 2011;25:72–7.

48. Myles P, Simons J, Leslie K. Anaesthetists' attitudes towards awareness and depth-of-anaesthesia monitoring. Anaesthesia. 2003;58:11–6.

49. Avidan MS, Jacobsohn E, Glick D, Burnside BA, Zhang L, Villafranca A, Karl L, Kamal S, Torres B, O'Connor M, Evers AS, Gradwohl S, Lin N, Palanca BJ, Mashour GA. Prevention of intraoperative awareness in a high-risk surgical population. N Engl J Med. 2011;365:591–600.

50. Mashour GA, Shanks A, Tremper KK, Kheterpal S, Turner CR, Ramachandran SK, Picton P, Schueller C, Morris M, Vandervest JC, Lin N, Avidan MS. Prevention of intraoperative awareness with explicit recall in an unselected surgical population: a randomized comparative effectiveness trial. Anesthesiology. 2012;117:717–25.

51. Enlund M, Hassan H. Intraoperative awareness: detected by the structured Brice interview. Acta Anaesthesiol Scand. 2002;46:345–9.

52. Xu L, Wu A, Yue Y. The incidence of intraoperative awareness during general anesthesia in China: a multicenter observational study. Acta Anesthesiol Scand. 2009;53:873–82.

53. Sury MR, Palmer JH, Cook TM, Pandit JJ. The state of UK anaesthesia: a survey of National Health Service activity in 2013. Br J Anaesth. 2014;113:575–84.

54. Absalom AR, Green D. NAP5: the tip of the iceberg, or all we need to know? Br J Anaesth. 2014;113:527–30.

55. Avidan MS, Sleigh JW. Beware the Boojum: the NAP5 audit of accidental awareness during intended general anaesthesia. Anaesthesia. 2014;69:1065–8.

56. Ye Z, Guo QL, Zheng H. Investigation and analysis of the incidence of awareness during general anesthesia. Zhong Nan Da Xue Xue Bao Yi Xue Ban. 2008;33:533–6.

57. Johansen J, Sebel P. Development and clinical application of electroencephalographic bispectrum monitoring. Anesthesiology. 2000;93:1336–44.

58. Barr G, Andersson R, Jakobsson J. A study of bispectral analysis and auditory evoked potential indices during propofol-induced hypnosis in volunteers. Anaesthesia. 2001;56:888–93.

59. VanNatta M, Rex D. Propofol alone titrated to deep sedation versus propofol in combination with opioids and/or benzodiazepines and titrated to moderate sedation for colonoscopy. Am J Gastroenterol. 2006;101:2209–17.

60. Allen M, Leslie K, Hebbard G, Jones I, Mettho T, Maruff P. A randomized controlled trial of light versus deep propofol sedation for elective outpatient colonoscopy: recall, procedural conditions, and recovery. Can J Anaesth. 2015;62(11):1169–78.

61. Ghoneim M. Incidence of and risk factors for awareness during anaesthesia. Best Pract Res Clin Anaesthesiol. 2007;21(3):327–43.

62. Bergman I, Kluger M, Short T. Awareness during general anaesthesia: a review of 81 cases from the Anaesthetic Incident Monitoring Study. Anaesthesia. 2002;57:549–56.

63. Domino K, Aitkenhead A. Medico-legal consequences of awareness during anesthesia. In: Ghoneim M, editor. Awareness during anesthesia. Oxford: Butterworth-Heinemann; 2001. p. 155–72.

64. Bennett C, Voss L, Barnard J, Sleigh J. Practical use of the electroencephalogram waveform during general anesthesia: the art and science. Anesth Analg. 2009;99:532–7.

65. Dahaba A. Different conditions that could result in the bispectral index indicating an incorrect hypnotic state. Anesth Analg. 2005;101:765–73.

66. Dahaba AA, Mattweber M, Fuchs A, Zenz W, Rehak PH, List WF, Metzler H. The effect of different stages of neuromuscular block on the bispectral index and the bispectral index-XP under remifentanil/propofol anesthesia. Anesth Analg. 2004;99:781–7.

67. Messner M, Beese U, Romstock J, Dinkel M, Tschaikowsky K. The bispectral index declines during neuromuscular blockage in fully awake persons. Anesth Analg. 2003;97:488–91.

68. Schuller PJ, Newell S, Strickland PA, Barry JJ. Response of bispectral index to neuromuscular block in awake volunteers. Br J Anaesth. 2015;115 Suppl 1:i95–103.

69. Osterman J, Hopper J, Heran W, Keane T, Van der Kolk B. Awareness during anesthesia and the development of post-traumatic stress disorder. Gen Hosp Psychiat. 2001;23:198–204.

70. Schwender D, Kunze-Kronawitter H, Dietrich P, Klasing S, Forst H, Madler C. Conscious awareness during anaesthesia patients' perceptions, emotions, cognition and reactions. Br J Anaesth. 1998;80:133–9.

71. Moerman N, Bonke B, Oosting J. Awareness and recall during general anesthesia. Facts and feelings. Anesthesiology. 1993;79:454–64.

72. Domino K, Posner K, Caplan R, Cheney F. Awareness during anesthesia: a closed claims analysis. Anesthesiology. 1999;90:1053–61.

73. Evans J. Patients' experiences of awareness during general anaesthesia. In: Rosen M, Lunn J, editors. Consciousness, awareness and pain in general anaesthesia. London: Butterworths; 1987. p. 184–92.

74. Laukkala T, Ranta S, Wennervirta J, Henriksson M, Suominen K, Hynynen M. Long-term psychosocial outcomes after intraoperative awareness with recall. Anesth Analg. 2014;119:86–92.

75. Lennmarken C, Bildfors K, Enlund G, Samuelsson P, Sandin R. Victims of awareness. Acta Anaesthesiol Scand. 2002;46:229–31.

76. Leslie K, Chan M, Myles P, Forbes A, McCulloch T. Post-traumatic stress disorder in aware patients from the B-Aware Trial. Anesth Analg. 2010;110:823–8.

77. Whitlock EL, Rodebaugh TL, Hassett AL, Shanks AM, Kolarik E, Houghtby J, West HM, Burnside BA, Shumaker E, Villafranca A, Edwards WA, Levinson CA, Langer JK, Fernandez KC, El-Gabalawy R, Zhou EY, Sareen J, Jacobsohn E, Mashour GA, Avidan MS. Psychological sequelae of surgery in a prospective cohort of patients from three intraoperative awareness prevention trials. Anesth Analg. 2015;120:87–95.

78. Kent CD, Mashour GA, Metzger NA, Posner KL, Domino KB. Psychological impact of unexpected explicit recall of events occurring during surgery performed under sedation, regional anaesthesia, and general anaesthesia: data from the Anesthesia Awareness Registry. Br J Anaesth. 2013;110:381–7.

79. Ranta S, Ranta V, Aromaa U. The claims for compensation for awareness with recall during general anaesthesia in Finland. Acta Anaesthesiol Scand. 1997;41:356–9.

80. Aranake A, Gradwohl S, Ben-Abdallah A, Lin N, Shanks A, Helsten DL, Glick DB, Jacobsohn E, Villafranca AJ, Evers AS, Avidan MS, Mashour GA. Increased risk of intraoperative awareness in patients with a history of awareness. Anesthesiology. 2013;119:1275–83.

81. ASA Task Force on Intraoperative Awareness. Practice advisory for intraoperative awareness and brain function monitoring: a report by the American Society of Anesthesiologists Task Force on Intraoperative Awareness. Anesthesiology. 2006;104:847–64.

82. Cook TM, Andrade J, Bogod DG, Hitchman JM, Jonker WR, Lucas N, Mackay JH, Nimmo AF, O'Connor K, O'Sullivan EP, Paul RG, Palmer JH, Plaat F, Radcliffe JJ, Sury MR, Torevell HE, Wang M, Hainsworth J, Pandit JJ. 5th National Audit Project (NAP5) on accidental awareness during general anaesthesia: patient experiences, human factors, sedation, consent, and medicolegal issues. Br J Anaesth. 2014;113:560–74.

83. Wang J, Ren Y, Zhu Y, Chen JW, Zhu MM, Xu YJ, Tan ZM. Effect of penehyclidine hydrochloride on the incidence of intraoperative awareness in Chinese patients undergoing breast cancer surgery during general anaesthesia. Anaesthesia. 2013;68:136–41.

84. Punjasawadwong Y, Phongchiewboon A, Bunchungmongkol N. Bispectral index for improving anaesthetic delivery and postoperative recovery. Cochrane Database Syst Rev. 2014;6, Cd003843.

85. Australian and New Zealand College of Anaesthetists. Recommendations on monitoring during anaesthesia (professional document PS18). Melbourne: Australian and New Zealand College of Anaesthetists; 2013.

86. Ben-Menachem E, Zalcberg D. Depth of anesthesia monitoring: a survey of attitudes and usage patterns among Australian anesthesiologists. Anesth Analg. 2014;119:1180–5.

87. Moerman N, Van Dam F, Oosting J. Recollections of general anaesthesia: a survey of anaesthesiological practice. Acta Anaesthesiol Scand. 1992;36:767–71.

88. Laurent S, Fry R, Nixon C. Serial failure of Diprifuser infusion pumps. Anaesthesia. 2001;56:596–7.

89. Nielsen T. A review of mentation in REM and NREM sleep: 'covert' REM sleep as a possible reconciliation of two opposing models. Behav Brain Sci. 2000;23:851–66.

90. Pace-Schott E, Gersh T, Silverstri R, Stickgold R, Salzman C, Hobson J. SSRI treatment suppresses dream recall frequency but increases subjective dream intensity in normal subjects. J Sleep Res. 2001;10:129–42.

91. Millar JM, Jewkes CF. Recovery and morbidity after daycase anaesthesia. A comparison of propofol with thiopentone-enflurane with and without alfentanil. Anaesthesia. 1988;43:738–43.

92. Galletly DC, Short TG. Total intravenous anaesthesia using propofol infusion–50 consecutive cases. Anaesth Intensive Care. 1988;16:150–7.

93. Ensink F, Schwabe K, Bittrich B, Kuhn U, Weingarten J, Schenk H. Comparison of anesthesia with bolus administration of propofol, methohexital or etomidate as a hypnotic in combination with alfentanil analgesia. Anaesthesist. 1989;38:333–40.

94. Oddby-Muhrbeck E, Jakobsson J. Recall of music: a comparison between anaesthesia with propofol and isoflurane. Acta Anaesthesiol Scand. 1993;37:33–7.

95. Oxorn D, Orser B, Ferris LE, Harrington E. Propofol and thiopental anesthesia: a comparison of the incidence of dreams and perioperative mood alterations. Anesth Analg. 1994;79:553–7.

96. Munte S, Kobbe I, Demertzis A, Lullwitz E, Munte TF, Piepenbrock S, Leuwer M. Increased reading speed for stories presented during general anaesthesia. Anesthesiology. 1999;90:662–9.

97. Aceto P, Congedo E, Lai C, Valente A, Gualtieri E. Dreams recall and auditory evoked potentials during propofol anaesthesia. Neuroreport. 2007;18:823–6.

98. Schaefer H, Marsch S. An unusual emergence after total intravenous anaesthesia. Anaesthesia. 1989;44:928–9.

99. Grace R. The effect of variable-dose diazepam on dreaming and emergence phenomena in 400 cases of ketamine-fentanyl anaesthesia. Anaesthesia. 2003;58:904–10.

100. Bogod D, Orton J, Oh T. Detecting awareness during general anaesthetic caesarian section. Anaesthesia. 1990;45:279–84.

101. Leslie K, Stonell C. Anaesthesia and sedation for gastrointestinal endoscopy. Curr Opin Anaesthesiol. 2005;18:431–6.

102. Stonell C, Leslie K, He C, Lee L. No sex differences in memory formation during general anesthesia. Anesthesiology. 2006;105:920–6.

Apoptosis and Neurocognitive Effects of IV Anesthetics

45

Sulpicio G. Soriano and Laszlo Vutskits

Introduction

Neuronal cell death and neurocognitive impairments after exposure to sedatives have been unequivocally demonstrated in laboratory animal models [1, 2]. Subsequently, the potential neurotoxic effects of these drugs have captured the attention of pediatric care providers [3, 4]. Personality changes have been historically documented in children receiving anesthetic and sedative drugs [5]. Despite this early observation, anesthetic and sedative have been routinely used to facilitate painful and distressing procedures on infants and children and is the standard of care. Two extensive reviews of the neurotoxic potential of sedation in neonatal and pediatric intensive care settings have been published [6, 7] Given the public health implications of this phenomenon, we will discuss relevance of these issues in the context of the use of intravenous sedatives in pediatric patients undergoing diagnostic and painful procedures and prolonged mechanical ventilation and circulatory support. These are disparate clinical conditions at the extremes of duration of exposure to sedative drugs, where the former can be minutes and the latter weeks.

Sedative and anesthetic drugs are potent modulators of the central nervous system and reversibly render patients insensate to painful and stressful procedures [8]. Although the exact molecular mechanisms that produce immobility,

analgesia, and amnesia are unknown, most are either γ-aminobutyrate (GABA) receptor agonists, N-methyl-D-aspartate (NMDA) glutamate receptor antagonists, or a combination of the two. Most intravenous drugs are specific agonists or antagonists of the GABA or NMDA receptors respectively, while volatile anesthetics have multiple molecular targets. Sedation is primarily produced by intravenous drugs.

Characterization of Sedative-Induced Developmental Neurotoxicity

Brain development is regulated by environmental cues, which shape subsequent neurocognitive function. Neuronal and glial cells are produced in excess, and the elimination of as much as 50–70 % of these cells is critical for achieving normal brain morphology and function [9]. This occurs by elimination of precursor cells and postmitotic programmed cell death of neurons and supporting glial cells [10]. Redundant neural progenitor cells and neurons that do not migrate properly or make synapses are physiologically pruned by apoptosis, which is an essential component of neural development [11].

The developing central nervous system is exquisitely sensitive to its internal milieu, and critical periods of plasticity during brain development are modulated by environmental cues and have been implicated in perceptual development [12]. Likewise, the perioperative environment has the potential to influence brain development. Peak synaptogenesis occurs between the third and seventh postnatal week in rats [13]. This is equivalent to the period between 25 gestational weeks and 1 year of age in humans. However, neurogenesis and context-dependent modulation of neural plasticity continue throughout life from the perinatal period to adulthood. The rate of neurogenesis peaks in different brain regions in an age-dependent fashion, with a majority of this process occurring primarily during the perinatal period and less

S.G. Soriano (✉)
Department of Anesthesiology, Perioperative and Pain Medicine, Harvard Medical School, Boston Children's Hospital, 300 Longwood Avenue, Boston, MA 02115, USA
e-mail: sulpicio.soriano@childrens.harvard.edu

L. Vutskits
Department of Anesthesiology, Pharmacology and Intensive Care, University Hospitals of Geneva, 4 rue Gabrielle-Perret-Gentil, 1205 Geneva 4, Switzerland

Department of Basic Neuroscience, University of Geneva Medical School, 1 rue Michel Servet, 1211 Geneva 4, Switzerland

© Springer International Publishing AG 2017
A.R. Absalom, K.P. Mason (eds.), *Total Intravenous Anesthesia and Target Controlled Infusions*,
DOI 10.1007/978-3-319-47609-4_45

during adulthood. Therefore, nonphysiologic exposure to stressors (painful stimuli, maternal deprivation, hypoglycemia, hypoxia, and ischemia) during this critical window may impact neural development. These findings beg the question of whether other confounding variables are involved in this process [14]. The potential contribution of coexisting medical conditions and undiagnosed genetic syndromes to neurodevelopmental has to be considered in light of the potential neurotoxic effects of drugs used for sedation [15].

Sedative drugs are powerful modulators of neuronal circuits and have an impact on the constant flux of CNS development and remodeling in both health and disease states [8]. It appears that newly born neurons are most vulnerable to the neuroapoptotic effect of anesthetic and sedative drugs [16, 17]. Since neurogenesis is ongoing throughout life, from the fetus to the elderly, these neural progenitor cells are vulnerable to the toxic effects of anesthetic and sedative drugs. For example, isoflurane has been shown to induce neuronal cell death in brain regions where neural progenitor cells reside [16]. Therefore, susceptibility to anesthetic-induced developmental neurotoxicity (AIDN) extends from the fetal period to late adulthood. Exposure to anesthetic and sedative drugs during the perinatal period leads to neuroapoptosis (cell death), aberrant morphogenesis, and subsequent neurocognitive deficits in laboratory rodent and monkey models [18, 19].

Pathological apoptosis is the primary hallmark of AIDN [20, 21]. Although it is an essential process in modulating neural development, the apoptotic pathway is also activated by cellular stress [22]. Stresses that can initiate this include glucocorticoids, heat, radiation, starvation, infection, hypoxia, pain, and sedative and anesthetic drugs. Exposure to sedative drugs during brain development not only induces neuronal cell death but can also impair neurogenesis and synaptogenesis in an age-dependent manner. Perinatal exposure to anesthetic and sedative drugs leads to neuroapoptosis and learning deficits [23, 24]. Of note, the pro-apoptotic effect depends on the developmental stage: being most pronounced at postnatal day 7 and inexistent in 15-day-old rodents. Postnatal rat pups had decreased neuronal progenitor proliferation and persistent deficits of hippocampal function, while older rats increased progenitor proliferation and neuronal differentiation, and this was correlated with improved memory function [25]. The administration of intravenous sedatives to juvenile rats leads to enhanced dendritic formation and synaptic density; the clinical significance for this finding is unknown [26]. However, similar dendritic morphology has been observed in psychiatric and neurological disorders [27].

Sedative drugs are primarily N-methyl-D-aspartate (NMDA) antagonists (ketamine) and γ-aminobutyric acid (GABA) agonists (midazolam, propofol, pentobarbital, and hloral hydrate). Transient pharmacological blockade of the NMDA receptor with the noncompetitive pharmacological antagonist MK801, phenylcyclidine, or ketamine induced developmental stage-dependent widespread apoptosis in the developing brain [20]. Using a similar experimental paradigm, the same laboratory group developed increased neurodegeneration in rat pups treated with the GABA agonists, diazepam, and pentobarbital [28]. Furthermore, subanesthetic doses of midazolam or propofol induce neuroapoptosis in neonatal mice [29, 30]. Propofol diminishes the survival and maturation of adult-born hippocampal neurons in a developmental stage-dependent manner by inducing a significant decrease in dendritic maturation and survival of newly born neurons that were 17 days but not at 11 days [17]. Likewise, 5 h exposure to propofol resulted in apoptosis of neurons and oligodendrocytes in fetal and neonatal nonhuman primates [31]. Chloral hydrate has been shown to induce neuroapoptosis in neonatal rats [32].

The neurotoxic potential of other drug classes used to provide sedation and analgesia has been reported. Opioids are the most commonly administered sedative and analgesic drug in the setting of mechanical ventilation and extracorporeal circulatory support. A single dose of morphine given to postnatal day 7 rat pups did not increase neuroapoptosis [33]. However, repeated morphine administration over 7 days is associated with increased apoptosis in the sensory cortex and amygdala of neonatal rats [34]. Furthermore, daily administration of morphine for 9 consecutive days did not alter dendritic morphology. These areas of the brain are not the areas of the brain that are affected by volatile and intravenous anesthetics which preferentially affect the learning and memory areas (hippocampus) of developing brains. Dexmedetomidine is a selective α₂-adrenergic agonist with sympatholytic, sedative, amnestic, and analgesic properties. When administered as an adjuvant to volatile anesthetics, it reduces minimum alveolar concentration [35] and has been shown to decrease isoflurane- and ketamine-induced neurotoxicity in neonatal rats [36–39]. Dexmedetomidine has been the only drug that has neuroprotective properties [36]. However, high doses of dexmedetomidine can induce neuroapoptosis [40].

These experimental paradigms were conducted in the absence of concurrent noxious stimulation, which does not account for the interaction of sedation and stressful/painful procedures. Recent reports of neonatal rats receiving ketamine during the application of noxious stimuli resulted in less neuronal cell death [41, 42]. These experimental paradigms do not reflect clinical conditions associated with procedural sedation in pediatric patients [43]. Taken together, these preclinical observations demonstrate causality between anesthetic exposure during a vulnerable developmental period with synaptic modeling and plasticity.

The behavioral impact of perinatal exposure to intravenous anesthetics has been investigated in laboratory animals.

Neonatal mice receiving ketamine, propofol, and thiopental not only developed increased levels of apoptotic and degeneration cells in brain slices but reduced spontaneous activity and impaired leaning as adults [44]. Juvenile rats with repeated exposures to ketamine-xylazine developed impaired motor learning and learning-dependent dendritic spine plasticity later in life [45]. Propofol administered over 6 h to neonatal rats had increased apoptosis in thalamic samples, but minor behavioral and learning activity at adolescence [46]. When compared to naïve rat pups, dexmedetomidine did not have a different response to a fear conditioning paradigm and actually mitigated deficits in isoflurane-treated cohorts [36]. Ketamine induces neuronal apoptosis in fetal and neonatal rhesus monkeys in a dose- and duration-dependent fashion [31, 47, 48]. A 3-h-long exposure to ketamine did not seem to affect cell death, while a 5-h-long exposure has been shown to induce apoptosis both in the fetal and early postnatal brain. This experimental paradigm resulted in persistent cognitive deficits assessed by an operant test battery [19]. Monkeys receiving a 24-h-long ketamine anesthesia at postnatal day 5 showed impaired motivation and learning but no problems with short-term memory when tested up to 3.5 years postexposure. These reports clearly demonstrate that intravenous sedative has an impact on cognition and behavior at a later age.

Mechanisms of Aberrant Neuronal Development from Sedative Drugs

Although the mechanisms of NMDA antagonists and GABA agonists are divergent, both clearly induce neurodegenerative and neurocognitive changes in animal models [18]. These preclinical reports clearly demonstrate that drugs that are routinely utilized to sedate pediatric patients have neurotoxic properties.

Several lines of investigation have implicated other neuronal cell death mechanisms such as excitotoxicity, mitochondrial dysfunction, aberrant cell cycle reentry, trophic factor dysregulation, and disruption of cytoskeletal assembly [49–55]. A combination of these and other parallel neurodegenerative pathways likely mediate the neurotoxic effect of anesthetic drugs.

The notion that sedative drugs can be excitotoxic can be a contradiction. However, GABA agonists stimulate immature neurons due to a developmental variation of the chloride channels [56]. While GABA is inhibitory in the mature brain, it has been found in many preclinical studies to be an excitatory agent during early stages of brain development [57, 58]. The immature NA/K/2CL transporter protein NKCC1 produces a chloride influx leading to neuron depolarization. As a consequence, GABA remains excitatory until the GABA neurons switch to the normal inhibitory mode when the mature chloride transporter, KCC2, actively transports chloride out of the cell [50]. This switch begins around 15th postnatal week in term human infants but is not complete until about 1 year of age. Subsequent reports on the mechanism of GABAergic-induced seizures in newborn rats revealed that the NKCC1 chloride channel blocker, bumetanide, attenuated the both neuroapoptosis and epileptiform activity [50]. Diazepam increased epileptiform activity in an immature neocortical organotypic slice model [59]. Prolonged exposure to a NMDA antagonist such as ketamine leads to an upregulation of the NMDA receptor, leading to an increased accumulation of excitotoxic intracellular calcium [49]. Excitotoxic insults are also linked to mitochondrial dysfunction in neurons, and prolonged exposure to sedative drugs may incite a comparable response [51]. The neuroprotective properties of selective α_2-adrenergic stimulation with dexmedetomidine have been attributed to an increased expression of the pro-survival kinases, phosphorylated extracellular signal-regulated protein kinase 1 and 2 (pERK1/2), and protein kinase B (AKT)-glycogen synthase kinase-3β (GSK-3β) [60–62].

Taken together, three factors appear to induce AIDN in laboratory models: 1. developmental susceptibility during synaptogenesis, 2. high dose of the anesthetic, and 3. prolonged duration of exposure. Given the low doses administered and brief exposure to the drugs, the relevance of AIDN in the setting of procedural sedation may be superfluous. However, the use of sedative drugs for prolonged ventilator and circulatory support can potentially increase the susceptibility of critically ill neonates and infants to this phenomenon.

Clinical Evidence for Sedative-Induced Neurological Sequelae

The preclinical evidence indicates that prolonged and repetitive exposure at a vulnerable age to sedatives causes the most neuroapoptosis and later developmental delays (Table 45.1). Most of clinical reports that examine the effect of anesthetic exposure on neurocognitive are based on retrospective observations on pediatric patients undergoing surgery and presumably general anesthesia. These reports do not specifically identify the classes of anesthetic and sedative drugs administered. Although most of the studies have attempted to control for obvious confounders but the retrospective nature of these investigations make it impossible to control for all the known and unknown confounders.

Several retrospective reports demonstrate an association between surgery and anesthesia and subsequent learning and behavioral disorders. In a series of retrospective reports, the Mayo Clinic group examined a cohort born from 1976 to

Table 45.1

Drug	Neurotoxicity/ Altered plasticity	Reference
Propofol	Yes	[26, 30, 31, 44, 86, 87]
Midazolam	Yes	[26, 29]
Pentobarbital	Yes	[44]
Chloral hydrate	Yes	[32, 74]
Ketamine	Yes	[19, 20, 26, 47, 48, 52]
Dexmedetomidine	No	[36]

1982 for learning disabilities. The patients who were exposed to surgery and anesthesia before the age of four had increased incidence of learning disability at age 19 years [63]. Risk factors included more than one anesthetic exposure and general anesthesia lasting longer than 2 h. A similar study was done using matched cohort revealed that children under the age of two who had more than one anesthetic were almost twice as likely to have speech and language disabilities than those who had a single or no anesthetic exposure [64]. In contrast, cohort study from a birth registry reported that even a single exposure to general anesthesia before age 3 years was related to decreased performance on receptive and expressive language and cognitive testing done at 10 years [65]. A similar retrospective report derived from Iowa revealed a negative correlation between the duration of surgery/anesthesia and scores on academic achievement tests [66]. Data analysis from the Medicaid database indicates that, even after adjustment for potential confounding factors, children who underwent hernia repair before the age of 3 years were twice as likely as children in the comparison group to be subsequently diagnosed with a developmental or behavioral disorder [67]. When this group was controlled for gender and birth weight, there was still a nearly twofold increase in these issues. A follow-up study that matched patients with non-anesthetic-exposed siblings found that the former had a 60 % greater association between exposure to anesthesia and later neurologic and developmental problems [68].

Meanwhile other investigators report no evidence of an association between exposure to general anesthesia at a young age and later school problems. An analysis of a twin-twin registry from the Netherlands compared with the educational achievements of identical twin pairs revealed that twin pairs exposed to general anesthesia had lower educational achievements than unexposed twin pairs [69]. However, when one twin was exposed and the other was not, there were no differences in educational achievements. These findings imply that exposure to general anesthesia was not associated with impaired educational performance. A Danish birth cohort compared average test scores at ninth grade in infants who have inguinal hernia study and reported no statistically significant differences from naïve cohorts

after adjusting for known confounders [70]. A similar analysis of infants undergoing pyloromyotomies revealed no difference in their educational performance to a surgery naïve cohort [71]. Since these retrospective reports are based on patients undergoing surgery and presumably general anesthesia, they may not be relevant in the setting of procedural sedation.

Several reports have been published on the effect of sedation on neurocognitive parameters in intensive care patients. In a review of premature neonates receiving sedation for mechanical ventilation, prolonged sedation was not associated with a poor neurological outcome [72]. A similar report examining the impact of perioperative administration of sedatives in pediatric cardiac surgery found no association between the dose and duration of these drugs and adverse neurodevelopmental outcome at 18–24 months [73]. A reevaluation of these children at kindergarten age demonstrated that the number of days on chloral hydrate was associated with lower performance intelligence quotient and the cumulative dose of benzodiazepines was associated with lower visual motor integration (VMI) scores [74]. The Beery-Buktenica VMI scores reflect the ability to integrate visual and motor abilities and screens for possible learning and neuropsychological and behavioral problems [75]. These sedation studies in the intensive care unit may reveal a mild association between GABA agonists and neurodevelopmental deficits. However, the overwhelming impact of severe illness and prolonged administration of the sedative drugs cannot be discounted [76].

The limitations of retrospective studies are well known and prompt the need for prospective investigations into the impact of sedative and anesthetic drugs on neurocognitive development in humans. There is at least one prospective ongoing study (the GAS study), which is comparing the neurodevelopmental outcomes of 2- and 5-year-old children who were randomized to either regional or general anesthesia for inguinal herniorrhaphies at age 6 months or less [77]. The 2-year neurocognitive interim results reveal no differences between infants exposed to either general anesthesia or regional anesthesia [78]. Other prospective studies are underway [79, 80]. The EUROPAIN consortium reported a prospective cohort study on sedation and analgesia in neonatal intensive care units [81]. They observed a wide variation in practice among the participating centers, which highlight the potential for confounding factors as the cause for altered neurocognition.

The acute effects of sedation have been investigated. A prospective comparison of preterm and term children undergoing procedural sedation revealed that the former had a twofold increased risk of an adverse event [82]. These include increased oxygen desaturations and apnea in the preterm patients. The overall rate of oxygen desaturation and apnea/upper airway obstruction were 154 and 575 per

10,000 respective in a general cohort of pediatric patients undergoing procedural sedation with propofol [83]. An intravenous bolus of propofol for procedural sedation in neonates undergoing brief painful intervention resulted in a period of hypotension up to 60 min with a transient decrease in cerebral tissue oxygenation index [84]. Morphine infusions and boluses administered to mechanically ventilated preterm neonates were associated with hypotension [85]. The impact of these transient events on neurocognitive is unknown but has the potential to affect neurocognition.

Conclusions from Preclinical and Clinical Investigations

Extrapolation of these preclinical and clinical studies to procedural sedation in pediatric patients is problematic. Since millions of young children undergo sedation every year worldwide, the public health impact of sedative-induced neurotoxicity, if existing, could be a major issue. The nature of the published clinical reports may have unaccounted confounders that may lead to neurological deficits. These studies cannot separate the effects of sedation from coexisting condition, surgery, or stress of hospitalization. Clearly, rigorous clinical research is needed to resolve this issue. Since the use of sedative drugs is a standard practice and unavoidable in pediatric patients, the clinician should be aware of the evolving investigations on AIDN and be up to date on the best clinical practices.

References

1. Lin EP, Soriano SG, Loepke AW. Anesthetic neurotoxicity. Anesthesiol Clin. 2014;32:133–55.
2. Vutskits L. General anesthesia: a gateway to modulate synapse formation and neural plasticity? Anesth Analg. 2012;115:1174–82.
3. Rappaport B, Mellon RD, Simone A, Woodcock J. Defining safe use of anesthesia in children. N Engl J Med. 2011;364:1387–90.
4. Rappaport BA, Suresh S, Hertz S, Evers AS, Orser BA. Anesthetic neurotoxicity—clinical implications of animal models. N Engl J Med. 2015;372:796–7.
5. Eckenhoff JE. Relationship of anesthesia to postoperative personality changes in children. AMA Am J Dis Child. 1953;86:587–91.
6. Durrmeyer X, Vutskits L, Anand KJS, Rimensberger PC. Use of analgesic and sedative drugs in the NICU: integrating clinical trials and laboratory data. Pediatr Res. 2010;67:117–27.
7. Loepke AW. Developmental neurotoxicity of sedatives and anesthetics: a concern for neonatal and pediatric critical care medicine? Pediatr Crit Care Med. 2010;11:217–26.
8. Rudolph U, Antkowiak B. Molecular and neuronal substrates for general anaesthetics. Nat Rev Neurosci. 2004;5:709–20.
9. Buss RR, Oppenheim RW. Role of programmed cell death in normal neuronal development and function. Anat Sci Int. 2004;79:191–7.
10. de la Rosa EJ, de Pablo F. Cell death in early neural development: beyond the neurotrophic theory. Trends Neurosci. 2000;23:454–8.
11. Buss RR, Sun W, Oppenheim RW. Adaptive roles of programmed cell death during nervous system development. Annu Rev Neurosci. 2006;29:1–35.
12. Hensch TK. Critical period plasticity in local cortical circuits. Nat Rev Neurosci. 2005;6:877–88.
13. Dobbing J, Sands J. Comparative aspects of the brain growth spurt. Early Hum Dev. 1979;3:79–83.
14. McCann ME, Soriano SG. Perioperative central nervous system injury in neonates. Br J Anaesth. 2012;109 Suppl 1:i60–7.
15. Homsy J, Zaidi S, Shen Y, Ware JS, Samocha KE, Karczewski KJ, DePalma SR, McKean D, Wakimoto H, Gorham J, Jin SC, Deanfield J, Giardini A, Porter Jr GA, Kim R, Bilguvar K, Lopez-Giraldez F, Tikhonova I, Mane S, Romano-Adesman A, Qi H, Vardarajan B, Ma L, Daly M, Roberts AE, Russell MW, Mital S, Newburger JW, Gaynor JW, Breitbart RE, Iossifov I, Ronemus M, Sanders SJ, Kaltman JR, Seidman JG, Brueckner M, Gelb BD, Goldmuntz E, Lifton RP, Seidman CE, Chung WK. De novo mutations in congenital heart disease with neurodevelopmental and other congenital anomalies. Science. 2015;350:1262–6.
16. Hofacer RD, Deng M, Ward CG, Joseph B, Hughes EA, Jiang C, Danzer SC, Loepke AW. Cell-age specific vulnerability of neurons to anesthetic toxicity. Ann Neurol. 2013;73(6):695–704.
17. Krzisch M, Sultan S, Sandell J, Demeter K, Vutskits L, Toni N. Propofol anesthesia impairs the maturation and survival of adult-born hippocampal neurons. Anesthesiology. 2013;118:602–10.
18. Stratmann G. Review article: neurotoxicity of anesthetic drugs in the developing brain. Anesth Analg. 2011;113:1170–9.
19. Paule MG, Li M, Allen RR, Liu F, Zou X, Hotchkiss C, Hanig JP, Patterson TA, Slikker Jr W, Wang C. Ketamine anesthesia during the first week of life can cause long-lasting cognitive deficits in rhesus monkeys. Neurotoxicol Teratol. 2011;33:220–30.
20. Ikonomidou C, Bosch F, Miksa M, Bittigau P, Vockler J, Dikranian K, Tenkova TI, Stefovska V, Turski L, Olney JW. Blockade of NMDA receptors and apoptotic neurodegeneration in the developing brain. Science. 1999;283:70–4.
21. Jevtovic-Todorovic V, Hartman RE, Izumi Y, Benshoff ND, Dikranian K, Zorumski CF, Olney JW, Wozniak DF. Early exposure to common anesthetic agents causes widespread neurodegeneration in the developing rat brain and persistent learning deficits. J Neurosci. 2003;23:876–82.
22. Blomgren K, Leist M, Groc L. Pathological apoptosis in the developing brain. Apoptosis. 2007;12:993–1010.
23. Li Y, Liang G, Wang S, Meng Q, Wang Q, Wei H. Effects of fetal exposure to isoflurane on postnatal memory and learning in rats. Neuropharmacology. 2007;53:942–50.
24. Palanisamy A, Baxter MG, Keel PK, Xie Z, Crosby G, Culley DJ. Rats exposed to isoflurane in utero during early gestation are behaviorally abnormal as adults. Anesthesiology. 2011;114:521–8.
25. Stratmann G, Sall JW, May LD, Bell JS, Magnusson KR, Rau V, Visrodia KH, Alvi RS, Ku B, Lee MT, Dai R. Isoflurane differentially affects neurogenesis and long-term neurocognitive function in 60-day-old and 7-day-old rats. Anesthesiology. 2009;110:834–48.
26. De Roo M, Klauser P, Briner A, Nikonenko I, Mendez P, Dayer A, Kiss JZ, Muller D, Vutskits L. Anesthetics rapidly promote synaptogenesis during a critical period of brain development. PLoS One. 2009;4, e7043.
27. Penzes P, Cahill ME, Jones KA, Vanleeuwen J-E, Woolfrey KM. Dendritic spine pathology in neuropsychiatric disorders. Nat Neurosci. 2011;14:285–93.
28. Ikonomidou C, Bittigau P, Ishimaru MJ, Wozniak DF, Koch C, Genz K, Price MT, Stefovska V, Horster F, Tenkova T, Dikranian K, Olney JW. Ethanol-induced apoptotic

neurodegeneration and fetal alcohol syndrome. Science. 2000;287:1056–60.

29. Young C, Jevtovic-Todorovic V, Qin YQ, Tenkova T, Wang H, Labruyere J, Olney JW. Potential of ketamine and midazolam, individually or in combination, to induce apoptotic neurodegeneration in the infant mouse brain. Br J Pharmacol. 2005;146:189–97.

30. Cattano D, Young C, Straiko MM, Olney JW. Subanesthetic doses of propofol induce neuroapoptosis in the infant mouse brain. Anesth Analg. 2008;106:1712–4.

31. Creeley C, Dikranian K, Dissen G, Martin L, Olney J, Brambrink A. Propofol-induced apoptosis of neurones and oligodendrocytes in fetal and neonatal rhesus macaque brain. Br J Anaesth. 2013;110 Suppl 1:i29–38.

32. Cattano D, Straiko MM, Olney JW. Chloral hydrate induces and lithium prevents neuroapoptosis in the infant mouse brain. Anesthesiology. 2008;109:A315.

33. Massa H, Lacoh CM, Vutskits L. Effects of morphine on the differentiation and survival of developing pyramidal neurons during the brain growth spurt. Toxicol Sci. 2012;130:168–79.

34. Bajic D, Commons KG, Soriano SG. Morphine-enhanced apoptosis in selective brain regions of neonatal rats. Int J Dev Neurosci. 2013;31:258–66.

35. Segal IS, Vickery RG, Walton JK, Doze VA, Maze M. Dexmedetomidine diminishes halothane anesthetic requirements in rats through a postsynaptic alpha 2 adrenergic receptor. Anesthesiology. 1988;69:818–23.

36. Sanders RD, Xu J, Shu Y, Januszewski A, Halder S, Fidalgo A, Sun P, Hossain M, Ma D, Maze M. Dexmedetomidine attenuates isoflurane-induced neurocognitive impairment in neonatal rats. Anesthesiology. 2009;110:1077–85.

37. Sanders RD, Sun P, Patel S, Li M, Maze M, Ma D. Dexmedetomidine provides cortical neuroprotection: impact on anaesthetic-induced neuroapoptosis in the rat developing brain. Acta Anaesthesiol Scand. 2010;54:710–6.

38. Duan X, Li Y, Zhou C, Huang L, Dong Z. Dexmedetomidine provides neuroprotection: impact on ketamine-induced neuroapoptosis in the developing rat brain. Acta Anaesthesiol Scand. 2014;58:1121–6.

39. Li Y, Zeng M, Chen W, Liu C, Wang F, Han X, Zuo Z, Peng S. Dexmedetomidine reduces isoflurane-induced neuroapoptosis partly by preserving PI3K/Akt pathway in the hippocampus of neonatal rats. PLoS One. 2014;9, e93639.

40. Pancaro C, Segal BS, Sikes RW, Almeer Z, Schumann R, Azocar R, Marchand JE. Dexmedetomidine and ketamine show distinct patterns of cell degeneration and apoptosis in the developing rat neonatal brain. J Matern Fetal Neonatal Med. 2016;29 (23):3827–33.

41. Anand KJ, Garg S, Rovnaghi CR, Narsinghani U, Bhutta AT, Hall RW. Ketamine reduces the cell death following inflammatory pain in newborn rat brain. Pediatr Res. 2007;62:283–90.

42. Liu JR, Liu Q, Li J, Baek C, Han XH, Athiraman U, Soriano SG. Noxious stimulation attenuates ketamine-induced neuroapoptosis in the developing rat brain. Anesthesiology. 2012;117(1):64–71.

43. Anand KJ, Soriano SG. Anesthetic agents and the immature brain: are these toxic or therapeutic? Anesthesiology. 2004;101:527–30.

44. Fredriksson A, Ponten E, Gordh T, Eriksson P. Neonatal exposure to a combination of N-methyl-D-aspartate and gamma-aminobutyric acid type A receptor anesthetic agents potentiates apoptotic neurodegeneration and persistent behavioral deficits. Anesthesiology. 2007;107:427–36.

45. Huang L, Yang G. Repeated exposure to ketamine-xylazine during early development impairs motor learning-dependent dendritic spine plasticity in adulthood. Anesthesiology. 2015;122:821–31.

46. Karen T, Schlager GW, Bendix I, Sifringer M, Herrmann R, Pantazis C, Enot D, Keller M, Kerner T, Felderhoff-Mueser U. Effect of propofol in the immature rat brain on short- and long-term neurodevelopmental outcome. PLoS One. 2013;8, e64480.

47. Slikker W, Zou X, Hotchkiss CE, Divine RL, Sadovova N, Twaddle NC, Doerge DR, Scallet AC, Patterson TA, Hanig JP, Paule MG, Wang C. Ketamine-induced neuronal cell death in the perinatal rhesus monkey. Toxicol Sci. 2007;98:145–58.

48. Brambrink AM, Evers AS, Avidan MS, Farber NB, Smith DJ, Martin LD, Dissen GA, Creeley CE, Olney JW. Ketamine-induced neuroapoptosis in the fetal and neonatal rhesus macaque brain. Anesthesiology. 2012;116:372–84.

49. Slikker Jr W, Paule MG, Wright LK, Patterson TA, Wang C. Systems biology approaches for toxicology. J Applied Toxicol. 2007;27:201–17.

50. Edwards DA, Shah HP, Cao W, Gravenstein N, Seubert CN, Martynyuk AE. Bumetanide alleviates epileptogenic and neurotoxic effects of sevoflurane in neonatal rat brain. Anesthesiology. 2010;112:567–75.

51. Sanchez V, Feinstein SD, Lunardi N, Joksovic PM, Boscolo A, Todorovic SM, Jevtovic-Todorovic V. General anesthesia causes long-term impairment of mitochondrial morphogenesis and synaptic transmission in developing rat brain. Anesthesiology. 2011;115:992–1002.

52. Soriano SG, Liu Q, Li J, Liu J-R, Han XH, Kanter JL, Bajic D, Ibla JC. Ketamine activates cell cycle signaling and apoptosis in the neonatal rat brain. Anesthesiology. 2010;112:1155–63.

53. Liu JR, Baek C, Han XH, Shoureshi P, Soriano SG. Role of glycogen synthase kinase-3beta in ketamine-induced developmental neuroapoptosis in rats. Br J Anaesth. 2013;110 Suppl 1:i3–9.

54. Lu LX, Yon J-H, Carter LB, Jevtovic-Todorovic V. General anesthesia activates BDNF-dependent neuroapoptosis in the developing rat brain. Apoptosis. 2006;11:1603–15.

55. Lemkuil BP, Head BP, Pearn ML, Patel HH, Drummond JC, Patel PM. Isoflurane neurotoxicity is mediated by p75NTR-RhoA activation and actin depolymerization. Anesthesiology. 2011;114:49–57.

56. Ben-Ari Y. Excitatory actions of gaba during development: the nature of the nurture. Nat Rev Neurosci. 2002;3:728–39.

57. Zhang LL, Pathak HR, Coulter DA, Freed MA, Vardi N. Shift of intracellular chloride concentration in ganglion and amacrine cells of developing mouse retina. J Neurophysiol. 2006;95:2404–16.

58. Dzhala VI, Talos DM, Sdrulla AD, Brumback AC, Mathews GC, Benke TA, Delpire E, Jensen FE, Staley KJ. NKCC1 transporter facilitates seizures in the developing brain. Nat Med. 2005;11:1205–13.

59. Glykys J, Staley KJ. Diazepam effect during early neonatal development correlates with neuronal Cl⁻. Ann Clin Transl Neurol. 2015;2:1055–70.

60. Dahmani S, Paris A, Jannier V, Hein L, Rouelle D, Scholz J, Gressens P, Mantz J. Dexmedetomidine increases hippocampal phosphorylated extracellular signal-regulated protein kinase 1 and 2 content by an alpha 2-adrenoceptor-independent mechanism: evidence for the involvement of imidazoline I1 receptors. Anesthesiology. 2008;108:457–66.

61. Zhu YM, Wang CC, Chen L, Qian LB, Ma LL, Yu J, Zhu MH, Wen CY, Yu LN, Yan M. Both PI3K/Akt and ERK1/2 pathways participate in the protection by dexmedetomidine against transient focal cerebral ischemia/reperfusion injury in rats. Brain Res. 2013;1494:1–8.

62. Dahmani S, Rouelle D, Gressens P, Mantz J. Characterization of the postconditioning effect of dexmedetomidine in mouse organotypic hippocampal slice cultures exposed to oxygen and glucose deprivation. Anesthesiology. 2010;112:373–83.

63. Wilder RT, Flick RP, Sprung J, Katusic SK, Barbaresi WJ, Mickelson C, Gleich SJ, Schroeder DR, Weaver AL, Warner DO. Early exposure to anesthesia and learning disabilities in a population-based birth cohort. Anesthesiology. 2009;110:796–804.

64. Flick RP, Katusic SK, Colligan RC, Wilder RT, Voigt RG, Olson MD, Sprung J, Weaver AL, Schroeder DR, Warner DO. Cognitive and behavioral outcomes after early exposure to anesthesia and surgery. Pediatrics. 2011;128:e1053–61.

65. Ing C, DiMaggio C, Whitehouse A, Hegarty MK, Brady J, von Ungern-Sternberg BS, Davidson A, Wood AJ, Li G, Sun LS. Long-term differences in language and cognitive function after childhood exposure to anesthesia. Pediatrics. 2012;130:e476–85.

66. Block RI, Thomas JJ, Bayman EO, Choi JY, Kimble KK, Todd MM. Are anesthesia and surgery during infancy associated with altered academic performance during childhood? Anesthesiology. 2012;117:494–503.

67. DiMaggio C, Sun LS, Kakavouli A, Byrne MW, Li G. A retrospective cohort study of the association of anesthesia and hernia repair surgery with behavioral and developmental disorders in young children. J Neurosurg Anesthesiol. 2009;21:286–91.

68. Dimaggio C, Sun L, Li G. Early childhood exposure to anesthesia and risk of developmental and behavioral disorders in a sibling birth cohort. Anesth Analg. 2011;113(5):1143–51.

69. Bartels M, Althoff RR, Boomsma DI. Anesthesia and cognitive performance in children: no evidence for a causal relationship. Twin Res Hum Genet. 2009;12:246–53.

70. Hansen TG, Pedersen JK, Henneberg SW, Pedersen DA, Murray JC, Morton NS, Christensen K. Academic performance in adolescence after inguinal hernia repair in infancy: a nationwide cohort study. Anesthesiology. 2011;114(5):1076–85.

71. Hansen TG, Pedersen JK, Henneberg SW, Morton NS, Christensen K. Educational outcome in adolescence following pyloric stenosis repair before 3 months of age: a nationwide cohort study. Paediatr Anaesth. 2013;23:883–90.

72. Roze JC, Denizot S, Carbajal R, Ancel PY, Kaminski M, Arnaud C, Truffert P, Marret S, Matis J, Thiriez G, Cambonie G, Andre M, Larroque B, Breart G. Prolonged sedation and/or analgesia and 5-year neurodevelopment outcome in very preterm infants: results from the EPIPAGE cohort. Arch Pediatr Adolesc Med. 2008;162:728–33.

73. Guerra GG, Robertson CM, Alton GY, Joffe AR, Cave DA, Dinu IA, Creighton DE, Ross DB, Rebeyka IM, Western Canadian Complex Pediatric Therapies Follow-up Group. Neurodevelopmental outcome following exposure to sedative and analgesic drugs for complex cardiac surgery in infancy. Paediatr Anaesth. 2011;21:932–41.

74. Guerra GG, Robertson CM, Alton GY, Joffe AR, Cave DA, Dinu IA, Creighton DE, Ross DB, Rebeyka IM, Western Canadian Complex Pediatric Therapies Follow-up Group. Neurotoxicity of sedative and analgesia drugs in young infants with congenital heart disease: 4-year follow-up. Paediatr Anaesth. 2014;24:257–65.

75. Beery KE, Buktenica NA. Beery-Buktenica developmental test of visual motor integration. 5th ed. Minneapolis, MN: NCS Pearson Inc.; 2004.

76. Moser JJ, Veale PM, McAllister DL, Archer DP. A systematic review and quantitative analysis of neurocognitive outcomes in children with four chronic illnesses. Paediatr Anaesth. 2013;23:1084–96.

77. Davidson AJ, McCann ME, Morton NS, Myles PS. Anesthesia and outcome after neonatal surgery: the role for randomized trials. Anesthesiology. 2008;109:941–4.

78. Davidson AJ, Disma N, de Graaff JC, Withington DE, Dorris L, Bell G, Stargatt R, Bellinger DC, Schuster T, Arnup SJ, Hardy P, Hunt RW, Takagi MJ, Giribaldi G, Hartmann PL, Salvo I, Morton NS, von Ungern Sternberg BS, Locatelli BG, Wilton N, Lynn A, Thomas JJ, Polaner D, Bagshaw O, Szmuk P, Absalom AR, Frawley G, Berde C, Ormond GD, Marmor J, McCann ME, GAS consortium. Neurodevelopmental outcome at 2 years of age after general anaesthesia and awake-regional anaesthesia in infancy (GAS): an international multicentre, randomised controlled trial. Lancet. 2015;387:239–50.

79. Sun LS, Li G, DiMaggio CJ, Byrne MW, Ing C, Miller TL, Bellinger DC, Han S, McGowan FX. Feasibility and pilot study of the Pediatric Anesthesia NeuroDevelopment Assessment (PANDA) project. J Neurosurg Anesthesiol. 2012;24:382–8.

80. Gleich SJ, Flick R, Hu D, Zaccariello MJ, Colligan RC, Katusic SK, Schroeder DR, Hanson A, Buenvenida S, Wilder RT, Sprung J, Voigt RG, Paule MG, Chelonis JJ, Warner DO. Neurodevelopment of children exposed to anesthesia: design of the Mayo Anesthesia Safety in Kids (MASK) study. Contemp Clin Trials. 2015;41:45–54.

81. Carbajal R, Eriksson M, Courtois E, Boyle E, Avila-Alvarez A, Andersen RD, Sarafidis K, Polkki T, Matos C, Lago P, Papadouri T, Montalto SA, Ilmoja ML, Simons S, Tameliene R, van Overmeire B, Berger A, Dobrzanska A, Schroth M, Bergqvist L, Lagercrantz H, Anand KJ, Group ESW. Sedation and analgesia practices in neonatal intensive care units (EUROPAIN): results from a prospective cohort study. Lancet Respir Med. 2015;3:796–812.

82. Havidich JE, Beach M, Dierdorf SF, Onega T, Suresh G, Cravero JP. Preterm versus term children: analysis of sedation/anesthesia adverse events and longitudinal risk. Pediatrics. 2016;137:1–9.

83. Cravero JP, Beach ML, Blike GT, Gallagher SM, Hertzog JH, Pediatric Sedation Research Consortium. The incidence and nature of adverse events during pediatric sedation/anesthesia with propofol for procedures outside the operating room: a report from the Pediatric Sedation Research Consortium. Anesth Analg. 2009;108:795–804.

84. Vanderhaegen J, Naulaers G, Van Huffel S, Vanhole C, Allegaert K. Cerebral and systemic hemodynamic effects of intravenous bolus administration of propofol in neonates. Neonatology. 2010;98:57–63.

85. Hall RW, Kronsberg SS, Barton BA, Kaiser JR, Anand KJ, Group NTI. Morphine, hypotension, and adverse outcomes among preterm neonates: who's to blame? Secondary results from the NEOPAIN trial. Pediatrics. 2005;115:1351–9.

86. Vutskits L, Gascon E, Tassonyi E, Kiss JZ. Clinically relevant concentrations of propofol but not midazolam alter in vitro dendritic development of isolated gamma-aminobutyric acid-positive interneurons. Anesthesiology. 2005;102:970–6.

87. Briner A, Nikonenko I, De Roo M, Dayer A, Muller D, Vutskits L. Developmental stage-dependent persistent impact of propofol anesthesia on dendritic spines in the rat medial prefrontal cortex. Anesthesiology. 2011;115:282–93.

Epilogues

Anthony R. Absalom, M.B.Ch.B., F.R.C.A., F.H.E.A., M.D.
Professor of Anesthesiology
University Medical Center Groningen
Groningen University
Groningen, The Netherlands

Ram M. Adapa, M.B.B.S., M.D., F.R.C.A., Ph.D.
Consultant Neuroanaesthetist
Addenbrooke's Hospital, Cambridge
Honorary Visiting Senior Research Fellow
Division of Anaesthesia
University of Cambridge
Cambridge, UK

Brian J. Anderson, M.B.Ch.B., Ph.D., F.A.N.Z.C.A., F.C.I.C.M.
Professor of Anesthesiology
Faculty of Medicine and Health Science
Department of Anesthesiology
University of Auckland
Auckland, New Zealand

Keith J. Anderson, M.B., Ch.B., F.R.C.A., Ph.D.
Assistant Clinical Professor of Anesthesiology
University of Calgary
Foothills Medical Centre
Calgary, AL, Canada

Fazil Ashiq, M.D.
Anesthesiology Institute
Cleveland Clinic Abu Dhabi
Abu Dhabi, UAE

Oliver Bagshaw, M.B.Ch.B., F.F.I.C.M.
Consultant Pediatric Anaesthetist
Birmingham Children's Hospital
Birmingham, UK

Thierry Beths, D.V.M., Cert. V.A., M.R.C.V.S., C.V.A., C.V.P.P., Ph.D.
Associate Professor in Veterinary Anaesthesiology and Pain Management
Head of Anaesthesia and Pain Management
U-Vet, University of Melbourne
Werribee, VIC, Australia

Arno G. A. Brouwers, M.D.
Department of Pediatrics, Pediatric Intensive Care Unit
Maastricht University Medical Centre
Maastricht, The Netherlands

Matthew T. V. Chan, M.B., B.S., Ph.D., F.A.N.Z.C.A., F.H.K.C.A., F.H.K.A.M. (Anaesthesiology)
Professor, Department of Anaesthesia and Intensive Care
The Chinese University of Hong Kong
Prince of Wales Hospital
Hong Kong Special Administrative Region
China

Isabelle Constant, M.D., Ph.D.
Professor of Anesthesiology and Intensive Care
Head of Department of Anesthesiology and Intensive Care
Head of Surgical and Medical Pediatric Department
Armand Trousseau Hospital, UPMC, APHP
Paris, France

Luis I. Cortínez, M.D.
Associate Professor of Anesthesiology
Hospital Clínico, Pontificia Universidad Católica de Chile
Santiago, Chile

Douglas J. Eleveld, Ph.D.
Assistant Professor
Department of Anesthesiology
University Medical Center Groningen
University of Groningen
The Netherlands

Frank H. M. Engbers, M.D., F.R.C.A.
Board Member European Society for Intravenous Anaesthesia
Staff Member Department of Anaesthesiology, Section Cardio Thoracic Anaesthesia
Leiden University Medical Centre
Leiden, The Netherlands

John B. Glen, B.V.M.S., Ph.D., F.R.C.A.
Retired Director
GlenPharma (Independent Pharmaceutical Consultancy)
Knutsford, Cheshire, UK
Former Project Leader and Clinical Scientist
ICI Pharmaceuticals/AstraZeneca
Alderley Park, Cheshire, UK

Christina J. Hayhurst, M.D.
Assistant Professor of Anesthesiology
Division of Anesthesiology Critical Care Medicine
Department of Anesthesiology
Vanderbilt University Medical Center
Nashville, TN, USA

© Springer International Publishing AG 2017
A.R. Absalom, K.P. Mason (eds.), *Total Intravenous Anesthesia and Target Controlled Infusions*,
DOI 10.1007/978-3-319-47609-4

Wolfgang Heinrichs, M.D.
Professor of Anesthesiology
AQAI Medical Simulation Center
Mainz, Germany

Stefan G. De Hert, M.D., Ph.D.
Professor of Anesthesiology
Ghent University
Director of Research
Department of Anesthesiology
Ghent University Hospital
Ghent, Belgium

Hugh C. Hemmings Jr., M.D., Ph.D., F.R.C.A.
Editor- in-Chief, British Journal of Anaesthesia
Joseph F. Artusio Professor and Chair of Anesthesiology
Professor of Pharmacology
Weill Cornell Medicine
Anesthesiologist-in-Chief
New York Presbyterian Hospital-Weill Cornell
New York, NY, USA

Karl F. Herold, M.D., Ph.D.
Department of Anesthesiology
Weill Cornell Medical College
New York, NY, USA

Christopher G. Hughes, M.D.
Associate Professor of Anesthesiology
Fellowship Director, Division of Anesthesiology Critical Care
Medicine
Department of Anesthesiology
Chair, VUMC Sedation Committee
Vanderbilt University Medical Center
Nashville, TN, USA

Ken B. Johnson, M.D.
Department of Anesthesiology
Vice Chair for Research
Carter M Ballinger Presidential Chair in Anesthesiology
Director, Center for Patient Simulation
Adjunct Faculty, Professor of Bioengineering
University of Utah, USA

Robert M. Kennedy, M.D.
Professor of Pediatrics
Associate Director, Education Affairs
Emergency Services
Washington University School of Medicine
Department of Pediatrics
St. Louis Children's Hospital
St. Louis, MO, USA

Ross R. Kennedy, M.B., Ch.B., Ph.D., F.A.N.Z.C.A.
Clinical Associate Professor and Specialist Anaesthetists
Department of Anaesthesia
Christchurch Hospital and University of Otago, Christchurch
Christchurch, New Zealand

**Gavin NC Kenny, B.Sc. (Hons), M.B., Ch.B., M.D.,
F.R.C.A., F.A.N.Z.C.A.**
Honorary Professor of Anaesthesiology
The University of Hong Kong
Professor Emeritus
Academic Unit of Anaesthesia, Pain and Critical Care
University of Glasgow

Susanne Koch, M.D.
Department of Anesthesiology and Intensive Care Medicine
Charité— Universitätsmedizin Berlin
Berlin, Germany

Massimo Lamperti, M.D., M.B.A.
Clinical Professor of Anesthesiology
Cleveland Clinic Lerner College of Medicine of Case Western
Reserve University
Neuroanesthesiology, Anesthesiology Institute
Cleveland Clinic Abu Dhabi
Abu Dhabi, UAE

Piet L. J. M. Leroy, M.D., Ph.D.
Associate Professor of Pediatrics
Department of Pediatrics
Division of Pediatric Critical Care
Pediatric Procedural Sedation Unit
Maastricht University Medical Centre
Maastricht, The Netherlands

**Kate Leslie, M.B.B.S., M.D., M.Epid., M.Hlth.Serv.Mt.,
F.A.N.Z.C.A., F.A.H.M.S., A.O.**
Department of Anaesthesia and Pain Management
Royal Melbourne Hospital
Parkville, VIC, Australia

Ngai Liu, M.D., Ph.D.
Associate Professor of Anesthesia and Critical Care
Hôpital Foch, Suresnes, France
Department of Anesthesiology
Director of Research
Outcomes Research Consortium
Cleveland, OH, USA

Mohamed Mahmoud, M.D.
Associate Professor of Pediatrics and Anesthesiology
Director, Radiology Anesthesia and Sedation
Department of Anesthesia
Cincinnati Children's Hospital Medical Center
University of Cincinnati
Cincinnati, OH, USA

Keira P. Mason, M.D.
Associate Professor of Anesthesia
Harvard Medical School
Department of Anesthesiology, Perioperative and Pain Medicine
Boston Children's Hospital
Boston, MA, USA

Kenichi Masui, M.D.
Junior Associate Professor
Department of Anesthesiology
National Defense Medical College
Tokorozawa, Saitama, Japan

Claude Meistelman, M.D.
Professor of Anesthesiology and Intensive Care Medicine
Chairman of the department of Anesthesiology and Intensive
Care Medicine
Hopital de Brabois, Vandoeuvre, France
Université de Lorraine, Nancy, France

Jane Montgomery, M.B., B.S., F.R.C.A., F.F.I.C.M.
Consultant Anaesthesiologist
Torbay Hospital
Devon, England, TQ2, 7AA

Pratik P. Pandharipande, M.D., M.S.C.I., F.C.C.M.
Professor of Anesthesiology and Surgery
Chief, Division of Anesthesiology Critical Care Medicine
Department of Anesthesiology
Co-Director Clinical and Translational Research, Medical Student
Research
Vanderbilt University Medical Center
Nashville, TN, USA

Johannes H. Proost, Pharm.D.
Associate Professor
Department of Anesthesiology
University Medical Center Groningen
University of Groningen
Groningen, The Netherlands

Johan Raeder, M.D., Ph.D.
Professor of Anesthesiology
University of Oslo
Director, Ambulatory Anesthesia
Department of Anesthesiology
Oslo University Hospital
Ullevaal, Oslo, Norway

Douglas E. Raines, M.D.
Edward Mallinckrodt, Jr. Professor of Anaesthesia
In the Field of Pharmacology and Innovation
Harvard Medical School
Anesthetist, Massachusetts General Hospital
Department of Anesthesia
Critical Care, and Pain Medicine
Massachusetts General Hospital
55 Fruit Street, Boston, MA, USA

Philippe Richebé, M.D., Ph.D.
Full Professor of Anesthesiology
Director of Research of the Department of Anesthesiology
of University of Montreal
Maisonneuve-Rosemont Hospital
University of Montréal
Montréal, QC, Canada

Mark G. Roback, M.D.
Professor of Pediatrics and Emergency Medicine
University of Minnesota Medical School
Co-Director, Pediatric Emergency Medicine
Department of Pediatrics
University of Minnesota Masonic Children's Hospital
Minneapolis, MN, USA

Janko Samardzic, M.D., Ph.D.
Medical Faculty, Institute of Pharmacology
Clinical Pharmacology and Toxicology
University of Belgrade, Belgrade, Serbia
Division of Paediatric Pharmacology and Pharmacometrics
University of Basel Children's Hospital
Basel, Switzerland

Jan N. M. Schieveld, M.D., Ph.D.
Consultant in Pediatric Neuropsychiatry
Maastricht University Medical Center+
Department of Psychiatry and Psychology
Division of Child and Adolescent Psychiatry and Psychology
Mutsaersstichting Venlo
European Graduate School For Neuroscience (EURON)
South Limbourg Mental Health Research & Teaching Network,
(SEARCH)
Maastricht, Limbourg, The Netherlands

Stefan Schraag, M.D., Ph.D., F.R.C.A., F.F.I.C.M.
Professor of Anaesthesia
Consultant Cardiothoracic Anaesthetist
Quality Audit and Research Coordinator
Department of Perioperative Medicine
Golden Jubilee National Hospital
Clydebank, Scotland, UK

**John W. Sear. M.A., B.Sc., M.B.B.S., Ph.D., F.F.A.R.C.S.,
F.A.N.Z.C.A.**
Emeritus Professor of Anaesthetics
University of Oxford
Green Templeton College
Oxford OX2 6HG, England, UK

Pablo O. Sepúlveda Voullième, Dr. Med., M.D.
Professor of Anestesia
Servicio De Anethesia
Clinica Alemana Santiago Chile
Santiago, Chile

Frederique S Servin, M.D., Ph.D.
Consultant anaesthesiologist
APHP – HUPNVS
Department of Anesthesiology and Critical Care
Hôpital Bichat
46, rue Henri Huchard, 75018 – Paris, France

Steven L. Shafer, M.D.
Professor of Anesthesiology
Perioperative and Pain Medicine
Stanford University, Stanford, CA, USA

Sulpicio G. Soriano, M.D., F.A.A.P.
Boston Children's Hospital Endowed Chair in Pediatric
Neuroanesthesia
Professor of Anaesthesia
Harvard Medical School
Boston, MA, USA

Claudia D. Spies, M.D.
Professor of Anesthesiology and Intensive Care Medicine
Director, CharitéCenter 7 (CC7) for Anesthesiology
and Intensive Care Medicine
Department of Anesthesiology
Charité Campus Mitte and Campus-Virchow Klinikum
Charité – Universitätsmedizin Berlin
Berlin, Germany

Mary E. Stocker, M.A. (Oxon), M.B.Ch.B., F.R.C.A.
Consultant Anaesthetist and President British Association
of Day Surgery (2016–2018)
Torbay and South Devon NHS Foundation Trust
Torquay, UK

Michael R. J. Sury, M.B.B.S., F.R.C.A., Ph.D.
Consultant Pediatric Anesthetist
Great Ormond Street Hospital for Children
Honorary Senior Lecturer in Anesthesia
PORTEX Unit of Pediatric Anesthesia
Institute of Child Health
University College of London
London, England

Nick Sutcliffe, M.B.,Ch.B., B.Sc.M.R.C.P., F.R.C.A.
Deputy Chairman
Department of Anesthesia
Pain and Perioperative Medicine
Hamed Medical Corporation
Doha, Qatar
Board Member European Society of Intravenous
Anaesthesia

Johannes N. van den Anker, M.D., Ph.D.
Vice Chair of Experimental Therapeutics and the Evan
and Cindy Jones Professor of Pediatric Clinical Pharmacology
Children's National Health System
Washington, DC, USA
Professor, Departments of Pediatrics
Integrative Systems Biology, Pharmacology & Physiology
The George Washington University School of Medicine
and Health Sciences
Division of Paediatric Pharmacology and Pharmacometrics
University of Base Children's Hospital
Basel, Switzerland
Intensive Care and Department of Pediatric Surgery
Erasmus Medical Center-Sophia Children's Hospital
Rotterdam, the Netherlands

Robert A. Veselis, M.D.
Professor of Anesthesiology
Weill Cornell Medical College
Director, Neuroanesthesiology Research Laboratory
Department of Anesthesiology/CCM
Memorial Sloan Kettering Cancer Center
New York, NY, USA

Gijs D. Vos, M.D., Ph.D.
Pediatric intensivist
Department of Pediatrics
Head of the Division of Pediatric Intensive Care
Maastricht University Medical Center
Maastricht, The Netherlands

Laszlo Vutskits, M.D., Ph.D.
Head of Pediatric Anesthesia
Department of Anesthesiology
Pharmacology and Intensive Care
Department of Fundamental Neuroscience
Geneva Neuroscience Center
University of Geneva
Geneva, Switzerland

Jaap Vuyk, M.D., Ph.D.
Associate Professor and Vice Chair
Department of Anesthesiology
Leiden University Medical Center (LUMC)
Leiden, The Netherlands

Michael Wang, Ph.D.
Emeritus Professor of Clinical Psychology
College of Medicine, Biological Science and Psychology
University of Leicester
England, UK

Craig S. Webster, B.Sc., M.Sc., Ph.D.
Senior Lecturer
Centre for Medical and Health Sciences Education and Department
of Anaesthesiology
School of Medicine
University of Auckland
Auckland, New Zealand

Vivian Man-ying Yuen, M.B.B.S., M.D., F.A.N.Z.C.A., F.H.K.C.A., F.H.K.A.M.
Consultant of University of Hong Kong-Shenzhen Hospital, Shenzhen, Guangdong, China
Honorary Clinical Associate Professor
Department of Anesthesiology
University of Hong Kong, Hong Kong
Honorary Consultant
Department of Anesthesiology
Queen Mary Hospital, Hong Kong

Index

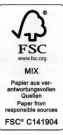

Druck:
Customized Business Services GmbH
im Auftrag der
KNV Zeitfracht GmbH
Ein Unternehmen der Zeitfracht - Gruppe
Ferdinand-Jühlke-Str. 7
99095 Erfurt